clinical examination

A systematic guide to physical diagnosis

8th edition

VOLUME ONE

NICHOLAS J TALLEY

MBBS (Hons)(NSW), MD (NSW), PhD (Syd), MMedSci (Clin Epi)(Newc.),
FRACP, FAFPHM, FAHMS, FRCP (Lond. & Edin.), FACP, FACG, AGAF, FAMS, FRCPI (Hon)
Laureate Professor and Pro Vice-Chancellor, Global Research, University of Newcastle, NSW, Australia
Senior Staff Specialist, John Hunter Hospital, Newcastle, NSW, Australia
Professor of Medicine, Professor of Epidemiology, Joint Supplemental Consultant Gastroenterology
and Health Sciences Research, Mayo Clinic, Rochester, MN, United States; Professor of Medicine,
University of North Carolina, United States; Foreign Guest Professor, Karolinska Institute, Sweden; Past
President, Royal Australasian College of Physicians

SIMON O'CONNOR

FRACP, DDU, FCSANZ
Cardiologist, The Canberra Hospital, Canberra, ACT, Australia
Clinical Senior Lecturer, Australian National University Medical School, Canberra, ACT, Australia

ELSEVIER

ELSEVIER

Elsevier Australia. ACN 001 002 357
(a division of Reed International Books Australia Pty Ltd)
Tower 1, 475 Victoria Avenue, Chatswood, NSW 2067

This edition ©2018 Elsevier Australia. 1st edition ©1988, 2nd edition ©1992, 3rd edition ©1996, 4th edition ©2001, 5th edition ©2006, 6th edition ©2010, 7th edition ©2014 Elsevier Australia

All rights reserved. No part of this publication may be reproduced or transmitted in any form or by any means, electronic or mechanical, including photocopying, recording, or any information storage and retrieval system, without permission in writing from the publisher. Details on how to seek permission, further information about the Publisher's permissions policies and our arrangements with organizations such as the Copyright Clearance Center and the Copyright Licensing Agency, can be found at our website: www.elsevier.com/permissions.

This book and the individual contributions contained in it are protected under copyright by the Publisher (other than as may be noted herein).

ISBN: 978-0-7295-4289-0

Notice

Practitioners and researchers must always rely on their own experience and knowledge in evaluating and using any information, methods, compounds or experiments described herein. Because of rapid advances in the medical sciences, in particular, independent verification of diagnoses and drug dosages should be made. To the fullest extent of the law, no responsibility is assumed by Elsevier, authors, editors or contributors for any injury and/or damage to persons or property as a matter of products liability, negligence or otherwise, or from any use or operation of any methods, products, instructions, or ideas contained in the material herein.

Although all advertising material is expected to conform to ethical (medical) standards, inclusion in this publication does not constitute a guarantee or endorsement of the quality or the value of such product or the claims made of it by its manufacturer.

National Library of Australia Cataloging-in-Publication Data

 A catalogue record for this book is available from the National Library of Australia

Senior Content Strategist: Larissa Norrie
Content Development Specialist: Lauren Santos
Project Manager: Devendran Kannan
Edited by Chris Wyard
Proofread by Annabel Adair
Design by Natalie Bowra
Index by Innodata Indexing
Typeset by Toppan BestSet Premedia Ltd.
Printed in China

Foreword

Clinical medicine is at its finest when demonstrated by the best exponents of the clinical examination. Like most doctors I could name five or so of my teachers and colleagues who made the clinical examination both a true art and finely honed diagnostic tool. They have had my enduring admiration and respect.

In the interests of open disclosure, and in order to protect the integrity of Nick Talley and Simon O'Connor, I am obliged to point out that I never perfected the art of a smooth, seamless, comprehensive physical examination.

I'm sure examiners could see me, and almost hear me, thinking through the cranial nerve examination nerve by nerve in much the same way that a novice dancer counts out loud the requisite steps while progressing through an uncomplicated routine.

I read, digested, wrote on and tried to memorise the other Talley and O'Connor text *Examination Medicine*, which was first published in 1985 and which I used for my clinical examination for my Fellowship in Emergency Medicine.

The first edition of this book, *Clinical Examination*, was published in 1988 and is aimed particularly at medical students. Perhaps if they had written this book a decade earlier when I was a student, as were they, I might have been more accomplished.

Of course a book alone, however well written, cannot confer proficiency in the art of history taking and physical examination. Only repeated practice, built on logical construction in the art, can achieve that. I suspect I could have done much better in my attitude to diligent practice but, failing that, Talley and O'Connor were extraordinarily helpful to me.

It was only in recent years that I met one of the authors, Nick Talley, and I greeted him with almost the same gratitude that a Harry Potter fan would greet J.K. Rowling. It fazed him not one iota. I suspect that he, and Simon O'Connor who, unfortunately, I have not met in spite of my spending five years in Canberra, are well used to such a reaction from the doctors they have assisted for the past 30 years.

This 8th edition of *Clinical Examination* has updated, peer-reviewed text with recent evidence, new images, clinical hints and guidance for OSCE.

The writing is clear. The richness and the potential of an understanding of a patient gained through the clinical examination shines through. The text encourages the reader to think logically about their approach and it does not impose a rote learning style. Nevertheless there are many aids throughout to encourage retention of what has been learned. Summary chapters, diagrams, tables, mnemonics, tips and tests will assist a quick revision.

Given my own interest in the art of medicine over the years, I found the chapter on clinical methods: an historical perspective, illuminating, grounding and reassuring. The art of the clinical examination is timeless and has not been forgotten by these authors.

Professor Chris Baggoley AO, BVSc(Hons), BM BS, BSocAdmin, FACEM, FRACMA, D.Univ (Flin)
EDMS, Southern Adelaide Local Health Network

Contents

Foreword — v
Preface — xix
Acknowledgements — xx
Clinical methods: an historical perspective — xxii
The Hippocratic oath — xxiv

VOLUME ONE

SECTION 1
THE GENERAL PRINCIPLES OF HISTORY TAKING AND PHYSICAL EXAMINATION — 1

CHAPTER 1
The general principles of history taking — 3

- T&O'C essentials — 3
  - Bedside manner and establishing rapport — 3
  - Obtaining the history — 5
  - Introductory questions — 6
- T&O'C essentials — 6
  - Presenting (principal) symptom — 7
  - History of the presenting illness — 7
    - Current symptoms — 7
    - Associated symptoms — 8
    - The effect of the illness — 12
  - Drug and treatment history — 12
  - Past history — 14
    - Additional history for the female patient — 15
  - Social history — 15
- T&O'C essentials — 15
  - Upbringing and education level — 15
  - Marital status, social support and living conditions — 15
  - Diet and exercise — 16
  - Occupation and hobbies — 16
  - Overseas travel — 16
  - Smoking — 16
  - Alcohol use — 17
  - Analgesics and street drugs — 18
  - Mood — 19
  - Sexual history — 19
- Family history — 19
- Systems review — 19
- Skills in history taking — 20
- T&O'C essentials — 20
- References — 21

CHAPTER 2
Advanced history taking — 22

- Taking a good history — 22
- The differential diagnosis — 22
- Fundamental considerations when taking the history — 22
- Personal history taking — 23
  - Common general symptoms — 24
  - Sexual history — 27
  - Reproductive history — 27
- Cross-cultural history taking — 28
- The 'uncooperative' or 'difficult' patient — 28
- Self-harming and Münchhausen's syndrome — 29
- History taking for the maintenance of good health — 29
- The elderly patient — 31
  - Activities of daily living — 31
  - Polypharmacy — 32
  - Adherence — 32
  - Mental state — 32
  - Specific problems in the elderly — 33
  - Advance care planning (advance health directives) — 33
- Patient confidentiality — 33
- Evidence-based history taking and differential diagnosis — 33
- The clinical assessment — 34
- Concluding the consultation — 34
- T&O'C essentials — 35
- References — 35

CHAPTER 3
The general principles of physical examination — 37

- Clinical examination — 38
- How to start — 38
  - Hand washing — 38
- First impressions — 39
  - *Vital signs* — 40
  - *Facies* — 40
  - *Jaundice* — 40
  - *Cyanosis* — 41
  - *Pallor* — 44
  - *Hair* — 45
- Weight, body habitus and posture — 45
- Hydration — 46
- The hands and nails — 48
- Temperature — 49
- Smell — 50
- Preparing the patient for examination — 51
- Advanced concepts: evidence-based clinical examination — 51
  - *Inter-observer agreement (reliability) and the κ-statistic* — 53
- **T&O'C essentials** — 54
- Introduction to the OSCE — 55
- **References** — 56

SECTION 2
THE CARDIOVASCULAR SYSTEM — 57

CHAPTER 4
The cardiovascular history — 59

- Presenting symptoms — 59
  - *Chest pain* — 59
  - *Dyspnoea* — 63
  - *Ankle swelling* — 64
  - *Palpitations* — 64
  - *Syncope, presyncope and dizziness* — 66
  - *Fatigue* — 67
  - *Intermittent claudication and peripheral vascular disease* — 67
- Risk factors for coronary artery disease — 68
- Drug and treatment history — 70
- Past history — 70
- Social history — 71
- Family history — 71
- **T&O'C essentials** — 71
- **OSCE example – CVS history** — 72
- **OSCE revision topics – CVS history** — 72
- **References** — 72

CHAPTER 5
The cardiac examination — 74

- Examination anatomy — 74
- Positioning the patient — 75
- General appearance — 76
- Hands — 79
- Arterial pulse — 81
  - *Rate of pulse* — 83
  - *Rhythm* — 83
  - *Radiofemoral and radial–radial delay* — 83
  - *Character and volume* — 84
  - *Condition of the vessel wall* — 84
- Blood pressure — 84
  - *Measuring the blood pressure with the sphygmomanometer* — 86
  - *Variations in blood pressure* — 88
  - *High blood pressure* — 88
  - *Postural blood pressure* — 88
- Face — 89
- Neck — 89
  - *Carotid arteries* — 89
  - *Jugular venous pressure* — 90
- Praecordium — 92
  - *Inspection* — 92
  - *Palpation* — 93
  - *Percussion* — 95
  - *Auscultation* — 95
  - *Abnormalities of the heart sounds* — 97
  - *Murmurs of the heart* — 100
  - *Auscultation of the neck* — 105
- The back — 106
- The abdomen and legs — 106
- **T&O'C essentials** — 107
- **OSCE example – CVS examination** — 107
- **OSCE revision topics – CVS examination** — 108
- **References** — 108

CHAPTER 6
The limb examination and peripheral vascular disease — 109

- Examination anatomy — 109
  - *Arms* — 109
  - *Legs* — 109
  - *Lower limbs* — 109
- Peripheral vascular disease — 113
- Acute arterial occlusion — 114
- Deep venous thrombosis — 115
- Varicose veins — 115
- Chronic venous disease — 116
- **T&O'C essentials** — 117
- **OSCE example – peripheral vascular disease** — 117

viii CONTENTS

OSCE revision topics	118
References	118

CHAPTER 7
Correlation of physical signs disease and cardiovascular disease — 119

Cardiac failure	119
Left ventricular failure (LVF)	*119*
Right ventricular failure (RVF)	*120*
Chest pain	121
Myocardial infarction or acute coronary syndrome	*121*
Pulmonary embolism	*122*
Acute aortic dissection	*122*
Pericardial disease	122
Acute pericarditis	*122*
Chronic constrictive pericarditis	*123*
Acute cardiac tamponade	*123*
Infective endocarditis	*123*
Systemic hypertension	124
Causes of systemic hypertension	*125*
Complications of hypertension	*125*
Malignant (accelerated) hypertension	*125*
Pulmonary hypertension	125
Causes of pulmonary hypertension	*126*
Innocent murmurs	126
Valve diseases of the left heart	126
Mitral stenosis	*126*
Mitral regurgitation (chronic)	*128*
Acute mitral regurgitation	*129*
Mitral valve prolapse (MVP, systolic-click murmur syndrome)	*130*
Aortic stenosis (AS)	*130*
Aortic regurgitation	*131*
Valve diseases of the right heart	135
Tricuspid stenosis	*135*
Tricuspid regurgitation (TR)	*136*
Pulmonary stenosis (in adults)	*137*
Pulmonary regurgitation	*137*
Prosthetic heart valves	*137*
Cardiomyopathy	137
Hypertrophic cardiomyopathy	*137*
Dilated cardiomyopathy	*139*
Restrictive cardiomyopathy	*139*
Acyanotic congenital heart disease	139
Ventricular septal defect	*139*
Atrial septal defect	*139*
Patent ductus arteriosus	*141*
Coarctation of the aorta	*141*
Ebstein's anomaly	*141*
Cyanotic congenital heart disease	142
Eisenmenger's syndrome (pulmonary hypertension and a right-to-left shunt)	*142*
Fallot's syndrome	*142*
'Grown-up' congenital heart disease	143
Fallot's syndrome	*143*
Transposition of the great arteries	*143*
T&O'C essentials	143
OSCE example – cardiovascular examination	144
OSCE revision topics – cardiovascular examination	144
References	144

CHAPTER 8
A summary of the cardiovascular examination and extending the cardiovascular examination — 145

Extending the cardiovascular physical examination	147
The chest X-ray: a systematic approach	*147*
The echocardiogram	*151*
T&O'C essentials	159
OSCE revision topics	159

SECTION 3
THE RESPIRATORY SYSTEM — 161

CHAPTER 9
The respiratory history — 163

Presenting symptoms	163
Cough and sputum	*163*
Haemoptysis	*165*
Breathlessness (dyspnoea)	*165*
Wheeze	*168*
Chest pain	*168*
Other presenting symptoms	168
Current treatment	169
Past history	171
Occupational history	171
Social history	172
Family history	173
T&O'C essentials	173
OSCE revision topics – the respiratory history	173
References	173

CHAPTER 10
The respiratory examination — 174

Examination anatomy	174
Positioning the patient	174
General appearance	174
Dyspnoea	*174*
Characteristic signs of COPD	*175*

Cyanosis	177	Bronchiectasis	194
Character of the cough	177	*Signs*	194
Sputum	177	*Causes*	194
Stridor	177	Bronchial asthma	194
Hoarseness	177	*Signs*	194
Hands	177	Chronic obstructive pulmonary disease	
Clubbing	178	(COPD)	195
Staining	178	*Signs*	195
Wasting and weakness	178	*Causes of generalised emphysema*	196
Pulse rate	178	Chronic bronchitis	196
Flapping tremor (asterixis)	178	*Signs*	196
Face	178	*Causes*	196
Trachea	179	Interstitial lung disease (ILD)	196
Chest	180	*Signs*	197
Inspection	180	*Causes*	197
Palpation	182	Tuberculosis (TB)	197
Percussion	184	*Primary tuberculosis*	197
Auscultation	184	*Postprimary tuberculosis*	197
The heart	188	*Miliary tuberculosis*	197
The abdomen	188	Mediastinal compression	197
Other	188	*Signs*	198
Pemberton's sign	188	Carcinoma of the lung	198
Legs	188	*Respiratory and chest signs*	198
Respiratory rate on exercise	188	*Apical (Pancoast's) tumour*	198
Temperature	188	*Distant metastases*	198
T&O'C essentials	**188**	*Non-metastatic extrapulmonary*	
OSCE revision topics – the respiratory		*manifestations*	198
examination	**189**	Sarcoidosis	199
References	**189**	*Pulmonary signs*	199
		Extrapulmonary signs	199
CHAPTER 11		Pulmonary embolism (PE)	199
Correlation of physical signs and		*Signs*	200
respiratory disease	**190**	**T&O'C essentials**	**200**
Respiratory distress: respiratory failure	190	**OSCE revision topics – respiratory**	
Consolidation (lobar pneumonia)	190	**disease**	**200**
Symptoms	191	**References**	**200**
Signs	191		
Causes of community-acquired		**CHAPTER 12**	
pneumonia	192	**A summary of the respiratory**	
Atelectasis (collapse)	192	**examination and extending the**	
Signs	192	**respiratory examination**	**201**
Causes	192	Extending the respiratory physical	
Pleural effusion	192	examination	203
Signs	192	*Bedside assessment of lung function*	203
Causes	192	*The chest X-ray and computed*	
Yellow nail syndrome	193	*tomography (CT) scan in*	
Pneumothorax	193	*respiratory medicine*	206
Signs	193	*Chest X-ray checklist*	206
Causes	193	**T&O'C essentials**	**213**
Tension pneumothorax	194	**OSCE revision topics – respiratory**	
Signs	194	**investigations**	**213**
Causes	194	**References**	**213**

SECTION 4
THE GASTROINTESTINAL SYSTEM — 215

CHAPTER 13
The gastrointestinal history — 217

- Presenting symptoms — 217
  - Abdominal pain — 217
  - Patterns of pain — 218
  - Appetite and weight change — 218
  - Early satiation and postprandial fullness — 218
  - Nausea and vomiting — 218
  - Heartburn and acid regurgitation (gastro-oesophageal reflux disease—GORD) — 219
  - Dysphagia — 220
  - Diarrhoea — 222
  - Constipation — 223
  - Mucus — 224
  - Bleeding — 224
  - Jaundice — 225
  - Pruritus — 225
  - Abdominal bloating and swelling — 225
  - Lethargy — 226
- Treatment — 226
- Past history — 227
- Social history — 227
- Family history — 227
- T&O'C essentials — 227
- OSCE revision topics – the gastrointestinal history — 228
- References — 228

CHAPTER 14
The gastrointestinal examination — 229

- Examination anatomy — 229
- Positioning the patient — 230
- General appearance — 230
  - Jaundice — 230
  - Weight and wasting — 231
  - Skin — 231
  - Mental state — 234
- Hands — 235
  - Nails — 235
  - Palms — 235
  - Hepatic flap (asterixis) — 236
- Arms — 237
- Face — 238
  - Eyes — 238
  - Salivary glands — 239
  - Mouth — 240
- Neck and chest — 243
- Abdomen — 244
  - Inspection — 244
  - Palpation — 248
  - Percussion — 257
  - Ascites — 258
  - Auscultation — 260
- Hernias — 261
  - Examination anatomy — 261
  - Hernias in the groin — 262
  - Epigastric hernia — 264
  - Incisional hernias — 264
- Rectal examination — 264
  - The pelvic floor—special tests for pelvic floor dysfunction — 267
  - Ending the rectal exam — 267
  - Testing of the stools for blood — 267
- Other — 268
- Examination of the gastrointestinal contents — 268
  - Faeces — 268
  - Vomitus — 269
- Urinalysis — 269
- T&O'C essentials — 271
- OSCE revision topics – the gastrointestinal examination — 271
- References — 271

CHAPTER 15
Correlation of physical signs and gastrointestinal disease — 272

- Examination of the acute abdomen — 272
- T&O'C essential — 273
  - Acute abdomen after blunt trauma — 274
- Liver disease — 274
  - Signs — 275
- Portal hypertension — 275
  - Signs — 275
  - Causes — 275
- Hepatic encephalopathy — 275
  - Grading — 275
  - Causes — 275
- Dysphagia — 276
  - Signs — 276
- Gastrointestinal bleeding — 276
  - Assessing degree of blood loss — 276
  - Determining the possible bleeding site — 277
- Inflammatory bowel disease — 277
  - Ulcerative colitis — 277
  - Crohn's disease — 279

Malabsorption and nutritional status	279
Signs	*280*
Causes	*280*
Classification of malabsorption	*280*
T&O'C essentials	**281**
References	**281**

CHAPTER 16
A summary of the gastrointestinal examination and extending the gastrointestinal examination — 282

Extending the gastrointestinal examination	284
Endoscopy	*284*
Biochemistry	*285*
Imaging the gastrointestinal system	285
Abdominal X-rays	*285*
Abdominal ultrasound	*287*
CT of the abdomen	*289*
T&O'C essentials	**294**
Revision OSCEs	**294**

SECTION 5
THE GENITOURINARY SYSTEM — **295**

CHAPTER 17
The genitourinary history — 297

Presenting symptoms	297
Change in appearance of the urine	*298*
Urinary tract infection	*298*
Urinary obstruction	*300*
Urinary incontinence	*300*
Chronic kidney disease	*300*
Menstrual and sexual history	303
Treatment	304
Past history	304
Social history	304
Family history	304
T&O'C essentials	**304**
OSCE revision topics – genitourinary history	**305**
References	**305**

CHAPTER 18
The genitourinary examination — 306

Examination anatomy	306
The examination	306
General appearance	306
Hands	306
Arms	307
Face	309
Neck	310
Chest	310
The abdominal examination	310
Inspection	*310*
Palpation	*310*
Ballotting	*311*
Percussion	*311*
Auscultation	*312*
Rectal and pelvic examination	*312*
The back	312
Legs	312
Blood pressure	313
Fundi	313
Male genitalia	313
Differential diagnosis of a scrotal mass	*314*
T&O'C essentials	**315**
OSCE revision topics – genitourinary examination	**316**
References	**316**

CHAPTER 19
A summary of the examination of chronic kidney disease and extending the genitourinary examination — 317

Extending the genitourinary examination	319
Investigations	*319*
T&O'C essentials	**326**
OSCE revision topics	**326**
Reference	**326**

SECTION 6
THE HAEMATOLOGICAL SYSTEM — **327**

CHAPTER 20
The haematological history — 329

Haematological disorders	329
Presenting symptoms	329
Red cell abnormalities	*329*
Clotting and bleeding	*330*
Recurrent infection	*333*
Treatment history to ask about	333
Past history	333
Social history	334
Family history	334
T&O'C essentials	**334**
OSCE revision topics	**334**

CHAPTER 21
The haematological examination — 335

Examination anatomy	335
General appearance	335
Hands	335

Forearms	339
Epitrochlear nodes	339
Axillary nodes	339
Face	340
Cervical and supraclavicular nodes	341
Bone tenderness	342
The abdominal examination	343
Inguinal nodes	345
Legs	345
Fundi	346
T&O'C essentials	**347**
References	**347**

CHAPTER 22
A summary of the haematological examination and extending the haematological examination — 348

Extending the haematological physical examination	350
Haematology tests	350
Examination of the peripheral blood film	350
Anaemia	350
Pancytopenia	354
Acute leukaemia	354
Chronic leukaemia	355
Myeloproliferative disease	355
Lymphoma	357
Multiple myeloma	358
Haematological imaging	358
T&O'C essentials	**360**
OSCE revision topics – the haematological system	**360**

SECTION 7
THE RHEUMATOLOGICAL SYSTEM — 361

CHAPTER 23
The rheumatological history — 363

Presenting symptoms	363
Peripheral joints	363
T&O'C essential	**365**
Back pain	365
Limb pain	366
Raynaud's phenomenon	367
Dry eyes and mouth	367
Red eyes	368
Systemic symptoms	368
Treatment history	368
Past history	368
Social history	369
Family history	369
T&O'C essentials	**369**
OSCE revision topics – the rheumatological history	**369**
References	**369**

CHAPTER 24
The rheumatological examination — 370

Examination anatomy	370
General inspection	370
Principles of joint examination	372
Look	372
Feel	373
Move	373
Measure	374
Assessment of individual joints	374
Hands and wrists	374
T&O'C essentials	**375**
Elbows	383
Shoulders	384
Temporomandibular joints	388
Neck	388
Thoracolumbar spine and sacroiliac joints	392
Hips	395
Knees	399
Ankles and feet	403
T&O'C essentials	**407**
OSCE revision topics – the rheumatological examination	**407**
References	**407**

CHAPTER 25
Correlation of physical signs with rheumatological and musculoskeletal disease — 408

Rheumatoid arthritis	408
General inspection	408
Hands	408
Wrists	408
Elbows	408
Shoulders and axillae	408
Eyes	408
Parotids	409
Mouth	409
Temporomandibular joints	410
Neck	410
Chest	410
Heart	410
Abdomen	410
Lower limbs	410
Ankles and feet	410

Seronegative spondyloarthritides	410
Ankylosing spondylitis	*411*
Reactive arthritis	*411*
Psoriatic arthritis	*412*
Enteropathic arthritis	*412*
Gouty arthritis	412
Calcium pyrophosphate arthritis (pseudogout)	413
Calcium hydroxyapatite arthritis	413
Osteoarthritis	413
Systemic lupus erythematosus	414
General inspection	*414*
Hands	*414*
Forearms	*414*
Head and neck	*414*
Chest	*415*
Abdomen	*415*
Hips	*416*
Legs	*416*
Urine and blood pressure	*416*
Temperature	*416*
Systemic sclerosis (scleroderma and CREST)	416
General inspection	*416*
Hands	*418*
Arms	*418*
Face	*419*
Chest	*419*
Legs	*419*
Urinalysis and blood pressure	*419*
The stool	*419*
Mixed connective tissue disease (MCTD)	420
Examination	*420*
Rheumatic fever	420
Examining the patient with suspected rheumatic fever	*420*
The vasculitides	420
Soft-tissue rheumatism	421
Shoulder syndromes	*421*
Elbow epicondylitis (tennis and golfer's elbow)	*423*
Tenosynovitis of the wrist	*423*
Bursitis	*424*
Nerve entrapment syndromes	424
Carpal tunnel syndrome	*425*
Meralgia paraesthetica	*425*
Tarsal tunnel syndrome	*425*
Morton's 'neuroma'	*425*
Fibromyalgia syndrome	*426*
T&O'C essentials	427
OSCE revision topics – rheumatological disease	427
References	427

CHAPTER 26
A summary of the rheumatological examination and extending the rheumatological examination — 428

Extending the rheumatological system examination	429
Rheumatology investigations	*429*
Imaging	*430*
T&O'C essentials	435
References	435

SECTION 8
THE ENDOCRINE SYSTEM — 437

CHAPTER 27
The endocrine history — 439

Presenting symptoms	439
Changes in appetite and weight	*439*
Changes in bowel habit	*439*
Changes in sweating	*439*
Changes in hair distribution	*439*
Lethargy	*440*
Changes in the skin and nails	*440*
Changes in pigmentation	*441*
Changes in stature	*441*
Erectile dysfunction (impotence)	*441*
Galactorrhoea	*441*
Menstruation	*441*
Polyuria	*441*
Risk factors for diabetes (metabolic syndrome)	442
Past history and treatment	442
Social history	443
Family history	443
T&O'C essentials	443
OSCE revision topics – the endocrine history	443

CHAPTER 28
The endocrine examination — 444

The thyroid	444
The thyroid gland	*444*
Hyperthyroidism (thyrotoxicosis)	*448*
Hypothyroidism (myxoedema)	*451*
The pituitary	453
Examination anatomy	*453*
Panhypopituitarism	*454*

xiv CONTENTS

Acromegaly	456
Other pituitary syndromes	458
The adrenals	458
Cushing's syndrome	458
Addison's disease	461
T&O'C essentials	462
OSCE revision topics – the endocrine examination	462
References	462

CHAPTER 29
Correlation of physical signs and endocrine disease — 463

Diabetes mellitus	463
Calcium metabolism	469
Primary hyperparathyroidism	469
The MEN syndromes	470
Hypoparathyroidism	470
Osteoporosis and osteomalacia	471
Syndromes associated with short stature	473
Turner's syndrome (45XO)	474
Down's syndrome (Trisomy 21)	475
Achondroplasia (dwarfism)	475
Rickets	475
Hirsutism	475
Gynaecomastia	476
Paget's disease	476
T&O'C essentials	478
OSCE revision topics – endocrine system	479
References	479

CHAPTER 30
A summary of the endocrine examination and extending the endocrine examination — 480

The endocrine examination: a suggested method	480
Extending the endocrine physical examination	480
Diagnostic testing	480
T&O'C essentials	486
OSCE revision topics – endocrine system	486

SECTION 9
THE NERVOUS SYSTEM — 487

CHAPTER 31
The neurological history — 489

Starting off	489
Presenting symptoms	489
Headache and facial pain	490
Faints and fits	492
T&O'C essential	494
Dizziness	495
Visual disturbances and deafness	496
Disturbances of gait	496
Disturbed sensation or weakness in the limbs	496
Tremor and involuntary movements	496
Speech and mental status	497
Past health	497
Medication history	497
Social history	498
Family history	498
T&O'C essentials	498
OSCE revision topics – the neurological history	499
References	499

CHAPTER 32
The neurological examination: general signs and the cranial nerves — 500

A preamble regarding the neurological examination	500
Examination anatomy	500
General signs	501
Consciousness	501
Neck stiffness	501
Handedness	501
Orientation	501
The cranial nerves	501
The first (olfactory) nerve	504
The second (optic) nerve	505
The third (oculomotor), fourth (trochlear) and sixth (abducens) nerves—the ocular nerves	510
The fifth (trigeminal) nerve	521
The seventh (facial) nerve	525
The eighth (vestibulocochlear) nerve	529
The ninth (glossopharyngeal) and tenth (vagus) nerves	531
The eleventh (accessory) nerve	533
The twelfth (hypoglossal) nerve	534
Multiple cranial nerve lesions	536
Carotid bruits	537
T&O'C essentials	538
OSCE example – introduction (STEM)	538
References	539

CHAPTER 33
The neurological examination: speech and higher centres — 540

Speech	540
Dysphasia	540
Dysarthria	542
Dysphonia	543

The cerebral hemispheres 543
   Parietal lobe function 543
   Temporal lobe function 545
   Frontal lobe function 546
T&O'C essentials 547
OSCE revision topics – speech and higher centres 547
References 547

CHAPTER 34
The neurological examination: the peripheral nervous system — 548

Limbs and trunk 548
   History 548
   Examination anatomy 549
   General examination approach 550
   General inspection 550
   Upper limbs 550
   Lower limbs 566
   Gait 577
T&O'C essentials 579
OSCE revision topics – the peripheral nervous system 579
References 579

CHAPTER 35
Correlation of physical signs and neurological syndromes and disease — 580

Upper motor neurone lesions 580
   Causes of hemiplegia (upper motor neurone lesion) 580
Lower motor neurone lesions 582
Motor neurone disease 583
Peripheral neuropathy 583
Guillain–Barré syndrome (acute inflammatory polyradiculoneuropathy) 583
Multiple sclerosis 584
Thickened peripheral nerves 585
Spinal cord compression 585
Important spinal cord syndromes 588
   Brown-Séquard syndrome 588
   Subacute combined degeneration of the cord (vitamin B_{12} deficiency) 588
   Dissociated sensory loss 589
   Syringomyelia (a central cavity in the spinal cord) 589
   An extensor plantar response plus absent knee and ankle jerks 590

Myopathy 590
Dystrophia myotonica 591
Myasthenia gravis 593
The cerebellum 595
Parkinson's disease 597
   Inspection 597
   Gait and movements 597
   Tremor 598
   Tone 598
   Face 598
   Writing 599
   Causes of Parkinson's syndrome 599
Other extrapyramidal movement disorders (dyskinesia) 600
   Chorea 600
   Dystonia 600
   Tics and de la Tourette's syndrome 601
The unconscious patient 601
   General inspection 601
   Level of consciousness 602
   Neck 603
   Head and face 603
   Upper and lower limbs 604
   Body 604
   Urine 604
   Blood glucose 604
   Temperature 604
   Stomach contents 604
T&O'C essentials 604
OSCE revision topics – neurological syndromes and disorders 604
References 605

CHAPTER 36
A summary of the neurological examination and extending the neurological examination — 606

Extending the neurological examination 608
   Handedness, orientation and speech 608
   Neck stiffness and Kernig's sign 608
   Cranial nerves 608
   Upper limbs 609
   Lower limbs 610
Diagnostic testing 611
   Lumbar puncture 611
   Neurological imaging 611
T&O'C essentials 615

VOLUME TWO

SECTION 10
PAEDIATRIC AND NEONATAL HISTORY AND EXAMINATION 617

CHAPTER 37
The paediatric history and examination 619

- Principles of paediatric history taking and examination 619
- Paediatric history taking 619
  - History-taking sequence 620
- General physical examination 622
  - Preparing for the examination 622
  - Examination 622
- T&O'C essentials 682
- OSCE revision topics – the paediatric history and examination 682
- References 683

CHAPTER 38
The neonatal history and examination 684

- The history 684
  - Maternal health 684
  - Other family history 685
  - History of the pregnancy, labour and delivery 685
- The physical examination 687
  - Preparing for the physical examination 688
  - Measurements 689
  - Head-to-toe assessment 696
  - Gestational age 723
- T&O'C essentials 723
- OSCE revision topics – the neonatal history and examination 724
- References 724

SECTION 11
WOMEN'S HEALTH HISTORY AND EXAMINATION 727

CHAPTER 39
The obstetric history and examination 729

- The obstetric history 729
- Early pregnancy symptoms 729
  - Amenorrhoea 729
  - Breast changes 730
  - Nausea and vomiting 730
- Minor symptoms in pregnancy 730
  - Hyperemesis gravidarum 730
  - Heartburn and acid regurgitation 730
  - Constipation 730
  - Back pain 731
  - Pubic symphysis pain 731
  - Vaginal discharge 731
  - Pruritus 731
  - Neuropathies 731
  - Tiredness 731
  - Breathlessness 731
  - Palpitations 731
- Major symptoms in pregnancy 731
  - Change in fetal movements 731
  - Vaginal bleeding 732
  - Rupture of membranes 732
  - Abdominal pain 732
  - Headache 732
  - Oedema 732
- History 732
  - Current pregnancy history 734
  - Past obstetric history 734
  - Past gynaecological history 734
  - Past medical history 734
  - Treatment history 734
  - Social history 735
  - Family history 736
- Examination anatomy 736
- Examination 736
  - Positioning the patient 736
  - General appearance 736
  - Observations 737
  - The abdomen: mother and fetal findings 737
  - The genitals 738
  - The lower limbs 740
  - Urinalysis 741
  - Obstetric ultrasound: a systematic approach 741
- T&O'C essentials 742
- OSCE revision topics – the obstetric history and examination 742
- References 742

CHAPTER 40
The gynaecological history and examination 743

- History 743
  - Presenting symptoms 743
  - Menstrual history 744
  - Sexual history 750
  - Previous gynaecological history 750
  - Previous medical history 750
  - Family and social history 750
- Examination 752
  - Examination of the breasts 752
  - Examination of the abdomen 752

Pelvic examination	752
Rectal examination	762
OSCE revision topics – the gynaecological history and examination	762
T&O'C essentials	762
References	762

CHAPTER 41
The breasts: history and examination — 763

Examination anatomy	763
History	763
Examination	764
Inspection	764
Palpation	765
Evaluation of a breast lump	766
T&O'C essentials	766
OSCE revision topics – the breasts	767
References	767

SECTION 12
SPECIALTY SYSTEM HISTORY AND EXAMINATION — 769

CHAPTER 42
The eyes, ears, nose and throat — 771

Eyes	771
Examination anatomy	771
History	772
Examination method	772
T&O'C essentials	775
T&O'C essentials	776
Diplopia	778
Horner's syndrome	778
Iritis	780
Glaucoma	780
Shingles	781
Eyelid	781
Ears	782
Examination anatomy	782
History	783
Examination method	785
T&O'C essentials	788
Nose and sinuses	788
Examination anatomy	788
History	789
Examination method	790
Sinusitis	790
Mouth and throat	791
Examination anatomy	791
History	792
Examination method	792
Pharyngitis	794
Supraglottitis (epiglottitis)	795
Common investigations	795
T&O'C essentials	796
OSCE examples	797
OSCE revision topics – eyes, ears, nose and throat	798
References	798

CHAPTER 43
The skin and lumps — 799

Examination anatomy	799
Dermatological history	800
General principles of physical examination of the skin	801
How to approach the clinical diagnosis of a lump	804
Correlation of physical signs and skin disease	806
Pruritus	806
Erythrosquamous eruptions	807
Blistering eruptions	809
Erythroderma	813
Livedo reticularis	814
Pustular and crusted lesions	814
Dermal plaques	815
Erythema nodosum	816
Erythema multiforme (EM)	816
Cellulitis and erysipelas	817
Folliculitis, furuncles and carbuncles	818
Other infections	818
Hyperpigmentation, hypopigmentation and depigmentation	819
Flushing and sweating	819
Skin tumours	821
The nails	823
T&O'C essentials	824
OSCE example – skin	825
References	825

CHAPTER 44
The older person assessment — 826

History taking in older persons: special considerations	826
Physical examination in older persons: special considerations	830
Dementia screening	833
OSCE revision topics – assessment of the geriatric patient	833
References	833

CHAPTER 45
Approaching infectious diseases — 834

- Pyrexia of unknown origin — 834
  - History — 835
  - Examination — 835
  - Clinical scenarios for unexplained fever — 836
- HIV infection and AIDS — 836
  - History — 837
  - Examination — 838
- T&O'C essentials — 840
- OSCE revision topics – infectious diseases — 841
- References — 841

SECTION 13
MENTAL HEALTH HISTORY AND EXAMINATION — 843

CHAPTER 46
The psychiatric history and mental state examination — 845

- The history — 845
- Obtaining the history — 846
  - Introductory questions — 846
  - History of the presenting illness — 846
  - Past history and treatment history — 851
  - Family history — 853
  - Social and personal history — 853
  - Premorbid personality — 854
- The mental state examination — 854
- The diagnosis — 854
- Examples of important psychiatric illnesses — 859
  - Disorders that lead to physical illness — 859
  - Schizophrenia — 860
  - Depression — 861
  - Anxiety disorders — 862
  - Post-traumatic stress disorder (PTSD) — 862
  - Obsessive–compulsive disorder (OCD) — 863
- T&O'C essentials — 863
- OSCE revision topics – the psychiatric history and the mental state examination — 863
- References — 863

SECTION 14
ACUTE CARE AND END OF LIFE — 865

CHAPTER 47
The acutely ill patient — 867

- Initial assessment — 867
- Level of consciousness — 867
- Delirium — 867
- Further examination — 868
- OSCE example – emergency care — 872
- References — 872

CHAPTER 48
The pre-anaesthetic medical evaluation (PAME) — 873

- The history — 873
  - Cardiovascular history — 873
  - The respiratory history — 874
  - Other — 874
- The examination — 874

CHAPTER 49
Assessment of death — 875

- Assessment — 875
  - Do-not-resuscitate (DNR) orders — 875
  - Do not misdiagnose death — 875
  - Examining a suspected death — 875
- Informing relatives — 876
- Completing the death certificate — 876
- Postmortem — 877
- Organ donation — 877

SECTION 15
ADULT HISTORY TAKING AND EXAMINATION IN THE WARDS AND CLINICS — 879

CHAPTER 50
Writing and presenting the adult history and physical examination — 881

- History — 881
- Physical examination (PE) — 882
- Provisional diagnosis — 882
- Problem list and plans — 882
- Continuation notes — 882
- Presentation — 882
- Reference — 885

CHAPTER 51
A suggested method for a rapid screening adult physical examination — 886

- Hands and arms — 886
- Face — 886
- Front of the neck — 886
- Chest — 886
- Back of the chest and neck — 886
- Abdomen — 887
- Legs — 887
- Neurological examination — 887
- Completing the examination — 888

Index — I-1

Preface

Acquire the art of detachment, the virtue of method, and the quality of thoroughness, but above all the grace of humility.

Ask not what disease the person has, but rather what person the disease has.

Sir William Osler

Welcome to the new edition of *Clinical Examination*, which has been carefully revised and updated. Clinical skills are the foundation of clinical medicine, most importantly history taking and physical examination. In most cases, a good history and physical examination will lead you to make the correct diagnosis, and this is critical—your diagnosis will more often than not seal the fate of your patient and, assuming you are correct, take them down the optimal management path.

In order to make a correct diagnosis you need to assemble all the facts at hand. Blindly ordering tests in the absence of the clinical history and relevant examination often leads to serious errors. It is distressingly common for tests to be ordered and referrals made without an adequate history or even a cursory examination of the patient. The wrong diagnosis can cause harm and distress that lasts a lifetime.

Clinical Examination is designed to take students on an exciting journey from acquiring core skills to an advanced level, applying a strong evidence-based focus. We have taken a systematic approach because recognition of all the facts aids accurate diagnosis. The patient presenting with, for example, heart disease may have not only objective changes of disease when listening to the heart but also relevant findings in the hands, arms, face, abdomen and legs that can guide identification of the underlying disease process and prognosis. Diagnosticians are great medical detectives who apply rigorous methodology to uncover the truth, solve a puzzle and commence the healing process.

Our book is not a traditional undergraduate textbook and we are proud of its distinctive features. Learning must be fun! Unlike most other similar textbooks, ours is deliberately laced with humour and historical anecdotes that generations of students have told us enhance the learning experience. Another distinguishing feature is that every chapter in this book has undergone peer review, just as you would expect would occur for any published journal article. We have believed from the beginning that peer review is integral to ensuring the highest possible standards and maximising the value of a core textbook. In this edition based on the peer review process we have made revisions, excluded irrelevant material and added updates where appropriate. Videos demonstrating techniques enhance the learning experience, and the e-book format supports learning from a tablet or computer anywhere and anytime. We are also proud of this book being current and as evidence based as is possible, with updated chapter references and annotations so readers can dive deeper into any of the literature that interests them. We want students at all levels to know there are many limitations and gaps (all crying out for more research), and to remain curious and excited about medicine as they learn.

Clinical skills can be mastered only by practice and you should aim to see as many cases as you can while studying from this or any book. You will learn from your patients your entire career if only you take the time to listen and observe.

Great clinicians are made not born, and everyone practising medicine needs to master clinical skills. Thank you to all those who have provided us with expert input as we have made our revisions. We also thank all of our colleagues and patients who educate us daily, and the legion of students who have written to us, including those who have pointed out omissions or mistakes (real or perceived).

Nicholas J. Talley
Simon O'Connor
Newcastle and Canberra, July 2017

Acknowledgements

This book provides an evidence-based account of clinical skills. We are very grateful for the reviews, comments and suggestions from the many outstanding colleagues over the years who have helped us to develop and refine this book. All chapters have again been peer reviewed, a hallmark of our books, and we have taken great care to revise the material based on the detailed reviews obtained. We take responsibility for any errors or omissions.

We would like to especially acknowledge **Professor Ian Symonds**, Dean of Medicine, University of Adelaide, and **Professor Kichu Nair**, Professor of Medicine and Associate Dean Continuing Medical Professional Development, University of Newcastle, for producing the videos for the OSCEs.

Dr Tom Wellings, Staff Specialist in Neurology, John Hunter Hospital, provided expert input into the neurology chapters for this edition. **Dr Philip McManis** provided invaluable input into neurology for earlier editions.

Dr A Manoharan and **Dr J Isbister** provided the original blood film photographs and the accompanying text. **Associate Professor L Schreiber** provided the original section on soft-tissue rheumatology. We have revised and updated all of these sections again.

We thank **Professor Alex Ford** (Leeds Teaching Hospitals Trust, UK) and his team for their systematic review of the evidence supporting (or refuting) key clinical signs that has been retained.

Professor Brian Kelly, Dean of Medicine at the University of Newcastle, provided valuable comments on the psychiatry chapter.

Thank you to **Dr Malcolm Thomson** who provided a number of the X-rays and scans for this title. Others have been provided by the Medical Imaging Department at the Canberra Hospital X-ray Library. We would like to thank **Associate Professor Lindsay Rowe**, Staff Specialist Radiologist at the John Hunter Hospital, for preparing the text and images within the gastrointestinal system section retained from the last edition.

Associate Professor S Posen, **Associate Professor IPC Murray**, **Dr G Bauer**, **Dr E Wilmshurst**, **Dr J Stiel** and **Dr J Webb** helped us obtain many of the original photographs in earlier editions. We would like to acknowledge and thank **Glenn McCulloch** for the photographs he supplied for this title. A set of photographs come from the Mayo Clinic library and from FS McDonald (editor), *Mayo Clinic images in internal medicine: self-assessment for board exam review* (Mayo Clinic Scientific Press, Rochester MN & CRC Press, Boca Raton FL, 2004). We would like to thank the following from Mayo Clinic College of Medicine for their kind assistance in selecting additional photographic material: **Dr Ashok M Patel**, **Dr Ayalew Tefferi**, **Dr Mark R Pittelkow** and **Dr Eric L Matteson**. We would also like to acknowledge **Coleman Productions** who provided new photographs.

Dr Michael Potter and **Dr Stephen Brienesse** provided assistance with the clinical examination photographs.

Elsevier Australia and the authors also extend their appreciation to the following reviewers for their comments and insights on the entire manuscript:

REVIEWERS

Jessica Bale, BMedRadSc, MBBS, Conjoint Lecturer (Dermatology), University of Newcastle, NSW, Australia

Andrew Boyle, MBBS, PhD, FRACP, Professor of Cardiovascular Medicine, University of Newcastle and John Hunter Hospital, Newcastle, NSW, Australia

Judi Errey, BSc, MBBS, MRACGP, Senior Lecturer and Clinical Coordinator, University of Tasmania, TAS, Australia

Tom Goodsall, BSc, MBBS (Hons), Advanced Trainee Gastroenterology and General Medicine, John Hunter Hospital, NSW, Australia

Hadia Haikal-Mukhtar, MBBS (Melb), BSc Hons (Melb), LLB Hons (Melb), FRACGP, Dip Ger Med (Melb), Grad Cert Health Prof Ed (Monash), Head of Auburn Clinical School, School of Medicine, Sydney, University of Notre Dame Australia, NSW, Australia

Adam Harris, MBChB, MMed, Conjoint lecturer at the University of Newcastle, NSW, Australia

Rohan Jayasinghe, MBBS (Sydney; 1st Class Honours), FRACP, FCSANZ, PhD (UNSW), MSpM(UNSW), MBA(Newcastle), Medical Director, Cardiology Department, Gold Coast University Hospital, QLD, Australia; Professor of Cardiology, Griffith University, QLD, Australia; Clinical Professor of Medicine, Macquarie University, Sydney, NSW, Australia

Kelvin Kong, BSc MBBS (UNSW), FRACS (OHNS), VMO John Hunter Hospital, NSW, Australia

Kypros Kyprianou, MBBS, FRACP, Grad Dip Med Ed., Consultant Paediatrician, Monash Children's Hospital and Senior Lecturer, University of Melbourne, VIC, Australia

Judy Luu, MBBS, FRACP, MIPH, Staff Specialist, John Hunter Hospital, NSW; Conjoint Lecturer, University of Newcastle, NSW, Australia

Joy Lyneham, PhD, Associate Professor, Faculty of Health and Medicine. University of Newcastle, NSW, Australia

Genevieve McKew, MBBS, FRACP, FRCPA, Staff Specialist, Concord Repatriation General Hospital and Clinical Lecturer, Concord Clinical School University of Sydney, NSW, Australia

Balakrishnan R Nair (Kichu), AM MBBS, MD (Newcastle) FRACP, FRCPE, FRCPG, FRCPI, FANZSGM, GradDip Epid, Professor of Medicine and Deputy Dean (Clinical Affairs), School of Medicine and Public Health, Newcastle, Australia; Director, Centre for Medical Professional Development HNE Local Health District, Adjunct Professor University of New England, Armidale, Australia

Christine O'Neill, MBBS(Hons), FRACS, MS, VMO General Surgeon, John Hunter Hospital, Newcastle, NSW, Australia

Steven Oakley, MBBS, FRACP, PhD, Staff Specialist Rheumatologist, John Hunter Hospital, Newcastle, Australia; Conjoint Associate Professor, School of Medicine and Public Health, University of Newcastle, Australia

Robert Pickles, BMed (Hons), FRACP, Senior Staff Specialist Infectious Diseases and General Medicine, John Hunter Hospital, NSW, Australia; Conjoint Associate Professor, School of Medicine and Public Health, University of Newcastle, NSW, Australia

Philip Rowlings, MBBS, FRACP, FRCPA, MS, Director of Haematology, Calvary Mater Newcastle and John Hunter Hospital, NSW, Australia; Senior Staff Specialist Pathology North-Hunter, Professor of Medicine, University of Newcastle, Australia

Josephine Thomas, BMBS, FRACP, Senior Lecturer, University of Adelaide, SA, Australia

Alicia Thornton, BSc, MBBS (Hons), Conjoint Lecturer (Dermatology), University of Newcastle, NSW, Australia

Scott Twaddell, BMed, FRACP, FCCP, Senior Staff Specialist, Department of Respiratory and Sleep Medicine, John Hunter Hospital, NSW, Australia

Martin Veysey, MBBS, MD, MRCP(UK), FRACP, MClinEd, Professor of Gastroenterology, Hull York Medical School, UK

Tom Wellings, BSc(Med), MBBS, FRACP, Staff Specialist Neurologist, John Hunter Hospital, NSW, Australia

CONTRIBUTORS

Joerg Mattes, MBBS, MD, PhD, FRACP, Senior Staff Specialist, John Hunter Children's Hospital and Professor of Paediatrics, University of Newcastle, NSW, Australia

Bryony Ross, B.Biomed.Sc, MBBS, FRACP, FRCPA, Staff Specialist, Calvary Mater Newcastle, John Hunter Children's Hospital and Pathology North, NSW, Australia; Conjoint Lecturer, School of Medicine and Public Health, University of Newcastle, NSW, Australia

Ian Symonds, MD, MMedSci, FRCOG, FRANZCOG, Dean of Medicine, University of Adelaide, SA, Australia

Clinical methods: an historical perspective

The best physician is the one who is able to differentiate the possible and the impossible.

Herophilus of Alexandria (335–280BC)

Since classical Greek times interrogation of the patient has been considered most important because disease was, and still is, viewed in terms of the discomfort it causes. However, the current emphasis on the use of history taking and physical examination for diagnosis developed only in the 19th century. Although the terms 'symptoms and signs' have been part of the medical vocabulary since the revival of classical medicine, until relatively recently they were used synonymously. During the 19th century, the distinction between *symptoms* (subjective complaints, which the clinician learns from the patient's account of his or her feelings) and *signs* (objective morbid changes detectable by the clinician) evolved. Until the 19th century, diagnosis was empirical and based on the classical Greek belief that all disease had a single cause: an imbalance of the four humours (yellow bile, black bile, blood and phlegm). Indeed the Royal College of Physicians, founded in London in 1518, believed that clinical experience without classical learning was useless, and physicians who were College members were fined if they ascribed to any other view. At the time of Hippocrates (460?–375BC), observation (inspection) and feeling (palpation) had a place in the examination of patients. The ancient Greeks, for example, noticed that patients with jaundice often had an enlarged liver that was firm and irregular. Shaking a patient and listening for a fluid splash was also recognised by the Greeks. Herophilus of Alexandria (335–280BC) described a method of taking the pulse in the 4th century BC. However, it was Galen of Pergamum (AD130–200) who established the pulse as one of the major physical signs, and it continued to have this important role up to the 18th century, with minute variations being recorded. These variations were erroneously considered to indicate changes in the body's harmony. William Harvey's (1578–1657) studies of the human circulation, published in 1628, had little effect on the general understanding of the value of the pulse as a sign. Sanctorius (1561–1636) was the first to time the pulse using a clock, while John Floyer (1649–1734) invented the pulse watch in 1707 and made regular observations of the pulse rate. Abnormalities in heart rate were described in diabetes mellitus in 1776 and in thyrotoxicosis in 1786. Fever was studied by Hippocrates and was originally regarded as an entity rather than a sign of disease. The thermoscope was devised by Sanctorius in 1625. In association with Gabriel Fahrenheit (1686–1736), Hermann Boerhaave (1668–1738) introduced the thermometer as a research instrument and this was produced commercially in the middle of the 18th century. In the 13th century Johannes Actuarius (d. 1283) used a graduated glass to examine the urine. In Harvey's time a specimen of urine was sometimes looked at (inspected) and even tasted, and was considered to reveal secrets about the body. Harvey recorded that sugar diabetes (mellitus) and dropsy (oedema) could be diagnosed in this way. The detection of protein in the urine, which Frederik Dekkers (1644–1720) first described in 1673, was ignored until Richard Bright (1789–1858) demonstrated its importance in renal disease. Although Celsus described and valued measurements such as weighing and measuring a patient in the 1st century AD, these methods became widely used only in the 20th century. A renaissance in clinical methods began with the concept of Battista Morgagni (1682–1771) that disease was not generalised but rather arose in organs, a conclusion published in 1761. Leopold Auenbrugger invented chest tapping (percussion) to detect disease in the same year. Van Swieten, his teacher, in fact used percussion to detect ascites. The technique was forgotten for nearly half a century until Jean Corvisart (1755–1821) translated Auenbrugger's work in 1808.

The next big step occurred with René Laënnec (1781–1826), a student of Corvisart. He invented the stethoscope in 1816 (at first merely a roll of stiff paper) as an aid to diagnosing heart and lung disease by listening (auscultation). This revolutionised chest examination, partly because it made the chest accessible in patients too modest to allow a direct application of the examiner's ear to the chest wall, as well as allowing accurate clinicopathological correlations. William Stokes (1804–78) published the first treatise in English on the use of the stethoscope in 1825. Josef Skoda's (1805–81) investigations of the value of these clinical methods led to their widespread and enthusiastic adoption after he published his results in 1839. These advances helped lead to a change in the practice of medicine. Bedside teaching was first introduced in the Renaissance by Montanus (1498–1552) in Padua in 1543. In the 17th century, physicians based their opinion on a history provided by an apothecary (assistant) and rarely saw the patients themselves. Thomas Sydenham (1624–89) began to practise more modern bedside medicine, basing his treatment on experience and not theory, but it was not until a century later that the scientific method brought a systematic approach to clinical diagnosis.

This change began in the hospitals of Paris after the French Revolution, with recognition of the work of Morgagni, Corvisart, Laënnec and others. Influenced by the philosophy of the Enlightenment, which suggested that a rational approach to all problems was possible, the Paris Clinical School combined physical examination with autopsy as the basis of clinical medicine. The methods of this school were first applied abroad in Dublin, where Robert Graves (1796–1853) and William Stokes worked. Later, at Guy's Hospital in London, the famous trio of Richard Bright, Thomas Addison (1793–1860) and Thomas Hodgkin (1798–1866) made their important contributions. In 1869 Samuel Wilks (1824–1911) wrote on the nail changes in disease and the signs he described remain important. Carl Wunderlich's (1815–77) work changed the concept of temperature from a disease in itself to a symptom of disease. Spectacular advances in physiology, pathology, pharmacology and the discovery of microbiology in the latter half of the 19th century led to the development of the new 'clinical and laboratory medicine', which is the rapidly advancing medicine of the present day. The modern systematic approach to diagnosis, with which this book deals, is still, however, based on taking the history and examining the patient by looking (inspecting), feeling (palpating), tapping (percussing) and listening (auscultating).

Suggested reading

Bordage G. Where are the history and the physical? *Can Med Assoc J* 1995; 152:1595–1598.

McDonald C. Medical heuristics: the silent adjudicators of clinical practice. *Ann Intern Med* 1996; 124:56–62.

Reiser SJ. The clinical record in medicine. Part I: Learning from cases. *Ann Intern Med* 1991; 114:902–907.

The Hippocratic oath

I swear by Apollo the physician, and Aesculapius, and Hygieia, and Panacea, and all the gods and goddesses that, according to my ability and judgment, I will keep this Oath and this stipulation: To reckon him who taught me this Art equally dear to me as my parents, to share my substance with him and relieve his necessities if required; to look upon his offspring in the same footing as my own brother, and to teach them this Art, if they shall wish to learn it, without fee or stipulation, and that by precept, lecture, and every other mode of instruction, I will impart a knowledge of the Art to my own sons and those of my teachers, and to disciples bound by a stipulation and oath according to the law of medicine, but to none others. I will follow that system of regimen which, according to my ability and judgment, I consider for the benefit of my patients, and abstain from whatever is deleterious and mischievous. I will give no deadly medicine to any if asked, nor suggest any such counsel; and in like manner I will not give a woman a pessary to produce abortion. With purity and with holiness I will pass my life and practise my Art. I will not cut persons laboring under the stone, but will leave this to be done by men who are practitioners of this work. Into whatever houses I enter I will go into them for the benefit of the sick and will abstain from every voluntary act of mischief and corruption; and further from the seduction of females or males, of freemen and slaves. Whatever, in connection with my professional practice, or not in connection with it, I may see or hear in the lives of men which ought not to be spoken of abroad I will not divulge, as reckoning that all such should be kept secret. While I continue to keep this Oath unviolated may it be granted to me to enjoy life and the practice of the Art, respected by all men, in all times! But should I trespass and violate this Oath, may the reverse be my lot!

Hippocrates, born on the Island of Cos (c.460–357 BC) is agreed by everyone to be the father of medicine. He is said to have lived to the age of 109. Many of the statements in this ancient oath remain relevant today, while others, such as euthanasia and abortion, remain controversial. The seduction of slaves, however, is less of a problem.

SECTION 1
The general principles of history taking and physical examination

CHAPTER 1
The general principles of history taking

CHAPTER 2
Advanced history taking

CHAPTER 3
The general principles of physical examination

CHAPTER 1
The general principles of history taking

Medicine is learned by the bedside and not in the classroom. SIR WILLIAM OSLER (1849–1919)

An extensive knowledge of medical facts is not useful unless a doctor is able to extract accurate and succinct information from a sick person about his or her illness, and then synthesise the data. This is how you make an accurate diagnosis. In all branches of medicine, the development of a rational plan of management depends on a correct diagnosis or a sensible, differential diagnosis (list of possible diagnoses). Except for patients who are extremely ill, taking a careful medical history should precede both examination and treatment.

Taking the medical history is the first step in making a diagnosis; it will be used to direct the physical examination and will usually determine what investigations are appropriate. More often than not, an accurate history suggests the correct diagnosis, whereas the physical examination and subsequent investigations merely serve to confirm this impression.[1,2] Text box 1.1 shows the consultation sequence.

Great diagnosticians have been feted by history and you will see their names live on in this book: Hippocrates, Osler, Mayo, Addison and Cushing, to name a few. History taking involves more than listening: you must observe actively (a part of physical examination). Noting the discomfort of a patient who has abdominal pain, for example, will influence the interpretation of the history. Remember that the history is the least-expensive way of making a diagnosis.

Changes in medical education mean that much student teaching is now conducted away from the traditional hospital ward. Students must learn how to take a medical history in any and every setting, but obviously adjustments to the technique must be made for patients seen in busy surgeries or outpatient departments. Much information about a patient's previous medical history may already be available in hospital or clinic records (some regrettably inaccurately recorded, so be on your guard); the detail needed will vary depending on the complexity of the presenting problem and on whether the visit is a follow-up or a new consultation.

T&O'C ESSENTIALS

All students must have a comprehensive understanding of how to take a complete medical history, which is usually essential for accurate diagnosis.

The consultation sequence

1. History
2. Examination
3. Explanation to patient of findings, differential diagnosis (possible diagnoses) and management plan (further tests and treatment)
4. Ordering of, and explanation of, appropriate tests
5. Commencement of treatment, if indicated

TEXT BOX 1.1

BEDSIDE MANNER AND ESTABLISHING RAPPORT

History taking requires practice and depends very much on the doctor–patient relationship.[3] It is important to learn an approach that helps put patients at ease. This is often best done by watching the way more senior colleagues work with their patients. Students need to develop their own methods of feeling easy with their patients. Once students learn how to establish this rapport with patients, the history taking and indeed all of the consultation is likely to be rewarding.

Successful doctors are able to imagine what it would be like to be in the position of the patient they are treating. Ask yourself the question 'How would I like to be treated if I were this patient?'

It is possible to be understanding and sympathetic about a patient's illness and circumstances but retain objectivity. Doctors who can become overwhelmed by their patients' problems cannot look after them properly.[a]

Hospitals and clinics all have rules and suggestions for students about how they should dress and identify themselves, and whose permission they need to see patients on wards. Make sure you are familiar with these rather than face ejection from the ward by a senior doctor or (more frightening) nurse.[b]

Remember that patients tell doctors and even medical students facts they would tell no one else. It is essential that these matters be kept confidential except when shared for clinical reasons and in accordance with privacy legislation. There should be no problem in discussing a patient with a colleague, but unless the colleague is directly involved in the patient's management the patient should not be identified. This applies to discussion of patients and their results at clinical meetings. In open meetings, the patient's name should be removed from displayed tests and documents.

There is no doubt that the treatment of a patient begins the moment one reaches the bedside or the patient enters the consulting rooms. The patient's first impressions of a doctor's professional manner will have a lasting effect. One of the axioms of the medical profession is *primum non nocere* (first, do no harm).[4] An unkind and thoughtless approach to questioning and examining a patient can cause harm before any treatment has had the opportunity to do so. You should aim to leave the patient feeling better for your visit.

Much has been written about the correct way to interview patients, but each doctor has to develop his or her own method, guided by experience gained from clinical teachers and patients themselves.[5–8] To help establish this good relationship, the student or doctor must make a deliberate point of introducing him- or herself and explaining his or her role. A student might say: 'Good afternoon, Mrs Evans. My name is Jane Smith. I am Dr Osler's medical student. She has asked me to come and see you.' A patient seen at a clinic should be asked to come and sit down, and be directed to a chair. The door should be shut or, if the patient is in the ward, the curtains drawn to provide some privacy. The clinician should sit down beside or near the patient so as to be close to eye level and give the impression that the interview will be an unhurried one.[9,10]

It is important here to address the patient respectfully, look at him or her (not the computer) and use his or her name and title (see Fig. 1.1). Some general remarks about the weather, hospital food or the crowded waiting

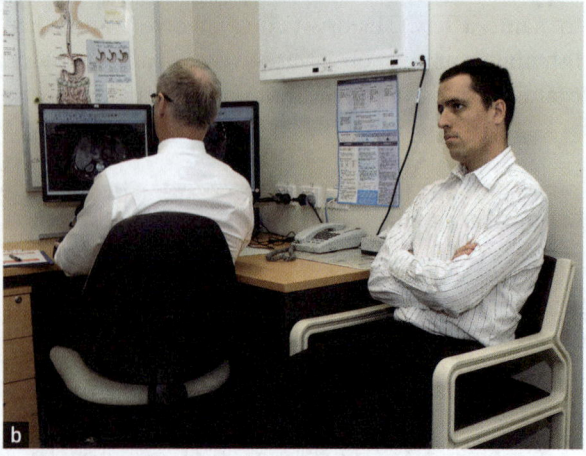

(a) Interviewing correctly. (b) Interviewing incorrectly

FIGURE 1.1

---

[a] Remember; 'the patient is the one with the disease', from the infamous *House of God* by Samuel Shem.
[b] Many hospitals have banned ties and long sleeves for their staff so as to prevent the spread of infection. Who knows where this trend for less and less clothing may end?

room may be appropriate to help put the patient at ease, but these must not be patronising.

OBTAINING THE HISTORY

Start with an open-ended question and listen actively—patients will 'tell you the diagnosis' if you take the time to listen to the story in their own words and synthesise what they are saying based on your knowledge of pathophysiology.

Allow the patient to tell the story first and avoid the almost overwhelming urge to interrupt. Encourage the patient to continue telling you about his or her main problem or problems from the beginning. Then ask specific questions to fill in all the gaps.

At the end of the history and examination, a detailed record is made. However, many clinicians find it useful to make rough notes during the interview. Tell patients you will be doing this but will also be listening to them. With practice, note taking can be done without any loss of rapport. Pausing to make a note of a patient's answer to a question and engaging his or her eyes directly can help, and indicates that the story is being taken seriously.

Many clinics and hospitals use computer records, which may be displayed on a computer screen on the desk. Notes are sometimes added to these during the interview via a keyboard. It can be very off-putting for a patient when the interviewing doctor looks entirely at the computer screen rather than at the patient. With practice it is possible to enter data while maintaining eye contact with a patient, but at first it is probably preferable to make written notes and transcribe or dictate them later.

The final record must be a sequential, accurate account of the development and course of the illness or illnesses of the patient (see Ch 50). There are a number of methods of recording this information. Hospitals may have printed forms with spaces for recording specific information. This applies especially to routine admissions (e.g. for minor surgical procedures). Follow-up consultation questions and notes will be briefer than those of the initial consultation; obviously, many questions are relevant only for the initial consultation. When a patient is seen repeatedly at a clinic or in a general practice setting, the current presenting history may be listed as an 'active' problem and the past history as a series of 'inactive' or 'still active' problems.

A sick patient will sometimes emphasise irrelevant facts and forget about very important symptoms. For this reason, a systematic approach to history taking and recording is crucial.[11] List 1.1 outlines a history-taking

---

HISTORY-TAKING SEQUENCE

1. **Presenting** (principal) **symptom** (PS)
2. **History of the presenting illness** (HPI)
   Details of current illnesses
   Details of previous similar episodes
   Extent of functional disability
   Effect of the illness
3. **Drug and treatment history**
   Current treatment
   Drug history (dose, duration, indication, side effects): prescription, over-the-counter and alternative therapies
   Past treatments
   Drug allergies or reactions
4. **Past history** (PH)
   Past illnesses
   Surgical operations (dates, indication, procedure)
   Menstrual and reproductive history for women
   Immunisations
   Blood transfusions (and dates)
5. **Social history** (SH)
   Upbringing and education level
   Marital status, social support, living conditions and financial situation
   Diet and exercise
   Occupation and hobbies
   Overseas travel (where and when)
   Smoking and alcohol use
   Analgesic and illicit (street) drug use
   Mood and sexual history
6. **Family history** (FH)
7. **Systems review** (SR)
   See Questions box 1.1 on pages 9–12

Also refer to Chapter 50.

LIST 1.1

sequence, but the detail required depends on the complexity of the presenting illness.

INTRODUCTORY QUESTIONS

In order to obtain a thorough history the clinician must establish a **good relationship**, interview in a **logical manner**, **listen** carefully, **interrupt** appropriately and usually only after allowing the patient to tell the initial story, note **non-verbal clues** and **correctly interpret** the information obtained.

The next step after introducing oneself should be to find out the patient's major symptoms or medical problems. Asking the patient 'What brought you here today?' can be unwise, as it often promotes the reply 'an ambulance' or 'a car'. This little joke wears thin after some years in clinical practice. It is best to attempt a conversational approach and ask the patient 'What has been the trouble or problem recently?' or 'When were you last quite well?' or 'What made you come to the hospital (or clinic) today?' For a follow-up consultation some reference to the last visit is appropriate, for example: 'How have things been going since I saw you last?' or 'It's been about … weeks since I saw you last, isn't it? What's been happening since then?' This lets the patient know the clinician hasn't forgotten him or her.

Some have suggested that the clinician begin with questions about more general aspects of the patient's life. There is a danger that this attempt to establish early rapport will seem intrusive to a person who has come for help about a specific problem, albeit one related to other aspects of life. This type of general and personal information may be better approached once the clinician has shown an interest in the presenting problem or as part of the social history—usually intrusive questions should be deferred to a subsequent consultation when the patient and clinician know each other better. The best approach and timing of this part of the interview will vary, depending on the nature of the presenting problem and the patient's and clinician's attitude.

> **T&O'C ESSENTIALS**
>
> Encourage patients to tell their story in their own words from the onset of the first symptom to the present time. Find out the full details of each problem and document them.

When a patient stops volunteering information, the question '**What else?**' will usually help start the conversation up again, and can be repeated several times if necessary.[8] On the other hand, some direction may be necessary to keep a garrulous patient on track later during the interview.

It is necessary to *ask specific questions to test diagnostic hypotheses*. For example, the patient may not have noticed an association between the occurrence of chest discomfort and exercise (typical of angina) unless asked specifically. It may also be helpful to give a list of possible answers. A patient with suspected angina who is unable to describe the symptom may be asked whether the sensation is sharp, dull, heavy or burning. The reply that it is sharp makes angina less likely.

Appropriate (but not exaggerated) reassuring gestures are of value to maintain the flow of conversation. If the patient stops giving the story spontaneously, it can be useful to provide a short summary of what has already been said and encourage him or her to continue.

The clinician must learn to listen with an open mind.[10] The temptation to leap to a diagnostic decision before the patient has had the chance to describe all the symptoms in his or her own words should be resisted. Avoid using pseudo-medical terms and if the patient uses them then find out exactly what is meant by them, as misinterpretation of medical terms is common.

Patients' descriptions of their symptoms may vary as they are subjected to repeated questioning by increasingly senior medical staff. The patient who has described his chest pain as sharp and left-sided to the medical student may tell the registrar that the pain is dull and in the centre of his chest. These discrepancies come as no surprise to experienced clinicians; they are sometimes the result of the patient having had time to reflect on his or her symptoms. This does mean, however, that very important aspects of the story should be checked by asking follow-up questions, such as: 'Can you show me exactly where the pain is?' and 'What do you mean by sharp?'

Some patients may have medical problems that make the interview difficult for them; these include deafness and problems with speech and memory. These must be recognised by the clinician if the interview is to be successful. See Chapter 2 for more details.

PRESENTING (PRINCIPAL) SYMPTOM

Not uncommonly, a patient has many symptoms. An attempt must be made to decide which symptom led the patient to present. It must be remembered that the patient's and the doctor's ideas of what constitutes a serious problem may differ. A patient with symptoms of a cold who also, in passing, mentions that he has recently coughed up blood (haemoptysis) may need more attention to his chest than to his nose. Find out what problem or symptom most concerns the patient. Patients are unlikely to be satisfied with their consultation if the issue that troubles them the most is not dealt with, even if it is a minor problem for which reassurance is all that is required. Record each presenting symptom or symptoms in the patient's own words, avoiding technical terms at this stage.

Whenever you identify a major complaint or symptom, think of the following as you are trying to unravel the story and ask questions to try to find out:

1. Where is the problem? (Probable anatomical diagnosis)
2. What is the nature of the symptom? (Likely pathological diagnosis)
3. How does it affect the patient? (Physiological and functional diagnosis)
4. Why did the patient develop it? (Aetiological diagnosis)

A diagnosis is not just about a name; you are trying to determine the likely disease process so that you can advise the patient of the prognosis and plan management.

HISTORY OF THE PRESENTING ILLNESS

Each of the presenting problems has to be talked about in detail with the patient, but in the first part of the interview the patient should lead the discussion. In the second part the doctor should take more control and ask specific questions. When writing down the history of the presenting illness, the events should be placed in chronological order; this might have to be done later when the whole history has been obtained. If numerous systems are affected, the events should be placed in chronological order for each system. Remember, patients may have multiple problems, of which some are interdependent and some not. In the older person, multiple problems are the rule, not the exception. Your job is to identify them all accurately and create a full medical picture of the individual.

Current symptoms

Certain information should routinely be sought for each current symptom if this hasn't been volunteered by the patient. The mnemonic **SOCRATES** summarises the questions that should be asked about most symptoms:

- **S** ite
- **O** nset
- **C** haracter
- **R** adiation (if the symptom is pain or discomfort)
- **A** lleviating factors
- **T** iming
- **E** xacerbating factors
- **S** everity.

Site

Ask where the symptom is exactly and whether it is localised or diffuse. Ask the patient to point to the actual site on the body.

Some symptoms are not localised. Patients who complain of dizziness do not localise this to any particular site—but vertigo may sometimes involve a feeling of movement within the head and to that extent is localised. Other symptoms that are not localised include cough, shortness of breath (dyspnoea) and change in weight.

Onset (mode of onset and pattern)

Find out whether the symptom came on rapidly, gradually or instantaneously. Some cardiac arrhythmias are of instantaneous onset and offset. Sudden loss of consciousness (syncope) with immediate recovery occurs with cardiac but not neurological disease. Ask whether the symptom has been present continuously or intermittently. Find out whether the symptom is getting worse or better, and, if so, when the change occurred. For example, the exertional breathlessness of chronic obstructive pulmonary disease (COPD) may come on with less and less activity as it worsens. Find out what the patient was doing at the time the symptom began. For example, severe breathlessness that wakes a patient from sleep is very suggestive of cardiac failure.

Character
Here it is necessary to ask the patient what is meant by the symptom, to describe its character. If the patient complains of dizziness, does this mean the room spins around (vertigo) or is it more a feeling of impending loss of consciousness? Does indigestion mean abdominal pain, heartburn, fullness after eating, excess wind or a change in bowel habit? If there is pain, is it sharp, dull, stabbing, boring, burning or cramp-like?

Radiation of pain or discomfort
Determine whether the symptom, if localised, radiates; this mainly applies if the symptom is pain. Certain patterns of radiation are typical of a condition or even diagnostic, for example the nerve root distribution of pain associated with herpes zoster (shingles).

Alleviating factors
Ask whether anything makes the symptom better. For example, the pain of pericarditis may be relieved when a patient sits up, whereas heartburn from acid reflux may be relieved by drinking milk or taking an antacid. Have analgesic medications been used to control the pain? Have narcotics been required?

Timing
Find out when the symptom first began and try to date this as accurately as possible. For example, ask the patient what the first thing was that he or she noticed was 'unusual' or 'wrong'. Ask whether the patient has had a similar illness in the past. It is often helpful to ask patients when they last felt entirely well. In a patient with long-standing symptoms, ask why he or she decided to see the doctor at this time.

Exacerbating factors
Ask whether anything makes the symptom worse. The slightest movement may exacerbate the abdominal pain of peritonitis or the pain in the big toe caused by gout.

Severity
This is subjective. The best way to assess severity is to ask the patient whether the symptom interferes with normal activities or sleep. Severity can be graded from mild to very severe. A mild symptom can be ignored by the patient, whereas a moderate symptom cannot be ignored but does not interfere with daily activities. A severe symptom interferes with daily activities, whereas a very severe symptom markedly interferes with most activities. Alternatively, pain or discomfort can be graded on a 10-point scale from 0 (no discomfort) to 10 (unbearable). (However, asking patients who are in severe pain to provide a number out of 10 seems at best a distraction and at worst rather unkind.) A face scale using pictures of different faces to represent pain severity from no pain (0) to very much pain (10) can be useful in practice.[12]

A number of other methods of quantifying pain are available (e.g. the visual analogue scale, whereby the patient is asked to mark the severity of pain on a 10-centimetre horizontal line). Note that all of these scales are more useful for comparing the subjective severity of pain over time than for absolute severity—for example, comparing before and after a certain treatment has been started.

The severity of some symptoms can be quantified more precisely; for example, shortness of breath on exertion occurring after walking 10 metres on flat ground is more severe than shortness of breath occurring after walking 90 metres up a hill. Central chest pain from angina occurring at rest is more significant than angina occurring while running 90 metres to catch a bus.

It is relevant to quantify the severity of each symptom—but also to remember that symptoms that a patient considers mild may be very significant.

Associated symptoms
Here an attempt is made to uncover in a systematic way those symptoms that might be expected to be associated with disease of a particular area. Initial and most thorough attention must be given to the system that includes the presenting problem (see Questions box 1.1). Remember that, although a single symptom may provide the clue that leads to the correct diagnosis, usually it is the combination of characteristic symptoms that most reliably suggests the diagnosis.

QUESTIONS BOX

The systems review
Enquire about common symptoms and three or four of the common disorders in each major system listed below. Not all of these questions should be asked of every patient. Adjust the detail of questions based on the presenting problem, the patient's age and the answers to the preliminary questions.

! denotes symptoms for the possible diagnosis of an urgent or dangerous (alarm) problem.

General
1. Have you had problems with tiredness? (Many physical and psychological causes)
2. Do you sleep well? (Insomnia and poor 'sleep hygiene', sleep apnoea)

Cardiovascular system
1. Have you had any pain or pressure in your chest, neck or arm? (Myocardial ischaemia)
2. Are you short of breath on exertion? How much exertion is necessary?
3. Have you ever woken up at night short of breath? (Cardiac failure)
4. Can you lie flat without feeling breathless?
5. Have you had swelling of your ankles?
6. Have you noticed your heart racing or beating irregularly?
! 7. Have you had blackouts without warning? (Stokes–Adams attacks)
! 8. Have you felt dizzy or blacked out when exercising? (Severe aortic stenosis or hypertrophic cardiomyopathy)
9. Do you have pain in your legs on exercise?
10. Do you have cold or blue hands or feet?
11. Have you ever had rheumatic fever, a heart attack or high blood pressure?

Respiratory system
1. Are you ever short of breath? Has this come on suddenly? (Pulmonary embolism)
2. Have you had any cough?
3. Is your cough associated with shivers and shakes (rigors) and breathlessness and chest pain? (Pneumonia)
4. Do you cough up anything?
! 5. Have you coughed up blood? (Bronchial carcinoma)
6. What type of work have you done? (Occupational lung disease)
7. Do you snore loudly? Do you fall asleep easily during the day? When? Have you fallen asleep while driving? Obtain a sleep history.
8. Do you ever have wheezing when you are short of breath?
9. Have you had fevers?
10. Do you have night sweats?
11. Have you ever had pneumonia or tuberculosis?
12. Have you had a recent chest X-ray?

Continued

QUESTIONS BOX continued

Gastrointestinal system
1. Are you troubled by indigestion? What do you mean by indigestion?
2. Do you have heartburn?
! 3. Have you had any difficulty swallowing? (Oesophageal cancer)
! 4. Have you had vomiting, or vomited blood? (Gastrointestinal bleeding)
5. Have you had pain or discomfort in your abdomen?
6. Have you had any abdominal bloating or distension?
7. Has your bowel habit changed recently? (Carcinoma of the colon)
8. How many bowel motions a week do you usually pass?
9. Have you lost control of your bowels or had accidents? (Faecal incontinence)
! 10. Have you seen blood in your motions? (Gastrointestinal bleeding)
! 11. Have your bowel motions been black? (Gastrointestinal bleeding)
! 12. Have you lost weight recently without dieting? (Malignancy)
13. Have your eyes or skin ever been yellow?
14. Have you ever had hepatitis, peptic ulceration, colitis or bowel cancer?
15. Tell me (briefly) about your diet recently.

Genitourinary system
1. Do you have difficulty or pain on passing urine?
2. Is your urine stream as good as it used to be?
3. Is there a delay before you start to pass urine? (Applies mostly to men)
4. Is there dribbling at the end?
5. Do you have to get up at night to pass urine?
6. Are you passing larger or smaller amounts of urine?
7. Has the urine colour changed?
! 8. Have you seen blood in your urine? (Urinary tract malignancy)
9. Have you any problems with your sex life? Difficulty obtaining or maintaining an erection?
10. Have you noticed any rashes or lumps on your genitals?
11. Have you ever had a sexually transmitted disease?
12. Have you ever had a urinary tract infection or kidney stone?

Haematological system
1. Do you bruise easily?
2. Have you had fevers, or shivers and shakes (rigors)?
! 3. Do you have difficulty stopping a small cut from bleeding? (Bleeding disorder)
! 4. Have you noticed any lumps under your arms, or in your neck or groin? (Haematological malignancy)
5. Have you ever had blood clots in your legs or in the lungs?

QUESTIONS BOX *continued*

Musculoskeletal system
1. Do you have painful or stiff joints?
2. Are any of your joints red, swollen and painful?
3. Have you had a skin rash recently?
4. Do you have any back or neck pain?
5. Have your eyes been dry or red?
6. Have you ever had a dry mouth or mouth ulcers?
7. Have you been diagnosed as having rheumatoid arthritis or gout?
8. Do your fingers ever become painful and become white and blue in the cold? (Raynaud's)

Endocrine system
1. Have you noticed any swelling in your neck?
2. Do your hands tremble?
3. Do you prefer hot or cold weather?
4. Have you had a thyroid problem or diabetes?
5. Have you noticed increased sweating?
6. Have you been troubled by fatigue?
7. Have you noticed any change in your appearance, hair, skin or voice?
8. Have you been unusually thirsty lately? Or lost weight? (New onset of diabetes)

Reproductive and breast history (women)
1. Are your periods regular?
2. Do you have excessive pain or bleeding with your periods?
3. How many pregnancies have you had?
4. Have you had any miscarriages?
5. Have you had high blood pressure or diabetes in pregnancy?
6. Were there any other complications during your pregnancies or deliveries?
7. Have you had a Caesarean section?
! 8. Have you had any bleeding or discharge from your breasts or felt any lumps there? (Carcinoma of the breast)

Neurological system and mental state
1. Do you get headaches?
! 2. Is your headache very severe and did it begin very suddenly? (Subarachnoid haemorrhage)
3. Have you had fainting episodes, fits or blackouts?
4. Do you have trouble seeing or hearing?
5. Are you dizzy?
6. Have you had weakness, numbness or clumsiness in your arms or legs?
7. Have you ever had a stroke or head injury?
8. Do you feel sad or depressed, or have problems with your 'nerves'?
9. Have you ever been sexually or physically abused?

Continued

QUESTIONS BOX continued

The elderly patient
1. Have you had problems with falls or loss of balance? (High fracture risk)
2. Do you walk with a frame or stick?
3. Do you take sleeping tablets or sedatives? (Falls risk)
4. Do you take blood pressure tablets? (Postural hypotension and falls risk)
5. Have you been tested for osteoporosis?
6. Can you manage at home without help?
7. Are you affected by arthritis?
8. Have you had problems with your memory or with managing things like paying bills? (Cognitive decline)
9. How do you manage your various tablets? (Risk of polypharmacy and confusion of doses)

Concluding the interview
Is there anything else you would like to talk about?

BOX 1.1

The effect of the illness

A serious illness can change a person's life—for example, a chronic illness may prevent work or further education. The psychological and physical effects of a serious health problem may be devastating and, of course, people respond differently to similar problems. Even after full recovery from a life-threatening illness, some people may be permanently affected by loss of confidence or self-esteem. There may be continuing anxieties about the capability of supporting a family. Try to find out how the patient and his or her family have been affected. How has the patient coped so far, and what are the expectations and hopes for the future with regard to health? What explanations of the condition has the patient been given or obtained (e.g. from the internet)?

Helping a patient to manage ill-health is a large part of the clinician's duty. This depends on sympathetic and realistic explanations of the probable future course of the disease and the effects of treatment.

DRUG AND TREATMENT HISTORY

Ask the patient whether he or she is currently taking any tablets or medicines (the use of the word 'drug' may cause alarm); the patient will often describe these by colour or size rather than by name and dose.[c] Then ask the patient to show you all his or her medications (see Fig. 1.2), if possible, and list them. Note the dose, length of use, indication for each drug and any side effects.

This drug list may provide a useful clue to chronic or past illnesses, otherwise forgotten. For example, a patient who denies a history of high blood pressure may remember when asked why he or she is taking an antihypertensive drug having an elevated blood pressure in the past. Remember that some drugs are prescribed as transdermal patches or subcutaneous implants (e.g. contraceptives and hormonal treatment of carcinoma of the prostate). Ask whether the drugs were taken as prescribed. Always ask specifically whether a woman is taking the contraceptive pill, because many who take it do not consider it a medicine or tablet. The same is true of inhalers, or what many patients call their 'puffers'.

To remind the patient, it is often worthwhile to ask about the use of classes of drugs. A basic list should include questions about treatment for:

- blood pressure
- high cholesterol

---

[c] If you ask a patient what size a tablet is (meaning how many milligrams) a common answer will be, 'Oh it is quite small'.

CHAPTER 1 THE GENERAL PRINCIPLES OF HISTORY TAKING   13

(a) Medications packed for hospital discharge. (b) A Webster packet; medications packed for the patient by the pharmacy by time and day of the week

FIGURE 1.2

- diabetes
- arthritis
- anxiety or depression
- erectile dysfunction (no longer called impotence)
- contraception
- hormone replacement
- epilepsy
- anticoagulation
- antibiotics.

Also ask whether the patient is taking any over-the-counter preparations (e.g. aspirin, antihistamines, vitamins). Aspirin and standard non-steroidal anti-inflammatory drugs (NSAIDs), but not paracetamol (acetaminophen), can cause gastrointestinal bleeding. Patients with chronic pain may consume large amounts of analgesics, including drugs containing opioids such as codeine and morphine. These may be used in the form of skin patches. A careful history of the period of use of opioids and the quantities used is important, because they are drugs of dependence.

Many patients have printed copies of parts of their electronic records with lists of drugs. Unless these are updated regularly, they tend to contain names of drugs the patient may no longer be using. Ask about each drug on the list—whether it is still being taken and what it is for. It is very common for patients to say they have not used certain drugs on their list for years. Update the list for the patient if you are in charge of his or her care.

There may be some medications or treatments the patient has had in the past that remain relevant. These include corticosteroids, chemotherapeutic agents (anticancer drugs) and radiotherapy. Often patients, especially those with a chronic disease, are very well informed about their condition and their treatment. However, some allowance must be made for patients' non-medical interpretation of what happened.[10]

Note any **adverse reactions** in the past. Also ask specifically about any **allergy to drugs** (often a skin reaction or episode of bronchospasm) and what the allergic reaction actually involved, to help decide whether it was really an allergic reaction.[13] Patients often confuse an allergy with a side effect of a drug.

Approximately 50% of people now use 'natural remedies' of various types.[14] They may not feel that these are a relevant part of their medical history, but these chemicals, like any drug, may have adverse effects. Indeed, some have been found to be adulterated with drugs such as steroids and NSAIDs. More information about these substances and their effects is becoming available and there is an increasing responsibility for clinicians to be aware of them and to ask about them directly.

Ask (where relevant—not the 90-year-old nursing home resident) about 'recreational' or street drug use (*vide infra*). The use of intravenous drugs has many implications for the patient's health. Ask whether any attempt has been made to avoid sharing needles. This may protect against the injection of viruses, but not against bacterial infection from the use of impure substances. Cocaine use has become a common cause of myocardial infarction in young people in some countries. Acutely ill patients may have taken overdoses of drugs whose purity has been underestimated (especially narcotics) or taken drugs without knowing what they are. The use of amphetamine-like drugs at parties can be associated with dehydration with electrolyte abnormalities and psychotic symptoms. Here an attempt to find out more detail from the patient or other party-goers is essential.

Not all medical problems are treated with drugs. Ask about courses of physiotherapy or rehabilitation for musculoskeletal problems or injuries, or to help recovery following surgery or a severe illness. Certain gastrointestinal conditions are treated with dietary supplements (e.g. pancreatic enzymes for chronic pancreatitis) or restrictions (e.g. avoidance of gluten for coeliac disease).

PAST HISTORY

Some patients may feel that questions about past problems and the more general questions asked in the systems review (p 19) are somewhat intrusive. It may be best to preface these questions by saying something like, 'I need to ask you some questions about your past medical problems and general health. These may affect your current investigations and treatment.'

Ask the patient whether he or she has had any serious illnesses, operations or admissions to hospital in the past, including any obstetric or gynaecological problems. Where relevant obtain the details. Do not forget to enquire about childhood illnesses. Ask about past blood transfusion (including when and what for). Serious or chronic childhood illnesses may have interfered with a child's education and social activities like sport. Ask what the patient remembers and thinks about this.

Previous illnesses or operations may have a direct bearing on current health. It is worth asking specifically about certain operations that have a continuing effect on the patient—for example, operations for malignancy, bowel surgery or cardiac surgery, especially valve surgery. Implanted prostheses are common in surgical, orthopaedic and cardiac procedures. These may involve a risk of infection of the foreign body, whereas magnetic metals—especially most cardiac pacemakers—are a contraindication to magnetic resonance imaging (MRI). Chronic kidney disease (CKD) may be a contraindication to X-rays using iodine contrast materials and MRI scanning using gadolinium contrast. Pregnancy is usually a contraindication to radiation exposure (X-rays and nuclear scans—remember that computed tomography [CT] scans cause hundreds of times the radiation exposure of simple X-rays).

The patient may believe that he or she has had a particular diagnosis made in the past, but careful questioning may reveal this as unlikely. For example, the patient may mention a previous duodenal ulcer, but not have had any investigations or treatment for it, which makes the diagnosis less certain. Therefore, it is important to obtain the particulars of each relevant past illness, including the symptoms experienced, tests performed and treatments prescribed. The mature clinician needs to maintain an *objective scepticism* about the information that is obtained from the patient.

Patients with chronic illnesses may have had their condition managed with the help of various doctors and at specialised clinics. For example, patients with diabetes mellitus are often managed by a team of health professionals including diabetic educators, nurses and dietitians. Find out what supervision and treatment these have provided. For example, who does the patient contact if there is a problem with the insulin dose, and does the patient know what to do (an **action plan**) if there is an urgent or a dangerous complication? Patients with chronic diseases are often very much involved in their own care and are very well informed about aspects of their treatment. For example, diabetics should keep records of their home-measured blood sugar levels, heart failure patients should monitor their weight daily and so on. These patients will often make their own adjustments to their medication doses. Assessing a patient's understanding of and confidence in making these changes should be part of the history taking.

It should be routine to find out whether the adult patient is up to date with the recommended immunisations (e.g. mumps, measles, rubella, tetanus, etc.) as well as other recent immunisations (e.g. for human papilloma virus [HPV], hepatitis B, pneumococcal disease, *Haemophilus influenzae* or influenza) (p 30).

Ask what other medical practitioners the patient sees and whether he or she wants copies of your report sent to them. Patients have the right not to have information sent to other doctors if they choose.

Additional history for the female patient

For women, a menstrual history should be obtained; it is particularly relevant for a woman with abdominal pain, a suspected endocrine disease or genitourinary symptoms. Write down the date of the last menstrual period. Ask about the age at which menstruation began, whether the periods are regular or whether menopause has occurred. Ask whether the symptoms occur at a particular time in the menstrual cycle. Do not forget to ask a woman of childbearing age if there is a possibility of pregnancy; this, for example, may preclude the use of certain investigations or drugs.[15] Observing the well-known axiom that 'every woman of childbearing years is pregnant until proven otherwise' can prevent unnecessary danger to the unborn child and avoid embarrassment for the unwary clinician. Ask about any miscarriages. Record *gravida* (the number of pregnancies) and *para* (the number of births of babies over 20 weeks' gestation).

SOCIAL HISTORY

This is the time to find out more about the patient as a person. The questions should be asked in an interested and conversational way and should not sound like a routine learned by rote. For example, chronic pain can affect relationships, employment, income and leisure activities, and it is your job to understand these matters in order to provide the best possible care plan.

> **T&O'C ESSENTIALS**
>
> *The social history includes the patient's economic, social, domestic and work situations.*

Upbringing and education level

Ask first about the places of birth and residence, and the level of education obtained (including problems with schooling caused by childhood illnesses). This can influence the way things need to be explained to the patient. Recent migrants may have been exposed to infectious diseases like tuberculosis; ethnic background is important in some diseases, such as thalassaemia and sickle cell anaemia.

Marital status, social support and living conditions

To determine the patient's marital status, ask who is living at home with the patient. Find out about the health of the spouse and any children. Check whether there are any other household members. If the patient is not able to look after him- or herself unaided, establish who the patient's main 'caregiver' is. 'Matter of fact' questions about sexual activity may be very relevant. For example, erectile dysfunction may occur in neurological conditions, debilitating illness or psychiatric disease. Questions about living arrangements are particularly important for chronic or disabling illnesses, where it is necessary to know what social support is available and whether the patient is able to manage at home (e.g. the number of steps required to get into the house, or the location of the toilet).

Ask whether the patient considers him- or herself to be a spiritual person. Spirituality is an important factor, especially in the care of dying patients, in the creation of living wills and in understanding the support network available for the patient.

The presence of pets in the home may be important if infections or allergies are suspected.

Ask about mobility (e.g. if an adult patient is still driving and how he or she gets to the shops and appointments).

Diet and exercise

Ask about the adequacy of the patient's diet, who does the cooking, the availability of 'meals on wheels' and other services such as house cleaning. Also ask how physically active the patient is.

Occupation and hobbies

Ask the patient about present occupation;[16] the **WHACS** mnemonic is useful here:[17]

W hat do you do?
H ow do you do it?
A re you concerned about any of your exposures or experiences?
C olleagues or others exposed?
S atisfied with your job?

Finding out exactly what the patient does at work can be helpful, as some occupations (and hobbies) are linked to disease (see Text box 1.2). Note particularly any work exposure to dusts, chemicals or disease; for example, mine and industrial workers may have the disease asbestosis. Find out whether any similar problems have affected fellow workers. Checking on hobbies can also be informative (e.g. bird fanciers and lung disease, use of solvents).

Occupations and hobbies linked to disease

1. Farmers: mouldy hay—hypersensitivity pneumonitis
2. Bird fanciers: birds—hypersensitivity pneumonitis, psittacosis
3. Welders: eye flash burns, pacemaker malfunction
4. Stone masons: silicosis
5. Shipyard workers, builders, emergency workers: asbestosis
6. Coal miners: pneumoconiosis and silicosis
7. Timber workers: asthma
8. Electronic workers: berylliosis
9. Healthcare workers: needle-stick HIV, hepatitis B, TB

HIV=human immunodeficiency virus; TB=tuberculosis.

TEXT BOX 1.2

Overseas travel

If an infectious disease is a possibility, ask about recent overseas travel, destinations visited and how the patient lived when away (e.g. did he or she drink unbottled water and eat local foods, or dine at expensive international hotels?). Note any hospitalisations or procedures overseas. Travel overseas, if hospitalised, may be associated with acquiring antibiotic-resistant bacteria. Ask about the patient's immunisation status (see Ch 2). Determine whether any prophylactic drugs (e.g. for malaria) were taken during the travel period.

Smoking

The patient may claim to be a non-smoker if he or she stopped smoking that morning. Therefore, ask whether the patient has ever smoked and, if so, how many cigarettes (or cigars or pipes) were smoked a day and for how many years. Find out whether the patient has stopped smoking and, if so, when this was. It is necessary to ask how many packets of cigarettes per day the patient has smoked and for how many years the patient has smoked. An estimate should be made of the number of packet-years of smoking. Remember that this estimate is based on 20-cigarette packets[d] and that packets of cigarettes are getting larger; curiously, most manufacturers now make packets of 30 or 35. More recently, giant packets of 50 have appeared: these are too large to fit into a pocket and must be carried in the hands as a constant reminder to the patient of his or her addiction.

Cigarette smoking is a risk factor for vascular disease, chronic lung disease, several cancers and peptic ulceration, and may damage the fetus (see List 1.2). The more recent the exposure and the greater the number of packet-years, the greater the risk of these problems becomes. Cigar and pipe smokers typically inhale less smoke than cigarette smokers and overall mortality rates are correspondingly lower in this group, except from carcinoma of the oral cavity, larynx and oesophagus.

As a routine this may be a good time to give a gentle reminder about smoking cessation. Suggesting 'This might be a good time to think about becoming a non-smoker' avoids giving the impression that the

---

[d] 20 cigarettes a day for a year=1 packet-year.

> **SMOKING AND CLINICAL ASSOCIATIONS***
>
> **Cardiovascular disease**
> Premature coronary artery disease
> Peripheral vascular disease, erectile dysfunction
> Cerebrovascular disease
>
> **Respiratory disease**
> Lung cancer
> Chronic obstructive pulmonary disease (chronic airflow limitation)
> Increased incidence of respiratory infection
> Increased incidence of postoperative respiratory complications
>
> **Other cancers**
> Larynx, oral cavity, oesophagus, nasopharynx, bladder, kidney, pancreas, stomach, uterine, cervix
>
> **Gastrointestinal disease**
> Peptic ulceration, Crohn's disease
>
> **Pregnancy**
> Increased risk of spontaneous abortion, fetal death, neonatal death, sudden infant death syndrome
>
> **Drug interactions**
> Induces hepatic microsomal enzyme systems, e.g. increased metabolism of propranolol, theophylline
>
> *Individual risk is influenced by the duration, intensity and type of smoke exposure, as well as by genetic and other environmental factors. Passive smoking is also associated with respiratory disease
>
> LIST 1.2

habit is condoned and the patient's thinking 'Smoking can't be a problem for me; the doctor hasn't suggested I stop.'

Alcohol use

Ask whether the patient drinks alcohol.[18] If so, ask what type, how much and how often. Excessive use of alcohol is common in the community; if the patient claims to be a social drinker, find out exactly what this means. Again a conversational approach may help keep the patient onside and seem less censorious—for example: 'Do you drink beer or wine or spirits?' and 'How many glasses of … would you have on most days?' In a glass of wine, a nip (or shot) of spirits, a glass of port or sherry or a 200 mL (7 oz) glass of beer there are approximately 8–10 g of alcohol (1 unit=8 g).

Guidelines for safe drinking levels vary around the world.[19] The National Health and Medical Research Council (NHMRC) in Australia recommends a maximum alcohol intake of no more than 2 standard drinks per day on average and no more than 4 standard drinks on a single day with 2 alcohol-free days per week for men and women.[20] In the United Kingdom, the current recommended safe limits are 21 units (168 g of ethanol) per week for men and 14 units (112 g of ethanol) for women; weekly consumption of more than 50 units for men and 35 units for women is considered to place the user in a high-risk group. In the United States, the National Institute on Alcohol Abuse and Alcoholism (NIAAA) suggests that the following alcohol levels are harmful: for men under the age of 65, an average of more than 14 standard drinks per week (or more than 4 drinks on any day); and for women and all adults 65 years and older an average of more than 7 standard drinks per week. Alcohol becomes a major risk factor for liver disease in men who consume more than 80 g daily and women who consume more than 40 g daily for 5 years or longer.

Alcoholics are notoriously unreliable about describing their alcohol intake, so it may be important to suspend belief and sometimes (with the patient's permission) talk to relatives.

Certain questions can be helpful in making a diagnosis of alcoholism; these are referred to as the CAGE questions:[21]

- Have you ever felt you ought to *Cut* down on your drinking?
- Have people *Annoyed* you by criticising your drinking?
- Have you ever felt bad or *Guilty* about your drinking?
- Have you ever had a drink first thing in the morning to steady your nerves or get rid of a hangover? (*Eye opener*)

If the patient answers 'yes' to any two of these questions, this suggests that he or she has a serious alcohol dependence problem (77% sensitivity, 79%

specificity), but the screening often misses unhealthy alcohol use.

A more useful screening test to identify unhealthy drinking comprises three simple questions (AUDIT-C):

1. How often do you have a drink containing alcohol?
2. How many drinks containing alcohol do you have on a typical day when you are drinking alcohol?
3. How often do you have 6 or more alcoholic drinks on one occasion?

Each question is scored from 0 (never) to 4 (4 or more times per week). Positive scores for unhealthy (excess) drinking are:

- 3 or more for women (73% sensitivity, 91% specificity)
- 4 or more for men (86% sensitivity, 89% specificity).[22]

An even simpler screening question is to ask, 'How many times in the past year have you had 5 (for men; 4 for women) or more drinks in a day?' A score of *over* 0 (or 'I don't remember') suggests alcohol use in the unhealthy range. This question performs almost as well as the AUDIT-C screening.[23]

The complications of alcohol abuse are summarised in List 1.3.

Analgesics and street drugs

Over-the-counter analgesics can cause harm—for example, if an alcoholic has just a bit too much paracetamol it may lead to acute liver failure.

ALCOHOL (ETHANOL) ABUSE: COMPLICATIONS

Gastrointestinal system
- Acute gastric erosions
- Gastrointestinal bleeding from varices, erosions, Mallory–Weiss tear, peptic ulceration
- Pancreatitis (acute, recurrent or chronic)
- Diarrhoea (watery, due to alcohol itself, or steatorrhoea from chronic alcoholic pancreatitis or, rarely, liver disease)
- Hepatomegaly (fatty liver, chronic liver disease)
- Chronic liver disease (alcoholic hepatitis, cirrhosis) and associated complications
- Cancer (oesophagus, cardia of stomach, liver, pancreas)

Cardiovascular system
- Cardiomyopathy
- Cardiac arrhythmias
- Hypertension

Nervous system
- 'Blackouts'
- Nutrition-related conditions, e.g. Wernicke's encephalopathy, Korsakoff's psychosis, peripheral neuropathy (thiamine deficiency), pellagra (dementia, dermatitis and diarrhoea from niacin deficiency)
- Withdrawal syndromes, e.g. tremor, hallucinations, 'rum fits', delirium tremens
- Cerebellar degeneration
- Alcoholic dementia
- Alcoholic myopathy
- Autonomic neuropathy

Haematopoietic system
- Anaemia (dietary folate deficiency, iron deficiency from blood loss, direct toxic suppression of the bone marrow, rarely B_{12} deficiency with chronic pancreatitis, or sideroblastic anaemia)
- Thrombocytopenia (from bone marrow suppression or hypersplenism)

Genitourinary system
- Erectile dysfunction (impotence), testicular atrophy in men
- Amenorrhoea, infertility, spontaneous abortion, fetal alcohol syndrome in women

Other effects
- Increased risk of fractures and osteonecrosis of the femoral head

LIST 1.3

Ask whether the patient has ever used marijuana, has tried other street drugs or has ever shot up. An excellent screening question that is 100% sensitive (and 74% specific) is to ask, 'How many times in the past year have you used an illegal drug or used a prescription medication for non-medical reasons?'[24] Asking about 'recreational' or street drug use, if not already known, is important.

Mood

Depression severe enough to cause distress to a patient is common: it has a prevalence of up to 8%.[25] Depression can be the result of any significant medical illness; in fact, the incidence of depression increases threefold for these patients. Patients with underlying depression may find illness more difficult to cope with. Questioning patients about depression can be difficult. A common approach is to ask first, 'How are things going at home and at work at the moment?' Questions about depressed mood (see p 25, Questions box 2.2) and *anhedonia* (loss of interest or pleasure in activities previously enjoyed) can be helpful. Major depression is unlikely if the answer to these questions is 'no'.

Certain medical conditions such as hypothyroidism or Cushing's disease can be direct causes of depression.

If depression seems likely, questions about suicide risk should be asked. There is no evidence that asking such questions increases the risk of suicide (see Ch 46, Volume 2).[26]

Sexual history

The sexual history may be relevant; if so, specific questions should be asked. Good judgement is necessary about the right time to ask very personal questions (see p 27).

FAMILY HISTORY

Many diseases run in families. For example, ischaemic heart disease that has developed at a young age in parents or siblings is a major risk factor for ischaemic heart disease in their offspring. Various malignancies, such as breast and large-bowel carcinoma, are more common in certain families. Both genetic and common environmental exposures may explain these familial associations. Some diseases (e.g. haemophilia) are directly inherited.[27] Patient reporting of a family history

> **FACTORS SUGGESTING AN INCREASED RISK TO A PATIENT BECAUSE OF GENETIC FACTORS**
>
> - Family history of numerous relatives affected by the disorder, e.g. three family members with bowel cancer
> - Disease occurring in less-often-affected sex, e.g. thyroid disease in male relatives
> - Earlier onset of disease than usual in relatives, e.g. premature coronary artery disease
> - Disease occurring despite absence in patient of the usual risk factors, e.g. hyperlipidaemia despite normal weight and excellent diet
> - Racial predisposition to a disease, e.g. haemochromatosis in people of Irish descent
> - Consanguinity of parents, e.g. cystic fibrosis
>
> LIST 1.4

of malignancy is not always accurate. However, two important cancers—bowel and breast—are accurately reported by patients.

Ask about any history of a similar illness in the family. Certain factors suggest an increased genetic risk (List 1.4).

Enquire about the health and, if relevant, the causes of death and ages of death of the parents and siblings. If there is any suggestion of a hereditary disease, a complete family tree should be compiled showing all members affected (see Fig. 1.3). Patients can be reluctant to mention that they have relatives with mental illness, epilepsy or cancer, so ask tactfully about these diseases. Consanguinity (usually first cousins marrying) increases the probability of autosomal recessive abnormalities in the children; ask about this if the pedigree is suggestive.

SYSTEMS REVIEW

As well as detailed questioning about the system likely to be diseased, it is essential to ask about important symptoms and disorders in other systems (see Questions box 1.1), as otherwise important diseases may be missed.[28,29] An experienced clinician will perform a targeted systems review, based on information already obtained from the patient; clearly it is not realistic to ask anyone all of the listed questions.

When recording the systems review, list important negative answers ('relevant negatives'). Remember: if

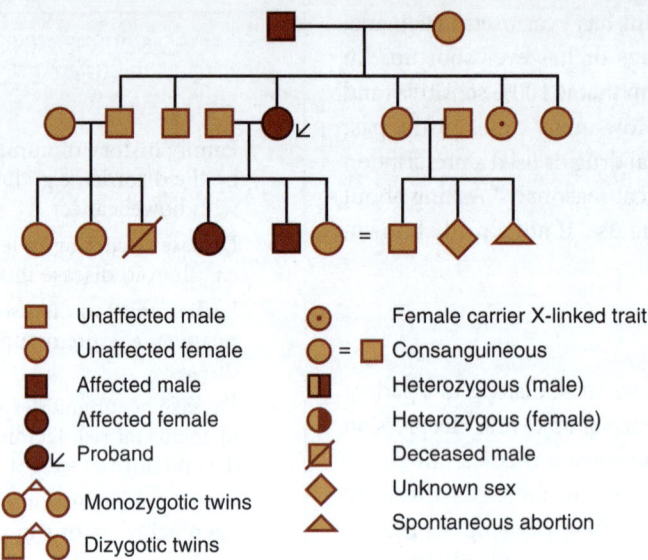

Preparing a family tree: note the symbols used for the documentation

FIGURE 1.3

other recent symptoms are unmasked, more details must be sought; relevant information is then added to the history of the presenting illness.

Before completing the history, it is often valuable to ask what the patient thinks is wrong and what he or she is most concerned about. General and sympathetic questions about the effect of a chronic or severe illness on the patient's life are important for establishing rapport and for finding out what else might be needed (both medical and non-medical) to help the patient.

Major presenting symptoms for each system are described in the following chapters. Examples of supplementary important questions to ask about past history, social history and family history are also given there for each system.

SKILLS IN HISTORY TAKING

> **T&O'C ESSENTIALS**
>
> 1. Several skills are important in obtaining a useful and accurate history.
>   a. Establish rapport and understanding.
>   b. Ask questions in a logical sequence. Start with open-ended questions. Listen to the answers and adjust your interview accordingly.
>   c. Observe and provide non-verbal clues carefully. Encouraging, sympathetic gestures and concentration on the patient that make it clear he or she has your undivided attention are most important and helpful, but are really a form of normal politeness.
>   d. Proper interpretation of the history is crucial.
> 2. A good grounding in history taking will stand you in good stead for the rest of your career in medicine.
> 3. A successful consultation with a patient, based on a good history-taking manner, is satisfying and even enjoyable for both parties.
> 4. Repeated practice in history taking makes it an accurate and quite rapid process (usually).
> 5. Not taking a proper history (a regrettably common event) can lead to an incorrect differential diagnosis, the wrong tests and often the wrong treatment.
> 6. No test is accurate enough (sensitive and specific enough) to be useful if it is ordered for the wrong reason (e.g. as a result of poor history taking).
> 7. Screen for alcohol and drug use using standard questions.

Your aim should be to obtain information that will help establish the likely anatomical and physiological disturbances present, the aetiology of the presenting symptoms and the impact of the symptoms on the patient's ability to function.[30] (In Ch 2, some advice on how to take the history in more challenging circumstances is considered.) This type of information will help you plan the diagnostic investigations and treatment, and to discuss the findings with, or present them to, a colleague if necessary. First, however, a comprehensive and systematic physical examination is required.

These skills can be obtained and maintained only by practice.[31]

References

1. Longson D. The clinical consultation. *J R Coll Physicians Lond* 1983; 17:192–195. Outlines the principles of hypothesis generation and testing during the clinical evaluation.
2. Nardone DA, Johnson GK, Faryna A et al. A model for the diagnostic medical interview: nonverbal, verbal and cognitive assessments. *J Gen Intern Med* 1992; 7:437–442. Verbal and non-verbal questions and diagnostic reasoning are reviewed in this useful article.
3. Bellet PS, Maloney MJ. The importance of empathy as an interviewing skill in medicine. *JAMA* 1991; 266:1831–1832. Distinguishes between empathy, reassurance and patient education.
4. Brewin T. Primum non nocere? *Lancet* 1994; 344:1487–1488. Reviews a key principle in clinical management.
5. Platt FW, McMath JC. Clinical hypocompetence: the interview. *Ann Intern Med* 1979; 91:898–902. A valuable review of potential flaws in interviewing, condensed into five syndromes: inadequate content, database flaws, defects in hypothesis generation, failure to obtain primary data and a controlling style.
6. Platt FW, Gaspar DL, Coulehan JL et al. 'Tell me about yourself': the patient-centred interview. *Ann Intern Med* 2001; 134:1079–1084.
7. Fogarty L, Curbow BA, Wingard JR et al. Can 40 seconds of compassion reduce patient anxiety? *J Clin Oncol* 1999; 17:371–379.
8. Barrier P, Li JT, Jensen NM. Two words to improve physician–patient communication: what else? *Mayo Clin Proc* 2003; 78:211–214. Ask 'What else?' whenever the interview pauses to obtain an optimal history.
9. Blau JN. Time to let the patient speak. *BMJ* 1999; 298:39. The average doctor's uninterrupted narrative with a patient lasts less than 2 minutes (and often much less!), which is too brief. Open interviewing is vital for accurate history taking.
10. Smith RC, Hoppe RB. The patient's story: integrating the patient- and physician-centered approaches to interviewing. *Ann Intern Med* 1991; 115:470–477. Patients tell stories of their illness, integrating both the medical and psychosocial aspects. Both need to be obtained, and this article reviews ways to do this and to interpret the information.
11. Beckman H, Markakis K, Suchman A, Frankel R. Getting the most from a 20-minute visit. *Am J Gastroenterol* 1994; 89:662–664. A lot of information can be obtained from a patient, even when time is limited, if the history is taken logically.
12. Tomlinson D, von Baeyer CL, Stinson JN, Sung L. A systematic review of faces scales for the self-report of pain intensity in children. *Pediatrics* 2010; 126(5):e1168–e1198.
13. Salkind AR, Cuddy PG, Foxworth JW. The rational clinical examination. Is this patient allergic to penicillin? An evidence-based analysis of the likelihood of penicillin allergy. *JAMA* 2001; 285(19):2498–2505.
14. Holtmann G, Talley NJ. Herbal medicines for the treatment of functional and inflammatory bowel disorders. *Clin Gastroenterol Hepatol* 2015; 13:422–432.
15. Ramosaka EA, Sacchetti AD, Nepp M. Reliability of patient history in determining the possibility of pregnancy. *Ann Emerg Med* 1989; 18:48–50. In this study, one in 10 women who denied the possibility of pregnancy had a positive pregnancy test.
16. Newman LS. Occupational illness. *N Engl J Med* 1995; 333:1128–1134. The importance of knowing the occupation for the diagnosis of an illness cannot be overemphasised.
17. Blue AV, Chessman AW, Gilbert GE et al. Medical students' abilities to take an occupational history: use of the WHACS mnemonic. *J Occup Environ Med* 2000; 42(11):1050–1053.
18. Kitchens JM. Does this patient have an alcohol problem? *JAMA* 1994; 272:1782–1787. A useful guide to making this assessment.
19. Friedmann PD. Clinical practice. Alcohol use in adults. *N Engl J Med* 2013; 368(4):365–373.
20. Australian Government. National Health and Medical Research Council. Alcohol guidelines. www.nhmrc.gov.au/your-health/alcohol-guidelines.
21. Beresford TP, Blow FC, Hill E et al. Comparison of CAGE questionnaire and computer-assisted laboratory profiles in screening for covert alcoholism. *Lancet* 1990; 336:482–485.
22. Bradley KA, DeBenedetti AF, Volk RJ et al. AUDIT-C as a brief screen for alcohol misuse in primary care. *Alcohol Clin Exp Res* 2007; 31:1208.
23. Smith PC, Schmidt SM, Allensworth-Davies D, Saitz R. Primary care validation of a single-question alcohol screening test. *J Gen Intern Med* 2009; 24:783–788.
24. Smith PC, Schmidt SM, Allensworth-Davies D, Saitz R. A single-question screening test for drug use in primary care. *Arch Intern Med* 2010; 170(13):1155–1160.
25. World Health Organization. Depression. www.who.int/mentalhealth/management/depression/definition/en.
26. Zimmerman M, Lish DT, Lush DT et al. Suicide ideation among urban medical outpatients. *J Gen Intern Med* 1995; 10(10):573–576.
27. Rich EC, Burke W, Heaton CJ et al. Reconsidering the family history in primary care. *J Gen Intern Med* 2004; 19(3):273–280.
28. Hoffbrand BI. Away with the system review: a plea for parsimony. *BMJ* 1989; 198:817–819. Presents the case that the systems review approach is not valuable. A focused review still seems to be useful in practice (see reference 29 below).
29. Boland BJ, Wollan PC, Silverstein MD. Review of systems, physical examination, and routine test for case-finding in ambulatory patients. *Am J Med Sci* 1995; 309:194–200. A systems review can identify unsuspected clinically important conditions.
30. Simpson M, Buchman R, Stewart M et al. Doctor–patient communication: the Toronto consensus statement. *BMJ* 1991; 303:1385–1387. Most complaints about doctors relate to failure of adequate communication. Encouraging patients to discuss their major concerns without interruption or premature closure enhances satisfaction and yet takes little time (average 90 seconds). Factors that improve communication include using appropriate open-ended questions, giving frequent summaries, and using clarification and negotiation. These skills can be learned but require practice.
31. Henderson MC, Tierney LM, Smetana GW (eds). *The patient history. An evidence-based approach to differential diagnosis*. McGraw-Hill Lange, New York: 2012.

CHAPTER 2
Advanced history taking

First the doctor told me the good news: I was going to have a disease named after me.[a] STEVE MARTIN

Most complaints about doctors relate to the failure of adequate communication.[1,2] Encouraging patients to discuss their major concerns without interruption enhances satisfaction and yet takes little time (on average only 90 seconds).[3,4] Giving premature advice or reassurance, or inappropriate use of closed questions, badly affects the interview.

Giving a patient the impression that you disapprove of some aspect of his or her life can put up a major barrier to the success of the interview. Avoid what might be seen as a judgemental attitude to anything you hear. This should not prevent you from giving sensible advice about activities that are dangerous to the patient's health. Expressing sympathy about the patient's problems (medical or otherwise) should be a normal human reaction on the part of the clinician.

TAKING A GOOD HISTORY

Communication and history-taking skills can be learned but require constant practice. Watch for signs that the patient is uncomfortable. For example, the sudden breaking off of eye contact or the crossing of arms or legs: this body language suggests that the patient is not comfortable with the questioning and you need to redirect or change tack.[5] Factors that improve communication include using appropriate open-ended questions, giving frequent summaries, and using clarification and negotiation.[3,4,6] (See List 2.1.)

THE DIFFERENTIAL DIAGNOSIS

As the interview proceeds, you will need to begin to consider the possible diagnosis or diagnoses—the **differential diagnosis**. This usually starts as a long and ill-defined mental list in your mind. As more detail of the symptoms emerges, the list becomes more defined. This mental list must be used as a guide to further questioning in the latter part of the interview. Specific questions should then be used to help confirm or eliminate various possibilities. The physical examination and investigations may then be directed to help further narrow the differential. At the end of the history and examination, a likely diagnosis and list of differential diagnoses should be drawn up. This will often be modified as results of tests emerge.

This method of history taking is called, rather grandly, the *hyopthetico-deductive approach*. It is in fact used by most experienced clinicians. History taking does not mean asking a series of set questions of every patient, but rather knowing what questions to ask as the differential diagnosis begins to become clearer.

FUNDAMENTAL CONSIDERATIONS WHEN TAKING THE HISTORY

As the medical interview proceeds, keep in mind four underlying principles:

1. *What is the probable diagnosis so far?* This is a basic differential diagnosis. As you complete the history of the presenting illness, ask yourself: 'For *this* patient based on *these* symptoms and what I know so far, what are the most likely diagnoses?' Think about the anatomical location, then the likely pathology or pathophysiology, then the possible causes, then direct additional questions accordingly.
2. *Could any of these symptoms represent an urgent or dangerous diagnosis—**red-flag** (alarm) symptoms?* Such diagnoses may have to be

---
[a] This does not happen often but **Christmas disease** is an example of a disease named after the patient rather than the clinician.

> **TAKING A BETTER HISTORY**
>
> - Ask open questions to start with (and resist the urge to interrupt), but finish with specific questions to narrow the differential diagnosis.
> - Do not hurry (or at least do not appear to be in a hurry, even if you have only limited time).
> - Ask the patient 'What else?' after he or she has finished speaking, to ensure that all problems have been identified. Repeat the 'What else?' question as often as required.
> - Maintain comfortable eye contact and an open posture. Do not cross your legs, and do not lean backwards.
> - Use the head nod appropriately, and use silences to encourage the patient to express him- or herself.
> - When there are breaks in the narrative, provide a summary for the patient by briefly restating the facts or feelings identified, to maximise accuracy and demonstrate active listening.
> - Clarify the list of chief or presenting complaints with the patient, rather than assuming that you know them.
> - If you are confused about the chronology of events or other issues, admit it and ask the patient to clarify.
> - Make sure the patient's story is internally consistent and, if not, ask more questions to verify the facts.
> - If emotions are uncovered, name the patient's emotion and indicate that you understand (e.g. 'You seem sad'). Show respect and express your support (e.g. 'It's understandable that you would feel upset').
> - Ask about any other concerns the patient may have, and address specific fears.
> - Express your support and willingness to cooperate with the patient to help solve the problems together.
>
> LIST 2.1

considered and acted upon even though they are not the most likely diagnosis for this patient. For example, the sudden occurrence of breathlessness in an asthmatic who has had surgery this week is more likely to be due to a worsening of asthma than to a pulmonary embolism, but an embolism must be considered because of its urgent seriousness. Ask yourself: 'What diagnoses must not be missed?'

3. *Could these symptoms be due to one of the mimicking diseases that can present with a great variety of symptoms in different parts of the body?* Tuberculosis used to be the great example of this, but HIV infection, syphilis, sarcoidosis and vasculitis are also important disease 'mimickers'. Anxiety and depression commonly present with many bodily (somatic) symptoms.

4. *Is the patient trying to tell me about something more than these symptoms alone?* Apparently trivial symptoms may be worrying to the patient because of an underlying anxiety about something else. Asking 'What is it that has made you concerned about these problems now?' or 'Is there anything else you want to talk about?' may help clarify this aspect. Ask the patient 'What else?' as natural breaks occur in the conversation.

PERSONAL HISTORY TAKING

Certain aspects of history taking go beyond routine questioning about symptoms. This part of the art needs to be learned by taking a lot of histories; practice is absolutely essential. With time you will gain confidence in dealing with patients whose medical, psychiatric or cultural situations make standard questioning difficult or impossible.[7,8]

Most illnesses are upsetting and can induce feelings of anxiety or depression. On the other hand, patients with primary psychiatric illnesses often present with physical rather than psychological symptoms. This brain–body interaction is bidirectional, and this must be understood as you obtain the story.

Discussion of *sensitive matters* may actually be therapeutic in some cases. *Sympathetic confrontation* can be helpful in some situations. For example, if the patient appears sad, angry or frightened, referring to this in a tactful way may lead to the patient volunteering appropriate information.

If you obtain an emotional response, use **emotion-handling skills** (**NURS**) to deal with this during the interview (see Text box 2.1).

The patient may be reluctant or initially unable to discuss sensitive problems with a stranger. Here, gaining the patient's confidence is critical. Although this type of history taking can be difficult, it can also be the

> **Emotion-handling skills—NURS**
>
> **N**ame the emotion
> Show **U**nderstanding
> Deal with the issue with great **R**espect
> Show **S**upport (e.g. 'It makes sense you were angry after your husband left you. This must have been very difficult to deal with. Can I be of any help to you now?')
>
> TEXT BOX 2.1

> **PERSONAL QUESTIONS TO CONSIDER ASKING A PATIENT**
>
> 1. Where do you live (e.g. a house, flat or hostel)?
> 2. What work do you do now, and what have you done in the past?
> 3. Do you get on well with people at home?
> 4. Do you get on well with people at work?
> 5. Do you have any money problems?
> 6. Are you married, or have a partner, or have you been married?
> 7. Could you tell me about your close relationships?
> 8. Would you describe your marriage (or living arrangements) as happy?
> 9. Has your partner ever hurt you?
> 10. Have you been hit, kicked or physically hurt by someone (physical abuse)?
> 11. Have you been forced to have sex (sexual abuse)?
> 12. Would you say you have a large number of friends?
> 13. Are you religious?
> 14. Do you feel you are too fat or too thin?
> 15. Has anyone in the family had problems with psychiatric illness?
> 16. Have you ever had a nervous breakdown?
> 17. Have you ever had any psychiatric problem?
>
> QUESTIONS BOX 2.1

most satisfying of all interviews, since interviewing can be directly therapeutic for the patient.

It is important for the history taker to maintain an objective demeanour, particularly when asking about delicate subjects such as sexual problems, grief reactions or abuse. It is not the clinician's role to appear to judge patients or their lives.

Any medical illness may affect the psychological status of a patient. Moreover, pre-existing psychological factors may influence the way a medical problem presents. Psychiatric disease can also present with medical symptoms. Therefore, an essential part of the history-taking process is to obtain information about psychological distress and the patient's mental state. A sympathetic, unhurried approach using open-ended questions will provide much information that can then be systematically recorded after the interview. If depression is a concern, it is safe to ask about suicidal ideation.[9]

The formal psychological or psychiatric interview differs from general medical history taking. It takes considerable time for patients to develop rapport with, and confidence in, the interviewer. There are certain standard questions that may give valuable insights into the patient's state of mind (see Questions boxes 2.1–2.3). It may be important to obtain much more detailed information about each of these problems, depending on the clinical circumstances (see Ch 46).

Common general symptoms

Fatigue

Up to 30% of people will report that they are often or always tired. Many patients will volunteer this information. Fatigue needs to be distinguished from sleepiness, muscle weakness and dyspnoea. Questions about the numerous possible causes uncover the underlying problem (List 2.2).

Chronic fatigue

Chronic fatigue syndrome is in the process of being renamed *systemic exertion intolerance disease* (SEID).[b]

---
[b] New names do not always catch on.

CHAPTER 2 ADVANCED HISTORY TAKING

> **QUESTIONS TO ASK THE PATIENT WHO MAY HAVE DEPRESSION**
>
> 1. Have you been feeling sad, down or blue?
> 2. Have you felt depressed or lost interest in things daily for two or more weeks in the past?
> 3. Have you ever felt like taking your own life? (Risk of self-harm)
> 4. Do you find you wake very early in the morning?
> 5. Has your appetite been poor recently?
> 6. Have you lost weight recently?
> 7. How do you feel about the future?
> 8. Have you had trouble concentrating on things?
> 9. Have you had guilty thoughts?
> 10. Have you lost interest in things you usually enjoy?
>
> **QUESTIONS BOX 2.2**

> **QUESTIONS TO ASK THE PATIENT WHO MAY HAVE ANXIETY**
>
> 1. Do you worry excessively about things?
> 2. Do you have trouble relaxing?
> 3. Do you have problems getting to sleep at night?
> 4. Do you feel uncomfortable in crowded places?
> 5. Do you worry excessively about minor things?
> 6. Do you feel suddenly frightened, or anxious or panicky, for no reason in situations in which most people would not be afraid?
> 7. Do you find you have to do things repetitively, such as washing your hands multiple times?
> 8. Do you have any rituals (such as checking things) that you feel you have to do, even though you know it may be silly?
> 9. Do you have recurrent thoughts that you have trouble controlling?
>
> **QUESTIONS BOX 2.3**

By definition these patients:[10]

1. have an inability to carry out normal activities because of severe fatigue that does not improve with rest
2. feel worse after any exertion (physical, cognitive or emotional)
3. find sleep unrefreshing
4. have symptoms that have lasted more than 6 months
5. have symptoms that worsen when they stand up (orthostatic intolerance)
6. often have associated symptoms such as pain syndromes, slow recovery from infections, sore throat, tender lymph nodes and food sensitivities
7. commonly have associated conditions including irritable bowel syndrome and fibromyalgia.

Insomnia

The inability to fall asleep or stay asleep for long enough to feel refreshed is common especially as people age—up to 30% of older adults are affected.[11]

Ask about:

1. the patient's current sleep pattern—regular or irregular bedtime
2. distractions—using computer or telephone in bed
3. alcohol, caffeine use before bed
4. large meal late at night
5. recent emotional upsets
6. use of sedatives
7. shift work
8. daytime sleepiness—especially when driving or at work
9. symptoms suggesting sleep apnoea
10. arthritis causing pain at night
11. restless legs
12. history of depression or main problem of early morning waking.

> **CAUSES OF FATIGUE**
>
> **Way of living**
> - Not enough sleep
> - Too much alcohol
> - Too much activity
> - Drug use e.g. alcohol
>
> **Psychological**
> - Anxiety
> - Worries
> - Depression
>
> **Medical**
> - Thyroid disease
> - Heart failure
> - Obesity
> - Obstructive sleep apnoea
> - Uncontrolled diabetes mellitus
> - Coeliac disease
> - Malignancy
> - Hypoxia (e.g. chronic lung disease)
> - Anaemia
> - HIV infection
> - Medications (e.g. beta-blockers, antidepressants, benzodiazepines)
>
> LIST 2.2

> **SOMATIC SYMPTOM DISORDER AND ILLNESS ANXIETY DISORDER**
>
> **Somatic symptom disorder**
> 1. At least one somatic symptom, present for over 6 months and interfering with normal life. The nature of the disorder may change within this time
> 2. Excessive thoughts, behaviours and feelings related to the symptoms
> 3. Disproportionate concern about seriousness of symptoms
> 4. Persistent anxiety about health
> 5. Excessive time and energy spent on health worries
>
> **Illness anxiety disorder**
> 1. Preoccupation about having or acquiring an illness
> 2. Somatic symptoms are absent or mild
>
> LIST 2.3

Medically unexplained symptoms (MUS)

It is quite common for patients to present with symptoms that cannot be explained. These people have often had years of distressing problems that have led to numerous investigations and visits to doctors.[12] Common symptoms of this sort include:

1. chest pain
2. fatigue
3. dizziness
4. abdominal pain
5. paraesthesiae and numbness
6. headache
7. back pain
8. dyspnoea.

Some of these patients meet the criteria for the diagnosis of *somatic symptom disorder* or *illness anxiety disorder* (List 2.3). These terms are replacing the previous terms: hypochondriasis, conversion disorder or functional disorder. This is because, although psychological problems can play a part in the development of these symptoms, psychological distress alone is not the cause of the problem.

Patients with MUS are more often women, have less education and have reported lower quality of life. A systematic approach to patients with suspected MUS can help both the patient and clinician with this frustrating problem (Questions box 2.4).

Patients with these chronic and often disabling symptoms need sympathetic medical help, but in many cases the patient's desire to have more investigations should be resisted and management moved towards reducing the symptoms with regular review of the patient as required.

Non-specific dizziness

Dizziness can be the result of a number of neurological, cardiac and ear abnormalities. These are described in the appropriate sections of the book. Sometimes, however, no specific cause can be found. These patients often describe light-headedness, a feeling of swimming or floating, being 'spaced out' or having a heavy head.

> **QUESTIONS TO ASK THE PATIENT WITH POSSIBLE MUS**
>
> 1. What are your main problems (symptoms) at the moment?
> 2. How long have they been going on? What seems to make them better or worse? (Exacerbating and relieving factors, etc.)
> 3. How badly do the symptoms affect you? What happens on a typical day?
> 4. What is your main worry about this symptom?
> 5. What made you come in today in particular?
> 6. Was there something you thought I could do in particular to help?
> 7. Consider asking about depression and mood.
> 8. What tests and treatment have you had for these symptoms in the past?
>
> QUESTIONS BOX 2.4

> **FEATURES OF CHRONIC SUBJECTIVE DIZZINESS**
>
> 1. Symptoms of dizziness or light-headedness for more than 3 months
> 2. No other diagnosis to explain the symptoms
> 3. Severity varies but worse when standing or walking and better when patient lies down
> 4. Worse with motion or moving environment e.g. in train or car
> 5. Worse when light is dim
> 6. Often associated with depression, anxiety, obsessive–compulsive traits
>
> LIST 2.4

When the sensation has been present for most days during a period of 3 months or more and the symptoms cannot be explained by an identifiable abnormality, a diagnosis of *chronic subjective dizziness (CSD)* might be considered (List 2.4). Conditions of this sort are not diagnoses of exclusion but should be diagnosed on the basis of their distinctive symptoms and signs.

Sexual history

The sexual history is important, but these questions are not appropriate for all patients, at least not at the first visit when the patient has not yet had time to develop confidence and trust. The patient's permission should be sought before questions of this sort are asked. This request should include some explanation as to why the questions are necessary.[13]

A sexual history is most relevant if the patient presents with a urethral discharge, painful urination (dysuria), vaginal discharge, a genital ulcer or rash, abdominal pain, pain on intercourse (dyspareunia) or anorectal symptoms, or if human immunodeficiency virus (HIV) or hepatitis is suspected.[14] Ask about the last date of intercourse, number of contacts, gender of partners and type of sexual activity and contacts with sex workers. Ask whether sexual intercourse was unprotected.

The type of sexual practice may also be important: for example, oro-anal contact may predispose to colonic infection, and rectal contact may predispose to hepatitis B or C or HIV.

It is also often relevant to ask diplomatic and matter-of-fact questions about a history of sexual abuse. One way to start is: 'You may have heard that some people have been sexually or physically victimised, and this can affect their illness. Has this ever happened to you?' Such events may have important and long-lasting physical and psychological effects.[15]

Accurate answers to some of these questions may not be obtained until the patient has had a number of consultations and has developed trust in the treating doctor. If an answer seems unconvincing, it may be reasonable to ask the question again at a later stage.

Reproductive history

Questions about a woman or couple's intentions about having a family may be appropriate. Ask 'Have there been problems with infertility or with contraceptive use?' Some drugs should be stopped before women become pregnant. Previous pregnancies and any problems associated with pregnancy or delivery should be discussed. (See Chapters 39 and 40 in Volume 2.)

CROSS-CULTURAL HISTORY TAKING

If the patient's first language is not the same as yours, he or she may find the medical interview very difficult. Maintain eye contact (unless this is considered rude in the cultural context) and be attentive as you ask questions.[16]

If language is an issue, an **interpreter** who is *not* a relative should be used to assist these patients. Some patients may be embarrassed to discuss medical problems in front of a relative, and relatives are often tempted to explain (or change) the patient's answers instead of just translating them. Professional translators are trained to avoid this and can often provide simultaneous and accurate translation, but not all patients feel comfortable with a third person present.

It is important to continue to make eye contact with the patient while asking questions, even though it will be the interpreter who responds; otherwise the patient may feel left out of the discussion. Questions should be directed as if going straight to the patient: 'Have you had any problems with shortness of breath?' rather than 'Has he had any breathlessness?' It always takes longer to interview a patient using an interpreter, and more time should be allowed for the consultation.

It is alarmingly common for relatives who accompany patients to interrupt and contradict the patient's version of events even when they are not acting as translators. The interposition of a relative between the clinician and the patient always makes the history taking less direct and the patient's symptoms more subject to 'filtering' or interpretation before the information reaches the clinician. Try tactfully to direct relatives to allow the patient to answer in his or her own words. Remember that relatives may be more anxious about the patient than the patient him- or herself.

Attitudes to illness and disease vary in different cultures. Problems considered shameful by the patient may be very difficult for him or her to discuss. In some cultures, women may object to being questioned or examined by male doctors or students. Male students may need to be accompanied by a female chaperone for the interview with sensitive female patients, and certainly should have one during the physical examination of the patient. It is most important that cultural sensitivities on either side are not allowed to prevent a thorough medical assessment.

Patients including those from an Indigenous background may have a large extended family. These relatives may be able to provide invaluable support to the patient, but their own medical or social problems may interfere with the patient's ability to manage his or her own health. Commitments to family members may make it difficult for the patient to attend medical appointments or to travel for specialist treatment. Detailed questioning about family contacts and responsibilities may help with the planning of the patient's treatment.

Recent concepts in Indigenous healthcare include the notions of cultural awareness, cultural sensitivity and cultural safety.[17] *Cultural awareness* can be thought of as the first step towards understanding the rituals, beliefs, customs and practices of a culture. *Cultural sensitivity* means accepting the importance and roles of these differences. *Cultural safety* means using this knowledge to protect patients and communities from danger, and making sure that there is a genuine partnership between health workers and their Indigenous patients. These skills have general application for all cultural groups but vary in detail from one to another.

All of these matters require an especially sensitive approach. You as a clinician need to be impartial and objective.

THE 'UNCOOPERATIVE' OR 'DIFFICULT' PATIENT

Most clinical encounters involve a cooperative effort on the part of the patient and the clinician. The patient wants help to find out what is wrong and to get better. This should make the meeting satisfying and friendly for both parties. However, interviews do not always run smoothly.[18]

Resentment may occur on both sides if the patient seems not to be taking the doctor's advice seriously, or will not cooperate with attempts at history taking or examination. Unless there is a serious psychiatric or neurological problem that impairs the patient's judgement, taking or not taking advice remains the patient's prerogative. The clinician's role is to give advice and explanation, not to dictate. Indeed, it must be realised that the advice may not always be correct. Keeping this in mind will help prevent that most unsatisfactory and unprofessional of outcomes—becoming angry with the patient. In all cases you should provide a proper, sympathetic and thorough explanation of the problem and the consequences of ignoring medical advice, to the extent that the patient will allow. A clinician whose advice is rarely accepted should begin to wonder about his or her clinical acumen.

Patients who are *aggressive* and *uncooperative* may have a medical reason for their behaviour. The possibilities to be considered include alcohol or drug withdrawal, an intracranial lesion such as a tumour or subdural haematoma, or a psychiatric disease such as paranoid schizophrenia. In other cases, resentment at the occurrence of illness may be the problem.

Some patients may seem difficult because they are *too cooperative*. The patient concerned about his blood pressure may have brought printouts of his own blood pressure measurements at half-hour intervals for several weeks. It is important to show restrained interest in these recordings, without encouraging excessive enthusiasm in the patient. Other patients may bring with them information about their symptoms or a diagnosis obtained from the internet. It is important to remember, and perhaps to point out, that information obtained in this way may not have been subjected to any form of peer review.

People with a chronic illness or rare disease, on the other hand, may know more about their condition than their medical attendants and they may seem difficult because they are knowledgeable. The best approach is to say that this is an unusual condition and you will need to find out more about the latest aspects of its management and get back to the patient. Accept gratefully material offered by the patient about the condition. Saying 'This is a complicated problem and we may need the help of a specialist in this area' is a very reasonable approach.

Sometimes the interests of the patient and the doctor are not the same. This is especially so in cases where there is the possibility of compensation for an illness or injury. These patients may, consciously or unconsciously, attempt to manipulate the encounter. This is a very difficult situation and can be approached only by rigorous application of clinical methods.

Occasionally, attempted manipulation takes the form of flattery or inappropriate personal interest directed at the clinician. This should be dealt with by carefully maintaining professional detachment. The clinician and the patient must be conscious that their meeting is a professional and not a social one. Sometimes patients offer inappropriate gifts.[19] This may be seen as a way of obtaining more attention or becoming more important. Valuable gifts should not be accepted and the patient should be told that it is not ethical to accept something of this sort. The danger of medical students finding themselves in this position is small, however.

SELF-HARMING AND MÜNCHHAUSEN'S SYNDROME

When patients give a history of contact with numerous doctors and of many investigations and procedures without definite diagnoses, you should think, 'Could this be a fictitious disorder?'[c] The assumption that patients who come to the doctor want help and do not deliberately try to deceive tends to delay the diagnosis in these cases. Careful history taking and consultation with colleagues previously involved in the patient's care may help avoid further unnecessary investigations and treatment.

HISTORY TAKING FOR THE MAINTENANCE OF GOOD HEALTH

There has never been more public awareness of the influence the way people live has on their health. Most people have some understanding of the dangers of smoking, excessive alcohol consumption and obesity. People have more varied views on what constitutes a healthy diet and exercise regimen, and many are ignorant of what constitutes risky sexual activity.

The first interview with a patient is an opportunity to make an assessment of the patient's knowledge of risk factors for a number of important medical conditions. Even when the patient has come about an unconnected problem, there is often the opportunity for a quick review. Constant matter-of-fact reminding about these can make a great difference to the way people protect themselves from ill-health.

Part of the thorough assessment of patients includes obtaining and conveying some idea of what measures

---

[c] Named after Baron von Münchhausen (Karl Friedrich Hieronymus Freiherr von Münchhausen, 1720–97). Baron von Münchhausen's improbable stories about himself were published by Rudolf Raspe as *The Surprising Adventures of Baron Münchhausen*.

may help them maintain good health (see Questions box 2.5). This includes a comprehensive approach to the combination of risk factors for various diseases, which is much more important than each individual risk factor. For example, advising a patient about the risk of premature cardiovascular disease will involve knowing about the patient's family history, smoking history, previous and current blood pressure, current and historical cholesterol levels, dietary history and assessment for diabetes mellitus and how much exercise the patient undertakes.

Depending on the patient's age, ask about screening tests being done for any serious illnesses, such as mammograms for breast cancer, Pap smears for cervical cancer or colonoscopy for colon cancer.[20]

The patient's awareness and understanding of basic measures for maintaining good health can be assessed throughout the interview. Even when they are unrelated to the presenting problem, serious examples of risky behaviour should be pointed out. This should not be done in an aggressive way. For example, you might say: 'This might be a good time to make a big effort to reduce your consumption of alcohol, because it's especially unwise for someone like you who has abnormal liver function.'

Certain questions can be helpful in making a diagnosis of alcoholism (see Ch 1). Another approach is to ask, 'Have you ever had a drinking problem?' and 'Did you have your last drink within the last 24 hours?' The patient who answers 'yes' to both questions is likely to be a high-risk drinker.

The patient's vaccination record should be reviewed regularly and brought up to date when indicated (Table 2.1).

Live vaccines are contraindicated for certain patients (List 2.5).

Travel to rural Asia and other exotic places may be an indication for additional vaccinations (e.g. Japanese encephalitis, typhoid).

> **QUESTIONS RELATED TO THE MAINTENANCE OF GOOD HEALTH FOR ADULTS**
>
> 1. Are you a smoker? When did you stop?
> 2. Do you know what your cholesterol level is?
> 3. Do you think you eat a healthy diet? Tell me about your diet.
> 4. Has your blood pressure been high?
> 5. Have you had diabetes or a raised blood sugar level?
> 6. Do you drink alcohol? Every day? How many drinks?
> 7. Do you do any sort of regular exercise?
> 8. Do you think you have engaged in any risky sexual activity? What was that?
> 9. Have you ever used illegal drugs? Which ones? Do you use over-the-counter or complementary medications?
> 10. What vaccinations have you had? Include specific questions about tetanus, influenza, pneumococcal and meningococcal vaccination and *Haemophilus influenzae* (these last three are essential for patients who have had a splenectomy as they are especially vulnerable to infection with these encapsulated organisms), hepatitis A and B, human papilloma virus (HPV) and travel vaccinations.
> 11. Have you had any regular screening for breast cancer (based on family history or from age 50 years)?
> 12. Have you had screening for colon cancer? (From age 50 or earlier if a relevant family history of colon cancer or inflammatory bowel disease.) What test was done?
>
> QUESTIONS BOX 2.5

> **CONTRAINDICATIONS TO LIVE VACCINES**
>
> 1. Pregnancy
> 2. HIV with CD4 count <200 / μL
> 3. Haematological malignancies—leukaemia, lymphoma
> 4. Solid organ transplant recipient
> 5. Haemopoietic stem cell transplant
> 6. Cellular immunodeficiency
>
> LIST 2.5

Vaccine recommendations for adults*

Disease	Vaccine	Indications
Influenza	Inactivated or live attenuated	Annually for all adults (especially health workers, pregnant women and patients with chronic disease)
Varicella	Live attenuated	2 doses 4 weeks apart if demonstrated lack of varicella immunity
Tetanus, diphtheria, pertussis	Inactivated	All unvaccinated adults, 10-year booster of tetanus vaccine
Herpes zoster	Live attenuated	Adults over 70 who are not immunocompromised
Pneumococcal	Inactivated	Adults over 65, smokers, splenectomy patient, patients with chronic illnesses
Measles, mumps, rubella	Live attenuated	Adults born in 1960 or later second dose as adult
Meningococcal	Inactivated	Unvaccinated adults before splenectomy or travel
Human papilloma virus	Inactivated	Unvaccinated women to age of 26, unvaccinated men to age of 26, immunocompromised people to age of 26
Hepatitis A	Inactivated	Any adult who asks for it, especially travellers to endemic areas
Hepatitis B	Inactivated	Any adult who asks for it, especially travellers to endemic areas

*Australian guidelines are updated regularly—visit: http://immunise.health.gov.au/internet/immunise/publishing.nsf/Content/Home.

TABLE 2.1

THE ELDERLY PATIENT

Patients who are in their seventies or older present with similar illnesses to younger patients but certain problems are more likely in older patients. History taking should address these potential problems as part of the 'maintenance of good health' aspect of history taking. The risk of complications of infections is increased, and most elderly people should have routine influenza vaccinations—ask if vaccinations are up to date. See Chapter 44 for more details.

Activities of daily living

For elderly patients and those with a chronic illness, ask some basic screening questions about **functional activity**. The appearance of the patient in the consulting room using a walking frame (see Fig. 2.1) or other aid should prompt detailed questions regarding activities of daily living (ADL). Ask specific questions about the patient's ability to bathe, walk, use the toilet, eat and dress. Find out whether the patient needs help to perform these tasks and who provides it. It may be necessary to ask, 'How do you manage?' or 'What do you do about that problem?' Help may come from relatives, neighbours, friends, the health service or charitable organisations. The proximity and availability

Walking frame (wheelie-walker)

FIGURE 2.1

of these services vary, and more details should be sought. Try to find out whether the patient is happy to accept help or not.

You should also ask questions about the instrumental activities of daily living (IADL), such as shopping, cooking and cleaning, the use of transport, and managing money and medications.

Establish whether the patient has ever been assessed by an occupational therapist or whether there has been a 'home visit'. Ask whether alterations have been made to the house (e.g. installation of ramps, railings in the bathroom, emergency call buttons).

Find out who lives with the patient and how they seem to be coping with the patient's illness. Obviously, the amount of detail required depends on the severity and chronicity of the patient's illness.

Polypharmacy

Try to find out what drugs the patient is taking, how long each drug has been used and what it is for. It is surprising how many people take medications apparently without knowing what they are for. (Other patients look up their prescribed drugs on the internet and then become too frightened to take them.) Drugs with particularly high risk in elderly people are shown in Table 2.2. In many cases, one drug may have been given to treat a side effect of another.

Up to 40% of people over the age of 60 take five or more different medications a day—by definition, polypharmacy. The risks of side effects and complications of drugs increase with age. Careful history taking will enable a comprehensive assessment of a patient's drugs and their potential effects. It may lead to a trial of ceasing drugs no longer needed. Good clinicians regularly review and stop drugs that are not beneficial.

Adherence

There is evidence that up to 50% of patients do not take their medications as prescribed.[21] Poor adherence (tactfully no longer known as *compliance*) is more likely when drug regimens are complicated (e.g. three-times-a-day medications), the disease is not associated with symptoms (e.g. hypertension), the drugs are expensive, the patient is young or old, or the treatment is for a psychiatric condition. When treatment seems ineffective, the problem may be adherence. Although elaborate ways of determining adherence have been developed (e.g. electronic pill dispensing, tracking of pharmacy dispensing) these are intrusive and expensive.

Careful questioning may be a helpful way of determining adherence with medications. Begin with a neutral remark and questions, such as: 'Yours is quite a complicated combination of tablets. Do you think you ever miss any of them? How often? Do you use a pill-dispensing device (like a Webster packet)?' (see Fig. 1.2(b), page 13).

In some cases the absence of predictable drug effects may be a clue. For example, a normal heart rate for a patient prescribed beta-blockers (drugs that reduce heart rate) or absence of dark bowel motions for a patient prescribed iron supplements suggests non-adherence to these drugs. It is possible to measure the blood concentrations of many drugs. For example, the level of anticonvulsants can be measured when a patient continues to have seizures despite treatment.

Assessing adherence, at least by careful questioning, is important before more treatment is added for patients who are apparently not responding to medications.

Mental state

Ask questions that may help to assess cognitive function. Is there a family history of dementia? Has the patient noticed problems with memory or with aspects of life, such as paying bills?

Ask about depression. Severe depression can affect cognitive function.

Delirium refers to confusion and altered consciousness. Do not confuse this with *dementia*, where

Common drug side effects in elderly people

Class of drug	Common side effects
Psychotropics	Sedation and falls, fractures, etc.
Diuretics	Hypokalaemia, renal dysfunction, gout
NSAIDs	Exacerbation of hypertension, heart failure, chronic kidney disease
Antihypertensives	Postural hypotension and falls

NSAID = non-steroidal anti-inflammatory drug.

TABLE 2.2

consciousness is not altered but there is progressive loss of long-term memory and other cognitive functions. If indicated, perform a formal mental state examination (see Ch 46).

Specific problems in the elderly

Falls and loss of balance are common and dangerous for elderly patients. Hip fractures and head injuries are life-threatening events. Ask about falls and near-falls. Does the patient use a stick or a frame? Are there hazards in the house that increase the risk (e.g. steep and narrow stairs)? The use of sedatives like sleeping tablets or antianxiety (anxiolytic) drugs and some antihypertensive drugs increases the risk of falls and must be assessed.

Screening for osteoporosis is recommended for all women over the age of 65 and all men aged 70 and older. Risk factors for osteoporosis include being underweight, heavy alcohol use, use of corticosteroids, early menopause and a history of previous fractures.

General questions about mobility should also include asking about reasons for immobility. These may include arthritis, obesity, general muscle weakness and proximal muscle weakness (sometimes due to corticosteroid use).

Elder abuse (emotional, physical and sexual) does occur; to detect it, it is important to understand the patient's social circumstances. Useful screening questions to ask (without the carer present) include:
- Do you feel safe where you live?
- Who makes your meals?
- Who handles your finances?[22,23]

Advance care planning (advance health directives)

Patients may have strong feelings about the extent of treatment they want if their condition deteriorates. These should be recorded before a deteriorating medical illness makes the patient incapable of expressing his or her wishes. In a *living will*, patients record their decisions about consenting to medical interventions and this legal document comes into effect when they can no longer make their own decisions. Encourage patients to discuss the plan with their doctor, appoint someone to make decisions on their behalf and provide copies of the legal documentation to the people who care for them at home and their doctors.

This can be a difficult area. If a patient expresses a wish not to have certain treatments, the clinician must make very sure that patient understands the nature and likely success of these treatments. For example, a patient who expresses a wish not to be revived if her heart stops after a myocardial infarct may not understand that early ventricular fibrillation is often successfully treated by cardioversion without long-term sequelae. Patients' decisions must be *informed* decisions.

PATIENT CONFIDENTIALITY

Patients have a right to expect that the things they say and the results of their tests will be kept confidential. This means not discussing patients, even with colleagues, in a way that enables them to be identified. Passing on information at hand-over rounds or as part of a referral is the exception to this. Referral information must be relevant to the patient's current problem and should not include unnecessary information that the patient does not want included.

The patient's right to privacy may have to give way to public health regulations. Certain infectious diseases and suspected sexual abuse must be notified. Doctors in most jurisdictions have a duty to warn patients with certain conditions (e.g. visual impairment, uncontrolled epilepsy, recurrent syncope) that they must not drive.[24]

EVIDENCE-BASED HISTORY TAKING AND DIFFERENTIAL DIAGNOSIS

The principles of evidence-based clinical examination are discussed in Chapter 3 in more detail, but they also have an application to history taking. The starting point of the differential diagnosis of a certain symptom is the likelihood (or probability) that a certain condition will occur in this patient. Most clinicians still rely on their own experience when making this assessment, although some information of disease prevalence in different populations is becoming available. Unfortunately, one person's experience is a relatively small sample, and past experience may bias the clinician in favour of or against a certain diagnosis.

Some diagnoses may largely be excluded from the differential diagnosis list at once. This may be based, for example, on the patient's age, sex or race or the extreme rarity of the disease in a particular country. For example, chronic obstructive pulmonary disease would be very unlikely in a 20-year-old non-smoker who presents with breathlessness.

The differential diagnosis is gradually narrowed as more information about the patient's symptoms comes from the patient directly, and as a result of specific questioning about features of the symptoms that will help to refine the list.

THE CLINICAL ASSESSMENT

After the physical examination, the interview with the patient concludes with your assessment of what the diagnosis or possible diagnoses are, in order of probability. Note that the history is the most powerful tool in your toolbox for identifying the likely diagnosis in the majority of cases![25] Diagnostic errors in clinical practice are usually related to a breakdown in the success of the clinical encounter.[26] Your assessment is, not unreasonably, the most important part of the whole process from the patient's point of view.

The explanation must relate to the patient's symptoms or perception of the problem. You should explain how the symptoms and any examination findings relate to the diagnosis. For example, if a patient presents with dyspnoea, you should begin by saying, 'I believe your shortness of breath is probably the result of pneumonia, but there are a few other possibilities.' The complexity of the explanation will depend on your understanding of the patient's ability to follow any technical aspects of the diagnosis. The patient's desire for a detailed explanation is also variable, and this must be taken into account.

If the diagnosis is fairly definite, then the prognosis and the implications of this must be outlined. A serious diagnosis must be discussed frankly but always in the context of the variability of outcome for most medical conditions and the benefits of correct treatment. When a patient seems unwilling to accept a serious diagnosis and seems likely to decline treatment, you must attempt to find out the reason for the patient's decision. Has the patient had previous bad experiences with medical treatment, or has a friend or relative had a similar diagnosis and a difficult time with treatment or complications?

Sometimes blunt language may be justified—for example, 'It is important for you to realise that this is a life-threatening illness that needs urgent treatment.' Patients who seem unable to accept advice of this sort should be offered a chance to discuss the matter with another doctor or with their family. This must be done sympathetically: 'This is obviously a difficult time for you. Would you like me to arrange for you to see someone else for another opinion about it? Or would you like to come back with some of your family to talk about it again?' The patient's response should be carefully documented in the notes.

Patients may need to be cautioned about certain activities until the condition is treated. For example, a patient with a possible first epileptic seizure must be told that he or she cannot legally drive a motor vehicle.

CONCLUDING THE CONSULTATION

After talking to the patient about the assessment and prognosis, the need for investigations and any urgency involved should be discussed. Admission to hospital may be recommended if the problem is a serious one. This may involve major inconvenience to the patient; the clinician must be ready to justify the recommendation and attempt to predict the likely length of stay. If the investigations are onerous or involve risk, this must also be explained and alternatives discussed, if they are available.

If drug treatment is being prescribed, the patient is entitled to know why this is necessary, what it is likely to achieve and what possible important adverse effects might occur. This is a complicated topic. On the clinician's part, it requires a comprehensive understanding of drug interactions and adverse effects, as well as an assessment of what it is reasonable to tell a patient without causing alarm or symptoms by suggestion. Patients must at least know what dangerous symptoms should lead to immediate cessation of the drug. Pharmacies often provide patients with long and unedited lists of possible adverse effects when they dispense drugs. Patients may be too frightened to take the prescription unless these are explained at the time of the consultation. Dealing with this difficult area takes time and experience.

There is no shame in telling a patient you will look up possible side effects and interactions of a drug before you prescribe it or if a patient expresses concern about it. You could say: 'I haven't heard of that problem with this drug but let me look it up and check.'

The patient must be given the opportunity to ask questions.[27] Few people, given a new diagnosis, can absorb everything that has been said to them. The patient should be reminded that there will be an opportunity to ask further questions at the next consultation, when the results of tests or the effects of treatment can be assessed.

Finally, you may find that the patient introduces a brand new problem, sometimes serious, at the end of the consultation. (Studies suggest that this happens in up to one in five consultations in primary care.[28]) Here is a real example: as one patient was walking towards the door, he said: 'Thank you. I feel much better now that I know my back pain is nothing to worry about. Oh, by the way, I've noticed a bit of yellow discharge from my penis this week. I'm sure it's nothing, isn't it?' The patient had gonorrhoea. Any new problems must not be dismissed and require you to obtain all the relevant details.

> diagnosis fits poorly, consider alternatives and seek more historical data. Do not close your mind early!
> 5. If language is a barrier, use a professional interpreter, not a relative.
> 6. Remember that questions about maintenance of good health are part of history taking.
> 7. Make a reassessment of the patient's medications at each visit.

References

1. Nardone DA, Johnson GK, Faryna A et al. A model for the diagnostic medical interview: nonverbal, verbal, and cognitive assessments. *J Gen Intern Med* 1992; 7:437–442.
2. Balint J. Brief encounters: speaking with patients. *Ann Intern Med* 1999; 131:231–234.
3. Simpson M, Buchman R, Stewart M et al. Doctor–patient communication: the Toronto consensus statement. *BMJ* 1991; 303:1385–1387.
4. Stewart MA. Effective physician–patient communication and health outcomes in review. *Can Med Assoc J* 1995; 152:1423–1433. The outcome of an illness can be affected by the first part of the medical intervention, the doctor's history taking.
5. Beck RS, Daughtridge R, Sloane PD. Physician–patient communication in the primary care office: a systematic review. *J Am Board Fam Pract* 2002; 15(1):25–38. Useful nonverbal behaviours may include head-nodding when appropriate, leaning forwards, facing the patient at his or her level and having uncrossed arms and legs.
6. Teutsch C. Patient–doctor communication. *Med Clin North Am* 2003; 87(5):1115–1145. Patient fears and concerns can be very broad; read this review to learn more.
7. Smith RC, Hoppe RB. The patient's story: integrating the patient- and physician-centered approaches to interviewing. *Ann Intern Med* 1991; 115:470–477. Patients tell stories of their illness, integrating both the medical and the psychosocial aspects. Both need to be obtained, and this article reviews ways to do this and to interpret the information.
8. Ness DE, Ende J. Denial in the medical interview: recognition and management. *JAMA* 1994; 272:1777–1781. Denial is not always maladaptive, but can be addressed using appropriate techniques. This is a good guide to the problem and the process.
9. Mathias CW, Michael Furr R, Sheftall AH et al. What's the harm in asking about suicidal ideation? *Suicide Life Threat Behav* 2012; 42(3):341–351. There is no identified harm in asking about this issue.
10. Smith ME, Haney E, McDonagh M et al. Treatment of myalgic encephalomyelitis / chronic fatigue syndrome: a systematic review for National Institutes of Health Pathways to Prevention workshop. *Ann Intern Med* 2015; 162(12):841–850.
11. Masters PA. In the clinic. Insomnia. *Ann Intern Med* 2014; 161(7).
12. Smith RC, Lyles JS, Gardiner JC et al. Primary care clinicians treat patients with medically unexplained symptoms: a randomised controlled trial. *J Gen Int Med* 2006; 21(7):671–677.
13. Ende J, Rockwell S, Glasgow M. The sexual history in general medicine practice. *Arch Intern Med* 1984; 144:558–561. This study emphasises the importance of obtaining the sexual history as a routine.
14. Furner V, Ross M. Lifestyle clues in the recognition of HIV infection. How to take a sexual history. *Med J Aust* 1993; 158:40–41. This review guides the shy medical student through this difficult task.

> ### T&O'C ESSENTIALS
>
> 1. Ask open questions to start with (and resist the urge to interrupt), but finish with specific questions to narrow the differential diagnosis.
> 2. Ask the patient 'What else?' after he or she has finished speaking, to ensure that all problems have been identified. Repeat the 'What else?' question as often as required.
> 3. If emotions are uncovered, name the patient's emotion and indicate that you understand (e.g. 'You seem sad'), show respect and express your support (e.g. 'It's understandable that you would feel upset').
> 4. Synthesise the history as you go: think about the likely anatomical site affected, the possible pathophysiology or pathology and common causes. As you make a diagnosis, look for the evidence for and against it in the story. If the

15. Drossman DA, Talley NJ, Leserman J et al. Sexual and physical abuse and gastrointestinal illness. *Ann Intern Med* 1995; 123:782–794. Abuse is common, occurs more often in women, causes a poorer adjustment to illness and usually remains a fact not discussed with the doctor.
16. Qureshi B. How to avoid pitfalls in ethnic medical history, examination, and diagnosis. *J R Soc Med* 1992; 85:65–66. This article provides information on transcultural issues, including taboos on anogenital examinations.
17. Nguyen T. Patient centered care. Cultural safety in indigenous health. *Aust Fam Physician* 2008; 37(12):900–904. Cultural awareness and competence are important issues discussed in this review.
18. Groves JE. Taking care of the hateful patient. *N Engl J Med* 1978; 298:833–837. This article describes groups of patients who induce negative feelings and provides important management insights.
19. Breen KJ, Greenberg PB. Difficult patient encounters. *Internal Med J* 2010; 40:682–688. Read this review! It provides advice on how to prevent and manage such encounters.
20. Heidelbaugh JJ, Tortorello M. The adult well male examination. *Am Fam Phys* 2012; 85(10):964–971. Ask routinely about depression, exercise and diet, substance abuse and risk factors for sexually transmitted infections in men and women. Look for obesity and hypertension.
21. Haynes RB, McKibbon KA, Kanani R. Systematic review of randomised trials of interventions to assist patients to follow prescriptions for medications. *Lancet* 1996; 348(9024):383–386. Counselling and written information may help prescription adherence, but this is a complex area and most interventions do not help.
22. Lachs MS, Pillemer K. Abuse and neglect of elderly persons. *N Engl J Med* 1995; 332(7):437–443. All older adults should be asked about family violence.
23. Fox AW. Elder abuse. *Med Sci Law* 2012; 52(3):128–136. Physical, psychological, sexual, neglect and financial abuse all occur in the elderly.
24. Assessing fitness to drive. AustRoads. National Transport Commission 2016. www.onlinepublications.austroads.com.au/items/AP-G56-16.
25. Hampton JR, Harrison MJG, Mitchell JAR et al. Relative contributions of history-taking, physical examination, and the laboratory to the diagnosis and management of medical outpatients. *BMJ* 1975; 2:486–489. In this study, in 66 out of 80 new patients the diagnosis based on the history was correct; physical examination was useful in only seven patients and laboratory tests in another seven. Take a good history: it's the key to success!
26. Singh H, Giardina TD, Meyer AN et al. Types and origins of diagnostic errors in primary care settings. *JAMA Intern Med* 2013; 173(6):418–425.
27. Judson TJ, Detsky AS, Press MJ. Encouraging patients to ask questions, how to overcome 'white-coat silence'. *JAMA* 2013; 309:2325–2326.
28. White J, Levinson W, Roter D. 'Oh, by the way …': the closing moments of the medical visit. *J Gen Intern Med* 1994; 9(1):24–28. In up to one in five consultations in primary care, a new problem is raised by the patient at the very end of the consultation.

CHAPTER 3
The general principles of physical examination

More mistakes are made from want of a proper examination than for any other reason.
RUSSELL JOHN HOWARD (1875–1942)

In an era of increasingly sophisticated testing, the physical examination (or 'laying on of hands') is not only about tradition—physical examination remains a key element in the diagnostic and healing process. Patients expect to be examined and this strengthens the doctor–patient relationship.[1,2] Even more importantly, failing to examine remains a common reason avoidable errors are made.[1,2] You must learn to become an expert in physical examination.

Students beginning their training in physical examination will be surprised at the formal way this examination is taught and performed.[3,4] There are, however, a number of reasons for this formal approach. The first is that it ensures the examination is thorough and that important signs are not overlooked because of a haphazard method.[5] The second is that the most convenient methods of examining patients in bed, and for particular conditions in various other postures, have evolved with time. By convention, patients are usually examined from the right side of the bed, even though this may be more convenient only for right-handed people. When students learn this, they often feel safer huddling on the left side of the bed with their colleagues in tutorial groups, but many tutors are aware of this strategy, particularly when they notice all students standing as far away from the right side of the bed as possible.

It should be pointed out here that there is only limited evidence-based information concerning the validity of clinical signs. Many parts of the physical examination are performed as a matter of tradition. As students develop their examination skills, experience and new evidence-based data will help them to refine their use of examination techniques. We have included information about the established usefulness of signs where it is available, but have also included signs that students will be expected to know about despite their unproven value.

This formal approach to the physical examination leads to the examination of the parts of the body by **body system**. For example, examination of the cardiovascular system, which includes the heart and all the major accessible blood vessels, begins with positioning the patient correctly. This is followed by a quick general inspection and then, rather surprisingly for the uninitiated, seemingly prolonged study of the patient's fingernails. From there, a set series of manoeuvres brings the doctor to the heart. This type of approach applies to all major systems, and is designed to discover peripheral signs of disease in the system under scrutiny. The attention of the examining doctor is directed particularly towards those systems identified in the history as possibly being diseased, but of course proper physical examination requires that all the systems be examined.

The danger of a systematic approach is that time is not taken to stand back and look at the patient's **general appearance**, which may give many clues to the diagnosis. Doctors must be observant, like a detective (Conan Doyle based his character Sherlock Holmes on an outstanding Scottish surgeon).[6] Taking the time to make an appraisal of the patient's general appearance, including the face, hands and body, conveys the impression to the patient (and to the examiners) that the doctor or student is interested in the person as much as the disease. This general appraisal usually occurs at the bedside when patients are in hospital, but for patients seen in the consulting room it should begin as the patient walks into the room and during the history taking, and continue at the start of the physical examination.

Diagnosis has been defined as 'the crucial process that labels patients and classifies their illnesses, that identifies (and sometimes seals) their likely fates or prognoses and that propels us towards specific treatments in the confidence (often unfounded) that they will do more good than harm'.[7]

In normal clinical practice, the detail of the physical examination performed will be 'targeted' and will depend on clues from the history and whether the consultation is a follow-up or a new consultation. Students, however, must know how to perform a complete examination of the body systems, even though they will not often perform this in practice.

CLINICAL EXAMINATION

In clinical examinations you will be expected to be able to demonstrate a polished and thorough examination method—this book will teach you how. The most common examination format is the objective structured clinical examination (OSCE), which is discussed later in this chapter. Other formats used include the long case (testing your ability to take the history, perform a thorough examination and plan management, just as people do in clinical practice) and the short case (testing your ability to examine a specific part or system and your diagnostic skills, without knowing the details of the history).

A high level of competency in history taking and physical examination remains central to the provision of effective and safe medical practice. Learn, practise and hone these core skills every day.

HOW TO START

A few simple steps will help put the patient at ease and assist you in completing the examination (see Text box 3.1). Always wash your hands before and after, to protect the patient and yourself.

Hand washing

Patients must come first and reducing the spread of infection is your responsibility as a healthcare professional. You must wash your hands both *before* touching a patient (to protect them) and *after* completing

---

A mnemonic for starting the physical examination: WIPER

Wash hands (before and after)—wear gloves where appropriate.

Introduce yourself to the patient and seek his or her consent.

Position the patient correctly.

Expose the patient as needed (e.g. 'Please take off your shirt for me now, if that is all right').

Right side of the bed.

TEXT BOX 3.1

---

your examination (to protect you) *every time without fail*. Follow the World Health Organization (WHO) guidelines:

- If there is any dirt or material on your hands, use soap and water, covering all hand surfaces for at least 40 seconds.
- If there is no soiling on your hands, use a palmful of alcohol-based formulation (alcohol rub) applied for at least 20 seconds (see Fig. 3.1).
- The correct sequence is to rub:
  - hands palm to palm
  - right palm over the left dorsum with interlaced fingers, then vice versa
  - palm to palm with interlaced fingers
  - back of the fingers to opposing palms with interlocked fingers
  - each thumb rotationally
  - the palms rotationally.
- Finally, if using soap and water, rinse your hands, dry with a towel and use the towel (or your elbow) to turn off the tap. If using alcohol rub, let it dry and proceed.
- Do not use alcohol rub if your hands are soiled or if there is an outbreak of *Clostridium difficile* infection; use soap and water instead.[2]
- Do not forget to clean your stethoscope bell and diaphragm with an alcohol wipe after every examination (see Fig. 3.2c).

Try to examine in a warm room that has good lighting so that you maximise your chances of seeing the signs. Introduce yourself and seek the patient's permission to examine him or her. For an examination of the genital or anal areas, ask whether the patient would like a

'For a long time I used to go to bed early.'

FIGURE 3.2

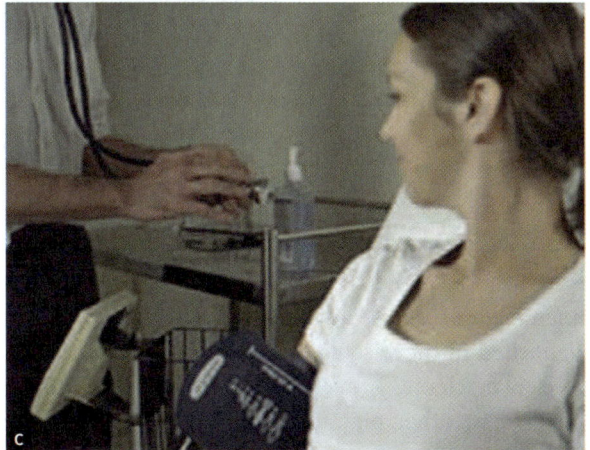

Examiner washing hands (a) and (b) and stethoscope (c)

(From Talley NJ, O'Connnor S. *Clinical examination essentials*, 4th edn. Chatswood, NSW: Elsevier, 2015, with permission.)

FIGURE 3.1

chaperone (and include the chaperone's name in the records, if you use one). Unless the adult patient requests that relatives stay, ask them to leave temporarily. Make sure the patient is positioned comfortably and adequately exposed (but not over-exposed—cover or recover areas not being directly examined). Start by standing on the right side of the bed. Be gentle and courteous.

FIRST IMPRESSIONS

First impressions of a patient's condition must be deliberately sought. Make a conscious point of assessing the patient's general condition right at the start. The specific changes that occur in particular illnesses (e.g. myxoedema) will be discussed in detail in the appropriate chapters. However, certain abnormalities should be obvious to the trained or training doctor.

First, decide how sick the patient seems to be—that is, does he or she look generally ill or well? The cheerful person sitting up in bed reading Proust (see Fig. 3.2) is unlikely to require urgent attention to save his life. At the other extreme, the patient on the verge of death may be described as *in extremis* or moribund. In this case the patient may be lying still in bed and seem unaware of the surroundings. The face may be sunken and expressionless, and respiration may be shallow and laboured. At the end of life, respiration often becomes slow and intermittent, with longer and longer pauses between rattling breaths.

When a patient walks into the consulting room or undresses for the examination, there is an opportunity to look for problems with mobility and breathlessness. Apart from gaining a general impression of a patient's state of health, certain general physical signs must be sought.

Vital signs

Certain important measurements must be made during the assessment of the patient. These relate primarily to cardiac and respiratory function and comprise:
- pulse
- blood pressure
- respiratory rate
- temperature.

For example, an increasing respiratory rate has been shown to be an accurate predictor of respiratory failure.[8] Patients in hospital may have continuous ECG and pulse oximetry monitoring on display on a monitor. These measurements may be considered an extension of the physical examination.

The vital signs must be assessed at once if a patient appears unwell. Patients in hospital have these measurements taken regularly and charted. They provide important basic physiological information.

Facies

A specific diagnosis can sometimes be made by inspecting the face, its appearance giving a clue to the likely diagnosis. Other physical signs must usually be sought to confirm the diagnosis. Some facial characteristics are so typical of certain diseases that they immediately suggest the diagnosis and are called the **diagnostic facies** (the Latin word *facies* means more than just *face*, including *form*, *shape*, *appearance* and *character*; see List 3.1 and Figs 3.3–3.12). Apart from these 'spot diagnoses', there are several other important abnormalities that must be looked for in the face.

Jaundice

When the serum bilirubin level rises to about twice the upper limit of normal, bilirubin is deposited in the tissues of the body. It then causes yellow discoloration of the skin (*jaundice*) and, more dramatically, the apparent discoloration of the sclerae. The usual term *scleral icterus* is misleading, as the bilirubin is actually deposited in the vascular conjunctiva rather than the avascular sclerae. The sclerae (conjunctivae) are rarely affected by other pigment changes. In fact, jaundice is the only condition causing yellow sclerae. Other causes of yellow discoloration of the skin, but where the sclerae remain normal, are carotenaemia (usually due to excess consumption of carotene, often from intemperate eating of carrots or mangoes), acriflavine, fluorescein[a] and picric acid ingestion.

SOME IMPORTANT DIAGNOSTIC FACIES

Acromegalic (see Fig. 3.5)
Amiodarone (antiarrhythmic drug)—deep blue discoloration around the malar area and nose (see Fig. 3.6)
Agitated faces—seen with anxiety, mania or hyperthyroidism
Cushing's syndrome (p 460)
Cyanosis (see Figs 3.3, 3.4)
Depression—flat expression and apathy if severe (also seen in hypothyroidism; p 452)
Down's syndrome (p 475)
Hippocratic (advanced peritonitis)—eyes are sunken, temples collapsed, nose is pinched with crusts on the lips and the forehead is clammy
Lipodystrophic—atrophy of fat (antiretroviral therapy) (see Fig. 3.7)
Marfan's syndrome (p 79)
Mitral facies (see Fig. 3.8)
Myopathic (see Fig. 3.9(a))
Myotonic (see Fig. 3.9(b))
Myxoedematous (severe hypothyroidism) (p 452)
Paget's disease (p 477)
Parkinson's disease (p 597)
Rickets (p 474)
Risus sardonicus* (tetanus; see Fig. 3.10)
SLE facies (see Fig. 3.11)
Thyrotoxicosis (p 449)
Turner's syndrome (p 474)
Virile facies (see Fig. 3.12)

*The translation of this Latin phrase is 'sardonic smile'.

LIST 3.1

---

[a] Used by ophthalmologists to stain the cornea for the detection of ulcers.

CHAPTER 3 THE GENERAL PRINCIPLES OF PHYSICAL EXAMINATION 41

Peripheral cyanosis:

(a) In lips; (b) in fingers

(From Zitelli BJ, Davis HW. *Atlas of pediatric physical diagnosis*, 5th edn. Maryland Heights, MO: Mosby, 2007.)

FIGURE 3.3

Central cyanosis

(Hutchinson's Clinical Methods, General patient examination and differential diagnosis: An integrated approach to clinical, William M. Drake, 2012, page 15–30.)

FIGURE 3.4

Jaundice may be the result of excess production of bilirubin, usually from excessive destruction of red blood cells (termed *haemolytic anaemia*), when it can produce a pale lemon-yellow scleral discoloration. Alternatively, jaundice may be due to obstruction of bile flow from the liver, which, if severe, produces a dark-yellow or orange tint. Scratch marks may be prominent due to associated itching (pruritus). The other main cause of jaundice is hepatocellular failure. Gilbert's disease is also a common cause of jaundice.[b] It causes a mild elevation of unconjugated bilirubin and is due to an inherited enzyme deficiency that limits bilirubin conjugation; it has a benign prognosis. (Jaundice is discussed in detail on p 225.)

Cyanosis

This refers to a blue discoloration of the skin and mucous membranes; it is due to the presence of deoxygenated haemoglobin in superficial blood vessels. The haemoglobin molecules change colour from blue to red when oxygen is added to them in the lungs. If more than about 50 g / L of deoxygenated haemoglobin is present in the capillary blood, the skin will have a bluish tinge.[9] Cyanosis does *not* occur in anaemic hypoxia because the total haemoglobin content is low. Cyanosis is more easily detected in fluorescent light than in daylight.

Central cyanosis means that there is an abnormal amount of deoxygenated haemoglobin in the arteries and that a blue discoloration is present in parts of the body with a good circulation, such as the tongue (see Fig. 3.4). This must be distinguished from *peripheral cyanosis*, which occurs when the blood supply to a certain part of the body is reduced and the tissues extract more oxygen than normal from the circulating

---

[b] Nicholas Augustin Gilbert (1858–1927), a Paris physician, described this condition in 1900. He was the author of a standard medical textbook.

Acromegalic facies

(Underwood JCE: *General and Systemic Pathology*, 3rd ed. Edinburgh, Churchill Livingstone, 2000, p. 413.)

FIGURE 3.5

Amiodarone facies (note the deep-blue discoloration)

FIGURE 3.6

Lipodystrophic facies

(Courtesy of Dr A Watson, Infectious Diseases Department, The Canberra Hospital.)

FIGURE 3.7

Mitral facies

(From Talley NJ, O'Connnor S. *Clinical examination essentials*, 4th edn. Chatswood, NSW: Elsevier, 2015, p 42.)

FIGURE 3.8

Risus sardonicus (tetanus)

(From Cook GC. *Manson's tropical diseases*, 22nd edn. Edinburgh: Saunders, 2008.)

FIGURE 3.10

Some neurological diagnostic facies:

(a) Myopathic; (b) myotonic

(From Mir MA. *Atlas of clinical diagnosis*, 2nd edn. Edinburgh: Saunders, 2003.)

FIGURE 3.9

(a) and (b) Systemic lupus erythematosus (SLE)

(From Zitelli BJ, McIntire SC, Nowalk AJ. *Zitelli and Davis' atlas of pediatric physical diagnosis*, 6th edn, Philadelphia: Saunders, 2012.)

FIGURE 3.11

> **CAUSES OF CYANOSIS**
>
> **Central cyanosis**
> 1. Decreased arterial oxygen saturation
>   - Decreased concentration of inspired oxygen: high altitude
>   - Hypoventilation: coma, airway obstruction
>   - Lung disease: chronic obstructive pulmonary disease (COPD) with cor pulmonale, massive pulmonary embolism
>   - Right-to-left cardiac shunt (cyanotic congenital heart disease)
> 2. Polycythaemia
> 3. Haemoglobin abnormalities (rare)
>   - Methaemoglobinaemia (ferrous [Fe^{2+}] ions of haem are oxidised to the ferric [Fe^{3+}] state, usually owing to drugs such as dapsone or topical anaesthetics in adults, which can be fatal if not immediately recognised and treated)*
>
> **Peripheral cyanosis**
> 1. All causes of central cyanosis cause peripheral cyanosis
> 2. Exposure to cold
> 3. Reduced cardiac output: left ventricular failure or shock
> 4. Arterial or venous obstruction
>
> *Antidote is methylene blue given intravenously.
>
> LIST 3.2

Virile facies

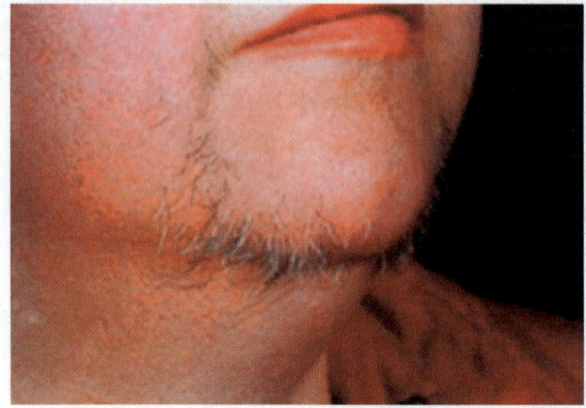

(From Talley NJ, O'Connnor S. *Clinical examination essentials*, 4th edn. Chatswood, NSW: Elsevier, 2015, p 43, with permission.)

FIGURE 3.12

blood (see Fig. 3.3). For example, the lips are often blue in cold weather, but the tongue is spared. The presence of central cyanosis should lead to a careful examination of the cardiovascular (Ch 5) and respiratory (Ch 10) systems (see also List 3.2).

Pallor

A deficiency of haemoglobin (*anaemia*) can produce pallor of the skin and should be noticeable, especially in the mucous membranes of the sclerae if the anaemia is severe (less than 70 g/L of haemoglobin). Pull the lower eyelid down and compare the colour of the anterior part of the palpebral conjunctiva (attached to the inner surface of the eyelid) with the posterior part where it reflects off the sclera. There is usually a marked difference between the red anterior and creamy posterior

CAUSES OF SHOCK

1. Hypovolaemia
   - External fluid loss (e.g. blood, vomitus, diarrhoea, urine, burns, excess sweating)
   - Sequestration of body fluids in the abdomen (e.g. ascites), chest (e.g. haemothorax) or limbs (e.g. fracture)
2. Cardiac
   - Pump failure (e.g. myocardial infarction, acute mitral regurgitation)
   - Cardiac tamponade
   - Dissecting aortic aneurysm
   - Arrhythmia
3. Massive pulmonary embolus
4. Sepsis (e.g. Gram-negative bacteria [endotoxin])
5. Anaphylaxis
6. Endocrine failure (e.g. adrenal failure)
7. Neuropathic—from drugs (e.g. antihypertensives, anaesthesia), spinal cord injury of autonomic neuropathy

LIST 3.3

parts (see Fig. 42.4 on p 776). This difference is absent when significant anaemia is present. Although this is at best a crude way of screening for anaemia, it can be specific (though not sensitive) when anaemia is suspected for other reasons. It should be emphasised that pallor is a sign, whereas anaemia is a diagnosis based on laboratory results.

Facial pallor may also be found in *shock*, which is usually defined as a reduction of cardiac output such that the oxygen demands of the tissues are not being met (see List 3.3). These patients usually appear clammy and cold and are significantly hypotensive (have low blood pressure). Pallor may also be a normal variant due to a deep-lying venous system and opaque skin.

Hair

Bearded or bald women and hairless men not uncommonly present to doctors. These conditions may be a result of more than the rich normal variations of life, and occasionally are due to endocrine disorders (see Ch 29).

WEIGHT, BODY HABITUS AND POSTURE

Look specifically for *obesity*,[10] and note the fat distribution. Is the patient apple (abdominal obesity) or pear shaped (generalised obesity including hips and thighs)? Obesity is most objectively assessed by calculating the body mass index (BMI), whereby the patient's weight in kilograms is divided by the height in metres squared. Normal is less than 25 kg/m^2. A BMI of ≥30 indicates frank obesity; *morbid* obesity is a BMI >40. Medical risks are increasingly recognised in association with obesity (see List 3.4). The risk of medical complications of obesity is increased in certain populations including Australian Aboriginals.

The waist–hip ratio (WHR) is also predictive of health risk. This measurement is of the circumference of the waist (at the midpoint between the costal margin and the iliac crest) divided by that at the hips (at the widest part around the buttocks). Increased risk occurs when this exceeds 1.0 for men and 0.85 for women. Simple waist measurement correlates with the risks of obesity. A waist circumference of more than 80 centimetres for females and 94 centimetres for males indicates an increased risk and more than 88 centimetres for females and 102 centimetres for males indicates a greatly increased risk. These measurements can usefully be made repeatedly and recorded.

Severe underweight (BMI <18.5) is called *cachexia*.[11] Look for wasting of the muscles, which may be due to neurological or debilitating disease, such as malignancy. There may be signs of vitamin deficiencies described later in this book (pp 279 and 346). For example, vitamin C deficiency causes scurvy, which is characterised by small bleeds around the hair follicles (perifollicular haemorrhages; see Fig. 3.13) as well as bruising. Vitamin K deficiency also causes bruising but not perifollicular haemorrhages.

Note excessively short or tall stature, which may be rather difficult to judge when the patient is lying in bed. Inspect for limb deformity or missing limbs (rather embarrassing if missed in viva examinations) and observe whether the physique is consistent with the patient's stated chronological age. A number of body shapes are almost diagnostic of different conditions (see List 3.5 and Fig. 3.14). If the patient walks into the examining room, the opportunity to examine gait

MEDICAL CONDITIONS ASSOCIATED WITH OBESITY (BMI >30)

Endocrine
Type 2 diabetes
Amenorrhoea
Dyslipidaemia
Infertility
Polycystic ovary syndrome
Hypogonadism

Respiratory
Sleep apnoea
Dyspnoea

Cardiovascular
Hypertension
Cardiac failure
Ischaemic heart disease
Cor pulmonale (right heart failure secondary to lung disease)
Pulmonary embolism

Musculoskeletal
Arthritis
Immobility

Skin
Skin abscesses; cellulitis; fungal infections
Venous stasis

Gut
Gastro-oesophageal reflux disease
Non-alcoholic steatohepatitis
Hernias

LIST 3.4

SOME BODY HABITUS* SYNDROMES

Endocrine
Acromegaly (see Fig. 28.9)
Cushing's syndrome (see Fig. 28.13)
Hypopituitarism (p 454)
Pseudohypoparathyroidism (see Fig. 29.10a and b)
Rickets (see Fig. 29.13)
Paget's disease (see Fig. 29.17)

Musculoskeletal
Marfan's syndrome (see Fig. 5.9)
Turner's syndrome (see Fig. 29.12)
Klinefelter's syndrome (see Fig. 29.16)
Achondroplasia (see Fig. 3.14)

*From the Latin word meaning condition or appearance.

LIST 3.5

Scurvy with perifollicular haemorrhages

(From Hoffbrand AV, Pettit JE, Vyas P. *Color atlas of clinical hematology*. Maryland Heights, MO: Mosby, 2010.)

FIGURE 3.13

should not be lost. The full testing of gait is described in Chapter 34.

HYDRATION

Although this is not easy to assess, all doctors must be able to estimate the approximate state of *hydration* of a patient.[12–14] For example, a severely dehydrated patient is at risk of death from developing acute renal failure, whereas an overhydrated patient may develop fluid overload and pulmonary oedema. Excessive oral

Achondroplasia

(*Journal of Pediatric Endocrinology*, 2005, Plate 8.3.)

FIGURE 3.14

Dehydration

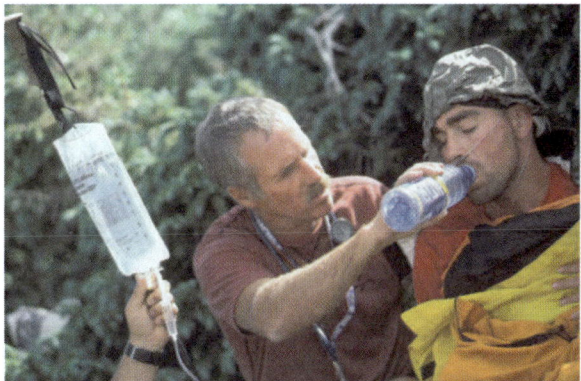

(*Journal of Wilderness Medicine*, 2007. Figure 91.6.)

FIGURE 3.15

> ### CLASSICAL PHYSICAL SIGNS OF DEHYDRATION (OF VARIABLE RELIABILITY)
>
> **Mild (<5%): =2.5 L deficit**
> Mild thirst
> Dry mucous membranes
> Concentrated urine
>
> **Moderate (5%–8%): =4 L deficit**
> As above
> Moderate thirst
> Reduced skin turgor (elasticity), especially arms, forehead, chest, abdomen
> Tachycardia
>
> **Severe (9%–12%): =6 L deficit**
> As above
> Great thirst
> Reduced skin turgor and decreased eyeball pressure
> Collapsed veins, sunken eyes, 'gaunt' face
> Postural hypotension
> Oliguria (<400 mL urine / 24 hours)
>
> **Very severe (>12%): >6 L deficit**
> As above
> Comatose
> Moribund
> Signs of shock
>
> *Note:* Total body water in a man of 70 kg is about 40 L.
>
> LIST 3.6

rehydration with water (e.g. during sporting events) can lead to reduced blood sodium levels and cause confusion and even loss of consciousness.

For a traditional assessment of dehydration (see List 3.6 and Fig. 3.15), inspect for sunken orbits, dry mucous membranes and the moribund appearance of severe dehydration. Reduced skin turgor (pinch the skin: normal skin returns immediately on being released) occurs in moderate and severe dehydration (this traditional test is not of proven value, especially in the elderly, whose skin may always be like that). The presence of dry axillae increases the likelihood of dehydration and a moist tongue reduces the likelihood, but look for a combination of signs for guidance.

Take the blood pressure and look for a fall in pressure when the patient sits or stands up after lying down. The patient should stand, if possible, for at least 1 minute before the blood pressure is taken again (the

Onychogryphosis: finger- or toenails shaped like a talon.

This deformity is due to repeated trauma or candida infection. The name derives from the mythological animal the griffin, which had the head, body and tail of a lion and an eagle's head, wings and talons

(Courtesy of Dr A Watson, Infectious Diseases Department, The Canberra Hospital.)

FIGURE 3.16

Beau's lines

(Courtesy of Dr A Watson, Infectious Diseases Department, The Canberra Hospital.)

FIGURE 3.17

Yellow tar staining due to cigarette smoking

FIGURE 3.18

patient's inability to stand because of postural dizziness is probably a more important sign than the blood pressure difference). This is called *postural hypotension*. An increase in the pulse rate of 30 beats per minute or more, when the patient stands, is also a sign of *hypovolaemia*.

Weigh the patient. Following the body weight daily is the best way to determine changes in hydration over time. For example, a 5% decrease in body weight over 24 hours indicates that about 5% of body water has been lost. Using the same set of scales improves the accuracy of these measurements. Assessment of the patient's jugular venous pressure is one of the most sensitive ways of judging intravascular volume overload, or overhydration (see Ch 5).

THE HANDS AND NAILS

Changes occur in the hands in many different diseases (see Figs 3.16–3.18). If culturally acceptable, it is useful as an introduction to shake a patient's hand when meeting him or her. Apart from being polite, this may help make the diagnosis of dystrophia myotonica, a rare muscle disease in which the patient may be unable to let go. Shaking hands is also an acceptable and gentle way of introducing the physical examination. The physical examination is an intrusive event that is tolerated only because of the doctor's (and even the medical student's) professional and cultural standing.

Examination of the hands by *looking*, *feeling* and *moving* is the gateway to diagnosis in many cases. There is no subspecialty of internal medicine in which examination of the hands is not rewarding. The shape of the nails may change in some cardiac and respiratory diseases, the whole size of the hand may increase in growth hormone excess (acromegaly; p 456), gross distortion of the hands' architecture occurs in some

Nails signs in systemic disease

Nail sign	Some causes	Page no.
Blue nails	Cyanosis, Wilson's disease, ochronosis	41
Red nails	Polycythaemia (reddish-blue), carbon monoxide poisoning (cherry-red)	355
Yellow nails	Yellow nail syndrome	193
Clubbing	Lung cancer, chronic pulmonary suppuration, infective endocarditis, cyanotic heart disease, congenital, HIV infection, chronic inflammatory bowel disease, etc.	81
Splinter haemorrhages	Infective endocarditis, vasculitis	82
Koilonychia (spoon-shaped nails)	Iron deficiency, fungal infection, Raynaud's disease	335
Onycholysis	Thyrotoxicosis, psoriasis, over-enthusiastic cleaning beneath the nails (quite common)	449
Non-pigmented transverse bands in the nail bed (Beau's lines;* see Fig. 3.17)	Fever, cachexia, malnutrition	48
Leuconychia (white nails)	Hypoalbuminaemia	235
Transverse opaque white bands (Muehrcke's lines)	Trauma, acute illness, hypoalbuminaemia, chemotherapy	306
Single transverse white band (Mees' lines)	Arsenic poisoning, chronic kidney disease, chemotherapy or severe illness	309
Nail fold erythema and telangiectasia	Systemic lupus erythematosus	414
'Half and half nails' (proximal portion white to pink and distal portion red or brown: Terry's nails)	Chronic renal failure, cirrhosis	235

Joseph Honoré Simon Beau (1806–65) first described this in 1846. The cause of Beau's lines is usually a serious systemic illness or treatment (e.g. septicaemia or chemotherapy), which stops growth of the nail plate. After recovery the nail grows again. The distance of the line from the cuticle can be measured to work out when the illness occurred. The fingernail plate grows at an average rate of 0.1 mm/day.

(Clinical Examination Essentials, Talley & O'Connor, 2015, pp 49–51.)

TABLE 3.1

forms of arthritis (p 433), tremor or muscle wasting may represent neurological disease and pallor of the palmar creases may indicate anaemia (see also Table 3.1). Yellow tar staining of the fingers indicates a cigarette smoker (see Fig. 3.18). These and other changes in the hands await you later in the book.

TEMPERATURE

The patient's temperature should always be recorded as part of the initial clinical examination. The normal temperature (in the mouth) ranges from 36.6°C to 37.2°C (98°F to 99°F). The rectal temperature is normally higher and the axillary and tympanic temperatures are lower than the oral temperature (see Table 3.2). In very hot weather the temperature may rise by up to 0.5°C. Patients who report they have a fever are usually correct, as is a mother who reports that her child's forehead is warm and that fever is present.[15]

There is a diurnal variation. Body temperature is lowest in the morning and reaches a peak between 6 pm and 10 pm. The febrile pattern of most diseases follows this diurnal variation. The pattern of the fever (pyrexia) may be helpful in diagnosis (see Table 3.3).

Average temperature values

	Normal	Fever
Mouth	36.8°C	>37.3°C
Axilla*	36.4°C	>36.9°C
Rectum	37.3°C	>37.7°C

*Tympanic temperatures are similar to axillary ones.

TABLE 3.2

Types of fever

Type	Character	Examples
Continued	Does not remit	Typhoid fever, typhus, drug fever, malignant hyperthermia
Intermittent	Temperature falls to normal each day	Pyogenic infections, lymphomas, miliary tuberculosis
Remittent	Daily fluctuations >2°C, temperature does not return to normal	Not characteristic of any particular disease
Relapsing	Temperature returns to normal for days before rising again	Malaria: Tertian—3-day pattern, fever peaks every other day (*Plasmodium vivax, P. ovale*); Quartan—4-day pattern, fever peaks every 3rd day (*P. malariae*) Lymphoma: Pel–Ebstein* fever of Hodgkin's disease (very rare) Pyogenic infection

*Pieter Pel (1859–1919), Professor of Medicine, Amsterdam; Wilhelm Ebstein (1836–1912), a German physician.
Note: *The use of antipyretic and antibiotic drugs has made these patterns unusual today.*

TABLE 3.3

Sepsis refers to a syndrome ranging from bacteria in the blood to multiple organ dysfunction (and death). The **systemic inflammatory response syndrome (SIRS)** refers to two or more features that often occur in sepsis, namely fever, a rapid pulse (tachycardia), a high respiratory rate (tachypnoea) and a high white cell blood count on testing. Look for an obvious source of infection such as a wound infection after surgery, oozing pus (and remember: increasing wound pain is an indicator of possible underlying infection).

SIRS can occur not only in infection but also after surgery and with pancreatitis, burns, pulmonary emboli or autoimmune disease.[16]

Very high temperatures (*hyperpyrexia*, defined as above 41.6°C) are a serious problem and may result in death. The causes include heat stroke from exposure or excessive exertion (e.g. in marathon runners), malignant hyperthermia (a group of rare genetically determined disorders in which hyperpyrexia occurs in response to various anaesthetic agents [e.g. halothane] or muscle relaxants [e.g. suxamethonium]), the neuroleptic malignant syndrome (a reaction to antipsychotic medication), and hypothalamic disease.

Hypothermia is defined as a temperature of less than 35°C. Normal thermometers do not record below 35°C and therefore special low-reading thermometers must be used if hypothermia is suspected. Causes of hypothermia include hypothyroidism and prolonged exposure to cold.

SMELL

Certain medical conditions are associated with a characteristic odour, but not all doctors can detect odour abnormalities (which may be genetically determined).[17] Notable odours include the sickly sweet acetone smell of the breath of patients with ketoacidosis, the sweet smell of the breath in patients with liver failure, the ammoniacal fish breath ('uraemic fetor') of end-stage chronic kidney disease and, of course, the stale cigarette smell of the patient who smokes. This smell will be on his or her clothes and even on the referral letter kept in a bag or pocket next to a packet of cigarettes. Recent consumption of alcoholic drinks may be obvious. 'Bad breath', although often of uncertain cause, may be related to poor dental hygiene, gingivitis (infection of the gums) or nasopharyngeal tumours. Chronic suppurative infections of the lung can make the breath and saliva foul smelling.

Skin abscesses may be very offensive, especially if caused by anaerobic organisms or *Pseudomonas* spp. Urinary incontinence is associated with the characteristic smell of stale urine, which is often more offensive if the patient has a urinary tract infection. The smell of bacterial vaginosis is usually just described as offensive. Severe bowel obstruction and the rare gastrocolic fistula can cause faecal contamination of the breath when the patient belches. The black faeces (*melaena*) caused by upper gastrointestinal bleeding and the breakdown of blood in the gut has a strong smell, familiar to those who have worked in a gastroenterology ward. The metallic smell of fresh blood, sometimes detectable during interventional cardiological procedures, is very mild by comparison.

PREPARING THE PATIENT FOR EXAMINATION

An accurate physical examination is best performed when the examining conditions are ideal. This means that, if possible, the patient should be in a well-lit room (preferably daylight) from which distracting noises and interruptions have been excluded (rarely possible in busy hospital wards). Screens must be drawn around patients before the examination. Consulting rooms and outpatient clinics should be set up to ensure privacy and comfort for patients.

Patients have a right to expect that students and doctors will have washed their hands or rubbed them with antimicrobial hand sanitisers before they perform an examination. This is as important in clinics and surgeries as in hospital wards. Many hospitals now have notices telling patients that they may ask their doctors whether their hands have been washed. The diaphragm and bell of the stethoscope should be cleaned with an antimicrobial wipe (see Fig. 3.1c) and any other equipment that touches a patient should be disposable (e.g. neurology pin) or wiped down.

The examination should not begin until permission has been asked of the patient and the nature of the examination has been explained.

The patient must be undressed so that the parts to be examined are accessible. Modesty requires that a woman's breasts be covered temporarily with a towel or sheet while other parts of the body are being examined. Male doctors and students should be accompanied by a female chaperone when they examine a woman's pelvis, rectum or breasts. Both men and women should have the groin covered, for example, during examination of the legs. Outpatients should be provided with a gown to wear. However, important physical signs will be missed in some patients if excessive attention is paid to modesty.

The position of the patient in bed or elsewhere should depend on what system is to be examined. For example, a patient's abdomen is best examined if he or she lies flat with one pillow placed so that the abdominal muscles are relaxed. This is discussed in detail in subsequent chapters.

Within each of the examining systems, four elements comprise the main parts of the physical examination: looking—*inspection*, feeling—*palpation*, tapping—*percussion*, and listening—*auscultation*.[c] For many systems a fifth element—*assessment of function*—is added. *Measuring* is also relevant in some systems. Each of these is discussed in detail in the following chapters.

ADVANCED CONCEPTS: EVIDENCE-BASED CLINICAL EXAMINATION

History taking and physical examination are late-comers to evidence-based medicine. There are intensive efforts in all areas of medicine to base practice on evidence of benefit.

By their nature, physical signs unless gross have an element of subjectivity and one examiner will not always agree with another. For example, the loudness of a murmur or the presence or absence of fingernail changes may be controversial. There are often different accepted methods of assessing the presence or absence of a sign, and experienced clinicians may disagree about whether, for example, the apex beat is in the normal position or not. Even apparently objective measurements such as blood pressure can vary depending on whether Korotkoff sound IV or V (p 87) is used, and from minute to minute for the same patient. Some physical signs are present only intermittently. The pericardial rub may disappear before students can be found to come and listen to it.

Many of the studies that have examined the reliability of physical signs have had problematic variations in disease severity and examiners' experience.[18] This is likely to have led to an underestimation of the reliability of signs.

One way of looking at the usefulness of a sign or a test is to measure or estimate its specificity and sensitivity:

- The **specificity** of a sign is the proportion of people *without* the disease who do *not* have the sign ('negative in health'). For example, an 80%

---

[c] Infectious diseases doctors add *prevent infection transmission* (wash hands) to these elements.

specificity means that 8 out of 10 people *without* that sign *do not have* the condition.

- The **sensitivity** of a sign is the proportion of people *with* the disease who *have* the sign—that is, those who are correctly identified by the test ('positive in disease'). A sensitivity of 80% means that assessment of the presence of that sign will pick up 80% of people with the condition (but will not pick up 20%).

You may find it helpful to use the following mnemonics to help you remember this:

SpIn = **S**pecific tests when **p**ositive help to rule **In** disease

SnOut = **S**ensitive tests when **n**egative help to rule **Out** disease.

The perfect test or sign (if there were such a thing) is 100% sensitive and 100% specific. A sign or test that is present or 'positive' in a person who does not have the condition is called a *false positive*. The absence of a sign, or a negative test, in a patient who has the condition is called a *false negative*. Another way of looking at this is the positive or negative predictive value of a test—that is, the probability that a positive result means the condition is present or that a negative result means it is absent. Table 3.4 lists the sensitivity and specificity of some common signs.

The likelihood that a test or sign result will be a true positive or negative depends on the prevalence of the disease in the practice setting (or alternatively, what is called the pretest probability of the condition). For example, if splinter haemorrhages (p 80) are found in the nails of a healthy manual labourer they are likely to represent a false-positive sign of infective endocarditis. This sign is not very sensitive or specific and in this case the pretest probability of the condition is low. If splinters are found in a sick patient with known valvular heart disease and a new murmur, the sign is likely to be a true positive in this patient with a high pretest probability of endocarditis. This pretest probability analysis of the false and true positive rates is based on Bayes' theorem.

A useful way to summarise sensitivity and specificity is the **likelihood ratio** (LR). A positive LR indicates that the presence of a sign is likely to occur that much more often in an individual with the disease than in one without it. The higher the positive LR, the more useful is a positive sign. A negative likelihood ratio increases the likelihood that the disease is absent if the sign is not present.

Examples of sensitivities and specificities for common clinical signs

Sign	Underlying condition	Sensitivity (%)	Specificity (%)
Shifting dullness	Ascites	85	50
Palpable spleen—specifically examined	Splenomegaly	58	92
Goitre	Thyroid disease	70	82
Abnormal foot pulses	Peripheral vascular disease	63–95	73–99
Third heart sound (S3)	Ejection fraction <50%	51	90
	Ejection fraction <30%	78	88
Trophic skin changes	Peripheral vascular disease	43–50	70
Hepatojugular reflux	Congestive cardiac failure	24–33	95
Initial impression	COPD	25	95
Femoral arterial bruit	Peripheral vascular disease	20–29	95
Prolonged capillary refill	Peripheral vascular disease	25–28	85
Tinel's sign	Carpal tunnel syndrome	25–75	75–90
Kernig's sign	Meningitis	5	95

COPD = chronic obstructive pulmonary disease.

(Anthony MJ, Celermajer DS, Stockler MR. Beauty is in the eye of the beholder: reaching agreement about physical signs and their value. *Internal Med J* 2005; 35(3):178–187, with permission from John Wiley & Sons.)

TABLE 3.4

$$\text{positive LR} = \frac{\text{sensitivity}}{1-\text{specificity}}$$

$$\text{negative LR} = \frac{1-\text{sensitivity}}{\text{specificity}}$$

Remember that if the LR is greater than 1, there is an increased probability of disease; if the LR is less than 1, there is a decreased probability of disease. For example, the presence of a third heart sound in a patient who might have heart failure (e.g. breathlessness on exertion) has a positive LR of 3.8 and a negative LR around 1. This means that a third heart sound is specific for heart failure (increases likelihood of the condition nearly four times) but not sensitive (the absence of a third heart sound does not reduce the likelihood).

All of these figures are calculated on a population suspected of disease; it would be quite incorrect to apply them to an asymptomatic group of people. Fagan's nomogram (see Fig. 3.19) can be used to apply LRs to clinical problems if the pretest probability of the condition is known or can be estimated. Remember, positive LRs of 2, 5 and 10 increase the probability of disease by 15%, 30% and 45% respectively. Similarly, negative LRs of 0.5, 0.2 and 0.1 decrease the probability of disease by 15%, 30% and 45% respectively.

When the pretest probability is very low, even a high positive LR does not make the disease very likely. A line is drawn from the pretest probability number through the known LR and ends up on the post-test probability number. For example, if the pretest probability of the condition is low, say 10 (10%) and a sign is present that has an LR of 2, the post-test probability of the condition being present is only about 20%. We have included example LRs in the Good signs guides in many chapters of this book.

Inter-observer agreement (reliability) and the κ-statistic

The LR of a sign assumes that the sign is present, but there is considerable variability in the agreement between observers about the presence of many signs. There are a number of reasons for this low reliability (see List 3.7).

The κ (kappa) statistic is a way of expressing the inter-observer variation for a sign or test. Values are between 0 and 1, where 0 means agreement about the sign is the same as it would be by chance and 1 means

Fagan's nomogram for interpreting a diagnostic test result

(Adapted from Sackett DL, Richardson WS, Rosenberg W, Haynes RB. *Evidence-based medicine: how to practice and teach EBM*. London: Churchill-Livingstone, 1997.)

FIGURE 3.19

complete (100%) agreement. Occasionally values of less than 0 are obtained when inter-observer agreement is worse than should occur by chance. By convention, a κ-value of 0.8 to 1 means almost perfect to complete agreement, 0.6 to 0.8 substantial agreement, 0.4 to 0.6 good agreement, 0.2 to 0.4 fair agreement and 0 to 0.2 slight agreement. A selection of signs and their κ-values is listed in Table 3.5. Remember that a high κ-value means agreement about the presence of a sign, *not* that the sign necessarily has a high positive LR. A low κ-value may be an indication that the sign is a difficult one to elicit accurately, especially for beginners, but it does not always mean that the sign is not useful. For example the detection of the typical fine crackles of

Comparisons of kappa values for common clinical signs (agreement between observers beyond that expected by chance alone)

Sign	Reliability	Kappa value
Abnormality of extraocular movements	Substantial	0.77
Size of goitre by examination	Substantial	0.74
Forced expiratory time	Substantial	0.70
Presence of wheezes	Substantial	0.69
Signs of liver disease, e.g. jaundice, Dupuytren's contracture, spider naevi	Substantial	0.65
Palpation of the posterior tibial pulse	Good	0.6
Dullness to percussion	Good	0.52
Tender liver edge	Good	0.49
Clubbing	Fair to almost perfect	0.39–0.90
Bronchial breath sounds	Fair	0.32
Hearing a systolic murmur	Fair to substantial	0.3–0.48
Tachypnoea	Fair	0.25
Clinical breast examination for cancer	Fair to substantial	0.22–0.59
Neck stiffness	Unreliable	−0.01

(Anthony MJ, Celermajer DS, Stockler MR. Beauty is in the eye of the beholder: reaching agreement about physical signs and their value. *Internal Med J* 2005; 35(3):178–187, with permission from John Wiley & Sons.)

TABLE 3.5

> **IMPORTANT REASONS FOR INTER-OBSERVER DISAGREEMENT**
>
> 1. The sign comes and goes; e.g. basal crackles in heart failure, a fourth heart sound.
> 2. Some of the observers' techniques may be imperfect; e.g. not asking the patient to cough before declaring the presence of lung crackles consistent with heart failure.
> 3. Some signs are intrinsically subjective; e.g. the grading of the loudness of a murmur.
> 4. Preconceptions about the patient based on other observations or the history may influence the observer; e.g. goitre may seem readily palpable when a patient is known to have thyroid disease.
>
> LIST 3.7

have also been calculated and are not much more impressive—for example, the reporting of cardiomegaly on a chest X-ray is 0.48, while cholestasis reported on a liver biopsy is 0.40.

In medical practice, multiple factors are taken into account when diagnostic decisions are made.[19] Only very rarely is one symptom, sign or test diagnostic of a condition. The evidence supporting the usefulness of most signs is based on looking at a sign in isolation. It is much more difficult to study the combined importance of the range of historical and physical findings that are present. However, the skilled and experienced clinician uses many pieces of information and is sceptical when an unexpected or illogical finding or test result is obtained.

interstitial lung disease may have a high κ-value when performed by a group of experienced chest doctors but a low value when assessed by a group of orthopaedic surgeons.

Although some of these values appear low, κ-values for the reporting of a number of diagnostic tests

> **T&O'C ESSENTIALS**
>
> 1. A systematic approach to the physical examination will ensure that the examination is complete.

2. Always take the time to make a general inspection of the patient.
3. The secret to successful physical examination (especially for student exams) is constant practice.
4. Position the patient correctly for the examination.
5. Ensure the patient has privacy during the examination.
6. Never hurt the patient during the examination.
7. Hand-washing and cleaning of equipment must be routine.

'How old are you?'

FIGURE 3.20

INTRODUCTION TO THE OSCE (see Intoduction to the OSCE video at Student CONSULT)

In most medical schools today, history taking and physical examination are examined using the OSCE (although long- and short-case testing may also be used). This comprises a series of stations (e.g. 10 minutes each) where particular history or physical examination skills are tested in front of one or two examiners. Students rotate through all of the stations and each station has different examiners. At each station, after a stem or introduction has been provided (e.g. patient's name, age and presenting symptom), the task to be completed is highly specific (e.g. 'Please take the blood pressure'). The questions are standardised and preset, and the scoring is predetermined, as is (usually) the pass mark. You gain a mark for each necessary step properly completed (e.g. introducing yourself: 1 mark; washing your hands: 1 mark). This means that you must have a system for examination in the OSCE setting and practise it until it becomes second nature.

At the end of most chapters of this text a list of sample OSCE cases and questions is provided to help with revision and as a preparation guide. Look up the answers in the chapter and use this as a way of revising.

At OSCE stations, candidates may be asked to take a specific history (e.g. the social history) or examine a particular body system or part (e.g. the praecordium for heart murmurs or the posterior chest for lung signs). Other stations, depending on the students' seniority, may test clinical skills such as prescription writing. Each medical school conducts these exams slightly differently, but there are certain general principles all students should understand (if they wish to pass).

Remember, the 'patient' in the exam may be an actor trained to answer questions in a certain way. Actors are also used for the physical examination to test that students complete their techniques properly. The idea of using trained actors is that answers to student questions will be standardised. The actor patients often come from local theatrical schools and there is a small risk that they will be tempted to overact (e.g. bursting into tears when asked their age; see Fig. 3.20). The good news is that all candidates will experience the same conditions.

There are a number of key points to keep in mind during this ordeal:

1. The examiners know how difficult it is to perform while being watched.
2. Their expectations are much lower for students in their first few years of the course.
3. You will be given a spoken or written introduction, or both. This will tell you what the examiners expect you to do, so don't do something different. For example, if the request is to examine the upper limbs of a patient with weakness in the arms, don't begin by testing sensation. Time is limited and the examiners will have directed you to where the abnormal signs

will be (if there are any, which often there are not in this type of exam).

4. As important to the examiners as a good technical approach is your attitude to the patient. You can expect to fail if you are rude and inconsiderate.

5. It is important to develop a routine when you practise for these exams. This includes introducing yourself and explaining at the start, and then with each step, what you are going to do. For example, if asked to examine the patient's abdomen, having introduced yourself, say something like 'I have been asked to examine your abdomen. I will need you to lie flat for me with just one pillow. Will you be comfortable like that? I will need to pull your underpants down a little lower. Is that all right? Are you sore anywhere? I'm sorry my hands are a little cold. Please let me know if this is at all uncomfortable for you.' Make it clear during the examination that you are watching the patient's face for any sign that the examination is painful. This type of approach to patients is really only normal politeness and should be routine (i.e. not just used during exams).

6. Remember to wash your hands before and after for an easy mark (and in practice you should always do this to protect the patient and you).

Video-recorded OSCE examinations are provided with this edition to help guide you further. They are marked with this reference guide from the appropriate chapter. There is more help online; for example, search for Wikiversity's OSCE review or Instamedic. There are also useful phone apps available.

References

1. Verghese A1, Brady E, Kapur CC, Horwitz Rl. The bedside evaluation: ritual and reason. *Ann Intern Med* 2011; 155(8):550–553. doi: 10.7326/0003-4819-155-8-201110180-00013.
2. Verghese A, Charlton B, Kassirer JP et al. Inadequacies of physical examination as a cause of medical errors and adverse events: a collection of vignettes. *Am J Med* 2015; 128(12):1322–1324.
3. Sacket DL. The science of the art of clinical examination. *JAMA* 1992; 267:2650–2652. This article examines the limitations of current research in the field of clinical examination.
4. Sackett DL. A primer on the precision and accuracy of the clinical examination (the rational clinical examination). *JAMA* 1992; 267:2638–2644. An important article examining the relevance of understanding both precision (reproducibility among various examiners) and accuracy (determining the truth) in clinical examination.
5. Wiener S, Nathanson M. Physical examination: frequently observed errors. *JAMA* 1976; 236:852–855. This article categorises errors, including poor skills, underreporting and over-reporting of signs, use of inadequate equipment and inadequate recording.
6. Fitzgerald FT, Tierney LM Jr. The bedside Sherlock Holmes. *West J Med* 1982; 137:169–175. Here deductive reasoning is discussed as a tool in clinical diagnosis.
7. Sackett DL, Haynes RB, Tugwell P. *Clinical epidemiology. A basic science for clinical medicine.* Boston: Little, Brown & Co, 1985. The perceived commonness of diseases affects our approach to their diagnosis.
8. Cretikos MA, Bellomo R, Hillman K et al. Respiratory rate: the neglected vital sign. *Med J Aust* 2008; 188(11):657–659.
9. Martin L, Khalil H. How much reduced hemoglobin is necessary to generate central cyanosis? *Chest* 1990; 97:182–185. This useful article explains the chemistry of haemoglobin and its colour change.
10. Moyer VA; U.S. Preventive Services Task Force. Screening for and management of obesity in adults: U.S. Preventive Services Task Force recommendation statement. *Ann Intern Med* 2012; 157(5):373–378.
11. Detsky AS, Smalley PS, Chang J. Is this patient malnourished? *JAMA* 1994; 271:54–58. Assessment of nutrition is an important part of the examination but needs a scientific approach.
12. Gross CR, Lindquist RD, Woolley AC et al. Clinical indicators of dehydration severity in elderly patients. *J Emerg Med* 1992; 10:267–274. This important and urgent assessment is more difficult in elderly sick patients.
13. Koziol-McLain J, Lowenstein SR, Fuller B. Orthostatic vital signs in emergency medicine department patients. *Ann Emerg Med* 1991; 20:606–610. These signs help in the assessment of the severity of illness in emergency patients, but there is a wide range of normal.
14. McGee S, Abernethy WB III, Simel DL. Is this patient hypovolemic? *JAMA* 1999; 281:1022–1029. The most sensitive clinical features for large-volume blood loss are severe postural dizziness and a postural rise in pulse rate of >30 beats per minute, not tachycardia or supine hypotension. A dry axilla supports dehydration. Moist mucous membranes and a tongue without furrows make hypovolaemia unlikely; assessing skin turgor, surprisingly, is not of proven value.
15. Coburn B, Morris AM, Tomlinson G, Detsky AS. Does this adult patient with suspected bacteremia require blood cultures? *JAMA* 2012; 308(5):502–511. doi: 10.1001/jama.2012.8262.
16. Reddy M1, Gill SS, Wu W et al. Does this patient have an infection of a chronic wound? *JAMA* 2012; 307(6):605–611.
17. Hayden GF. Olfactory diagnosis in medicine. *Postgrad Med* 1980; 67:110–115, 118. Describes characteristic patient odours and their connections with disease, although the diagnostic accuracy is uncertain.
18. Benbassat J, Baumal R. Narrative review: should teaching of the respiratory physical examination be restricted only to signs with proven reliability and validity? *J Gen Intern Med* 2010; 25(8):865–872. Physical signs in respiratory disease generally have lower than ideal reliability and sensitivity, but some signs have high specificity. While physical examination of the chest should not be ignored, more research is needed!
19. Wets DM, Dupras DM. 5 ways statistics can fool you—tips for practising clinicians. *Vaccine* 2013; 31(12):1550–1552.

SECTION 2
The cardiovascular system

CHAPTER 4
The cardiovascular history

CHAPTER 5
The cardiac examination

CHAPTER 6
The lower limb examination and peripheral vascular disease

CHAPTER 7
Correlation of physical signs and cardiovascular disease

CHAPTER 8
A summary of the cardiovascular examination and extending the cardiovascular examination

CHAPTER 4
The cardiovascular history

The heart ... moves of itself and does not stop unless for ever. LEONARDO DA VINCI (1452–1519)

The following chapters deal with the history and the examination of the heart and blood vessels, as well as other parts of the body where symptoms and signs of heart disease may appear. Not only is this fundamental to the assessment of any patient, but the cardiovascular system is also one of the most commonly tested systems in OSCEs and viva voce examinations. It is believed by cardiologists to be the most important system in the body.

PRESENTING SYMPTOMS
Chest pain

Rather to the satisfaction of cardiologists, the mention of chest pain by a patient (see Table 4.1) tends to provoke more urgent attention than other symptoms. The surprised patient may find him- or herself whisked into an emergency ward with the rapid appearance of worried-looking doctors. This is because ischaemic

Causes (differential diagnosis) of chest pain and typical features

Pain	Causes	Typical features
Cardiac pain	Myocardial ischaemia or infarction	Central, tight or heavy; may radiate to the jaw or left arm
Vascular pain	Aortic dissection	Very sudden onset, radiates to the back
Pleuropericardial pain	Pericarditis ± myocarditis Infective pleurisy Pneumothorax Pneumonia Autoimmune disease Mesothelioma Metastatic tumour	Pleuritic pain, worse when patient lies down Pleuritic pain Sudden onset, sharp, associated with dyspnoea Often pleuritic, associated with fever and dyspnoea Pleuritic pain Severe and constant Severe and constant, localised
Chest wall pain	Persistent cough Muscular strains Intercostal myositis Thoracic zoster Coxsackie B virus infection Thoracic nerve compression or infiltration Rib fracture Rib tumour, primary or metastatic Tietze's syndrome	Worse with movement, chest wall tender Worse with movement, chest wall tender Sharp, localised, worse with movement Severe, follows nerve root distribution, precedes rash Pleuritic pain Follows nerve root distribution History of trauma, localised tenderness Constant, severe, localised Costal cartilage tender
Gastrointestinal pain	Gastro-oesophageal reflux Diffuse oesophageal spasm	Not related to exertion, may be worse when patient lies down—common Relieved by swallowing e.g. of warm water

TABLE 4.1

Continued

Causes (differential diagnosis) of chest pain and typical features—cont'd

Pain	Causes	Typical features
Airway pain	Tracheitis Central bronchial carcinoma Inhaled foreign body	Pain in throat, breathing painful
Central pain	Panic attacks	Often preceded by anxiety, associated with breathlessness and hyperventilation symptoms (dizziness, perioral paraesthesia)
Mediastinal pain	Mediastinitis Sarcoid adenopathy, lymphoma	

TABLE 4.1

Differential diagnosis of chest pain

Favours angina	Favours pericarditis or pleurisy	Favours oesophageal (acid) reflux pain
Tight or heavy	Sharp or stabbing	Burning
Onset predictable with exertion	Not exertional	Not exertional
Relieved by rest	Present at rest	Present at rest
Relieved rapidly by nitrates	Unaffected by nitrates	Unaffected unless spasm
Not positional	Worse supine (pericarditis)	Onset may be when supine
Not affected by respiration	Worse with respiration Pericardial or pleural rub	Unaffected by respiration

TABLE 4.2A

Differential diagnosis of chest pain

Favours myocardial infarction (acute coronary syndrome)	Favours angina
Onset at rest	Onset with exertion
Severe pain	Moderate pain or discomfort
Sweating	No sweating
Anxiety (angor)	Mild or no anxiety
No relief with nitrates	Rapid relief with nitrates
Associated symptoms (nausea and vomiting)	Associated symptoms absent

Favours myocardial infarction	Favours aortic dissection*
Central chest pain	Radiates to back
Subacute onset (minutes)	Instantaneous onset
Severe pain	Very severe pain, tearing quality

Favours myocardial ischaemia	Favours chest wall pain
Exertional	Positional
Occurs with exertion	Often worse at rest
Brief episodes	Prolonged
Diffuse	Localised
No chest wall tenderness (only discriminates between infarction and chest wall pain)	Chest wall tenderness

*+ve LR of dissection of 66 if all three characteristics or two plus history of hypertension.

(Adapted from Simel DL, Rennie D. *The rational clinical examination: evidence-based diagnosis*. New York: McGraw-Hill, 2009.)

TABLE 4.2B

heart disease, which may be a life-threatening condition, often presents in this manner (see List 4.1).

The pain of *angina* and *myocardial infarction* tends to be similar in character; both are due to the accumulation of metabolites from ischaemic muscle following complete or partial obstruction of a coronary artery, which leads to stimulation of the cardiac sympathetic nerves.[1,2] Patients with cardiac transplants who develop coronary disease in the transplanted heart may not feel angina, presumably because the heart is denervated. Similarly, patients with diabetes are more likely to be diagnosed with 'silent infarcts'.

To help determine the cause of chest pain (see Tables 4.2A and B), it is important to ascertain the duration,

> **THE CARDIOVASCULAR HISTORY: PRESENTING SYMPTOMS**
>
> **Major symptoms**
>
> Chest pain or heaviness
>
> Dyspnoea: exertional (note degree of exercise necessary), orthopnoea, paroxysmal nocturnal dyspnoea
>
> Ankle swelling
>
> Palpitations
>
> Syncope
>
> Intermittent claudication
>
> Fatigue
>
> **Past history**
>
> History of ischaemic heart disease: myocardial infarction, coronary artery bypass grafting (CABG), coronary angioplasty, rheumatic fever, chorea, sexually transmitted disease, recent dental work, thyroid disease
>
> Prior medical examination revealing heart disease (e.g. military, school, insurance)
>
> Drugs
>
> **Social history**
>
> Tobacco and alcohol use
>
> Occupation
>
> **Family history**
>
> Myocardial infarcts, cardiomyopathy, congenital heart disease, mitral valve prolapse, Marfan's syndrome
>
> **Coronary artery disease risk factors**
>
> Previous coronary disease
>
> Smoking
>
> Hypertension
>
> Hyperlipidaemia
>
> Family history of coronary artery disease (first-degree relatives)
>
> Diabetes mellitus
>
> Rheumatoid arthritis and chronic inflammatory rheumatological disease
>
> Obesity and physical inactivity
>
> Male sex and advanced age
>
> Erectile dysfunction
>
> **Functional status in established heart disease**
>
> Class I—disease present, angina* does not occur during ordinary physical activity or cardiac dysfunction, but no symptoms of dyspnoea present[†]
>
> Class II—angina or dyspnoea during ordinary activity
>
> Class III—angina or dyspnoea during less than ordinary activity
>
> Class IV—angina or dyspnoea at rest
>
> *Canadian Cardiovascular Society (CCVS) classification.
> [†]New York Heart Association (NYHA) classification.
>
> LIST 4.1

location, quality and precipitating and aggravating factors (the **four cardinal features**), as well as means of relief and accompanying symptoms (the SOCRATES questions; see Ch 1).[3] The term angina[a] was coined by Heberden from the Greek and Latin words meaning 'choking' or strangling, and the patient may complain of crushing pain, heaviness, discomfort or a choking sensation in the retrosternal area or in the throat. It is best to ask whether the patient experiences chest 'discomfort' rather than 'pain', because angina is often dull and aching in character and may not be perceived as pain (see Questions box 4.1, Fig. 4.1).

The pain or discomfort is usually central rather than left-sided. The patient may dismiss the pain as non-cardiac because it is not felt over the heart on the left side. It may radiate to the jaw or to the arms, but very rarely travels below the umbilicus. The severity of the pain or discomfort is variable.

Angina characteristically occurs with exertion, with rapid relief once the patient rests or slows down. The

---

[a] William Heberden's (1710–1801) description of angina (1768) is difficult to improve upon: 'They who are afflicted with it, are seized while they are walking (more especially if it be up hill and soon after eating) with a painful and most disagreeable sensation in the breast, which seems as if it would extinguish life, if it were to increase or continue; but the moment they stand still, all this uneasiness vanishes.' Heberden did not realise that angina was a result of coronary artery narrowing.

62 SECTION 2 THE CARDIOVASCULAR SYSTEM

QUESTIONS TO ASK THE PATIENT WITH SUSPECTED ANGINA

! denotes symptoms for the possible diagnosis of an urgent or dangerous problem.

1. Can you tell me what the pain or discomfort is like? Is it sharp or dull, heavy or tight?
2. When do you get the pain? Does it come out of the blue, or does it come on when you do physical things? Is it worse if you exercise after eating?
3. How long does it last?
4. Where do you feel it?
5. Does it make you stop or slow down?
6. Does it go away quickly when you stop exercising?
! 7. Is it coming on with less effort or at rest? (Unstable symptoms)
8. Have you had angina before, and is this the same?

QUESTIONS BOX 4.1

Clinical classification of angina from the European Society of Cardiology

Typical angina	Meets **all three** of the following characteristics: 1. Characteristic retrosternal chest discomfort—typical quality and duration 2. Provoked by exertion or emotion 3. Relieved by rest or GTN (glyceryl trinitrate) or both
Atypical angina	Meets **two** of the above characteristics
Non-cardiac chest pain	Meets **one** or **none** of the above characteristics

TABLE 4.3

amount of exertion necessary to produce the pain may be predictable to the patient. A change in the pattern of onset of previously stable angina must be taken very seriously.

These features constitute *typical angina* (see Table 4.3).[3,4] Although angina typically occurs on exertion, it may also occur at rest or wake a patient from sleep. Ischaemic chest pain is usually unaffected by respiration. The use of sublingual nitrates characteristically brings relief within a couple of minutes, but this is not specific as nitrates may also relieve oesophageal spasm and have a pronounced placebo effect.

The pain associated with an acute coronary syndrome (ST elevation—STEMI, or non-ST elevation—non-STEMI myocardial infarction) often comes on at rest, is usually more severe and lasts much longer. Certain features make an acute coronary syndrome more likely (Good symptoms guide 4.1).[5] Acute coronary syndromes are usually caused by the rupture of a coronary artery plaque, which leads to the formation of thrombus in the arterial lumen. Stable exertional angina is a result of a fixed coronary narrowing.

Pain present for more than half an hour is more likely to be due to an acute coronary syndrome than to stable angina, but pain present continuously for many days is unlikely to be either. Associated symptoms of myocardial infarction include dyspnoea, sweating, anxiety, nausea and faintness.

Other causes of retrosternal pain are listed in Tables 4.1 and 4.2A. Chest pain made worse by inspiration is called *pleuritic pain*. This may be due to pleurisy or pericarditis (p 310). Pleurisy may occur because of

Locations of symptoms of angina

FIGURE 4.1

> **GOOD SYMPTOMS GUIDE 4.1**
> **Clinical factors and positive likelihood ratios for chest pain and diagnosis of an acute coronary syndrome**
>
> | Symptom | Likelihood ratio |
> | --- | --- |
> | Radiation to right arm or shoulder | 4.7 |
> | To both arms | 4.1 |
> | History of association with exertion | 2.4 |
> | Radiation to left arm | 2.3 |
> | Sweating | 2.0 |
> | Nausea or vomiting | 1.9 |
> | Worse than previous angina | 1.8 |
> | Pressure feeling | 1.3 |
> | Known abnormal exercise test | 3.1 |
> | Peripheral vascular disease | 2.7 |

inflammation of the pleura as a primary problem (usually due to viral infection), or secondary to pneumonia or pulmonary embolism. Pleuritic pain is not usually brought on by exertion and is often relieved by sitting up and leaning forwards. It is caused by the movement of inflamed pleural or pericardial surfaces on one another.

Chest wall pain is usually localised to a small area of the chest wall, is sharp and is associated with respiration or movement of the shoulders rather than with exertion. It may last only a few seconds or be present for prolonged periods. Disease of the *cervical or upper thoracic spine* may also cause pain associated with movement. This pain tends to radiate around from the back towards the front of the chest.

Pain due to a *dissecting aneurysm* of the aorta is usually very severe and may be described as tearing. This pain is often greatest at the moment of onset and radiates to the back. These three features—quality, rapid onset and radiation—are very specific for aortic dissection. A proximal dissection causes anterior chest pain and involvement of the descending aorta causes interscapular pain. A history of hypertension or of a connective tissue disorder such as Marfan's syndrome or Ehlers–Danlos syndrome puts the patient at increased risk of this condition.

Massive pulmonary embolism causes pain of very sudden onset, which may be retrosternal and associated with collapse, dyspnoea and cyanosis (p 199). It is often pleuritic, but can be identical to anginal pain, especially if associated with right ventricular ischaemia.

Spontaneous pneumothorax may result in pain and severe dyspnoea (p 193). The pain is sharp and localised to one part of the chest.

Gastro-oesophageal reflux commonly causes angina-like pain without heartburn. It is important to remember that these two relatively common conditions may coexist. *Oesophageal spasm* may cause retrosternal chest pain or discomfort and can be quite difficult to distinguish from angina but is uncommon; the pain may radiate to the jaw and is often relieved by swallowing warm water or by the use of nitrates.

Cholecystitis can cause chest pain and be confused with myocardial infarction. Right upper quadrant abdominal tenderness is usually present (p 253).

The cause of severe, usually unilateral, chest pain may not be apparent until the typical vesicular rash of *herpes zoster* appears in a thoracic nerve root distribution.

Dyspnoea

Shortness of breath may be due to cardiac disease. Dyspnoea (from the Greek *dys* 'bad', *pnoia* 'breathing') is often defined as an unexpected awareness of breathing. It occurs whenever the work of breathing is excessive, but the mechanism is uncertain. It is probably due to a sensation of increased force required of the respiratory muscles to produce a volume change in the lungs, because of a reduction in compliance of the lungs or increased resistance to air flow.

Cardiac dyspnoea is typically chronic and occurs with exertion because of failure of the left ventricular output to rise with exercise; this in turn leads to an acute rise in left ventricular end-diastolic pressure, raised pulmonary venous pressure, interstitial fluid leakage and thus reduced lung compliance. However, the dyspnoea of chronic cardiac failure does not correlate well with measurements of pulmonary artery pressures, and clearly the origin of the symptom of cardiac dyspnoea is complicated.[6] Left ventricular function may be impaired because of ischaemia (temporary or permanent reduction in myocardial blood supply), previous infarction (damage) or hypertrophy (often related to hypertension). As it becomes more severe, cardiac dyspnoea occurs at rest. Cardiac dyspnoea may begin suddenly as a result of myocardial infarction,

> **CAUSES OF ORTHOPNOEA**
>
> Cardiac failure
>
> **Uncommon causes**
> Massive ascites
> Pregnancy
> Bilateral diaphragmatic paralysis
> Large pleural effusion
> Severe pneumonia
>
> LIST 4.2

pulmonary oedema or sudden mitral regurgitation due to rupture of a chorda tendineae or papillary muscle infarction.

Orthopnoea (from the Greek *ortho* 'straight'; see List 4.2), or dyspnoea that develops when a patient is supine, occurs because in an upright position the patient's interstitial oedema is redistributed; the lower zones of the lungs become worse and the upper zones better. This allows improved overall blood oxygenation. Patients with severe orthopnoea spend the night sitting up in a chair or propped up on numerous pillows in bed. The absence of orthopnoea suggests that left ventricular failure is unlikely to be the cause of a patient's dyspnoea (negative likelihood ratio [LR] = 0.04[7]).

Paroxysmal[b] *nocturnal dyspnoea* (PND) is severe dyspnoea that wakes the patient from sleep so that he or she is forced to get up gasping for breath. This occurs because of a sudden failure of left ventricular output with an acute rise in pulmonary venous and capillary pressures; this leads to transudation of fluid into the interstitial tissues, which increases the work of breathing. The sequence may be precipitated by resorption of peripheral oedema at night while supine. Acute cardiac dyspnoea may also occur with acute pulmonary oedema or a pulmonary embolus.

Cardiac dyspnoea can be difficult to distinguish from that due to lung disease or other causes (p 165).[8] One should enquire particularly about a history of any cardiac disease that could be responsible for the onset of cardiac failure. For example, a patient with a number of known previous myocardial infarctions who develops dyspnoea is more likely to have decreased left ventricular contractility. A patient with a history of hypertension or a very heavy alcohol intake may have hypertensive heart disease or an alcoholic cardiomyopathy. The presence of orthopnoea or paroxysmal nocturnal dyspnoea is more suggestive of cardiac failure than of lung disease.

Dyspnoea is also a common symptom of anxiety. These patients often describe an inability to take a big enough breath to fill the lungs in a satisfying way. Their breathing may be deep and punctuated with sighs.

Ankle swelling

The presence of *oedema* alone is poorly correlated with heart failure (there are many more common causes), but some heart failure patients present with bilateral ankle swelling due to oedema. Unlike the swelling that occurs with inflammatory conditions, the area is not painful or red. Patients with the recent onset of oedema and who take a serious interest in their weight may have noticed a weight gain of 3 kg or more.

Ankle oedema of cardiac origin is usually symmetrical and worse in the evenings, with improvement during the night. It may be a symptom of biventricular failure or right ventricular failure secondary to a number of possible underlying aetiologies. As failure progresses, oedema ascends to involve the legs, thighs, genitalia and abdomen. There are usually other symptoms or signs of heart disease.

It is important to find out whether the patient is taking a vasodilating drug (e.g. a calcium channel blocker), which can cause peripheral oedema.[9] There are other (more) common causes of ankle oedema than heart failure that also need to be considered; see List 6.2 on p 112). Oedema that affects the face is more likely to be related to kidney disease, from the nephrotic syndrome (p 321).

Palpitations

This is not a very precise term (see Table 4.4). It is usually taken to mean an unexpected awareness of the heartbeat.[10] Ask the patient to describe exactly what he or she notices and whether the palpitations are slow or fast, regular or irregular, and how long they last (see Questions box 4.2).

There may be the sensation of a missed beat followed by a particularly heavy beat; this can be due to an *atrial* or *ventricular ectopic beat* (see the ECG Library at Student CONSULT) (which produces little cardiac output) followed by a compensating pause and then a normally conducted beat (which is more forceful than usual because there has been a longer diastolic filling period for the ventricle).

---
[b] Paroxysmal symptoms or signs occur suddenly and intermittently.

If the patient complains of a rapid heartbeat, it is important to find out whether the palpitations are of sudden or gradual onset and offset. Cardiac arrhythmias are usually instantaneous in onset and offset, whereas the onset and offset of *sinus tachycardia* is more gradual. A completely irregular rhythm is suggestive of *atrial fibrillation* (see the ECG Library at Student CONSULT), particularly if it is rapid.

It may be helpful to ask the patient to tap the rate and rhythm of the palpitations with his or her finger. Associated features including pain, dyspnoea or faintness must be enquired about. The awareness of rapid palpitations followed by syncope suggests *ventricular tachycardia* (see the ECG Library at Student CONSULT). These patients usually have a past history of significant heart disease. Any rapid rhythm may precipitate angina in a patient with ischaemic heart disease.

Patients may have learned manoeuvres that will return the rhythm to normal. Attacks of *supraventricular tachycardia* (SVT) (see the ECG Library at Student CONSULT) may be suddenly terminated by increasing vagal tone with the Valsalva manoeuvre (p 91), by carotid massage, coughing or swallowing cold water or ice cubes.[c]

Palpitations: differential diagnosis	
Feature	**Suggests**
Heart misses and thumps	Ectopic beats
Worse at rest	Ectopic beats
Very fast, regular	SVT (VT)
Instantaneous onset	SVT (VT)
Offset with vagal manoeuvres	SVT
Fast and irregular	AF
Forceful and regular—not fast	Awareness of sinus rhythm (anxiety)
Severe dizziness or syncope	VT
Pre-existing heart failure	VT

SVT = supraventricular tachycardia; VT = ventricular tachycardia; AF = atrial fibrillation.

TABLE 4.4

[c] Testicular traction is a potent vagal manoeuvre but not in common use. Carotid massage (whereby the carotid artery is compressed below the angle of the jaw for several seconds) can be dangerous for people with carotid disease because of the risk of precipitating a stroke.

QUESTIONS TO ASK THE PATIENT WITH PALPITATIONS

! denotes symptoms for the possible diagnosis of an urgent or dangerous problem.

1. Is the sensation one of the heart beating abnormally, or something else?
2. Does the heart seem fast or slow? Have you counted how fast? Is it faster than it ever goes at any other time, e.g. with exercise?
3. Does the heart seem regular or irregular: stopping and starting? If it is irregular, is this the feeling of normal heart beats interrupted by missed or strong beats—ectopic beats; or is it completely irregular? (Atrial fibrillation)
4. How long do the episodes last?
! 5. Is it accompanied by chest tightness or dyspnoea?
6. Do the episodes start and stop very suddenly? (Supraventricular tachycardia [SVT])
7. Can you terminate the episodes by deep breathing or holding your breath? (SVT)
8. Is there a sensation of pounding in the neck? (Some types of SVT[12])
9. Has an episode ever been recorded on an ECG?
! 10. Have you lost consciousness during an episode? (Ventricular arrhythmias)
! 11. Have you had other heart problems such as heart failure or a heart attack in the past? (Ventricular arrhythmias?)
12. Is there heart trouble of this sort or of people dying suddenly in the family? (Sudden death syndromes, e.g. Brugada syndrome or a long QT interval syndrome)

QUESTIONS BOX 4.2

Syncope, presyncope and dizziness

Syncope is a transient loss of consciousness resulting from cerebral anoxia, usually due to inadequate blood flow (see List 4.3). Presyncope is a transient sensation of weakness without loss of consciousness. (See Questions box 31.4 on p 493.)

Syncope may represent a simple faint or be a symptom of cardiac or neurological disease. One must establish whether the patient actually loses consciousness and under what circumstances the syncope occurs—for example, on standing for prolonged periods or standing up suddenly (*postural syncope*), while passing urine (*micturition syncope*), on coughing (*tussive syncope*) or with sudden emotional stress (*vasovagal syncope*). Find out whether there is any warning, such as dizziness or palpitations, and how long the episodes last. Recovery may be spontaneous or the patient may require attention from bystanders.

If the patient's symptoms appear to be postural, enquire about the use of antihypertensive or antianginal drugs and other medications that may induce postural hypotension. If the episode is vasovagal, it may be precipitated by something unpleasant like the sight of blood or occur in a crowded, hot room; patients often sigh and yawn and feel nauseated and sweaty before fainting and may have previously had similar

---

DIFFERENTIAL DIAGNOSIS OF SYNCOPE AND DIZZINESS

Favours vasovagal syncope (most common cause)
Onset in teens or 20s
Occurs in response to emotional distress, e.g. sight of blood
Associated with nausea and clamminess
Injury uncommon
Unconsciousness brief, no neurological signs on waking

Favours orthostatic hypotension
Brief duration
Injury uncommon
More common when fasted or dehydrated
Known low systolic blood pressure
Use of antihypertensive medications

Favours 'situational syncope'
Occurs during micturition
Occurs with prolonged coughing

Favours syncope due to left ventricular outflow obstruction (AS, HCM)
Occurs during exertion

Favours cardiac arrhythmia
Family history of sudden death (Brugada or long or short QT syndrome)
Antiarrhythmic medication (prolonged QT)
History of cardiac disease (ventricular arrhythmias)
History of rapid palpitations
No warning (heart block—Stokes–Adams attack)

Favours vertigo
No loss of consciousness
Worse when turning head
Head or room seems to spin

Favours seizure
Prodrome—aura
Tongue bitten
Jerking movements during episode
Head turns during episode
Cyanosis during episode
Sleepiness afterwards
Muscle pain afterwards
Follows emotional stress

Favours metabolic cause of syncope (coma)
Hypoglycaemic agents, low blood sugar

AS=aortic stenosis; HCM=hypertrophic cardiomyopathy.

LIST 4.3

episodes, especially during adolescence and young adulthood.[11]

If syncope is due to an *arrhythmia*, there is a sudden loss of consciousness regardless of the patient's posture; chest pain may precede the syncopal episode if the patient has ischaemic heart disease or aortic stenosis.[13] Recovery is equally quick. Exertional syncope may occur with obstruction to left ventricular outflow by *aortic stenosis* or *hypertrophic cardiomyopathy*. Profound and sudden slowing of the pulse (bradycardia), usually a result of complete heart block, causes sudden and recurrent syncope (Stokes–Adams[d] attacks[e]). These patients may have a history of atrial fibrillation. Typically they have periods of tachycardia (fast heart rate) as well as periods of bradycardia (slow heart rate). This condition is called the *sick sinus syndrome*. The patient must be asked about drug treatment that could cause bradycardia (e.g. beta-blockers, digoxin, calcium channel blockers).

It is important to ask about a family history of sudden death. An increasing number of *ion channelopathies* are being identified as a cause of syncope and sudden death. These rare inherited conditions include the long and short QT syndromes and the Brugada syndrome[f,14] (see the ECG Library at Student CONSULT). They are often diagnosed from typical ECG changes. In addition, certain drugs can cause the acquired long QT syndrome (see the ECG Library at Student CONSULT) (see List 4.4).

Neurological causes of syncope are associated with a slow recovery and often residual neurological symptoms or signs. Bystanders may also have noticed abnormal movements if the patient has epilepsy, although cerebral hypoxia caused by a cardiac arrhythmia can also cause tonic and clonic movements. Dizziness that occurs even when the patient is lying down or that is made worse by movements of the head is more likely to be of neurological origin, although recurrent tachyarrhythmias may occasionally cause dizziness in any position. One should attempt to decide whether the dizziness is really *vertiginous* (where the world seems to be turning around) or is a presyncopal (impending loss of consciousness) feeling.

> **DRUGS AND SYNCOPE**
>
> **Associated with QT interval prolongation and ventricular arrhythmias**
>
> Antiarrhythmics; flecainide, quinidine, sotalol, procainamide, amiodarone
>
> Gastric motility promoter; cisapride, domperidone
>
> Antibiotics; clarithromycin, erythromycin
>
> Antipsychotics; chlorpromazine, haloperidol
>
> **Associated with bradycardia**
>
> Beta-blockers
>
> Some calcium channel blockers (verapamil, diltiazem)
>
> Digoxin
>
> **Associated with postural hypotension**
>
> Most antihypertensive drugs, but especially prazosin and calcium channel blockers
>
> Anti-Parkinsonian drugs
>
> LIST 4.4

Fatigue

Fatigue is a common symptom of cardiac failure. It may be associated with a reduced cardiac output and poor blood supply to the skeletal muscles. There are many other causes of fatigue, including lack of sleep, anaemia and depression.

Intermittent claudication and peripheral vascular disease

The word *claudication*[g] comes from the Latin, meaning to limp. Patients with claudication notice pain in one or both calves, thighs or buttocks when they walk more than a certain distance. This distance is called

---

[d] William Stokes (1804–78) succeeded his father as Regius professor of physic in 1840. He was a member of the 'Dublin School' of medicine along with famous physicians like Graves, Cheyne, Adams and Corrigan. He was an art lover, and insisted his students have an arts degree before studying medicine.
  Robert Adams (1791–1875) was Regius professor of surgery in Dublin, and became Queen Victoria's surgeon. He was affected by gout, and wrote a famous paper on it.

[e] Stokes–Adams attacks were probably described first by Gerbezius in 1691 and then by Morgagni in 1761; the latter was a pupil of Valsalva and also described Turner's syndrome 170 years before Turner.

[f] Joseph, Philip and Raoul Brugada are three brothers who are contemporary Spanish electrophysiologists.

[g] The Roman Emperor Tiberius Claudius Drusus Nero Germanicus (10 BC–AD 54) limped owing to some form of paralysis. 'Claudication' and 'Claudius', however, are etymologically unrelated, which seems rather a cruel coincidence for Claudius. 'Claudicant' first appeared in English in 1624.

the *claudication distance*. The claudication distance may be shorter when patients walk up hills. A history of claudication suggests peripheral vascular disease with a poor blood supply to the affected muscles. The most important risk factors are smoking, diabetes, hypertension and a history of vascular disease elsewhere in the body, including cerebrovascular disease and ischaemic heart disease (see Questions box 4.3). More severe disease causes the feet or legs to feel cold, numb and finally painful at rest. Rest pain is a symptom of severely compromised arterial supply. Remember the six Ps of peripheral vascular disease:

- **P** ain
- **P** allor
- **P** ulselessness
- **P** araesthesias
- **P** erishingly cold
- **P** aralysed.

Popliteal artery entrapment can occur, especially in young men with intermittent claudication on walking but *not* running. Also, *lumbar spinal stenosis* causes pseudo-claudication: unlike vascular claudication, the pain in the calves is not relieved by standing still, but is relieved by sitting (flexing the spine) and may be exacerbated by extending the spine (e.g. walking downhill).

RISK FACTORS FOR CORONARY ARTERY DISEASE

An essential part of the cardiac history involves obtaining detailed information about a patient's risk factors—the patient's cardiovascular risk factor profile (see Questions box 4.4).

Previous ischaemic heart disease is the most important risk factor for further ischaemia. The patient may know of previous infarcts or have had a diagnosis of angina in the past.

Hypercholesterolaemia is the next most important risk factor for ischaemic heart disease. Many patients now know their serum cholesterol levels because widespread testing has become fashionable. The total serum cholesterol is a useful screening test, and levels above 5.2 mmol/L are considered undesirable. Cholesterol measurements (unlike triglyceride measurements) are accurate even when a patient has not been fasting. Patients with established coronary artery disease benefit from lowering of total cholesterol to below 4 mmol/L with the low-density lipoprotein (LDL) of 1.8 mmol/L or less. An elevated total cholesterol level is even more significant if the high-density lipoprotein (HDL) level is low (less than 1.0 mmol/L). Significant elevation of the triglyceride level is a coronary risk factor in its own right and also adds further to the risk if the total cholesterol is high. If a patient already has coronary disease, *hyperlipidaemia* is even more important. Control of risk factors for these patients is called secondary prevention. Patients who have multiple risk factors for ischaemic heart disease (e.g. diabetes and hypertension) should have their cholesterol controlled aggressively. If the patient's cholesterol is known to be

---

QUESTIONS TO ASK THE PATIENT WITH SUSPECTED PERIPHERAL VASCULAR DISEASE

! denotes symptoms for the possible diagnosis of an urgent or dangerous problem.

1. Have you had problems with walking because of pains in the legs?
2. Where do you feel the pain?
3. How far can you walk before it occurs?
4. Does it make you stop?
5. Does it go away when you stop walking?
! 6. Does the pain ever occur at rest? (Severe ischaemia may threaten the limb)
7. Have there been changes in the colour of the skin over your feet or ankles?
8. Have you had any sores or ulcers on your feet or legs that have not healed?
9. Have you needed treatment of the arteries of your legs in the past?
10. Have you had diabetes, high blood pressure or problems with stroke or heart attacks in the past?
11. Have you been a smoker?

QUESTIONS BOX 4.3

> ### QUESTIONS TO ASK ABOUT POSSIBLE CARDIOVASCULAR RISK FACTORS
>
> 1. Have you had angina or a heart attack in the past?
> 2. Do you know what your cholesterol level is? Before or after treatment?
> 3. Are you a diabetic? How well controlled is your diabetes?
> 4. Have you had high blood pressure and has it been treated?
> 5. Are you now or have you been a smoker? How long since you stopped?
> 6. Have you had kidney problems?
> 7. Do you have rheumatoid arthritis?
> 8. Do you drink alcohol? How much?
> 9. For men: Have you had any problems with sex? Obtaining erections?
> 10. Have people in your family had angina or heart attacks? Who? How old were they?
>
> QUESTIONS BOX 4.4

Hypertension[h] is another important risk factor for coronary artery disease. Find out when hypertension was first diagnosed and what treatment, if any, has been instituted (see Questions box 4.4). Treatment of hypertension reduces the risk of ischaemic heart disease, hypertensive heart disease, cardiac failure and cerebrovascular disease (stroke). Treatment of hypertension has also been shown to reverse left ventricular hypertrophy.

A family history of coronary artery disease increases a patient's risk, particularly if it has been present in first-degree relatives (parents or siblings) and if it has affected these people before the age of 60. Not all heart disease, however, is ischaemic; a patient whose relatives suffered from rheumatic heart disease is at no greater risk of ischaemic heart disease than anybody else.

A history of *diabetes mellitus* increases the risk of ischaemic heart disease very substantially. A diabetic without a history of ischaemic heart disease has the same risk of myocardial infarction as a non-diabetic who has had an infarct. It is important to find out how long a patient has been diabetic and whether insulin treatment has been required. Good control of the blood sugar level in diabetes mellitus may reduce this risk. An attempt should therefore be made to find out how well a patient's diabetes has been controlled.

Chronic kidney disease is associated with a very high risk of vascular disease. This is possibly related to high calcium-×-phosphate product. The risk may be reduced by dietary intervention, 'phosphate binders', efficient dialysis or renal transplant. Ischaemic heart disease is the most common cause of death in patients with kidney disease on dialysis.

Chronic inflammatory diseases such as rheumatoid arthritis, psoriasis, poor dentition and gingivitis, and HIV infection significantly increase the risk of vascular disease too.

Erectile dysfunction is a sensitive indicator of arterial endothelial abnormality and is a risk factor for, or indicator of, vascular disease.

The presence of multiple risk factors makes control of each one more important. Aggressive control of risk factors is often indicated in these patients.

It is interesting to note that in the diagnosis of angina the patient's description of typical symptoms is more

high, it is worth obtaining a dietary history. This can be very trying. It is important to remember that not only foods containing cholesterol but also those containing saturated fats contribute to the serum cholesterol level. High alcohol consumption and obesity are associated with hypertriglyceridaemia.

Smoking is probably the next most important risk factor for cardiovascular disease and peripheral vascular disease. Some patients describe themselves as non-smokers even though they stopped smoking only a few hours ago. The number of years the patient has smoked and the number of cigarettes smoked per day are both very important (and are recorded as packet-years; p 16). The significance of a history of smoking for a patient who has not smoked for many years is controversial. The risk of symptomatic ischaemic heart disease falls gradually over the years after smoking has been stopped. After about 2 years the risk of myocardial infarction falls to the same level as for those who have never smoked. After 10 years the risk of developing angina falls close to that of non-smokers.

---

[h] Hypertension is more important as a risk factor for stroke and cholesterol for ischaemic heart disease.

discriminating than is the presence of risk factors, which only marginally increase the likelihood that chest pain is ischaemic.[4] Previous ischaemic heart disease is an exception. Certainly a patient who has had angina before and says he or she has it again is usually right.

A history of dental decay or infection is important for patients with valvular heart disease, as it puts them at risk of infective endocarditis. Ask about the regularity of visits to the dentist and the patient's awareness of the need for antibiotic prophylaxis[i] before dental (and some surgical) procedures. Cardiac surgeons will not replace heart valves for people with infected teeth or gums for fear of infection on the artificial valve.

DRUG AND TREATMENT HISTORY

The medications a patient is taking often give a good clue to the diagnosis. Find out about any ill-effects from current or previous medications. Ask about previous procedures or interventions including angioplasty or coronary artery bypass grafting. If the patient is unable to provide a history, a midline sternotomy scar and leg scars (consistent with previous saphenous vein harvesting) support this diagnosis.

Patients with heart failure may have been advised to restrict their total daily fluid intake. Ask what volume has been recommended (often 1500 mL). They may also have been advised to weigh themselves daily and to increase their diuretic drug dose if their weight has increased. Ask what advice has been given about this.

Street drug use is relevant. The use of cocaine or amphetamines is an important cause of myocardial infarction in young people.

PAST HISTORY

Patients with a history of definite previous angina or myocardial infarction remain at high risk of further ischaemic events. It is very useful at this stage to find out how a diagnosis of ischaemic heart disease was made and in particular what investigations were undertaken. The patient may well remember exercise testing or a coronary angiogram, and some patients can even remember how many coronary arteries were narrowed, and how many coronary bypasses were performed (having more than three grafts often leads to a certain amount of boasting). The angioplasty patient may know how many arteries were dilated and whether stents (often called coronary stunts by patients and cardiac surgeons) were inserted. Acute coronary syndromes are now usually treated with early coronary angioplasty.

Patients may recall a diagnosis of rheumatic fever in their childhood, but many were labelled as having 'growing pains'.[15] A patient who was put to bed for a long period as a child or who received many painful buttock injections (of penicillin) may well have had rheumatic fever. A history of *chorea* (quick abnormal involuntary dance-like movements; p 600) is strongly associated with rheumatic fever in girls. A history of rheumatic fever places patients at risk of rheumatic valvular disease.

Hypertension may be caused or exacerbated by aspects of the patient's activities and diet (see Questions box 4.5). A high salt intake, moderate or greater alcohol

---

QUESTIONS TO ASK THE PATIENT WITH HYPERTENSION

1. Do you use much salt in your diet, or eat salty prepared or snack foods?
2. Have you put on weight recently?
3. How much alcohol do you drink?
4. What sort of exercise do you do and how much?
5. Do you take your blood pressure at home? What readings do you get?
6. Are you taking any blood pressure tablets now? Have you taken these medications in the past? Do the tablets cause you any problems?
7. Are you taking arthritis drugs (NSAIDs)? Steroids?
8. Have you had any kidney problems? Blood in the urine? Ankle swelling? Shortness of breath?

QUESTIONS BOX 4.5

---

[i] This means the use of one or more doses of antibiotics given before and after a procedure, which may lead to bacteraemia (circulation of microorganisms in the blood) and potential infection of a heart valve (endocarditis). Having a level of antibiotics present in the blood at the time of such procedures is thought (but not proven) to prevent endocarditis.

use, lack of exercise, obesity and kidney disease may all be factors contributing to high blood pressure. Non-steroidal anti-inflammatory drugs (NSAIDs) cause salt and fluid retention and may also worsen blood pressure. Ask about these, about previous advice to modify these factors and about any drug treatment of hypertension when interviewing any patient with high blood pressure.

SOCIAL HISTORY

Both ischaemic heart disease and rheumatic heart disease are chronic conditions that may affect a patient's ability to function normally. It is therefore important to find out whether the patient's condition has prevented him or her from working and over what period. Patients with severe cardiac failure, for example, may need to make adjustments to their living arrangements so that they are not required to walk up and down stairs at home.

Most hospitals run cardiac rehabilitation programs for patients with ischaemic heart disease or chronic heart failure. They provide exercise classes that help patients to regain their confidence and physical fitness, along with information classes about diet and drug treatment, and can help with psychological problems. Find out whether the patient has been enrolled in one of these and whether it has been helpful. Is this service used as a point of contact for the patient if he or she has concerns about new symptoms or the management of medications?

The return of confidence and self-esteem is a very important matter for patients and for their families after a life-threatening illness.

FAMILY HISTORY

Certain heart diseases are genetic. Onset of heart disease at a young age (e.g. as a result of familial hypercholesterolaemia) or sudden death in the family (e.g. hypertrophic cardiomyopathy, Brugada syndrome) should raise the spectre of genetic disease.

T&O'C ESSENTIALS

1. Breathlessness can be a result of cardiac, respiratory or other problems. A careful history will often help sort this out. Cardiac dyspnoea (i.e. breathlessness due to cardiac failure) is worse on exertion or when the patient lies flat (orthopnoea).
2. Chest pain can be the result of non-cardiac problems but the history often contains vital clues that help sort out the diagnosis.
3. Ischaemic heart disease should be suspected from the history. When angina is stable, the pain or discomfort occurs with a predictable amount of exertion and is relieved by rest. A recent increase in the frequency or the occurrence of pain at rest suggests worsening angina.
4. Dizziness and syncope can have cardiac and non-cardiac causes. Proper history taking will give the correct diagnosis in many cases and indicate the best investigations in others.
5. Assessment of cardiac risk factors takes little time and should be routine.
6. Patients know that cardiac disease can be life threatening and that it sometimes causes sudden death. The history should include sympathetic questions about the effect of the illness.

OSCE EXAMPLE – CVS HISTORY (see the OSCE video at Student CONSULT: history taking from a patient with angina)

1. Mr Smith is 56 years old and is complaining of chest pain. Please take a history of the presenting illness.
2. Introduce yourself and explain that you will be asking some questions about the patient's recent problem.
3. Ask what the pain or discomfort is like. If necessary, give some alternatives; for example 'Is it sharp or dull, or heavy or tight?'
4. 'Where do you feel the pain? Show me.'
5. 'Does it go anywhere else? To your arm or jaw?'
6. 'When do you get it? Is it when you are walking or exercising? Is it worse if you walk after a meal or in the cold weather?'
7. 'Does it go away when you stop or slow down? How long does it take to settle down?'
8. 'Is it getting worse or coming on with less activity?'
9. 'Have you had it when you are not doing anything?'
10. 'Have you used tablets or spray (nitrates) under the tongue for it? Does that help take it away? If so, how long does it take for it to become effective?'
11. 'Have you had any heart trouble before? What sort? What treatment did you have?'
12. 'Have you had high blood pressure or cholesterol? Has it been treated?'
13. 'Are you a smoker? Have you smoked in the past?'
14. 'Have there been problems in your family with heart disease? Who was affected and how old were they?'
15. 'Have any recent heart tests been done: an ECG or a stress test? Do you know what the results were?'

OSCE REVISION TOPICS – CVS HISTORY

Use these topics, which commonly occur in the OSCE examination, to help with revision.

1. Question this patient about ischaemic heart disease risk factors. (p 68)
2. This man has had problems with chest pain. Please take a history from him. (p 59)
3. This woman has been increasingly short of breath over the last 3 months. Please take a history from her. (p 63)
4. Please take a history from this woman who has had palpitations. (p 64)
5. This man may have claudication. Please take a history from him. (p 67)
6. This young woman has had blackouts. Please take a history from her. (p 66)
7. This man has been diagnosed recently with hypertension. Please take a history from him. (pp 70, 88, 124)

References

1. Albert JS. The patient with angina: the importance of careful listening. *J Am Col Cardiol* 1988; 11:27. The history further distinguishes cardiac events even if a coronary angiogram is available.
2. Panju AA, Hemmegan BR, Guyatt GH, Simel DL. Is this patient having a myocardial infarction? *JAMA* 1995; 273:1211–1218. A focused history and examination (and an ECG) can aid subdivision of patients into those highly likely and those highly unlikely to be having a myocardial infarction.
3. Evan AT. Sensitivity and specificity of the history and physical examination for coronary artery disease. *Ann Intern Med* 1994; 120:344–345.
4. Chun AA, McGee SR. Bedside diagnosis of coronary artery disease: a systematic review. *Am J Med* 2004; 117:334–343.
5. Fanaroff AC, Rymer JA, Goldstein SA et al. Does this patient with chest pain have acute coronary syndrome?: The rational clinical examination systematic review. *JAMA* 2015; 314(18):1955–1965.
6. Poole-Wilson P. The origin of symptoms in patients with chronic heart failure. *Eur Heart J* 1998; 9 (supplement H):49–53. This article discusses the lack of correlation between symptoms of heart failure and haemodynamic measurements.
7. McGee S. *Evidence-based physical diagnosis*, 3rd edn. St Louis: Saunders, 2012.
8. Wang CS, FitzGerald JS, Schulzer M et al. Does this dyspneic patient in the emergency department have congestive heart failure? *JAMA* 2005; 294(15):1944–1956.
9. Makani H, Bangalore S, Romero J et al. Peripheral oedema associated with calcium channel blockers; incidence and withdrawal rate a meta-analysis of randomised trials. *J Hypertens* 2011; 29(7)1270–1280.
10. Brugada P, Gursoy S, Brugada J, Ardries E. Investigation of palpitations. *Lancet* 1993; 341:1254–1258. Emphasises the role of history taking and examination as well as the ECG in sorting out the patient presenting with palpitations.

11. Task Force for the Diagnosis and Management of Syncope; European Society of Cardiology; Moya A, Sutton J, Ammirati F et al. Guidelines for the diagnosis and management of syncope. *Eur Heart J* 2009; 30(21):2631–2671.
12. Gursoy S, Steurer G, Brugada J et al. The hemodynamic mechanism of pounding in the neck in atrioventricular nodal reentrant tachycardia. *N Engl J Med* 1992; 327:772–774.
13. Calkins H, Shyr Y, Frumin H et al. The value of the clinical history in the differentiation of syncope due to ventricular tachycardia, atrioventricular block, and neurocardiogenic syncope. *Am J Med* 1995; 98:365–373. Describes useful historical features in differential diagnosis.
14. Brugada J, Brugada P, Brugada R. The syndrome of right bundle branch block ST segment elevation in V1 to V3 and sudden death: the Brugada syndrome. *Europace* 1999; 1(3):156–166.
15. Special Writing Group of the Committee on Rheumatic Fever, Endocarditis and Kawasaki Disease of the Council on Cardiovascular Disease in the Young of the American Heart Association. Guidelines for the diagnosis of rheumatic fever. Jones Criteria, 1992 Update. *JAMA* 1992; 268:2069–2073.

CHAPTER 5
The cardiac examination

A man is as old as his arteries. THOMAS SYDENHAM

EXAMINATION ANATOMY

The contraction of the heart results in a wringing or twisting movement that is often palpable (the *apex beat*) and sometimes visible on the part of the chest that lies in front of it—the *praecordium*.[a] The passage of blood through the heart and its valves and on into the great vessels of the body produces many interesting sounds, and causes pulsation in arteries and movement in veins in remote parts of the body. Signs of cardiac disease may be found by examining the praecordium and the many accessible arteries and veins of the body.

The surface anatomy of the heart and of the cardiac valves (see Fig. 5.1) and the positions of the palpable arteries (see Fig. 5.2) must be kept in mind during the examination of the cardiovascular system. In addition, the physiology of blood flow through the systemic and pulmonary circuits needs to be understood if the cardiac cycle and causes of cardiac murmurs are to be understood (see Fig. 5.3).

The cardiac valves separate the atria from the ventricles (the atrioventricular [AV] or mitral and tricuspid valves) and the ventricles from their corresponding great vessels. Fig. 5.4 shows the fibrous skeleton that supports the four valves and their appearance during systole (cardiac contraction) and diastole (cardiac relaxation).[b]

The myocardium (cardiac muscle) is supplied by the three coronary[c,1] arteries (see Fig. 5.5). The left main coronary artery arises from the left coronary sinus

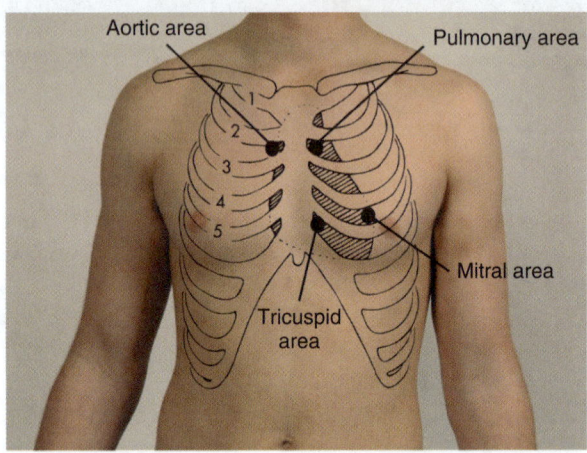

The areas best suited for auscultation do not exactly correlate with the anatomical location of the valves

FIGURE 5.1

of Valsalva and divides into the left anterior descending (LAD) artery, which supplies the anterior wall of the heart, and the circumflex (Cx) artery, which supplies the back of the heart. The right coronary artery (RCA) arises from the right sinus of Valsalva and supplies the inferior wall of the left ventricle and the right ventricle. The coronaries are often described as the *epicardial coronary arteries*. They must run over the surface of the heart or they would be squashed during ventricular systole.

The filling of the right side of the heart from the systemic veins can be assessed by inspection of the jugular veins in the neck (see Fig. 5.6) and by palpation of the liver.[2] These veins empty into the right atrium.

The internal jugular vein is deep in the sternocleidomastoid muscle, whereas the external jugular vein is lateral to it. Traditionally, use of the

---

[a] This is derived from the plural Latin word *praecordia*, meaning the parts of the body below the heart (the entrails), but also the seat of feelings and emotions. In Latin medical writing it means the same as in English: the part of the body over the heart.
[b] Systole comes from the Greek word meaning a contraction and originally applied to a vowel sound usually pronounced long, shortened so as to scan. Diastole means the opposite.
[c] The name is from the Latin *corona*, which means a garland or crown. The coronaries look like a garland draped over the surface of the heart.

CHAPTER 5 THE CARDIAC EXAMINATION 75

Palpable arteries

FIGURE 5.2

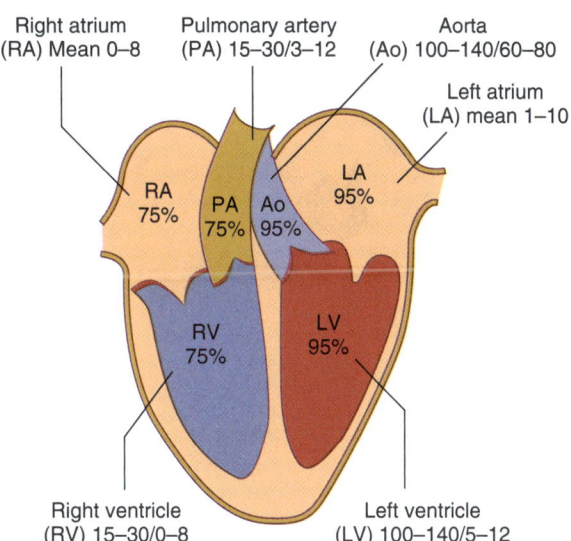

Normal pressures (mmHg) and saturations (%) in the heart

FIGURE 5.3

external jugular vein to estimate venous pressure is discouraged, but the right internal and external jugular veins usually give consistent readings. The left-sided veins are less accurate because they cross from the left side of the chest before entering the right atrium. Pulsations that occur in the right-sided veins reflect movements of the top of a column of blood that extends directly into the right atrium. This column of blood may be used as a manometer and enables us to observe pressure changes in the right atrium. By convention, the sternal angle is taken as the zero point, and the maximum height of pulsations in the internal jugular vein, which are visible above this level when the patient is at 45°, is measured in centimetres. In the average person, the centre of the right atrium lies 5 centimetres below this zero point (see Figs 5.6a and 5.7).[d,1]

POSITIONING THE PATIENT

The cardiovascular system lends itself particularly well to the formal examination approach (see the OCSE CVS examination video at Student CONSULT). There are a number of equally satisfactory methods, but the precise approach used is not as important as having a

---

[d] This is the *method of Lewis*. Sir Thomas Lewis (1881–1945), a pioneering British cardiologist, described the bedside use of assessment of the JVP as a way of estimating the central venous pressure in 1930.

SECTION 2 THE CARDIOVASCULAR SYSTEM

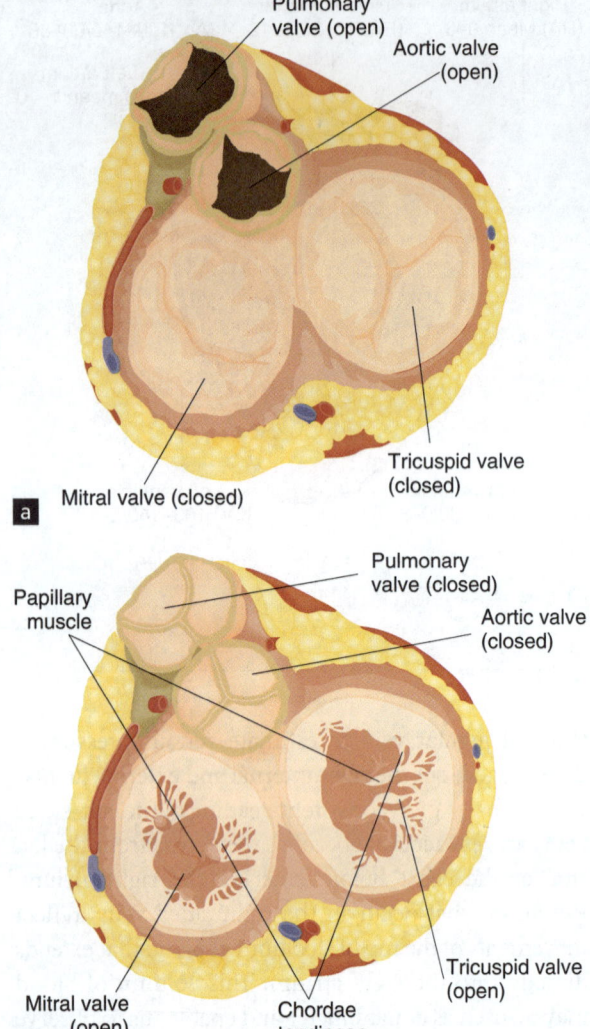

The cardiac valves in systole (a) and diastole (b) Semilunar (aortic, pulmonary); atrioventricular (mitral, tricuspid)

FIGURE 5.4

The three coronary arteries.

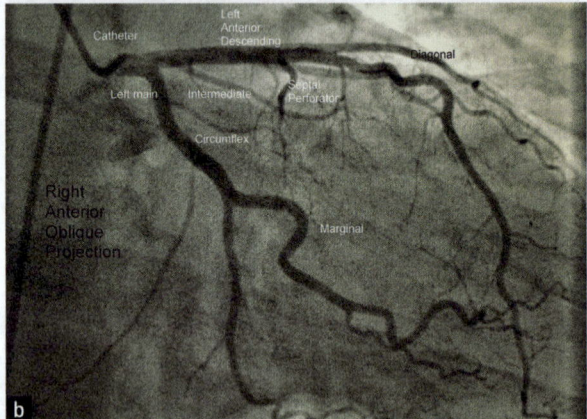

(a) An angiogram of the right coronary artery; (b) an angiogram of the left and circumflex coronary arteries

FIGURE 5.5

method that is comprehensive, gives the impression of being (and is) proficient, and ensures that no important part of the examination is omitted.[3]

First, appropriately expose and position the patient properly and pause to get an impression of the patient's general appearance. Then begin the detailed examination with the patient's hands and pulses and progress smoothly to the neck, face and onto the praecordium. A summary of a suggested method of examination can be found in Text box 8.1 on page 145.

It is important to have the patient lying in bed with enough pillows to support him or her at 45° (see Fig. 5.8). This is the usual position in which the jugular venous pressure (JVP) is assessed.[2] Even a 'targeted' cardiovascular examination in an outpatients' clinic or surgery can be performed adequately only if the patient is lying down and an examination couch should be available. During auscultation, optimal examination requires further positioning of the patient, as discussed later.

GENERAL APPEARANCE

Look at the patient's general state of health. Does he or she appear to be ill? If so, try to decide why you

The jugular venous pressure (JVP).

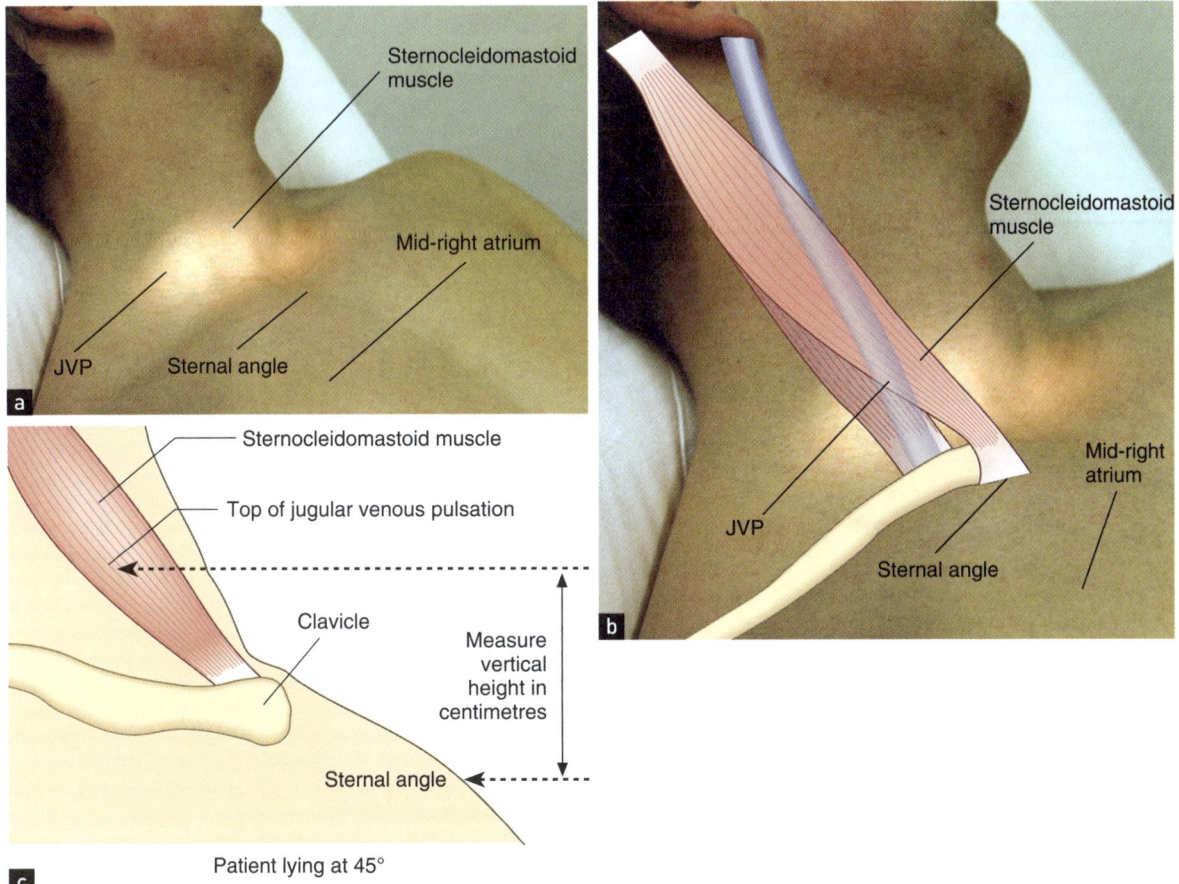

(a) Assessment of the JVP. The patient should lie at 45°. The relationships between the sternocleidomastoid muscle, the JVP, the sternal angle and the mid-right atrium are shown (b, c). The anatomy of the neck showing the relative positions of the main vascular structures, clavicle and sternocleidomastoid muscle. (See also Fig. 5.7.)

(Figures (b) and (c) adapted from Douglas G, Nicol F, Robertson C. *Macleod's clinical examination*, 11th edn. Edinburgh: Churchill Livingstone, 2005.)

FIGURE 5.6

---

have formed that impression. Note whether the patient at rest has rapid and laboured respiration, suggesting dyspnoea (see Table 9.4, p 170).

The patient may look *cachectic*—that is, there may be severe loss of weight and muscle wasting. This is commonly caused by malignant disease, but severe cardiac failure may also have this effect (*cardiac cachexia*). It probably results from a combination of anorexia (due to congestive enlargement of the liver), impaired intestinal absorption (due to congested intestinal veins) and increased levels of inflammatory cytokines such as tumour necrosis factor alpha (TNF-α).

There are also some syndromes that are associated with specific cardiac disease. Marfan's[e] syndrome (see

---

[e] Bernard-Jean Antonin Marfan (1858–1942), a French physician and first professor of hygiene in Paris.

Changes in the height of the JVP as the patient sits up

(Adapted from McGee S. *Evidence-based physical diagnosis*, 2nd edn. St Louis, MO: Saunders, 2007.)

FIGURE 5.7

Cardiovascular examination: positioning the patient at 45°

FIGURE 5.8

CHAPTER 5 **THE CARDIAC EXAMINATION**   79

(a) Marfan's syndrome: tall stature, thoracic kyphosis, pectus excavatum, arachnodactyly (spider fingers), long limbs, aortic regurgitation and a high-arched palate; (b) high-arched palate

FIGURE 5.9

Fig. 5.9), Down's[f] syndrome (p 475) and Turner's[g] syndrome (p 474) are important examples.

HANDS

Pick up the patient's right hand. Look first at the nails. Now is the time for a decision as to the presence or absence of *clubbing*.[4] Clubbing is an increase in the soft tissue of the distal part of the fingers or toes. The causes of clubbing are surprisingly varied (see List 5.1). The mechanism is unknown but there are, of course, several theories. A popular one is that platelet-derived growth factor (PDGF), released from megakaryocyte and platelet emboli in the nail beds, causes fibrovascular proliferation. Megakaryocytes and clumps of platelets do not normally reach the arterial circulation. Their large size (up to 50 μm) prevents their passing through the pulmonary capillaries when they are released from the bone marrow. In conditions where platelets may clump in the arterial circulation (infected cardiac valve) or bypass the pulmonary capillaries (right-to-left shunt associated with congenital heart disease), they can reach the systemic circulation and become trapped in the terminal capillaries of the fingers and toes. Damage to pulmonary capillaries from various lung disorders can have the same effect.

Proper examination for clubbing involves inspecting the fingernails (and toenails) from the side to determine

---

[f] John Langdon Down (1828–96), Assistant Physician to the London Hospital and founder of the Normansfield Mental Hospital. He described the clinical picture of 'mongolism' in 1866.
[g] Henry Hubert Turner (1892–1970), Clinical Professor of Medicine at Oklahoma University. He described the syndrome in 1938.

CAUSES OF CLUBBING

Common

CARDIOVASCULAR
Cyanotic congenital heart disease
Infective endocarditis

RESPIRATORY
Lung carcinoma (usually not small-cell carcinoma)
Chronic pulmonary suppuration:
- Bronchiectasis
- Lung abscess
- Empyema

Idiopathic pulmonary fibrosis

Uncommon

RESPIRATORY
Cystic fibrosis
Asbestosis
Pleural mesothelioma (benign fibrous type) or pleural fibroma

GASTROINTESTINAL
Cirrhosis (especially biliary cirrhosis)
Inflammatory bowel disease
Coeliac disease

THYROTOXICOSIS
Familial (usually before puberty) or idiopathic

Rare
Neurogenic diaphragmatic tumours
Pregnancy
Secondary parathyroidism

UNILATERAL CLUBBING
Bronchial arteriovenous aneurysm
Axillary artery aneurysm

LIST 5.1

whether there is any loss of the angle between the nail bed and the finger—the *hyponychial angle* (see Fig. 5.10). Schamroth's sign is the disappearance of the diamond-shaped space that is formed when the nails of two similar fingers are held facing each other (see Fig. 5.11).[h] One accepted measurement is the *interphalangeal depth ratio*. The anteroposterior (AP) dimension of the finger is measured at the distal interphalangeal joint and compared with the AP diameter at the level of the point where the skin joins the nail. A ratio of more than 1 means clubbing.[4,i] Eventually the distal phalanx becomes enlarged, owing to soft-tissue swelling. Patients hardly ever notice that they have clubbing, even when it is severe. They often express surprise at their doctor's interest in such an unlikely part of their anatomy.

Before leaving the nails, look for *splinter haemorrhages* in the nail beds (see Fig. 5.12). These are linear haemorrhages lying parallel to the long axis of the nail. They are most often due to trauma, particularly in manual workers.[j] However, an important cause is infective endocarditis, which is a bacterial or other infection of the heart valves or part of the endocardium. In this disease splinter haemorrhages are probably the result of a vasculitis in the nail bed, but this is controversial. Other rare causes of splinter haemorrhages include vasculitis as in rheumatoid arthritis, polyarteritis nodosa or the antiphospholipid syndrome, sepsis elsewhere in the body, haematological malignancy or profound anaemia.

Osler's[k] *nodes* are a rare manifestation of infective endocarditis. These are red, raised, tender palpable nodules on the pulps of the fingers (or toes), or on the thenar or hypothenar eminences. They are reported to have occurred in 50% of patients before antibiotic treatment of endocarditis became available. Currently

---

[h] The eminent South African cardiologist Leo Schamroth developed clubbing as a result of endocarditis in 1976. As the condition advanced, he observed this in his own fingers, only for the space to reappear as he improved.
[i] This angle can be measured with a *shadowgraph*, which projects the silhouette of the finger so that it can be measured with a protractor. It is not in common use. If the angle is greater than 190°, clubbing is generally agreed to be present.
[j] It is said that gardening is the most common cause of splinter haemorrhages.
[k] Sir William Osler (1849–1919), a Canadian physician, Professor of Medicine at McGill University at 25, and later famous Regius professor of medicine at Oxford and renowned medical historian. He was made a baronet. His only son was killed at Ypres. There was no treatment for endocarditis until antibiotics became available.

Finger clubbing.

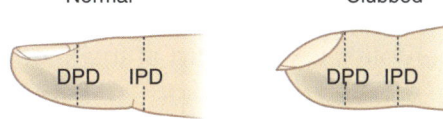

DPD = distal phalangeal depth
IPD = interphalangeal depth

(a) Appearance; (b) phalangeal depth ratio (**not** routinely measured)

FIGURE 5.10

(a) Schamroth's sign; (b) normal

(Figure (a) from Brown MA, von Mutius EM, Wayne J. Clinical assessment and diagnostic approach to common problems. *Pediatric respiratory medicine*. St Louis, MO: Mosby, 1999.)

FIGURE 5.11

they are seen in fewer than 5% of patients. *Janeway*[l] *lesions* (see Fig. 5.13) are non-tender erythematous maculopapular lesions containing bacteria, which occur very rarely on the palms or pulps of the fingers in patients with infective endocarditis.[m]

Tendon xanthomata are yellow or orange deposits of lipid in the tendons that occur in type II hyperlipidaemia. These can be seen over the tendons of the hand and arm. *Palmar xanthomata* and *tuboeruptive xanthomata* over the elbows and knees are characteristic of type III hyperlipidaemia (see Fig. 5.14).[n]

ARTERIAL PULSE

The accomplished clinician is able, while inspecting the patient's hands, to palpate the radial artery at the wrist. Patients expect to have their pulse taken as part of a proper medical examination. The clinician can feel the pulse while talking to the patient and while looking for other signs. When this traditional part of

---

[l] Edward Janeway (1841–1911), an American physician.
[m] These signs are now mostly of historical interest. They date from the period when endocarditis could be diagnosed but not treated. Physicians were able to describe and name interesting signs but were unable to provide treatment (cf. the eponymous signs of aortic regurgitation). They are much less commonly seen now because patients are treated.

[n] These hyperlipidaemias are classified according to the lipid-carrying protein (lipoprotein) that is elevated. In type II this is low-density lipoprotein (LDL) or very-low-density lipoprotein (VLDL), and cholesterol alone or both cholesterol and triglycerides are elevated.

SECTION 2 THE CARDIOVASCULAR SYSTEM

Splinter haemorrhages in the fingernails of a patient with staphylococcal aortic valve endocarditis

(From Baker T, Nikolić G, O'Connor S. *Practical cardiology*, 2nd edn. ©2008, Sydney: Elsevier Australia.)

FIGURE 5.12

Tuboeruptive xanthomata of the knee

FIGURE 5.14

Janeway lesion

FIGURE 5.13

Taking the radial pulse

FIGURE 5.15

the examination is performed with some ceremony, it may help to establish rapport between patient and doctor.

Although the radial pulse is distant from the central arteries, certain useful information may be gained from examining it. The pulse is usually felt just medial to the radius, using the forefinger and middle finger pulps of the examining hand (see Fig. 5.15). The following observations should be made: (1) rate of pulse, (2) rhythm and (3) presence or absence of delay of the femoral pulse compared with the radial pulse (*radiofemoral delay*; see Fig. 5.17). The character and volume of the pulse are better assessed from palpation of the brachial or carotid arteries.

Rate of pulse

Practised observers can estimate the rate quickly. Formal counting over 30 seconds is accurate and requires only simple mathematics to obtain the rate per minute. The normal resting heart rate in adults is usually said to be between 60 and 100 beats per minute but a more sensible range is probably 55 to 95 (95% of normal people). *Bradycardia* (from the Greek *bradys* 'slow', *kardia* 'heart') is defined as a heart rate of less than 60 beats per minute. *Tachycardia* (from the Greek *tachys* 'swift', *kardia* 'heart') is defined as a heart rate over 100 beats per minute (see the OSCE ECGs nos 2, 3 and 4 at Student CONSULT). The causes of bradycardia and tachycardia are listed in Table 5.1.

Rhythm

The rhythm of the pulse can be regular or irregular. An irregular rhythm can be completely irregular with no pattern (*irregularly irregular* or *chaotic* rhythm); this is usually due to atrial fibrillation (see Table 5.1). In atrial fibrillation coordinated atrial contraction is lost, and chaotic electrical activity occurs with bombardment of the atrioventricular node with impulses at a rate of over 600 per minute. Only a variable proportion of these is conducted to the ventricles because (fortunately) the AV node is unable to conduct at such high rates. In this way, the ventricles are protected from very rapid rates, but beat irregularly, usually at rates between 150 and 180 per minute (unless the patient is being treated with drugs to slow the heart rate [see the OCSE ECG no. 8 at Student CONSULT]). The pulse also varies in amplitude from beat to beat in atrial fibrillation because of differing diastolic filling times. This type of pulse can occasionally be simulated by frequent irregularly occurring supraventricular or ventricular ectopic beats.

Patients with atrial fibrillation or frequent ectopic beats may have a detectable *pulse deficit*. This means that the heart rate when counted by listening to the heart with the stethoscope is higher than the rate obtained when the radial pulse is counted at the wrist. In these patients the heart sounds will be audible with every systole, but some early contractions preceded by short diastolic filling periods will not produce enough cardiac output for a pulse to be palpable at the wrist.

An irregular rhythm can also be *regularly irregular*. For example, in patients with sinus arrhythmia the pulse rate increases with each inspiration and decreases with each expiration (see the OCSE ECG no. 7 at Student CONSULT); this is a normal finding. It is associated with changes in venous return to the heart.

Patterns of irregularity (see Fig. 5.16) can also occur when patients have frequent ectopic beats. These may arise in the atrium (atrial ectopic beats, AEBs) or in the ventricle (ventricular ectopic beats, VEBs [see the OCSE ECG no. 6 at Student CONSULT]) Ectopic beats quite commonly occur in a fixed ratio to normal beats. When every second beat is an ectopic one, the rhythm is called *bigeminy*. A bigeminal rhythm caused by ectopic beats has a characteristic pattern: normal pulse, weak (or absent) pulse, delay, normal pulse and so on. Similarly, every third beat may be ectopic—*trigeminy*. A pattern of irregularity is also detectable in the Wenckebach° phenomenon. Here the AV nodal conduction time increases progressively until a non-conducted atrial systole occurs. Following this, the AV conduction time shortens and the cycle begins again.

Radiofemoral and radial–radial delay

Radiofemoral delay is an important sign, especially in a young patient with hypertension. While palpating the radial pulse, place the fingers of your other hand over the femoral pulse, which is situated below the inguinal ligament, one-third of the way up from the pubic tubercle (see Fig. 5.17). A noticeable delay in the arrival of the femoral pulse wave suggests the diagnosis of *coarctation of the aorta*, where a congenital narrowing in the aortic isthmus occurs at the level where the ductus arteriosus joins the descending aorta. This is just distal to the origin of the subclavian artery. This lesion can cause upper limb hypertension.

You can palpate both radial pulses together to detect radial–radial inequality in timing or volume, which is usually due to a large arterial occlusion by an atherosclerotic plaque or aneurysm, or to subclavian artery stenosis on one side. It can also be a sign of dissection of the thoracic aorta.

° Marel Frederik Wenckebach (1864–1940), a Dutch physician who practised in Vienna. He worked out the mechanism of this arrhythmia without having ECGs.

Common pulse patterns.

Bigeminal rhythm

Trigeminal rhythm

Frequent ectopic beats – when 2 ectopics occur in a row this is called a couplet

Sinus arrhythmia

Irregularly irregular (chaotic rhythm)

N=normal; E=ectopic; C=couplet

FIGURE 5.16

Feeling for radiofemoral delay

FIGURE 5.17

Character and volume

Character and volume are poorly assessed by palpating the radial pulse; the carotid or brachial arteries should be used to determine the character and volume of the pulse, as these more accurately reflect the form of the aortic pressure wave. However, the collapsing (bounding) pulse of *aortic regurgitation*, and *pulsus alternans* (alternating strong and weak pulse) of advanced left ventricular failure, may be readily apparent in the radial pulse.

Condition of the vessel wall

Only changes in the medial layer of the radial artery can be assessed by palpation. Thickening or tortuosity will be detected commonly in the arteries of elderly people. These changes, however, do not indicate the presence of luminal narrowing due to atherosclerosis. Therefore, this sign is of little clinical value.

BLOOD PRESSURE

Measurement of the arterial blood pressure[p] is an essential part of the examination of almost any patient. (See the OCSE video Taking the blood pressure and examining the hypertensive patient at Student CONSULT .) Usually, indirect measurements

---

[p] Blood pressure was first measured in a horse in 1708 by Stephen Hales, an English clergyman. Measurement of the blood pressure was the last of the traditional vital signs measurements to come into regular use. It was not until early in the 20th century that work by Korotkoff and Janeway led to its routine use.

Causes of bradycardia and tachycardia

Bradycardia

Regular rhythm	Irregular rhythm
Physiological (athletes, during sleep: due to increased vagal tone) Drugs (e.g. beta-blockers, digoxin, amiodarone) Hypothyroidism (decreased sympathetic activity secondary to thyroid hormone deficiency) Hypothermia Raised intracranial pressure (due to an effect on central sympathetic outflow)—a late sign Third-degree atrioventricular (AV) block, or second-degree (type 2) AV block Myocardial infarction Paroxysmal bradycardia: vasovagal syncope Jaundice (in severe cases only, due to deposition of bilirubin in the conducting system)	**Irregularly irregular** Atrial fibrillation (in combination with conduction system disease or AV nodal blocking drugs) due to: • alcohol, post-thoracotomy, idiopathic • mitral valve disease or any cause of left atrial enlargement Frequent ectopic beats **Regularly irregular rhythm** Sinus arrhythmia (normal slowing of the pulse with expiration) Second-degree AV block (type 1) **Apparent** Pulse deficit* (atrial fibrillation, ventricular or atrial bigeminy)

Tachycardia

Regular rhythm	Irregular rhythm
Hyperdynamic circulation, due to: • exercise or emotion (e.g. anxiety) • fever (allow 15–20 beats per minute per °C above normal) • pregnancy • thyrotoxicosis • anaemia • arteriovenous fistula (e.g. Paget's disease or hepatic failure) • beri-beri (thiamine deficiency) Congestive cardiac failure Constrictive pericarditis Drugs (e.g. salbutamol and other sympathomimetics, atropine) Normal variant Denervated heart, e.g. diabetes mellitus (resting rate of 106–120 beats per minute) Hypovolaemic shock Supraventricular tachycardia (usually >150) Atrial flutter with regular 2:1 AV block (usually 150) Ventricular tachycardia (often >150) Sinus tachycardia, due to: • thyrotoxicosis • pulmonary embolism • myocarditis • myocardial ischaemia • fever, acute hypoxia or hypercapnia (paroxysmal) Multifocal atrial tachycardia Atrial flutter with variable block	Atrial fibrillation, due to: • myocardial ischaemia • mitral valve disease or any cause of left atrial enlargement • thyrotoxicosis • hypertensive heart disease • sick sinus syndrome • pulmonary embolism • myocarditis • fever, acute hypoxia or hypercapnia (paroxysmal) • other: alcohol, post-thoracotomy, idiopathic Multifocal atrial tachycardia Atrial flutter with variable block

*This is the difference between the heart rate counted over the heart (praecordium) and that observed at the periphery. In beats where diastole is too short for adequate filling of the heart, too small a volume of blood is ejected during systole for a pulse to be appreciated at the wrist. Automatic home blood pressure machines (popular with patients who have an intense interest in their blood pressure) will often report an alarmingly low pulse rate in patients with frequent ectopic beats and precipitate unnecessary alarm.

TABLE 5.1

A classification of blood pressure readings		
Category	Systolic (mmHg)	Diastolic (mmHg)
Optimal	<120	<80
Normal	120–129	80–84
High normal	130–139	85–89
Mild hypertension (grade 1)	140–159	90–99
Moderate hypertension (grade 2)	160–179	100–109
Severe hypertension (grade 3)	>180	>110

(2013 ESH/ESC Guidelines for the management of arterial hypertension. The Task Force for the management of arterial hypertension of the European Society of Hypertension (ESH) and of the European Society of Cardiology (ESC). Reprinted with permission of Oxford University Press.)

TABLE 5.2

Measuring the blood pressure, with the patient lying at 45°

FIGURE 5.18

of the systolic and diastolic pressures are obtained with a sphygmomanometer (from the Greek *sphygmos* 'pulsing', *manos* 'thin').[5,6] The systolic blood pressure is the peak pressure that occurs in the artery following ventricular systole, and the diastolic blood pressure is the level to which the arterial blood pressure falls during ventricular diastole. Normal blood pressure is defined as a systolic reading of less than 130 mmHg *and* a diastolic reading of less than 85 mmHg. High normal is 130–39 mmHg systolic and 85–9 mmHg diastolic. In some circumstances, lower pressures may be considered normal (e.g. in pregnancy) or desirable (e.g. for diabetics) (Table 5.2).

Measuring the blood pressure with the sphygmomanometer

The usual blood pressure cuff width is 12.5 centimetres. This is suitable for a normal-sized adult upper arm. However, in obese patients with large arms (up to 30% of the adult population) the normal-sized cuff will overestimate the blood pressure and therefore a large cuff must be used. A range of smaller sizes is available for children. Use of a cuff that is too large results in only a small underestimate of blood pressure.

Traditionally the blood pressure is not measured using the arm on the side of a previous mastectomy (especially if the axillary nodes have been removed) for fear of further upsetting lymphatic drainage. Modern mastectomies are less radical and the risk of causing trouble is very small. It should not be taken from an arm that has had an arteriovenous fistula inserted for renal dialysis for fear of damaging the fistula and enraging the patient's renal physician and vascular surgeon.

The cuff is wrapped around the upper arm with the bladder centred over the brachial artery (see Fig. 5.18). This is found in the antecubital fossa, one-third of the way over from the medial epicondyle. For an approximate estimation of the systolic blood pressure, the cuff is fully inflated and then deflated slowly (3–4 mmHg per second) until the radial pulse returns. Then, for a more accurate estimation of the blood pressure, this manoeuvre is repeated with the diaphragm of the stethoscope placed over the brachial artery, slipped underneath the distal end of the cuff's bladder.

Korotkoff sounds.

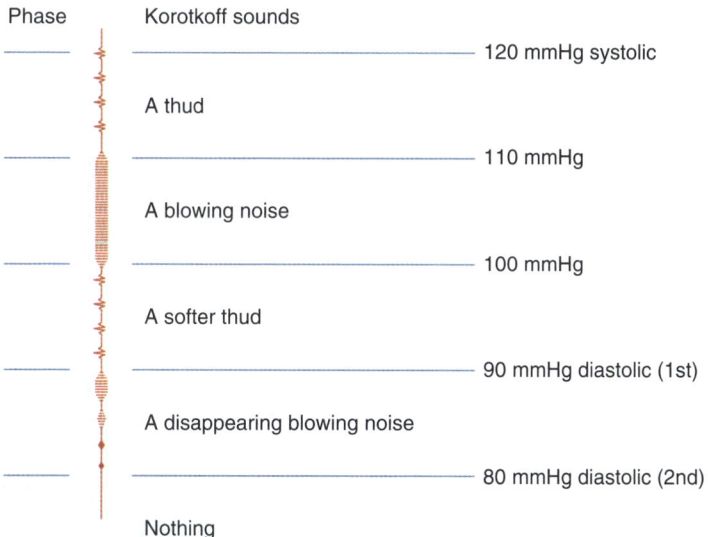

Systolic pressure is determined by the appearance of the first audible sound, and diastolic pressure is determined by its disappearance

FIGURE 5.19

The patient's brachial artery should be at about the level of the heart, which is at the level of the fourth intercostal space at the sternum. If the arm is too high—for example, at the level of the supraclavicular notch—the blood pressure reading will be about 5 mmHg lower; if the arm is too low, the reading will be higher than is accurate.

Five different sounds will be heard as the cuff is slowly released (see Fig. 5.19). These are called the Korotkoff[q] sounds. The pressure at which a sound is first heard over the artery is the systolic blood pressure (Korotkoff I, or KI). As deflation of the cuff continues, the sound increases in intensity (KII), then decreases (KIII), becomes muffled (KIV) and disappears (KV). Different observers have used KIV and KV to indicate the level of the diastolic pressure. KV is probably the best measure. However, this provides a slight underestimate of the arterial diastolic blood pressure. Although diastolic pressure usually corresponds most closely to KV, in severe aortic regurgitation KIV is a more accurate indication. KV is absent in some normal people and KIV must then be used.

Occasionally, there will be an auscultatory gap (the sounds disappear just below the systolic pressure and reappear before the diastolic pressure) in healthy people. This can lead to an underestimate of the systolic blood pressure if the cuff is not pumped up high enough.

The systolic blood pressure may normally vary between the arms by up to 10 mmHg (the mean difference has been reported as almost 5 mmHg).[6] In the legs the blood pressure is normally up to 20 mmHg higher than in the arms, unless the patient has coarctation of the aorta. Measurement of the blood pressure in the legs is more difficult than in the arms. It requires a large cuff that is placed over the mid-thigh. The patient lies prone and the stethoscope is placed in the popliteal fossa, behind the knee.

During inspiration, the systolic and diastolic blood pressures normally decrease (because intrathoracic pressure becomes more negative, blood pools in the pulmonary vessels, so left-heart filling is reduced). When this normal reduction in blood pressure with inspiration is exaggerated, it is termed *pulsus paradoxus*. Kussmaul meant by this that there was a fall in blood pressure and a paradoxical rise in pulse rate. A fall in arterial pulse pressure on inspiration of more than 10 mmHg is abnormal and may occur with *constrictive*

---

[q] Nikolai Korotkoff (1874–1920), a St Petersburg surgeon, described the auscultatory method of determining blood pressure in 1905, although his findings were scoffed at.

pericarditis, *pericardial effusion* or severe asthma. To detect this, lower the cuff pressure slowly until KI sounds are heard intermittently (expiration) and then until KI is audible with every beat. The difference between the two readings represents the level of the pulsus paradoxus.

Variations in blood pressure

When blood pressure is measured with an intra-arterial catheter it becomes clear that blood pressure varies from minute to minute in normal people. Short-term changes of 4 mmHg in the systolic and 3 mmHg in the diastolic readings are common. Hour-to-hour and day-to-day variations are even greater. The standard deviation between visits is up to 12 mmHg for systolic pressure and 8 mmHg for diastolic. This means that when there is concern about an abnormal reading, repeat measurements are necessary.

When the heart is very irregular (most often because of atrial fibrillation), the cuff should be deflated slowly, and the point at which most of the cardiac contractions are audible (KI) taken as the systolic pressure and the point at which most have disappeared (KV) taken as diastole.

High blood pressure

High blood pressure is difficult to define.[5] The most helpful definitions of hypertension are based on an estimation of the level associated with an increased risk of vascular disease. There have been many classifications of blood pressure, because what is considered normal or abnormal changes as more information comes to hand. Table 5.2 gives a useful guide to current definitions. If recordings above 140/90 mmHg are considered abnormal, high blood pressure may occur in up to 20% of the adult population.[r] Blood pressure measured by the patient at home, or by a 24-hour monitor, should be up to 10/5 mmHg less than that measured in the surgery (the so-called 'white coat phenomenon').[7]

Postural blood pressure

The blood pressure should routinely be taken with the patient both lying down and standing (see Fig. 5.20).[8] A fall of more than 15 mmHg in systolic blood pressure or 10 mmHg in diastolic blood pressure after the patient has stood up for 1 minute is abnormal and is called *postural hypotension* (see Text box 5.1). It may cause dizziness or not be associated with symptoms. The most common cause is the use of antihypertensive drugs, α-adrenergic antagonists in particular.

Measuring the blood pressure, with patient standing

FIGURE 5.20

Causes of postural hypotension (HANDI)

H ypovolaemia (e.g. dehydration, bleeding); hypopituitarism

A ddison's* disease (adrenal gland failure)

N europathy—autonomic (e.g. diabetes mellitus, amyloidosis, Shy–Drager syndrome)

D rugs (e.g. vasodilators and other antihypertensives, tricyclic antidepressants, diuretics, antipsychotics)

I diopathic orthostatic hypotension (rare progressive degeneration of the autonomic nervous system, usually in elderly men)

*Thomas Addison (1793–1860), a London physician.

TEXT BOX 5.1

---

[r] *Pseudohypertension* means the blood pressure, as measured by the sphygmomanometer, is artificially high because of arterial wall calcification. Osler's manoeuvre traditionally detects this condition: inflate the cuff above systolic pressure and palpate the radial artery, which in pseudohypertension may be palpable despite being pulseless. However, the value of Osler's manoeuvre has been questioned.[9]

(a) and (b) Xanthelasmata

(Figure b from McDonald FS, ed. *Mayo Clinic images in internal medicine*, with permission. © Mayo Clinic Scientific Press and CRC Press. Reproduced by permission of Taylor and Francis Group, LLC, a division of Informa plc.)

FIGURE 5.21

FACE

Inspect the sclerae for yellow *jaundice* (p 239). This can occur with severe congestive cardiac failure and hepatic congestion. Prosthetic heart valve-induced haemolysis of red blood cells, due to excessive turbulence, is an uncommon but cardiac cause of jaundice. *Xanthelasmata* (see Fig. 5.21) are intracutaneous yellow cholesterol deposits around the eyes and are relatively common. These may be a normal variant or may indicate type II or III hyperlipidaemia, though they are not always associated with hyperlipidaemia.

Look at the pupils for an *arcus senilis* (see Fig. 5.22). This half or complete grey circle is seen around the outer perimeter of the pupil and is probably associated with some increase in cardiovascular risk.[s]

---

[s] The connection of arcus senilis with old age and cardiovascular disease has been made from early in the 19th century. The pathologist Virchow was convinced it was an indicator of vascular disease.

Arcus senilis

FIGURE 5.22

Next look for the presence of a *mitral facies*, which refers to rosy cheeks with a bluish tinge due to dilation of the malar capillaries (see Fig. 3.8 on p 43). This is associated with pulmonary hypertension and a low cardiac output such as occurs in severe mitral stenosis, and is now rare.

Look in the patient's mouth using a torch to see if there is a *high-arched palate*. This occurs in Marfan's syndrome, a condition that is associated with congenital heart disease, including aortic regurgitation secondary to aortic root dilation, and also mitral regurgitation due to mitral valve prolapse. Notice whether the teeth look diseased, as they can be a source of organisms responsible for infective endocarditis. Look at the tongue and lips for central cyanosis. Inspect the mucosa for petechiae that may indicate infective endocarditis.

NECK

Oddly enough, this small area of the body is packed with cardiovascular signs that must be elicited with great care and skill.

Carotid arteries

The carotids are not only easily accessible, medial to the sternocleidomastoid muscles (see Fig. 5.23), but also provide a great deal of information about the wave form of the aortic pulse, which is affected by many cardiac abnormalities. Never palpate both carotid arteries simultaneously as they provide much of the blood supply to the *brain* (a vital organ).

Palpating the carotid pulse

FIGURE 5.23

Arterial pulse character	
Type of pulse	**Cause(s)**
Anacrotic (small volume, slow uptake, notched wave on upstroke)	Aortic stenosis
Plateau (slow upstroke)	Aortic stenosis
Bisferiens (anacrotic and collapsing)	Aortic stenosis and regurgitation
Collapsing	Aortic regurgitation Hyperdynamic circulation Patent ductus arteriosus Peripheral arteriovenous fistula Arteriosclerotic aorta (elderly patients in particular)
Small volume	Aortic stenosis Pericardial effusion
Alternans (alternating strong and weak beats)	Left ventricular failure

TABLE 5.3

Evaluation of the pulse wave form (the amplitude, shape and volume) is important in the diagnosis of various underlying cardiac diseases and in assessing their severity. It takes considerable practice to distinguish between the different important types of carotid wave forms (see Table 5.3). Auscultation of the carotids may be performed now or in association with auscultation of the praecordium.

Jugular venous pressure

Just as the carotid pulse tells us about the aorta and left ventricular function, the JVP (see Fig. 5.6) tells us about right atrial and right ventricular function.[2,10,11] The positioning of the patient and lighting are important for this examination to be done properly. The patient must be lying down at 45° to the horizontal with his or her head on pillows and in good lighting conditions (see Fig. 5.8). It is usual to ask the patient to turn the head slightly to the left so that the base of the neck is exposed. However, if the head is turned too far, the sternocleidomastoid muscle will contract and obscure the view. This is a difficult examination and there is considerable inter- (and intra-) observer variation in the findings.

When the patient is lying at 45°, the sternal angle is also roughly in line with the base of the neck (see Fig. 5.6(c)). This provides a convenient zero point from which to measure the vertical height of the column of blood in the jugular vein. The jugular venous pulsation (movement) can be distinguished from the arterial pulse because: (1) it is visible but not palpable and has a more prominent *inward* movement than the artery, (2) it has a complex wave form, usually seen to flicker twice with each cardiac cycle (if the patient is in sinus rhythm), (3) it moves on respiration—normally the JVP decreases on inspiration, and (4) it is at first obliterated and then filled from above when light pressure is applied at the base of the neck.

JVP must be assessed for *height* and *character*. When the JVP is more than 3 centimetres above the zero point, the right-heart filling pressure is raised (a normal reading is less than 8 centimetres of water: 5 centimetres + 3 centimetres). This is a sign of right ventricular failure, volume overload or some types of pericardial disease.

The assessment of the character of JVP is difficult, even for experienced clinicians. There are two positive waves in the normal JVP.[t] The first is called the *a wave* and coincides with right atrial systole.[u] It is due to atrial

---

[t] The waves visible in the JVP were named by Sir James Mackenzie (1853–1925), a British physician and one of the founders of the specialty of cardiology.
[u] Sir James Mackenzie first applied these labels to the jugular wave forms in the late 19th century.

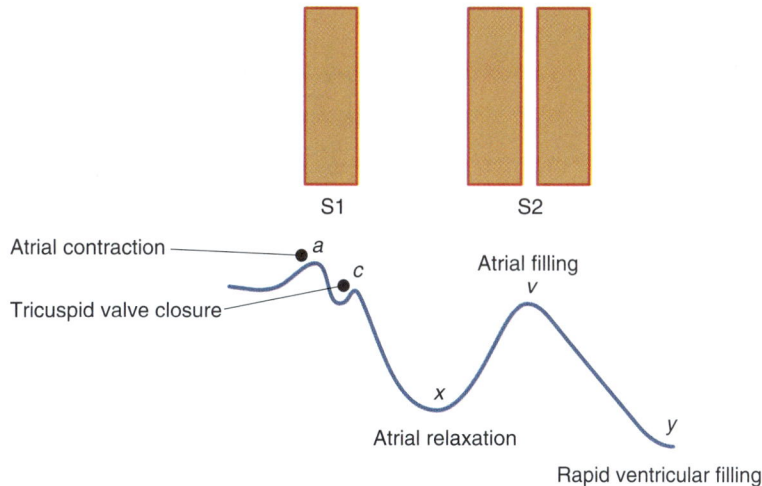

JVP and its relationship to the first (S1) and second (S2) heart sounds

FIGURE 5.24

contraction. The *a* wave also coincides with the first heart sound and precedes the carotid pulsation. The second impulse is called the *v wave* and is due to atrial filling, in the period when the tricuspid valve remains closed during ventricular systole. Between the *a* and the *v* waves there is a trough caused by atrial relaxation. This is called the *x descent*. It is interrupted by the *c point*, which is due to transmitted carotid pulsation and coincides with tricuspid valve closure; it is not usually visible. Following the *v* wave, the tricuspid valve opens and rapid ventricular filling occurs; this results in the *y descent* (see Fig. 5.24).

In List 5.2, characteristic changes in JVP are described. Any condition in which right ventricular filling is limited (e.g. *constrictive pericarditis*, *cardiac tamponade* or *right ventricular infarction*) can cause elevation of the venous pressure, which is more marked on inspiration when venous return to the heart increases. This rise in JVP on inspiration, called *Kussmaul's*[v] sign, is the opposite of what normally happens. This sign is best elicited with the patient sitting up at 90° and breathing quietly through the mouth.

The *abdominojugular reflux* test (hepatojugular reflux) is a way of testing for right or left ventricular failure or reduced right ventricular compliance.[12] It is important that the patient be relaxed, breathe through the mouth and not perform a Valsalva manoeuvre. The examiner should press firmly with the palm over the upper abdomen. It is not necessary to apply pressure for more than 10 seconds. Pressure exerted over the upper abdomen for 10 seconds will increase venous return to the right atrium. The JVP normally rises transiently following this manoeuvre.[w] *If there is right ventricular failure or if left atrial pressures are elevated (left ventricular failure), the JVP will remain elevated (>4 centimetres) for the duration of the compression—a positive abdominojugular reflux test.* The sudden fall in JVP (>4 centimetres) as the pressure is released may be easier to see than the initial rise. It is not necessary to compress the liver and so the older name, hepatojugular reflux, is not so appropriate.

Cannon a waves occur when the right atrium contracts against the closed tricuspid valve. This occurs intermittently in complete heart block where the two chambers beat independently.

Giant a waves are large but not explosive *a* waves with each beat. They occur when right atrial pressures are raised because of elevated pressures in the pulmonary circulation or obstruction to outflow (tricuspid stenosis).

The *large v waves* of tricuspid regurgitation should never be missed (LR+ 10.9).[12] They are a reliable sign of tricuspid regurgitation and are visible welling up

---

[v] Adolf Kussmaul (1822–1909), a German physician who also described laboured breathing ('air hunger') in diabetic coma (1874) and was the first to use an oesophagoscope. He coined the word hemiballismus.

[w] First described by Louis Pasteur in 1885.

SECTION 2 THE CARDIOVASCULAR SYSTEM

> ### JUGULAR VENOUS PRESSURE (JVP)
>
> **Causes of an elevated central venous pressure (CVP)**
> Right ventricular failure
> Tricuspid stenosis or regurgitation
> Pericardial effusion or constrictive pericarditis
> Superior vena caval obstruction
> Fluid overload
> Hyperdynamic circulation
>
> **Wave form**
> CAUSES OF A DOMINANT *A* WAVE
> Tricuspid stenosis (also causing a slow *y* descent)
> Pulmonary stenosis
> Pulmonary hypertension
>
> CAUSES OF CANNON *A* WAVES
> Complete heart block
> Paroxysmal nodal tachycardia with retrograde atrial conduction
> Ventricular tachycardia with retrograde atrial conduction or atrioventricular dissociation
>
> CAUSES OF A DOMINANT *V* WAVE
> Tricuspid regurgitation
>
> *X* DESCENT
> Absent: atrial fibrillation
> Exaggerated: acute cardiac tamponade, constrictive pericarditis
>
> *Y* DESCENT
> Sharp: severe tricuspid regurgitation, constrictive pericarditis
> Slow: tricuspid stenosis, right atrial myxoma
>
> LIST 5.2

(a) Simultaneous ECG and pressure recordings from the right (RV) and left (LV) ventricles. Right ventricular pressures are elevated. (b) Recordings from the right atrium

(From Ragosta M. *Textbook of clinical hemodynamics*, 1st edn. Philadelphia: Saunders, ©2008.)

FIGURE 5.25

into the neck during each ventricular systole (see Fig. 5.25). If you see distended neck veins but cannot see any venous pulsation, sit the patient at 90° and reassess.[2]

PRAECORDIUM

Now at last you have reached the praecordium.

Inspection

Inspect first for scars. Previous cardiac operations will have left scars on the chest wall. The position of the scar can be a clue to the valve lesion that has been operated on. Most valve surgery requires cardiopulmonary bypass and for this a median sternotomy (a cut down the middle of the sternum) is very commonly used. This type of scar is occasionally hidden under a forest of chest hair. It is not specifically helpful, as it may also be a result of previous coronary artery bypass grafting. Alternatively, left- or even right-sided lateral thoracotomy scars, which may be hidden under a pendulous breast, may indicate an old (usually more than 30 years old) previous closed mitral valvotomy (now very rare). In this operation a stenosed mitral valve is opened through an incision made in the left atrial appendage; cardiopulmonary bypass is not required. Coronary artery bypass grafting and even valve surgery are now sometimes performed using small lateral 'port' incisions for video-assisted instruments.

Skeletal abnormalities such as *pectus excavatum* (funnel chest; p 181) or *kyphoscoliosis* (from the Greek *kyphos* 'hunchbacked', *skolios* 'curved'), a curvature of the vertebral column, may be present. Skeletal abnormalities such as these, which may be part of Marfan's syndrome, can cause distortion of the position of the heart and great vessels in the chest and thus alter the position of the apex beat. Severe deformity can interfere with pulmonary function and cause pulmonary hypertension (p 125).

Another surgical 'abnormality' that must not be missed, if only to avoid embarrassment, is a pacemaker or cardioverter-defibrillator box (see the OCSE ECGs nos 17–19 showing paced rhythm at Student CONSULT). These are usually under the right or left pectoral muscle just below the clavicle, are usually easily palpable and obviously metallic. The pacemaker leads may be palpable under the skin, leading from the top of the box. The box is normally mobile under the skin. Fixation of the skin to the box or stretching of the skin over the box may be an indication for repositioning. Erosion of the box through the skin is a serious complication because of the inevitable infection that will occur around this foreign body. Rarely, a loose lead connection will lead to twitching of the muscles of the chest wall around the box. Penetration of the right ventricular lead into or through the right ventricular wall may lead to disconcerting paced diaphragmatic contractions (hiccups) at whatever rate the pacemaker is set. Defibrillator boxes are larger than pacemakers.

The apex beat.

The coin is over the apex. The intercostal spaces are numbered. Vertical lines show right and left midclavicular line. Care must be taken in identifying the midclavicular line; the inter-observer variability can be as much as 10 centimetres!

FIGURE 5.26

They are currently about 10×5 centimetres and a little less than 1 centimetre thick.

Look for the apex beat. Its normal position is in the fifth left intercostal space, 1 centimetre medial to the midclavicular line (see Fig. 5.26). It is due primarily to recoil of the heart as blood is expelled in systole. There may be other visible pulsations—for example, over the pulmonary artery in cases of severe pulmonary hypertension.

Palpation

Palpate the *apex beat* (see Fig. 5.27).[13] Count down the number of interspaces (see Fig. 5.26). The first palpable interspace is the second. It lies just below the manubriosternal angle. The position of the apex beat is defined as the most lateral and inferior point at which the palpating fingers are raised with each systole. The normal apex is felt over an area the size of a 20 cent (50 p) coin. Use firm pressure with the tips of your fingers in the rib interspaces. Lift the heel of your hand off the patient's sternum. Note that the apex beat is palpable in only about 50% of adults.

Feeling for the apex beat

FIGURE 5.27

Feeling for the parasternal impulse

FIGURE 5.28

It is worth noting that the palpable apex beat is not the anatomical apex of the heart but a point above it. At the time the apex beat is palpable,[x] the heart is assuming a more spherical shape and the apex is twisting away from the chest wall. The area above the apex, however, is moving closer to the chest and is palpable. If the apex beat is displaced laterally or inferiorly, or both, this usually indicates enlargement,[13] but may sometimes be due to chest wall deformity, or pleural or pulmonary disease (p 182).

The character of the apex beat may provide vital diagnostic clues. The normal apex beat gently lifts the palpating fingers. There are a number of types of abnormal apex beats:

- The *pressure loaded* (heaving, hyperdynamic or systolic overloaded) apex beat is a forceful and sustained impulse. This occurs with aortic stenosis or hypertension.
- The *volume-loaded* (thrusting) apex beat is a displaced, diffuse, non-sustained impulse. This occurs most commonly in advanced mitral regurgitation or dilated cardiomyopathy.
- The *dyskinetic* apex beat is an uncoordinated impulse felt over a larger area than normal in the praecordium and is usually due to left ventricular dysfunction (e.g. in anterior myocardial infarction).
- The *double-impulse* apex beat, where two distinct impulses are felt with each systole, is characteristic of hypertrophic cardiomyopathy (p 137).
- The *tapping* apex beat will be felt when the first heart sound is actually palpable (heart sounds are not palpable in health) and indicates mitral or very rarely tricuspid stenosis.

The character, but not the position, of the apex beat may be more easily assessed when the patient lies on the left side.

In many patients the apex beat may not be palpable. This is most often due to a thick chest wall, emphysema, pericardial effusion, shock (or death) and rarely to dextrocardia (where there is inversion of the heart and great vessels). The apex beat will be palpable to the right of the sternum in many cases of dextrocardia.

Other praecordial impulses may be palpable in patients with heart disease. A *parasternal impulse* may be felt when the heel of the hand is rested just to the left of the sternum with the fingers lifted slightly off the chest (see Fig. 5.28). Normally no impulse or a slight inward impulse is felt. In cases of right ventricular enlargement or severe left atrial enlargement, where the right ventricle is pushed anteriorly, the heel of the hand is lifted off the chest wall with each systole. Palpation with the fingers over the pulmonary area may reveal the palpable tap of pulmonary valve closure

---

[x] James Hope was the first to demonstrate (in 1830) that the apex beat was caused by ventricular contraction. Jean-Nicholas Corvisant (Napoleon's personal doctor) was the first to associate abnormal palpation of the heart with cardiac chamber enlargements.

Palpating the base of the heart

FIGURE 5.29

Auscultation in the mitral area with the bell of the stethoscope: listening for mitral stenosis in the left lateral position

FIGURE 5.30

(*palpable P2*) in cases of pulmonary hypertension (see Fig. 5.29).

Turbulent blood flow, which causes cardiac murmurs on auscultation, may sometimes be palpable. These palpable murmurs are called *thrills*. The praecordium should be systematically palpated for thrills with the flat of the hand, first over the apex and left sternal edge, and then over the base of the heart (this is the upper part of the chest and includes the aortic and pulmonary areas; see Fig. 5.29).

Apical thrills can be more easily felt with the patient rolled over to the left side (the left lateral position) as this brings the apex closer to the chest wall. Thrills are best felt with the patient sitting up, leaning forwards and in full expiration. In this position the base of the heart is moved closer to the chest wall. A thrill that coincides in time with the apex beat is called a *systolic thrill*; one that does not coincide with the apex beat is called a *diastolic thrill*.

The presence of a thrill usually indicates a severe valve lesion. Careful palpation for thrills is a useful, but often neglected, part of the cardiovascular examination.

Percussion

It is possible to define the cardiac outline by means of percussion,[y] but this is not routinely performed (p 184).[14] Percussion is most accurate when performed in the fifth intercostal space. The patient should lie supine and the examiner percusses from the anterior axillary line towards the sternum. The point at which the percussion note becomes dull represents the left heart border. A distance of more than 10.5 centimetres between the border of the heart and the middle of the sternum indicates cardiomegaly. The sign is not useful in the presence of lung disease.

Auscultation

Now at last the stethoscope is required.[15] However, in some cases the diagnosis should already be fairly clear. In the viva voce and OSCE examination, the examiners will occasionally amuse themselves by stopping a candidate before auscultation and ask for an opinion.

Auscultation of the heart (reference to heart sounds recordings) begins in the mitral area with the bell of the stethoscope (see Figs 5.1 and 5.30). The bell is designed as a resonating chamber and is particularly efficient in amplifying low-pitched sounds, such as the diastolic murmur of mitral stenosis or a third heart sound. It must be applied lightly to the chest wall, because forceful application will stretch the skin under the bell so that it forms a diaphragm. Some modern stethoscopes do not have a separate bell: the effect of a bell is produced when the diaphragm is placed lightly

---

[y] Percussion of the heart and other organs was enthusiastically promoted by Pierre Poiry, a student of Laënnec, in the early 19th century. He performed indirect percussion using an ivory plate instead of his left middle finger.

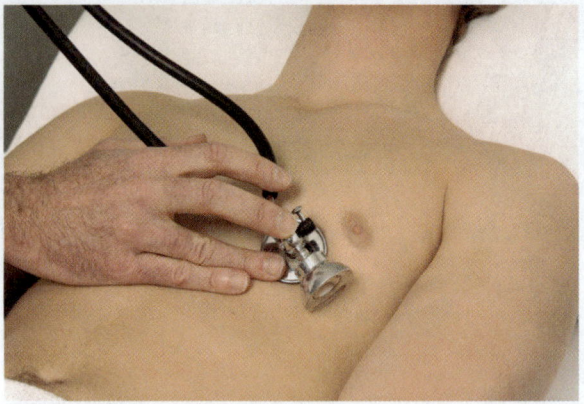

Auscultation at the apex with the diaphragm of the stethoscope

FIGURE 5.31

Auscultation at the base of the heart (pulmonary area)

FIGURE 5.32

on the chest, and of a diaphragm when it is pushed more firmly.

Next, listen in the mitral area with the diaphragm of the stethoscope (see Fig. 5.31), which best reproduces higher-pitched sounds, such as the systolic murmur of mitral regurgitation or a fourth heart sound. Then place the stethoscope in the tricuspid area (fifth left intercostal space) and listen. Next inch up the left sternal edge to the pulmonary (second left intercostal space) and aortic (second right intercostal space) areas (see Figs 5.32 and 5.33), listening carefully in each position with the diaphragm.

For accurate auscultation, experience with what is normal is important. This can be obtained only through constant practice. Auscultation of the normal heart reveals two sounds called, not surprisingly, the first and second heart sounds. The explanation for the origin of these noises changes from year to year; the sounds are probably related to vibrations caused by the closing of the heart valves in combination with rapid changes in blood flow and tensing within cardiac structures that occur as the valves close.

The *first heart sound* (S1) has two components corresponding to mitral and tricuspid valve closure. Mitral closure occurs slightly before tricuspid, but usually only one sound is audible. The first heart sound indicates the beginning of ventricular systole.

The *second heart sound* (S2), which is softer, shorter and at a slightly higher pitch than the first and marks

Auscultation at the base of the heart (aortic area)

FIGURE 5.33

the end of systole, is made up of sounds arising from aortic and pulmonary valve closures. In normal cases, although left and right ventricular systole end at the same time, the lower pressure in the pulmonary circulation compared with the aorta means that flow continues into the pulmonary artery after the end of left ventricular systole. As a result, closure of the pulmonary valve occurs later than that of the aortic valve. These components are usually (in 70% of normal adults) sufficiently separated in time so that splitting of the second heart sound is audible. Because the pulmonary component of the second heart sound (P2) may not be audible throughout the praecordium, splitting of the second heart sound may best be appreciated in the pulmonary area and along the left sternal edge. Pulmonary valve closure is further delayed (by 20 or 30 milliseconds) with inspiration because of increased venous return to the right ventricle; thus, splitting of the second heart sound is wider on inspiration. The second heart sound marks the beginning of diastole, which is usually longer than systole.

It can be difficult to decide which heart sound is which. Palpation of the carotid pulse will indicate the timing of systole and enable the heart sounds to be more easily distinguished. It is obviously crucial to define systole and diastole during auscultation so that cardiac murmurs and abnormal sounds can be placed in the correct part of the cardiac cycle. Students are often asked to time a cardiac murmur; this is not a request to measure its length, but rather to say in which part of the cardiac cycle it occurs. Even the experts can mistake a murmur if they do not time it. It is important, during auscultation, to concentrate separately on the components of the cardiac cycle: attempt to identify each and listen for abnormalities. There can be more than 12 components to identify in patients with heart disease. An understanding of the cardiac cycle is helpful when interpreting the auscultatory findings (see Fig. 5.34).

Abnormalities of the heart sounds

Alterations in intensity

The first heart sound (S1) is *loud* when the mitral or tricuspid valve cusps remain wide open at the end of diastole and shut forcefully with the onset of ventricular systole. This occurs in mitral stenosis because the narrowed valve orifice limits ventricular filling so that there is no diminution in flow towards the end of diastole. The normal mitral valve cusps drift back towards the closed position at the end of diastole as ventricular filling slows down. Other causes of a loud S1 are related to reduced diastolic filling time (e.g. tachycardia or any cause of a short atrioventricular conduction time).

Soft first heart sounds can be due to a prolonged diastolic filling time (as with first-degree heart block) or a delayed onset of left ventricular systole (as with left bundle branch block), or to failure of the leaflets to coapt normally (as in mitral regurgitation).

The second heart sound (S2) may have a *loud* aortic component (A2) in patients with systemic hypertension. This results in forceful aortic valve closure secondary to high aortic pressures. Congenital aortic stenosis is another cause, because the valve is mobile but narrowed and closes suddenly at the end of systole. The pulmonary component of the second heart sound (P2) is traditionally said to be *loud* in pulmonary hypertension, where the valve closure is forceful because of the high pulmonary pressure. In fact, a palpable P2 correlates better with raised pulmonary pressures than a loud P2.[16]

A *soft* A2 will be found when the aortic valve is calcified and leaflet movement is reduced, and in aortic regurgitation when the leaflets cannot coapt.

Splitting

Splitting of the heart sound is usually most obvious during auscultation in the pulmonary area. Splitting of the first heart sound is usually not detectable clinically; however, when it occurs it is most often due to the cardiac conduction abnormality known as complete right bundle branch block (see the OCSE ECG library no. 22 at Student CONSULT).

Increased normal splitting (wider on inspiration) of the second heart sound occurs when there is any delay in right ventricular emptying, as in right bundle branch block (delayed right ventricular depolarisation), pulmonary stenosis (delayed right ventricular ejection), ventricular septal defect (increased right ventricular volume load) and mitral regurgitation (because of earlier aortic valve closure, due to more rapid left ventricular emptying).

In the case of *fixed splitting* of the second heart sound, there is no respiratory variation (as is normal) and splitting tends to be wide. This is caused by an atrial septal defect where equalisation of volume loads between the two atria occurs through the defect. This results in the atria acting as a common chamber.

Reversed splitting is present when P2 occurs first and splitting occurs in expiration. This can be due to delayed left ventricular depolarisation (left bundle branch block [see the OCSE ECG library no. 23 at

The cardiac cycle.

Normally, the onset of left ventricular systole precedes the onset of pressure rise in the right ventricle. The mitral valve therefore closes before the tricuspid valve. Because the pulmonary artery diastolic pressure is lower than the aortic diastolic pressure, the pulmonary valve opens before the aortic valve. Therefore, pulmonary ejection sounds occur closer to the first heart sound than do aortic ejection sounds. During systole the pressure in the ventricles slightly exceeds the pressure in the corresponding great arteries. Towards the end of systole, the ventricular pressure falls below the pressure in the great arteries, and when diastolic pressure is reached the semilunar valves close. Normally, aortic valve closure precedes pulmonary valve closure. The mitral and tricuspid valves begin to open at the point at which the ventricular pressures fall below the corresponding atrial pressures.

(Adapted from Swash M, ed. *Hutchison's clinical methods*, 20th edn. Philadelphia: Baillière Tindall, 1995.)

FIGURE 5.34

 Student CONSULT]), delayed left ventricular emptying (severe aortic stenosis, coarctation of the aorta) or increased left ventricular volume load (large patent ductus arteriosus). However, in the last-mentioned, the loud machinery murmur means that the second heart sound is usually not heard.

Extra heart sounds

The *third heart sound* (S3) is a low-pitched (20–70 Hz) mid-diastolic sound that is best appreciated by listening for a triple rhythm.[17] Its low pitch makes it more easily heard with the bell of the stethoscope. It has been likened (rather accurately) to the galloping of a horse and is often called a **gallop rhythm**. Its cadence is similar to that of the word 'Kentucky'. It is more likely to be appreciated if the clinician listens not to the individual heart sounds but to the rhythm of the heart. It is probably caused by tautening of the mitral or tricuspid papillary muscles at the end of rapid diastolic filling, when blood flow temporarily stops.

A pathological S3 is due to reduced ventricular compliance, so that a filling sound is produced even when diastolic filling is not especially rapid. It is strongly associated with increased atrial and ventricular end-diastolic pressure.

A *left ventricular* S3 is louder at the apex than at the left sternal edge, and is louder on expiration. It can be physiological when it is due to very rapid diastolic filling, associated with an increased cardiac output, as occurs in pregnancy and thyrotoxicosis and in some children. Otherwise, it is an important sign of left ventricular failure and dilation, but may also occur in aortic regurgitation, mitral regurgitation, ventricular septal defect and patent ductus arteriosus.[18]

A new third heart sound after a myocardial infarction is an indicator of increased mortality risk (LR+, 8.0).[19]

A *right ventricular* S3 is louder at the left sternal edge and with inspiration. It occurs in right ventricular failure or constrictive pericarditis.

The *fourth heart sound* (S4) is a late diastolic sound pitched slightly higher than the S3.[20] The cadence of an S4 is similar to that of the word 'Tennessee'. Again, this is responsible for the impression of a triple (gallop) rhythm. It is due to a high-pressure atrial wave reflected back from a poorly compliant ventricle. It does not occur if the patient is in atrial fibrillation, because the sound depends on effective atrial contraction, which is lost when the atria fibrillate. Its low pitch means that, unlike a split first heart sound, it disappears if the bell of the stethoscope is pressed firmly onto the chest.

A *left ventricular* S4 may be audible when left ventricular compliance is reduced owing to aortic stenosis, acute mitral regurgitation, systemic hypertension, ischaemic heart disease or advanced age. It is sometimes present during an episode of angina or with a myocardial infarction, and may be the only physical sign of that condition.

A *right ventricular* S4 occurs when right ventricular compliance is reduced as a result of pulmonary hypertension or pulmonary stenosis.

If the heart rate is greater than 120 beats per minute, S3 and S4 may be superimposed, resulting in a **summation gallop**. In this case, two inaudible sounds may combine to produce an audible one. This does not necessarily imply ventricular stress, unless one or both of the extra heart sounds persists when the heart rate slows or is slowed by carotid sinus massage. When both S3 and S4 are present, the rhythm is described as a quadruple rhythm. It usually implies severe ventricular dysfunction.

Additional sounds

An **opening snap** is a high-pitched sound that occurs in mitral stenosis at a variable distance after S2. It is due to the sudden opening of the mitral valve and is followed by the diastolic murmur of mitral stenosis. It can be difficult to distinguish from a widely split S2, but normally occurs rather later in diastole than the pulmonary component of the second heart sound. It is pitched higher than a third heart sound and so is not usually confused with this. It is best heard at the lower left sternal edge with the diaphragm of the stethoscope. Use of the term *opening snap* implies the diagnosis of mitral stenosis or, rarely, tricuspid stenosis.

A **systolic ejection click** is an early systolic high-pitched sound that is heard over the aortic or pulmonary and left sternal edge areas, and that may occur in cases of congenital aortic or pulmonary stenosis where the valve remains mobile; it is followed by the systolic ejection murmur of aortic or pulmonary stenosis. It is due to the abrupt doming of the abnormal valve early in systole.

A **non-ejection systolic click** is a high-pitched sound heard during systole that is best appreciated at the mitral area. It is a common finding. It may be followed by a systolic murmur. The click may be due to prolapse of one or more redundant mitral valve leaflets during systole. Non-ejection clicks may also be heard in patients with atrial septal defects or Ebstein's anomaly (p 141).

An atrial myxoma[z] is a very rare tumour that may occur in either atrium. During atrial systole a loosely pedunculated tumour may be propelled into the mitral or tricuspid valve orifice, causing an early diastolic

---

[z] This gelatinous tumour's name is derived from the Greek word meaning mucus.

GOOD SIGNS GUIDE 5.1
LRs of signs suggesting that a systolic murmur is significant (abnormal)

Sign	LR+	LR−
Systolic thrill	12	0.73
Pansystolic murmur	8.7	0.19
Loud murmur	6.5	0.08
Plateau-shaped murmur	4.1	0.48
Loudest at apex	2.5	0.84
Radiation to carotid	0.91	1.0

(Adapted from Etchells EE, Bell C, Robb K. Does this patient have an abnormal systolic murmur? *JAMA* 1997; 277(7):564–571.)

plopping sound: a **tumour plop**. This sound is only rarely heard, even in patients with a myxoma (about 10%).

A **diastolic pericardial knock** may occur when there is sudden cessation of ventricular filling because of constrictive pericardial disease.[21]

Prosthetic heart valves produce characteristic sounds (p 138).[22] Rarely, a right ventricular pacemaker produces a late diastolic high-pitched click due to contraction of the chest wall muscles (the **pacemaker sound**).

Murmurs of the heart

Murmurs are continuous sounds caused by turbulent blood flow. Some turbulence is inevitable as the blood is accelerated through the aortic and pulmonary valves during ventricular systole. Increased turbulence across normal valves occurs in association with anaemia and thyrotoxicosis. The normal velocity of flow through these valves is about 1 metre per second. This may be enough to produce a soft swishing sound audible with the stethoscope, an innocent murmur. Greater turbulence—flow velocities of 4 metres per second or more across narrowed aortic valves and even higher velocities when the mitral valve leaks—lead to more prominent murmurs. Certain features have been shown to indicate a likelihood that a murmur is significant (see Good signs guide 5.1[aa]).

In deciding the origin of a cardiac murmur, a number of different features must be considered. These are: associated features (peripheral signs), timing, the area of greatest intensity and radiation (see Fig. 5.35), the loudness and pitch and the effect of dynamic manoeuvres, including respiration and the Valsalva manoeuvre. The presence of a characteristic murmur is very reliable for the diagnosis of certain valvular abnormalities, but for others less so.

Associated features

As already mentioned, the cause of a cardiac murmur can sometimes be elicited by careful analysis of the peripheral signs.

Timing

Systolic murmurs (which occur during ventricular systole) may be pansystolic, midsystolic (ejection systolic) or late systolic (see Table 5.4).

The *pansystolic murmur* extends throughout systole, beginning with the first heart sound and going right up to the second heart sound. Its loudness and pitch do not vary during systole. Pansystolic murmurs occur when a ventricle leaks to a lower-pressure chamber or vessel. As there is a pressure difference from the moment the ventricle begins to contract (S1), blood flow and the murmur both begin at the first heart sound and continue until the pressures equalise (S2). Causes of pansystolic murmurs include mitral regurgitation,[bb] tricuspid regurgitation, ventricular septal defect and aortopulmonary shunts.

The *midsystolic ejection murmur* does not begin right at the first heart sound; its intensity is greatest in midsystole or later, and wanes again late in systole. This is described as a *crescendo–decrescendo* murmur. These murmurs are usually produced by turbulent flow through the aortic or pulmonary valve orifices or by greatly increased flow through a normal-sized orifice or outflow tract. Causes include aortic or pulmonary stenosis, hypertrophic cardiomyopathy and atrial septal defect.

When it is possible to distinguish an appreciable gap between the first heart sound and the murmur, which then continues right up to the second heart sound,

---

[aa] The same study showed that if a cardiologist thought a murmur was significant the LR+ was 38, but if an emergency doctor thought so it was only 14—very cheering.

[bb] The older term *incompetence* is synonymous with regurgitation, but the latter better describes the pathophysiology and changes to terminology of this sort keep non-cardiologists on the back foot.

CHAPTER 5 THE CARDIAC EXAMINATION 101

Sites of maximum intensity and radiation of murmurs and heart sounds (2–5 refer to intercostal spaces).

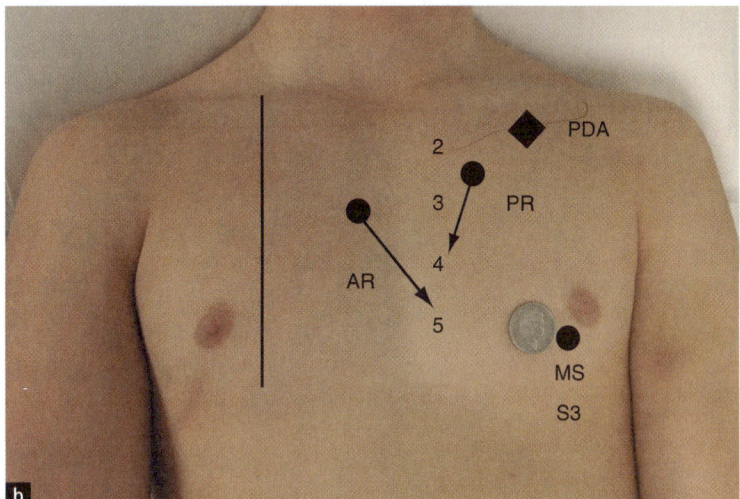

(a) Systolic murmurs:
   AS=aortic stenosis
   MR=mitral regurgitation
   HCM=hypertrophic cardiomyopathy
   PS=pulmonary stenosis
   VSD=ventricular septal defect
   I=innocent.
(b) Diastolic murmurs and sounds:
   AR=aortic regurgitation
   MS=mitral stenosis
   S3=third heart sound
   PR=pulmonary regurgitation
   PDA=patent ductus arteriosus (continuous murmur).

FIGURE 5.35

Cardiac murmurs	
Timing	**Lesion**
Pansystolic	Mitral regurgitation Tricuspid regurgitation Ventricular septal defect Aortopulmonary shunts
Midsystolic	Aortic stenosis or sclerosis (most common cause) Pulmonary stenosis Hypertrophic cardiomyopathy Pulmonary flow murmur of an atrial septal defect
Late systolic	Mitral valve prolapse Papillary muscle dysfunction (due usually to ischaemia or hypertrophic cardiomyopathy)
Early diastolic	Aortic regurgitation Pulmonary regurgitation
Mid-diastolic	Mitral stenosis Tricuspid stenosis Atrial myxoma Austin Flint* murmur of aortic regurgitation Carey Coombs† murmur of acute rheumatic fever
Presystolic	Mitral stenosis Tricuspid stenosis Atrial myxoma
Continuous	Patent ductus arteriosus Arteriovenous fistula (coronary artery, pulmonary, systemic) Aortopulmonary connection (e.g. congenital, Blalock‡ shunt) Venous hum (usually best heard over right supraclavicular fossa and abolished by ipsilateral internal jugular vein compression) Rupture of sinus of Valsalva into right ventricle or atrium 'Mammary soufflé' (in late pregnancy or early postpartum period: high-pitched, superficial, heard over one or both breasts)

Note: The combined murmurs of aortic stenosis and aortic regurgitation, or mitral stenosis and mitral regurgitation, may sound as if they fill the entire cardiac cycle, but are not continuous murmurs by definition.
*See footnote k, page 133.
†Carey F Coombs (1879–1932), Bristol physician.
‡Alfred Blalock (1899–1965), Baltimore physician.

TABLE 5.4

the murmur is described as a *late systolic murmur*. This is typical of mitral valve prolapse or papillary muscle dysfunction where mitral regurgitation begins in midsystole.

Diastolic murmurs (always abnormal) occur during ventricular diastole. They are more difficult for students to hear than systolic murmurs and are usually softer. A loud murmur is unlikely to be diastolic.

The *early diastolic murmur* begins immediately with the second heart sound and has a decrescendo quality (it is loudest at the beginning and extends for a variable distance into diastole). These early diastolic murmurs are typically high-pitched and are due to regurgitation through leaking aortic or pulmonary valves. The murmur is loudest at the beginning because this is when aortic and pulmonary artery pressures are highest.

The *mid-diastolic murmur* begins later in diastole and may be short or extend right up to the first heart sound. It has a much lower-pitched quality than early diastolic murmurs. It is due to impaired flow during ventricular filling and can be caused by mitral stenosis and tricuspid stenosis, where the valve is narrowed, or rarely by an atrial myxoma, where the tumour mass obstructs the valve orifice, or mitral valvulitis from acute rheumatic fever.

In severe aortic regurgitation, the regurgitant jet from the aortic valve may cause the anterior leaflet of the mitral valve to shudder, producing a diastolic murmur. Occasionally, normal mitral or tricuspid valves can produce flow murmurs, which are short and mid-diastolic, and occur when there is torrential flow across the valve. Causes include a high cardiac output or intracardiac shunting (atrial or ventricular septal defects).

The *presystolic murmur* may be heard when atrial systole increases blood flow across the valve just before the first heart sound. It is an extension of the mid-diastolic murmurs of mitral stenosis, tricuspid stenosis and atrial myxoma, and usually does not occur when atrial systole is lost in atrial fibrillation.

As the name implies, **continuous murmurs** extend throughout systole and diastole. They are produced when a communication exists between two parts of the circulation with a permanent pressure gradient so that blood flow occurs continuously. They can usually be distinguished from combined systolic and diastolic murmurs (due, for example, to aortic stenosis and aortic regurgitation), but this may sometimes be difficult. The various causes are presented in Table 5.4.

A **pericardial friction rub** is a superficial scratching sound; there may be up to three distinct components occurring at any time during the cardiac cycle. They are not confined to systole or diastole. A rub is caused by movement of inflamed pericardial surfaces; it is a result of pericarditis. The sound can vary with respiration and posture; it is often louder when the patient is sitting up and breathing out. It tends to come and go, and is often absent by the time students can be found to come and listen for it. It has been likened to the crunching sound made when walking on snow.

A **mediastinal crunch** (Hamman's[cc] sign) is a crunching sound heard in time with the heartbeat but with systolic and diastolic components. It is caused by the presence of air in the mediastinum, and once heard it is not forgotten. It is very often present after cardiac surgery and may occur associated with a pneumothorax or after aspiration of a pericardial effusion (if air has been let into the pericardium).

Area of greatest intensity

Although the place on the praecordium where a murmur is heard most easily is a guide to its origin, this is not a particularly reliable physical sign. For example, mitral regurgitation murmurs are usually loudest at the apex, over the mitral area, and tend to radiate towards the axillae (see Fig. 5.35, Good signs guide 5.2), but they may be heard widely over the praecordium and even right up into the aortic area or over the back. Conduction of an ejection murmur up into the carotid arteries strongly suggests that this arises from the aortic valve.

Loudness and pitch

The *loudness* of the murmur may be helpful in deciding the severity of the valve lesion; for example, for mitral regurgitation (see Good signs guide 5.3).[23]

The loudness and harshness of the murmur (and the presence of a thrill) correlate with the severity of aortic stenosis except in the severest forms of valve stenosis, when murmurs may be soft because cardiac output has fallen. Cardiologists most often use a classification with six grades (Levine's grading system):[24]

[cc] Louis Hamman (1877–1946), a physician at Johns Hopkins Hospital, Baltimore.

GOOD SIGNS GUIDE 5.2
Mitral regurgitation (MR)

1. Radiation to anterior axillary line	MR moderate or worse +ve LR 6.8*
2. Known mitral valve prolapse, absence of pansystolic or late systolic murmur (according to cardiologist)	−ve LR of moderate or worse MR 0 to 0.8†

*McGee S. Etiology and diagnosis of systolic murmurs in adults. *Am J Med* 2010; 123:913–921.
†Panidis IP, McAllister M, Ross J, Mintz GS. Prevalence and severity of mitral regurgitation in the mitral valve prolapse syndrome; a Doppler echocardiographic study of 80 patients. *J Am Cardiol* 1986; 7;975–981.

GOOD SIGNS GUIDE 5.3
Loudness of severe mitral regurgitation (MR)

Loudness of systolic murmur	LR+ for severe MR
Grade 4 or more	14
Grade 3	3.5
Grade 0–2	0.12

(Desjardins VA, Enriquz-Sarano M, Tajik AJ et al. Intensity of murmurs correlates with severity of valvular regurgitation. *Am J Med* 1996; 100(2):149–156.)

Grade 1/6   Very soft and not heard at first (often audible only to consultants and to those students who have been told the murmur is present)
Grade 2/6   Soft, but can be detected almost immediately by an experienced auscultator
Grade 3/6   Moderate; there is no thrill
Grade 4/6   Loud; thrill just palpable
Grade 5/6   Very loud; thrill easily palpable
Grade 6/6   Very, very loud; can be heard even without placing the stethoscope right on the chest (rare nowadays).

This grading is useful, particularly because a change in the intensity of a murmur may be of great significance—for example, after a myocardial infarction.

It requires practice to appreciate the *pitch* of the murmur, but this may be of use in identifying its type. In general, low-pitched murmurs indicate turbulent flow under low pressure, as in mitral stenosis, and high-pitched murmurs indicate a high velocity of flow, as in mitral regurgitation.

Dynamic manoeuvres

All patients with a newly diagnosed murmur should undergo dynamic manoeuvre testing (see Table 5.5 and Good signs guide 5.4).[25]

- **Respiration:** murmurs that arise on the right side of the heart become louder during inspiration as this increases venous return and therefore blood flow to the right side of the heart. Left-sided murmurs are either unchanged or become softer. Expiration has the opposite effect. This can be a sensitive and specific way of differentiating right- and left-sided murmurs.
- **Left lateral position:** the low-pitched murmur of mitral stenosis is more easily heard (using the bell of the stethoscope) when the patient is rolled onto the left side (Fig. 5.36). If mitral stenosis is still difficult to hear, exercise the patient by getting him or her to sit up and down several times and then go back quickly onto the side, and listen again.
- **Deep expiration:** a routine part of the examination of the heart (see Fig. 5.37) includes leaning the patient forwards in full expiration and listening to the base of the heart for aortic regurgitation, which may otherwise be missed. In this case, the manoeuvre brings the base of the heart closer to the chest wall. The scraping sound

GOOD SIGNS GUIDE 5.4
Dynamic auscultation and systolic murmurs

Sign	Sensitivity (%)	Specificity (%)
Louder on inspiration—right-sided murmur	100	88
Softer with expiration—right-sided murmur	100	88
Louder squatting to standing—hypertrophic cardiomyopathy	95	84
Softer with isometric handgrip—hypertrophic cardiomyopathy	85	75
Louder with isometric handgrip—mitral regurgitation/ventricular septal defect	68	92
Louder with Valsalva strain—hypertrophic cardiomyopathy	65	96

(Adapted from Anthony MJ, Celermajer DS, Stockler MR. Beauty is in the eye of the beholder: reaching agreement about physical signs and their value. *Internal Med J* 2005; 35(3):178–187.)

Dynamic manoeuvre: left lateral position

FIGURE 5.36

Dynamic manoeuvres and systolic cardiac murmurs

	Lesion			
Manoeuvre	Hypertrophic cardiomyopathy	Mitral valve prolapse	Aortic stenosis	Mitral regurgitation
Valsalva strain phase (decreases preload)	Louder	Longer	Softer	Softer
Squatting or leg raise (increases preload)	Softer	Shorter	Louder	Louder
Handgrip (increases afterload)	Softer	Shorter	Softer	Louder

TABLE 5.5

Dynamic auscultation for aortic regurgitation or a pericardial friction rub; the patient sitting up in deep expiration

FIGURE 5.37

of a pericardial friction rub is also best heard in this position.
- **The Valsalva manoeuvre:**[dd] this is forceful expiration against a closed glottis. Ask the patient to hold his or her nose with the fingers, close the mouth, breathe out hard and completely so as to pop the eardrums, and hold this for as long as possible. Listen over the left sternal edge during this manoeuvre for changes in the systolic murmur of hypertrophic cardiomyopathy, and over the apex for changes when mitral valve prolapse is suspected.

  The Valsalva manoeuvre has four phases. In phase 1 (beginning the manoeuvre), a rise in intrathoracic pressure and a transient increase in left ventricular output and blood pressure occur. In phase 2 (the straining phase), systemic venous return falls, filling of the right and then the left side of the heart is reduced, and stroke volume and blood pressure fall while the heart rate increases. *As stroke volume and arterial blood pressure fall, most cardiac murmurs become softer; however, because the left ventricular volume is reduced, the systolic murmur of hypertrophic cardiomyopathy becomes louder and the systolic click and murmur of mitral valve prolapse begin earlier.* In phase 3 (the release of the manoeuvre), first right-sided and then left-sided cardiac murmurs become louder briefly before returning to normal. Blood pressure falls further because of pooling of blood in the pulmonary veins. In phase 4, the blood pressure overshoots as a result of increased sympathetic activity as a response to the previous hypotension. Changes in heart rate are opposite to the blood pressure changes.
- **Standing to squatting:** when the patient squats rapidly from the standing position, venous return and systemic arterial resistance increase simultaneously, causing a rise in stroke volume and arterial pressure. This makes most murmurs louder. However, left ventricular size is increased, which reduces the obstruction to outflow and therefore reduces the intensity of the systolic murmur of hypertrophic cardiomyopathy, while the midsystolic click and murmur of mitral valve prolapse are delayed.
- **Squatting to standing:** when the patient stands up quickly after squatting, the opposite changes in the loudness of these murmurs occur.
- **Isometric exercise:** sustained handgrip or repeated sit-ups for 20–30 seconds increases systemic arterial resistance, blood pressure and heart size. The systolic murmur of aortic stenosis may become softer because of a reduction in the pressure difference across the valve but often remains unchanged. Most other murmurs become louder, except the systolic murmur of hypertrophic cardiomyopathy, which is softer, and the mitral valve prolapse murmur, which is delayed because of an increased ventricular volume.

Auscultation of the neck

This is often performed as a part of dynamic auscultation for valvular heart disease, but certain aspects of the examination may be considered here. Abnormal sounds heard over the arteries are called **bruits**. These sounds are low-pitched and may be more easily heard with the bell of the stethoscope. Carotid artery bruits are most easily heard over the anterior part of the

---

[dd] Antonio Valsalva (1666–1723), Professor of Anatomy at Bologna, was noted for his studies of the ear. He described his manoeuvre in 1704. Forced expiration against the closed glottis causes discharge of pus into the external auditory canal in cases of chronic otitis media. Friedrich Weber rediscovered the manoeuvre in 1859 and demonstrated that he could slow his pulse at will. He stopped demonstrating this after he caused himself to faint and have convulsions.

Neck auscultation: carotid artery bruits

FIGURE 5.38

sternocleidomastoid muscle above the medial end of the clavicle (Fig. 5.38). Ask the patient to stop breathing for a brief period to remove the competing noise of breath sounds. It may be prudent to ask the patient not to speak. The amplified voice is often painfully loud when heard through the stethoscope.

A systolic bruit may be a conducted sound from the heart. The murmur of aortic stenosis is always audible in the neck and a soft carotid bruit is sometimes audible in patients with severe mitral regurgitation or pulmonary stenosis. A bruit due to carotid stenosis will not be audible over the base of the heart. Move the stethoscope from point to point onto the chest wall; if the bruit disappears, it is likely the sound arises from the carotid. It is not possible to exclude a carotid bruit in a patient with a murmur of aortic stenosis that radiates to the neck. Carotid artery stenosis is an important cause of a carotid bruit.

More severe stenosis is associated with a noise that is longer and of increased pitch. Total obstruction of the vessel leads to disappearance of the bruit. It is not possible to exclude significant (>60% obstruction) carotid stenosis clinically. The upshot is that a carotid bruit poorly predicts significant carotid stenosis or stroke risk.

Thyrotoxicosis can result in a systolic bruit due to the increased vascularity of the gland.

A continuous noise is sometimes audible at the base of the neck. This is usually a venous hum, a result of audible venous flow. It disappears if light pressure is applied to the neck just above the stethoscope. Haemodialysis patients frequently have an audible bruit transmitted from their arteriovenous fistula.

THE BACK

It is now time to leave the praecordium. Percussion and auscultation of the *lung bases* (Ch 10) are also part of the cardiovascular examination. Signs of cardiac failure may be detected in the lungs; in particular late or pan-inspiratory crackles or a pleural effusion may be present. The murmur associated with coarctation of the aorta may be prominent over the upper back.

While the patient is sitting up, feel for pitting oedema of the sacrum, which occurs in severe right heart failure, especially in patients who have been in bed.[26] This is because the sacrum then becomes a dependent area and oedema fluid tends to settle under the influence of gravity.

THE ABDOMEN AND LEGS

Lay the patient down flat (on one pillow) and examine the abdomen (Ch 14). You are looking particularly for an enlarged tender *liver*, which may be found when the hepatic veins are congested in the presence of right heart failure. Distension of the liver capsule is said to be the cause of liver tenderness in these patients. When tricuspid regurgitation is present the liver may be *pulsatile*, as the right ventricular systolic pressure wave is transmitted to the hepatic veins—this is a very reliable sign. Test for hepatojugular reflux.[12,27] *Ascites* may occur with severe right heart failure. *Splenomegaly*, if present, may indicate infective endocarditis.

Feel for the pulsation of the abdominal aorta, to the left of the middle line. It is often palpable in normal thin people but the possibility of an abdominal aortic aneurysm should always be considered when the aorta's pulsations are palpable and expansile.[28,29]

The cardiovascular examination is not complete until the legs have been examined (in particular test for pitting ankle oedema) as set out in Chapter 6.

T&O'C ESSENTIALS

1. The cardiovascular examination is important even when patients have no cardiac symptoms (e.g. when patients are assessed before surgery).
2. If the examination is to be thorough, the patient must be positioned correctly and undressed adequately.
3. Students should develop their own examination method and become familiar with it.
4. A systematic examination will ensure that nothing is left out.
5. Pay particular attention when examining the cardiovascular system to the rate, rhythm and character of the pulse, the level of the blood pressure, elevation of the JVP, the position of the apex beat and the presence of the heart sounds, any extra sounds or murmurs.
6. Many cardiac signs are diagnostic or nearly so, which can make the examination very satisfying.
7. Practice and experience are essential if students are to recognise significant cardiac murmurs and distinguish them from innocent ones.
8. The position and timing of cardiac murmurs give important clues about the underlying valve lesion.
9. The most useful cardiac signs of left ventricular failure are a third heart sound and a displaced and dyskinetic apex beat.
10. The diastolic murmur of aortic regurgitation is characteristic and has high diagnostic utility—the only differential diagnosis is pulmonary regurgitation.

OSCE EXAMPLE – CVS EXAMINATION (see the OSCE VIDEO video no. 2 at Student CONSULT)

Please examine Mrs Keith, who has high blood pressure.

1. Introduce yourself to the patient, and wash your hands as usual.
2. Inspect the patient for abnormal facies and body habitus (e.g. Cushing's syndrome, virilisation).
3. Check the pulse (rate and rhythm) and for radiofemoral delay (coarctation of the aorta).
4. Make sure the cuff size is correct and position the patient correctly (elbow at heart level, lying).
5. Take the patient's systolic blood pressure by the palpation method on one arm.
6. Take the blood pressure by auscultation on the same arm, then the other arm (a difference between the arms of more than 10 mmHg suggests vascular disease).
7. Take the blood pressure standing (ask permission first) to look for a postural change.
8. Examine the cardiovascular system for signs of heart failure (raised JVP, displaced apex beat, S3) and for left ventricular hypertrophy and S4.
9. Examine the abdomen for enlarged kidneys, an abdominal aortic aneurysm and renal bruits (see p 310).
10. Look into the fundi (for hypertensive changes; see p 124).
11. Examine the urine for blood (red cell casts) (see p 321).

OSCE REVISION TOPICS – CVS EXAMINATION

Use these topics, which commonly occur in the OSCE, to help with revision.

1. This woman has orthopnoea. Please examine her. (p 119)
2. This man has a murmur. Please examine him. (p 145)
3. This man has had previous cardiac surgery. Please examine him. (p 145)
4. This woman has palpitations. Please examine her. (p 145)
5. This woman has hypertension. Please examine her. (p 124)
6. This man has suspected endocarditis. Please examine him. (p 123)

References

1. Lewis T. Early signs of cardiac failure of the congestive type. *BMJ* 1930; 1(3618):849–852.
2. Elder A, Nair K. The jugular veins: gateway to the heart. *Med J Aust* 2016; 205(5):204–205.
3. Elder A, Japp A, Verghese A. Abstract: 'How valuable is physical examination of the cardiovascular system?' *BMJ* 2016; 354; i3309.
4. Myers KA. Does this patient have clubbing? *JAMA* 2001; 286(3):341–347. Clubbing is a sign you will miss if you do not look.
5. Reeves RA. Does this patient have hypertension? *JAMA* 1995; 273:15. An important review of technique and of the errors to avoid.
6. Weinberg I, Gona P, O'Donnell CJ et al. The systolic blood pressure difference between the arms and cardiovascular disease in the Framingham heart study. *Am J Med* 2014; 127(3):209–215.
7. Turner JR, Viera AJ, Shimbo D. Ambulatory blood pressure monitoring in clinical practice: a review. *Am J Med* 2015; 128(1):14–20.
8. Jansen RWMM, Lipsitz LA. Postprandial hypotension: epidemiology, pathophysiology and clinical management. *Ann Intern Med* 1995; 122:186–195. It is important to recognise that blood pressure decreases postprandially and that this can affect interpretation of the blood pressure reading and the management of hypertension.
9. Bellman J, Visintin JM, Salvatore R et al. Osler's manoeuvre: absence of usefulness for the detection of pseudohypertension in an elderly population. *Am J Med* 1995; 98:42–49. Although it is reproducible, the manoeuvre failed to identify pseudohypertension compared with intra-arterial measurements.
10. From AM, Lam CS, Pitta SR et al. Bedside assessment of cardiac haemodynamics: the impact of noninvasive testing and examiner experience. *Am J Med* 2011; 124(11):1051–1057.
11. Cook DC. Does this patient have abnormal central venous pressure? *JAMA* 1996; 275:8. A useful review that explains how to examine the veins and conduct the hepatojugular reflux test.
12. Maisel AS, Attwood JE, Goldberger AL. Hepatojugular reflux: useful in the bedside diagnosis of tricuspid regurgitation. *Ann Intern Med* 1984; 101:781–782. This test has excellent sensitivity and specificity.
13. O'Neill TW, Barry M, Smith M, Graham IM. Diagnostic value of the apex beat. *Lancet* 1989; 1:410–411. Palpation of the apex beat beyond the left midclavicular line is specific (59%) for identifying true cardiomegaly.
14. Heckerling PS, Wiener SL, Wolfkiel CJ et al. Accuracy and reproducibility of precordial percussion and palpation for detecting increased left ventricular end-diastolic volume and mass. *JAMA* 1993; 270:16. Percussion has a high sensitivity but low specificity for detecting left ventricular enlargement. Therefore this manoeuvre may have some value despite being previously discredited.
15. Harvey WP. Cardiac pearls. *Disease-a-Month* 1994; 40:41–113. A good review of auscultatory findings that helps demystify the many noises heard when auscultating the heart.
16. Sutton G, Harris A, Leatham A. Second heart sound in pulmonary hypertension. *Br Heart J* 1968; 30:743–756.
17. Timmis AJ. The third heart sound. *BMJ* 1987; 294:326–327.
18. Folland ED, Kriegel BJ, Henderson WG et al. Implications of third heart sounds in patients with valvular heart disease. *N Engl J Med* 1992; 327:458–462. An analysis of patients with valvular regurgitation shows that a third heart sound may occur before cardiac failure has supervened.
19. Ramani S, Weber BN. Detecting the gallop: the third heart sound and its significance. *Med J Aust* 2017; in press.
20. Benchimol A, Desser KB. The fourth heart sound in patients with demonstrable heart disease. *Am Heart J* 1977; 93:298–301. In 60 out of 100 consecutive patients with normal studies, an S4 was heard. An S4 can be a normal finding, although a loud sound is more likely to be pathological.
21. Tyberg TI, Goodyer AVN, Langou RA. Genesis of pericardial knock in constrictive pericarditis. *Am J Cardiol* 1980; 46:570–575. Sudden cessation of ventricular filling generates this sound.
22. Smith ND, Raizada V, Abrams J. Auscultation of the normally functioning prosthetic valve. *Ann Intern Med* 1981; 95:594–598. Provides clear information on auscultatory changes with prosthetic valves.
23. Desjardins VA, Enriquz-Sarano M, Tajik AJ et al. Intensity of murmurs correlates with severity of valvular regurgitation. *Am J Med* 1996; 100(2):149–156.
24. Levine SA. Notes on the gradation of the intensity of cardiac murmurs. *JAMA* 1961; 177:261.
25. Lembo NJ, Dell'Italia LJ, Crawford MH, O'Rourke RA. Bedside diagnosis of systolic murmurs. *N Engl J Med* 1988; 318:24. This well-conducted study describes the predictive value of bedside manoeuvres during auscultation.
26. Whiting E, McCready ME. Pitting and non-pitting oedema. *Med J Aust* 2016; 205:157–158. Pitting oedema can be graded from 1 (up to 2 mm that disappears immediately) to 4 (deep pit over 6 mm that takes 2–5 minutes to disappear).
27. Ewy GA. The abdominojugular test. *Ann Intern Med* 1988; 109:56–60. Note that an abnormal abdominal–jugular test can occur as a result of left heart disease (i.e. elevated pulmonary–capillary wedge pressure).
28. Lederle FA, Walker JM, Reinke DB. Selective screening for abdominal aortic aneurysms with physical examination and ultrasound. *Arch Intern Med* 1988; 148:1753–1756. In fat patients, palpation of aneurysms is unlikely but in thin ones the technique is valuable.
29. Lederle FA, Simel DL. Does this patient have an abdominal aortic aneurysm? *JAMA* 1999; 281:77–82. The only clinical sign of definite value is palpation to detect widening of the aorta. The sensitivity of this sign for aneurysms 5 centimetres or larger is 76%.

CHAPTER 6
The limb examination and peripheral vascular disease

Leg; the limb by which we walk; particularly the part between the knee and the foot.
SAMUEL JOHNSON, A Dictionary of the English Language *(1775)*

EXAMINATION ANATOMY

The arteries are normally palpable where they run close to the surface. Figs 5.2 and 6.1 show their basic anatomy.

Arms

Most of the blood supply of the arm is provided by the axillary artery, which, after giving off some small branches in the upper arm, becomes the brachial artery. This divides into the radial and ulnar arteries, which run down the forearm following their bones. Both continue to the wrist where they go on to supply the hands and fingers. The radial artery is very superficial at the wrist and easily palpable. The veins of the arm include the digital veins of the hands, the cephalic and median vein of the forearm and the basilica vein, which runs the whole length of the arm. In the upper arm the brachial and cephalic veins run to the shoulder. These veins drain via the axillary vein into the superior vena cava.

Legs

The main blood supply to the leg is from the external iliac artery, which becomes the femoral artery in the groin. Its main branches are the profunda femoris (deep femoral) artery in the thigh and the anterior and posterior tibial arteries in the lower leg. The posterior tibial artery is usually palpable behind the medial malleolus and the continuation of the anterior tibial—the dorsalis pedis is palpable over the dorsum of the foot. The veins of the leg include the longest vein in the body: the great saphenous vein. This superficial vein drains via perforating veins to the deep veins, which contain valves assisting return of blood to the heart. Damage to these valves, for example by venous thromboses, can lead to venous varicosities. The leg veins drain into the external iliac veins and then into the inferior vena cava.

Lower limbs

See List 6.1 and Fig. 6.2. Palpate behind the medial malleolus of the tibia and the distal shaft of the tibia for *oedema* by compressing the area for at least 15 seconds with the thumb. This latter area is often tender in normal people, and gentleness is necessary. Oedema occurs when fluid leaks from capillaries into the interstitial space. There are a number of causes. Oedema may be pitting (the skin is indented and only slowly refills—Fig. 6.3) or non-pitting. Oedema due to hypoalbuminaemia often refills more quickly.[1]

The oedema that occurs in cardiac failure is pitting unless the condition has been present for a long time and secondary changes in the lymphatic vessels have occurred. If oedema is present, note its upper level (e.g. 'pitting oedema to mid-calf' or 'pitting oedema to mid-thigh'). Severe oedema can involve the skin of the abdominal wall and the scrotum as well as the lower limbs. Oedema secondary to fluid retention suggests about 6 litres or more is retained. Differential diagnosis and causes of oedema are listed in Lists 6.2 and 6.3 respectively.

Non-pitting oedema suggests chronic lymphoedema that is due to lymphatic obstruction (see Fig. 6.4). Myxoedema that occurs in thyroid disease is due to the accumulation of hydrophilic molecules in subcutaneous tissue.

The venous system

FIGURE 6.1

LOWER LIMB EXAMINATION

1. Inspection—anterior and lateral surfaces, sole of foot, between toes:
   - Amputation
   - Ulcers
   - Erythema
   - Varicosities
   - Atrophy
   - Scars
   - Discoloration (e.g. venous staining; see Fig. 6.2)
   - Loss of hair.
2. Palpation:
   - Temperature: run the dorsum of the hand from the hips to the foot on each side. Note any reduction in temperature peripherally and compare left and right.
   - Test capillary refill: press on the great toenail and release. The blanched nail bed should turn pink within 3 seconds.
   - Test venous filling: occlude the dorsal venous arch of each foot in turn using two fingers; release the distal finger and look for venous refilling. Absence of venous refilling suggests poor arterial supply to the foot.
   - Pulses: feel for an abdominal aortic aneurysm, femoral pulses, the popliteal pulses (flex the patient's leg), then the posterior tibial and dorsalis pedis pulses.
3. Auscultation:
   - Listen for abdominal, renal and femoral bruits.
4. Perform Buerger's test (see text).
5. Measure the ankle–brachial index.
6. Test lower limb sensation. Diabetes may cause sensory loss in a 'stocking' distribution.
7. Test for glucose in the urine.

LIST 6.1

Venous staining

(Courtesy of Dr A Watson, Infectious Diseases Department, The Canberra Hospital.)

FIGURE 6.2

Severe pitting oedema of the legs

FIGURE 6.3

ANKLE OEDEMA—DIFFERENTIAL DIAGNOSIS

Favours heart failure
History of cardiac failure
Other symptoms of heart failure
Jugular venous pressure elevated

Favours hypoproteinaemia
Jugular venous pressure normal
Oedema pits and refills rapidly, 2–3 s

Favours deep venous thrombosis or cellulitis
Unilateral
Skin erythema
Calf tenderness

Favours drug-induced oedema
Patient takes calcium channel blocker

Favours lymphoedema
Not worse at end of day
Not pitting when chronic

Favours lipoedema
Not pitting
Spares foot
Obese woman

(Khan NA, Rahim SA, Avand SS et al. Does the clinical examination predict lower extremity peripheral arterial disease? *JAMA* 2006; 295(5):536–546.)

LIST 6.2

CAUSES OF OEDEMA

Pitting lower limb oedema
Cardiac: congestive cardiac failure, constrictive pericarditis
Hepatic: cirrhosis causing hypoalbuminaemia
Renal: nephrotic syndrome causing hypoalbuminaemia
Gastrointestinal tract: malabsorption, starvation, protein-losing enteropathy causing hypoalbuminaemia (may be facial oedema)
Drugs: calcium antagonists
Joint disease in, or injury to, the leg
Venous abnormalities in the legs (e.g. varicose veins) including:
- Increased intravascular hydrostatic pressure (e.g. insufficiency of venous valves, cardiac failure)
- Reduced oncotic pressure (e.g. hypoalbuminaemia)
- Increased vessel wall permeability (e.g. inflammation or infection)

Beri-beri (wet)
Cyclical oedema

Pitting unilateral lower limb oedema
Deep venous thrombosis
Compression of large veins by tumour or lymph nodes

Non-pitting lower limb oedema
Hypothyroidism
Lymphoedema:
- Infectious (e.g. filariasis)
- Malignant (tumour invasion of lymphatics)
- Congenital (lymphatic development arrest)
- Allergy
- Milroy's* disease (unexplained lymphoedema that appears at puberty and is more common in females)

Myxoedema

*William Milroy (1855–1914), Professor of Medicine, University of Nebraska, described the disease in 1928.

LIST 6.3

Lymphoedema (elephantiasis)
(Courtesy of Dr A Watson, Infectious Diseases Department, The Canberra Hospital.)

FIGURE 6.4

Lipoedema is a term used to describe fat deposition in the ankles. It typically spares the feet and affects obese women.

Look for evidence of Achilles[a] tendon xanthomata due to hyperlipidaemia. Also look for cyanosis and clubbing of the toes (this may occur without finger clubbing in a patient with a patent ductus arteriosus, because a rise in pulmonary artery pressures sufficient to reverse the direction of flow in the shunt has occurred).

PERIPHERAL VASCULAR DISEASE

Examine both *femoral arteries* by palpating and then auscultating them. A bruit may be heard if the artery is narrowed. Next palpate the following pulses: *popliteal* (behind the knee—see Fig. 6.5(a): if this is difficult to feel when the patient is supine, try the method shown in Fig. 6.5(b)), *posterior tibial* (under the medial malleolus, see Fig. 6.6(a)) and *dorsalis pedis* (on the forefoot, Fig. 6.6(b)) on both sides.[2]

Patients with exertional calf pain (intermittent claudication) are likely to have disease of the peripheral arteries. More severe disease can lead to pain even at rest and to ischaemic changes in the legs and feet (see Good signs guide 6.1). Look for atrophic skin and loss of hair, colour changes of the feet (blue or red) and ulcers at the lower end of the tibia.[3] Venous and diabetic ulcers can be distinguished from arterial ulcers (see Figs 6.7–6.9).

Look for reduced capillary return (compress the toenails—the return of the normal red colour is slow).[4] In such cases, perform *Buerger's*[b] *test* to help confirm your diagnosis: elevate the legs to 45° (pallor is rapid if there is a poor arterial supply), then place them dependent at 90° over the edge of the bed (cyanosis occurs if the arterial supply is impaired). Normally there is no change in colour in either position.

Palpating the popliteal artery.

(a) Patient supine; (b) patient prone

FIGURE 6.5

The **ankle–brachial index** (ABI) is a measure of arterial supply to the lower limbs; an abnormal index indicates increased cardiovascular risk.[5] The systolic blood pressure in the dorsalis pedis or posterior tibial artery is measured using a Doppler probe and a blood pressure cuff over the calf. This is divided by the systolic blood pressure measured in the normal way at the brachial artery. An ABI of less than 0.9 indicates significant arterial disease and an ABI of between 0.4 and 0.9 is associated with claudication. An ABI of less than 0.4 is associated with critical limb ischaemia. An ABI greater than 1.3 occurs with a calcified (non-compressible) artery. A reduced ABI is also considered a risk factor for arterial disease elsewhere.

---

[a] Achilles, mythical Greek hero, whose body was invulnerable except for his heels, by which he was held when dipped in the River Styx as a baby to make him immortal. He was killed by Paris, who shot an arrow into his heel.
[b] Leo Buerger (1879–1943), New York physician, born in Vienna, who described thromboangiitis obliterans. He was obsessed with expensive cars.

114 SECTION 2 THE CARDIOVASCULAR SYSTEM

Feeling (a) the posterior tibial artery and (b) the dorsalis pedis artery

FIGURE 6.6

Venous ulcer.

This venous ulcer has an irregular margin, pale surrounding neoepithelium (new skin) and a pink base of granulation tissue. There is often a history of deep venous thrombosis. The skin is warm and oedema is often present. (See List 6.4.)

(From McDonald FS, ed. *Mayo Clinic images in internal medicine*, with permission. © Mayo Clinic Scientific Press and CRC Press. Reproduced by permission of Taylor and Francis Group, LLC, a division of Informa plc.)

FIGURE 6.7

GOOD SIGNS GUIDE 6.1
Peripheral vascular disease

Sign	LR+	LR−
Sores or ulcers on feet	5.9	0.98
Feet pale, red or blue	2.3	0.80
Atrophic skin	1.65	0.72
Absent hair	1.6	0.71
One foot cooler	5.9	0.92
Absent femoral pulse	5.8	0.94
Absent dorsalis pedis or posterior tibial pulse	3.7	0.37
Limb bruit present	5.7	0.58
Capillary refill time >5 seconds	1.9	0.84
Venous refill time >20 seconds	3.6	0.83
LR=likelihood ratio.		

ACUTE ARTERIAL OCCLUSION

Acute arterial occlusion of a major peripheral limb artery results in a painful, pulseless, pale, 'paralysed' limb that is perishingly cold and has paraesthesias (the six Ps). It can be the result of embolism, thrombosis or injury. Peripheral arterial embolism usually arises from thrombus in the heart, where it may be secondary to:

1. atrial fibrillation
2. myocardial infarction
3. dilated cardiomyopathy, or
4. infective endocarditis.[6]

DEEP VENOUS THROMBOSIS

Deep venous thrombosis (DVT) is a difficult clinical diagnosis.[7] The patient may complain of calf pain. On examination, the clinician should look for swelling of the calf and the thigh, and dilated superficial veins. Feel then for increased warmth and squeeze the calf (gently) to determine whether the area is tender. Homans'[c] sign (pain in the calf when the foot is sharply dorsiflexed, i.e. pushed up) is of limited diagnostic value and is theoretically dangerous because of the possibility of dislodgement of loose thrombus.

The causes of thrombosis were described by Virchow[d] in 1856 under three broad headings (the famous *Virchow's triad*):

1. changes in the vessel wall
2. changes in blood flow
3. changes in the constitution of the blood.

Deep venous thrombosis is usually caused by prolonged immobilisation (particularly after lower limb orthopaedic surgery), cardiac failure (stasis) or trauma (vessel wall damage), but may also result from neoplasm, sepsis, chronic inflammatory bowel disease, disseminated intravascular coagulation, the contraceptive pill, pregnancy and a number of inherited defects of coagulation (the *thrombophilias*: e.g. antithrombin III deficiency or the factor V Leiden mutation).

VARICOSE VEINS

If a patient complains of 'varicose veins', ask him or her to *stand* with the legs fully exposed.[8] *Inspect* the front of the whole leg for tortuous, dilated branches of the long saphenous vein (below the femoral vein in the groin to the medial side of the lower leg). Then inspect the back of the calf for varicosities of the short saphenous vein (from the back of the calf and lateral malleolus to the popliteal fossa). Look to see whether

Arterial ulcer.

This arterial ulcer has a regular margin and 'punched out' appearance. The surrounding skin is cold. The peripheral pulses are absent. (See List 6.4.)

(From McDonald FS, ed. *Mayo Clinic images in internal medicine*, with permission. © Mayo Clinic Scientific Press and CRC Press. Reproduced by permission of Taylor and Francis Group, LLC, a division of Informa plc.)

FIGURE 6.8

Diabetic (neuropathic) ulcer.

Neuropathic ulcers are painless and are associated with reduced sensation in the surrounding skin.

(From McDonald FS, ed. *Mayo Clinic images in internal medicine*, with permission. © Mayo Clinic Scientific Press and CRC Press. Reproduced by permission of Taylor and Francis Group, LLC, a division of Informa plc.)

FIGURE 6.9

---

[c] John Homans (1877–1954), a professor of surgery at Harvard University, Boston. He described his sign in 1941, originally in cases of thrombophlebitis. He later became disenchanted with the sign and is reputed to have asked why if a sign were to be named after him it couldn't be a useful one.

[d] Rudolph Virchow (1821–1902), a brilliant German pathologist, regarded as the founder of modern pathology, professor of pathological anatomy in Berlin. He provided the first description of leukaemia. He died aged 81 after fracturing his femur jumping from a moving tram.

the leg is inflamed, swollen or pigmented (subcutaneous haemosiderin deposition secondary to venous stasis).

Palpate the veins. Hard leg veins suggest thrombosis, whereas tenderness indicates thrombophlebitis. Perform the *cough impulse test*. Put the fingers over the long saphenous vein opening in the groin, medial to the femoral vein. (Do not forget the anatomy—femoral vein [medial], artery [your landmark], nerve [lateral].) Ask the patient to cough: a fluid thrill is felt if the saphenofemoral valve is incompetent.

The following supplementary tests are occasionally helpful (and surgeons like to quiz students on them in examinations):

- **Trendelenburg**[e] **test:** with the patient lying down, the leg is elevated. Firm pressure is placed on the saphenous opening in the groin, and the patient is instructed to stand. The sign is positive if the veins stay empty until the groin pressure is released (incompetence at the saphenofemoral valve). If the veins fill despite groin pressure, the incompetent valves are in the thigh or calf, and Perthes'[f] test is performed.
- **Perthes' test:** repeat the Trendelenburg test, but when the patient stands, allow some blood to be released and then get him or her to stand up and down on the toes a few times. The veins will become less tense if the perforating calf veins are patent and have competent valves (the muscle pump is functioning).

If the pattern of affected veins is unusual (e.g. pubic varices), try to exclude secondary varicose veins. These may be due to an intrapelvic neoplasm that has obstructed deep venous return. Rectal and pelvic examinations should then be performed.

CHRONIC VENOUS DISEASE

Chronic venous stasis is a common cause of leg oedema. It is a result of increased pressure in the venous system. There may be a history of previous deep venous thrombosis or of varicose veins. These are associated with incompetence of the valves of the perforating veins, which connect the deep and superficial veins of the legs. This can lead to dilation of the upper part of the long saphenous veins and make their valves incompetent. Failure of the muscle pump mechanism that directs blood up the veins can have similar effects. It is common in elderly inactive patients. Chronic venous stasis leads to oedema and a rise in tissue pressure, which causes thinning of skin and subcutaneous tissue. Skin ulceration and necrosis may occur.

Typically ulcers occur above the medial malleoli. Eventual healing often has inadequate circulation and skin will often break down again. The indurated skin is often stained a purple black colour; this is a result of staining with haemosiderin from red blood cells that have been extravasated into the tissues. Chronic venous eczema may complicate the condition. The legs appear more swollen and erythematous (Fig. 6.10). This is often misdiagnosed as cellulitis (skin infection), but cellulitis is never bilateral.

This chronic oedema is described as *brawny*. It will pit only slowly and unwillingly on compression. Signs of right heart failure (raised JVP and pulsatile liver, ascites) are absent.

The differential diagnosis of leg ulcers is summarised in List 6.4.

Chronic venous disease

(From Sieggreen M. *Nurs Clin North Am* 2005; 40(2):391–410, Fig 6. Philadelphia: Elsevier, June 2005, with permission.)

FIGURE 6.10

---

[e] Friedrich Trendelenburg (1844–1924), a professor of surgery in Leipzig.
[f] Georg Clemens Perthes (1869–1927), a German surgeon and professor of surgery at Tübingen. He was the first to use radiotherapy for the treatment of cancer (in 1903).

CAUSES OF LEG ULCERS

1. Venous stasis ulcer—most common (see Fig. 6.7)
   Site: around malleoli
   Character: irregular margin, granulation tissue in the floor. Surrounding tissue inflammation and oedema
   Associated pigmentation, stasis eczema
2. Ischaemic ulcer (see Fig. 6.8)
   - Large-artery disease (atherosclerosis, thromboangiitis obliterans): usually lateral side of leg (pulses absent)
   - Small-vessel disease (e.g. leucocytoclastic vasculitis): palpable purpura
   Site: over pressure areas, lateral malleolus, dorsum and margins of the feet and toes
   Character: smooth, rounded, 'punched out' pale base that does not bleed
3. Malignant ulcer, e.g. basal cell carcinoma (pearly translucent edge), squamous cell carcinoma (hard everted edge), melanoma, lymphoma, Kaposi's sarcoma
4. Infection, e.g. *Staphylococcus aureus*, syphilitic gumma, tuberculosis, atypical *Mycobacterium*, fungal
5. Neuropathic (painless penetrating ulcer on sole of foot: peripheral neuropathy, e.g. diabetes mellitus, tabes [tertiary syphilis], leprosy) (see Fig. 6.9)
6. Underlying systemic disease
   - Diabetes mellitus: vascular disease, neuropathy or necrobiosis lipoidica (front of leg)
   - Pyoderma gangrenosum
   - Rheumatoid arthritis
   - Lymphoma
   - Haemolytic anaemia (small ulcers over malleoli), e.g. sickle cell anaemia

LIST 6.4

T&O'C ESSENTIALS

1. Peripheral oedema is not a specific sign of cardiac failure.
2. Always consider non-cardiac causes of oedema: venous abnormalities, calcium antagonist drugs, hypoalbuminaemia.
3. Claudication (calf pain when walking a certain distance) should prompt assessment of the peripheral pulses.
4. Failure of a leg ulcer to heal should lead to a suspicion of peripheral vascular disease or diabetes, or both.
5. A painless ulcer is very suggestive of the presence of a peripheral neuropathy, often as a result of diabetes.

OSCE EXAMPLE – PERIPHERAL VASCULAR DISEASE

Mr Claude has had pain in his calves when walking more than 100 metres. Please examine his lower limbs.

1. Wash your hands, introduce yourself and explain that you would like to examine Mr Claude's legs.
2. Ask whether you may expose them from the upper thighs to the feet.
3. Inspect for cyanosis, muscle wasting, loss of hair or nails, and ulcers.
4. Note oedema or venous staining and the presence of varicose veins.
5. Feel the temperature of the legs and feet, and compare each side, using the back of your hand.
6. Feel for the posterior tibial and dorsalis pedis pulses on each side (remember which is which).
7. If these are absent or reduced, feel the popliteal pulses and if necessary the femoral pulses.
8. Thank the patient.
9. Wash your hands.
10. Describe your findings.

OSCE REVISION TOPICS

1. Examine this woman, who has varicose veins. (p 115)
2. Examine this woman, who has peripheral oedema. (p 109)
3. This man has a leg ulcer; please examine him. (pp 109, 117)

References

1. Whiting E, McCready M. Pitting and non-pitting oedema. *Med J Aust* 2016; 205(4):157–158.
2. Magee TR, Stanley P, Mufti R et al. Should we palpate foot pulses? *Ann Roy Coll Surg Eng* 1992; 74:166–168. Elderly patients who do not have a palpable dorsalis pedis pulse will often have adequate perfusion (unless there is clinical evidence of claudication or foot ulcers). Palpation of the dorsalis pedis is more helpful than the posterior tibial.
3. Khan NA, Rahim SA, Avand SS et al. Does the clinical examination predict lower extremity peripheral arterial disease? *JAMA* 2006; 295(5):536–546.
4. McGee SR, Boyko EJ. Physical examination and chronic lower-extremity ischemia: a critical review. *Arch Intern Med* 1998; 158:1357–1364. The presence of peripheral arterial disease is positively predicted by abnormal pedal pulses, a unilaterally cool extremity, prolonged venous filling time and a femoral bruit.
5. Organ N. How to perform the ankle brachial index (ABI) in clinical practice. *MJA* 2017; in press. Provides practical advice and the likelihood ratios for this bedside test.
6. O'Keefe ST, Woods BO, Breslin DJ, Tsapatsaris NP. Blue toe syndrome. Causes and management. *Arch Intern Med* 1992; 152:2197–2202. Explains how to identify the cause by clinical methods and directed investigations.
7. Anand SS, Wells PS, Hunt D et al. Does this patient have deep venous thrombosis? *JAMA* 1998; 279:1094–1099. The sensitivity of individual symptoms and signs is 60%–96% and the specificity 20%–72%. Patients can be subdivided into those with a low, intermediate or high pretest probability, based on risk factors and clinical features.
8. Butie A. Clinical examination of varicose veins. *Dermat Surg* 1995; 21:52–56. Techniques are outlined and compared with Doppler ultrasound assessment.

CHAPTER 7
Correlation of physical signs disease and cardiovascular disease

When a disease is named after some author, it is very likely that we don't know much about it.
AUGUST BIER (1861–1949)

CARDIAC FAILURE

Cardiac failure is one of the most common syndromes: the signs of cardiac failure should be sought in all patients admitted to hospital, especially if there is a complaint of dyspnoea (see Questions box 9.2, p 167).[1] Cardiac failure has been defined as a reduction in cardiac function such that cardiac output is reduced relative to the metabolic demands of the body and compensating mechanisms have occurred. The specific signs depend on whether the left, right or both ventricles are involved. It is important to note that the absence of definite signs of cardiac failure may not exclude the diagnosis. Patients with compensated, chronic cardiac failure may be normal on cardiac examination.

Findings that favour heart failure as the cause of dyspnoea

History of myocardial infarction
No wheeze
Paroxysmal nocturnal dyspnoea (PND)
Orthopnoea
Cough only on lying down
Abnormal apex beat
Third heart sound (S3)
Mitral regurgitant murmur
Early and mid-inspiratory crackles

LIST 7.1

Left ventricular failure (LVF)

- **Symptoms:** exertional dyspnoea, orthopnoea, paroxysmal nocturnal dyspnoea.
- **General signs:** tachypnoea, due to raised pulmonary pressures; central cyanosis, due to pulmonary oedema; Cheyne–Stokes breathing (see Table 9.4, p 170), especially in sedated elderly patients; peripheral cyanosis, due to low cardiac output; hypotension, due to low cardiac output; cardiac cachexia (see List 7.1).
- **Arterial pulse:** sinus tachycardia, due to increased sympathetic tone; low pulse pressure (low cardiac output); pulsus alternans (alternate strong and weak beats; it is unlike a bigeminal rhythm caused by regular ectopic beats, in that the beats are regular; see Fig. 7.1)—this is a rare but specific sign of unknown aetiology.

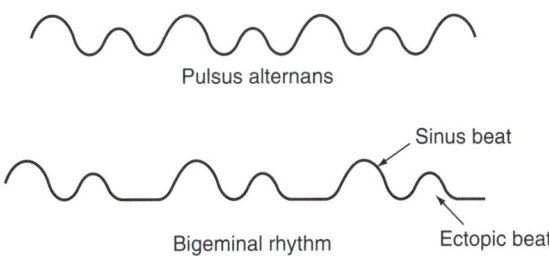

Pulsus alternans

FIGURE 7.1

- **Apex beat:** displaced, with dilation of the left ventricle; it may feel dyskinetic if the patient has had an anterior myocardial infarction or has a dilated cardiomyopathy; a gallop rhythm may be palpable. The absence of these signs does not exclude left ventricular failure.

- **Auscultation:** left ventricular S3 (an important sign); functional mitral regurgitation (secondary to valve ring dilation).
- **Lung fields:** signs of pulmonary congestion (basal inspiratory crackles) or pulmonary oedema (crackles and wheezes throughout the lung fields), due to raised venous pressures (increased preload). The typical middle-to-late inspiratory crackles at the lung bases may be absent in chronic, compensated heart failure, and there are many other causes of basal inspiratory crackles. This makes crackles a rather non-specific and insensitive sign of heart failure.
- **Other signs:** positive abdominojugular reflux test; signs of RVF, which may complicate or accompany LVF, especially if this is severe and chronic.
- **Signs of the underlying or precipitating cause:**
  - *Causes of LVF:* (1) myocardial disease (ischaemic heart disease, cardiomyopathy); (2) volume overload (aortic regurgitation, mitral regurgitation (occasionally acute—ruptured cord), patent ductus arteriosus); (3) pressure overload (systolic hypertension, aortic stenosis).
  - *Signs of a precipitating cause:* anaemia, systemic infection, thyrotoxicosis (p 448), rapid arrhythmia (usually atrial fibrillation). (See Good signs guide 7.1.)

Right ventricular failure (RVF)

- **Symptoms:** ankle, sacral or abdominal swelling, anorexia, lethargy, nausea.
- **General signs:** peripheral cyanosis, due to low cardiac output.
- **Arterial pulse:** low volume, due to low cardiac output.
- **Jugular venous pressure (JVP):** raised, due to the raised venous pressure (right heart preload); Kussmaul's sign, due to poor right ventricular compliance (e.g. right ventricular myocardial infarction); large *v* waves (functional tricuspid regurgitation secondary to valve ring dilation).
- Praecordial palpation; parasternal impulse (right ventricular heave).

GOOD SIGNS GUIDE 7.1
Left ventricular failure in a patient with dyspnoea

General signs	LR+	LR−
Heart rate >100 beats per minute at rest	5.5	NS
Abdominojugular reflux test	6.4	0.79
LUNGS		
Crackles	2.8	0.5
CARDIAC EXAMINATION		
JVP elevated	5.1	0.66
S4 (4th heart sound)	NS	NS
Apex displaced lateral to midclavicular line	5.8	NS
S3 (3rd heart sound)	11	0.88
Any murmur	2.6	0.81
OTHER FINDINGS		
Oedema	2.3	0.64
Wheezing	0.22	1.3
Ascites	0.33	1.0
THE HISTORY (GOOD SYMPTOMS GUIDE)		
PND	2.6	0.7
Orthopnoea	2.2	0.65
Dyspnoea on exertion	1.3	0.48
Fatigue and weight gain	1.0	0.99
Previous heart failure	5.8	0.45
Previous myocardial infarction	3.1	0.69
Hypertension	1.4	0.7
COPD	0.81	1.1

COPD=chronic obstructive pulmonary disease; LR=likelihood ratio; NS=not significant; PND=paroxysmal nocturnal dyspnoea.

- **Auscultation:** right ventricular S3; pansystolic murmur of functional tricuspid regurgitation (absence of a murmur does not exclude tricuspid regurgitation).
- **Abdomen:** tender hepatomegaly, due to increased venous pressure transmitted via the hepatic veins; pulsatile liver (a useful sign), if tricuspid regurgitation is present.
- **Oedema:** due to sodium and water retention plus raised venous pressure; may be manifested by pitting ankle and sacral oedema, ascites or pleural effusions (small).

- **Signs of the underlying cause:**
  - *Causes of RVF:* (1) chronic obstructive pulmonary disease (most common cause of cor pulmonale); (2) LVF (severe chronic LVF causes raised pulmonary pressures resulting in secondary RVF); (3) volume overload (atrial septal defect, primary tricuspid regurgitation); (4) other causes of pressure overload (pulmonary stenosis, idiopathic pulmonary hypertension); (5) myocardial disease (right ventricular myocardial infarction, cardiomyopathy).

CHEST PAIN

Many of the causes of chest pain represent a medical (or surgical) emergency. The appropriate diagnosis or differential diagnosis is often suggested by the history, and urgent investigations (e.g. ECG [see the OCSE ECGs 31, 33, 34, 35, 37, 39, 49 at Student CONSULT], chest X-ray, lung scan or computed tomography pulmonary angiogram [CTPA]) may be indicated. However, a careful and rapid physical examination may add important information in many cases. In all cases the general inspection and measurement of the vital signs will help with the assessment of the severity and urgency of the problem. Certain specific signs may help with the diagnosis.[2,3]

Myocardial infarction or acute coronary syndrome

- **General signs:** there are few specific signs of myocardial infarction but many patients appear obviously unwell and in distress from their chest pain. Sweating (often called diaphoresis by accident and emergency staff), an appearance of anxiety (*angor animi* or sense of impending doom) and restlessness may be obvious. It is important that all of this information be recorded so that changes to the patient's condition can be assessed as the infarct evolves.
- **Pulse and blood pressure (BP):** tachycardia and/or hypotension (25% with anterior infarction from sympathetic hyperactivity); bradycardia and/or hypotension (up to 50% with inferior infarction from parasympathetic hyperactivity). Other arrhythmias including atrial fibrillation (due to atrial infarction), ventricular tachycardia and heart block may be present.
- **Jugular venous pressure (JVP):** increased with right ventricular infarction; Kussmaul's sign is a specific and sensitive sign of right ventricular infarction in patients with a recent inferior infarct.
- **Apex beat:** dyskinetic in patients with large anterior infarction.
- **Auscultation:** S4; S3; decreased intensity of heart sounds; transient apical midsystolic or late-systolic murmur (in 25% from mitral regurgitation secondary to papillary muscle dysfunction), or a pericardial friction rub (usually occurs only some days later).
- **Complications:** arrhythmias (ventricular tachycardia, atrial fibrillation, ventricular fibrillation or heart block); heart failure; cardiogenic shock; rupture of a papillary muscle; perforation of the ventricular septum; ventricular aneurysm; thromboembolism or cardiac rupture. Signs of these complications (which do not usually occur for a few days after the infarct) include the development of a new murmur, recurrent chest pain, dyspnoea, sudden hypotension or sudden death.

The **Killip**[a] **Class** can be calculated from the examination. It gives considerable prognostic information:[2]

Killip Class I	No evidence of heart failure.
Killip Class II	Mild heart failure; crackles over lower third or less of the lungs; systolic BP >90 mmHg.
Killip Class III	Pulmonary oedema, crackles more than one-third of chest; systolic BP >90 mmHg.
Killip Class IV	Cardiogenic shock, pulmonary oedema, crackles more than one-third of chest, systolic BP <90 mmHg.

Killip Class III or IV is associated with a greater than fivefold mortality risk and Class II with a greater than threefold risk compared with Class I.

---

[a] T Killip, a New Zealand cardiologist, published his classification in 1967.

Pulmonary embolism

There may be no physical signs of this condition, but dyspnoea (which may be profound and make the patient exhausted) is often the most common sign of a large pulmonary embolism. There is usually a resting tachycardia. Signs of shock—hypotension and cyanosis—indicate a very large and life-threatening embolus. There may be signs of deep vein thrombosis (DVT) in the legs, but absence of these by no means excludes the diagnosis.

Acute aortic dissection

Acute aortic dissection is a difficult diagnosis that cannot usually be excluded on clinical grounds. A tear in the intima leads to blood surging into the aortic media separating the intima and adventitia; this may present acutely or chronically. There are three different types: *type I* begins in the ascending aorta and extends proximally and distally, *type II* is limited to the ascending aorta and aortic arch (this is particularly associated with Marfan's syndrome), and *type III* begins distal to the left subclavian artery and has the best prognosis.

- **Symptoms:**
  - Chest pain (typically very severe, it radiates to the back and is maximal in intensity at the time of onset due to either the aortic tear or associated myocardial infarction).
  - Stroke.
  - Syncope (associated with tamponade); symptoms of left ventricular failure.
  - Rarely, limb pain (ischaemia), paraplegia (spinal cord ischaemia) or abdominal pain (mesenteric ischaemia).
- **Signs:** the examination can reveal signs that make the diagnosis very likely (specific but not sensitive).
  - There may be signs of a body habitus associated with dissection (e.g. Marfan's or Ehlers–Danlos syndrome).
  - A diminution of the radial pulse on one side or a difference in blood pressure of 20 mmHg or more between the arms is significant and suggests dissection has progressed to involve the origin of the arm vessels.
  - Examine the patient for signs of pericardial tamponade (p 123), which occurs if the aorta ruptures into the pericardial sac. Examine the heart for signs of aortic regurgitation caused by disruption of the aortic valve annulus. A neurological examination may reveal signs of hemiplegia, due to dissection of one of the carotid arteries. Rare signs that have been described include a pulsatile sternoclavicular joint, hoarseness (recurrent laryngeal nerve compression) and dysphagia (oesophageal compression). A tracheal tug (p 179; Oliver's sign) may be present if there is already an aneurysm of the aortic arch.[b] The dilated vessel crosses the left main bronchus and pulls the trachea down during systole.

PERICARDIAL DISEASE

Acute pericarditis

- **Signs:** fever; dyspnoea; pericardial friction rub—sit the patient up and listen to the heart with the patient holding his or her breath in deep expiration (see the OCSE ECG 38 at Student CONSULT).
- **Causes of acute pericarditis:**
  1. Viral infection (coxsackie virus A or B, influenza).
  2. After myocardial infarction—early, or late (10–14 days, termed Dressler's syndrome[c]).
  3. After pericardiotomy (cardiac surgery).
  4. Chronic kidney disease.
  5. Neoplasia—tumour invasion (e.g. bronchus, breast, lymphoma) or after irradiation for tumour.
  6. Connective tissue disease (e.g. systemic lupus erythematosus, rheumatoid arthritis).
  7. Hypothyroidism.
  8. Other infections (e.g. tuberculosis, pyogenic pneumonia or septicaemia).
  9. Acute rheumatic fever.

---

[b] Although described now chiefly in association with severe asthma and chronic obstructive pulmonary disease (COPD), this sign was originally described by William Oliver (1836–1908), a Canadian military surgeon, in 1878 as a sign of a thoracic aortic aneurysm; it has been taken over by the chest doctors and paediatricians.

[c] William Dressler (1890–1969), a New York cardiologist, described this syndrome in 1956.

Chronic constrictive pericarditis

- **General signs:** cachexia.
- **Pulse and blood pressure:** pulsus paradoxus (more than the normal 10 mmHg fall in the arterial pulse pressure on inspiration, because increased right ventricular filling compresses the left ventricle); low blood pressure.
- **JVP:** raised; Kussmaul's sign—lack of a fall or even increased distension on inspiration (50%); prominent x and y descents (brisk collapse during diastole).
- **Apex beat:** impalpable.
- **Auscultation:** heart sounds distant, early S3; early pericardial knock (rapid ventricular filling abruptly halted).
- **Abdomen:** hepatomegaly, due to raised venous pressure; splenomegaly, due to raised venous pressure; ascites.
- **Peripheral oedema.**
- **Causes of chronic constrictive pericarditis include:**
  1. cardiac operation or trauma
  2. tuberculosis, histoplasmosis or pyogenic infection
  3. neoplastic disease
  4. mediastinal irradiation
  5. connective tissue disease (especially rheumatoid arthritis)
  6. chronic kidney disease.

Acute cardiac tamponade

- **General signs:** tachypnoea; anxiety and restlessness; syncope. Patients look very ill.
- **Pulse and blood pressure:** rapid pulse rate; pulsus paradoxus; hypotension.
- **JVP:** raised; prominent x but an absent y descent.
- **Apex beat:** impalpable.
- **Auscultation:** soft (muffled) heart sounds.
- **Lungs:** dullness and bronchial breathing at the left base, due to lung compression by the distended pericardial sac.

Example of an intravenous drug addict's forearm

FIGURE 7.2

Infective endocarditis

- **General signs:** fever; weight loss; pallor (anaemia).
- **Hands:** splinter haemorrhages; clubbing (within 6 weeks of onset); Osler's nodes (rare); Janeway lesions (very rare).
- **Arms:** evidence of intravenous drug use (see Fig. 7.2)—right (and left) heart endocarditis can result from this.
- **Eyes:** pale conjunctivae (anaemia); retinal or conjunctival haemorrhages—Roth's spots[d] are fundal vasculitic lesions with a yellow centre surrounded by a red ring (see Fig. 7.3).
- **Heart**—signs of *underlying heart disease*:
  1. acquired (mitral regurgitation, mitral stenosis, aortic stenosis, aortic regurgitation)
  2. congenital (patent ductus arteriosus, ventricular septal defect, coarctation of the aorta)
  3. prosthetic valves.
- **Abdomen:** splenomegaly.
- **Peripheral evidence of embolisation** to limbs or central nervous system. This may manifest as mycotic aneurysms or erythematous nodules on the skin (toes, ankles, buttocks), while large emboli may cause an ischaemic limb or stroke.
- **Urinalysis:** haematuria (a fresh urine specimen will then show dysmorphic red cells and red cell casts on microscopy).

---

[d] Moritz von Roth (1839–1914), a Swiss physician and pathologist, described these changes in 1872.

124 SECTION 2 THE CARDIOVASCULAR SYSTEM

Roth's spot on fundoscopy
(Courtesy of Dr Chris Kennedy and Professor Ian Constable ©Lions Eye Institute, Perth.)

FIGURE 7.3

Hypertensive retinopathy grade 3.

Note the flame-shaped haemorrhages and cottonwool spots
(Courtesy of Dr Chris Kennedy and Professor Ian Constable ©Lions Eye Institute, Perth.)

FIGURE 7.4

SYSTEMIC HYPERTENSION

It is important to have in mind a method for the examination of a patient with systemic hypertension (see the OSCE CVS examination video at Student CONSULT). The examination aims to measure the blood pressure level, determine whether there is an underlying cause present and assess the severity as determined by signs of end-organ damage. It is a common clinical problem.

On **general inspection** the signs of the rare causes of secondary hypertension must be sought—for example, Cushing's[e] syndrome, acromegaly, polycythaemia or chronic kidney disease.

Take the **blood pressure**, with the patient lying and standing, using an appropriately sized cuff. A rise in diastolic pressure on standing occurs typically in essential hypertension; a fall on standing may suggest a secondary cause, but is usually an effect of antihypertensive medications.

- Palpate for radiofemoral delay, and check the blood pressure in the legs if coarctation of the aorta is suspected or if severe hypertension is discovered before 30 years of age.

- Next examine the **fundi** for retinal changes of hypertension (see Figs 7.4 and 7.5), which can be classified from grades 1 to 4:

  Grade 1 'Silver wiring' of the arteries only (sclerosis of the vessel wall reduces its transparency so that the central light streak becomes broader and shinier).

  Grade 2 Grade 1 plus arteriovenous nipping or nicking (indentation or deflection of the veins where they are crossed by the arteries).

  Grade 3 Grade 2 plus haemorrhages (flame-shaped) and exudates (soft—cottonwool spots due to ischaemia; or hard—lipid residues from leaking vessels).

  Grade 4 Grade 3 plus papilloedema.

Describe the changes present rather than just giving a grade.

---

[e] Harvey Cushing (1869–1939), a professor of surgery at Harvard University and 'founder of neurosurgery', friend of Osler and prize-winning writer of Osler's biography in 1925.

Hypertensive retinopathy grade 4.

Note arteriovenous nipping, silver wiring and papilloedema

(Courtesy of Dr Chris Kennedy and Professor Ian Constable ©Lions Eye Institute, Perth.)

FIGURE 7.5

Causes of systemic hypertension

Hypertension may be essential or idiopathic (more than 95% of cases), or secondary (less than 5%). Immoderate alcohol and salt consumption and obesity (see Questions box 4.5, p 70) are associated with hypertension. Obstructive sleep apnoea is also an association.

Secondary causes include:

1. renal disease—renal artery stenosis, chronic pyelonephritis, analgesic nephropathy, connective tissue disease, glomerulonephritis, polycystic disease, diabetic nephropathy, reflux nephropathy
2. endocrine disorders—Cushing's syndrome, Conn's syndrome (primary aldosteronism), phaeochromocytoma, acromegaly, thyrotoxicosis, hypothyroidism, hyperparathyroidism
3. coarctation of the aorta
4. other, such as the contraceptive pill, amphetamine, cocaine, polycythaemia rubra vera, toxaemia of pregnancy, neurogenic causes (increased intracranial pressure, lead poisoning, acute porphyria), hypercalcaemia.

Now examine the **rest of the cardiovascular system** for signs of left ventricular failure secondary to hypertension and for coarctation of the aorta. A fourth heart sound is frequently detectable if the blood pressure is greater than 180/110 mmHg.

Then go to the **abdomen** to palpate for renal or adrenal masses (possible causes) and for the presence of an abdominal aortic aneurysm (a possible complication). Auscultate for a renal bruit (p 261) due to renal artery stenosis.[4] Remember that most left-sided abdominal bruits arise from the splenic artery and are of no significance. A bruit is less likely to be significant if it is short, soft and midsystolic. A loud systolic–diastolic bruit that is prominent in the epigastrium is more likely to be associated with renal artery stenosis.

Examine the **central nervous system** for signs of previous cerebrovascular accidents, and palpate and auscultate the **carotid arteries** for bruits (however, see pp 105 and 537 for a discussion of the accuracy of this examination). Stenosis may be a manifestation of vascular disease, and may be associated with renal artery stenosis. **Urinalysis** should also be performed to look for evidence of renal disease.

Complications of hypertension

These include left ventricular failure, cerebrovascular ischaemic events (strokes), renal failure and eye disease (blindness). Hypertension is also a risk factor for ischaemic heart disease and peripheral vascular disease, including abdominal aortic aneurysm and arterial dissections (see the OCSE ECG 43 at Student CONSULT).

Malignant (accelerated) hypertension

This can be defined as the presence of flame-shaped haemorrhages, cottonwool spots and/or papilloedema (≥grade 3 retinal changes) as a result of severe hypertension. These patients need admission to hospital for urgent treatment.

PULMONARY HYPERTENSION

Mean pulmonary artery pressures higher than 25 mmHg and systolic pressures of more than 50 mmHg are abnormal and constitute pulmonary hypertension. Symptoms of pulmonary hypertension do not usually occur until the pressures are about twice normal (i.e. >50 mmHg). Exertional dyspnoea and fatigue are then common, and chest pain possibly due to right ventricular ischaemia occurs in up to 50% of patients. It is important to know what signs to look for in a patient who may have pulmonary hypertension.

- **General signs** (usually only in patients with severe pulmonary hypertension): tachypnoea; peripheral cyanosis and cold extremities, due to low cardiac output; hoarseness (very rare, due to pulmonary artery compression of the left recurrent laryngeal nerve).
- **Pulse:** usually of small volume, due to the low cardiac output (only in severe disease).
- **JVP:** prominent *a* wave, due to forceful right atrial contraction.
- **Apex beat/praecordium:** right ventricular heave; palpable P2.
- **Auscultation:** systolic ejection click, due to dilation of the pulmonary artery; loud P2,[f] due to forceful valve closure because of high pulmonary artery pressures; S4; pulmonary ejection murmur, due to dilation of the pulmonary artery resulting in turbulent blood flow; murmur of pulmonary regurgitation if dilation of the pulmonary artery occurs.
- **Signs of right ventricular failure** (late: termed *cor pulmonale*).

Causes of pulmonary hypertension

Pulmonary hypertension may be idiopathic (primary) or rarely hereditary or secondary. Secondary causes include:

1. pulmonary emboli—e.g. blood clots, tumour particles, fat globules
2. lung disease—COPD (p 195), obstructive sleep apnoea, interstitial lung disease (ILD)
3. connective tissue disease (with or without ILD), e.g. scleroderma
4. left ventricular failure resulting in back-pressure into the pulmonary circulation or mitral stenosis
5. congenital heart disease causing a large left-to-right shunt—atrial septal defect, ventricular septal defect, patent ductus arteriosus
6. severe kyphoscoliosis.

INNOCENT MURMURS

The detection of a systolic murmur on routine examination is a common problem. It can cause considerable alarm to both the patient and the examining clinician. These murmurs in asymptomatic people are often the result of normal turbulence within the heart and great vessels. When no structural abnormality of the heart or great vessels is present these are called *innocent*, *functional* or *organic* murmurs. They probably arise from vibrations within the aortic arch near the origins of the head and neck vessels or from the right ventricular outflow tract. They are more common in children and young adults. They are louder just after exercise and during febrile illnesses (a common time for them to be detected).

Innocent murmurs are always systolic. (A venous hum, which is not really a murmur, has both systolic and diastolic components.) They are usually soft and ejection-systolic in character. Those arising from the aortic arch may radiate to the carotids and be heard in the neck. Those arising from the right ventricular outflow tract are loudest in the pulmonary area and may have a scratchy quality. These outflow tract murmurs must be distinguished from the pulmonary flow murmur of an atrial septal defect. Therefore it is important to listen carefully for wide or fixed splitting of the second heart sound before pronouncing a murmur innocent (see Questions box 7.1).

VALVE DISEASES OF THE LEFT HEART

(See Table 7.1.)

Mitral stenosis

The normal area of the mitral valve is 4 to 6 cm². Reduction of the valve area to half normal or less causes significant obstruction to left ventricular filling, and

---

[f] This traditional sign is not very helpful. A loud P2 is more likely to mean the patient is thin rather than that there is pulmonary hypertension; a palpable P2 is more significant.

blood will flow from the left atrium to the left ventricle only if the left atrial pressure is raised.

- **Symptoms:** dyspnoea, orthopnoea, paroxysmal nocturnal dyspnoea (increased left atrial pressure); haemoptysis (ruptured bronchial veins); ascites, oedema, fatigue (pulmonary hypertension).

- **General signs:** tachypnoea; 'mitral facies'; peripheral cyanosis (severe mitral stenosis).
- **Pulse and blood pressure:** normal or reduced in volume, due to a reduced cardiac output; atrial fibrillation may be present because of left atrial enlargement.
- **JVP:** normal; prominent *a* wave if pulmonary hypertension is present; loss of the *a* wave if the patient is in atrial fibrillation.
- **Palpation:** tapping quality of the apex beat (palpable S1); right ventricular heave (parasternal impulse) and palpable P2 if pulmonary hypertension is present; diastolic thrill rarely (lay patient on the left side).
- **Auscultation** (see Fig. 7.6): loud S1 (valve cusps widely apart at the onset of systole)—this also indicates that the valve cusps remain mobile; loud or perhaps rather palpable P2 if pulmonary hypertension is present; opening snap (high left atrial pressure forces the valve cusps apart, but the valve cone is halted abruptly); low-pitched rumbling diastolic murmur (best heard with the bell of the stethoscope with the patient in the left lateral position, and quite different in quality and timing from the murmur of aortic regurgitation); a late diastolic accentuation of the diastolic murmur may occur if the patient is in sinus rhythm, but is usually absent if atrial fibrillation has supervened—this is best heard in the left

> ### QUESTIONS TO ASK THE PATIENT WITH A HEART MURMUR
>
> 1. Has anyone noticed this murmur before? Were any tests done?
> 2. Did you have rheumatic fever as a child?
> 3. Have you been told you need antibiotics before dental work or surgical operations?
> 4. Have you become breathless when you exert yourself?
> 5. Have you had chest tightness during exercise? (Aortic stenosis)
> 6. Have you had dizziness or a blackout during heavy exercise? (Severe aortic stenosis)
> 7. Have you been breathless lying flat? (Heart failure complicating valve disease)
>
> QUESTIONS BOX 7.1

Mitral stenosis.

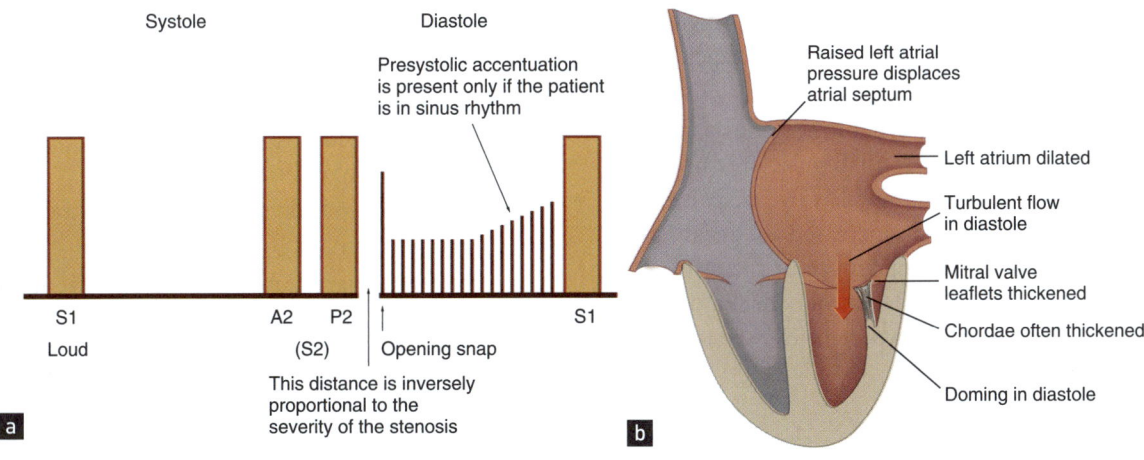

(a) Murmur, at the apex; (b) anatomy

FIGURE 7.6

Features of important valve lesions and congenital abnormalities

	Site	Timing	Radiation	Character	Accentuation and manoeuvres	Other features
Aortic regurgitation	Aortic area	Early diastolic	Lower left sternal edge	Decrescendo	Expiration, patient leaning forwards	Wide pulse pressure, eponymous signs
Aortic stenosis	Aortic area	Systolic	Carotids	Ejection	Expiration	Separate from heart sounds, slow-rising pulse
Mitral stenosis	Apex	Middle and late diastolic	—	Low-pitched (use stethoscope bell)	Presystolic accentuation, left lateral position, exercise	Loud S1, opening snap
Mitral regurgitation	Apex	Pansystolic or middle and late systolic (mitral valve prolapse)	Axilla or left sternal edge	Blowing (MVP)	Longer and louder with Valsalva (MVP)	Parasternal impulse (enlarges left atrium)
Ventricular septal defect	Lower left sternal edge	Pansystolic	None	Localised	—	Often associated with a thrill
Tricuspid regurgitation	Lower left and right sternal edge	Pansystolic	—	—	Louder on inspiration	Big *v* waves, pulsatile liver
Hypertrophic cardiomyopathy	Apex and left sternal edge	Late systolic at left sternal edge, pansystolic at apex	—	—	Louder with Valsalva, softer with squatting	S4, double-impulse apex beat, jerky carotid pulse

MVP = mitral valve prolapse.

TABLE 7.1

lateral position; exercise accentuates the murmur (ask the patient to sit up and down quickly in bed several times).[g]
- **Signs indicating severe mitral stenosis** (valve area less than 1 cm^2): small pulse pressure; soft first heart sound (immobile valve cusps); early opening snap (due to increased left atrial pressure); long diastolic murmur (persists as long as there is a gradient); diastolic thrill at the apex; signs of pulmonary hypertension (see the OCSE ECG 45 at Student CONSULT).

- **Causes of mitral stenosis include:**
  1. rheumatic (following acute rheumatic fever)
  2. severe mitral annular calcification, sometimes associated with hypercalcaemia and hyperparathyroidism
  3. rarely after mitral valve repair for mitral regurgitation
  4. congenital parachute valve (all chordae insert into one papillary muscle—rare).

Mitral regurgitation (chronic)

A regurgitant mitral valve allows part of the left ventricular stroke volume to regurgitate into the left atrium, imposing a volume load on both the left atrium and the left ventricle.

---

[g] This murmur is famously difficult to identify. Fewer than 10% of medical students identified the murmur on a standardised audiotape.

- **Symptoms:** dyspnoea (increased left atrial pressure); fatigue (decreased cardiac output).
- **General signs:** tachypnoea.
- **Pulse:** normal, or sharp upstroke due to rapid left ventricular decompression; atrial fibrillation is relatively common.
- **Palpation:** the apex beat is displaced, diffuse and hyperdynamic; a pansystolic thrill is occasionally present at the apex; a parasternal impulse may be present (owing to left atrial enlargement behind the right ventricle—the left atrium is often larger in mitral regurgitation than in mitral stenosis and can be enormous).
- **Auscultation** (see Fig. 7.7): soft or absent S1 (by the end of diastole, atrial and ventricular pressures have equalised and the valve cusps have drifted back together); left ventricular S3, which is due to rapid left ventricular filling in early diastole and, when soft, does not imply severe regurgitation; pansystolic murmur maximal at the apex and usually radiating towards the axilla.
- **Signs indicating severe chronic mitral regurgitation:** small volume pulse; enlarged left ventricle; loud S3; soft S1; A2 is early, because rapid left ventricular decompression into the left atrium causes the aortic valve to close early; early diastolic rumble; signs of pulmonary hypertension; signs of left ventricular failure.
- **Causes of chronic mitral regurgitation include:**
  1. mitral valve prolapse
  2. 'degenerative'—associated with ageing
  3. rheumatic
  4. papillary muscle dysfunction, due to left ventricular failure or ischaemia
  5. cardiomyopathy—hypertrophic, dilated or restrictive cardiomyopathy
  6. connective tissue disease (e.g. Marfan's syndrome, rheumatoid arthritis, ankylosing spondylitis)
  7. congenital (e.g. atrioventricular canal defect).

Acute mitral regurgitation

In this case patients can present with pulmonary oedema and cardiovascular collapse. The murmur may be softer and lower pitched than that of severe chronic mitral regurgitation. It tends to be short and may be decrescendo (i.e. declines in intensity towards the end of systole) because atrial pressure is increased.

With anterior leaflet chordae rupture the murmur radiates to the axilla and back; with posterior leaflet rupture the murmur radiates to the cardiac base and carotids.

Mitral regurgitation.

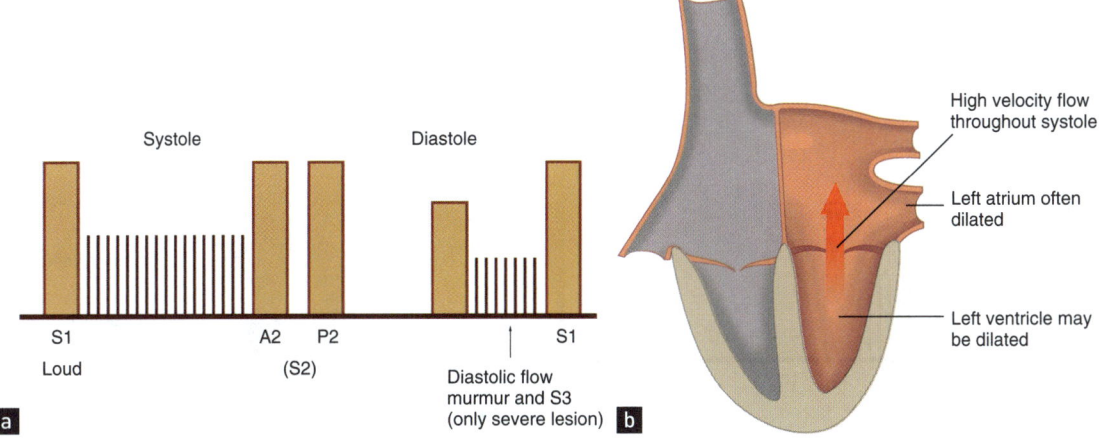

(a) Murmur, at the apex; (b) anatomy

FIGURE 7.7

- **Causes of acute mitral regurgitation include:**
  1. myocardial infarction (dysfunction or rupture of papillary muscles)
  2. infective endocarditis
  3. trauma or surgery
  4. spontaneous rupture of a myxomatous cord (sometimes during exercise).

Mitral valve prolapse (MVP, systolic-click murmur syndrome)

This syndrome can cause a systolic murmur or click, or both, at the apex. The presence of the murmur indicates that there is some mitral regurgitation present.

- **Auscultation** (see Fig. 7.8): typically there is a midsystolic click followed by a middle and late systolic murmur that extends to the second heart sound. It often has a blowing quality. There may, however, be a click and no murmur (suggests little or no regurgitation) or a typical murmur without an audible click.
- **Dynamic auscultation:** murmur and click occur earlier and may become louder with the Valsalva manoeuvre and with standing (unlike the ejection click of aortic or pulmonary stenosis), but with squatting and isometric exercise both murmur and click occur later and may become softer.
- **Causes of mitral valve prolapse:**
  1. Myxomatous degeneration of the mitral valve tissue—it is very common, especially in women, and the severity may increase with age, particularly in men, so that significant mitral regurgitation may supervene.
  2. May be associated with atrial septal defect (secundum), hypertrophic cardiomyopathy or Marfan's syndrome.

Aortic stenosis (AS)

The normal area of the aortic valve is more than 2 cm². Significant narrowing of this valve restricts left ventricular outflow and imposes a pressure load on the left ventricle.

- **Symptoms:** exertional chest pain (50% do not have coronary artery disease), exertional dyspnoea and exertional syncope.
- **General signs:** usually there is nothing remarkable about the general appearance.
- **Pulse:** there may be a plateau or anacrotic pulse, or the pulse may be late peaking (*tardus*) and of small volume (*parvus*).[5]

Mitral valve prolapse (MVP).

(a) Murmur, at the apex; (b) anatomy

FIGURE 7.8

- **Palpation:** the apex beat is hyperdynamic and may be slightly displaced; systolic thrill at the base of the heart (aortic area).
- **Auscultation** (see Fig. 7.9): a narrowly split or reversed S2 because of delayed left ventricular ejection; a harsh midsystolic ejection murmur, maximal over the aortic area and extending into the carotid arteries (see Fig. 7.10), is characteristic. However, it may be heard widely over the praecordium and may extend to the apex. The murmur is loudest with the patient sitting up and in full expiration; associated aortic regurgitation is common; in congenital aortic stenosis where the valve cusps remain mobile and the dome of the valve comes to a sudden halt, an ejection click may precede the murmur—the ejection click is absent if the valve is calcified or if the stenosis is not at the valve level but above or below it (supra- or subvalvular stenosis).
- **Signs indicating severe aortic stenosis** (see Good signs guide 7.2; valve area less than 1 cm^2, or valve gradient greater than 50 mmHg): plateau pulse, carotid pulse reduced in force; thrill in the aortic area; length of the murmur and lateness of the peak of the systolic murmur; soft or absent A2; left ventricular failure (very late sign); pressure-loaded apex beat. These signs are not reliable for distinguishing between moderate and severe disease. It is important to remember that the signs of severity of aortic stenosis are less reliable in the elderly.[6]
- **Causes of aortic stenosis include:**
  1. degenerative calcific aortic stenosis, particularly in elderly patients
  2. calcific in younger patients, usually on a congenital bicuspid valve
  3. rheumatic.
- **Other types of aortic outflow obstruction are also possible:**
  1. Supravalvular obstruction, where there is narrowing of the ascending aorta or a fibrous diaphragm just above the aortic valve—this is rare and may be associated with a characteristic facies (a broad forehead, widely set eyes and a pointed chin); there is a loud A2 and often a thrill in the area of the sternal notch.
  2. Subvalvular obstruction, where there is a membranous diaphragm or fibrous ridge just below the aortic valve—aortic regurgitation is associated and is due to a jet lesion affecting the coronary cusp of the valve.
  3. Dynamic left ventricular outflow tract obstruction may occur in hypertrophic cardiomyopathy—here there may be a double apical impulse. Atrial contraction into a stiff left ventricle may be palpable before the left ventricular impulse (only in the presence of sinus rhythm, of course).

Aortic sclerosis presents in the elderly; there are none of the peripheral signs of aortic stenosis. The term implies the absence of a gradient across the aortic valve despite some thickening and a murmur.

Aortic regurgitation

The incompetent aortic valve allows regurgitation of blood from the aorta to the left ventricle during diastole for as long as the aortic diastolic pressure exceeds the left ventricular diastolic pressure.[7,8]

- **Symptoms:** occur in the late stages of disease and include exertional dyspnoea, fatigue, palpitations (hyperdynamic circulation) and exertional angina.
- **General signs:** Marfan's syndrome, ankylosing spondylitis or one of the other seronegative

GOOD SIGNS GUIDE 7.2
Severe aortic stenosis

Sign	LR+	LR−
Delayed carotid upstroke	9.2	0.56
Diminished carotid pulse on palpation	2.0	0.64
Absent or decreased A2	7.5	0.5
Murmur over right clavicle	3.0	0.1
Any systolic murmur	2.6	0
Murmur radiates to the right carotid artery	8.1	0.29

LR=likelihood ratio; A2=aortic component 2nd heart sound. (Adapted from Etchells E, Glenns V, Shadowitz S et al. A bedside clinical prediction rule for detecting moderate or severe aortic stenosis. *J Gen Intern Med* 1998; 13(10):699–704.)

Aortic stenosis (AS).

(a) Murmur, at the aortic area; (b) anatomy

FIGURE 7.9

Aortic stenosis: listening over the carotid

FIGURE 7.10

arthropathies or, rarely, Argyll Robertson pupils may be obvious.
- **Pulse and blood pressure:** the pulse is characteristically collapsing, a 'water hammer'[h] pulse (see Table 7.2); there may be a wide pulse pressure. This sign is most obvious if the clinician raises the patient's arm while feeling the radial pulse with the web spaces of the lifting hand. A *bisferiens* pulse (from the Latin, to beat twice) may be a sign of severe aortic regurgitation or of combined aortic regurgitation and aortic stenosis. It is best assessed at the carotid artery, where two beats can be felt in each cardiac cycle. It is probably caused by a Venturi effect in the aorta related to rapid ejection of blood and brief in-drawing of the aortic wall, leading to a diminution of the pulse followed by a rebound increase. It was a particular favourite of Galen's.[i]
- **Neck:** prominent carotid pulsations (Corrigan's sign).[j]

- **Palpation:** the apex beat is characteristically displaced and hyperkinetic. A diastolic thrill may be felt at the left sternal edge when the patient sits up and breathes out.
- **Auscultation** (see Fig. 7.11): A2 (the aortic component of the second heart sound) may be soft; there is a decrescendo high-pitched diastolic murmur beginning immediately after the second heart sound and extending for a variable time into diastole—it is loudest at the third and fourth left intercostal spaces; a systolic ejection murmur is usually present (due to associated aortic stenosis or to torrential flow across an aortic valve of normal diameter).

Aortic stenosis is distinguished from an aortic flow murmur by the presence of the peripheral signs of significant aortic stenosis, such as a plateau pulse. However, the harsher and louder the murmur (and especially if there is a thrill), the more likely it is to be aortic stenosis.

An *Austin Flint murmur*[k] may be present. This is a low-pitched rumbling mid-diastolic and presystolic murmur audible at the apex (the regurgitant jet from the aortic valve causes the anterior mitral valve leaflet to shudder). It can be distinguished from mitral stenosis because S1 (the first heart sound) is not loud and there is no opening snap. Many other signs have been described, but they are interesting rather than helpful (see Table 7.2 and Good signs guide 7.3).

- **Signs indicating severe chronic aortic regurgitation include:**
  - collapsing pulse; wide pulse pressure (systolic pressure 80 mmHg more than the diastolic)
  - long decrescendo diastolic murmur
  - left ventricular S3 (third heart sound)
  - soft A2
  - Austin Flint murmur
  - signs of left ventricular failure.
- **Causes of aortic regurgitation:** disease may affect the valvular area or aortic root, and may be acute or chronic.

---

[h] This Victorian children's toy consisted of a sealed tube half-filled with fluid, with the other half being a vacuum. Inversion of the tube caused the fluid to fall rapidly without air resistance and strike the other end with a noise like a hammer blow. It is not easy to imagine a child today being entertained by this for very long.
[i] Claudius Galen (AD 130–200). Born in Pergamum, he worked as a gladiator's surgeon but moved to Rome in AD 164 to become the city's most famous physician. He was the first to describe the cranial nerves. He never performed dissection on human bodies, but his often-erroneous anatomical teachings were regarded as infallible for 15 centuries.
[j] This is probably the most useful of all these eponymous signs; the diagnosis may be strongly suspected from the end of the bed when it is present.

[k] Austin Flint (1812–86), a New York physician and professor of medicine at the New Orleans Medical School, described this murmur in 1862. Author of *The principles and practice of medicine*, he was very much opposed to the naming of signs after people.

Eponymous signs of aortic regurgitation

Quincke's sign	Capillary pulsation in the nail beds—it is of no value, as this sign occurs normally.
Corrigan's sign	Prominent carotid pulsations; the Corrigan water hammer pulse sign is present when the patient lies supine with the arms beside the body; the radial pulse is compressed until it disappears, the arm is then lifted perpendicular to the body and the pulse becomes palpable again even though the same pressure has been maintained on the radial artery.
De Musset's sign	Head nodding in time with the heartbeat.
Hill's sign	Increased blood pressure (>20 mmHg) in the legs compared with the arms.
Mueller's sign	Pulsation of the uvula in time with the heartbeat.
Duroziez's sign	Systolic and diastolic murmurs over the femoral artery on gradual compression of the vessel. The vessel is compressed with the diaphragm of the stethoscope. A systolic murmur will always be heard. As the compression is increased a diastolic murmur will be heard in patients with significant aortic regurgitation and is due to retrograde flow of blood back towards the heart in diastole. Tilting the diaphragm towards the patient's head will make the diastolic bruit softer if the patient has aortic regurgitation, but louder if the bruit is due to an increased cardiac output (e.g. due to thyrotoxicosis).
Traube's sign	A double sound heard over the femoral artery on compressing the vessel distally; this is not a 'pistol shot' sound that may be heard over the femoral artery with very severe aortic regurgitation.
Mayne's sign	A decrease in diastolic pressure of 15 mmHg when the patient's arm is held above the head compared with that when the arm is at the level of the heart.
Rosenbach's liver pulsation sign	Pulsation of the liver in time with the heartbeat (in the absence of tricuspid regurgitation).
Austin Flint murmur	Short rumbling diastolic murmur, thought by Flint to be due to functional mitral stenosis caused by impinging of the aortic regurgitant jet on the anterior mitral valve leaflet.
Becker's sign	Accentuated retinal artery pulsations.
Gerhard's sign	Pulsatile spleen.
Landolfi's sign	Prominent alternating constriction and dilation of the pupils (hippus, from the Greek *hippos*—'horse'—and its rhythmical galloping).
Lincoln's sign (see Fig. 7.11(c))	Exaggerated movement of the ankle when one leg is crossed over the other; said to have been described by Abraham Lincoln from a photograph of himself (he did not know the cause).
Sherman's sign	An easily palpable dorsalis pedis pulse in a patient over the age of 75 years.
Watson's water hammer pulse	See page 133.
Ashrafian's sign	Pulsatile pseudoproptosis.

Note: These signs are amusing, but not often helpful. The signs were named after the following people: Heinrich Quincke (1842–1922), a German neurologist; Dominic Corrigan (1802–80), an Edinburgh graduate who worked in Dublin and is credited with discovering aortic regurgitation; Alfred de Musset, a 19th-century French poet who suffered from aortic regurgitation (the sign was noticed by his brother, a physician); Sir Leonard Hill (1866–1952), an English physiologist who also described the physiology of the cerebral circulation; Frederick Von Mueller (1858–1941), a German physician who also noted an increase in metabolism in exophthalmic goitre; Paul Duroziez (1826–97), a French physician; Ludwig Traube (1818–76), a Hungarian physician who worked in Germany; Otto Heinrich Becker (1828–90), a professor of ophthalmology at University of Heidelberg, who also described this sign in patients with Graves' disease; Lincoln's sign is like de Musset's sign in being named after the patient with the condition; Thomas Watson, an English physician, who described this sign in 1844; Hutan Ashrafian, a cardiothoracic surgeon at St Mary's Hospital, London, who described this sign in 2006—proof that the hunt for more signs of aortic regurgitation goes on.

(Babu AN, Kymes SM, Carpenter Fryer SM. Eponyms and the diagnosis of aortic regurgitation: What says the evidence? *Ann Intern Med* 2003: 138:736–745.)

TABLE 7.2

Aortic regurgitation.

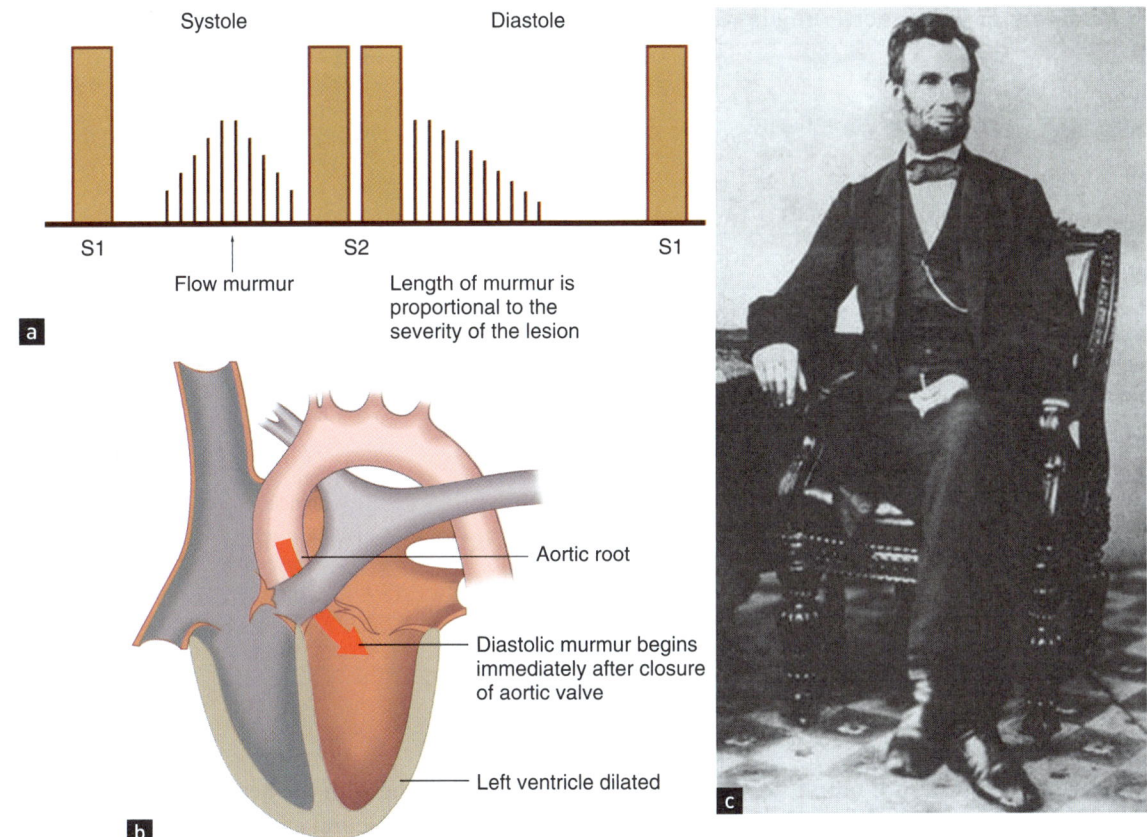

(a) Murmur, at the left sternal edge; (b) anatomy; (c) Lincoln's sign: left foot is blurred by motion

FIGURE 7.11

- **Causes of chronic aortic regurgitation include:**
  1. valvular—rheumatic (rarely the only murmur in this case), congenital (e.g. bicuspid valve; ventricular septal defect—an associated prolapse of the aortic cusp is not uncommon), seronegative arthropathy, especially ankylosing spondylitis
  2. aortic root dilation (murmur may be maximal at the right sternal border)—Marfan's syndrome, aortitis (e.g. seronegative arthropathies, rheumatoid arthritis, tertiary syphilis), dissecting aneurysm.
- **Acute aortic regurgitation:** presents differently—there is no collapsing pulse (blood pressure is low) and the diastolic murmur is short.

- **Causes of acute aortic regurgitation include:**
  1. valvular—infective endocarditis
  2. aortic root—Marfan's syndrome, dissecting aneurysm of the aortic root.

VALVE DISEASES OF THE RIGHT HEART
Tricuspid stenosis
This is very rare.
- **JVP:** raised; giant *a* waves with a slow *y* descent may be seen.
- **Auscultation:** a diastolic murmur audible at the left sternal edge, accentuated by inspiration, very

GOOD SIGNS GUIDE 7.3
Moderate or worse aortic regurgitation

Finding	LR+	LR−
Typical murmur	4.0–8.3	0.1
Grade 1 murmur (moderate to severe AR)	0.0	NA
Grade 2 murmur (moderate to severe AR)	1.1	NA
Murmur grade 3 or more (moderate to severe AR)	4.5	NA
S3	5.9	
PULSE PRESSURE		
>80 mmHg	10.9	
OTHER SIGNS—DISTINGUISHING MILD FROM MODERATE TO SEVERE AR		
Duroziez's sign, pistol shot femorals, water hammer pulse	NS	NS

AR=aortic regurgitation; LR=likelihood ratio; NS=not significant; NA=not applicable.
(Adapted from Simel DL, Rennie D. *The rational clinical examination: evidence-based diagnosis*. New York: McGraw-Hill, 2009, Table 32-3.)

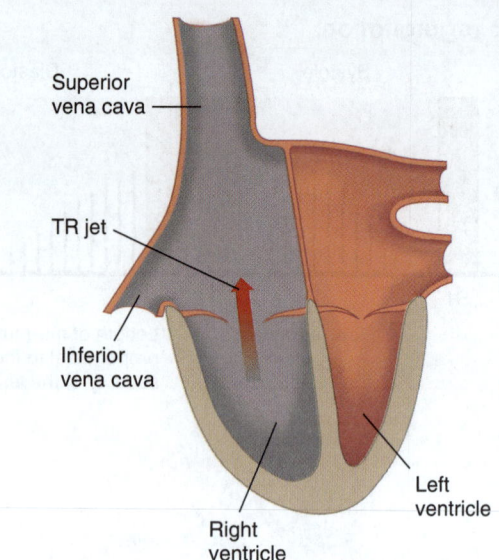

Tricuspid regurgitation (TR): anatomy

FIGURE 7.12

similar to the murmur of mitral stenosis except for the site of maximal intensity and the effect of respiration (louder on inspiration); tricuspid regurgitation and mitral stenosis are often present as well; no signs of pulmonary hypertension.
- **Abdomen:** presystolic pulsation of the liver, caused by forceful atrial systole.
- **Cause of tricuspid stenosis:** rheumatic heart disease.

Tricuspid regurgitation (TR)
(see Fig. 7.12)

- **JVP:** large *v* waves; the JVP is elevated if right ventricular failure has occurred.
- **Palpation:** parasternal impulse.
- **Auscultation:** there may be a pansystolic murmur maximal at the lower end of the sternum that increases on inspiration, but the diagnosis can be made on the basis of the peripheral signs alone.
- **Abdomen:** a pulsatile, large and tender liver is usually present and may cause the right nipple to dance in time with the heartbeat;[l] ascites, oedema and pleural effusions may also be present.
- **Legs:** dilated, pulsatile veins.
- **Causes of tricuspid regurgitation include:**[m]
  1. functional (no disease of the valve leaflets)—right ventricular failure
  2. rheumatic—only very rarely does rheumatic tricuspid regurgitation occur alone, usually mitral valve disease is also present
  3. infective endocarditis (right-sided endocarditis in intravenous drug addicts)
  4. tricuspid valve prolapse
  5. right ventricular papillary muscle infarction
  6. trauma (usually caused by a steering wheel injury to the sternum)
  7. congenital—Ebstein's anomaly.[n]

---

[l] A sign described by Dr Gaston Bauer, an Australian cardiologist, who trained Nick Talley.
[m] Doppler echocardiography has shown that trivial tricuspid regurgitation is very common and is then considered physiological. Christian Doppler (1803–53) was an Austrian physicist and mathematician.
[n] Wilhelm Ebstein (1836–1912), a professor of medicine at Göttingen in Germany, who invented and developed palpation.

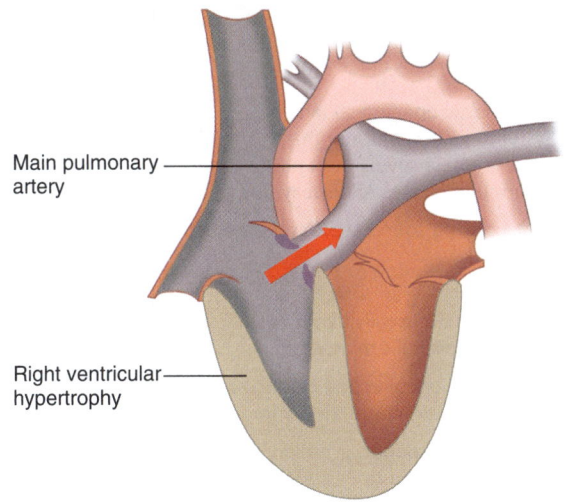

Valvar pulmonary stenosis: anatomy

FIGURE 7.13

Pulmonary stenosis (in adults)

(See Fig. 7.13.)

- **General signs:** peripheral cyanosis, due to a low cardiac output, but only in severe cases.
- **Pulse:** normal or reduced if cardiac output is low.
- **JVP:** giant *a* waves because of right atrial hypertrophy; the JVP may be elevated.
- **Palpation:** parasternal impulse; thrill over the pulmonary area.
- **Auscultation:** the murmur may be preceded by an ejection click; a harsh and usually loud ejection systolic murmur, heard best in the pulmonary area and with inspiration, is typically present; right ventricular S4 may be present (owing to right atrial hypertrophy). It is not well heard over the carotid arteries.
- **Abdomen:** presystolic pulsation of the liver may be present.
- **Signs of severe pulmonary stenosis include:**
  1. an ejection systolic murmur peaking late in systole
  2. absence of an ejection click (also absent when the pulmonary stenosis is infundibular—i.e. below the valve level)
  3. presence of S4
  4. signs of right ventricular failure.

- **Causes of pulmonary stenosis include:**
  1. congenital
  2. carcinoid syndrome (rare).

Pulmonary regurgitation

This is an uncommon pathological condition; trivial pulmonary regurgitation is often found at echocardiography and is considered physiological.

- **Auscultation:** a decrescendo diastolic murmur that is high-pitched and audible at the left sternal edge is characteristic—this typically but not always increases on inspiration (unlike the murmur of aortic regurgitation). It is called the Graham Steell murmur[o] when it occurs secondary to pulmonary artery dilation caused by pulmonary hypertension.
- **Causes of pulmonary regurgitation include:**
  1. pulmonary hypertension
  2. infective endocarditis
  3. following balloon valvotomy for pulmonary stenosis or surgery for pulmonary atresia
  4. congenital absence of the pulmonary valve.

Prosthetic heart valves

The physical signs with common types of valves are presented in Table 7.3. Mechanical prosthetic valves should have a crisp sound.[p] Muffling of the mechanical sounds may be a sign of thrombotic obstruction of the valve or chronic tissue ingrowth (pannus). After replacement of the aortic valve the presence of audible aortic regurgitation may indicate a *paravalvular leak*, often through a stitching hole in the valve sewing ring. As tissue valves age and degenerate they may develop signs of regurgitation or stenosis, or both.

CARDIOMYOPATHY
Hypertrophic cardiomyopathy

(See Fig. 7.14.)

This is abnormal hypertrophy of the muscle in the left ventricular or right ventricular outflow tract,

---

[o] Graham Steell (1851–1942), a Manchester physician, described this murmur in 1888.
[p] Modern leaflet valves are much less noisy than ball-in-cage valves, which can be heard from the other side of a crowded room. When patients complain of the noise, reassure them that they should worry only if the noise stops.

Prosthetic heart valves: physical signs

Type	Mitral	Aortic
Ball valve (e.g. Starr–Edwards)*	Sharp mitral opening sound after S2, sharp closing sound at S1. Systolic ejection murmur, no diastolic murmur	Sharp aortic opening sound. Systolic ejection murmur (harsh), no diastolic murmur unless a paravalvular leak has occurred, early diastolic murmur indicates AR usually due to a paravalvular leak**
Disc valve (e.g. Bjork–Shiley)†	Sharp closing sound at S1, soft systolic ejection murmur and diastolic rumble (diastolic murmur occasionally)	Sharp closing sound at S2, systolic ejection murmur (soft)
Porcine or bovine pericardial valve‡	Usually sound normal, diastolic rumble mitral opening sound occasionally	Closing sound usually heard, systolic ejection murmur (soft), no diastolic murmur
Bileaflet valve (e.g. St Jude)	—	Aortic valve opening and closing sounds common, soft systolic ejection murmur common
Homograft (human) valve		Normal heart sounds, occasional soft systolic murmur; early diastolic murmur if AR has occurred

*Modern mechanical valves (e.g. St Jude) make softer opening and closing sounds than do older valves. The Starr–Edwards valve is often very noisy and sounds like a ball rattling around in a cage (which is what it is).
**An aortic regurgitation murmur present after aortic valve replacement suggests regurgitation of the valve ring. It is not uncommon. Less often, a mitral regurgitation murmur suggests the same problem with a prosthetic mitral valve.
†Severe prosthetic dysfunction causes absence of the opening or closing sounds. Ball and cage valves cause more haemolysis than do other types and make the most noise, whereas disc valves are more thrombogenic.
‡Bioprosthetic obstruction or patient–prosthetic mismatch causes diastolic rumbling. These valves are used less often in the mitral position because they often have a very limited life there. A degenerated bioprosthetic valve may cause murmurs of regurgitation or stenosis, or both.
AR = aortic regurgitation.

(Modified from Smith ND, Raizada V, Abrams J. Auscultation of the normally functioning prosthetic valve. *Ann Intern Med* 1981; 95:594.)

TABLE 7.3

---

or both. It can obstruct outflow from the left ventricle late in systole when the hypertrophied area contracts. Systolic displacement of the mitral valve apparatus into the left ventricular outflow tract also occurs, causing mitral regurgitation and contributing to the outflow obstruction. Although the outflow tract is narrowed by the hypertrophied septum, the major contribution to the dynamic increase in obstruction comes from the systolic movement of the mitral valve. Variants of hypertrophic cardiomyopathy may involve the mid-ventricle or apex with varying degrees of obstruction.

- **Symptoms:** dyspnoea (increased left ventricular end-diastolic pressure due to abnormal diastolic compliance), angina, syncope or sudden death on exertion (secondary to ventricular fibrillation or a sudden increase in outflow obstruction).
- **Pulse:** sharp rising and jerky or double (bisferiens). Rapid ejection by the hypertrophied ventricle early in systole is followed by obstruction caused by the displacement of the mitral valve into the outflow tract. This is quite different from the pulse of aortic stenosis.
- **JVP:** there is usually a prominent *a* wave, due to forceful atrial contraction against a non-compliant right ventricle.
- **Palpation:** double or triple apical impulse, due to presystolic expansion of the ventricle caused by atrial contraction.
- **Auscultation:** late systolic murmur at the lower left sternal edge and apex (due to the obstruction) and a pansystolic murmur at the apex (due to mitral regurgitation); S4.
- **Dynamic manoeuvres:** the outflow murmur is increased by the Valsalva manoeuvre, by standing and by isotonic exercise; it is decreased by squatting and isometric exercise.

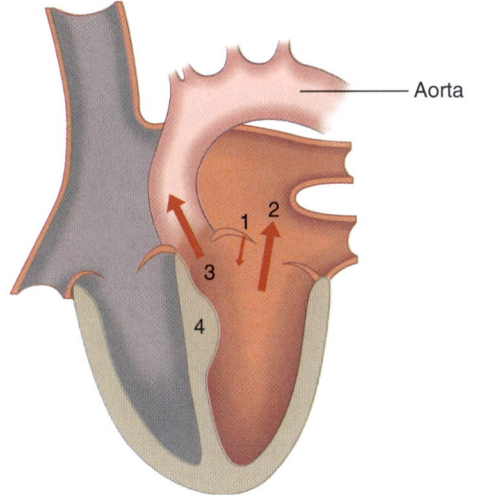

1 Systolic anterior motion
of anterior mitral valve leaflet
2 Jet of mitral regurgitation
3 Left ventricular outflow tract
4 Septal hypertrophy

Hypertrophic cardiomyopathy: anatomy

FIGURE 7.14

- Causes of hypertrophic cardiomyopathy include:
  1. autosomal dominant (sarcomeric heavy chain or troponin gene mutation) with variable expressivity
  2. Friedreich's ataxia[q] (p 597).

Dilated cardiomyopathy

This heart muscle abnormality results in a global reduction in cardiac function. Coronary artery disease is excluded as a cause by definition. (Ischaemic cardiomyopathy is a term often used to describe severe myocardial dysfunction secondary to recurrent ischaemic events.) The signs are those of congestive cardiac failure, including those of mitral and tricuspid regurgitation. The heart sounds themselves may be very quiet. Ventricular arrhythmias are common. It is a common indication for cardiac transplantation.

- Causes of dilated cardiomyopathy include:
  1. idiopathic and familial
  2. alcohol
  3. postviral
  4. postpartum
  5. drugs (e.g. doxorubicin)
  6. dystrophia myotonica
  7. haemochromatosis.

Restrictive cardiomyopathy

This causes similar signs to those caused by constrictive pericarditis, but Kussmaul's sign is more common and the apex beat is usually easily palpable.

- Causes of restrictive cardiomyopathy include:
  1. idiopathic
  2. eosinophilic endomyocardial disease
  3. endomyocardial fibrosis
  4. infiltrative disease (e.g. amyloid)
  5. granulomas (e.g. sarcoid).

ACYANOTIC CONGENITAL HEART DISEASE

Ventricular septal defect

In this condition one or more holes are present in the membranous or muscular ventricular septum.

- **Palpation:** hyperkinetic displaced apex if the defect is large; a thrill at the left sternal edge.
- **Auscultation** (see Fig. 7.15): a harsh pansystolic murmur maximal at, and almost confined to, the lower left sternal edge with a third or fourth heart sound—the murmur is louder on expiration; sometimes a mitral regurgitation murmur is associated. There is often a palpable systolic thrill. The murmur is often louder and harsher when the defect is small.
- Causes of ventricular septal defect include:
  1. congenital
  2. acquired (e.g. myocardial infarction involving the septum).

Atrial septal defect

There are two main types: *ostium secundum* (90%), where there is a defect in the part of the septum

---

[q] Nikolaus Friedreich (1825–82), a German physician, described this disease in 1863. He succeeded Virchow as professor of pathological anatomy at Würzburg at the age of 31.

Ventricular septal defect (VSD).

(a) Murmur, at the left sternal edge; (b) anatomy

FIGURE 7.15

Atrial septal defect (ASD).

(a) Murmur, at the left sternal edge; (b) anatomy

FIGURE 7.16

that does not involve the atrioventricular valves, and *ostium primum*, where the defect does involve the atrioventricular valves.
- **Palpation:** normal or right ventricular enlargement.
- **Auscultation** (see Fig. 7.16): fixed splitting of S2; the defect produces no murmur directly, but increased flow through the right side of the heart can produce a low-pitched diastolic tricuspid flow murmur and more often a pulmonary systolic ejection murmur—these are both louder on inspiration.
- **Signs:** the signs of an ostium primum defect are the same as for an ostium secundum defect, but associated mitral regurgitation, tricuspid regurgitation or a ventricular septal defect may be present. The left ventricular impulse is often impalpable (see the OCSE ECG 26 at Student CONSULT).

Patent ductus arteriosus: anatomy

FIGURE 7.17

Coarctation of the aorta: anatomy

FIGURE 7.18

Patent ductus arteriosus

(See Fig. 7.17.)

This is a persistent embryonic vessel that connects the pulmonary artery and the aorta. The shunt is from the aorta to the pulmonary artery unless pulmonary hypertension has supervened.

- **Pulse and blood pressure:** a collapsing pulse with a sharp upstroke (due to ejection of a large volume of blood into the empty aorta with systole); low diastolic blood pressure (due to rapid decompression of the aorta).
- **Palpation:** often there is a hyperkinetic apex beat.
- **Auscultation:** if the shunt is of moderate size a single second heart sound is heard, but if the shunt is of significant size then reversed splitting of the second heart sound occurs (due to a delayed A2 because of an increased volume load in the left ventricle); a continuous loud 'machinery' murmur maximal at the first left intercostal space is usually present; flow murmurs through the left side of the heart, including a mitral mid-diastolic murmur, may be heard.

Note: the transmitted sound from an arteriovenous fistula in the arm, used for dialysis, can cause a similar continuous murmur—to avoid embarrassment, look at the arm.

Coarctation of the aorta

(See Fig. 7.18.)

This is congenital narrowing of the aorta usually just distal to the origin of the left subclavian artery. It is more common in males. The underlying cause is uncertain but seems related to abnormal placement of tissue involved in the closing of the ductus arteriosus. There is an association with bicuspid aortic valve and Turner's syndrome.

- **Signs:** the upper body may be better developed than the lower; radiofemoral delay is present, and the femoral pulses are weak; hypertension occurs in the arms but not in the legs; a midsystolic murmur is usually audible over the praecordium and the back, owing to blood flow through collateral chest vessels and across the coarct itself.

Ebstein's anomaly

This is a very rare lesion. The abnormality is a downward displacement of the tricuspid valve apparatus into the right ventricle so that the right atrium becomes very large and consists partly of ventricular muscle, while the right ventricle becomes small. An atrial septal defect is commonly associated. Characteristically, multiple clicks occur owing to asynchronous closure of the tricuspid valve. Tricuspid regurgitation is usually present.

> **CLASSIFICATION OF CONGENITAL HEART DISEASE**
>
> **Acyanotic**
> WITH LEFT-TO-RIGHT SHUNT
> Ventricular septal defect
> Atrial septal defect
> Patent ductus arteriosus
>
> WITH NO SHUNT
> Bicuspid aortic valve, congenital aortic stenosis
> Coarctation of aorta
> Dextrocardia
> Pulmonary stenosis, tricuspid stenosis
> Ebstein's anomaly
>
> **Cyanotic**
> Eisenmenger's syndrome (pulmonary hypertension and a right-to-left shunt)
> Tetralogy of Fallot
> Ebstein's anomaly (if an atrial septal defect and right-to-left shunt are also present)
> Truncus arteriosus
> Transposition of the great vessels
> Tricuspid arteria
> Total anomalous pulmonary venous drainage
>
> LIST 7.2

CYANOTIC CONGENITAL HEART DISEASE

This is a difficult area. The causes of congenital heart disease are listed in List 7.2. The important point to determine is whether or not signs of pulmonary hypertension are present. Congenital heart disease in which a shunt from the left to the right side of the circulation occurs leads to an increase in pulmonary blood flow. This can cause reactive pulmonary hypertension so that pulmonary pressures eventually exceed systemic pressures. When that happens, the systemic to pulmonary (left to right) shunt will reverse. This right-to-left shunt leads to deoxygenated blood being mixed in the systemic circulation, resulting in cyanosis. This is called Eisenmenger's syndrome.[r]

Eisenmenger's syndrome (pulmonary hypertension and a right-to-left shunt)

- **Signs:** central cyanosis; clubbing; polycythaemia; signs of pulmonary hypertension.

It may be possible to decide at what level the shunt occurs by listening to the second heart sound (S2). If there is wide fixed splitting, this suggests an atrial septal defect. If a single second heart sound is present, this suggests truncus arteriosus or a ventricular septal defect. A normal or reversed S2 suggests a patent ductus arteriosus.

Fallot's syndrome[s]

There are four features that are due to a single developmental abnormality (tetralogy of Fallot):

1. ventricular septal defect
2. right ventricular outflow obstruction, which determines the severity of the condition, and can be at the pulmonary valve or infundibular level
3. an aorta that overrides the ventricular septal defect and is responsible for the cyanosis, and
4. right ventricular hypertrophy secondary to outflow obstruction.

- **Signs:** central cyanosis—this occurs without pulmonary hypertension because venous mixing is possible at the ventricular level, where pressures are balanced. The aorta overrides both ventricles and so receives right and left ventricular blood. Clubbing and polycythaemia are usually present. There may be evidence of right ventricular enlargement—a parasternal impulse at the left sternal edge. A systolic thrill caused by pulmonary valve or right ventricular outflow obstruction may be present. There is no overall cardiomegaly. On auscultation the second heart sound is single and there are no signs of pulmonary hypertension; a pulmonary systolic ejection murmur is present.

---

[r] Victor Eisenmenger (1864–1932), a German physician, described this syndrome in 1897.

[s] Etienne-Louis Fallot (1850–1911), a professor of hygiene at Marseilles, described this in 1888.

'GROWN-UP' CONGENITAL HEART DISEASE

Patients who have been treated for serious congenital cardiac conditions now frequently survive into adult life. Many of the surgical procedures undertaken for these conditions, especially 20 years ago, were palliative rather than curative. The patients present with specific symptoms and signs.

Fallot's syndrome

Patients who have had repair of this condition in infancy may present with particular problems. Repair of the right ventricular outflow obstruction and enlargement of the pulmonary valve annulus may leave severe pulmonary regurgitation. This may lead eventually to exertional dyspnoea. The surgery itself has, until recently, required a right ventriculotomy (cutting into the right ventricle). This leaves a scar that can be associated with cardiac rhythm abnormalities in later life. Patients may present with palpitations or syncope.

- Signs may include:
  - a median sternotomy scar
  - a long diastolic murmur of pulmonary regurgitation
  - signs of right ventricular enlargement (parasternal impulse)
  - later signs of tricuspid regurgitation (big *v* waves in the neck and a pulsatile liver).

Transposition of the great arteries

Most adults who have had surgery for this abnormality have had a palliative operation called a *Mustard procedure*. Younger adults are more likely to have had a more definitive *switch* operation. In this abnormality, the pulmonary artery is connected to the left ventricle and the aorta to the right ventricle. Thus the systemic and pulmonary circulations are in parallel. This is not compatible with life unless some connection between the two circulations is present. Neonates with the condition will have had an atrial septal defect created soon after birth with a catheter-based balloon (balloon septostomy). This allows mixing of the circulations. Later, 'baffles' will be created surgically in the atria to direct blood returning from the body into the right atrium across the atrial septal defect and into the left atrium, where it is pumped into the pulmonary artery and into the lungs. Blood returning from the lungs into the left atrium is directed across into the right atrium and into the morphological right ventricle and on into the aorta. This means that the morphological right ventricle is working as the systemic ventricle. This arrangement works very well, but there are long-term concerns about the ability of the right ventricle to cope with systemic workloads.

- **Symptoms:** commonly include palpitations caused by supraventricular arrhythmias, dizziness caused by bradycardias and breathlessness related to failure of the systemic ventricle. Occasionally, obstruction of the baffles may occur. The most common problem is with the superior vena caval baffle, which leads to facial swelling and flushing.
- **Signs include:** the usual scar, facial flushing and oedema, cyanosis, peripheral oedema from inferior caval baffle obstruction and signs of tricuspid regurgitation. On auscultation there may be a gallop rhythm and the murmurs of mitral and tricuspid regurgitation.

T&O'C ESSENTIALS

1. Careful examination of the heart can lead to an accurate diagnosis in most cases of valvular heart disease.
2. Proper history taking and examination will prevent the ordering of expensive and inappropriate cardiac tests.
3. It is not necessary to memorise the entire list of eponymous signs of aortic regurgitation (in fact, you can forget them all).
4. The presence of specific signs of heart failure (e.g. a third heart sound and abnormal apex beat) makes the diagnosis almost certain; their absence does not rule out heart failure.
5. There are few specific signs of myocardial infarction and the diagnosis depends on the history and ECG.

OSCE EXAMPLE – CARDIOVASCULAR EXAMINATION (see the OSCE CVS examination video at Student CONSULT)

Please examine this 75-year-old woman with dyspnoea and suspected heart failure.

1. Wash your hands.
2. Introduce yourself to the patient and explain the purpose and nature of the examination. (e.g. 'I'm going to examine your heart if that is all right?')
3. Stand back to look for breathlessness and tachypnoea, cyanosis, elevated JVP, use of supplementary oxygen. Does the patient look unwell?
4. Position the patient at 45°, and loosen the patient's gown to allow access to the front of the chest but keep a female's breasts covered.
5. Take the patient's pulse (consider rate and possible AF).
6. Take the blood pressure.
7. Look at the JVP again (especially big *v* waves). Perform an abdominojugular reflux test.
8. Loosen the patient's gown further and inspect the chest for scars (previous valve surgery).
9. Look for the apex beat; feel carefully for the apex beat, thrills and parasternal impulse.
10. Listen for a gallop rhythm and valvular disease (mitral regurgitation may occur as a result of, or be the cause of, heart failure).
11. Listen to the lung bases (medium inspiratory crackles—not specific); look for sacral oedema.
12. Look at the legs for oedema (not specific).
13. Collect your thoughts while washing your hands.
14. Present the positive and negative findings associated with heart failure.

OSCE REVISION TOPICS – CARDIOVASCULAR EXAMINATION

Use these topics, which commonly occur in the OSCE, to help with revision.

1. Please examine this man, who has previous cardiac valve surgery. (p 126)
2. This man has aortic regurgitation. Please examine him and estimate the severity of the condition. (p 131)
3. This woman has had a diagnosis of pulmonary hypertension. Please examine her. (p 125)

References

1. Stevenson LW, Perluff JK. The limited reliability of physical signs for estimating hemodynamics in chronic heart failure. *JAMA* 1989; 261:884–888. Physical signs poorly predict haemodynamic changes in heart failure. However, some signs are useful.
2. Khot U, Jia G, Moliterno DJ et al. Prognostic value of physical examination for heart failure in non-ST elevation acute coronary syndromes. *JAMA* 2003; 290:2174–2181. This analysis of the Killip classification for patients with acute coronary syndromes expands the relevance of the classification from its original use for patients with ST elevation infarction in the pre-thrombolytic era.
3. Klompas M. Does this patient have an acute thoracic dissection? *JAMA* 2002; 287(17):2262–2272.
4. Turnbull JM. Is listening for abdominal bruits useful in the evaluation of hypertension? The rational clinical examination. *JAMA* 1995; 274:16. If an abdominal bruit extends into diastole, this has a high predictive value for a clinically important bruit. The pitch and intensity are not helpful.
5. Etchells E, Bell C, Robb K. Does this patient have an abnormal systolic murmur? *JAMA* 1997; 277:564–571. The most useful positive predictive features for aortic stenosis appear to be a slow rate of rise of the carotid pulse, a mid-to-late peak intensity of the murmur and a decreased second heart sound; absence of radiation to the right carotid helps rule it out.
6. Aronow WS. Prevalence and severity of valvular aortic stenosis determined by Doppler echocardiography, and its association with echocardiographic and electrocardiographic left ventricular hypertrophy and physical signs of aortic stenosis in elderly patients. *Am J Cardiol* 1991; 67:776–777. Analysis of the signs of severity of aortic stenosis in elderly patients shows that they are less reliable than in younger patients.
7. Choudhry NK, Etchells EE. The Rational Clinical Examination. Does this patient have aortic regurgitation? *JAMA* 1999; 281:2231–2238. It is easy if you listen carefully: the presence of an early diastolic murmur at the left sternal edge best rules in AR; the absence of an early diastolic murmur essentially rules out AR.
8. Aronow WS, Kronzon I. Correlation of prevalence and severity of aortic regurgitation detected by pulsed Doppler echocardiography with the murmur of aortic regurgitation in elderly patients in a long-term health care facility. *Am J Cardiol* 1989; 63:128–129.

CHAPTER 8

A summary of the cardiovascular examination and extending the cardiovascular examination

Never forget to look at the back of the patient. Always look at the feet. Looking at a woman's legs has often saved her life. SIR WILLIAM OSLER (1849–1919)

> **The cardiovascular examination: a suggested method (see the OCSE CVS examination video at Student CONSULT)**
>
> 1. **General inspection**
>   Marfan's, Turner's, Down syndromes
>   Rheumatological disorders, e.g. ankylosing spondylitis (aortic regurgitation)
>   Dyspnoea
> 2. **Hands**
>   Radial pulses—right and left
>   Radiofemoral delay
>   Clubbing
>   Signs of infective endocarditis—splinter haemorrhages, etc.
>   Peripheral cyanosis
>   Xanthomata
> 3. **Blood pressure**
> 4. **Face**
>   Eyes
>   Sclerae—pallor, jaundice
>   Pupils—Argyll Robertson (aortic regurgitation)
>   Xanthelasmata
>   Malar flush (mitral stenosis, pulmonary stenosis)
>   Mouth
>   Cyanosis
>   Palate (high arched—Marfan's syndrome)
>   Dentition
> 5. **Neck (at 45 degrees)**
>   Jugular venous pressure
>   Central venous pressure height
>   Wave form (especially large *n* waves)
>   Carotids—pulse character
> 6. **Praecordium**
>   *Inspect*
>   Scars—whole chest, back
>   Deformity
>   Apex beat—position, character
>   Abnormal pulsations
>   *Palpate*
>   Apex beat—position, character
>   Thrills
>   Abnormal impulses
> 7. **Auscultate**
>   Heart sounds
>   Murmurs
>   Position patient
>   Left lateral position
>   Sitting forwards (forced expiratory apnoea)
>   NB: Palpate for thrills again after positioning
>   Dynamic auscultation
>   Respiratory phases
>   Valsalva
>   Exercise (isometric, e.g. handgrip)
>   Carotids
> 8. **Back (sitting forwards)**
>   Scars, deformity
>   Sacral oedema
>   Pleural effusion (percuss)
>   Left ventricular failure (auscultate)
> 9. **Abdomen (lying flat—1 pillow only)**
>   Palpate liver (pulsatile, etc.), spleen, aorta
>   Percuss for ascites (right heart failure)
>   Femoral arteries—palpate, auscultate
> 10. **Legs**
>   Peripheral pulses
>   Cyanosis, cold limbs, trophic changes, ulceration (peripheral vascular disease)
>   Oedema
>   Xanthomata
>   Calf tenderness

TEXT BOX 8.1

Continued

The cardiovascular examination: a suggested method continued

Cardiovascular system.

Patient lying at 45°

FIGURE 8.1

11. **Other**
    Urine analysis (infective endocarditis)
    Fundi (endocarditis)
    Temperature chart (endocarditis)

Position the patient at 45° and make sure his or her chest and neck are fully exposed (Fig. 8.1). Cover the breasts of a female patient with a towel or loose garment.

Inspect while standing back for the appearance of Marfan's, Turner's or Down syndromes. Also look for dyspnoea, cyanosis, jaundice and cachexia.

Pick up the patient's right **hand**. Feel the radial pulse. At the same time inspect the hands for clubbing. Also look for the peripheral stigmata of infective endocarditis: splinter haemorrhages are common (and are also caused by trauma), whereas Osler's nodes and Janeway lesions are rare. Look quickly, but carefully, at each nail bed, of both hands, otherwise it is easy to miss these signs. Note any tendon xanthoma (type II hyperlipidaemia).

The **pulse** at the wrist should be timed for rate and rhythm. Feel for radiofemoral delay (which occurs in coarctation of the aorta) and radial–radial inequality. Pulse character is best assessed at the carotids.

Take the **blood pressure** (lying and standing or sitting—postural hypotension).

Next inspect the face. Look at the eyes briefly for jaundice (e.g. valve haemolysis) or xanthelasmata (type II or type III hyperlipidaemia*). You may also notice the classical mitral facies. Then inspect the mouth using a torch for a high-arched palate (Marfan's syndrome), petechiae and the state of dentition (endocarditis). Look at the tongue or lips for central cyanosis.

The **neck** is very important. The jugular venous pressure (JVP) must be assessed for height and character. Use the right internal jugular vein for this assessment. Look for a change with inspiration (Kussmaul's sign). Now feel each carotid pulse separately. Assess the pulse character.

Proceed to the **praecordium**. Always begin by inspecting for scars, deformity, site of the apex beat and visible pulsations. Do not forget about pacemaker boxes. Mitral valvotomy scars (usually under the left breast) (see Fig. 8.11) can be quite lateral and very easily missed.

Palpate for the position of the **apex beat**. Count down the correct number of interspaces. The normal position is the fifth left intercostal space, 1 cm medial to the midclavicular line. The character of the apex beat is important. There are a number of types. A *pressure-loaded* (hyperdynamic, systolic overloaded) apex beat is a forceful and sustained impulse that is not displaced (e.g. aortic stenosis, hypertension). A *volume-loaded* (hyperkinetic, diastolic overloaded) apex beat is a forceful but unsustained impulse that is displaced down and laterally (e.g. aortic regurgitation, mitral regurgitation). A *dyskinetic* apex beat (cardiac failure) is palpable over a larger area than normal and moves in an uncoordinated way under the examiner's hand. Do not miss the tapping apex beat of mitral stenosis (a palpable first heart sound). The double or triple apical impulse of hypertrophic cardiomyopathy is very important too. Feel also for an apical thrill, and time it.

Then palpate with the heel of your hand for a left parasternal impulse (which indicates right ventricular enlargement or left atrial enlargement) and for thrills. Now feel at the base of the heart for a palpable pulmonary component of the second heart sound (P2) and aortic thrills. Percussion may be helpful if there is uncertainty about cardiac enlargement.

TEXT BOX 8.1

The cardiovascular examination: a suggested method *continued*

Auscultation begins in the mitral area with both the bell and the diaphragm. Listen for each component of the cardiac cycle separately. Identify the first and second heart sounds, and decide whether they are of normal intensity and whether the second heart sound is normally split. Now listen for extra heart sounds and murmurs. Do not be satisfied at having identified one abnormality.

Repeat the approach at the left sternal edge and then the base of the heart (aortic and pulmonary areas). Time each part of the cycle with the carotid pulse. Listen over the carotids.

It is now time to **reposition** the patient. First put him or her in the left lateral position. Again feel the apex beat for character (particularly tapping) and auscultate. Sit the patient up and palpate for thrills (with the patient in full expiration) at the left sternal edge and base. Then listen in those areas, particularly for aortic regurgitation or a pericardial rub.

Dynamic auscultation should be done if there is any doubt about a systolic murmur. The Valsalva manoeuvre should be performed whenever there is a pure systolic murmur. Hypertrophic cardiomyopathy is easily missed otherwise.

The patient is now sitting up. Percuss the **back** quickly to exclude a pleural effusion (e.g. due to left ventricular failure) and auscultate for inspiratory crackles (left ventricular failure). If there is a radiofemoral delay, listen for a coarctation murmur over the back. Feel for sacral oedema and note any back deformity (e.g. ankylosing spondylitis with aortic regurgitation).

Next have the patient lie flat and examine the **abdomen** properly for hepatomegaly (right ventricular failure) and a pulsatile liver (tricuspid regurgitation). Test for the abdominojugular reflux sign if relevant. Feel for splenomegaly (endocarditis) and an aortic aneurysm.

Move on to the **legs**. Palpate both femoral arteries and auscultate here for bruits. Go on and examine all the peripheral pulses. Look for signs of peripheral vascular disease, peripheral oedema, clubbing of the toes, Achilles tendon xanthomata and stigmata of infective endocarditis.

Finally, examine the **fundi** (for hypertensive changes, and Roth's spots in endocarditis) and the **urine** (haematuria in endocarditis). Take the **temperature**.

---

*In type III, which is rare, chylomicrons and intermediate-density lipoproteins (IDLs) are elevated.

TEXT BOX 8.1

EXTENDING THE CARDIOVASCULAR PHYSICAL EXAMINATION

Just as analysis of the chest X-ray has long been considered an extension of the patient's physical examination, electrocardiography (see the OCSE ECG library at Student CONSULT) and echocardiography are now essential parts of cardiac assessment. It is not possible to order even basic tests without knowing how a test might be helpful and what it is able to detect. In addition, students must have a basic understanding of electrocardiography and be able to diagnose important cardiac rhythm disturbances and recognise electrocardiogram (ECG) abnormalities suggesting myocardial ischaemia or infarction.

The chest X-ray: a systematic approach

Interpretation of the chest X-ray is not easy. It requires knowledge of anatomy and pathology, appreciation of the whole range of normal appearances (see Fig. 8.2) and knowledge of the likely X-ray changes occurring with pathological processes. The clinician should feel personally responsible for viewing a patient's radiographs.

Most medical students faced with giving their interpretation of a chest X-ray either opt for a 'spot diagnosis' (usually wrong) or raise their eyes to heaven, hoping for divine inspiration. However, a systematic approach is generally more useful! More is missed by not looking than by not knowing.

Normal chest X-ray.

(a) The posteroanterior view shows: (1) aortic knuckle, (2) left heart border formed by the lateral border of the left ventricle, (3) left hilum formed mostly by the left main pulmonary artery and partly by the left upper pulmonary veins, (4) right heart border formed by the right atrium, (5) inferior angle of the scapula, (6) right basal pulmonary artery, (7) medial aspect of the left clavicle, (8) spine of the scapula, (9) right cardiophrenic angle, and (10) superimposition of the right lateral margins of the superior vena cava and the ascending aorta.

(b) The lateral view shows: (11) anterior border of the trachea, (12) pulmonary vein, entering the left atrium, (13) oblique fissure, (14) left hemidiaphragm, and (15) right hemidiaphragm

FIGURE 8.2

Frontal film

Name, date and projection

First, it is important to check the name and date, to be sure that it is the correct patient's film. The film markings also indicate the projection and patient position. The standard frontal film is taken by a posteroanterior (PA; back to front) projection of an erect patient. Anteroposterior (AP) and supine films are only second best. On a supine film there is distension of all the posterior (gravity-dependent) vessels and thus the lung fields appear more plethoric. A small pleural effusion may not be visible if it is lying posteriorly, and the heart often appears large on a supine film.

Centring

The medial ends of the clavicles should be equidistant from the midline spinous processes. If the patient is rotated, this will accentuate the hilum that is turned forwards.

Exposure

There should be enough X-ray penetration for the spine to be just seen through the mediastinum, otherwise the film will be too white. With good radiographic technique, the scapulae are projected outside the lung fields.

The film needs to be exposed on full inspiration so that there is no basal crowding of the pulmonary vessels and estimation of the cardiothoracic ratio is accurate. On full inspiration, the diaphragm lies at the level of the tenth or eleventh rib posteriorly or at the level of the sixth costal cartilage anteriorly. The right hemidiaphragm usually lies about 2 centimetres higher than the left.

Correct orientation

Do not miss dextrocardia—the heart apex will be to the right and the stomach gas to the left. Do not be misled by left or right markers wrongly placed by a radiographer.

Systematic film interpretation

Mediastinum

The trachea should lie in the middle line. It may be deviated by a goitre or mediastinal mass. It is normally deviated a little to the left as it passes the aortic knuckle. (The aortic arch becomes wider and unfolded with age because of loss of elasticity.)

The mediastinum, including the trachea, can be deviated by a large pleural effusion, a tension pneumothorax or pulmonary collapse.

Rotation of the patient may make the mediastinum appear distorted.

Hila

The hila are mostly formed by the pulmonary arteries with the upper lobe veins superimposed. The left hilum is higher than the right. The left has a squarish shape whereas the right has a V shape.

A hilum can become more prominent if the patient is rotated. Lymphadenopathy or a large pulmonary artery will cause hilar enlargement.

Heart

The heart shape is ovoid with the apex pointing to the left. Characteristically, about two-thirds of the heart projects to the left of the spine.

The right heart border is formed by the outer border of the right atrium, and the left heart border by the left ventricle. The left margin of the right ventricle lies about a thumb's breadth in from the left heart border. (On the surface of the heart, this is marked by the left anterior descending coronary artery.)

The cardiothoracic diameter is a rather approximate way of determining whether the heart is enlarged. If the heart size is more than 50% of the transthoracic diameter, enlargement may be present. Apparent slight cardiac enlargement can occur because of a relatively small AP diameter of the chest. A cardiothoracic ratio at the upper limit of normal should not cause alarm if the patient has no reason to have cardiac failure and no symptoms of it.

Valve calcification, if present, is better seen on the lateral view. On the frontal view, valve calcification cannot be visualised over the spine.

Diaphragm

The hemidiaphragms visualised on the frontal films are the top of the domes seen tangentially. Much lung in the posterior costophrenic angles is not seen on the frontal film.

If the hemidiaphragms are low and flat, emphysema may be present. A critical look must be made beneath the diaphragm to see whether there is free peritoneal gas.

Lung fields

On the frontal field, it is convenient to divide the lung fields into zones. It is easy then to compare one zone with another for density differences and the distribution of the vascular 'markings'.

The apices lie above the level of the clavicles. The upper zones include the apices and pass down to the level of the second costal cartilages. The mid zones lie between the second and fourth costal cartilage levels. The lower zones lie between the fourth and sixth costal cartilages.

The radiolucency of the lung fields is due to the air filling the lung. The 'greyness' is due to blood in the pulmonary vessels.

The upper zones of the lungs are normally less well perfused, resulting in smaller blood vessels. When left atrial pressure is elevated, there is upper zone blood diversion and the vessels are congested.

An increase in lung radiolucency occurs when the lungs are over-inflated (e.g. as a result of chronic obstructive pulmonary disease [COPD]). Lung radiolucency is reduced in the presence of an effusion or consolidation.

Terms such as 'opacity', 'consolidation' and 'patchy shadowing' are used to describe the lung fields. It is usually unwise to attempt to make too precise a diagnosis of the underlying pathology.

The lungs are divided into lobes by reflections of the visceral pleura. The right lung is composed of the upper, middle and lower lobes. On the left, there are only the upper and lower lobes.

The right upper lobe has three segments:
- anterior
- posterior
- apical.

The right middle lobe has a lateral and medial segment. Apical, medial basal, lateral basal, anterior basal and posterior basal segments compose the lower lobe.

There are three differences in the segmental anatomy of the left lung (see Fig. 12.6, p 207). The left upper lobe has four segments: an apicoposterior, an anterior and two lingular segments. The superior and inferior lingular segments are the equivalent of the right middle lobe. The left lower lobe has four segments: it does not contain a medial basal segment.

The fissures are seen as hairline shadows. The horizontal fissure is at the level of the right fourth costal cartilage. The oblique fissures are not seen on the frontal view.

Bones and soft tissue

Nipple shadows are often seen over the lower zones and are about 5 millimetres in diameter. They can be confused with a 'coin' lesion. In such a case, nipple markers may be helpful.

Look carefully for a missing breast shadow in a female patient. A mastectomy may provide a diagnostic clue to explain bony or pulmonary metastases, or upper zone postradiation fibrosis.

Soft-tissue gas may accompany a pneumothorax or be present after a thoracotomy.

Calcified tuberculous glands in the neck should be looked for in patients with lung scarring or calcified hilar lymph nodes.

Check that there are no rib fractures (these are difficult to see and a normal chest X-ray does not exclude rib fractures) or space-occupying lesions. Look for rib notching, due to increased blood flow through intercostal vessels (e.g. coarctation of the aorta). Cervical ribs or thoracic scoliosis should be noted. Erosions or arthritis around the shoulder joints should be looked for.

Review

Certain parts of the film should be double-checked if the radiograph appears normal.

The retrocardiac region should be looked at again. A collapsed left lower lobe will reveal itself as a triangular opacity behind the heart shadow.

Both apices should be rechecked for lesions, especially Pancoast's tumours or tuberculosis.

Has the patient a pneumothorax? There will be a difference between the translucency of the two lungs.

Lateral film

The lateral view is used largely for localisation of an already visible lesion on the frontal film. Examine it just as carefully. Sometimes a lesion is seen only on the lateral view. If there is clinical evidence of heart or lung disease, frontal and lateral views should always be obtained.

- Points to remember:
  1. The retrosternal and retrocardiac triangles are normally of a similar radiodensity.
  2. The thoracic vertebrae become less opaque lower down the spine, unless there is pulmonary or pleural disease.
  3. The posterior costophrenic angle is sharp unless there is fluid or adjacent consolidation.

The hemidiaphragms are well defined unless there is pleural or pulmonary disease.

The oblique fissure placement is '4 to 4'. It passes from approximately 4 centimetres behind the anterior costophrenic angle through the hilum to the T4 vertebral bodylevel.

Heart

The right ventricle forms the anterior heart border on the lateral film. The left atrium forms the upper posterior border.

Mitral valve calcification is seen below an imaginary line drawn from the anterior costophrenic angle to the hilum, whereas aortic valve calcification lies above this line.

Examples of chest X-rays in cardiac disease (see also the OCSE X-ray and imaging library at Student CONSULT)

The radiological changes seen in pulmonary venous congestion, interstitial pulmonary oedema and alveolar pulmonary oedema are shown in Figs 8.3 to 8.5 respectively. Mitral valve disease is shown in Fig. 8.6, while a ventricular aneurysm is seen in Fig. 8.7. The characteristic notching of the inferior aspects of the ribs, due to hypertrophy of the intercostal arteries, appears in Fig. 8.8, while the pulmonary plethora that

Pulmonary venous congestion.

The heart is enlarged owing to failure. This failure is not severe enough to cause pulmonary oedema. However, the increased pulmonary venous pressure has caused upper zone blood diversion so that the vessels above the hilum appear wider than those below. (The mechanism of the blood diversion is not fully understood.) These changes are seen when the pulmonary venous pressure is about 15–20 mmHg. The cardiothoracic ratio A:B is a useful indicator of cardiac enlargement if it is greater than 50%. The thoracic measurement (T) is the widest diameter above the costophrenic angles, usually at the level of the right hemidiaphragm. The cardiac diameter is the addition of the two widths A and B

FIGURE 8.3

Interstitial pulmonary oedema.

The heart is moderately enlarged. The interstitial oedema causes fine, diffuse shadowing in the lung fields with blurring of the vessel margins. The escape of fluid into the interstitial tissue occurs when the capillary pressure exceeds the plasma osmotic pressure of 25 mmHg. The interstitial oedema is characterised by Kerley 'B' lines, which are oedematous interlobular septa. They are best seen peripherally in the right costophrenic angle (arrow), where they lie horizontally, and are about 1 cm long. They contain the engorged lymphatics, which were originally thought by Kerley to be the sole cause of the 'B' lines.

Sternal sutures are present from previous cardiac surgery

FIGURE 8.4

is characteristic of a left-to-right shunt is obvious in Fig. 8.9. Marfan's syndrome is illustrated in Fig. 8.10; a pacemaker and defibrillators are shown in Fig. 8.11.

The echocardiogram

Echocardiography is now an essential and basic part of cardiac assessment and can be performed at the bedside. It does not expose the patient to radiation. Small hand-held models are available that can be used almost as readily as a stethoscope. Although these devices will result in the temptation not to bother listening to the heart, any test used without an adequate history and examination is likely to be misleading.

Students and junior doctors need to understand when an echocardiogram is likely to be a helpful test (List 8.1) and not order one simply as a delaying tactic to help avoid making a decision about the patient's diagnosis.

Most echocardiographic studies involve four modalities:

- In *M mode*, detailed information is provided from a single line of ultrasound. It is used to study motion in detail and to make

Alveolar pulmonary oedema.

When the pulmonary venous pressure reaches 30 mmHg, oedema fluid will pass into the alveoli. This causes shadowing (patchy to confluent depending on the extent) in the lung fields. This usually occurs first around the hila and gives a bat's wing appearance. These changes are usually superimposed on the interstitial oedema.

A lamellar pleural effusion (arrow) is seen at the right costophrenic angle where Kerley 'B' lines are also evident

FIGURE 8.5

Ventricular aneurysm.

There is a bulge of the left cardiac border (arrow), which indicates an aneurysm of the left ventricular wall. The most common cause is weakness following myocardial infarction

FIGURE 8.7

Mitral valve disease.

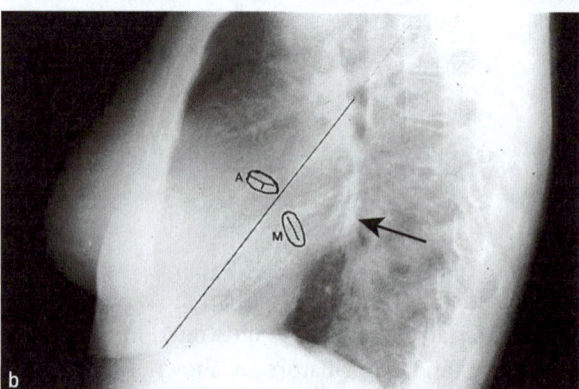

The left atrium enlarges because of the pressure and volume load. It bulges posteriorly and to both sides (blue arrows show the left atrial appendage). The atrial appendage bulges out below the left hilum. The prominent right border of the atrium causes the 'double right heart border' appearance.

To distinguish the valves if calcification is present, draw imaginary lines. On the PA view (a) the line passes from the right cardiophrenic angle to the inferior aspect of the left hilum. The line on the lateral view (b) passes from the anteroinferior angle through the midpoint of the hilum. The aortic valve (A) lies above this line, whereas the mitral valve (M) lies below it

FIGURE 8.6

Aortic coarctation.

The classical sign in aortic coarctation is notching of the inferior aspects of the ribs (arrow on left). This is due to hypertrophy of the intercostal arteries in which retrograde flow from the axillary collaterals is taking blood back to the descending aorta.

Because of the increased resistance to the left heart flow, left ventricular hypertrophy and then failure can occur. Failure causing cardiac enlargement has not yet occurred in this patient. The arrow on the right indicates a smaller-than-normal aortic knuckle

FIGURE 8.8

Atrial septal defect (ASD).

The most important thing to recognise is that there is pulmonary plethora indicating a left-to-right shunt. Left-to-right shunts occur in ASD, ventricular septal defect (VSD) and patent ductus arteriosus (PDA).

The shunted flow causes enlargement of the main pulmonary artery and its branches. The right hilum is enlarged because of the very dilated right pulmonary artery. The left hilum is hidden by the very dilated main pulmonary artery (arrow).

The ascending aorta is small (in contrast to its enlargement in PDA). The left atrium and ventricle are not enlarged, as they are in VSD and PDA

FIGURE 8.9

measurements of chamber sizes (see Figs 8.12–8.14).

- In *two-dimensional or sector scanning*, ultrasound information is assembled into a moving picture that shows the relationship between different areas of the heart in a series of two-dimensional slices (see Figs 8.15 and 8.16 below). This gives information about valve appearance, cardiac function and the presence of congenital abnormalities.
- In *continuous and pulsed wave Doppler*, interrogation of the returning ultrasound signal enables calculation of the Doppler shift caused by reflection of the beam from moving columns of blood. This means that the velocity and direction of blood flow from different parts of the heart can be measured. The Doppler signal can be displayed as a velocity wave. By superimposing the Doppler callipers on the two-dimensional image, the echocardiographer is able to measure the velocity of jets of blood from a particular area (e.g. in the ascending aorta just beyond the aortic valve cusps; see Fig. 8.17).
- In *colour flow mapping*, it is possible for echo machines to solve the Doppler equations for sectors of the two-dimensional scan in real time,

Marfan's syndrome.

The mediastinum is widened by uniform dilation of the ascending aorta, the aortic arch and the descending aorta. This patient had Marfan's syndrome. Dissecting aneurysms can also occur and have a similar appearance

FIGURE 8.10

Pacemaker and defibrillators

(From Baker T, Nikolić G, O'Connor S. *Practical cardiology*, 2nd edn. ©2008, Sydney: Elsevier Australia.)

FIGURE 8.11

IMPORTANT INDICATIONS FOR ECHOCARDIOGRAPHY

1. Assessment of cardiac function—patient with symptoms or signs of heart failure
2. Following myocardial infarction—assess left ventricular damage
3. Assessment of valvular heart disease—patient has a murmur
4. Atrial fibrillation—look for causes or effects: mitral valve disease, left atrial size, left ventricular function, left ventricular wall thickness
5. Known or suspected congenital heart disease—cardiac structure
6. Family history of inherited cardiac disease—e.g. cardiomyopathy, hypertrophic cardiomyopathy
7. Ventricular arrhythmia—left and right ventricular function
8. Suspected increase in LV wall thickness—abnormal ECG, severe hypertension, storage disease or amyloidosis
9. Possible myocardial ischaemia—stress echo
10. Endocarditis—transoesophageal echo
11. Suspected cardiac source of embolic stroke—intracardiac mass, atrial septal defect, dilated left atrium, mitral stenosis

ECG=electrocardiogram; LV=left ventricular.

LIST 8.1

Normal long-axis M-mode measurements.

Both the fractional shortening (change in the dimensions between systole and diastole; normally >27%) and the ejection fraction have been calculated

(From Baker T, Nikolić G, O'Connor S. *Practical cardiology*, 2nd edn. ©2008, Sydney: Elsevier Australia.)

FIGURE 8.12

M-mode echo from a 34-year-old man with 2 months of increasing dyspnoea, diagnosed initially as asthma.

The left ventricle is very dilated. The end-diastolic dimension is 70 mm (<57). The fractional shortening is only 14% (>25–27). Contraction of the septum and posterior wall are equally reduced, typical of dilated cardiomyopathy (p 139)

(From Baker T, Nikolić G, O'Connor S. *Practical cardiology*, 2nd edn. ©2008, Sydney: Elsevier Australia.)

FIGURE 8.13

M-mode measurements in a patient with hypertension.

There is symmetrical thickening of the left ventricular wall

(From Baker T, Nikolić G, O'Connor S. *Practical cardiology*, 2nd edn. ©2008, Sydney: Elsevier Australia.)

FIGURE 8.14

Normal long-axis view of the heart.

The mitral valve leaflets can be seen wide open in this diastolic frame. The apex of the heart is on the left and the right ventricle is at the top of the picture

(From Baker T, Nikolić G, O'Connor S. *Practical cardiology*, 2nd edn. ©2008, Sydney: Elsevier Australia.)

FIGURE 8.15

Normal four-chamber view of the heart.

The left atrium and ventricle are on the right side of the picture. The AV (mitral and tricuspid) valves are closed in this systolic frame

(From Baker T, Nikolić G, O'Connor S. *Practical cardiology*, 2nd edn. ©2008, Sydney: Elsevier Australia.)

FIGURE 8.16

(a) Four-chamber view of a patient with prolapse of both mitral valve leaflets. This systolic frame shows the closed mitral leaflets (anterior on the left) bowing back into the left atrium as they face the full force of left ventricular systole. (b) Four-chamber view of a 50-year-old woman with a middle and late systolic murmur. A brightly coloured (high-velocity) jet is seen in this systolic frame, extending from the centre of the mitral valve well back into the left atrium

(From Baker T, Nikolić G, O'Connor S. *Practical cardiology*, 2nd edn. ©2008, Sydney: Elsevier Australia.)

FIGURE 8.17

assign a colour code depending on the direction and velocity of flow and superimpose this on the two-dimensional image. In this way, flow within the heart is visible in relation to the anatomy and abnormal jets of blood can be more easily detected (see Fig. 8.18).

Information commonly available from an echocardiogram

1. **Structural and functional measurements.** Assessment of left ventricular function by echo involves measurement of the left ventricular end-diastolic dimension (normally less than about 57 mm) and the end-systolic dimension. Fig. 8.12 shows echo views of the heart in the long axis. It shows some of the measurements and structures that can be assessed in this standard view.

    The echo also allows the left ventricle to be examined for areas of segmental hypokinesis (reduced wall motion), the presence of which suggests previous infarction as the cause of the cardiac failure. Fig. 8.16 shows the structures seen in the four-chamber view of the heart.

    Here the echo transducer scans the heart from the position of the apex beat.

2. **Blood flow measurements.** Sector scanning and M-mode pictures can provide information about valve morphology, for example

Colour Doppler showing a jet of mitral regurgitation extending from the valve back into the left atrium

FIGURE 8.18

Short-axis view of the aortic valve in a patient with severe aortic stenosis. The valve cusps are heavily calcified

(From Baker T, Nikolić G, O'Connor S. *Practical cardiology*, 2nd edn. Sydney: Churchill Livingstone, ©2008.)

FIGURE 8.19

Aortic regurgitation

(From Baker T, Nikolić G, O'Connor S. *Practical cardiology*, 2nd edn. Sydney: Churchill Livingstone, ©2008.)

FIGURE 8.20

thickening or prolapse of the leaflets (see Fig. 8.17). Doppler echo can reveal abnormal jets of blood, for example regurgitant jets, and can measure flow velocity across valves. This measurement can be used to estimate the valve gradient (the difference in pressure across the valve).

3. **Mitral regurgitation and mitral valve prolapse.** Here the mitral valve may appear abnormal and abnormal coaptation of the leaflets may be visible (see Figs 8.17, 8.18).
4. **Aortic stenosis.** Thickening and calcification (bright echoes) of the aortic valve are usually visible (see Fig. 8.19). The movement of the valve cusps may appear reduced. The anatomy of the valve may be apparent. Doppler interrogation of the jet of blood in the ascending aorta will enable its velocity to be measured. A simple formula enables estimation of the pressure gradient to be made from this measurement.
5. **Aortic regurgitation.** The valve may look thickened or occasionally a cusp may be seen to prolapse (see Fig. 8.20). The aortic root size may be increased, especially if this is the cause of the aortic regurgitation. Left ventricular dilation is often present and the size of the ventricle may be used as an indication of severity. Doppler interrogation will show the regurgitant jet for a variable distance into the left ventricle.
6. **Tricuspid regurgitation.** This is more often secondary to abnormalities of right ventricular function or to raised right ventricular (RV) pressure than to primary tricuspid valve

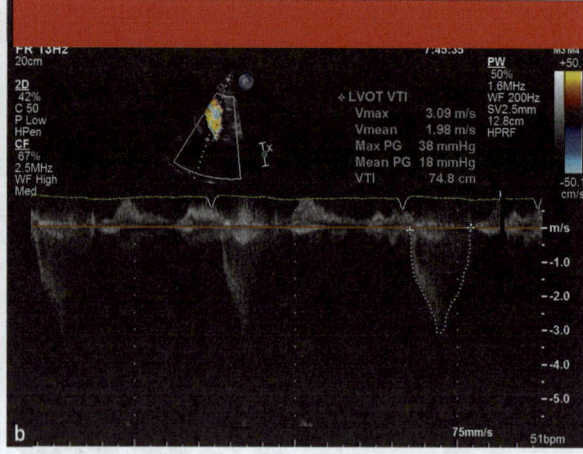

(a) and (b) Hypertrophic cardiomyopathy
(From Baker T, Nikolić G, O'Connor S. *Practical cardiology*, 2nd edn. Sydney: Churchill Livingstone, ©2008.)

FIGURE 8.21

disease. The valve will appear normal. Doppler interrogation will show a jet of blood in the right atrium.

7. **Hypertrophic cardiomyopathy.** Certain anatomical abnormalities are characteristic of this condition (see Fig. 8.21). There is asymmetrical septal hypertrophy (ASH). The normal interventricular septum measures up to 11 millimetres in thickness. This may be considerably increased to 40 millimetres or even more. Doppler interrogation may reveal a gradient in the left ventricular outflow tract or mitral regurgitation, or both.

8. **Ventricular septal defect.** The defect may be visible in the muscular or membranous septum. The diameter of the opening can be measured. Indirect measurements of the effect of the defect include signs of RV dilation caused by left-to-right shunting.

    Doppler interrogation, especially with colour mapping, will usually show left-to-right shunting across the septum, even if the defect itself is not visible. Measurement of the velocity of this jet gives an indication of right ventricular pressures. If the gradient across the defect is large, RV pressure must be much lower than left ventricular (LV) pressure, as is normal. A large ventricular septal defect may cause pulmonary hypertension and elevation of RV pressures.

9. **Atrial septal defect.** The atrial septum can often be seen well enough to reveal a defect, although this is sometimes difficult. There may be indirect indications of left-to-right shunting at the atrial level, including enlargement of the right ventricle and abnormal motion of the interventricular septum.

    Doppler interrogation may show shunting across the defect. If there is doubt, a transoesophageal echo may be needed for accurate definition of the anatomy of the atrial septum.

10. **Patent ductus arteriosus.** The main pulmonary artery will appear large. The ductus itself may be visible. Doppler interrogation reveals continuous flow in the main pulmonary artery at the point where the duct empties.

T&O'C ESSENTIALS

1. *Chest X-ray, ECG and echocardiography are extensions of the cardiovascular examination.*
2. *ECGs and echocardiograms lead to no radiation exposure and can be repeated as required.*
3. *Students need to have an approach to interpreting chest X-rays and ECGs and an understanding of the information that can be obtained from an echocardiogram.*
4. *The initial diagnosis of myocardial infarction should be based on the history, physical examination and ECG and should not be delayed until blood test results are to hand.*

OSCE REVISION TOPICS

1. This woman has been breathless. Please assess her chest X-ray. (p 147)
2. Look at this normal chest X-ray and point out the cardiac borders and the positions of the cardiac chambers. Indicate where the aortic and mitral valve lie. (p 152)
3. Perform a standard cardiovascular examination on this patient. Explain what you are doing as you go along. (p 146)

SECTION 3
The respiratory system

CHAPTER 9

The respiratory history

CHAPTER 10

The respiratory examination

CHAPTER 11

Correlation of physical signs and respiratory disease

CHAPTER 12

A summary of the respiratory examination and extending the respiratory examination

CHAPTER 9
The respiratory history

A medical chest specialist is long winded about the short winded. KENNETH T BIRD (b.1917)

PRESENTING SYMPTOMS

(See List 9.1.)

PRESENTING SYMPTOMS

Major symptoms
Cough
Sputum
Haemoptysis
Dyspnoea (acute, progressive or paroxysmal)
Wheeze
Chest pain
Fever
Hoarseness
Night sweats

LIST 9.1

Cough and sputum

Cough is a common presenting respiratory symptom. It occurs when deep inspiration is followed by explosive expiration. Flow rates of air in the trachea approach the speed of sound during a forceful cough. Coughing enables the airways to be cleared of secretions and foreign bodies.

The duration of a cough is important (see Questions box 9.1). Find out when the cough first became a problem. A cough of recent origin, particularly if associated with fever and other symptoms of respiratory tract infection, may be due to acute bronchitis or pneumonia. A chronic cough (of more than 8 weeks duration) associated with wheezing may be due to asthma; sometimes asthma can present with just cough alone. A change in the character of a chronic cough may indicate the development of a new and serious underlying problem (e.g. infection or lung cancer).

QUESTIONS TO ASK THE PATIENT WITH A COUGH

! denotes symptoms for the possible diagnosis of an urgent or dangerous problem.

1. How long have you had the cough?
2. Do you cough up anything? What? How much?
3. Have you had sinus problems?
! 4. Is the sputum clear or discoloured? Is there any blood in the sputum?
5. Have you had high temperatures?
6. Does coughing occur particularly at night (acid reflux)?
7. Have you become short of breath?
8. Have you had lung problems in the past?
9. Have you been a smoker? Do you still smoke?
10. Have you noticed wheezing? (Asthma, chronic obstructive pulmonary disease [COPD])
11. Do you take any tablets? (e.g. ACE inhibitors)

QUESTIONS BOX 9.1

A differential diagnosis of cough based on its character is shown in Table 9.1 and on its duration is shown in List 9.2.

A cough associated with a postnasal drip or sinus congestion or headaches may be due to the upper airway cough syndrome, which is the single most common cause of chronic cough. Although patients with this

Differential diagnosis of cough based on its character

Origin	Character	Causes
Nasopharynx/larynx	Throat clearing, chronic	Postnasal drip, acid reflux
Larynx	Barking, painful, acute or persistent	Laryngitis, pertussis (whooping cough), croup
Trachea	Acute, painful	Tracheitis
Bronchi	Intermittent, sometimes productive, worse at night	Asthma
	Worse in morning	COPD
	With blood	Bronchial malignancy
Lung parenchyma	Dry then productive	Pneumonia
	Chronic, very productive	Bronchiectasis
	Productive, with blood	Tuberculosis
	Irritating and dry, persistent	Interstitial lung disease
	Worse on lying down, sometimes with frothy sputum	Pulmonary oedema
ACE inhibitors	Dry, scratchy, persistent	Medication induced

ACE = angiotensin-converting enzyme; COPD = chronic obstructive pulmonary disease.

TABLE 9.1

DIFFERENTIAL DIAGNOSIS OF COUGH BASED ON ITS DURATION

Acute cough (<3 weeks duration): differential diagnosis

Upper respiratory tract infection
   Common cold, sinusitis
Lower respiratory tract infection
   Pneumonia, bronchitis, exacerbation of COPD
Irritation—inhalation of bronchial irritant (e.g. smoke or fumes)

Chronic cough: differential diagnosis and clues

COPD—smoking history
Asthma—wheeze, relief with bronchodilators
Gastro-oesophageal reflux—occurs when lying down, burning central chest pain
Upper airway cough syndrome—history of rhinitis, postnasal drip, sinus headache and congestion
Bronchiectasis—chronic, very productive
ACE inhibitor medication—drug history
Carcinoma of the lung—smoking, haemoptysis
Cardiac failure—dyspnoea, PND
Psychogenic—variable, prolonged symptoms, usually mild

ACE = angiotensin-converting enzyme; COPD = chronic obstructive pulmonary disease; PND = paroxysmal nocturnal dyspnoea.

LIST 9.2

---

problem often complain of a cough, when asked to demonstrate their cough they sometimes do not cough but rather clear the throat. An irritating, chronic dry cough can result from oesophageal reflux and acid irritation of the airway. There is some controversy about these as causes of true cough. A dry cough may be a feature of late interstitial lung disease or associated with the use of the angiotensin-converting enzyme (ACE) inhibitors—drugs used in the treatment of hypertension and cardiac failure. Cough that wakes a patient from sleep may be a symptom of cardiac failure or of the reflux of acid from the oesophagus into the upper airway that can occur when a person lies down. A chronic cough that is productive of large volumes of purulent sputum may be due to bronchiectasis. Chronic cough is associated with: postnasal drip, bronchiectasis, pulmonary fibrosis, asthma and gastro-oesophageal reflux disease.

Patients' descriptions of their cough may be helpful.

- In children, a cough associated with inflammation of the epiglottis may have a muffled quality and cough related to viral croup is often described as 'barking'. In adults a barking cough may indicate a condition of flaccid trachea and large bronchi, known as tracheomalacia.
- Cough caused by tracheal compression by a tumour may be loud and brassy. Cough associated with recurrent laryngeal nerve palsy has a hollow sound because the vocal cords are unable to close completely; this has been described as a bovine cough.

- A cough that is worse at night is suggestive of asthma or heart failure, while coughing that comes on immediately after eating or drinking may be due to incoordinate swallowing or oesophageal reflux or, rarely, a tracheo-oesophageal fistula.

An immunocompromised patient with a cough often has an infectious cause. Infections such as tuberculosis, *Cryptococcus* spp., Cytomegalovirus, Varicella and *Aspergillosis* spp. should be considered.

Some patients feel the need to cough after an ectopic heartbeat. There may be an associated sensation of a missed heartbeat.

It is an important (though perhaps a somewhat unpleasant task) to enquire about the type of sputum produced and then to look at it, if it is available. Be warned that some patients have more interest in their sputum than others and may go into more detail than you really want. A large volume of purulent (yellow or green) sputum suggests the diagnosis of bronchiectasis or lobar pneumonia. Foul-smelling dark-coloured sputum may indicate the presence of a lung abscess with anaerobic organisms. Pink frothy secretions from the trachea, which occur in pulmonary oedema, should not be confused with sputum. It is best to rely on the patient's assessment of the taste of the sputum, which, not unexpectedly, is foul in conditions like bronchiectasis or lung abscess.

Haemoptysis

Haemoptysis (coughing up of blood) can be a sinister sign of lung disease (see Table 9.2) and must always be investigated. It must be distinguished from haematemesis (vomiting of blood) and from nasopharyngeal bleeding (see Table 9.3).

Ask how much blood has been produced. Mild haemoptysis usually means less than 20 mL in 24 hours. It appears as streaks of blood discolouring sputum. Massive haemoptysis is more than 250 mL of blood in 24 hours and represents a medical emergency; its most common causes are carcinoma, cystic fibrosis, bronchiectasis and tuberculosis.

Breathlessness (dyspnoea)

The awareness that an abnormal amount of effort is required for breathing is called dyspnoea. It can be due to respiratory or cardiac disease, or lack of physical fitness or sometimes to anxiety (see List 9.3). Careful questioning about the timing of onset, severity and pattern of dyspnoea is helpful in making the diagnosis (see Questions box 9.2 and List 9.4).[1] The patient may be aware of this only on heavy exertion or have much more limited exercise tolerance. Dyspnoea can be

Causes (differential diagnosis) of haemoptysis and typical histories

Respiratory	
Bronchitis	Small amounts of blood with sputum
Bronchial carcinoma	Frank blood, history of smoking, hoarseness
Bronchiectasis	Large amounts of sputum with blood
Pneumonia	Fever, recent onset of symptoms, dyspnoea
(The above four account for about 80% of cases)	
Pulmonary infarction	Pleuritic chest pain, dyspnoea
Cystic fibrosis	Recurrent infections
Lung abscess	Fever, purulent sputum
Tuberculosis (TB)	Previous TB, contact with TB, HIV-positive status
Foreign body	History of inhalation, cough, stridor
Anti-glomerular basement membrane (GBM) antibody disease*	Pulmonary haemorrhage, glomerulonephritis, antibody to basement membrane antigens
Wegener's granulomatosis†	History of sinusitis, saddle-nose deformity
Systemic lupus erythematosus	Pulmonary haemorrhage, multisystem involvement
Rupture of a mucosal blood vessel after vigorous coughing	History of severe cough preceding haemoptysis
Cardiovascular	
Mitral stenosis (severe)	
Acute left ventricular failure	
Bleeding diatheses	

Note: *Exclude spurious causes, such as nasal bleeding or haematemesis.*
*Ernest W Goodpasture (1886–1960), pathologist at Johns Hopkins, Baltimore described this in 1919.
†Better named GPA: granulomatosis with polyangiitis.

TABLE 9.2

Features distinguishing haemoptysis from haematemesis and nasopharyngeal bleeding

Favours haemoptysis	Favours haematemesis	Favours nasopharyngeal bleeding
Mixed with sputum	Follows nausea	Blood appears in mouth
Occurs immediately after coughing	Mixed with vomitus; follows dry retching	

TABLE 9.3

graded from I to IV based on the New York Heart Association classification:

Class I   Disease present but no dyspnoea or dyspnoea only on heavy exertion
Class II Dyspnoea on moderate exertion
Class III Dyspnoea on minimal exertion
Class IV Dyspnoea at rest.

It is more useful, however, to determine the amount of exertion that actually causes dyspnoea—that is, the distance walked or the number of steps climbed.

The association of dyspnoea with wheeze suggests *airways disease*, which may be due to asthma or chronic obstructive pulmonary disease (COPD; see List 9.5). The duration and variability of the dyspnoea are important.

CAUSES OF DYSPNOEA

Respiratory

1. AIRWAYS DISEASE
Chronic bronchitis and emphysema (COPD)
Asthma
Bronchiectasis
Cystic fibrosis
Laryngeal or pharyngeal tumour
Bilateral cord palsy
Tracheal obstruction or stenosis
Tracheomalacia
Cricoarytenoid rheumatoid arthritis

2. PARENCHYMAL DISEASE
Interstitial lung diseases (diffuse parenchymal lung diseases, e.g. idiopathic pulmonary fibrosis, sarcoidosis, connective tissue disease, inorganic or organic dusts)
Diffuse infections
ARDS
Infiltrative and metastatic tumour
Pneumothorax
Pneumoconiosis

3. PULMONARY CIRCULATION
Pulmonary embolism
Chronic thromboembolic pulmonary hypertension
Pulmonary arteriovenous malformation
Pulmonary arteritis

4. CHEST WALL AND PLEURA
Effusion or massive ascites
Pleural tumour
Fractured ribs
Ankylosing spondylitis
Kyphoscoliosis
Neuromuscular diseases
Bilateral diaphragmatic paralysis

Cardiac
Left ventricular failure
Mitral valve disease
Cardiomyopathy
Pericardial effusion or constrictive pericarditis
Intracardiac shunt

Anaemia

Non-cardiorespiratory
Psychogenic
Acidosis (compensatory respiratory alkalosis)
Hypothalamic lesions

ARDS=acute respiratory distress syndrome; COPD=chronic obstructive pulmonary disease.

LIST 9.3

QUESTIONS TO ASK THE BREATHLESS PATIENT

! denotes symptoms for the possible diagnosis of an urgent or dangerous problem.

1. How long have you been short of breath? Has it come on quickly?
2. How much exercise can you do before your shortness of breath stops you or slows you down? Can you walk up a flight of stairs?
! 3. Have you been woken at night by breathlessness or had to sleep sitting up? (Paroxysmal nocturnal dyspnoea [PND], orthopnoea)
4. Have you had heart or lung problems in the past?
! 5. Have you had a temperature?
6. Do you smoke?
! 7. Is there a feeling of tightness in the chest when you feel breathless? (Angina)
8. Do you get wheezy in the chest? Cough?
9. Is the feeling really one of difficulty getting a satisfying breath? (Anxiety)
10. Is it painful to take a big breath? (Pleurisy or pericarditis)
! 11. Did the shortness of breath come on very quickly or instantaneously? (Pulmonary embolus [very quick onset] or pneumothorax [instantaneous onset])
12. Are you often short of breath when you are anxious? Do you feel numbness and tingling around your lips when you are breathless? (Hyperventilation associated with anxiety)

QUESTIONS BOX 9.2

DIFFERENTIAL DIAGNOSIS OF DYSPNOEA BASED ON TIME COURSE OF ONSET

Seconds to minutes—favours:
Asthma
Pulmonary embolism
Pneumothorax
Pulmonary oedema
Anaphylaxis
Foreign body causing airway obstruction

Hours or days—favours:
Exacerbation of COPD
Cardiac failure
Asthma
Respiratory infection
Pleural effusion
Metabolic acidosis

Weeks or longer—favours:
Pulmonary fibrosis
COPD
Interstitial lung disease
Pleural effusion
Anaemia

COPD = chronic obstructive pulmonary disease.

LIST 9.4

CHARACTERISTICS OF CHRONIC OBSTRUCTIVE PULMONARY DISEASE

History
History of smoking
Breathlessness and wheeze

Examination (p 175)
Increased respiratory rate
Pursed-lips breathing
Cyanosis
Leaning forwards—arms on knees
Intercostal and supraclavicular in-drawing
Hoover's sign
Tracheal tug

LIST 9.5

- Dyspnoea that worsens progressively over a period of weeks, months or years may be due to *interstitial lung disease* (ILD).
- Dyspnoea of more rapid onset may be due to an *acute respiratory infection* (including bronchopneumonia or lobar pneumonia) or to *pneumonitis* (which may be infective or secondary to a hypersensitivity reaction).
- Dyspnoea that varies from day to day or even from hour to hour suggests a diagnosis of *asthma*.
- Dyspnoea of very rapid onset associated with sharp chest pain suggests a *pneumothorax* (see List 9.6).
- Dyspnoea that is described by the patient as inability to take a breath big enough to fill the lungs and associated with sighing suggests *anxiety*.
- Dyspnoea that occurs on moderate exertion may be due to the combination of *obesity* and a *lack of physical fitness* ('deconditioning', a not uncommon occurrence).

Wheeze

A number of conditions can cause a continuous whistling noise that comes from the chest (rather than the throat) during breathing. These include asthma or COPD, infections such as bronchiolitis and airways obstruction by a foreign body or tumour. Wheeze is usually maximal during expiration and is accompanied by prolonged expiration. This must be differentiated from *stridor* (see below), which can have a similar sound, but is loudest over the trachea and occurs during inspiration.

Chest pain

Chest pain due to respiratory disease is usually different from that associated with myocardial ischaemia (p 121). The parietal pleura has pain fibres and may be the source of respiratory pain. Pleural pain is characteristically *pleuritic* in nature: sharp and made worse by deep inspiration and coughing. It is typically localised to one area of the chest. It may be of sudden onset in patients with:

- lobar pneumonia
- pulmonary embolism and infarction, or
- pneumothorax

and is often associated with dyspnoea.

The sudden onset of pleuritic chest pain and dyspnoea is an urgent diagnostic problem, as all three of these conditions may be life-threatening if not treated promptly.

OTHER PRESENTING SYMPTOMS

Bacterial pneumonia is an acute illness in which prodromal symptoms (fever, malaise and myalgia) occur for a short period (hours) before pleuritic pain and dyspnoea begin.

Viral pneumonia is often preceded by a longer (days) prodromal illness. Patients may occasionally present with episodes of *fever at night*.

Tuberculosis, pneumonia and lymphoma should always be considered in these cases. Occasionally,

---

DIFFERENTIAL DIAGNOSIS OF DYSPNOEA OF SUDDEN ONSET BASED ON OTHER FEATURES

Presence of pleuritic chest pain—favours:
Pneumothorax
Pleurisy/pneumonia
Pulmonary embolism

Absence of chest pain—favours:
Pulmonary oedema
Metabolic acidosis
Pulmonary embolism

Presence of central chest pain—favours:
Myocardial infarction and cardiac failure
Large pulmonary embolism

Presence of cough and wheeze—favours:
Asthma
Bronchial irritant inhalation
COPD

COPD=chronic obstructive pulmonary disease.

LIST 9.6

patients with tuberculosis may present with episodes of *drenching sweating* at night.

Hoarseness or *dysphonia* (an abnormality of the voice) may sometimes be considered a respiratory system symptom. It can be due to transient inflammation of the vocal cords (laryngitis), vocal cord tumour or recurrent laryngeal nerve palsy.

Sleep apnoea is an abnormal increase in the periodic cessation of breathing during sleep. Patients with *obstructive sleep apnoea* (OSA, where airflow stops during sleep for periods of at least 10 seconds and sometimes for more than 2 minutes, despite persistent respiratory efforts) typically present with:

- daytime somnolence
- chronic fatigue
- morning headaches
- personality disturbances.

Very loud snoring may be reported by anyone within earshot. However, snoring is very common among patients without sleep apnoea and nocturnal choking or gasping is a more reliable sign (LR 3.3).[2] These patients are often obese and hypertensive. The Epworth sleepiness scale is a way of quantifying the severity of sleep apnoea (see List 9.7). Patients with *central sleep apnoea* (where there is cessation of inspiratory muscle activity) may also present with somnolence but do not snore excessively (see Table 9.4).

Some patients respond to anxiety by increasing the rate and depth of their breathing. This is called *hyperventilation*. The result is an increase in CO_2 excretion and the development of alkalosis—a rise in the pH of the blood. These patients may complain of variable dyspnoea; they have more difficulty breathing in than out. The alkalosis results in paraesthesias of the fingers and around the mouth, light-headedness, chest pain and a feeling of impending collapse.

CURRENT TREATMENT

It is important to find out what drugs the patient is using (see List 9.8), how often they are taken and whether they are inhaled or swallowed. The patient's previous and current medications may give a clue to the current diagnosis. Bronchodilators and inhaled steroids are prescribed for COPD and asthma. A patient's increased use of bronchodilators suggests poor control of asthma and the need for review of treatment.

Chronic respiratory disease, including sarcoidosis, hypersensitivity pneumonias and asthma, may have been treated with oral steroids.

Oral steroid use may predispose to tuberculosis or pneumocystis pneumonia. Patients with chronic lung conditions like cystic fibrosis or bronchiectasis will often be very knowledgeable about their treatment and can describe the various forms of physiotherapy that are essential for keeping their airways clear.

Find out whether *home oxygen* has been prescribed. An oxygen concentrator or oxygen cylinder may be used and the oxygen administered by a mask or with nasal prongs. The flow rate is usually 2 L/minute or more and oxygen may be prescribed for 24 hours a day in some cases. Portable oxygen cylinders and rechargeable portable concentrators are available. Home oxygen is expensive and the rules for its prescription are quite strict. Usually arterial blood gas measurements that show low oxygen concentrations are required before oxygen can be prescribed. For safety reasons patients must have given up smoking before home oxygen can be allowed.

Pulmonary rehabilitation courses are now commonly prescribed for patients with chronic lung disease. They involve graded exercise programs and information

---

THE EPWORTH SLEEPINESS SCALE

'How easily would you fall asleep in the following circumstances?'*

0 = never
1 = slight chance
2 = moderate chance
3 = high chance

- Sitting reading
- Watching television
- At a meeting or at the theatre
- As a passenger in a car on a drive of more than an hour
- Lying down in the afternoon to rest
- Sitting talking to someone
- Sitting quietly after lunch (no alcohol)
- When driving and stopped at traffic lights

*A normal score is between 0 and 9. Severe sleep apnoea scores from 11 to 20.

LIST 9.7

Abnormal patterns of breathing

Type of breathing	Cause(s)
1. Sleep apnoea—cessation of airflow for more than 10 seconds more than 10 times a night during sleep	Obstructive (e.g. obesity with upper airway narrowing, enlarged tonsils, pharyngeal soft-tissue changes in acromegaly or hypothyroidism)
2. Cheyne–Stokes* breathing—periods of apnoea (associated with reduced level of consciousness) alternate with periods of hyperpnoea (lasts 30 s on average and is associated with agitation); this is due to a delay in the medullary chemoreceptor response to blood gas changes	Left ventricular failure Brain damage (e.g. trauma, cerebral haemorrhage) High altitude
3. Kussmaul's breathing (air hunger)—deep, rapid respiration due to stimulation of the respiratory centre	Metabolic acidosis (e.g. diabetes mellitus, chronic renal failure)
4. Hyperventilation, which results in alkalosis, tetany and perioral paraesthesias	Anxiety
5. Ataxic (Biot†) breathing—irregular in timing and depth	Brainstem damage
6. Apneustic breathing—a postinspiratory pause in breathing	Brain (pontine) damage
7. Paradoxical respiration—the abdomen sucks inwards with inspiration (it normally pouches outwards due to diaphragmatic descent)	Diaphragmatic paralysis

*John Cheyne (1777–1836), Scottish physician who worked in Dublin, described this in 1818. William Stokes (1804–78), Irish physician, described it in 1854.
†Camille Biot (1878–1936), French physician.

TABLE 9.4

DRUGS AND THE LUNGS

Cough
ACE inhibitors
Beta-blockers

Wheeze
Beta-blockers
Aspirin (aspirin sensitivity)
Other NSAIDs
Tamoxifen, dipyridamole (idiosyncratic)
Morphine sulfate
Succinylcholine

Interstitial lung disease (pulmonary fibrosis)
Amiodarone
Hydralazine
Anti-tumour necrosis factor (anti-TNF)—alpha-blockers
Bleomycin
Nitrofurantoin
Methotrexate

Pulmonary embolism
Oestrogens
Tamoxifen
Raloxifene

Non-cardiogenic pulmonary oedema
Hydrochlorothiazide

Pleural disease / effusion
Nitrofurantoin
Phenytoin, hydralazine (induction of systemic lupus erythematosus)
Methotrexate
Methysergide

ACE = angiotensin-converting enzyme; NSAIDs = non-steroidal anti-inflammatory drugs.

LIST 9.8

about ways of dealing with chronic respiratory symptoms. Find out whether this has been recommended and whether it has been helpful.

Almost every class of drug can produce lung toxicity. Examples include:

- pulmonary embolism from use of the oral contraceptive pill
- interstitial lung disease from cytotoxic agents (e.g. methotrexate, cyclophosphamide, bleomycin)

- bronchospasm from beta-blockers or non-steroidal anti-inflammatory drugs (NSAIDs), and
- cough from ACE inhibitors.

Some medications known to cause lung disease may not be mentioned by the patient because they:

- are illegal (e.g. cocaine)
- are used sporadically (e.g. hydrochlorothiazide)
- can be obtained over the counter (e.g. tryptophan), or
- are not taken orally (e.g. timolol, beta-blocker eye drops for glaucoma).

The clinician therefore needs to ask about these types of drugs specifically.

PAST HISTORY

Always ask about previous respiratory illness, including pneumonia, tuberculosis or chronic bronchitis, or abnormalities of the chest X-ray that have previously been reported to the patient. Many previous respiratory investigations may have been memorable, such as bronchoscopy, lung biopsy and video-assisted thoracoscopy. Spirometry, with or without challenge testing for asthma, may have been performed. Many severe asthmatics perform their own regular peak flow testing (p 203). Ask about the results of any of these investigations. Patients with the acquired immunodeficiency syndrome (AIDS) have a high risk of developing *Pneumocystis jiroveci* pneumonia and indeed other chest infections, including tuberculosis.

OCCUPATIONAL HISTORY

In no other body system assessment are the patient's present and previous occupations of more importance (see Table 9.5).[3] A detailed occupational history is essential. The occupational lung diseases or pneumoconioses cause interstitial lung disease by damaging the alveoli and small airways. Prolonged exposure to substances whose use is now heavily restricted is usually required. Cigarette smoking has an additive effect for these patients. These occupational conditions are now rare, and the most common occupational lung disease is asthma.

Ask about exposure to dusts in mining industries and factories:

Occupational lung disease (pneumoconioses)

Substance	Disease
Coal	Coal worker's pneumoconiosis
Silica	Silicosis
Asbestos	Asbestosis
Talc	Talcosis

TABLE 9.5

POSSIBLE OCCUPATIONAL EXPOSURE TO ASBESTOS

Asbestos mining, including relatives of miners

Naval dockyard workers and sailors—lagging of pipes

Builders—asbestos in fibreboard (particles are released during cutting or drilling)

Factory workers—manufacture of fibro-sheets, brake linings, some textiles

Building maintenance workers—asbestos insulation

Building demolition workers

Home renovation

Emergency workers—cleaning up after floods and fires

LIST 9.9

- asbestos
- coal
- silica
- iron oxide
- tin oxide
- cotton
- beryllium
- titanium oxide
- silver
- nitrogen dioxide
- anhydrides.

Heavy exposure to asbestos can lead to asbestosis (see List 9.9), but even trivial exposure can result in mesothelioma (malignant disease of the pleura). The patient may be unaware that his or her occupation involved exposure to dangerous substances; for example, factories making insulating cables and boards very often used asbestos until 25 years ago. Asbestos exposure can result in the development of asbestosis, pleural plaques, mesothelioma or carcinoma of the lung up to 30 years later. Relatives of people working with asbestos may be exposed when handling work clothes. Only very minor exposure is required for patients to develop the disease (although only a small minority of exposed people develop the disease) and sometimes considerable detective work is needed to work out the source of exposure. Finding the source of exposure can be important as a public health matter.

Work or household exposure to animals, including birds, is also relevant (e.g. Q fever or psittacosis, which are infectious diseases caught from animals).

Exposure to organic dusts can cause a local immune response to organic antigens and result in extensive *allergic alveolitis*. Within a few hours of exposure, patients develop flu-like symptoms. These often include:

- fever
- headache
- muscle pains
- dyspnoea without wheeze, and
- dry cough.

The culprit antigens may come from mouldy hay, humidifiers or air conditioners, among others (see Table 9.6).

It is most important to find out what the patient actually does when at work, the duration of any exposure, use of protective devices and whether other workers have become ill. An improvement in symptoms over the weekend is a valuable clue to the presence of occupational lung disease, particularly occupational asthma. This can occur as a result of exposure to spray paints or plastic or soldering fumes.

SOCIAL HISTORY

A smoking history must be routine, as it is the major cause of COPD[4] and lung cancer (see List 1.2, p 17). It also increases the risk of interstitial lung disease, spontaneous pneumothorax and of Goodpasture's syndrome. It is necessary to ask how many packets of cigarettes per day the patient has smoked and how many years the patient has smoked. An estimate should be made of the number of packet-years of smoking (see Ch 1). Occupation may further affect cigarette smokers; for example, asbestos workers who smoke are at an especially high risk of lung cancer. Passive smoking is now regarded as a significant risk for lung disease and the patient should be asked about exposure to other people's cigarette smoke at home and at work.

Many respiratory conditions are chronic and may interfere with the ability to work and exercise as well as interfering with normal family life. In some cases involving occupational lung disease there may be compensation matters affecting the patient.

- Ask about these problems and whether the patient has been involved in a pulmonary rehabilitation program.
- Housing conditions may be inappropriate for a person with a limited exercise tolerance or an infectious disease.
- Ask about the patient's alcohol consumption. Drinking large amounts of alcohol in binges can sometimes result in aspiration pneumonia, and alcoholics are more likely to develop pneumococcal or *Klebsiella* pneumonia.
- Intravenous drug users are at risk of lung abscess and drug-related pulmonary oedema.
- Unsafe sexual practices or history of intravenous drug use may be related to an increased risk of HIV infection and susceptibility to infection.

Such information may influence the decision about whether to advise treatment at home or in hospital.

Allergic alveolitis: sources	
Disorder	**Source**
Bird fancier's lung	Bird feathers and excreta
Farmer's lung	Mouldy hay or straw (*Aspergillus fumigatus*)
Byssinosis	Cotton or hemp dust
Cheese worker's lung	Mouldy cheese (*Aspergillus clavatus*)
Malt worker's lung	Mouldy malt (*Aspergillus clavatus*)
Humidifier fever	Air-conditioning (thermophilic *Actinomycetes*)

TABLE 9.6

FAMILY HISTORY

A family history of asthma or other atopic diseases, cystic fibrosis, lung cancer or emphysema should be sought. Alpha$_1$-antitrypsin deficiency, for example, is an inherited disease, and those affected are extremely susceptible to the development of emphysema. A family history of infection with tuberculosis is also important. A number of pulmonary diseases may have a familial or genetic association. These include carcinoma of the lung and pulmonary hypertension.

T&O'C ESSENTIALS

1. A careful history will often help in deciding if dyspnoea is due to cardiac or respiratory causes.
2. The diagnosis of COPD can be made based on the smoking history.
3. A careful occupational history is more important for the respiratory system assessment than for any other body system assessment.
4. Haemoptysis in a smoker—you must rule out lung cancer.
5. Take a drug history, an important cause of lung disease.
6. Anxious patients who complain of breathlessness often describe an inability to take a satisfying breath. Their symptoms often occur at rest.

OSCE REVISION TOPICS – THE RESPIRATORY HISTORY

Use these topics, which commonly occur in the OSCE, to help with revision.

1. This man has been found on X-ray to have pleural plaques. Please take a respiratory and occupational history from him. (p 171)
2. This man has been troubled by asthma. Please take a history from him. (p 165)
3. Find out if this woman's history is consistent with COPD. (p 165)
4. This woman has a cough. Ask her about it and take a respiratory history. (p 163)
5. Assess this man for possible sleep apnoea. (p 169)

References

1. Schmitt BP, Kushner MS, Wiener SL. The diagnostic usefulness of the history of the patient with dyspnea. *J Gen Intern Med* 1986; 1:386–393. History alone was correct three out of four times when deciding the cause of dyspnoea in defined circumstances.
2. Myers KA, Mrkobrada M, Simel DL. Does this patient have obstructive sleep apnoea?: The Rational Clinical Examination systematic review. *JAMA* 2013; 310(7):731–741.
3. Anonymous. Obtaining an exposure history. Agency for Toxic Substances and Disease Registry. United States Department of Health and Human Services, Public Health Service, Atlanta, Georgia. *Am Fam Phys* 1993; 48:483–491.
4. Broekhuizen BD, Sachs AP, Oostvogels R et al. The diagnostic value of history and physical examination for COPD in suspected or known cases: a systematic review. *Fam Pract* 2009; 26(4):260–268. Items of diagnostic value for COPD included a history of dyspnoea, wheezing and smoking. Items of value on examination included audible wheezing and forced expiratory time. However, the data were heterogeneous.

CHAPTER 10
The respiratory examination

More would I, but my lungs are wasted so, That strength of speech is utterly denied me.
WILLIAM SHAKESPEARE, Henry IV, Part 2

EXAMINATION ANATOMY

The **lungs** are paired asymmetrical organs protected by the cylinder composed of the ribs, vertebrae and diaphragm. The surface of the lungs is covered by the visceral **pleura**, a thin membrane, and a similar outer layer (the parietal pleura) lines the rib cage. These membranes are separated by a thin layer of fluid and enable the lungs to move freely during breathing. Various diseases of the lungs and of the pleura themselves, including infection and malignancy, can cause accumulation of fluid within the pleural cavity (a pleural effusion) (Fig. 10.1).

The heart, trachea, oesophagus and the great blood vessels and nerves sit between the lungs and make up the structure called the **mediastinum**. The left and right pulmonary arteries supply their respective lung. Gas exchange occurs in the pulmonary capillaries that surround the alveoli, the tiny air sacs that lie beyond the terminal bronchioles. Oxygenated blood is returned via the pulmonary veins to the left atrium. Abnormalities of the pulmonary circulation, such as raised pulmonary venous pressure resulting from heart failure or pulmonary hypertension, can interfere with gas exchange.

The position of the heart, whose apex points to the left, means that the **left lung** is smaller than the right and has only two lobes, which are separated by the oblique fissure. The **right lung** has both horizontal (upper) and oblique (lower) fissures dividing it into three lobes (see Fig. 10.2).

The muscles of respiration are the **diaphragm**, upon which the bases of the lungs rest, and the **intercostal muscles**. During inspiration, the diaphragm flattens and the intercostal muscles contract to elevate the ribs. Intrathoracic pressure falls as air is forced under atmospheric pressure into the lungs. Expiration is a passive process resulting from elastic recoil of the muscles. Abnormalities of lung function or structure may change the normal anatomy and physiology of respiration, for example as a result of over-inflation of the lungs (chronic obstructive pulmonary disease [COPD]). Muscle and neurological diseases can also affect muscle function adversely, and abnormalities of the control of breathing in the respiratory centres of the brain in the pons and medulla can interfere with normal breathing patterns.

During the respiratory examination, keep in mind the **surface anatomy** of the lungs and try to decide which lobes are affected.

POSITIONING THE PATIENT

The patient should be undressed to the waist.[1] Women should wear a gown or have a towel or some clothing to cover their breasts when the front of the chest is not being examined. If the patient is not acutely ill, the examination may be easiest to perform with him or her sitting over the edge of the bed or on a chair.

GENERAL APPEARANCE

If the patient is an inpatient in hospital, look around the bed for nasal prongs or a mask, metered dose inhalers (puffers) and other medications. Then make a deliberate point of looking for the following signs before beginning the detailed examination.

Dyspnoea

Watch the patient for signs of dyspnoea at rest. Count the respiratory rate; the normal rate at rest should not exceed 25 breaths per minute (range 16–25). The frequently quoted normal value of 14 breaths per

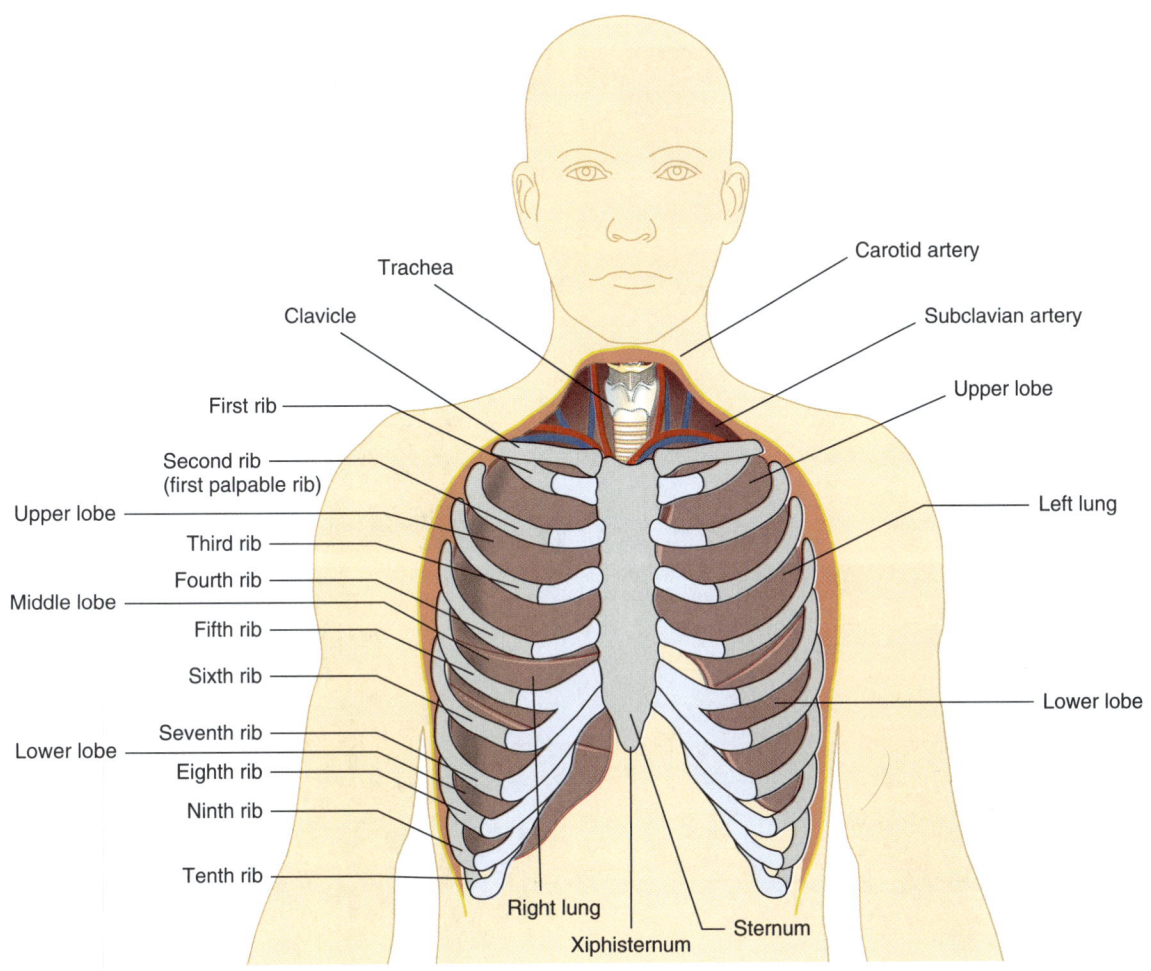

Basic anatomy of the lungs

FIGURE 10.1

minute is probably too low; normal people can have a respiratory rate of up to 25, and the average is 20 breaths per minute. It is traditional to count the respiratory rate surreptitiously while affecting to count the pulse. The respiratory rate is the only vital sign that is under direct voluntary control. *Tachypnoea* refers to a rapid respiratory rate of greater than 25. *Bradypnoea* is defined as a rate below 8, a level associated with sedation and adverse prognosis. In normal relaxed breathing, the diaphragm is the only active muscle and is active only in inspiration; expiration is a passive process.

Characteristic signs of COPD

Look to see whether the accessory muscles of respiration are being used. This is a sign of an increase in the work of breathing, and COPD[a] is an important cause. These muscles include the sternocleidomastoids, the platysma and the strap muscles of the neck. Characteristically, the accessory muscles cause elevation of the shoulders with inspiration, and aid respiration by increasing chest expansion. Contraction of the abdominal muscles may occur in expiration in patients with obstructed airways. Patients with severe COPD often have in-drawing

---

[a] This condition has undergone many changes in nomenclature, and it is pleasing to think that experts have something to keep them occupied. The term COPD encompasses emphysema, chronic bronchitis, chronic obstructive lung disease (COLD) and chronic airflow limitation (CAL). This term seems quite firmly established (at least for now). The diagnosis of COPD depends on clinical, radiographic and lung function assessment. There may be components of what used to be called chronic bronchitis and emphysema.

Lobes of the lung.

(a) Anterior; (b) posterior; (c) lobes of the right lung; (d) lobes of the left lung. Refer to Fig. 12.6, page 207, for a list of the segments in each lobe

FIGURE 10.2

of the intercostal and supraclavicular spaces during inspiration. This is due to a delayed increase in lung volume despite the generation of large negative pleural pressures.

In some cases, the pattern of breathing is helpful diagnostically (see Table 9.4, p 170). Look for pursed-lips breathing, which is characteristic of patients with severe COPD. This manoeuvre reduces the patient's breathlessness, possibly by providing continuous positive airways pressure and helping to prevent airways collapse during expiration. Patients with severe COPD may feel more comfortable leaning forwards with their arms on their knees. This position compresses the abdomen and pushes the diaphragm upwards. This partly restores its normal domed shape and improves its effectiveness during inspiration. Increased diaphragmatic movements may cause downward displacement of the trachea during inspiration—tracheal tug (this is also a sign of severe asthma, especially in children—see Ch 37).[b]

Cyanosis

Central cyanosis is best detected by inspecting the tongue. Examination of the tongue differentiates central from peripheral cyanosis. Lung disease severe enough to result in significant ventilation–perfusion imbalance (such as pneumonia, COPD and pulmonary embolism) may cause reduced arterial oxygen saturation and central cyanosis. Cyanosis becomes evident when the absolute concentration of deoxygenated haemoglobin is 50 g/L of capillary blood. Cyanosis is usually obvious when the arterial oxygen saturation falls below 90% in a person with a normal haemoglobin level. Central cyanosis is therefore a sign of severe hypoxaemia. In patients with anaemia, cyanosis does not occur until even greater levels of arterial desaturation are reached. The absence of obvious cyanosis does not exclude hypoxia. The detection of cyanosis is much easier in good (especially fluorescent) lighting conditions and don't be fooled if the patient's bed is surrounded by cheerful pink curtains.

Character of the cough

Coughing is a protective response to irritation of sensory receptors in the submucosa of the upper airways or bronchi. Ask the patient to cough several times. *Lack of the usual explosive beginning* may indicate vocal cord paralysis (the 'bovine' cough). A *muffled, wheezy, ineffective cough* suggests obstructive pulmonary disease. A *very loose productive cough* suggests excessive bronchial secretions due to chronic bronchitis, pneumonia or bronchiectasis. A *dry, irritating cough* may occur with chest infection, asthma or carcinoma of the bronchus and sometimes with left ventricular failure or interstitial lung disease (ILD). It is also typical of the cough produced by angiotensin-converting enzyme (ACE) inhibitor drugs. A *barking* or *croupy cough* may suggest a problem with the upper airway—the pharynx and larynx, or pertussis infection.

> **IMPORTANT CAUSES OF STRIDOR IN ADULTS**
>
> **Sudden onset (minutes)**
> Anaphylaxis
> Toxic gas inhalation
> Acute epiglottitis
> Inhaled foreign body
>
> **Gradual onset (days, weeks)**
> Laryngeal or pharyngeal tumours
> Cricoarytenoid rheumatoid arthritis
> Bilateral vocal cord palsy
> Tracheal carcinoma
> Paratracheal compression by lymph nodes
> Post-tracheostomy or intubation granulomata
>
> LIST 10.1

Sputum

Sputum should be inspected. Sputum mugs have disappeared but you may find a specimen jar at the bedside. Study of the sputum is an essential part of the physical examination. The colour, volume and type (purulent, mucoid or mucopurulent), and the presence or absence of blood, should be recorded.

Stridor

Obstruction of the larynx or trachea (the extrathoracic airways) may cause stridor, a rasping or croaking noise loudest on inspiration. This can be due to a foreign body, a tumour, infection (e.g. epiglottitis) or inflammation (see List 10.1). It is a sign that requires urgent attention.

Hoarseness

Listen to the patient's voice for hoarseness (dysphonia), as this may indicate recurrent laryngeal nerve palsy associated with carcinoma of the lung (usually left-sided), or laryngeal carcinoma. However, the most common cause is laryngitis and the use of inhaled corticosteroids for asthma. Non-respiratory causes include hypothyroidism.

HANDS

As usual, examination in detail begins with the hands.

---

[b] When the trachea moves in time with the pulse, the sign suggests an aneurysm of the thoracic aorta—this is the original meaning of *tracheal tug*.

Finger clubbing

FIGURE 10.3

Clubbing

Look for clubbing, which is due to respiratory disease in up to 80% of cases (see Fig. 10.3 and List 5.1 on p 80). An uncommon but important association with clubbing is *hypertrophic pulmonary osteoarthropathy* (HPO). HPO is characterised by the presence of periosteal inflammation at the distal ends of the long bones, the wrists, the ankles and the metacarpal and the metatarsal bones. There is swelling and tenderness over the wrists and other involved areas. Rarely HPO may occur without clubbing. The causes of HPO include primary lung carcinoma and pleural fibromas. It is important to note that clubbing does *not* occur as a result of COPD.

Staining

Look for staining of the fingers (actually caused by tar, as nicotine is colourless), a sign of cigarette smoking (see Fig. 3.18 on p 48). The density of staining does not indicate the number of cigarettes smoked, but depends rather on the way the cigarette is held in the hand.

Wasting and weakness

Compression and infiltration by a peripheral lung tumour of a lower trunk of the T1 nerve root results in wasting of the small muscles of the hand and weakness of finger abduction.

Pulse rate

Tachycardia and pulsus paradoxus (p 87) are important signs of severe asthma. Tachycardia is a common side effect of the treatment of asthma with beta-agonist drugs, and accompanies dyspnoea or hypoxia of any cause.

Flapping tremor (asterixis)

Ask the patient to dorsiflex the wrists with the arms outstretched and to spread out the fingers. A flapping tremor with a 2- to 3-second cycle may occur with severe CO_2 retention, which is usually due to severe COPD.[2] The problem is an inability to maintain a posture. Asterixis[c] can also be demonstrated by asking the patient to protrude his or her tongue or lift the leg and keep the foot dorsiflexed. However, this is a late and unreliable sign and can also occur in patients with liver or renal failure. Patients with severe CO_2 retention may be confused, and typically have warm peripheries and a bounding pulse.

FACE

The *nose* is sited conveniently in the centre of the face. In this position it may readily be inspected inside and out (see Ch 42). Ask the patient to tilt the head back. It may be necessary to use a nasal speculum to open the nostrils, and a torch. Look for polyps (associated with asthma), engorged turbinates (various allergic conditions) and a deviated septum (nasal obstruction).

As already discussed, look at the *tongue* for central cyanosis. Look in the *mouth* for:

- evidence of an upper respiratory tract infection (a reddened pharynx and tonsillar enlargement, with or without a coating of pus)
- 'crowding' of the pharynx, which is associated with sleep apnoea; it means a reduction in the size of the velopharyngeal lumen, which is the space between the soft palate, the tonsils and the back of the tongue
- a broken tooth or a rotten tooth stump, which may predispose to lung abscess or pneumonia
- severe periodontal disease, which may predispose to lung abscess.

Those who use a sleep apnoea mask at night often have marks from the mask on the face and puffiness around the eyes. They tend to be obese and have a short thick

---

[c] The word is derived from the Greek word *sterigma*, which means to support, and refers to a flapping tremor.

Feeling for the position of the trachea—a similar gap should be palpable on each side

FIGURE 10.4

neck and a small pharynx; sometimes the maxilla and mandible appear retracted (receding chin).

Sinusitis is suggested by tenderness over the *sinuses* on palpation (see Ch 42).[3]

Look at the patient's *face* for the red, leathery, wrinkled skin of the smoker.[4] There may be facial plethora or cyanosis if superior vena caval obstruction is present. Look for the characteristics of obstructive sleep apnoea (see above).

Inspect the *eyes* for evidence of the rare Horner's[d] syndrome (a constricted pupil, partial ptosis and loss of sweating), which can be due to an apical lung carcinoma (Pancoast's[e] tumour) compressing the sympathetic nerves in the neck. There may be skin changes on the face that suggest scleroderma or connective tissue disease.

TRACHEA

The position of the trachea is most important, and time should be spent establishing it accurately. This examination is uncomfortable for the patient, so you must be gentle. From in front of the patient push the forefinger of your right hand up and backwards from the suprasternal notch until the trachea is felt (see Fig. 10.4). If the trachea is displaced to one side, its edge

---

[d] Johann Horner (1831–86), a professor of ophthalmology in Zurich, described this syndrome in 1869.
[e] Henry Khunrath Pancoast (1875–1939), a professor of roentgenology at the University of Pennsylvania, described this in 1932.

> **CAUSES OF TRACHEAL DISPLACEMENT**
>
> 1. **Towards the side of the lung lesion**
>   Upper lobe collapse
>   Upper lobe fibrosis
>   Pneumonectomy
> 2. **Away from the side of the lung lesion (uncommon)**
>   Massive pleural effusion
>   Tension pneumothorax
> 3. **Upper mediastinal masses, such as retrosternal goitre**
>
> LIST 10.2

rather than its middle will be felt and a larger space will be present on one side than on the other. Slight displacement to the right is fairly common in normal people. Significant displacement of the trachea suggests, but is not specific for, disease of the upper lobes of the lung (see List 10.2).

A tracheal tug is demonstrated when the finger resting on the trachea feels it move inferiorly with each inspiration. This is a sign of gross overexpansion of the chest because of airflow obstruction. This movement of the trachea may be visible, and it is worth spending time inspecting the trachea when COPD is suspected.

If the patient appears dyspnoeic and use of the accessory muscles of respiration is suspected, place your fingers in the supraclavicular fossae. When the scalene muscles are recruited, they can be felt to contract under the fingers. Even more severe dyspnoea will result in use of the sternomastoid muscles. Their contraction is also easily felt with inspiration. Use of these muscles for long periods is exhausting and a sign of impending respiratory failure.

CHEST

The chest should be examined anteriorly and posteriorly by inspection, palpation, percussion and auscultation.[1] Compare the right and left sides during each part of the examination.

Inspection

Shape and symmetry of chest

When the anteroposterior (AP) diameter is increased compared with the lateral diameter, the chest is described as barrel-shaped (see Fig. 10.5). An increase in the AP diameter compared with the lateral diameter

Barrel chest

(From McDonald FS, ed. *Mayo Clinic images in internal medicine*, with permission. © Mayo Clinic Scientific Press and CRC Press. Reproduced by permission of Taylor and Francis Group, LLC, a division of Informa plc.)

FIGURE 10.5

(the thoracic ratio) beyond 0.9 is abnormal and is often seen in patients with severe asthma or emphysema. It is not always a reliable guide to the severity of the underlying lung disease and may be present in normal elderly people. It is sometimes an illusion when the abdomen is relatively small in thin people.

A **funnel chest (pectus excavatum)** is a developmental defect involving a localised depression of the lower end of the sternum (see Fig. 10.6(a)). The problem is usually an aesthetic one, but in severe cases lung capacity may be restricted.

A **pigeon chest (pectus carinatum)** is a localised prominence (an outward bowing of the sternum and costal cartilages; see Fig. 10.6(b)). It may be a manifestation of chronic childhood respiratory illness, in which case it is thought to result from repeated strong contractions of the diaphragm while the thorax is still pliable. It also occurs in rickets.[f]

Harrison's[g] sulcus is a linear depression of the lower ribs just above the costal margins at the site of attachment of the diaphragm. It can result from severe asthma in childhood, or rickets.

Kyphosis refers to an exaggerated forward curvature of the spine, whereas scoliosis is lateral bowing. **Kyphoscoliosis** can cause asymmetrical chest deformity; it may be idiopathic (80%), secondary to poliomyelitis or associated with Marfan's syndrome. It is often seen in elderly patients or those on corticosteroids as a result of wedge fractures of thoracic vertebral bodies. Severe thoracic kyphoscoliosis may reduce the lung capacity and increase the work of breathing.

Lesions of the chest wall may be obvious. Look for *scars* from previous thoracic operations or from chest drains for a previous pneumothorax or pleural effusion. Surgical removal of a lung (pneumonectomy) or of the lobe of a lung (lobectomy) leaves a long diagonal posterior scar on the thorax. The presence of three 2–3 centimetre scars suggests previous video-assisted thoracoscopic surgery, which can be performed to biopsy lymph nodes or carry out lung reduction surgery or pleurodesis. Thoracoplasty causes severe chest deformity; this operation was performed for tuberculosis and involved removal of a large number of ribs on one side of the chest to achieve permanent collapse of the affected lung.

---

[f] Bone disease caused by vitamin D deficiency in childhood.
[g] Edward Harrison (1766–1838), a British general practitioner in Lincolnshire, described this deformity in rickets in 1798. The sign has also been ascribed to Edwin Harrison (1779–1847), a London physician.

(a) Funnel chest (pectus excavatum); (b) pigeon chest (pectus carinatum)
(From Mir MA. *Atlas of clinical diagnosis*, 2nd edn. Edinburgh: Saunders, 2003.)

FIGURE 10.6

It is no longer performed because of the availability of effective antituberculous chemotherapy.

Radiotherapy may cause erythema and thickening of the skin over the irradiated area. There is sharp demarcation between abnormal and normal skin. There may be small tattoo marks indicating the limits of the irradiated area. Signs of radiotherapy usually indicate that the patient has been treated for carcinoma of the lung or breast or, less often, for lymphoma.

Subcutaneous emphysema is a crackling sensation felt on palpating the skin of the chest or neck. On inspection, there is often diffuse swelling of the chest wall and neck. It is caused by air tracking from the lungs and is usually due to a pneumothorax; less commonly it can follow rupture of the oesophagus or a pneumomediastinum (air in the mediastinal space).

Prominent veins may be seen in patients with superior vena caval obstruction. It is important to determine the direction of blood flow (p 246).

Movement of the chest wall should be noted. Look for asymmetry of chest wall movement anteriorly and posteriorly. Assessment of expansion of the upper lobes is best achieved by inspection from behind the patient, looking down at the clavicles during moderate respiration (see Fig. 10.7). Diminished movement indicates underlying lung disease. The affected side will show delayed or decreased movement. For assessment of lower lobe expansion, the chest should be inspected posteriorly.

Reduced chest wall movement on one side may be due to localised lung fibrosis, consolidation, collapse, pleural effusion or pneumothorax.

Bilateral reduction of chest wall movement indicates a diffuse abnormality such as COPD or diffuse interstitial lung disease (ILD). Unilateral reduced chest excursion or splinting may be present when patients have pleuritic chest pain or injuries such as rib fractures.

Inspecting upper lobe expansion.

(a) Expiration; (b) inspiration—note symmetrical elevation of the clavicles

FIGURE 10.7

Look for paradoxical inward motion of the abdomen during inspiration when the patient is supine (indicating diaphragmatic paralysis).

Palpation

Chest expansion

Place your hands firmly on the patient's chest wall with your fingers extending around the sides of the chest. Your thumbs should almost meet in the middle line and should be lifted slightly off the chest so that they are free to move with respiration (see Fig. 10.8). As the patient takes a big breath in, your thumbs should move symmetrically apart at least 5 centimetres. Reduced expansion on one side indicates a lesion on that side. The causes have already been discussed.

If COPD is suspected, Hoover's[h] sign may be sought (see Fig. 10.9). Place your hands along the costal margins with your thumbs close to the xiphisternum. Normally inspiration causes them to separate, but the overinflated chest of the COPD patient cannot expand in this way and the diaphragm pulls the ribs and your thumbs closer together[5] (LR+ 4.2).[6]

Lower lobe expansion is assessed from the back in this way. Some idea of upper and middle lobe expansion is possible when the manoeuvre is repeated on the front of the chest, but this is better gauged by inspection.

Apex beat

When the patient is lying down, establishing the position of the apex beat may be helpful, as displacement towards the side of the lesion can be caused by collapse of the lower lobe or by localised ILD. Movement of the apex beat away from the side of the lung lesion can be caused by pleural effusion or tension pneumothorax. The apex beat is often impalpable in a chest that is hyperexpanded secondary to COPD.

Vocal (tactile) fremitus

This is a palpable vibration felt by the examiner's hands on a patient's chest wall when the patient is speaking (or singing[i]). Palpate the chest wall with the palm of the hand while the patient repeats 'ninety-nine'. The front and back of the chest are each palpated in two comparable positions, with the palm of one hand on each side of the chest. In this way differences in vibration on the chest wall can be detected. This can be a difficult sign to interpret, with considerable inter-observer variability, and it is no longer a routine part of the examination. It depends on the recognition of changes

---

[h] Charles Hoover (1865–1927), a professor of medicine in Cleveland from 1907. He also described Hoover's test for non-organic limb weakness.

[i] Probably not to be encouraged during an OSCE exam.

Palpation for lower lobe expansion.

(a) Expiration; (b) inspiration

FIGURE 10.8

(a) Normal inspiration; (b) normal expiration; (c) Hoover's inspiration; (d) Hoover's expiration

FIGURE 10.9

in vibration conducted to the examiner's hands while the patient speaks. Practice is needed to appreciate the difference between normal and abnormal. Vocal fremitus is more obvious in men because of their lower-pitched voices. It may be absent in normal people (high-pitched voice or thick chest wall). It is only abnormal if different on one side from the other. The causes of change in vocal fremitus are the same as those for vocal resonance (p 187).

Ribs

Gently compress the chest wall anteroposteriorly and laterally. Localised pain suggests a rib fracture, which may be secondary to trauma or may be spontaneous as a result of tumour deposition, bone disease or sometimes the result of severe and prolonged coughing. Tenderness over the costochondral junctions suggests the diagnosis of costochondritis as the cause of chest pain.

Regional lymph nodes

The axillary and cervical and supraclavicular nodes must be examined (see Ch 21); they may be enlarged in lung malignancies and some infections.

Percussion

With your left hand on the patient's chest wall and fingers slightly separated and aligned with the patient's ribs, press your middle finger firmly against the patient's chest. Use the pad of your right middle finger (the *plexor*) to strike firmly the middle phalanx of the middle finger of your left hand (the *pleximeter*).[j] Remove the percussing finger quickly so that the note generated is not dampened (this may be less important if the pleximeter finger is held firmly on the chest wall, as it should be). The percussing finger must be held partly flexed and a loose swinging movement should come from the wrist and not from the forearm. Medical students soon learn to keep the right middle fingernail short.

Percussion of symmetrical areas of the anterior, posterior and axillary regions is necessary (see Fig. 10.10). Percussion in the supraclavicular fossa over the apex of the lung and direct percussion of the clavicle with the percussing finger are a traditional part of the examination. For percussion posteriorly, the scapulae should be moved out of the way by asking the patient to move the elbows forwards across the front of the chest; this rotates the scapulae anteriorly.

The feel of the percussion note is as important as its sound. The note is affected by the thickness of the chest wall, as well as by underlying structures. Percussion over a solid structure, such as the liver or a consolidated or collapsed area of lung, produces a dull note. Percussion over a fluid-filled area, such as a pleural effusion, produces an extremely dull (stony dull) note. Percussion over the normal lung produces a resonant note and percussion over hollow structures, such as the bowel or a pneumothorax, produces a hyperresonant note.

Considerable practice is required before expert percussion can be performed, particularly in front of an audience. The ability to percuss well is usually obvious in clinical examinations and counts in a student's favour, as it indicates a reasonable amount of experience in the wards.

Liver dullness

The upper level of liver dullness is determined by percussing down the anterior chest in the midclavicular line. Normally, the upper level of liver dullness is the sixth intercostal space in the right midclavicular line. If the chest is resonant below this level, it is a sign of hyperinflation, usually due to emphysema or asthma. This is a sign with considerable inter-observer variability.

Cardiac dullness

The area of cardiac dullness usually present on the left side of the chest may be decreased in emphysema or asthma.

Auscultation
Breath sounds

Using the diaphragm of the stethoscope, listen front and back (Fig. 10.11).[7-9] Ask the patient to take big breaths in and out through the mouth. It is important to compare each side with the other. Remember to listen high up into the axillae and, using the bell of the stethoscope applied above the clavicles, to listen to the lung apices. A number of observations must be made while auscultating and, as with auscultation of

---

[j] This was often a piece of wood, ivory or a coin in the 19th century but is now always the examiner's finger.

Percussion of the chest.

(a) Percussing (plexor) finger poised; inset: plexor finger strikes pleximeter finger; (b) direct percussion of the clavicle for upper lobe resonance

FIGURE 10.10

Normal and bronchial breath sounds.

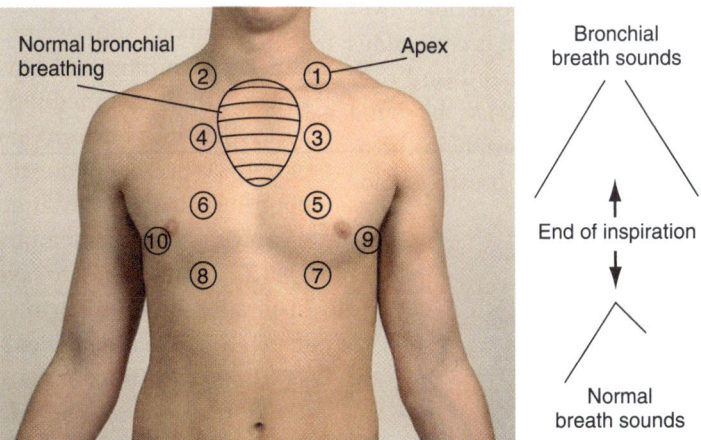

Auscultate in each area shown (the numbers represent a suggested order). Distinguish normal breath sounds from bronchial breathing

FIGURE 10.11

the heart, different parts of the cycle must be considered. Listen for the quality of the breath sounds, the intensity of the breath sounds and the presence of additional (adventitious) sounds.

Quality of breath sounds

Normal breath sounds are heard with the stethoscope over nearly all parts of the chest. The patient should be asked to breathe in and out through the mouth so that added sounds from the nasopharynx do not interfere.[k] During expiration these sounds are produced in the large airways rather than in the alveoli. However, inspiratory sounds are probably produced close to where they are heard, in the peripheral parts of the lungs. Since both sounds were once thought to arise in the alveoli, or vesicles of the lungs, they are called vesicular sounds. They have rather fancifully been compared by Laënnec to the sound of wind rustling in leaves. Their intensity is related to total airflow at the mouth and to regional airflow. Normal (vesicular) breath sounds are louder and longer on inspiration than on expiration and there is no gap between the inspiratory and expiratory sounds.

Bronchial breath sounds are present when turbulence in the large airways is heard without being filtered by the alveoli. Bronchial breath sounds have a hollow, blowing quality. They are audible throughout expiration and there is often a gap between inspiration and expiration. The expiratory sound has a higher intensity and pitch than the inspiratory sound. Bronchial breath sounds are more easily remembered than described. They are audible in normal people, posteriorly over the right upper chest where the trachea is contiguous with the right upper bronchus. They are heard over areas of consolidation, as solid lung conducts the sound of turbulence in main airways to peripheral areas without filtering. Causes of bronchial breath sounds are shown in List 10.3.

Occasionally, breath sounds over a large cavity have an exaggerated bronchial quality. This very hollow or *amphoric*[l] sound has been likened to that heard when air passes over the top of a hollow jar.

> ### CAUSES OF BRONCHIAL BREATH SOUNDS
>
> **Common**
>
> Lung consolidation (lobar pneumonia)
>
> **Uncommon**
>
> Localised pulmonary fibrosis
>
> Pleural effusion (above the fluid)
>
> Collapsed lung (e.g. adjacent to a pleural effusion)
>
> *Note:* The large airways must be patent.
>
> LIST 10.3

Intensity of the breath sounds

It is better to describe breath sounds as being of normal or reduced intensity than to speak about *air entry*. The entry of air into parts of the lung cannot be directly gauged from the breath sounds. Asymmetrical reduction of breath sounds is a sign of bronchial obstruction, for example by carcinoma or a foreign body on the side where breath sounds are reduced. Causes of reduced breath sounds include COPD (especially emphysema), pleural effusion, pneumothorax, pneumonia, a large neoplasm and pulmonary collapse. Breath sounds are generally louder if a patient breathes more deeply, for example after exercise.

Added (adventitious) sounds

There are two types of added sounds: continuous (wheezes) and interrupted (crackles).

Continuous sounds are called *wheezes*. They are abnormal findings and have a musical quality. The wheezes must be timed in relation to the respiratory cycle. They may be heard in expiration or inspiration, or both. Wheezes are due to continuous oscillation of opposing airway walls and imply significant airway narrowing. Wheezes tend to be louder on expiration. This is because the airways normally dilate during inspiration and are narrower during expiration. An inspiratory wheeze implies severe airway narrowing.

The pitch (frequency) of wheezes varies. It is determined only by the velocity of the air jet and is not related to the length of the airway. High-pitched wheezes are produced in the smaller bronchi and have a whistling quality, whereas low-pitched wheezes (sometimes called rhonchi) arise from the larger bronchi.

---

[k] Many people when asked to take big breaths, breathe in, and then, for some reason, stop. Although it is tempting to amuse oneself by waiting patiently for the patient to realise that expiration is also a part of breathing, this tends to waste time.

[l] From the Greek *amphiphoreus* meaning a 'vase with a narrow neck'.

Wheezes are usually the result of acute or chronic airflow obstruction due to asthma (often high-pitched) or COPD (often low-pitched), secondary to a combination of bronchial muscle spasm, mucosal oedema and excessive secretions. Wheezes are a poor guide to the severity of airflow obstruction. In severe airway obstruction, wheeze can be absent because ventilation is so reduced that the velocity of the air jet is reduced below a critical level necessary to produce the sound.

A fixed bronchial obstruction, usually due to a carcinoma of the lung, tends to cause a localised wheeze, which has a single musical note (monophonic) and does not clear with coughing.

Wheezes must be distinguished from *stridor* (p 177), which sounds very similar to wheeze but is louder over the trachea and is always inspiratory (wheezes usually occur in expiration—but can occur in both inspiration and expiration).

Interrupted non-musical sounds are best called *crackles*.[10,11] There is a lot of confusion about the naming of these sounds, perhaps as a result of mistranslations of Laënnec. Some authors describe low-pitched crackles as râles and high-pitched ones as crepitations, but others do not make this distinction. The simplest approach is to call all these sounds crackles, but also to describe their timing and pitch. Crackles are sometimes present in normal people but these crackles will always clear with coughing.

Crackles are probably the result of loss of stability of peripheral airways that collapse on expiration. With high inspiratory pressures, there is rapid air entry into the distal airways. This causes the abrupt opening of alveoli and of small- or medium-sized bronchi containing secretions in regions of the lung deflated to residual volume. More compliant (distensible) areas open up first, followed by the increasingly stiff areas. Fine- and medium-pitched crackles are not caused by air moving through secretions as was once thought, but rather by the opening and closing of small airways.

The timing of crackles is of great importance. *Early inspiratory crackles* (which cease before the middle of inspiration) suggest disease of the small airways and are characteristic of COPD.[10] The crackles are heard only in early inspiration and are of medium coarseness. They are different from those heard in left ventricular failure, which occur later in the respiratory cycle.

Late or *pan-inspiratory crackles* suggest disease confined to the alveoli. They may be fine, medium or coarse in quality. *Fine crackles* have been likened to the sound of hair rubbed between the fingers, or to the sound Velcro makes when pulled apart. They are typically caused by ILD (pulmonary fibrosis). Characteristically, more crackles are heard in each inspiration when they are due to fibrosis—up to 14 compared with 1 to 4 for COPD and 4 to 9 for cardiac failure. As ILD becomes more severe the crackles extend earlier into inspiration and are heard further up the chest.[m] *Medium crackles* are usually due to left ventricular failure. Here the presence of alveolar fluid disrupts the function of the normally secreted surfactant. *Coarse crackles* are characteristic of pools of retained secretions and have an unpleasant gurgling quality. They tend to change with coughing, which also has an unpleasant gurgling quality. Bronchiectasis is a common cause, but any disease that leads to retention of secretions may produce these features.

Pleural friction rub: when thickened, roughened pleural surfaces rub together as the lungs expand and contract, a continuous or intermittent grating sound may be audible. A pleural rub indicates pleurisy, which may be secondary to pulmonary infarction or pneumonia. Rarely, malignant involvement of the pleura, a spontaneous pneumothorax or pleurodynia may cause a rub.

Vocal resonance

Auscultation over the chest while a patient speaks gives further information about the lungs' ability to transmit sounds. Over normal lung, the low-pitched components of speech are heard with a booming quality and high-pitched components are attenuated. Consolidated lung, however, tends to transmit high frequencies so that speech heard through the stethoscope takes on a bleating quality (called *aegophony*[n] by Laënnec[12]). When a patient with aegophony says 'e' as in 'bee' it sounds like 'a' as in 'bay'.

Increased vocal resonance is a helpful sign in confirming consolidation but may not be necessary as a routine. Ask the patient to say 'ninety-nine' while you listen over each part of the chest. Over consolidated

---

[m] Expiratory crackles may also occur with lung fibrosis.
[n] From the Greek *aix* meaning 'goat' and *phone* meaning 'voice'.

lung the numbers will become clearly audible, while over normal lung the sound is muffled. If vocal resonance is present, bronchial breathing is likely to be heard (see List 10.3). Sometimes vocal resonance is increased to such an extent that whispered speech is distinctly heard; this is called whispering pectoriloquy.

If a localised abnormality is found at auscultation, try to determine the lobe involved (see Fig. 10.2).

THE HEART

Cardiac examination is an essential part of the respiratory assessment and vice versa. These two systems are intimately related.

Lay the patient down at 45° and measure the jugular venous pressure (JVP) for evidence of right heart failure. Next examine the praecordium. It is important to pay close attention to the pulmonary component of the second heart sound (P2). This is best heard at the second intercostal space on the left. It should not be louder than the aortic component, best heard at the right second intercostal space. If the P2 is louder (and especially if it is palpable), pulmonary hypertension should be strongly suspected. There may be signs of right ventricular failure or hypertension. Pulmonary hypertensive heart disease (cor pulmonale) may be primary or due to COPD, ILD, pulmonary thromboembolism, marked obesity, sleep apnoea or severe kyphoscoliosis.

THE ABDOMEN

Palpate the liver for ptosis,º due to emphysema, or for enlargement from secondary deposits of tumour in cases of lung carcinoma (see Ch 14).

OTHER

Pemberton's[p] sign

Ask the patient to lift the arms over the head and wait for 1 minute.[13] Note the development of facial plethora, cyanosis, inspiratory stridor and non-pulsatile elevation of the JVP. This occurs in superior vena caval obstruction.

Legs

Inspect the patient's legs for swelling (oedema) or cyanosis, which may be clues to cor pulmonale, and look for evidence of deep venous thrombosis.

Respiratory rate on exercise

Patients complaining of dyspnoea should have their respiratory rate measured at rest, at maximal tolerated exertion (e.g. after climbing one or two flights of stairs or during a treadmill exercise test) and supine. If dyspnoea is not accompanied by tachypnoea when the patient climbs the stairs, consider the possibility of anxiety or malingering.

Temperature

Fever may occur with any acute or chronic chest infection.

T&O'C ESSENTIALS

1. It is often easiest to examine the lungs with the patient sitting over the edge of the bed.
2. As always, a general inspection should precede the detailed examination. Note especially signs of respiratory distress and cyanosis.
3. Ask the patient to cough and look at the contents of the sputum mug.
4. Remember that lung disease may be associated with peripheral signs such as clubbing and Horner's syndrome.
5. Upper lobe signs can be difficult to elicit but look especially for tracheal deviation and compare movement of the clavicles from above and behind.
6. The fine late inspiratory crackles of interstitial lung disease are very characteristic and once heard are easily remembered.

º From the Greek word for falling, this was once mostly applied to the eyelid but now seems accepted as a description of the displacement of any organ.
p Hugh Pemberton (1891–1956), a physician in Liverpool, UK.

> **OSCE REVISION TOPICS – THE RESPIRATORY EXAMINATION** (see OSCE video no. 2 The respiratory exam at Student CONSULT)
>
> *Use these topics, which commonly occur in the OSCE, to help with revision.*
>
> 1. This man has had haemoptysis. Please examine him. (p 177)
> 2. This woman has a cough. Please examine her. (p 177)
> 3. This man has had pleuritic chest pain. Please examine his chest. (p 181)
> 4. This man has been a heavy smoker. Please examine him. (p 178)

References

1. Mulrow CD, Dolmatch BL, Delong ER et al. Observer variability in the pulmonary examination. *J Gen Intern Med* 1986; 1:364–367. Documents the poor reliability of many respiratory signs.
2. Conn HO. Asterixis: its occurrence in chronic obstructive pulmonary disease, with a commentary on its general mechanism. *N Engl J Med* 1958; 259:564–569.
3. Williams JW Jr, Simel DL, Roberts LR, Samsa GP. Clinical evaluation for sinusitis; making the diagnosis by history and physical examination. *Ann Intern Med* 1992; 117:705–710. The doctor's impression of the likelihood of sinusitis was superior to findings of a purulent nasal discharge, history of maxillary toothache, poor response to nasal decongestants and abnormal transillumination.
4. Model D. Smokers' face: an underrated clinical sign? *BMJ* 1985; 291:1760–1762. A red face with leathery skin and excessive wrinkling, associated with a gaunt look, may help identify up to half of chronic smokers.
5. Garcia-Pachon E. Paradoxical movement of the lateral rib margin (Hoover sign) for detecting obstructive airway disease. *Chest* 2002; 12:651–655.
6. McGee S. *Evidence-based physical diagnosis*, 3rd edn. St Louis: Saunders, 2012.
7. Kraman SS. Lung sounds for the clinician. *Arch Intern Med* 1986; 146:411–412. Describes the physiological evidence for many auscultatory findings.
8. Earis J. Lung sounds. *Thorax* 1992; 47:671–672.
9. Forgacs P. The functional basis of lung sounds. *Chest* 1978; 73:399–405.
10. Nath AR, Caple LH. Respiratory crackles: early and late. *Thorax* 1974; 29:223–227. Severe airways obstruction causes crackles in the first half of inspiration. In contrast, late crackles are not associated with airways obstruction.
11. Walshaw MJ, Nissa M, Pearson MG et al. Expiratory lung crackles in patients with fibrosing alveolitis. *Chest* 1990; 97:407–409. Inspiratory crackles are usually considered more important, but this report suggests that expiratory crackles occur intermittently in fibrosing alveolitis, usually in mid-expiration.
12. Shapira JD. About egophony. *Chest* 1995; 108:865–867.
13. Wallace C, Siminoski K. The Pemberton sign. *Ann Intern Med* 1996; 125:568–569. Discusses the mechanism of this useful sign, which is present when a large retrosternal goitre compresses the thoracic inlet.

CHAPTER 11
Correlation of physical signs and respiratory disease

Life cannot be maintained without respiration, neither can respiration be performed without motion. CROOKE, Body of Man *(1615)*

RESPIRATORY DISTRESS: RESPIRATORY FAILURE

A severe respiratory illness may be a medical emergency. Many of the respiratory illnesses discussed below and some non-respiratory illnesses (see List 11.1) can result in acute respiratory problems and it is important to recognise signs that suggest there is an urgent problem. These signs include:

- cyanosis, or low peripheral arterial oxygen saturation (S_pO_2) on oximetry
- use of accessory muscles of respiration
- inability to speak
- greatly increased or reduced respiratory rate
- signs of exhaustion
- silent lung fields
- stridor (airway obstruction)
- drowsiness
- chest injury
- tachycardia
- pulsus paradoxus.

There may be signs of an underlying respiratory illness (see Table 11.1).

CAUSES OF ACUTE RESPIRATORY DISTRESS OR FAILURE

Lung disease
COPD or asthma
Very large pleural effusion
Pneumonia
Non-cardiogenic pulmonary oedema (e.g. from toxic gas inhalation)
Pulmonary embolism
Chest injury or pneumothorax

Airways obstruction
Inhaled foreign body
Facial or neck injury
Angio-oedema
Epiglottitis or quinsy
Unconsciousness and aspiration—loss of airway protecting reflexes

Non-respiratory causes
Anaemia
Diabetic ketoacidosis
Anxiety and hyperventilation

COPD = chronic obstructive pulmonary disease.

LIST 11.1

CONSOLIDATION (LOBAR PNEUMONIA)

Pneumonia is defined as inflammation of the lung that is characterised by exudation into the alveoli (see Good signs guide 11.1). X-ray changes of new shadowing in one or more lung segments (lobes) are present. Pneumonia is classified as:

1. community acquired (CAP)
2. hospital acquired
3. occurring in a damaged lung (e.g. as a result of aspiration)
4. occurring in an immunocompromised host.

This classification allows prediction of the likely pathogens and assists in the choice of antibiotics for treatment.

CHAPTER 11 CORRELATION OF PHYSICAL SIGNS AND RESPIRATORY DISEASE

Comparison of the chest signs in common respiratory disorders

Disorder	Mediastinal displacement	Chest wall movement	Percussion note	Breath sounds	Added sounds
Consolidation	None	Reduced over affected area	Dull	Bronchial	Crackles
Collapse	Ipsilateral shift	Decreased over affected area	Dull	Absent or reduced	Absent
Pleural effusion	Heart displaced to opposite side (trachea displaced only if massive)	Reduced over affected area	Stony dull	Absent over fluid; may be bronchial at upper border	Absent; pleural rub may be found above effusion
Pneumothorax	Tracheal deviation to opposite side if under tension	Decreased over affected area	Resonant	Absent or greatly reduced	Absent
Bronchial asthma	None	Decreased symmetrically	Normal or decreased	Normal or reduced	Wheeze
Interstitial pulmonary fibrosis	None	Decreased symmetrically (minimal)	Normal unaffected by cough or posture	Normal	Fine, late or pan-inspiratory crackles over affected lobes

TABLE 11.1

GOOD SIGNS GUIDE 11.1
Pneumonia

Sign	LR+	LR−
GENERAL APPEARANCE		
Dementia	4.0	NS
Vital signs	3.4	0.94
Temperature >37.8°C	2.4	0.58
Respiratory rate >25/minute	1.5	0.8
HEART RATE		
>100 beats/minute	2.3	0.49
LUNG FINDINGS		
Percussion dullness	4.3	0.79
Reduced breath sounds	2.5	0.6
Bronchial breath sounds	3.5	0.9
Aegophony	5.3	0.76
Crackles	3.5	0.62
Wheezes	1.4	0.76

NS = not significant.
(Heckerling PS, Tape TG, Wigton RS et al. Clinical prediction rule for pulmonary infiltrates. *Ann Intern Med* 1990; 113(9):664–670.)

The signs of lobar pneumonia are characteristic and are referred to clinically as *consolidation*.[1]

There may be a history of the sudden onset of malaise, chest pain, dyspnoea and fever. Patients may appear very ill and the vital signs—including the temperature, respiratory rate and blood pressure—must be recorded. There may be signs of cyanosis and exhaustion in sick patients. The term *bronchopneumonia* refers to lung infection characterised by more patchy X-ray changes that often affect both lower lobes. The clinical signs of consolidation may be absent.

Symptoms

- Cough (painful and dry at first).
- Fever and rigors (shivers).
- Pleuritic chest pain.
- Dyspnoea.
- Tachycardia.
- Confusion.

Signs

- **Expansion:** reduced on the affected side.
- **Vocal fremitus:** increased on the affected side (in other chest disease this sign is of very little use!).

- **Percussion:** dull, but not stony dull.
- **Breath sounds:** bronchial.
- **Additional sounds:** medium, late or pan-inspiratory crackles as the pneumonia resolves.
- **Vocal resonance:** increased.
- **Pleural rub:** may be present.

Causes of community-acquired pneumonia

- *Streptococcus pneumoniae* (>30%).
- *Chlamydia pneumoniae* (10%).
- *Mycoplasma pneumoniae* (10%).
- *Legionella pneumoniae* (5%).

ATELECTASIS (COLLAPSE)

If a bronchus is obstructed by a tumour mass, retained secretions or a prolonged presence of a foreign body, the air in the part of the lung supplied by the bronchus is absorbed and the affected part of the lung collapses.

Signs

- **Trachea:** displaced towards the collapsed side.
- **Expansion:** reduced on the affected side with flattening of the chest wall on the same side.
- **Percussion:** dull over the collapsed area.
- **Breath sounds:** reduced, often without bronchial breathing above the area of atelectasis when a tumour is the cause, because the airways are not patent.

Note: (1) There may be no signs with complete lobar collapse. (2) The early changes after the inhalation of a foreign body may be over-inflation of the affected side.

Causes

- **Intraluminal:** mucus (e.g. postoperative, asthma, cystic fibrosis), foreign body, aspiration.
- **Mural:** bronchial carcinoma.
- **Extramural:** peribronchial lymphadenopathy, aortic aneurysm.

PLEURAL EFFUSION

This is a collection of fluid in the pleural space. Note that pleural collections consisting of blood (haemothorax), chyle (chylothorax) or pus (empyema) have specific names and are not called pleural effusions, although the physical signs are similar.

Signs

- **Trachea and apex beat:** displaced away from a massive effusion.
- **Expansion:** reduced on the affected side.
- **Percussion:** stony dullness over the fluid.
- **Breath sounds:** reduced or absent. There may be an area of bronchial breathing audible above the effusion due to compression of overlying lung.
- **Vocal resonance:** reduced.

Causes

- **Transudate** (Light's criteria)[a]:
  - cardiac failure
  - hypoalbuminaemia from the nephrotic syndrome or chronic liver disease
  - hypothyroidism.
- **Exudate** (Light's criteria[a]—LR for exudate if Light's criteria negative −0.04)[2]:
  - pneumonia
  - neoplasm—bronchial carcinoma, metastatic carcinoma, mesothelioma
  - tuberculosis
  - pulmonary infarction
  - subphrenic abscess
  - acute pancreatitis
  - connective tissue disease such as rheumatoid arthritis, systemic lupus erythematosus
  - drugs such as methysergide, cytotoxics
  - irradiation
  - trauma
  - Meigs' syndrome[b] (ovarian fibroma causing pleural effusion and ascites).

---

[a] The formal definition of an exudate is that the fluid has at least one of the following (Light's) criteria; (1) fluid protein/serum protein >0.5; (2) pleural fluid lactate dehydrogenase (LDH)/serum LDH >0.6; (3) pleural fluid LDH >2/3 normal upper limit of LDH in serum. The fluid is otherwise a transudate.
[b] Joe Vincent Meigs (1892–1963), Professor of Gynaecology at Harvard, described this in 1937.

- **Haemothorax** (blood in the pleural space):
  - severe trauma to the chest
  - rupture of a pleural adhesion containing a blood vessel.
- **Chylothorax** (milky-appearing pleural fluid due to leakage of lymph):
  - trauma or surgery to the thoracic duct
  - carcinoma or lymphoma involving the thoracic duct.
- **Empyema** (pus in the pleural space):
  - pneumonia
  - lung abscess
  - bronchiectasis
  - tuberculosis
  - penetrating chest wound.

Yellow nail syndrome

This is a rare condition that is caused by hypoplasia of the lymphatic system. The nails are thickened and yellow (see Fig. 11.1) and there is separation of the distal nail plate from the nail bed (onycholysis). It may be associated with a pleural effusion and bronchiectasis, and usually with lymphoedema of the legs.

PNEUMOTHORAX

Leakage of air from the lung or a chest wall puncture into the pleural space causes a pneumothorax.

Signs

- **Expansion:** reduced on the affected side.
- **Percussion:** hyperresonance if the pneumothorax is large.
- **Breath sounds:** greatly reduced or absent.
- There may be subcutaneous emphysema.
- There may be no signs if the pneumothorax is small (less than 30%).

Causes
Primary

- **'Spontaneous':** subpleural bullae rupture, usually in tall, healthy young males.

Yellow nail syndrome: (a) hands; (b) feet

(From McDonald FS, ed. *Mayo Clinic images in internal medicine*, with permission. © Mayo Clinic Scientific Press and CRC Press. Reproduced by permission of Taylor and Francis Group, LLC, a division of Informa plc.)

FIGURE 11.1

Secondary

- **Traumatic:** rib fracture, penetrating chest wall injury, or during pleural or pericardial aspiration.
- **Iatrogenic**[c] (caused by medical intervention): following the insertion of a central venous catheter.
- Emphysema with rupture of bullae, usually in middle-aged or elderly patients with generalised emphysema.
- Rarer causes include asthma, lung abscess, bronchial carcinoma, eosinophilic granuloma,

---

[c] *Iatros* means physician in Greek.

lymphangioleiomyomatosis (LAM—premenopausal women), end-stage fibrosis or Marfan's syndrome.

TENSION PNEUMOTHORAX

This occurs when there is a communication between the lung and the pleural space, with a flap of tissue acting as a valve, allowing air to enter the pleural space during inspiration and preventing it from leaving during expiration. A tension pneumothorax results from air accumulating under increasing pressure in the pleural space; it causes considerable displacement of the mediastinum with obstruction and kinking of the great vessels, and represents a medical emergency.

Signs

- The patient is often tachypnoeic and cyanosed, and may be hypotensive.
- **Trachea and apex beat:** displaced away from the affected side.
- **Expansion:** reduced or absent on affected side.
- **Percussion:** hyperresonant over the affected side.
- **Breath sounds:** absent.
- **Vocal resonance:** absent.

Causes

- Trauma.
- Mechanical ventilation at high pressure.
- Spontaneous (rare cause of tension pneumothorax).

BRONCHIECTASIS

This is a pathological dilation of the bronchi, resulting in impaired clearance of mucus and chronic infection. A history of chronic cough and of (usually voluminous) purulent sputum since childhood is virtually diagnostic.

Signs

Most likely during an exacerbation of the condition.

- **Systemic signs:** fever, cachexia; sinusitis (70%).
- **Sputum:** voluminous, purulent, foul-smelling, sometimes bloodstained.
- **Breath sounds:** Coarse pan-inspiratory or late inspiratory crackles over the affected lobe.
- **Signs of severe bronchiectasis:** very copious amounts of sputum and haemoptysis, clubbing, cyanosis, widespread crackles, signs of airways obstruction, signs of respiratory failure and cor pulmonale, signs of secondary amyloidosis (e.g. oedema from proteinuria, cardiac failure, enlarged liver and spleen, carpal tunnel syndrome).

Causes

- **Congenital:**
  - primary ciliary dyskinesia (including the immotile cilia syndrome)
  - cystic fibrosis
  - congenital hypogammaglobulinaemia.
- **Acquired:**
  - infections in childhood, such as whooping cough, pneumonia or measles
  - localised disease such as a foreign body, a bronchial adenoma or tuberculosis
  - allergic bronchopulmonary aspergillosis—this causes proximal bronchiectasis.

BRONCHIAL ASTHMA

This may be defined as paroxysmal recurrent attacks of wheezing (or in childhood of cough) due to airways narrowing, which changes in severity over short periods of time.

Signs

- Wheezing.
- Dry or productive cough.
- Tachypnoea.
- Tachycardia.
- Prolonged expiration.
- Prolonged forced expiratory time (decreased peak flow, decreased forced expiratory volume [FEV_1]).
- Use of accessory muscles of respiration.
- Hyperinflated chest (increased anteroposterior diameter with high shoulders and, on percussion, decreased liver dullness).

- Inspiratory and expiratory wheezes.
- **Signs of severe asthma:**
  - appearance of exhaustion and fear
  - inability to speak because of breathlessness
  - drowsiness due to hypercapnia (preterminal)
  - cyanosis (a very sinister sign)
  - tachycardia (pulse above 130 beats/minute correlates with significant hypoxaemia)
  - pulsus paradoxus (more than 20 mmHg)
  - reduced breath sounds or a 'silent' chest.

CHRONIC OBSTRUCTIVE PULMONARY DISEASE (COPD)

Chronic obstructive pulmonary disease (chronic airflow limitation; see Good signs guide 11.2) represents a spectrum of abnormalities from predominantly emphysema, where there i s pathologically an increase beyond normal in the size of the air spaces distal to the terminal bronchioles, to chronic bronchitis, where there is mucous gland hypertrophy, increased numbers of goblet cells and hypersecretion of mucus in the bronchial tree resulting in a chronic cough and sputum. COPD does *not* cause clubbing or haemoptysis. Some 50% of patients with chronic bronchitis have emphysema, so there may be considerable overlapping of signs.[3]

The diagnosis[4] can often be made on the basis of three findings:

1. a history of heavy smoking (more than 40 packet-years, LR 12; less than 20 packet-years, LR 0.5[5])
2. reduced breath sounds
3. previous diagnosis of emphysema or COPD.

If two or three of these are present, the positive LR of COPD is 25.7.

Signs

Patients are usually not cyanosed but are dyspnoeic, and used to be called 'pink puffers'. The signs result from hyperinflation.

- Barrel-shaped chest with increased anteroposterior diameter.
- Pursed-lip breathing (this occurs in emphysema and not in chronic bronchitis): expiration through partly closed lips increases the end-expiratory pressure and keeps airways open, helping to minimise air trapping.
- Use of accessory muscles of respiration and drawing in of the lower intercostal muscles with inspiration.
- Drowsiness or even coma may be a sign of CO_2 retention indicating a worsening of the patient's chronically increased CO_2 levels. It may be caused by the administration of oxygen supplements (look for the oxygen mask), which further diminishes the patient's respiratory drive.[d] This is type II respiratory failure.
- CO_2 retention also leads to warm peripheries, bounding pulses and sometimes a flapping tremor.
- **Palpation:** reduced expansion and a hyperinflated chest, Hoover's sign, tracheal tug.
- **Percussion:** hyperresonant with decreased liver dullness.
- **Breath sounds:** decreased, early inspiratory crackles.

GOOD SIGNS GUIDE 11.2
Chronic obstructive pulmonary disease

Sign	LR+	LR−
Hoover's sign (on inspiration the chest moves *in* and the abdomen *out*)	4.2	0.5
Early inspiratory crackles	NS	NS
Unforced wheeze	4.4	0.88
Greatly reduced breath sounds	2.6	0.66
Forced expiratory time:		
<6 s	0.6	—
6–9 s	1.8	—
>9 s	6.7	—

NS = not significant.
Note: A self-reported smoking history of >40 packet-years has an LR of 8.3 for COPD.
(Adapted from Simel DL, Rennie D. *The rational clinical examination: evidence-based diagnosis.* New York: McGraw-Hill, 2009, Table 32.3.)

---

[d] This is called type II respiratory failure. Type I failure is associated with a normal or low PCO_2 and can be due to acute lung problems (asthma, pneumonia, pneumothorax) or chronic conditions (ILD).

- Wheeze is often absent.
- Signs of right heart failure may occur, but only late in the course of the disease.

Causes of generalised emphysema

- Usually, smoking.
- Occasionally, alpha$_1$-antitrypsin deficiency.

CHRONIC BRONCHITIS

This is defined clinically as the daily production of sputum for 3 months a year for at least 2 consecutive years. It is not now diagnosed as a separate entity from COPD and is probably of mostly historical interest.

Signs

The signs are the result of bronchial hypersecretion and airways obstruction.

- Loose cough and sputum (mucoid or mucopurulent), particularly in the morning shortly after wakening, and lessening as the day progresses.
- **Cyanosis:** these patients were sometimes called 'blue bloaters' because of the cyanosis present in the latter stages and associated oedema from right ventricular failure.
- **Palpation:** hyperinflated chest with reduced expansion.
- **Percussion:** increased resonance.
- **Breath sounds:** reduced with end-expiratory high- or low-pitched wheezes and early inspiratory crackles.
- Signs of right ventricular failure.

Causes

Smoking is the major cause, but recurrent bronchial infection may cause progression of the disease.

INTERSTITIAL LUNG DISEASE (ILD)[e]

Diffuse fibrosis of the lung parenchyma impairs gas transfer and causes ventilation–perfusion mismatching.

---
[e] Sometimes still called pulmonary fibrosis.

INTERSTITIAL LUNG DISEASE

Secondary to alveolitis (previously called fibrosing alveolitis)

UNKNOWN CAUSE
- Idiopathic pulmonary fibrosis
- Connective tissue disease (e.g. SLE, rheumatoid arthritis, ankylosing spondylitis, systemic sclerosis)
- Pulmonary haemorrhage syndromes (e.g. Goodpasture's syndrome)
- Graft versus host disease
- Gastrointestinal or liver diseases (primary biliary cirrhosis, chronic active hepatitis)

KNOWN CAUSE
- Asbestosis
- Radiation injury
- Aspiration pneumonia
- Drugs (e.g. amiodarone)
- Exposure to gases or fumes

Secondary to granulomatous disease

UNKNOWN CAUSE
- Sarcoidosis
- GPA (granulomatosis with polyangiitis)
- Eosinophilic granulomatosis with polyangiitis (Churg–Strauss disease)

KNOWN CAUSE
- Hypersensitivity pneumonitis to organic or inorganic dusts (silica, beryllium)

SLE = systemic lupus erythematosus.

LIST 11.2

This fibrosis may be the result of inflammation (alveolitis and interstitial inflammation) or granulomatous disease (see List 11.2). It has often no known cause (idiopathic interstitial fibrosis) or is secondary to a disease of unknown aetiology (e.g. sarcoidosis, connective tissue disease). It can result from inhalation of mineral dusts (focal fibrosis), replacement of lung tissue following disease that damages the lungs (e.g. aspiration pneumonia, tuberculosis). Connective tissue diseases and vasculitis are important causes.

Signs

Remember the three Cs:
- **C**ough (dry)
- **C**lubbing
- **C**rackles.

- **General:** dyspnoea, cyanosis and clubbing may be present.
- **Palpation:** expansion is slightly reduced.
- **Auscultation:** fine (Velcro-like) late inspiratory or pan-inspiratory crackles heard over the affected lobes.
- **Signs of associated connective tissue disease:** rheumatoid arthritis, systemic lupus erythematosus, scleroderma, Sjögren's[f] syndrome, polymyositis and dermatomyositis.

Causes

- Upper lobe predominant—SCART:
  - **S** ilicosis (progressive massive fibrosis), sarcoidosis
  - **C** oal workers' pneumoconiosis (progressive massive fibrosis), cystic fibrosis, chronic allergic alveolitis, chronic eosinophilic pneumonitis
  - **A** nkylosing spondylitis, allergic bronchopulmonary aspergillosis, alveolar haemorrhage syndromes
  - **R** adiation
  - **T** uberculosis.
- Lower lobe predominant—RASIO:
  - **R** heumatoid arthritis, other collagen vascular diseases
  - **A** sbestosis, acute allergic alveolitis, acute eosinophilic pneumonitis
  - **S** cleroderma (systemic sclerosis)
  - **I** diopathic interstitial fibrosis
  - **O** ther (drugs, e.g. busulfan, bleomycin, nitrofurantoin, hydralazine, methotrexate, amiodarone).

TUBERCULOSIS (TB)

Primary tuberculosis

Usually no abnormal chest signs are found, but segmental collapse, due to bronchial obstruction by the hilar lymph nodes, occasionally occurs. Erythema nodosum (p 278) is an important associated sign, but is rare. In children the diagnosis may be made on chest X-ray, when a Ghon[g] focus with hilar lymphadenopathy is seen.

Postprimary tuberculosis

The causes of postprimary or adult tuberculosis are reactivation of a primary lesion or occasionally reinfection. Immune suppression (e.g. as a result of HIV infection) and malnutrition predispose to reactivation of tuberculosis.

There are often no chest signs. The clues to the diagnosis are the classical symptoms of cough, haemoptysis, weight loss, night sweats and malaise.

Miliary tuberculosis

Widespread haematogenous dissemination of tubercle bacilli causes multiple millet-seed tuberculous nodules in various organs—spleen, liver, lymph nodes, kidneys, brain or joints. Miliary tuberculosis may complicate both childhood and adult tuberculosis.

Fever, anaemia and cachexia are the general signs. The patient may also be dyspnoeic, and pleural effusions, lymphadenopathy, hepatosplenomegaly or signs of meningitis may be present.

MEDIASTINAL COMPRESSION

Mediastinal structures may be compressed by a variety of pathological masses, including carcinoma of the lung (90%), other tumours (lymphoma, thymoma, dermoid cyst), a large retrosternal goitre or, rarely, an aortic aneurysm.

---

[f] Henrik Samuel Conrad Sjögren (1899–1986), a Stockholm ophthalmologist. He described the syndrome in 1933.

[g] Anton Ghon (1866–1936), an Austrian pathologist and Professor of Anatomical Pathology in Prague. He described the lesion in 1912.

Superior vena caval obstruction (a) from the front (b) from the side

(From Mangione S. *Physical diagnosis secrets*, 2nd edn. Philadelphia: Mosby Elsevier, 2007.)

FIGURE 11.2

Signs

- **Superior vena caval obstruction:**[h] the face is plethoric and cyanosed with periorbital oedema (see Fig. 11.2); the eyes may show exophthalmos, conjunctival injection and venous dilation in the fundi; in the neck the JVP is raised but not pulsatile, the thyroid may be enlarged and there may be supraclavicular lymphadenopathy and a positive Pemberton's sign; the chest may show dilated collateral vessels or signs of lung carcinoma.
- **Tracheal compression:** stridor, usually accompanied by respiratory distress.
- **Recurrent laryngeal nerve involvement:** hoarseness of the voice.
- **Horner's syndrome**.
- **Paralysis of the phrenic nerve:** dullness to percussion at the affected base, which does not change with deep inspiration (abnormal tidal percussion), and absent breath sounds suggest a paralysed diaphragm due to phrenic nerve involvement.

[h] First described by William Hunter (1718–83, brother of John Hunter) in a patient with a syphilitic aortic aneurysm.

CARCINOMA OF THE LUNG

Many patients have no signs.

Respiratory and chest signs

- Haemoptysis.
- Clubbing, sometimes with hypertrophic pulmonary osteoarthropathy (usually not small cell carcinoma).
- Lobar collapse or volume loss.
- Pneumonia.
- Pleural effusion.
- Fixed inspiratory wheeze.
- Tender ribs (secondary deposits of tumour in the ribs).
- Mediastinal compression, including signs of nerve involvement.
- Supraclavicular or axillary lymphadenopathy.

Apical (Pancoast's) tumour

- **Signs:** Horner's syndrome, recurrent laryngeal nerve palsy (hoarseness) due to a C8/T1 nerve root lesion.

Distant metastases

The brain, liver and bone are most often affected.

Non-metastatic extrapulmonary manifestations

- Anorexia, weight loss, cachexia, fever.
- **Endocrine changes:**
  - hypercalcaemia, due to secretion of parathyroid hormone-like substances, occurs in squamous cell carcinoma
  - hyponatraemia—antidiuretic hormone is released by small (oat) cell carcinomas
  - ectopic adrenocorticotrophic hormone (ACTH) syndrome (small cell carcinoma)
  - carcinoid syndrome[i]

[i] This rare neuroendocrine tumour may arise in the bronchi but most often begins in the gut, usually the small bowel. It may secrete 5-hydroxytryptophan (5-HT). This is normally cleared from the circulation in the liver, but when hepatic metastases are present it reaches the systemic circulation and can cause wheezing and flushing: carcinoid syndrome.

- gynaecomastia (gonadotrophins—rare; more often squamous cell)
- hypoglycaemia (insulin-like peptide from squamous cell carcinoma).
- Neurological manifestations:
  - Eaton–Lambert[j] syndrome (progressive muscle weakness) and retinal blindness (small cell carcinoma)
  - peripheral neuropathy
  - subacute cerebellar degeneration
  - polymyositis
  - cortical degeneration.
- **Haematological features:** migrating venous thrombophlebitis, disseminated intravascular coagulation, anaemia.
- **Skin:** acanthosis nigricans (p 232), dermatomyositis (rare) (p 593).
- **Renal:** nephrotic syndrome due to membranous glomerulonephritis (rare).

SARCOIDOSIS

This is a systemic disease, characterised by the presence of non-caseating granulomas that commonly affect the lungs, skin, eyes, lymph nodes, liver, spleen and the nervous system. The aetiology is unknown. There may be no pulmonary signs. Lung involvement is staged from 0 to 4 (List 11.3).

Pulmonary signs

- **Lungs:** no signs usually, although 80% of patients have lung involvement. In severe disease there may be signs of ILD.

Extrapulmonary signs

- **Skin:** lupus pernio (violaceous patches on the face, especially the nose, fingers or toes), pink nodules and plaques (granulomata) in old scars, erythema nodosum on the shins.
- **Eyes:** ciliary injection, anterior uveitis.
- **Lymph nodes:** generalised lymphadenopathy.
- **Liver and spleen:** enlarged (uncommon).

> **LUNG DISEASE IN SARCOIDOSIS**
>
> 0 = no involvement
> 1 = BHL alone (DLCO may be reduced)
> 2 = BHL and pulmonary infiltrate on X-ray
> 3 = infiltrate with signs of fibrosis—no lymphadenopathy
> 4 = end-stage ILD
>
> BHL = bilateral hilar lymphadenopathy; DLCO = diffusing capacity of the lungs for carbon monoxide; ILD = interstitial lung disease.
>
> LIST 11.3

> **RISK FACTORS FOR PULMONARY EMBOLISM (PE)**
>
> Previous PE
> Immobilisation (long aeroplane or car trip or especially after surgery—highest risk with lower limb orthopaedic operations)
> Known clotting-factor abnormalities
> Known malignancy
>
> LIST 11.4

- **Parotids:** gland enlargement (uncommon).
- **Central nervous system:** cranial nerve lesions, peripheral neuropathy (uncommon).
- **Musculoskeletal system:** arthralgia, swollen fingers, bone cysts (rare).
- **Heart:** heart block or ventricular arrhythmias presenting as palpitations or syncope, cor pulmonale (both rare).
- Signs of hypercalcaemia.

PULMONARY EMBOLISM (PE)

Embolism to the lungs often occurs without symptoms or signs. One should always entertain this diagnosis if there has been sudden and unexplained dyspnoea when a patient has risk factors for embolism (see List 11.4). Pleuritic chest pain and haemoptysis occur only when there is infarction. Syncope or the sudden onset of severe substernal pain can occur with massive embolism.

---

[j] ML Eaton (1905–58), a 20th-century American physician, and EH Lambert (1915–2003), an American neurologist.

Signs

- **General signs:** tachycardia, tachypnoea, fever (with infarction).
- **Lungs:** pleural friction rub if infarction has occurred.
- **Massive embolism:** elevated JVP, right ventricular gallop, right ventricular heave, tricuspid regurgitation murmur, palpable pulmonary component of the second heart sound (P2), gallop (S3 and/or S4).
- **Signs of deep venous thrombosis:** fewer than 50% of patients have clinical evidence of a source.

Clinical assessment is improved with a clinical scoring system;[6] clinical signs or symptoms of DVT (3.0), heart rate >100 beats / minute (1.5), immobilisation for 3 or more days or surgery in last 4 weeks (1.5), previous DVT or pulmonary embolus (1.5), haemoptysis (1.0), known cancer (1.0) or another diagnosis less likely than a pulmonary embolus (3.0); if over 4.0 points a pulmonary embolus is likely.

T&O'C ESSENTIALS

1. Respiratory failure is a medical emergency.
2. Pulmonary embolism must be considered a possibility in any unexplained sudden dyspnoea, especially if it is associated with pleuritic pain.
3. The signs of severe asthma must be recognised without delay. This is a life-threatening illness.

OSCE REVISION TOPICS – RESPIRATORY DISEASE

Use these topics, which commonly occur in the OSCE, to help with revision.

1. This woman's chest X-ray shows a pleural effusion. Please outline the physical findings you would expect. (p 192)
2. This man has clubbing. Please examine his respiratory system. What are you looking for in particular? (p 198)
3. This man's chest X-ray shows consolidation. What findings would you expect on examination? (p 190)
4. Please examine this man with COPD and attempt to assess its severity. (p 195)

References

1. Metlay JP, Kappor WN, Fine MJ. Does this patient have community-acquired pneumonia? Diagnosing pneumonia by history and physical examination. *JAMA* 1997; 278:1440–1445. Normal vital signs and normal chest auscultation substantially reduce the likelihood of pneumonia, but a chest X-ray is required for a firm diagnosis.
2. Wilcox ME, Chong CA, Stanbrook MB et al. Does this patient have an exudative pleural effusion? *JAMA* 2014; 311(23):2422–2431.
3. Global Initiative for Chronic Obstructive Lung Disease (GOLD). Global strategy for diagnosis, management and prevention of chronic obstructive pulmonary disease. 2016. Available from: goldcopd.org/global-strategy-diagnosis-management-prevention-copd-2016.
4. Holloman DR, Simmel DL, Goldberg JS. Diagnosis of obstructive airways disease from the clinical examination. *J Gen Intern Med* 1993; 8:63–68. A history of smoking, self-reported wheezing and wheezing detected at auscultation combined had a high predictive value for chronic obstructive airways disease. The forced expiratory time added little additional information to these predictors.
5. Holleman DR, Simel DL. Does the clinical examination predict airflow limitation? *JAMA* 1995; 273(4):313–319.
6. van Belle A, Buller HR, Huisman MV et al. Effectiveness of managing suspected pulmonary embolism using an algorithm combining clinical probability, D-dimer testing, and computer tomography. *JAMA* 2006; 295:172–179.

CHAPTER 12

A summary of the respiratory examination and extending the respiratory examination

Investigation; the act of the mind by which unknown truths are discovered. SAMUEL JOHNSON, *A Dictionary of the English Language (1775)*

The respiratory examination: a suggested method (see the OSCE video Respiratory examination at Student CONSULT)

 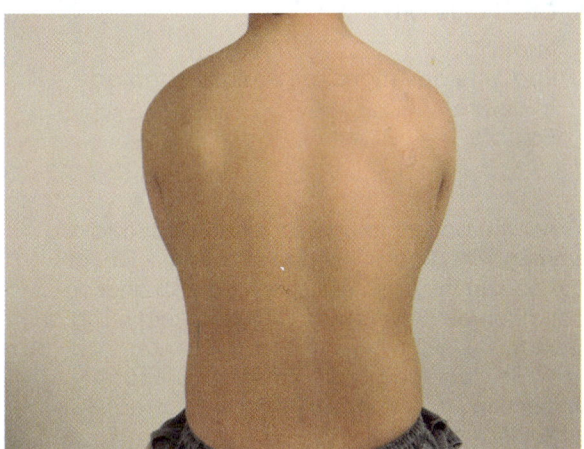

Respiratory system

FIGURE 12.1

Sitting up (if not acutely ill)

1. General inspection
  Sputum mug contents (blood, pus, etc.)
  Type of cough
  Rate and depth of respiration, and breathing pattern at rest
  Accessory muscles of respiration

2. Hands
  Clubbing
  Cyanosis (peripheral)
  Nicotine staining
  Wasting, weakness—finger abduction and adduction (lung cancer involving the brachial plexus)
  Wrist tenderness (hypertrophic pulmonary osteoarthropathy)
  Pulse (tachycardia, pulsus paradoxus)
  Flapping tremor (CO_2 narcosis)

3. Face
  Eyes—Horner's syndrome (apical lung cancer), anaemia
  Mouth—central cyanosis
  Voice—hoarseness (recurrent laryngeal nerve palsy)
  Facial plethora—smoker, SVC obstruction

4. Trachea

5. Chest posteriorly
  Inspect

TEXT BOX 12.1

Continued

> **The respiratory examination: a suggested method** *continued*

    Shape of chest and spine
    Scars
    Prominent veins (determine direction of flow)
    Palpate
    Cervical lymph nodes
    Expansion
    Vocal fremitus
    Percuss
    Supraclavicular region
    Back
    Axillae
    Tidal percussion (diaphragm paralysis)
    Auscultate
    Breath sounds
    Adventitious sounds
    Vocal resonance

6. Chest anteriorly
    Inspect
    Radiotherapy marks, other signs as noted above
    Palpate
    Supraclavicular nodes
    Expansion
    Vocal fremitus
    Apex beat
    Percuss
    Auscultate
    Pemberton's sign (SVC obstruction)

7. Cardiovascular system (lying at 45°)
    Jugular venous pressure (SVC obstruction, etc.)
    Cor pulmonale

8. Forced expiratory time

9. Other
    Lower limbs—oedema, cyanosis
    Breasts
    Temperature chart (infection)
    Evidence of malignancy or pleural effusion: examine the breasts, abdomen, rectum, lymph nodes, etc.
    Respiratory rate after exercise

Ask the patient to undress to the waist (provide women with a gown) and to sit over the side of the bed. In the clinic or surgery the examination can often be performed with the patient sitting on a chair.

While standing back to make your usual **inspection** (does the patient appear breathless while walking into the room or undressing?), ask whether sputum is available for inspection. Purulent sputum always indicates respiratory infection, and a large volume of purulent sputum is an important clue to bronchiectasis. Haemoptysis is also an important sign. Look for dyspnoea at rest and count the respiratory rate. Note any paradoxical inward motion of the abdomen during inspiration (diaphragmatic paralysis). Look for use of the accessory muscles of respiration, and any intercostal in-drawing of the lower ribs anteriorly (a sign of emphysema). Look for general cachexia.

Pick up the patient's **hands**. Look for clubbing, peripheral cyanosis, tar staining and anaemia. Note any wasting of the small muscles of the hands and weakness of finger abduction (lung cancer involving the brachial plexus). Palpate the wrists for tenderness (hypertrophic pulmonary osteoarthropathy). While holding the patient's hand, palpate the radial pulse for obvious pulsus paradoxus (dramatic fall in pulse pressure on normal inspiration). Take the blood pressure if indicated.

Go on to the **face**. Look closely at the eyes for constriction of one of the pupils and for ptosis (Horner's syndrome from an apical lung cancer). Inspect the tongue for central cyanosis.

Palpate the position of the **trachea**. This is an important sign, so spend time on it. If the trachea is displaced, you must concentrate on the upper lobes for physical signs. Also look and feel for a tracheal tug, which indicates severe airflow obstruction, and feel for the use of the accessory muscles. Now ask the patient to speak (hoarseness) and then cough, and note whether this is a loose cough, a dry cough or a bovine cough. Next measure the forced expiratory time (FET).[a] Tell the patient to take a maximal inspiration and blow out as rapidly and forcefully as possible while you listen. Note audible wheeze and prolongation of the time beyond 3 seconds as evidence of chronic obstructive pulmonary disease.[1]

The next step is to examine the **chest**. You may wish to examine the front first, or go to the back to start. The advantage of the latter is that

---

[a] There is good correlation between clinicians for the results of this test: κ-value 0.7. It is most accurate if performed with a stopwatch.

TEXT BOX 12.1

> **The respiratory examination: a suggested method** *continued*

there are often more signs there, unless the trachea is obviously displaced.

Inspect the **back**. Look for kyphoscoliosis. Do not miss ankylosing spondylitis, which causes decreased chest expansion and upper lobe fibrosis. Look for thoracotomy scars and prominent veins. Also note any skin changes from radiotherapy.

Palpate first from behind for the cervical nodes. Then examine for expansion—first upper lobe expansion, which is best seen by looking over the patient's shoulders at clavicular movement during moderate respiration. The affected side will show a delay or decreased movement. Then examine lower lobe expansion by palpation. Note asymmetry and reduction of movement.

Now ask the patient to bring his or her elbows together in the front to move the scapulae out of the way. Examine for vocal fremitus and then **percuss** the back of the chest.

Auscultate the chest. Note breath sounds (whether normal or bronchial) and their intensity (normal or reduced). Listen for adventitious sounds (crackles and wheezes). Finally examine for vocal resonance. If a localised abnormality is found, try to determine the abnormal lobe and segment.

Return to the **front of the chest**. Inspect again for chest deformity, distended veins, radiotherapy changes and scars. Palpate the supraclavicular nodes carefully. Then proceed with percussion and auscultation as before. Listen high up in the axillae too. Before leaving the chest feel the axillary nodes and examine the breasts (see Ch 36).

Lay the patient down at 45° and measure the jugular venous pressure. Then examine the praecordium and lower limbs for signs of cor pulmonale. Finally examine the **liver** and take the **temperature**.

Remember that most respiratory examinations are 'targeted'.[b] Not every part of the examination is necessary for every patient.

---

[b] If during an OSCE you forget to perform part of the examination you could try telling the examiner you had performed a 'targeted examination'—you might be lucky.

SVC=superior vena cava.

TEXT BOX 12.1

EXTENDING THE RESPIRATORY PHYSICAL EXAMINATION

Bedside assessment of lung function

Forced expiratory time

Physical examination can be complemented with an estimate of the forced expiratory time (FET).[1] Measure the time taken by the patient to exhale forcefully and completely through the open mouth after taking a maximum inspiration. It may be necessary to demonstrate this to the patient. The normal forced expiratory time is 3 seconds or less. Note any audible wheeze or cough. An increased FET indicates airways obstruction. The combination of a significant smoking history and an FET of 9 seconds or more is predictive of chronic obstructive pulmonary disease (COPD) (LR+ 9.6).[2] A peak flow meter or spirometer, however, will provide a more accurate measurement of lung function.

Peak flow meter

A peak flow meter is a simple gauge that is used to measure the maximum flow rate of expired air (Fig. 12.2). Again the patient is asked to take a full breath in but, rather than a prolonged expiration, a rapid forced maximal expiratory puff is made through the mouth.[c] The value obtained (the peak expiratory flow [PEF]) depends largely on airways diameter. Normal values are approximately 600 litres per minute for young men and 400 litres per minute for young women. The value depends on age, sex and height, so tables of normal values should be consulted. Airways obstruction, such as that caused by asthma or COPD, results in a reduced and variable PEF. It is a simple way of assessing and following patients with airways obstruction, but is rather effort dependent. The PEF is most useful when used for serial estimates of lung function.

---

[c] Students are advised to practise this so as to be able to demonstrate it without embarrassment.

Spirometry

The spirometer records graphically or numerically the forced expiratory volume and the forced vital capacity (see Fig. 12.3).[3]

- The *forced expiratory volume* (FEV) is the volume of air expelled from the lungs after maximum inspiration using maximum forced effort, and is measured in a given time.[d] Usually this is 1 second (FEV_1).
- The *forced vital capacity* (FVC) is the total volume of air expelled from the lungs after maximum inspiratory effort followed by maximum forced expiration.

The FVC is often nearly the same as the vital capacity, but in airways obstruction it may be less because of premature airways closure. It is usual to record the best of three attempts and to calculate the FEV_1/FVC ratio as a percentage. In healthy youth, the normal value is 80%, but this may decline to as little as 60% in old age. Normal values also vary with sex, age, height and race.

Reversibility of a reduced FEV_1/FVC after the use of bronchodilators is an important test for distinguishing asthma from COPD.

Obstructive ventilatory defect

When the FEV_1/FVC ratio is reduced (<70%) this is referred to as an obstructive defect. Both values tend to be reduced, but the FEV_1 is disproportionately low. The causes are loss of elastic recoil or airways narrowing, as in asthma or COPD.

Restrictive ventilatory defect

When the FEV_1/FVC ratio is normal or higher than normal, but both values are reduced, the pattern is described as a restrictive defect. This occurs in parenchymal lung disease, such as interstitial lung disease (ILD), sarcoidosis or when lung expansion is reduced by pneumonia or chest wall abnormalities.

Flow volume curve

As a part of spirometric assessment, the flow volume curve may be measured using a portable electronic device. This measures expiratory and inspiratory flow as a function of exhaled volume rather than against

---

[d] Ask the patient to breathe in as far as possible and then to breathe out as hard and fast as possible until the lungs are apparently empty.

Peak flow meter
(Shutterstock/Ugorenkov Aleksandr.)

FIGURE 12.2

Spirometry tracings

FIGURE 12.3

CHAPTER 12 A SUMMARY OF THE RESPIRATORY EXAMINATION AND EXTENDING THE RESPIRATORY EXAMINATION

time. It is a simple and reproducible test easily performed in the respiratory laboratory or at the bedside. The FVC, FEV$_1$ and various flow measurements (e.g. peak flow) can be calculated from the curve (see Fig. 12.4).

Pulse oximetry

Continuous measurement of a patient's arterial blood oxygen saturation (S_pO_2) is now possible with readily available oximetry devices (see Fig. 12.5). These simple devices can be used as an extension of the physical

Flow volume curves.

a

b

c

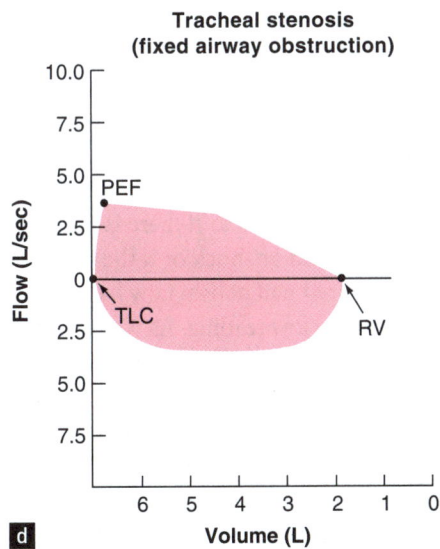
d

Look at the shape of the loop in each case ((a) to (d)). A normal flow volume curve is convex and symmetrical. In COPD, all flow routes are reduced and there is prolonged expiration (creating a 'scooped out' shape). In restrictive lung disease (e.g. pulmonary fibrosis), the loop is narrow but the shape normal (like a witch's hat). In fixed airway obstruction (e.g. tracheal stenosis), the loops look flattened as both expiration and inspiration are limited.

PEF=peak expiratory flow; TLC=total lung capacity; RV=residual volume

FIGURE 12.4

Pulse oximeter

(From Sanders MJ: *Mosby's paramedic textbook*, revised ed 3, St Louis, 2007, MosbyJems, Figure 1.32.)

FIGURE 12.5

examination, especially for patients who appear to be in respiratory distress. A fall in the reading may indicate a deteriorating respiratory problem such as exhaustion in a patient with severe asthma. This measurement is helpful for any patient who appears in respiratory distress or who has become cyanosed or drowsy.

The probe is attached to the patient's finger or earlobe. False readings may occur if there is poor tissue perfusion because of cold or shock or if the fingernails are coated with coloured nail polish. Low haemoglobin may cause a deceptively low reading. As with the results of any test it is important to ensure that the result is consistent with the clinical findings. A low S_pO_2 picked up in a patient who looks and feels perfectly well is likely to be a false reading. Generally, a reading of ≥95% is satisfactory. A reading of <90% is very abnormal and indicates respiratory failure or another critical illness (e.g. septic shock or a large pulmonary embolism).

The 6-minute walking test (6MWT)

Lung function can be tested during exertion with this relatively simple test. The patient is asked to walk at a normal pace along a measured course and the distance covered in 6 minutes is recorded. The walked distance can be compared with what the patient can achieve after treatment or the passage of time. Oxygen saturation, heart rate and apparent level of dyspnoea can also be added to the test. A reduction of oxygen saturation of more than 5% during exercise is abnormal. This test is a simple way of measuring exercise tolerance, the response to treatment and changes in the severity of the condition over time. It has been shown to predict mortality and morbidity.

The chest X-ray and computed tomography (CT) scan in respiratory medicine
(see the OSCE X-ray library at Student CONSULT)

The radiological appearance of a normal lung, with the lung segments labelled, is shown in Fig. 12.6.

The radiological changes of consolidation, pleural effusion, pneumothorax and hydropneumothorax are shown in Figs 12.7–12.10, respectively.

A pulmonary mass is obvious in Fig. 12.11, while multiple metastases are seen in Fig. 12.12. Primary tuberculosis is shown in Fig. 12.13, and Fig. 12.14 illustrates the features of emphysema.

Chest X-ray checklist

Airway (midline, no obvious deformities, no paratracheal masses).
Bones and soft tissue (no fractures, subcutaneous emphysema, median sternotomy wires, metal clips following lung resection or coronary artery bypass grafting).
Cardiac size, silhouette and retrocardiac density normal.
Diaphragms (right above left by 1–3 centimetres, costophrenic angles sharp, diaphragmatic contrast with lung sharp).
Equal volume (count ribs, look for mediastinal shift).
Fine detail (pleura and lung parenchyma).
Gastric bubble (above the air bubble one shouldn't see an opacity of any more than 0.5 centimetres width).

Text continued on p 210

Lung segments.

(a) Posteroanterior view. (b) CT scan through lung bases. (c) Left lateral view. (d) Right lateral view.

Right upper lobe: ä=apical segment; a=anterior segment, p=posterior segment.

Left upper lobe: ä – p=apicoposterior segment, s=anterior segment, sl=superior lingular segment, il=inferior lingular segment.

Right middle lobe (rml): m=medial segment, l=lateral segment.

Right lower lobe: äl=apical segment, mb=medial basal segment, lb=lateral basal segment, ab=anterior basal segment, pb=posterior basal segment.

Left lower lobe: äl=apical segment, lb=lateral basal segment, ab=anterior basal segment, pb=posterior basal segment

FIGURE 12.6

(a) and (b) Right upper lobe consolidation.
The right upper lobe is opacified and is limited inferiorly by the horizontal fissure (arrows). There must be some collapse as well, as the fissure shows some elevation. These changes could be due to a bacterial lobar pneumonia per se, but a central bronchostenotic lesion should be considered. If the pneumonia persists, a bronchoscopy is indicated to search for a central carcinoma

FIGURE 12.7

Pleural effusion.

The upper margin of the effusion is curved ('meniscus sign'). The left hemidiaphragm is not seen because there is no adjacent aerated lung for contrast. The heart shows some deviation to the right. It is unlikely that this is caused by an effusion of this size; it is probably related to the lower thoracic scoliosis

FIGURE 12.8

Pneumothorax.

(a) There is a massive right pneumothorax with collapsed lung seen against the hilum (arrow). There is increased translucency because of the absence of vascular shadows. (b) Different patient with a smaller pneumothorax. Small pneumothoraces are easier to see on an expiratory film as the pneumothorax volume remains constant, surrounding the partly deflated lung. The visceral pleural surface is marked (arrow)

FIGURE 12.9

Hydropneumothorax.

An air–fluid level is seen in the upper portion of the right hemithorax. When air and fluid are present in the pleural space, the fluid no longer forms a meniscus at its upper margin. Some aerated lung is seen deep in the fluid

FIGURE 12.10

A pulmonary mass.

There is a large solitary mass lesion in the left lower zone. The differential diagnosis is primary or secondary neoplasm, hydatid cyst or large abscess. No air–fluid level is seen within it to indicate cavitation

FIGURE 12.11

Pulmonary metastases.

Multiple rounded opacities are seen in both lung fields, mainly at the left base and around the right hilum. The most likely cause is multiple pulmonary metastases. Other rare possibilities are hydatid cysts, large sarcoid nodules or large rheumatoid nodules. Multiple abscesses are extremely unlikely in the absence of cavitation

FIGURE 12.12

Primary tuberculosis.

Two small rounded areas of shadowing are seen in the right upper zone (solid arrow). The right hilum is enlarged by the enlarged draining lymph nodes (open arrow). This combination of focal shadowing and enlarged lymph nodes is the primary (Ghon) complex of tuberculosis. With healing, calcification may occur in the parenchymal and nodal lesions. In contrast, in tuberculosis reactivation or reinfection, cavitation may occur and there is no lymphadenopathy

FIGURE 12.13

Hilum (left normally above right by up to 3 centimetres, no larger than a thumb), hardware (especially in the intensive care unit: endotracheal tube, central venous catheters, pacemaker).

High-resolution CT scans give more detailed information about the lungs but expose the patient to more radiation. They are particularly useful for diagnosing interstitial lung disease, pulmonary haemorrhage (see Fig. 12.15) and bronchiectasis (see Fig. 12.16). Primary and secondary lung tumours are best imaged with CT and tuberculous involvement of the lungs can be quantified (see Fig. 12.17).

Emphysema.

The lungs are overinflated with low, flat hemidiaphragms. The level of the hemidiaphragms is well below the anterior aspects of the sixth ribs. The diaphragm normally projects over the sixth rib anteriorly and the tenth intercostal space posteriorly. Count the ribs anteriorly (1–6). There is increased translucency of both upper zones with loss of the vascular markings due to bulla formation (arrow). This increased translucency is not due to overexposure. The hila are prominent because of the enlarged central pulmonary arteries. In contrast, the smaller peripheral pulmonary arteries (the lung markings) are decreased in size and number. This is due to actual destruction, displacement around bullae and decreased perfusion through emphysematous areas

FIGURE 12.14

Pulmonary haemorrhage

(From Hansell D. *Imaging of diseases of the chest*, 5th edn. Maryland Heights, MO: Mosby, 2009.)

FIGURE 12.15

(a) to (c) Bronchiectasis
(From Mettler FA. *Essentials of radiology*, 2nd edn. Philadelphia: Saunders, 2005.)

FIGURE 12.16

CHAPTER 12 A SUMMARY OF THE RESPIRATORY EXAMINATION AND EXTENDING THE RESPIRATORY EXAMINATION

CT of interstitial lung disease

(From Sellke F, del Nido PJ, Swanson SJ. *Sabiston & Spencer's surgery of the chest*, 8th edn. Philadelphia: Saunders, 2009.)

FIGURE 12.17

OSCE REVISION TOPICS – RESPIRATORY INVESTIGATIONS

Use these topics, which commonly occur in the OSCE, to help with revision.

1. What would be the typical findings on spirometry of a patient with severe COPD? (p 203)

2. This man's chest X-ray shows consolidation. What findings would you expect on examination? (p 190)

3. This CT scan of the chest shows changes of bronchiectasis. What physical examination findings would you expect? (p 194)

4. Demonstrate the use of this spirometer with this patient and explain the results you would expect in a patient with asthma and in one with interstitial lung disease. (p 203)

T&O'C ESSENTIALS

1. The chest X-ray is considered by chest physicians to be an extension of the physical examination.
2. Use a checklist to help you to systematically review a chest X-ray so that no abnormality is missed.
3. Always compare the physical findings with the X-ray changes: this will also help improve your examination technique.
4. The CT scan has improved sensitivity and specificity compared with the chest X-ray, but at the expense of enormously increased radiation exposure.
5. Bedside tests such as oximetry and peak flow measurements can be very helpful in quickly assessing a patient's status.

References

1. Schapira RM, Schapira MM, Funahashi A et al. The value of the forced expiratory time in the physical diagnosis of obstructive airways disease. *JAMA* 1993; 270:731–736. In patients with chronic obstructive airways who have a low pretest probability, an appropriate low-end cut-off is required (e.g. 3 seconds).
2. McGee S. *Evidence-based physical diagnosis*, 3rd edn. St Louis: Saunders, 2012.
3. Miller MR, Hankinson J et al; ATS/ERS Task force. Standardisation of spirometry. *Eur Respir J* 2005; 26(2):319–338.

SECTION 4
The gastrointestinal system

CHAPTER 13
The gastrointestinal history

CHAPTER 14
The gastrointestinal examination

CHAPTER 15
Correlation of physical signs and gastrointestinal disease

CHAPTER 16
A summary of the gastrointestinal examination and extending the gastrointestinal examination

CHAPTER 13
The gastrointestinal history

To study the phenomena of disease without books is to sail an uncharted sea, while to study books without patients is not to go to sea at all. SIR WILLIAM OSLER (1849–1919)

Gastroenterologists and gastrointestinal surgeons concern themselves with the entire length of the gut, the exocrine pancreas, the liver and the peripheral effects of alimentary disease.

PRESENTING SYMPTOMS

(See List 13.1.)

GASTROINTESTINAL HISTORY

Major symptoms
Abdominal pain
Appetite and/or weight change
Postprandial fullness or early satiation, or both
Nausea and/or vomiting
Heartburn and/or acid regurgitation
Waterbrash
Dysphagia
Disturbed defecation (diarrhoea, constipation, faecal incontinence)
Bloating or visible distension, or both
Bleeding (haematemesis, melaena, rectal bleeding)
Jaundice
Dark urine, pale stools
Pruritus
Lethargy
Fever

LIST 13.1

Abdominal pain

There are many causes of abdominal pain, and careful history taking will often lead to the correct diagnosis. The following should be considered.

Frequency and duration

Is the pain acute or chronic, when did it begin and how often does it occur?

Site and radiation

The site of the pain is important. Ask the patient to point to the area affected by pain and to the point of maximum intensity. Parietal peritoneal inflammation that causes pain usually does so in a localised area. Ask about radiation of pain.

- Pain that radiates through to the back suggests pancreatic disease or a penetrating peptic ulcer.
- Pain due to diaphragmatic irritation may radiate to the shoulder.
- Pain due to oesophageal reflux or spasm may radiate to the throat.

Character and pattern

The pain may be colicky (coming and going in waves and related to peristaltic movements) or steady. Colicky pain comes from obstruction of the bowel or the ureters. Colicky pain arises because of complete or partial blockage of the bowel, which triggers intestinal pain receptors. If the pain is chronic, ask about its daily pattern.

Aggravating and relieving factors

- Pain due to peptic ulceration may occur after meals (when acid increases).
- Eating may precipitate ischaemic pain in the gut (a result of a reduction of blood supply to the bowel caused by arterial disease or embolism).

- Vomiting or the use of antacids may relieve peptic ulcer pain or that of gastro-oesophageal reflux.
- Defecation or passage of flatus may temporarily relieve the pain of colonic disease.
- Patients who obtain some relief by rolling around vigorously are more likely to have a colicky pain (e.g. from bowel obstruction), while those who lie perfectly still are more likely to have peritonitis.

Patterns of pain

Peptic ulcer disease

This is classically a dull or burning pain in the epigastrium that is relieved to a degree by food or antacids. It is typically episodic and may occur at night, waking the patient from sleep. This combination of symptoms is suggestive of the diagnosis. The pain is not always related to meals, despite classical teaching to the contrary. It is not possible to distinguish duodenal ulceration from gastric ulceration clinically. Many patients with epigastric pain related to meals have no evidence of peptic ulcer on investigation (referred to as *non-ulcer* or *functional dyspepsia*).

Pancreatic pain

This is a steady epigastric pain that may be partly relieved by sitting up and leaning forwards. There is often radiation of the pain to the back, and vomiting is common.

Biliary pain

Although usually called 'biliary colic', this pain is rarely colicky. Obstruction of the cystic duct often causes epigastric pain. It is usually a severe, constant pain that can last for hours. There may be a history of episodes of similar pain in the past; although pain episodes can occur after fatty meals, they are usually unpredictable. If cholecystitis develops, the pain typically shifts to the right upper quadrant and becomes more severe. Biliary colic is often associated with nausea and vomiting.

Renal colic

This is a colicky pain superimposed on a background of constant pain in the renal angle, often with radiation towards the groin. It can be very severe indeed.

Bowel obstruction

This is colicky pain. Periumbilical pain suggests a small-bowel origin but colonic pain can occur anywhere in the abdomen. Small-bowel obstruction tends to cause more frequent colicky pain (with a cycle every 2–3 minutes) than does large-bowel obstruction (every 10–15 minutes). Obstruction is often associated with vomiting, constipation and abdominal distension.

Appetite and weight change

Loss of appetite (anorexia) and weight loss are important gastrointestinal symptoms. The presence of both anorexia and weight loss should make one suspicious of an underlying malignancy, but they may also occur with depression and in other diseases. The combination of weight loss with an increased appetite suggests malabsorption of nutrients or a hypermetabolic state (e.g. thyrotoxicosis). It is important to document when the symptoms began and how much weight loss has occurred over this period. Liver disease can sometimes cause disturbance of taste. This may cause smokers with acute hepatitis and jaundice to give up smoking.

Early satiation and postprandial fullness

Inability to finish a normal meal (early satiation) may be a symptom of gastric diseases, including gastric cancer and peptic ulcer. A feeling of inappropriate fullness after eating can also be a symptom of functional dyspepsia.

Nausea and vomiting

Nausea is the sensation of wanting to vomit.[a] Heaving and retching may occur but there is no expulsion of gastric contents. Vomiting refers to the explosive ejection of stomach contents through the mouth; it is involuntary.

There are many possible causes:
- gastrointestinal tract infections (e.g. from food poisoning by *Staphylococcus aureus*) or
- small-bowel obstruction

can cause acute symptoms.

---

[a] The word *nauseous* can mean either nauseated (i.e. feeling like vomiting) or repulsive (i.e. likely to make other people vomit). It is probably best to use the word *nauseated* to describe a patient who feels like vomiting in order to avoid this unfortunate ambiguity. (The Latin word has only the second meaning.)

In patients with chronic symptoms:
- pregnancy and
- drugs (e.g. digoxin, opiates, dopamine agonists, chemotherapy)

should always be considered.

In the gastrointestinal tract itself:
- peptic ulcer disease with gastric outlet obstruction
- motor disorders (e.g. gastroparesis from diabetes mellitus, or after gastric surgery)
- acute hepatobiliary disease and
- alcoholism

are important causes.

Finally, psychogenic vomiting, eating disorders (e.g. bulimia) and, rarely, increased intracranial pressure are possible causes of chronic unexplained nausea and vomiting.

Asking about the timing of the vomiting (see Questions box 13.1) can be helpful; vomiting delayed more than 1 hour after the meal is typical of gastric outlet obstruction or gastroparesis, whereas early morning vomiting before eating is characteristic of pregnancy, alcoholism and raised intracranial pressure. Also ask about the contents of the vomitus (e.g. bile indicates an open connection between the duodenum and stomach, old food suggests gastric outlet obstruction, while blood suggests ulceration). Vomiting due to bowel obstruction may occur with little or no nausea.

Vomiting is different from rumination. Rumination is effortless regurgitation of food into the mouth after eating; patients often call this vomiting when asked to describe what they mean. The food is spat out or reswallowed; the taste is, apparently, not unpleasant.

Heartburn and acid regurgitation (gastro-oesophageal reflux disease—GORD)

Heartburn refers to the presence of a burning pain or discomfort in the retrosternal area. Typically, this sensation travels up towards the throat and occurs after meals or is aggravated by bending, stooping or lying supine (see Questions box 13.2). Antacids usually relieve the pain, at least transiently. This symptom is due to regurgitation of stomach contents into the oesophagus. Usually these contents are acidic, although occasionally alkaline reflux can induce similar problems. Associated with gastro-oesophageal reflux may be *acid regurgitation*, in which the patient experiences a sour or bitter-tasting fluid coming up into the mouth. This symptom strongly suggests that reflux is occurring.

QUESTIONS TO ASK A PATIENT PRESENTING WITH RECURRENT VOMITING

! denotes symptoms for the possible diagnosis of an urgent or dangerous problem.

1. Describe what happens during a typical episode (rule out rumination).
2. How long have you been having attacks of vomiting (distinguish acute from chronic)?
3. Does the vomiting occur with nausea preceding it, or does it occur without any warning?
4. Is the vomiting usually immediately after a meal or hours after a meal?
5. Do you have vomiting early in the morning or late in the evening?
! 6. What does the vomit look like? Is it bloodstained, bile-stained or feculent? (Gastrointestinal bleeding or bowel obstruction)
7. Do you have specific vomiting episodes followed by feeling completely well for long periods before the vomiting episode occurs again? (Cyclical vomiting syndrome)
8. Is there any abdominal pain associated with the vomiting?
! 9. Have you been losing weight?
10. What medications are you taking?
11. Do you have worsening headaches? (Neurological symptoms suggest a central cause)

QUESTIONS BOX 13.1

> **QUESTIONS TO ASK THE PATIENT WITH ACID REFLUX OR SUSPECTED GASTRO-OESOPHAGEAL REFLUX DISEASE (GORD)**
>
> ❗ denotes symptoms for the possible diagnosis of an urgent or dangerous problem.
>
> 1. Do you have heartburn (a burning pain under the sternum radiating up towards the throat)? How often does this occur? (More than once a week suggests GORD)
> 2. Does your heartburn occur after meals or when you lean forwards or lie flat in bed? (Typical of acid reflux)
> ❗ 3. Does the pain radiate across your chest down your left arm or into your jaw? (Suggests myocardial ischaemia)
> 4. Is the pain relieved by antacids or acid-blocking drugs? (Typical of acid reflux)
> 5. Do you experience suddenly feeling bitter-tasting fluid in your mouth? (Acid regurgitation; typical of acid reflux)
> 6. Have you experienced the sudden appearance of a salty tasting or tasteless fluid in your mouth? (Waterbrash, not GORD)
> ❗ 7. Have you had trouble swallowing? (Dysphagia; see Questions box 13.3)
> 8. Have you been troubled by a cough when you lie down?
>
> QUESTIONS BOX 13.2

Some patients complain of a cough that troubles them when they lie down. In patients with gastro-oesophageal reflux disease, the lower oesophageal sphincter muscle relaxes inappropriately. Reflux symptoms may be aggravated by:

- alcohol
- chocolate
- caffeine
- a fatty meal
- theophylline
- calcium channel blockers, and
- anticholinergic drugs, as these lower the oesophageal sphincter pressure.

The diagnosis can usually be made confidently on the basis of typical symptoms as long as alarm features for malignancy

- dysphagia
- unintentional weight loss
- melaena or
- haematemesis

are *not* present.

Waterbrash refers to excessive secretion of saliva into the mouth and should not be confused with regurgitation; it may occur, uncommonly, in patients with peptic ulcer disease or oesophagitis.

Dysphagia

Dysphagia is difficulty in swallowing. Swallowing involves two phases:

1. The oropharyngeal component—food passes from mouth to hypopharynx and on to upper oesophagus.
2. The oesophageal component—the food bolus passes through the oesophagus to the stomach.

Such difficulty may occur with solids or liquids. The causes of dysphagia are listed in List 13.2. If a patient complains of difficulty swallowing, it is important to differentiate painful swallowing from actual difficulty.[1] Painful swallowing is termed *odynophagia* and occurs with any severe inflammatory process involving the oesophagus. Causes include infectious oesophagitis (e.g. *Candida*, herpes simplex), peptic ulceration of the oesophagus, caustic damage to the oesophagus or, rarely, oesophageal perforation.

If the patient complains of difficulty initiating swallowing (see Questions box 13.3), fluid regurgitating into the nose or choking on trying to swallow, this suggests that the cause of the dysphagia is in the pharynx (oropharyngeal dysphagia). Causes of oropharyngeal dysphagia can include neurological disease (e.g. motor neurone disease, resulting in bulbar or pseudobulbar palsy).

If the patient complains of food sticking in the oesophagus, it is important to consider a number of anatomical causes of oesophageal blockage.[1] Ask the patient to point to the site where the solids stick. If

CAUSES OF DYSPHAGIA

Mechanical obstruction
INTRINSIC (WITHIN OESOPHAGUS)
Reflux oesophagitis with stricture formation
Carcinoma of oesophagus or gastric cardia
Eosinophic oesophagitis
Pharyngeal or oesophageal web
Pharyngeal pouch
Schatzki (lower oesophageal) ring
Foreign body

EXTRINSIC (OUTSIDE OESOPHAGUS)
Goitre with retrosternal extension
Mediastinal tumours, bronchial carcinoma, vascular compression (rare)

Neuromuscular motility disorders
(Hints from the history: solids and liquids equally difficult, symptoms intermittent)
Achalasia
Diffuse oesophageal spasm
Scleroderma

Oropharyngeal dysphagia
(Hints: aspiration, fluid regurgitation into the nose)
Cricopharyngeal dysfunction—Zenker's diverticulum
Neurological disease: bulbar or pseudobulbar palsy, myasthenia gravis, polymyositis, myotonic dystrophy

LIST 13.2

QUESTIONS TO ASK A PATIENT WHO REPORTS DIFFICULTY SWALLOWING

! denotes symptoms for the possible diagnosis of an urgent or dangerous problem.

1. Do you have trouble swallowing solids or liquids, or both? (Solids and liquids suggests a motor problem, e.g. achalasia; solids only suggests a mechanical problem like cancer or a stricture)
2. Where does the hold-up occur (please point to the area)? (Pointing to the lower oesophagus suggests mechanical obstruction in the lower oesophagus)
3. Is the trouble swallowing intermittent or persistent? (Intermittent suggests eosinophilic oesophagitis [EoE], a lower oesophageal ring or a motor problem; EoE also causes acute food impaction)
4. Has the problem been getting progressively worse? (This suggests cancer or a stricture)
5. Do you cough or choke on starting to swallow? (This suggests oropharyngeal dysphagia)
6. Is it painful to swallow (odynophagia)? (This suggests acute inflammation of the oesophagus)
7. Do you have any heartburn or acid regurgitation? (Yes suggests GORD)
! 8. Have you been losing weight? (Worry about cancer)
9. Do you have asthma or hay fever? (This would be further supportive of EoE)

QUESTIONS BOX 13.3

there is a mechanical obstruction at the lower end of the oesophagus, most often the patient will localise the dysphagia to the lower retrosternal area. However, obstruction higher in the oesophagus may be felt anywhere in the retrosternal area. If heartburn is also present, for example, this suggests that gastro-oesophageal reflux with or without stricture formation may be the cause of the dysphagia.

The actual course of the dysphagia is also a very important part of the history to obtain.

- If the patient states that the dysphagia is **intermittent** or is present only with the first few swallows of food, this suggests the presence of a lower oesophageal ring, eosinophilic oesophagitis or, rarely, diffuse oesophageal spasm.
- However, if the patient complains of **progressive** difficulty swallowing, this suggests a stricture, carcinoma or achalasia.
- If the patient states that **both** solids and liquids stick, then a motor disorder of the oesophagus

such as achalasia or diffuse oesophageal spasm is more likely.

Diarrhoea

The symptom diarrhoea can be defined in a number of different ways. Patients may complain of frequent stools (more than three per day or a change from previous frequency is abnormal) or they may complain of a change in the consistency of the stools, which have become loose or watery. There are a large number of possible causes of diarrhoea.

Ask about the frequency and volume. Some patients pass small amounts of formed stool more than three times a day because of an increased desire to defecate. The stools are not loose and stool volume is not increased. This is not true diarrhoea. It can occur because of local rectal pathology, incomplete rectal emptying or a psychological disturbance that leads to an increased interest in defecation.

When a history of diarrhoea is obtained (see Questions box 13.4), it is also important to determine whether this has occurred acutely or it is a chronic problem. Acute diarrhoea is more likely to be infectious in nature, while chronic diarrhoea has a large number of causes.

Clinically, diarrhoea can be divided into a number of different groups based on the likely disturbance of physiology.[2]

1. If the stools are watery and of high volume consider the following:
   - *Secretory diarrhoea* when the diarrhoea is of high volume (commonly more than 1 litre per day) and persists when the patient fasts; there is no pus or blood, and the stools are not excessively fatty. Secretory diarrhoea occurs when net secretion in the colon or small bowel exceeds absorption; some of the causes include infections (e.g. *E. coli*, *S. aureus*, *Vibrio cholerae*), hormonal conditions (e.g.

QUESTIONS TO ASK THE PATIENT PRESENTING WITH DIARRHOEA

! denotes symptoms for the possible diagnosis of an urgent or dangerous problem.

1. How many stools per day do you pass now normally?
2. What do the stools look like (stool form, e.g. loose and watery)?
3. Do you have to run to the bathroom to have a bowel movement? (Urgency in colonic disease)
4. Have you been woken from sleep during the night by diarrhoea? (Organic cause more likely)
! 5. Have you seen any bright-red blood in the stools, or mucus or pus? (Suggests colonic disease)
6. Are you passing large volumes of stool every day? (Suggests small-bowel disease if non-bloody)
7. Are your stools pale, greasy, smelly and difficult to flush away (steatorrhoea)?
8. Have you seen oil droplets in the stool? (Chronic pancreatitis)
9. Have you had problems with leakage of stool (faecal incontinence)?
! 10. Have you lost weight? (e.g. cancer, malabsorption)
11. Have you had treatment with antibiotics recently? (Consider *Clostridium difficile* infection)
12. Have you had any recent travel? Where to? (Consider infections such as *Giardia*)
13. Have you a personal history of inflammatory bowel disease or prior gastrointestinal surgery?
14. Have you any history in the family of coeliac disease or inflammatory bowel disease?
15. Have you had any problems with arthritis? (e.g. inflammatory bowel disease, Whipple's disease)
! 16. Have you had recent fever, rigors or chills? (e.g. infection, lymphoma)
17. Have you had frequent infections? (Immunoglobulin deficiency)

QUESTIONS BOX 13.4

vasoactive intestinal polypeptide-secreting tumour, Zollinger–Ellison[b] syndrome, carcinoid syndrome) and villous adenoma.
- *Osmotic diarrhoea* when diarrhoea disappears with fasting and there are large-volume stools related to the ingestion of food. Osmotic diarrhoea occurs due to excessive solute drag; causes include lactose intolerance (disaccharidase deficiency), magnesium antacids or gastric surgery.
- *Abnormal intestinal motility* if the patient has thyrotoxicosis or the irritable bowel syndrome.

2. If the stools contain blood consider the following:
   - *Exudative diarrhoea* when there is inflammation in the colon. Typically the stools are of small volume but frequent, and there may be associated blood or mucus (e.g. inflammatory bowel disease, colon cancer).
3. If the stools are fatty consider the following:
   - *Malabsorption* of nutrients and steatorrhoea. Here the stools are fatty, pale-coloured, extremely smelly, float in the toilet bowel and are difficult to flush away. Steatorrhoea is defined as the presence of more than 7 g of fat in a 24-hour stool collection. There are many causes of steatorrhoea (p 280).

Constipation

It is important to determine what patients mean if they say they are constipated.[3] Constipation is a common symptom and can refer to the infrequent passage of stools (fewer than three times per week), hard stools or stools that are difficult to evacuate.

This symptom may occur acutely or may be a chronic problem (see Questions box 13.5). In many patients, chronic constipation arises because of habitual neglect of the impulse to defecate, leading to the accumulation of large, dry faecal masses. With constant rectal distension from faeces, the patient may grow less aware of rectal fullness, and this leads to chronic constipation.

QUESTIONS TO ASK A PATIENT PRESENTING WITH CONSTIPATION

! denotes symptoms for the possible diagnosis of an urgent or dangerous problem.

1. How often do you have a bowel movement?
2. Are your stools hard or difficult to pass?
3. What do the stools look like (stool form, e.g. small pellets)?
4. Do you strain excessively on passing stool?
5. Do you feel there may be a blockage at the anus area when you try to pass stool?
6. Do you ever press your finger in around the anus (or vagina) to help stool pass?
! 7. Has your bowel habit changed recently?
8. Any recent change in your medication?
! 9. Any blood in the stools?
10. Any abdominal pain? Is pain made better by a bowel movement?
! 11. Any recent weight loss?
12. Do you ever have diarrhoea?
! 13. Do you have a history of colon polyps or cancer? Any family history of colon cancer?

QUESTIONS BOX 13.5

Ask about medications and the past history. Constipation may arise from ingestion of drugs (e.g. codeine, antidepressants, or aluminium or calcium antacids) and with various metabolic or endocrine diseases (e.g. hypothyroidism, hypercalcaemia, diabetes mellitus, phaeochromocytoma, porphyria, hypokalaemia) and neurological disorders (e.g. aganglionosis, Hirschsprung's[c] disease, autonomic neuropathy, spinal cord injury, multiple sclerosis).

Constipation can also arise after partial colonic obstruction from carcinoma; it is therefore very

---

[b] Robert Milton Zollinger (1903–92), an American surgeon, and Edwin H Ellison (1918–70), an American physician. This syndrome is characterised by gastric acid hypersecretion, peptic ulceration and in 40% of cases diarrhoea, due to a gastrinoma (gastrin-secreting tumour). It was described in 1955.

[c] Harold Hirschsprung (1830–1916), a physician at Queen Louise Hospital for Children, Copenhagen, described this disease in 1888. It had previously been described by Caleb Parry, English physician, in 1825.

important to determine whether there has been a recent change in bowel habit, as this may indicate development of a malignancy. Patients with very severe constipation in the absence of structural disease may be found on a transit study to have slow colonic transit; such slow-transit constipation is most common in young women.

Constipation is common throughout pregnancy but especially in the later stages.

Ask about excessive straining or a feeling of stool being blocked during attempted bowel movements. Difficulty with evacuation of faeces may occur with disorders of the pelvic floor muscles or nerves, or anorectal disease (e.g. fissure or stricture). Patients with this problem may complain of straining, a feeling of anal blockage or even the need to self-digitate to perform manual evacuation of faeces.

Patients confined to bed in hospital or who have had abdominal operations are often constipated. Starvation and changes in diet can be other causes.

Irritable bowel syndrome (IBS)

A chronic but erratic disturbance in defecation (typically alternating constipation and diarrhoea) associated with abdominal pain, in the absence of any structural or biochemical abnormality, is very common; such patients are classified as having the *irritable bowel syndrome*.[4,5] Patients who report abdominal pain plus two or more of the following symptoms—abdominal pain relieved by defecation, looser or more frequent stools with the onset of abdominal pain, passage of mucus per rectum, a feeling of incomplete emptying of the rectum following defecation and visible abdominal distension—are more likely to have the irritable bowel syndrome than organic disease. The diagnosis is no longer considered one of exclusion but should be based on diagnostic criteria (List 13.3).

Mucus

The passage of mucus (white slime) may occur because of a solitary rectal ulcer, fistula or villous adenoma, or in the irritable bowel syndrome.

Bleeding

Patients may present with the problem of haematemesis (vomiting blood), melaena (passage of jet-black stools)

> **ROME IV DIAGNOSTIC CRITERIA FOR THE IRRITABLE BOWEL SYNDROME (IBS)**
>
> Recurrent abdominal pain at least 1 day a week on average in the last 3 months, and 2 or more of the following:
> 1. Improvement or aggravation with defecation
> 2. Associated with a change in the frequency of stool (more or less frequent)
> 3. Associated with a change in the appearance of stool[d] (looser or firmer stools)
>
> [d]You can observe this yourself if so desired. This is why we think so many want to be gastroenterologists!
>
> LIST 13.3

or haematochezia (passage of bright-red blood per rectum). Sometimes patients may present because routine testing for occult blood in the stools is positive (p 268). It is important to try to find out, if vomiting of blood is reported, that this is not the result of bleeding from a tooth socket or the nose, or the coughing up of blood.

Haematemesis indicates that the site of the bleeding is proximal to, or within, the duodenum (see Table 13.1). Ask about symptoms of peptic ulceration; haematemesis is commonly due to bleeding chronic peptic ulceration, particularly from a duodenal ulcer. Peptic ulcers often bleed without causing abdominal pain.

Ask whether the blood came up with the first vomit or not (see Questions box 13.6). A Mallory–Weiss tear usually occurs with repeated vomiting; typically the patient reports first the vomiting of clear gastric contents and then the vomiting of blood.

Ask if there is blood in the stool, and whether it is on top or mixed in. Haemorrhoids and local anorectal diseases such as fissures will commonly present with passing small amounts of bright-red blood per rectum. The blood is normally not mixed in the stools but is on the toilet paper, on top of the stools or in the toilet bowl.

Melaena (black tarry stools) usually results from bleeding from the upper gastrointestinal tract, although right-sided colonic and small-bowel lesions can occasionally be responsible. Massive bright-red rectal bleeding can occur from the distal colon or rectum, or

Causes of acute gastrointestinal bleeding	
Upper gastrointestinal tract MORE COMMON 1. Chronic peptic ulcer: duodenal ulcer, gastric ulcer 2. Acute peptic ulcer (erosions) LESS COMMON 3. Mallory–Weiss* syndrome (tear at the gastro-oesophageal junction) 4. Oesophageal and/or gastric varices 5. Erosive or ulcerative oesophagitis 6. Gastric carcinoma, polyp, other tumours 7. Dieulafoy's† ulcer (single defect that involves an ectatic submucosal artery) 8. Watermelon stomach (antral vascular ectasias) 9. Aortoenteric fistula (usually aortoduodenal and after aortic surgery) 10. Vascular anomalies—angiodysplasia, arteriovenous malformations, blue rubber bleb naevus syndrome, hereditary haemorrhagic telangiectasia, CRST syndrome 11. Pseudoxanthoma elasticum, Ehlers–Danlos‡ syndrome 12. Amyloidosis	13. Vasculitis 14. Ménétrier's§ disease 15. Bleeding diathesis 16. Pseudohaematemesis (nasopharyngeal origin) **Lower gastrointestinal tract** MORE COMMON 1. Angiodysplasia 2. Diverticular disease 3. Colonic carcinoma or polyp 4. Haemorrhoids or anal fissure LESS COMMON 5. Massive upper gastrointestinal bleeding 6. Inflammatory bowel disease 7. Ischaemic colitis 8. Meckel's# diverticulum 9. Small-bowel disease (e.g. tumour, diverticula, intussusception) 10. Haemobilia (bleeding from the gallbladder) 11. Solitary colonic ulcer

*George Kenneth Mallory (1900–86), professor of pathology, Boston, and Soma Weiss (1898–1942), professor of medicine, Boston City Hospital, described this syndrome in 1929.
†Georges Dieulafoy (1839–1911), Paris physician.
‡Edvard Ehlers (1863–1937), German dermatologist, described the syndrome in 1901, and Henri Alexandre Danlos (1844–1912), French dermatologist, described the syndrome in 1908.
§Pierre Ménétrier (1859–1935), French physician.
#Johann Friedrich Meckel the younger (1781–1833), Professor of Surgery and Anatomy at Halle. His father and grandfather were also professors of anatomy.
CRST = calcinosis, Raynaud's phenomenon, sclerodactyly and telangiectasia.

TABLE 13.1

from a major bleeding site higher in the gastrointestinal tract. When there is substantial lower gastrointestinal tract bleeding, it is important to consider the possibility of angiodysplasia or diverticular disease. Even though diverticula are more common in the left colon, bleeding more often occurs from those on the right side of the colon.

Spontaneous bleeding into the skin, or from the nose or mouth, can be a problem for patients with coagulopathy resulting from liver disease.

Jaundice

Usually the relatives notice a yellow discoloration of the sclerae or skin before the patient does. Jaundice is due to the presence of excess bilirubin being deposited in the conjunctivae and skin. The causes of jaundice are described on page 270. If there is jaundice, ask about the colour of the urine and stools; pale stools and dark urine occur with obstructive or cholestatic jaundice because urobilinogen is unable to reach the intestine. Also ask about abdominal pain; gallstones, for example, can cause biliary pain and jaundice.[6] (See Questions box 13.7.)

Pruritus

This symptom means itching of the skin, and may be either generalised or localised. Cholestatic liver disease can cause pruritus that tends to be worse over the extremities. Other causes of pruritus are discussed on pages 237 and 806.

Abdominal bloating and swelling

A feeling of swelling (bloating) may be a result of excess gas or a hypersensitive intestinal tract (as occurs in

> **QUESTIONS TO ASK THE PATIENT WHO PRESENTS WITH VOMITING BLOOD (HAEMATEMESIS)**
>
> ❗ denotes symptoms for the possible diagnosis of an urgent or dangerous problem.
>
> ❗ 1. Was there fresh blood in the vomitus? Or was the vomitus coffee-grain stained?
> ❗ 2. Have you passed any black stools or blood in the stools?
>   3. Before any blood was seen in the vomitus, did you experience intense retching or vomiting? (Mallory–Weiss tear)
>   4. Have you been taking aspirin, non-steroidal anti-inflammatory drugs or steroids?
>   5. Do you drink alcohol? Do you have liver disease?
>   6. Have you ever had a peptic ulcer?
> ❗ 7. Have you lost weight?
>
> QUESTIONS BOX 13.6

> **QUESTIONS TO ASK THE PATIENT PRESENTING WITH JAUNDICE**
>
> ❗ denotes symptoms for the possible diagnosis of an urgent or dangerous problem.
>
>   1. Is your urine dark? Are your stools pale? (Obstructive jaundice)
>   2. Do you have any skin itching (pruritus)?
> ❗ 3. Have you had any fever? (Cholangitis)
> ❗ 4. Have you had a change in your appetite or weight? (Malignancy)
>   5. Have you had any abdominal pain or change in bowel habit?
> ❗ 6. Have you had any vomiting of blood or passage of dark stools?
>   7. Do you drink alcohol? How much? How long? (CAGE questions, p 17)
>   8. Have you ever used intravenous drugs?
>   9. Do you have any tattoos?
> 10. Have you ever had a blood transfusion?
> 11. Have you started any new medications recently?
> 12. Have you had any recent contact with patients with jaundice or liver problems?
> 13. Have you any history of recent high-risk sexual behaviours?
> 14. Have you travelled overseas to areas where hepatitis A is endemic?
> 15. Have you been immunised against hepatitis B?
> 16. Have you any history of inflammatory bowel disease? (Primary sclerosing cholangitis)
> 17. Have you had any surgeries (e.g. pancreatic or biliary)?
> 18. What is your occupation? (Contact with hepatotoxins)
> 19. Is there any family history of liver disease?
>
> QUESTIONS BOX 13.7

the irritable bowel syndrome). Persistent swelling can be due to ascitic fluid accumulation; this is discussed on page 258; it may be associated with ankle oedema.

Lethargy

Tiredness and easy fatigability are common symptoms for patients with acute or chronic liver disease, but the mechanism is not known. They can also occur because of anaemia due to gastrointestinal or chronic inflammatory disease. Lethargy is very common in the general population and is not a specific symptom.

TREATMENT

The treatment history is very important. Traditional non-steroidal anti-inflammatory drugs (NSAIDs), including aspirin, can induce bleeding from acute or chronic damage to the gastrointestinal tract. As described above, many drugs can result in disturbed defecation. A large number of drugs are also known to affect the liver.

- Acute hepatitis can occur with halothane, phenytoin or chlorothiazide.
- Cholestasis may occur from a hypersensitivity reaction to chlorpromazine or other phenothiazines, sulfonamides, sulfonylureas, phenylbutazone, rifampicin or nitrofurantoin.
- Anabolic steroids and the contraceptive pill can cause dose-related cholestasis.
- Fatty liver can occur with alcohol use, tetracycline, valproic acid or amiodarone.
- Large blood-filled cavities in the liver called peliosis hepatis can occur with anabolic steroid use or the contraceptive pill.
- Acute liver cell necrosis can occur if an overdose of paracetamol (acetaminophen) is taken.

PAST HISTORY

Surgical procedures can result in jaundice from the anaesthesia (e.g. multiple uses of halothane), hypoxaemia of liver cells (hypotension during the operative or postoperative period) or direct damage to the bile duct during abdominal surgery. A history of relapsing and remitting epigastric pain in a patient who presents with severe abdominal pain may indicate that a peptic ulcer has perforated. A past history of inflammatory bowel disease (either ulcerative colitis or Crohn's disease) is important as these are chronic diseases that tend to flare up.

SOCIAL HISTORY

The patient's occupation may be relevant (e.g. healthcare workers may be exposed to hepatitis). Toxin exposure can also be important in chronic liver disease (e.g. carbon tetrachloride, vinyl chloride). If a patient has symptoms suggestive of liver disease, ask about recent travel to countries where hepatitis is endemic.

The alcohol history is very important, particularly as alcoholics often deny or understate the amount they consume (see List 1.3, p 18). Contact with anybody who has been jaundiced should always be noted.

The sexual history should be obtained. A history of any injections (e.g. intravenous drugs, plasma transfusions, dental treatment or tattooing) in a patient who presents with symptoms of liver disease is important, particularly as hepatitis B or C may be transferred in this way. Risk factors for viral hepatitis include sexual activity (e.g. between men), intravenous drug use, blood transfusion and tattoos.

FAMILY HISTORY

A family history of colon cancer, especially of familial polyps, or inflammatory bowel disease is important. Ask about coeliac disease in the family. A positive family history of jaundice, anaemia, splenectomy or cholecystectomy may occur in patients with haemolytic anaemia (due to haemoglobin abnormalities or autoimmune disease) or congenital or familial hyperbilirubinaemia.

T&O'C ESSENTIALS

1. Eliciting individual gastrointestinal symptoms and the pattern of presentation will often lead to the correct diagnosis.
2. Ask what the patient means if he or she uses terms like vomiting (could it really be rumination?), constipation or diarrhoea.
3. Intermittent dysphagia and food impaction suggests eosinophilic oesophagitis.
4. Dysphagia, bleeding and weight loss are alarm symptoms: investigation is needed.
5. Heartburn and acid regurgitation typically arise from gastro-oesophageal reflux disease.
6. Could this abdominal pain be biliary pain? Biliary pain ('colic') is due to gallstones or acute cholecystitis; it is acute, severe constant (not colicky) pain that often lasts for hours, usually arises in the epigastrium or right upper quadrant and occurs unpredictably.
7. Chronic or recurrent abdominal pain associated with constipation or diarrhoea, or both, plus bloating, in the absence of alarm symptoms, is usually due to the irritable bowel syndrome. A positive diagnosis can be made from the history.

OSCE REVISION TOPICS – THE GASTROINTESTINAL HISTORY

Use these topics, which commonly occur in the OSCE, to help with revision.

1. This woman has been troubled by abdominal pain for many years. Please take a history from her. (p 217)

2. This man has a recent history of jaundice. Please ask him about that. (pp 226, 229)

3. This man has had diarrhoea for the last 3 months. Please take a history from him. (p 222)

4. This man has noticed black bowel motions. Please ask him about this. (pp 224, 276)

5. This woman has been diagnosed with biliary colic. Please ask her about the symptoms she experienced. (p 218)

References

1. Hendrix TR. Art and science of history taking in the patient with difficulty swallowing. *Dysphagia* 1993; 8:69–73. A very good review of the key historical features that must be obtained when a patient presents with trouble swallowing.
2. Talley NJ. Chronic unexplained diarrhea: what to do when the initial workup is negative? *Rev Gastroenterol Disord* 2008; 8(3):178–185.
3. Talley NJ, Lasch KL, Baum CL. A gap in our understanding: chronic constipation and its comorbid conditions. *Clin Gastroenterol Hepatol* 2009; 7(1):9–19.
4. Ford AC, Talley NJ, Veldhuyzen van Zanten SJ et al. Will the history and physical examination help establish that irritable bowel syndrome is causing this patient's lower gastrointestinal tract symptoms? *JAMA* 2008; 300(15):1793–1805.
5. Mearin F, Lacy BE, Chang L et al. Bowel disorders. *Gastroenterology* 2016 Feb 18. pii: S0016-5085(16)00222-5. doi: 10.1053/j.gastro.2016.02.031. [Epub ahead of print.]
6. Theodossi A, Knill-Jones RP, Skene A. Interobserver variation of symptoms and signs in jaundice. *Liver* 1981; 1:21–32. The history and examination permitted a correct clinical diagnosis in jaundiced patients two-thirds of the time.

CHAPTER 14

The gastrointestinal examination

This lord wears his wit in his belly, and his guts in his head. WILLIAM SHAKESPEARE, Troilus and Cressida

Examination of the gastrointestinal system includes a complete examination of the abdomen. It is also important to search for the peripheral signs of gastrointestinal and liver disease. Some signs are more useful than others.[1]

EXAMINATION ANATOMY

An understanding of the structure and function of the gastrointestinal tract and abdominal organs is critical for the diagnosis of gastrointestinal disease (see Fig. 14.1). The mouth is the gateway to the gastrointestinal tract. It and the anus and rectum are readily accessible to the examiner, and both must be examined carefully in any patient with suspected abdominal disease. The position of the abdominal organs can be quite variable, but there are important surface markings that should be kept in mind during the examination.

The **liver** is the largest organ in the abdomen; it comprises a large right lobe and smaller left lobe divided into eight segments, including the caudate lobe (segment I) squeezed in between. The lower border of the liver

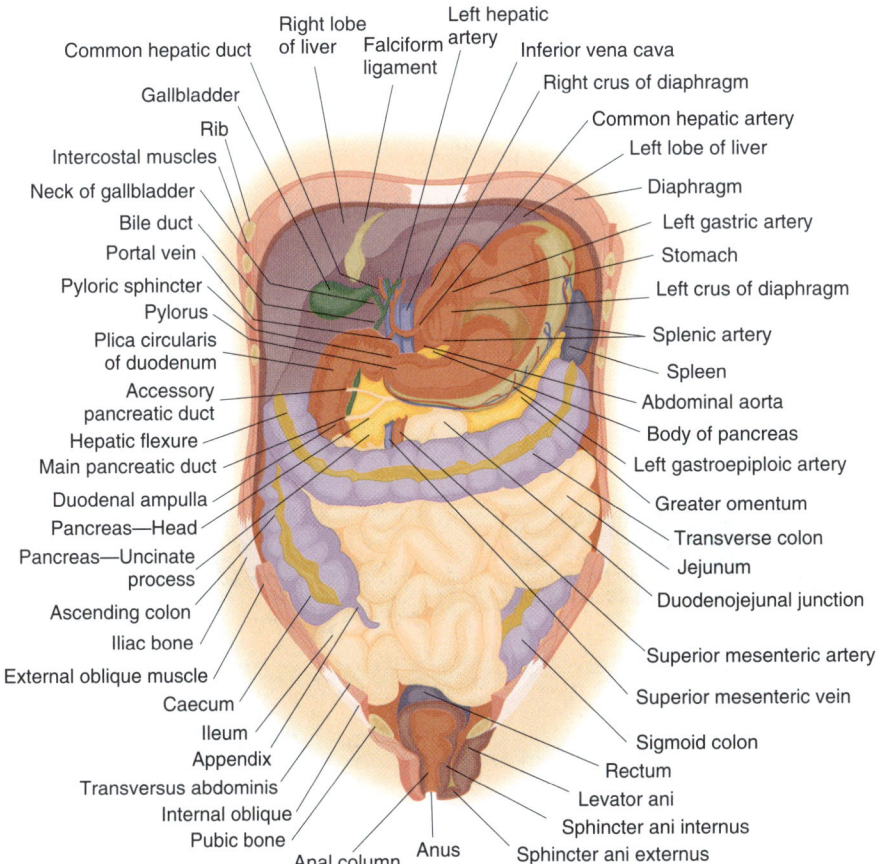

Anatomy of the gut

(Talley NJ, O'Connor S. *Pocket clinical examination*, 3rd edn. Sydney: Churchill Livingstone, 2009.)

FIGURE 14.1

extends from the tip of the right tenth rib to just below the left nipple. Normally the liver is not palpable, but it may just be possible to feel the lower edge in healthy people.

The **spleen** is a lymphoid organ that underlies the ninth, tenth and eleventh ribs posteriorly on the left. It is usually not palpable in health (see Ch 21).

The **kidneys** lie anteriorly four finger-breadths from the midline and posteriorly under the twelfth rib. Normally, the right kidney extends 2.5 centimetres lower than the left. The lower pole of the right kidney may be palpable in thin healthy people.

The **gallbladder** is a pear-shaped organ and the fundus (top) is at the tip of the right ninth costal cartilage; it cannot be felt in health. The **pancreas** is situated in the retroperitoneum (behind the peritoneum), with the head tucked into the C-shaped duodenum and the tail snuggling into the spleen. A huge pancreatic mass may rarely be large enough to be palpable.

The **aorta** lies in the midline and terminates just to the left of the midline at the level of the iliac crest. A pulsatile mass in the middle of the abdomen is likely to be arising from the aorta and may indicate an aneurysm.

The **stomach** is usually J-shaped and lies in the left upper part of the abdomen over the spleen and pancreas; it connects with the duodenum. The **small intestine** ranges from 3 to 10 metres in length and comprises the upper half (duodenum and jejunum) and the lower half (ileum). The small intestine lies over the middle section of the abdomen but is usually impalpable.

The **colon** is approximately 1.5 metres in length, and from right to left consists of the caecum, ascending colon, hepatic flexure, transverse colon, splenic flexure, descending colon, sigmoid colon, rectum and anal canal (anorectum). The **appendix** usually lies in the right lower abdominal area, arising posterior-medially from the caecum. The caecum and ascending colon lie on the right side of the abdomen, the transverse colon runs across the upper abdomen from right to left, and then the descending colon, sigmoid and rectum lie on the left side of the abdomen. Rarely, masses arising from the colon will be felt in the abdomen.

Other important anatomical areas include the **inguinal canal** and the **anorectum**, which are described later in this chapter in relation to examination of hernias and the rectal examination.

POSITIONING THE PATIENT

For proper examination of the abdomen it is important that the patient lies flat with the head resting on a single pillow (see Fig. 14.2). This relaxes the abdominal muscles and facilitates abdominal palpation. Helping the patient into this position affords the opportunity to make a general inspection.

GENERAL APPEARANCE

Jaundice

The yellow discoloration of the sclerae (conjunctivae) and the skin that results from hyperbilirubinaemia is best observed in natural daylight (p 40). Whatever the

Gastrointestinal examination: positioning the patient

FIGURE 14.2

underlying cause, the depth of jaundice can be quite variable.

Weight and wasting

The patient's weight must be recorded. Failure of the gastrointestinal tract to absorb food normally may lead to loss of weight and cachexia. This may also be the result of gastrointestinal malignancy or alcoholic cirrhosis. Folds of loose skin may be visible hanging from the abdomen and limbs; these suggest recent weight loss. Obesity can cause fatty infiltration of the liver (non-alcoholic steatohepatitis) and result in abnormal liver function tests. Anabolic steroid use can induce increase in muscle bulk (sometimes considered desirable) and various liver tumours, including adenomas or hepatocellular carcinomas.

Skin

The gastrointestinal tract and the skin have a common origin from the embryoblast. A number of diseases can present with both skin and gut involvement (see Figs 14.3–14.8 and Table 14.1).[2]

Pigmentation

Generalised skin pigmentation can result from chronic liver disease, especially in haemochromatosis (due to haemosiderin stimulating melanocytes to produce melanin). Malabsorption may result in Addisonian-type pigmentation ('sunkissed' pigmentation) of the nipples, palmar creases, pressure areas and mouth.

Peutz–Jeghers[a] syndrome

Freckle-like spots (discrete, brown-black lesions) around the mouth and on the buccal mucosa (see Fig. 14.5) and on the fingers and toes are associated with hamartomas of the small bowel (50%) and colon (30%), which can present with bleeding or intussusception. In this autosomal dominant condition the incidence of gastrointestinal adenocarcinoma is increased.

Acanthosis nigricans

These are brown-to-black velvety elevations of the epidermis due to confluent papillomas and are usually

Dermatitis herpetiformis in coeliac disease

(From McDonald FS, ed. *Mayo Clinic images in internal medicine*, with permission. © Mayo Clinic Scientific Press and CRC Press. Reproduced by permission of Taylor and Francis Group, LLC, a division of Informa plc.)

FIGURE 14.3

Glucagonoma: migratory rash involving the groin (very rare)

(From McDonald FS, ed. *Mayo Clinic images in internal medicine*, with permission. © Mayo Clinic Scientific Press and CRC Press. Reproduced by permission of Taylor and Francis Group, LLC, a division of Informa plc.)

FIGURE 14.4

---

[a] John Peutz (1886–1957), a physician at St John's Hospital, The Hague, The Netherlands, first described this condition in 1921. Harold Jeghers (1904–90), a professor of medicine at Boston City Hospital, USA, described it in 1949.

Acanthosis nigricans.

(a) Axilla; (b) chest wall

(From McDonald FS, ed. *Mayo Clinic images in internal medicine*, with permission. © Mayo Clinic Scientific Press and CRC Press. Reproduced by permission of Taylor and Francis Group, LLC, a division of Informa plc.)

FIGURE 14.6

Peutz–Jeghers syndrome, with discrete brown-black lesions of the lips

(Figure (a) from Jones DV et al, in Feldman M et al. *Sleisenger & Fordtran's gastrointestinal disease*, 6th edn. Philadelphia: WB Saunders, 1998, with permission. Figure (b) from McDonald FS, ed. *Mayo Clinic images in internal medicine*, with permission. © Mayo Clinic Scientific Press and CRC Press. Reproduced by permission of Taylor and Francis Group, LLC, a division of Informa plc.)

FIGURE 14.5

found in the axillae and nape of the neck (see Fig. 14.6). Acanthosis nigricans is associated rarely with gastrointestinal carcinoma (particularly stomach) and lymphoma, as well as with acromegaly, diabetes mellitus and other endocrinopathies.

Hereditary haemorrhagic telangiectasia (Rendu–Osler–Weber syndrome[b])

Multiple small telangiectasias occur in this disease. They are often present on the lips and tongue (see Fig. 14.7), but may be found anywhere on the skin. When they are present in the gastrointestinal tract they can cause chronic blood loss or even, occasionally, torrential bleeding. Associated arteriovenous malformations may occur. This is an autosomal dominant condition and is uncommon.

---

[b] Henri Rendu (1844–1902), a French physician. Frederick Weber (1863–1962), an English physician. The condition was described in 1907.

CHAPTER 14 THE GASTROINTESTINAL EXAMINATION

Hereditary haemorrhagic telangiectasia involving the lips

(From McDonald FS, ed. *Mayo Clinic images in internal medicine*, with permission. © Mayo Clinic Scientific Press and CRC Press. Reproduced by permission of Taylor and Francis Group, LLC, a division of Informa plc.)

FIGURE 14.7

Porphyria cutanea tarda

FIGURE 14.8

The skin and the gut

Disease	Skin	Gut	Other associations
Gastrointestinal polyposis syndromes			
Peutz–Jeghers syndrome (autosomal dominant)	Pigmented macules on hands, feet, lip	Hamartomatous polyps (rarely adenocarcinoma) in stomach, small bowel, large bowel	
Gardner's* syndrome (autosomal dominant)	Cysts, fibromas, lipomas (multiple)	Polyps, adenocarcinoma in large bowel	Bone osteomata
Cronkhite–Canada syndrome	Alopecia, hyperpigmentation, glossitis, dystrophic nails	Hamartomatous polyps, diarrhoea, exocrine pancreatic insufficiency	
Hormone-secreting tumours			
Carcinoid syndrome	Flushing, telangiectasias	Watery diarrhoea, hepatomegaly	Wheeze, right heart murmurs
Systemic mastocytosis (due to mast cell proliferation and histamine release)	Telangiectasias, flushing, pigmented papules, pruritus, dermographism, Darier's† sign (rub skin lesion with the blunt end of a pen: a palpable red wheal occurs minutes later)	Peptic ulcer, diarrhoea, malabsorption	Asthma, headache, tachycardia
Glucagonoma (glucagon-secreting tumour)	Migratory necrolytic rash (on flexural and friction areas)	Glossitis, weight loss, diabetes mellitus	
Vascular and other disorders			
Hereditary haemorrhagic telangiectasia (autosomal dominant)	Telangiectasias (especially nail beds, palms, feet)	Gastrointestinal bleeding	Nasopharyngeal bleeding, pulmonary arteriovenous fistulas, high output cardiac failure

TABLE 14.1

Continued

The skin and the gut—cont'd

Disease	Skin	Gut	Other associations
Pseudoxanthoma elasticum (autosomal recessive)	Yellow plaques/papules in flexural areas	Bowel bleeding, ischaemia	Angioid streaks in fundus
Blue rubber bleb syndrome	Haemangiomas (e.g. tongue)	Bleeding into bowel or liver	
Degos' disease (malignant atrophic papulosis)	Dome-shaped red papules (early), small porcelain white atrophic scars (late)	Intestinal perforation, infarction (primarily in young men—very rare)	
Acanthosis nigricans	Brown to black skin papillomas (usually axillae)	Carcinoma	Acromegaly, diabetes mellitus
Dermatitis herpetiformis	Pruritic vesicles—typically on knees, elbows, buttocks	Coeliac disease	
Zinc deficiency	Red, scaly, crusting lesions around mouth, eyes, genitalia; white patches on tongue	Diarrhoea (zinc deficiency occurs particularly in setting of Crohn's disease with fistulas, cirrhosis, parenteral nutrition, pancreatitis)	
Porphyria cutanea tarda	Vesicles on exposed skin (e.g. hands)	Alcoholic liver disease	
Inflammatory bowel disease	Pyoderma gangrenosum Erythema nodosum Clubbing Mouth ulcers	Ulcerative colitis or Crohn's disease	
Haemochromatosis (autosomal recessive)	Skin pigmentation (bronze)	Hepatomegaly, signs of chronic liver disease	Diabetes mellitus, heart failure (cardiomyopathy), arthropathy, testicular atrophy
Systemic sclerosis	Skin that is thick and bound down, calcinosis, Raynaud's[‡] phenomenon, sclerodactyly, telangiectases	Gastro-oesophageal reflux, oesophageal dysmotility, small-bowel bacterial overgrowth with malabsorption	

*Eldon John Gardner (1909–89), an American geneticist.
[†]Ferdinand Jean Darier (1856–1938), a Paris dermatologist.
[‡]Maurice Raynaud (1834–81), a Paris physician.

TABLE 14.1

Porphyria cutanea tarda

Fragile vesicles appear on exposed areas of the skin and heal with scarring (see Fig. 14.8). The urine is dark in this chronic disorder of porphyrin metabolism associated with alcoholism and hepatitis C.

Systemic sclerosis

Tense tethering of the skin in systemic sclerosis is often associated with gastro-oesophageal reflux and gastrointestinal motility disorders (p 416).

Mental state

Assess orientation (p 501). The syndrome of hepatic encephalopathy, due to decompensated advanced cirrhosis (chronic liver failure) or fulminant hepatitis (acute liver failure), is an organic neurological disturbance. The features depend on the aetiology and the precipitating factors. Patients eventually become stuporous and then comatose. The combination of hepatocellular damage and portosystemic shunting due to disturbed hepatic structure (both extrahepatic and intrahepatic) causes this syndrome. It is probably related to the liver's failure to remove toxic metabolites from the portal blood. These toxic metabolites may include ammonia, mercaptans, short-chain fatty acids and amines.

HANDS

Even experienced gastroenterologists must restrain their excitement and begin the examination of the gastrointestinal tract with the hands. The signs that may be elicited here give a clue to the presence of chronic liver disease. Whatever its aetiology, permanent diffuse liver damage results in similar peripheral signs. However, none of these signs alone is specific for chronic liver disease.

Nails

Leuconychia

When chronic liver or other disease results in hypoalbuminaemia, the nail beds opacify (the abnormality is of the nail bed and not of the nail), often leaving only a rim of pink nail bed at the top of the nail (Terry's nails;[c] see Fig. 14.9). The thumb and index nails are most often involved. The underlying mechanism may be compression of capillary flow by extracellular fluid.

Muehrcke's lines (transverse white lines) can also occur in hypoalbuminaemic states, including cirrhosis. Blue lunulae may be seen in patients with Wilson's disease (hepatolenticular degeneration).

Clubbing

Up to one-third of patients with cirrhosis may have finger clubbing. In at least some cases, this may be related to arteriovenous (AV) shunting in the lungs, resulting in arterial oxygen desaturation. Cyanosis may be associated with severe long-standing chronic liver disease. The cause of this pulmonary AV shunting is unknown. Conditions such as inflammatory bowel disease and coeliac disease, which cause long-standing nutritional depletion, can also cause clubbing.

Leuconychia—Terry's nails

(From McDonald FS, ed. *Mayo Clinic images in internal medicine*, with permission. © Mayo Clinic Scientific Press and CRC Press. Reproduced by permission of Taylor and Francis Group, LLC, a division of Informa plc.)

FIGURE 14.9

Palmar erythema

(From Goldman L, Schafer AI. *Goldman's Cecil medicine*, 24th edn. Philadelphia: Saunders, 2011.)

FIGURE 14.10

Palms

Palmar erythema ('liver palms')

Palmar erythema is reddening of the palms of the hands affecting the thenar and hypothenar eminences (see Fig. 14.10). Often the soles of the feet are also affected. This can be a feature of chronic liver disease. While the finding has been attributed to raised oestrogen

---

[c] These changes were first described by Dr Richard Terry in 1954 in association with cirrhosis. They are also found in patients with cardiac failure and become more common in normal people with age. In a patient under the age of 50, their presence indicates cirrhosis, heart failure or diabetes, with a likelihood ratio of 5.3.

levels, it has not been shown to be related to plasma oestradiol levels, so the aetiology remains uncertain. Palmar erythema can also occur with thyrotoxicosis, rheumatoid arthritis, polycythaemia and, rarely, with chronic febrile diseases or chronic leukaemia. It may also be a normal finding, especially in women, and like spider naevi can occur in pregnancy.

Anaemia

Inspect the palmar creases for pallor suggesting anaemia, which may result from gastrointestinal blood loss, malabsorption (folate, vitamin B_{12}), haemolysis (e.g. hypersplenism) or chronic disease.

Dupuytren's contracture

Dupuytren's contracture[d] is a visible and palpable thickening and contraction of the palmar fascia causing permanent flexion, most often of the ring finger (see Fig. 14.11). It is often bilateral and occasionally affects the feet. It is associated with alcoholism (not liver disease), but is also found in some manual workers; it is often familial. The palmar fascia of these patients contains abnormally large amounts of xanthine, and this may be related to the pathogenesis.

Hepatic flap (asterixis[e])

Before leaving the hands ask the patient to stretch out his or her arms in front, separate the fingers and extend the wrists for 15 seconds. Push on the patient's fingers to keep them extended (see Fig. 14.12). Jerky, irregular flexion–extension movements at the wrist and metacarpophalangeal joints, often accompanied by lateral movements of the fingers, constitute the flapping of hepatic encephalopathy (asterixis).

Asterixis is thought to be due to interference with the inflow of joint position sense information to the reticular formation in the brainstem. This results in rhythmical lapses of postural muscle tone. Occasionally the arms, neck, tongue, jaws and eyelids can also be involved. It can sometimes be demonstrated if the patient is asked to close the eyes forcefully or to protrude the tongue.

(a) Dupuytren's contracture of the palm.
(b) Dupuytren's contracture of the sole of the foot

(Waldman SD. *Pain management*, 2nd edn. Philadelphia: Saunders, 2011.)

FIGURE 14.11

The flap is bilateral, tends to be absent at rest and is brought on by sustained posture. The rhythmic movements are not synchronous on each side and the flap is absent when coma supervenes.

Although this flap is a characteristic and early sign of liver failure, it is not diagnostic: it can also occur in cardiac, respiratory and renal failure, as well as in hypoglycaemia, hypokalaemia, hypomagnesaemia or barbiturate intoxication.

---

[d] Baron Guillaume Dupuytren (1777–1835), Surgeon-in-Chief at the Hotel-Dieu in Paris. A cold, rude, ambitious and arrogant man, he was called 'the Napoleon of surgery'. He saw 10,000 private patients a year.
[e] From Greek *a*, 'not' and *sterixis*, 'fixed position'.

Testing for asterixis

FIGURE 14.12

Petechiae

(From Marks JG, Miller JJ. *Lookingbill & Marks' principles of dermatology*, 4th edn. Philadelphia: Saunders, 2006.)

FIGURE 14.13

An apparent tremor (really a form of choreoathetosis) may occur in Wilson's disease. A fine resting tremor is common in alcoholism.

ARMS

Inspect the upper limbs for *bruising*. Large bruises (ecchymoses) may be due to clotting abnormalities. Hepatocellular damage can interfere with protein synthesis and therefore the production of all the clotting factors (except factor VIII, which is made elsewhere in the reticuloendothelial system). Obstructive jaundice results in a shortage of bile acids in the intestine and therefore may reduce absorption of vitamin K (a fat-soluble vitamin), which is essential for the production of clotting factors II (prothrombin), VII, IX and X.

Petechiae (pinhead-sized bruises) may also be present (see Fig. 14.13). Chronic excessive alcohol consumption can sometimes result in bone marrow depression, causing thrombocytopenia, which may be responsible for petechiae. In addition, splenomegaly secondary to portal hypertension can cause hypersplenism, with resultant excessive destruction of platelets in the spleen; in severe liver disease (especially acute hepatic necrosis), diffuse intravascular coagulation can occur.

Look for muscle wasting, which is often a late manifestation of malnutrition in alcoholic patients (see Text box 14.1). Alcohol can also cause a proximal myopathy (p 590).

Scratch marks due to severe itch (pruritus) are often prominent in patients with obstructive or cholestatic jaundice. This is commonly the presenting feature of primary biliary cirrhosis[f] before other signs are apparent. The mechanism of pruritus is thought to be retention of an unknown substance normally excreted in the bile, rather than bile salt deposition in the skin as was earlier thought.

Spider naevi[g] (see Fig. 14.14) consist of a central arteriole from which radiate numerous small vessels that look like spiders' legs. They range in size from just visible to half a centimetre in diameter. Their usual distribution is in the area drained by the superior vena cava, so they are found on the arms, neck and chest

---

[f] Primary biliary cirrhosis (PBC) is an uncommon chronic non-suppurative destructive cholangitis of unknown aetiology; 90% of affected patients are female.
[g] Spider naevi were first described in 1867 by Sir Erasmus Wilson (1809–84), an English surgeon and dermatologist.

> **Physical examinations for malnutrition in chronic liver disease**
>
> 1. **Subcutaneous fat:** look for looseness of the skin over the subcutaneous tissues and loss of fullness. The changes may be most obvious over the triceps muscles, on the chest at the costal margin in the midaxillary line and in the hands.
> 2. **Muscle wasting:** look at the deltoids and the quadriceps femoris muscles. Loss of deltoid mass gives the shoulders a squared-off appearance. Remember that muscle wasting also occurs in neurological disease.
> 3. **Movement of fluid from the intravascular to the extravascular space** (associated with inability of the liver to manufacture normal serum proteins): look for ascites and peripheral oedema.
> 4. **Micronutrient deficiencies e.g. bruising** (vitamin K, C), glossitis (folate, vitamin B_{12}, niacin), dermatitis (vitamin A).
>
> TEXT BOX 14.1

A large crop of spider naevi

FIGURE 14.14

wall. They can occasionally bleed profusely. Pressure applied with a pointed object to the central arteriole causes blanching of the whole lesion. Rapid refilling from the centre to the legs occurs on release of the pressure. The finding of more than two spider naevi anywhere on the body is likely to be abnormal. They can be caused by cirrhosis, most frequently due to alcohol. In patients with cirrhosis their number may increase or decrease as the patient's condition changes, as does the prominence of palmar erythema. Spider naevi may occur transiently in viral hepatitis. During the second to fifth months of pregnancy, they frequently appear, only to disappear again within days of delivery. It is not known why they occur only in the upper part of the body, but it may be related to the fact that this is the part of the body where flushing usually occurs. Like palmar erythema they are traditionally attributed to oestrogen excess. Part of the normal hepatic function is the inactivation of oestrogens, which is impaired in chronic liver disease. Oestrogens are known to have a dilating effect on the spiral arterioles of the endometrium, and this has been used to explain the presence of spider naevi, but changes in plasma oestradiol levels have not been found to correlate with the appearance and disappearance of spider naevi.

The differential diagnosis of spider naevi includes *Campbell de Morgan*[h] *spots*, venous stars and hereditary haemorrhagic telangiectasia. Campbell de Morgan spots are elevated red circular lesions that occur on the abdomen or the front of the chest. They do not blanch on pressure and are very common and benign. *Venous stars* are 2- to 3-centimetre lesions that can occur on the dorsum of the feet, legs, back and lower chest. They are due to elevated venous pressure and are found overlying the main tributary to a large vein. They are not obliterated by pressure. The blood flow is from the periphery to the centre of the lesion, which is the opposite of the flow in the spider naevus. Lesions of *hereditary haemorrhagic telangiectasia* (p 232) occasionally resemble spider naevi.

Palpate the axillae for lymphadenopathy (p 340). Look in the axillae for acanthosis nigricans.

FACE

Eyes

Look first at the sclerae for signs of *jaundice* (see Fig. 14.15) or *anaemia* (pale conjunctiva). *Bitot's*[i] *spots* are yellow keratinised areas on the sclera (see Fig. 14.16). They are the result of severe vitamin A deficiency due to malabsorption or malnutrition. Retinal damage and blindness may occur as a later

---

[h] Campbell de Morgan (1811–76), a London surgeon, was one of the 300 original Fellows of the Royal College of Surgeons. He described his spots in 1872 and believed them to be a sign of cancer (which they are not).
[i] Pierre Bitot (1822–88) described this in 1863.

CHAPTER 14 THE GASTROINTESTINAL EXAMINATION 239

Scleral icterus

FIGURE 14.15

Kayser–Fleischer rings in Wilson's disease

(From McDonald FS, ed. *Mayo Clinic images in internal medicine*, with permission. © Mayo Clinic Scientific Press and CRC Press. Reproduced by permission of Taylor and Francis Group, LLC, a division of Informa plc.)

FIGURE 14.17

Bitot spot: focal area of conjunctival xerosis with a foamy appearance

(From Mir MA. *Atlas of clinical diagnosis*, 2nd edn. Edinburgh: Saunders, 2003.)

FIGURE 14.16

development. *Kayser–Fleischer rings*[j] (see Fig. 14.17) are brownish-green rings occurring at the periphery of the cornea, affecting the upper pole more than the lower. They are due to deposits of excess copper in Descemet's membrane[k] of the cornea. Slit-lamp examination is often necessary to show them. They are typically found in Wilson's disease,[l] a copper storage disease that causes cirrhosis and neurological disturbances. Kayser–Fleischer rings are usually present by the time neurological signs have appeared. Patients with other cholestatic liver diseases, however, can also have these rings. *Iritis* may be seen in inflammatory bowel disease (p 279).

Xanthelasmata are yellowish plaques in the subcutaneous tissues in the periorbital region and are due to deposits of lipids (see Fig. 5.21, p 89). They may indicate protracted elevation of the serum cholesterol. In patients with cholestasis, an abnormal lipoprotein (lipoprotein X) is found in the plasma and is associated with elevation of the serum cholesterol. Xanthelasmata are common in patients with primary biliary cirrhosis.

Periorbital purpura following proctosigmoidoscopy ('black eye syndrome') is a characteristic sign of amyloidosis (perhaps related to factor X deficiency) but is exceedingly rare (see Fig. 14.18).

Salivary glands

Next inspect and palpate the cheeks over the parotid area for *parotid enlargement* (see List 14.1, Fig. 14.19). Ask the patient to clench his or her teeth so that the

---

[j] Bernhard Kayser (1869–1954), a German ophthalmologist, described these rings in 1902. Bruno Fleischer (1848–1904), a German ophthalmologist, described them in 1903.
[k] Jean Desçemet (1732–1810), a professor of surgery and anatomy in Paris. He described the membrane in 1785.

[l] Samuel Alexander Wilson (1878–1937), a London neurologist at Queen Square. His colleagues there included Gowers and Hughlings Jackson. He described his disease in 1912 in his MD thesis. He also described the glabellar tap sign in Parkinson's disease, which is sometimes called Wilson's sign. He did not, however, describe the Kayser–Fleischer rings.

Amyloidosis causing periorbital purpura.

Note the periorbital purpura that followed a proctoscopic examination, a characteristic (albeit rare) sign

(From McDonald FS, ed. *Mayo Clinic images in internal medicine*, with permission. © Mayo Clinic Scientific Press and CRC Press. Reproduced by permission of Taylor and Francis Group, LLC, a division of Informa plc.)

FIGURE 14.18

Palpating for parotid enlargement

FIGURE 14.19

CAUSES OF PAROTID ENLARGEMENT

Bilateral
1. Mumps (can be unilateral)
2. Sarcoidosis or lymphoma, which may cause painless bilateral enlargement
3. Mikulicz* syndrome: bilateral painless enlargement of all three salivary glands; this disease is probably an early stage of Sjögren's syndrome
4. Alcohol-associated parotiditis
5. Malnutrition
6. Severe dehydration: as occurs in renal failure, terminal carcinomatosis and severe infections

Unilateral
7. Mixed parotid tumour (occasionally bilateral)
8. Tumour infiltration, which usually causes painless unilateral enlargement and may cause facial nerve palsy
9. Duct blockage (e.g. salivary calculus)

*Johann von Mikulicz-Radecki (1850–1905), a professor of surgery in Breslau, described this condition in 1892.

LIST 14.1

---

masseter muscle is palpable; the normal parotid gland is impalpable but the enlarged gland is best felt behind the masseter muscle and in front of the ear.

Bimanual palpation will enable the parotid duct to be felt. Feel in the mouth for a parotid calculus, which may be present at the parotid duct orifice (opposite the upper second molar). Parotidomegaly that is bilateral is associated with alcoholism rather than liver disease per se. It is due to fatty infiltration, perhaps secondary to alcohol toxicity with or without malnutrition. A tender, warm, swollen parotid suggests the diagnosis of parotiditis following an acute illness or surgery. A mixed parotid tumour (a pleomorphic adenoma) is the most common cause of a lump. Parotid carcinoma may cause facial nerve palsy (p 525). Mumps also causes acute parotid enlargement, which is usually bilateral.

Submandibular gland enlargement is most often due to a calculus. This may be palpable bimanually (see Fig. 14.20). Place your gloved index finger on the floor of the patient's mouth beside the tongue, feeling between it and your fingers placed behind the body of the mandible. It may also be enlarged in chronic liver disease.

Mouth
Teeth and breath

The very beginning of the gastrointestinal tract is, like the very end of the tract, accessible to inspection without elaborate equipment.[3] Look first briefly at the state of the teeth and note whether they are real or false. False

Examination of the submandibular gland

FIGURE 14.20

teeth will have to be removed for a complete examination of the mouth. Note whether there is gum hypertrophy (see List 14.2) or pigmentation (see List 14.3). Loose-fitting false teeth may be responsible for ulcers and decayed teeth may be responsible for fetor[m] (bad breath).

Other causes of fetor are listed in List 14.4. These must be distinguished from *fetor hepaticus*, which is a rather sweet smell of the breath. It is an indication of severe hepatocellular disease and may be due to methylmercaptans. These substances are known to be exhaled in the breath and may be derived from methionine when this amino acid is not demethylated by a diseased liver. Severe fetor hepaticus that fills the patient's room is a bad sign and indicates a precomatose condition in many cases. The presence of fetor hepaticus in a patient with a coma of unknown cause may be a helpful clue to the diagnosis.

Unless the smell is obvious, ask the patient to exhale through the mouth while you sniff a little of the exhaled air.

Tongue

Thickened epithelium with bacterial debris and food particles commonly causes a *coating* over the tongue, especially in smokers. It is rarely a sign of disease and is more marked on the posterior part of the tongue where there is less mobility and the papillae desquamate

---

[m] The Latin word means a stench.

CAUSES OF GUM HYPERTROPHY

1. Phenytoin
2. Pregnancy
3. Scurvy (vitamin C deficiency: the gums become spongy, red, bleed easily and are swollen and irregular)
4. Gingivitis, e.g. from smoking, calculus, plaque, Vincent's* angina (fusobacterial membranous tonsillitis)
5. Leukaemia (usually monocytic)

*Jean Hyacinthe Vincent (1862–1950), a professor of forensic medicine and French Army bacteriologist, described this in 1898.

LIST 14.2

CAUSES OF PIGMENTED LESIONS IN THE MOUTH

1. Heavy metals: lead or bismuth (blue-black line on the gingival margin), iron (haemochromatosis—blue-grey pigmentation of the hard palate)
2. Drugs: antimalarials, the oral contraceptive pill (brown or black areas of pigmentation anywhere in the mouth)
3. Addison's disease (blotches of dark brown pigment anywhere in the mouth)
4. Peutz–Jeghers syndrome (lips, buccal mucosa or palate)
5. Malignant melanoma (raised, painless black lesions anywhere in the mouth)

LIST 14.3

CAUSES OF FETOR (BAD BREATH)

1. Faulty oral hygiene
2. Fetor hepaticus (a sweet smell)
3. Ketosis (diabetic ketoacidosis results in excretion of ketones in exhaled air, causing a sickly sweet smell)
4. Uraemia (fish breath: an ammoniacal odour)
5. Alcohol (distinctive)
6. Paraldehyde
7. Putrid (due to anaerobic chest infections with large amounts of sputum)
8. Cigarettes

LIST 14.4

Leucoplakia

(From Weidner N et al. *Modern surgical pathology*, 2nd edn. Philadelphia: Saunders, 2009.)

FIGURE 14.21

Glossitis

(From Kanski JJ. *Clinical diagnosis in ophthalmology*, 1st edn. Maryland Heights, MO: Mosby, 2006.)

FIGURE 14.22

more slowly. It occurs frequently in respiratory tract infections, but is in no way related to constipation or any serious abdominal disorder.

Lingua nigra (black tongue) is due to elongation of papillae over the posterior part of the tongue, which appears dark brown because of the accumulation of keratin. Apart from its aesthetic problems it is symptomless. Bismuth compounds may also cause a black discoloration of the tongue.

Geographical tongue is a term used to describe slowly changing red rings and lines that occur on the surface of the tongue. It is not painful, and the condition tends to come and go. It is not usually of any significance, but can be a sign of riboflavin (vitamin B_2) deficiency.

Leucoplakia (see Fig. 14.21) is white-coloured thickening of the mucosa of the tongue and mouth; the condition is premalignant. Most of the causes of leucoplakia begin with 'S': sore teeth (poor dental hygiene), smoking, spirits, sepsis or syphilis, but often no cause is apparent. Leucoplakia may also occur on the larynx, anus and vulva.

The term *glossitis* (see Fig. 14.22) is generally used to describe a smooth appearance of the tongue, which may also be erythematous. The appearance is due to atrophy of the papillae, and in later stages there may be shallow ulceration. These changes occur in the tongue often as a result of nutritional deficiencies to which the tongue is sensitive because of the rapid turnover of mucosal cells. Deficiencies of iron, folate and the vitamin B group, especially vitamin B_{12}, are common causes. Glossitis is common in alcoholics and can also occur in the rare carcinoid syndrome. However, many cases, especially those in elderly people, are impossible to explain.

Enlargement of the tongue (*macroglossia*) may occur in congenital conditions such as Down syndrome or in endocrine disease, including acromegaly. Tumour infiltration (e.g. haemangioma or lymphangioma) or infiltration of the tongue with amyloid material in amyloidosis can also be responsible for macroglossia.

Mouth ulcers

This is an important topic because a number of systemic diseases can present with ulcers in the mouth (see List 14.5). *Aphthous ulceration* is the most common type seen (see Fig. 14.23). This begins as a small painful vesicle on the tongue or mucosal surface of the mouth, which may break down to form a painful, shallow ulcer. These ulcers heal without scarring. The cause is completely unknown. They usually do not indicate any serious underlying systemic disease, but may occur in Crohn's[n] disease or coeliac disease. HIV infection may be associated with a number of mouth lesions (p 836). *Angular stomatitis* (see Fig. 14.24) refers to cracks at

---

[n] Burrill Bernard Crohn (1884–1983), an American gastroenterologist at Mount Sinai Hospital, New York, described this disease in 1932. It had previously been described by Giovanni Battista Morgagni (1682–1771) in 1769.

CHAPTER 14 THE GASTROINTESTINAL EXAMINATION 243

Aphthous ulceration

(From McDonald FS, ed. *Mayo Clinic images in internal medicine*, with permission. © Mayo Clinic Scientific Press and CRC Press. Reproduced by permission of Taylor and Francis Group, LLC, a division of Informa plc.)

FIGURE 14.23

Angular stomatitis

(From Sproat C, Burke G, McGurk M. *Essential human disease for dentists*. London: Churchill Livingstone, 2006.)

FIGURE 14.24

> ### CAUSES OF MOUTH ULCERS
>
> **Common**
> Aphthous
> Trauma
> Drugs (e.g. steroids)
>
> **Uncommon**
> Gastrointestinal disease: Crohn's disease, ulcerative colitis, coeliac disease
> Rheumatological disease: Behçet's* syndrome, Reiter's† syndrome
> Erythema multiforme
> Infection: viral—herpes zoster, herpes simplex; bacterial—syphilis (primary chancre, secondary snail track ulcers, mucous patches), tuberculosis
> Self-inflicted
>
> *Halusi Behçet (1889–1948), a Turkish dermatologist, described the disease in 1937.
> †Hans Reiter (1881–1969), a Berlin bacteriologist, described this in 1916.
>
> LIST 14.5

the corners of the mouth; causes include deficiencies in vitamin B_6, vitamin B_{12}, folate and iron.

Candidiasis (moniliasis)

Fungal infection with *Candida albicans* (thrush) causes creamy white curd-like patches in the mouth that are removed only with difficulty and leave a bleeding surface (see Fig. 43.33 on page 820). The infection may spread to involve the oesophagus, causing dysphagia or odynophagia. Moniliasis is associated with immunosuppression (steroids, tumour chemotherapy, alcoholism or an underlying immunological abnormality such as HIV infection, or haematological malignancy), where it is due to decreased host resistance. Broad-spectrum antibiotics, which inhibit the normal oral flora, are also a common cause because fungal overgrowth is permitted. Faulty oral hygiene, iron deficiency and diabetes mellitus can also be responsible. Chronic mucocutaneous candidiasis is a distinct syndrome comprising recurrent or persistent oral thrush, fingernail or toenail bed infection and skin involvement. It is usually the result of T-cell immunodeficiency. In about half of these patients, endocrine diseases such as hypoparathyroidism, hypothyroidism or Addison's disease are associated.

NECK AND CHEST

Palpate the cervical lymph nodes (p 341, Ch 21). These may be enlarged as a result of infection in the mouth or pharynx or of oropharyngeal malignancy. They can be felt from in front of the patient (see Fig. 14.25) or from behind (see Fig.14.26). Feel for the supraclavicular nodes, especially on the left side. They are best examined

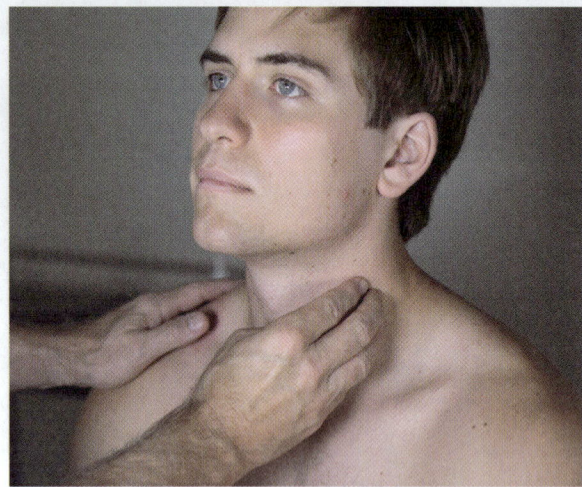

Palpating the cervical nodes from in front

FIGURE 14.25

Gynaecomastia with prominent breasts and unassociated with confounding obesity

(From Mir MA. *Atlas of clinical diagnosis*, 2nd edn. Edinburgh: Saunders, 2003.)

FIGURE 14.27

Palpating the supraclavicular nodes from behind—'Shrug your shoulders for me'

FIGURE 14.26

from in front after the patient has been asked to shrug his or her shoulders.

The most common cause of palpable nodes in developing countries is tuberculosis. These may also be enlarged as a result of advanced gastric or other gastrointestinal malignancy, or with lung cancer. The presence of a large left supraclavicular node (Virchow's node) in combination with carcinoma of the stomach is called Troisier's[o] sign.

Look for spider naevi.

In males, *gynaecomastia* (enlargement of the male breasts) may be a sign of chronic liver disease. Gynaecomastia may be unilateral or bilateral and the breasts may be tender (see Fig. 14.27). This may be a sign of cirrhosis, particularly alcoholic cirrhosis, or of chronic autoimmune hepatitis. In chronic liver disease, changes in the oestradiol-to-testosterone ratio may be responsible. In cirrhotic patients, spironolactone, used to treat ascites, is also a common cause. In addition, gynaecomastia may occur in alcoholics without liver disease because of damage to the Leydig[p] cells of the testis from alcohol. A number of other drugs may rarely cause gynaecomastia (e.g. digoxin, cimetidine).

ABDOMEN

Self-restraint is no longer required and it is now time to examine the abdomen itself.

Inspection

The patient should lie flat, with one pillow under the head and the abdomen exposed from the nipples to the pubic symphysis (see Fig. 14.2). It may be preferable to expose this area in stages to preserve the patient's dignity.

---

[o] Charles Émile Troisier (1844–1919), a professor of pathology in Paris, described this sign in 1886.

[p] Franz von Leydig (1821–1908), a Bonn anatomist and zoologist, Germany.

Does the patient appear unwell? The patient with an *acute abdomen* may be lying very still and have shallow breathing (p 272).

Inspection begins with a careful look for abdominal *scars*, which may indicate previous surgery or trauma (see Fig. 14.28). Look in the area around the umbilicus for laparoscopic surgical scars. Older scars are white and recent scars are pink because the tissue remains vascular. Note the presence of stomata (end-colostomy, loop colostomy, ileostomy or ileal conduit) or fistulae. There may be visible abdominal striae following weight loss.

Generalised abdominal *distension* (see Fig. 14.29) may be present. All the causes of this begin with the

Abdominal scars.

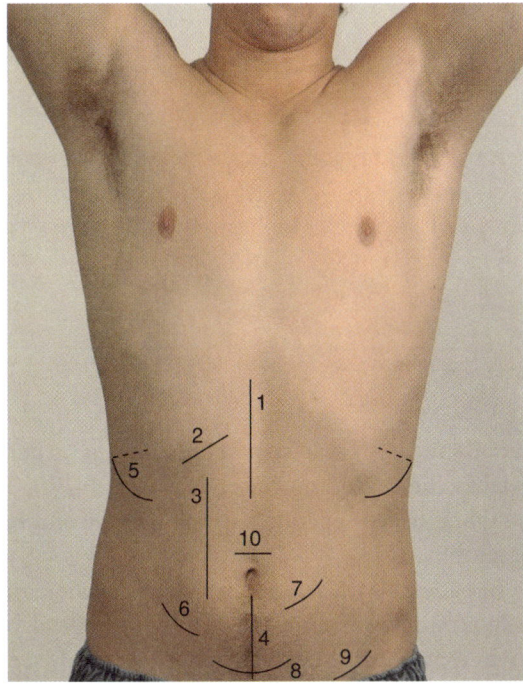

Note: Laparoscopic surgical scars are now common. Most of these procedures include a port about 2 cm in length, just above the umbilicus.

1. Upper midline
2. Right subcostal (Kocher's)
3. Right paramedian
4. Lower midline
5. Nephrectomy
6. Appendicectomy (Gridiron)
7. Transplanted kidney
8. Suprapubic (Pfannensteil)
9. Left inguinal
10. Umbilical port—laparoscopic surgery

FIGURE 14.28

(a) Abdomen distended with ascites (patient supine): umbilicus points downwards, unlike cases of distension due to a pelvic mass. (b) Gross ascites (patient sitting)

(Courtesy of Dr A Watson, Infectious Diseases Department, The Canberra Hospital.)

FIGURE 14.29

Detecting the direction of flow of a vein.

(a) Two fingers are placed firmly on the vein. (b) The second finger is moved along the vein to empty it of blood and keep it occluded. (c) The second finger is removed but the vein does not refill. (d) At repeat testing and removing the first finger, filling occurs, indicating the direction of flow

(Adapted from Swash M, ed. *Hutchison's clinical methods*, 20th edn. Philadelphia: Baillière Tindall, 1995.)

FIGURE 14.30

---

sound 'F': fat (gross obesity), fluid (ascites), fetus, flatus (gaseous distension due to bowel obstruction), faeces, 'filthy' big tumour (e.g. ovarian tumour or hydatid cyst) or 'phantom' pregnancy. Look at the shape of the umbilicus, which may give a clue to the underlying cause. An umbilicus buried in fat suggests that the patient eats too much. However, when the peritoneal cavity is filled with large volumes of fluid (ascites) from whatever cause, the abdominal flanks and wall appear tense and the umbilicus is shallow or everted and points downwards. In pregnancy the umbilicus is pushed upwards by the uterus enlarging from the pelvis. This appearance may also result from a huge ovarian cyst.

Local *swellings* may indicate enlargement of one of the abdominal or pelvic organs. A hernia is a protrusion of an intra-abdominal structure through an abnormal opening; this may occur because of weakening of the abdominal wall by previous surgery (incisional hernia), a congenital abdominal wall defect or chronically increased intra-abdominal pressure.

Prominent *veins* may be obvious on the abdominal wall. If these are present, the direction of venous flow should be elicited at this stage. Use one finger to occlude the vein and then empty blood from the vein below the occluding finger with a second finger. Remove the second finger; if the vein refills, flow is occurring towards the occluding finger (see Fig. 14.30). Flow should be tested separately in veins above and below the umbilicus.

In patients with severe portal hypertension, portal to systemic flow occurs through the umbilical veins, which may become engorged and distended (see Fig. 14.31). The direction of flow then is away from the umbilicus. Because of their engorged appearance they have been likened to the mythical Medusa's hair after Minerva had turned it into snakes; this sign is called a *caput Medusae* (head of Medusa[q]) but is very rare (see Fig. 14.32). Usually only one or two veins (often epigastric) are visible. Engorgement can also occur because of inferior vena caval obstruction, usually due to a tumour or thrombosis but sometimes because of tense ascites. In this case the abdominal veins enlarge to provide collateral blood flow from the legs, avoiding the blocked inferior vena cava. The direction of flow is then upwards towards the heart. Therefore, to distinguish caput Medusae from inferior vena caval obstruction, determine the direction of flow *below* the

---

[q] In Greek mythology Medusa was the only mortal among the three Gorgons. She had live snakes for hair and people who met her gaze were turned to stone (unless they looked at her in a mirror or polished shield).

CHAPTER 14 THE GASTROINTESTINAL EXAMINATION   247

Distended abdominal veins in a patient with portal hypertension

(From Mir MA. *Atlas of clinical diagnosis*, 2nd edn. Edinburgh: Saunders, 2003.)

FIGURE 14.31

Prominent veins on the abdominal wall.

1=thin veins over the costal margin—not of clinical relevance; 2=caput Medusae; 3=inferior vena caval obstruction

(Based on Swash M, ed. *Hutchison's clinical methods*, 20th edn. Philadelphia: Baillière Tindall, 1995.)

FIGURE 14.32

umbilicus; it will be towards the legs in the former and towards the head in the latter. Prominent superficial veins can occasionally be congenital.

Pulsations may be visible. An expanding central pulsation in the epigastrium suggests an abdominal aortic aneurysm. However, the abdominal aorta can often be seen to pulsate in normal thin people.

Visible peristalsis may occur occasionally in very thin normal people; however, it usually suggests intestinal obstruction. Pyloric obstruction due to peptic ulceration or tumour may cause visible peristalsis, seen as a slow wave of movement passing across the upper abdomen from left to right. Obstruction of the distal small bowel can cause similar movements in a ladder pattern in the centre of the abdomen.

Skin lesions should also be noted on the abdominal wall. These include the vesicles of herpes zoster, which occur in a radicular pattern (they are localised to only one side of the abdomen in the distribution of a single nerve root). Herpes zoster may be responsible for severe abdominal pain that is of mysterious origin until the rash appears. The Sister Joseph[r] nodule is a metastatic tumour deposit in the umbilicus, the anatomical region where the peritoneum is closest to the skin. Discoloration of the umbilicus where a faintly bluish hue is present is found rarely, in cases of extensive haemoperitoneum and acute pancreatitis (Cullen's sign[s]—the umbilical 'black eye'; see Fig. 14.33). Skin discoloration may also rarely occur in the flanks in severe cases of acute pancreatitis (Grey-Turner's sign[t]).

Stretching of the abdominal wall severe enough to cause rupture of the elastic fibres in the skin produces

---

[r] Sister Joseph of St Mary's Hospital, Rochester, Minnesota, described this sign to Dr William Mayo (1861–1939) of the Mayo Clinic.

[s] Thomas S Cullen (1869–1953), a professor of gynaecology at Johns Hopkins University, Baltimore, originally described this sign as an indication of a ruptured ectopic pregnancy.

[t] George Grey-Turner (1877–1951), a surgeon at Royal Victoria Infirmary, Newcastle-on-Tyne, England.

(a) Grey–Turner's sign and (b) Cullen's sign (umbilicus) in severe acute pancreatitis

(From Jarnagin, W et al. *Blumgart's surgery of the liver, pancreas and biliary tract*, 5th edn. Philadelphia: Saunders, 2012.)

FIGURE 14.33

pink linear marks with a wrinkled appearance, which are called *striae*. When these are wide and purple coloured, Cushing's syndrome may be the cause (p 460). Ascites, pregnancy or recent weight gain are much more common causes of striae.

Next, squat down beside the bed so that the patient's abdomen is at eye level (Fig. 14.34). Ask him or her to take slow deep breaths through the mouth and watch for evidence of asymmetrical movement, indicating the presence of a mass. In particular a large liver may be seen to move below the right costal margin or a large spleen below the left costal margin.

Palpation

This part of the examination often reveals the most information. Successful palpation is possible only if the patient's abdominal muscles are relaxed. To this end, reassure the patient that the examination will not be painful and use hands that are *gentle* and *warm*. Ask the patient whether any particular area is tender and examine this area last. Encourage the patient to breathe gently through the mouth. If necessary, ask him or her to bend the knees to relax the abdominal wall muscles.

Watch from eye level for abdominal masses that move with respiration

FIGURE 14.34

For descriptive purposes the abdomen has been divided into nine areas or regions (see Fig. 14.35). Palpation in each region is performed with the

CHAPTER 14 THE GASTROINTESTINAL EXAMINATION 249

 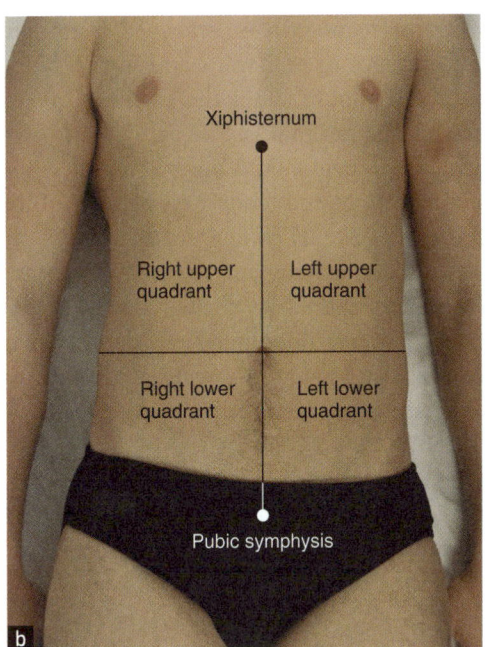

- Mid-clavicular lines
1. Right hypochondrium
2. Epigastrium
3. Left hypochondrium
4. Right lumbar region
5. Umbilical region
6. Left lumbar region
7. Right iliac fossa
8. Hypogastrium
9. Left iliac fossa

Xiphisternum
Right upper quadrant
Left upper quadrant
Right lower quadrant
Left lower quadrant
Pubic symphysis

(a) Regions of the abdomen. (b) Quadrants of the abdomen

FIGURE 14.35

palmar surface of the fingers acting together. For palpation of the edges of organs or masses, the lateral surface of the forefinger is the most sensitive part of the hand.

Palpation should begin with *light pressure* in each region. All the movements of the hand should occur at the metacarpophalangeal joints and the hand should be moulded to the shape of the abdominal wall. Note the presence of any tenderness or lumps in each region. As you move your hand over each region, consider the anatomical structures that underlie it. *Deep palpation* of the abdomen is performed next, though care should be taken to avoid the tender areas until the end of the examination. Deep palpation is used to detect deeper masses and to define those already discovered. Any mass must be carefully characterised and described (see List 14.6).

Guarding of the abdomen (when resistance to palpation occurs due to contraction of the abdominal muscles) may result from tenderness or anxiety, and is voluntary. It may be overcome by reassurance and gentleness. *Rigidity* is a constant involuntary reflex contraction of the abdominal muscles always associated

> **DESCRIPTIVE FEATURES OF INTRA-ABDOMINAL MASSES**
>
> For any abdominal mass all the following should be determined:
> - Site: the region involved
> - Tenderness
> - Size (which must be measured) and shape
> - Surface, which may be regular or irregular
> - Edge, which may be regular or irregular
> - Consistency, which may be hard or soft
> - Mobility and movement with inspiration
> - Whether it is pulsatile or not
> - Whether one can get above the mass
>
> LIST 14.6

with tenderness and indicates peritoneal irritation or inflammation (peritonitis).

Rebound tenderness is said to be present when the abdominal wall, having been compressed slowly, is released rapidly and a sudden stab of pain results. This may make the patient wince, so watch his or her face while this manoeuvre is performed. It strongly suggests the presence of peritonitis and should be performed if there is doubt about the presence of localised or generalised peritonitis. The patient with a confirmed acute abdomen should *not* be subjected to repeated testing of rebound tenderness because of the distress this can cause. Be careful not to surprise the patient by a sudden jabbing and release movement: rebound tenderness should be elicited slowly. If you suspect the patient may be feigning a tender abdomen, test for rebound with your stethoscope after telling the patient to lie still and quiet so that you can hear.

Liver

Feel for hepatomegaly (see Fig. 14.36).[4] With your examining hand aligned parallel to the right costal margin, and beginning in the right iliac fossa, ask the patient to breathe in and out slowly through the mouth. With each expiration advance your hand by 1 or 2 centimetres closer to the right costal margin. During inspiration the hand is kept still and the lateral margin of the forefinger waits expectantly for the liver edge to strike it.

The edge of the liver and the surface itself may be hard or soft, tender or non-tender, regular or irregular and pulsatile or non-pulsatile. The normal liver edge may be just palpable below the right costal margin on deep inspiration, especially in thin people. The edge is then felt to be soft and regular with a fairly sharply defined border and the surface of the liver itself is smooth. Sometimes only the left lobe of the liver may be palpable (to the left of the midline) in patients with cirrhosis.

If the liver edge is palpable the total *liver span* can be measured. Remember that the liver span varies with height and is greater in men than women, and that inter-observer error is quite large for this measurement. The normal upper border of the liver is level with the sixth intercostal space in the midclavicular line. At this point the percussion note over the chest changes from resonant to dull (see Fig. 14.37(a)). To estimate the liver span (see Fig. 14.37(b)), percuss down along the right midclavicular line until the liver dullness is encountered and measure from here to the palpable liver edge. Careful assessment of the position of the midclavicular line will improve the accuracy of this measurement. The normal span is less than 13 centimetres. Note that the clinical estimate of the liver span usually underestimates its actual size by 2 to 5 centimetres.

Other causes of a normal but palpable liver include ptosis due to emphysema, asthma or a subdiaphragmatic collection, or a Riedel's lobe.[u] The Riedel's lobe is a tongue-like projection of the liver from the right lobe's inferior surface; it can be quite large and rarely extends as far as the right iliac fossa. It can be confused with an enlarged gallbladder or right kidney.

Many diseases cause hepatic enlargement and these are listed in List 14.7. Detecting the liver edge below the costal margin clinically is highly specific (100%) but insensitive (48% for enlargement)—positive LR

Abdominal examination: the liver

FIGURE 14.36

[u] Bernhard Riedel (1846–1916), a German surgeon, described this in 1888.

Percussing the liver span.

(a) Upper border; (b) lower border

FIGURE 14.37

2.5, negative LR 0.5.[4,5] Remember, the diseased liver is not always enlarged; a small liver is common in advanced cirrhosis, and the liver shrinks rapidly with acute hepatic necrosis (due to liver cell death and collapse of the reticulin framework).

Spleen

The spleen enlarges inferiorly and medially (see Fig. 14.38). Its edge should be sought below the umbilicus in the midline initially. A two-handed technique is recommended. Place your left hand posterolaterally over the patient's left lower ribs and your right hand on the abdomen below the umbilicus, parallel to the left costal margin (see Fig. 14.39(a)). Do not start palpation too near the costal margin or a large spleen will be missed. As you advance your right hand closer to the left costal margin, compress your left hand firmly over the rib cage so as to produce a loose fold of skin (see Fig. 14.39(b)); this removes tension from the abdominal wall and enables a slightly enlarged soft spleen to be felt as it moves down towards the right iliac fossa at the end of inspiration (see Fig. 14.39(c)).

If the spleen is not palpable, roll the patient onto the right side towards you (the right lateral decubitus[v] position) and repeat palpation. Begin close to the left costal margin (see Fig. 14.39(d)). As a general rule, splenomegaly becomes just detectable if the spleen is

---

[v] From the Latin *accubitus*—reclining at table. Remember how the Romans lay on their sides to eat their dinners.

DIFFERENTIAL DIAGNOSIS IN LIVER PALPATION

Hepatomegaly

1. Massive
   - Metastases
   - Alcoholic liver disease with fatty infiltration
   - Myeloproliferative disease
   - Right heart failure
   - Hepatocellular cancer
2. Moderate
   - The above causes
   - Haemochromatosis
   - Haematological disease (e.g. chronic leukaemia, lymphoma)
   - Fatty liver (secondary to e.g. diabetes mellitus, obesity, toxins)
   - Infiltration (e.g. amyloid)
3. Mild
   - The above causes
   - Hepatitis
   - Biliary obstruction
   - Hydatid disease
   - Human immunodeficiency virus (HIV) infection

Firm and irregular liver

Hepatocellular carcinoma
Metastatic disease
Cirrhosis
Hydatid disease, granuloma (e.g. sarcoid), amyloid, cysts, lipoidoses

Tender liver

Hepatitis
Rapid liver enlargement (e.g. right heart failure, Budd–Chiari* syndrome [hepatic vein thrombosis])
Hepatocellular cancer
Hepatic abscess
Biliary obstruction cholangitis

Pulsatile liver

Tricuspid regurgitation
Hepatocellular cancer
Vascular abnormalities

*George Budd (1808–82), a professor of medicine at King's College Hospital, London, described this in 1845. Hans Chiari (1851–1916), a professor of pathology in Prague, described it in 1898.

LIST 14.7

one-and-a-half to two times enlarged. Palpation for splenomegaly is only moderately sensitive but highly specific. The positive LR of splenomegaly when the spleen is palpable is 9.6 and the negative LR of splenomegaly if the spleen is not palpable is 0.6.[5] Examination of the spleen is discussed further in Chapter 21. The causes of splenomegaly are listed in List 21.6 (p 344). The causes of hepatosplenomegaly are listed in List 14.8.

Kidneys

The first important differential diagnosis to consider, if a right or left subcostal mass is palpable, must be a kidney. An attempt to palpate the kidney should be a routine part of the examination. The bimanual method

CAUSES OF HEPATOSPLENOMEGALY

Chronic liver disease with portal hypertension
Haematological disease (e.g. myeloproliferative disease, lymphoma, leukaemia, pernicious anaemia, sickle cell anaemia)
Infection (e.g. acute viral hepatitis, infectious mononucleosis, cytomegalovirus)
Infiltration (e.g. amyloid, sarcoid)
Connective tissue disease (e.g. systemic lupus erythematosus)
Acromegaly
Thyrotoxicosis

LIST 14.8

Massive splenomegaly: note the splenic notch (tropical splenomegaly)

FIGURE 14.38

may be palpable in thin, healthy people. Both kidneys move downwards with inspiration.

It is particularly common to confuse a large left kidney with splenomegaly. The major distinguishing features are: (1) the spleen has no palpable upper border—the space between the spleen and the costal margin, which is present in renal enlargement, cannot be felt; (2) the spleen, unlike the kidney, has a notch that may be palpable; (3) the spleen moves inferomedially on inspiration whereas the kidney moves inferiorly; (4) the spleen is not usually ballottable unless gross ascites is present, but the kidney is, again because of its retroperitoneal position; (5) the percussion note is dull over the spleen but is usually resonant over the kidney, as the latter lies posterior to loops of gas-filled bowel; and (6) a friction rub may occasionally be heard over the spleen, but never over the kidney because it is too posterior.

Other abdominal masses

The causes of a mass in the abdomen, excluding the liver, spleen and kidneys, are summarised in List 14.9.

Gallbladder

The gallbladder is occasionally palpable below the right costal margin where this crosses the lateral border of the rectus muscles. If biliary obstruction or acute cholecystitis is suspected, the examining hand should be oriented perpendicular to the costal margin, feeling from medial to lateral. Unlike the liver edge, the gallbladder, if palpable, will be a bulbous, focal, rounded mass that moves downwards on inspiration. The causes of an enlarged gallbladder are listed in List 14.10.

Murphy's[w] *sign* should be sought if cholecystitis is suspected. On taking a deep breath, the patient catches his or her breath when an inflamed gallbladder presses on the examiner's hand, which is lying at the costal margin. Other signs are less helpful. An alternative technique is to stand behind the patient and place your right hand under the right costal margin while the patient takes a deep breath in.

When examining for an enlarged gallbladder always be mindful of *Courvoisier's*[x] *law*, which states that, if

is the best. The patient lies flat on his or her back. To palpate the right kidney, slide your left hand underneath the patient's back to rest with the heel of the hand under the right loin. The fingers remain free to flex at the metacarpophalangeal joints in the area of the renal angle. The flexing fingers can push the contents of the abdomen anteriorly. Place your right hand over the right upper quadrant.

First an attempt should be made to capture the kidney between both hands. It is more often possible to feel a kidney by bimanual palpation (this is traditionally called *ballotting*, although this term should probably be reserved for palpation of an organ or a mass in a fluid medium). In this case the renal angle is pressed sharply by the flexing fingers of the posterior hand (Fig. 14.40). It is important that the posterior hand is placed almost as far posterior as the spine and not just in the flank. The kidney can be felt to float upwards and strike the anterior hand. The opposite hands are used to palpate the left kidney.

When palpable, the kidney feels like a swelling with a rounded lower pole and a medial dent (the hilum). However, it is unusual for a normal kidney to be felt as clearly as this. The lower pole of the right kidney

---

[w] John Murphy (1857–1916), an American surgeon and professor of surgery at Rush Medical College, Chicago, described this in 1912.
[x] Ludwig Courvoisier (1843–1918), a professor of surgery in Switzerland, described this principle in 1890. He was a keen natural historian and wrote 21 papers on entomology.

Palpation of the spleen.

(a) Palpation begins in the lower mid-abdomen and finishes up under the left costal margin.
(b) The examiner's hand supports the patient's side …
(c) … and then rests over the lower costal margin to reduce skin resistance.
(d) If the spleen is not palpable when the patient is flat, he or she should be rolled towards the examiner

FIGURE 14.39

the gallbladder is enlarged and the patient is jaundiced, the cause is unlikely to be gallstones. Rather, carcinoma of the pancreas or lower biliary tree resulting in obstructive jaundice is likely to be present. This is because the gallbladder with stones is usually chronically fibrosed and therefore incapable of enlargement. Note that if the gallbladder is not palpable, and the patient is jaundiced, some cause other than gallstones is still possible, as at least 50% of dilated gallbladders are impalpable (see Good signs guide 14.1).

GOOD SIGNS GUIDE 14.1
Gallbladder: Courvoisier's sign

Sign	LR+	LR−
PALPABLE GALLBLADDER		
Detecting obstructed bile ducts in patients with jaundice	26.0	0.70
Detecting malignant obstruction in patients with obstructive jaundice	3.4	0.73

Balloting the kidney (bimanual palpation)

FIGURE 14.40

Stomach and duodenum

Although many clinicians palpate the epigastrium to elicit tenderness in patients with suspected peptic ulcer, the presence or absence of tenderness is not helpful in making this diagnosis.

With gastric outlet obstruction due to a peptic ulcer or gastric carcinoma, the 'succussion splash' (the sign of Hippocrates) may occasionally be present. In a case of suspected gastric outlet obstruction, after warning the patient what is to come, grasp one iliac crest with each hand, place your stethoscope close to the epigastrium and shake the patient vigorously from side to side. The listening ears eagerly await a splashing noise due to excessive fluid retained in an obstructed stomach. The test is not useful if the patient has just drunk a large amount of milk or other fluid for his or her ulcer; the clinician must then return 4 hours later, having forbidden the patient to drink anything further.

Pancreas

A pancreatic pseudocyst following acute pancreatitis may occasionally, if large, be palpable as a rounded swelling above the umbilicus. It is characteristically tense, does not descend with inspiration and feels fixed. Occasionally a pancreatic carcinoma may be palpable in thin patients.

Aorta

Arterial pulsation from the abdominal aorta may be present, usually in the epigastrium, in thin healthy people. The problem is to determine whether such

---

CAUSES OF ABDOMINAL MASSES

Right iliac fossa
Appendiceal abscess or mucocele of the appendix
Carcinoma of the caecum or caecal distension due to distal obstruction
Crohn's disease (usually when complicated by an abscess)
Ovarian tumour or cyst
Hernia
Transplanted kidney

Left iliac fossa
Faeces (*note:* can often be indented)
Carcinoma of sigmoid or descending colon
Ovarian tumour or cyst
Psoas abscess
Hernia
Transplanted kidney

Upper abdomen
Retroperitoneal lymphadenopathy (e.g. lymphoma, teratoma)
Left lobe of the liver
Abdominal aortic aneurysm (expansile)
Carcinoma of the stomach
Pancreatic pseudocyst or tumour
Gastric dilation (e.g. pyloric stenosis, acute dilation in diabetic ketoacidosis or after surgery)

Pelvis
Bladder
Ovarian tumour or cyst
Uterus (e.g. pregnancy, tumour, fibroids)
Small-bowel obstruction

LIST 14.9

---

a pulsation represents an aortic aneurysm (usually due to atherosclerosis) or not. Measure the width of the pulsation gently with two fingers by aligning these parallel to the aorta and placing them at the outermost palpable margins. With an aortic aneurysm, the pulsation is expansile (i.e. it enlarges appreciably with systole; see Fig. 14.41). If an abdominal aortic aneurysm is larger than 5 centimetres in diameter, it usually merits repair. The sensitivity of examination for finding an aneurysm of 5 centimetres or larger i

82%.[6,7] The sensitivity of the examination for detecting an aneurysm increases *pari passu* with the size of the aneurysm.

Bowel
Particularly in severely constipated patients with soft abdominal walls and retained faeces, the sigmoid colon is often palpable. Unlike other masses, faeces can usually be indented by the examiner's finger. Rarely, carcinoma of the bowel may be palpable, particularly in the caecum where masses can grow to a large size before they cause obstruction. Such a mass does not move on respiration. In the examination of children or adults with chronic constipation and a megarectum, the enlarged rectum containing impacted stool may be felt above the symphysis pubis, filling a variable part of the pelvis in the midline.

Bladder
An empty bladder is impalpable. If there is urinary retention, the full bladder may be palpable above the pubic symphysis. It forms part of the differential diagnosis of any swelling arising out of the pelvis. It is characteristically impossible to feel the bladder's lower border. The swelling is typically regular, smooth, firm and oval shaped. The bladder may sometimes reach as high as the umbilicus. It is unwise to make a definite diagnosis concerning a swelling coming out of the pelvis until you are sure the bladder is empty. This may require the insertion of a urinary catheter.

Inguinal lymph nodes
These are described on page 345.

Testes
Palpation of the testes should be considered if indicated during the abdominal examination (p 313). Testicular atrophy occurs in chronic liver disease (e.g. alcoholic liver disease, haemochromatosis); its mechanism is believed to be similar to that responsible for gynaecomastia.

Anterior abdominal wall
The skin and muscles of the anterior abdominal wall are prone to the same sorts of lumps that occur anywhere on the surface of the body (see List 14.11). So to avoid embarrassment it is important not to confuse these

---

> **GALLBLADDER ENLARGEMENT WITH JAUNDICE**
>
> **With jaundice**
> - Carcinoma of the head of the pancreas
> - Carcinoma of the ampulla of Vater*
> - In-situ gallstone formation in the common bile duct
> - Mucocele of the gallbladder due to a stone in Hartmann's† pouch and a stone in the common bile duct (very rare)
>
> **Without jaundice**
> - Mucocele or empyema of the gallbladder
> - Carcinoma of the gallbladder (stone hard, irregular swelling)
> - Acute cholecystitis
>
> *Abraham Vater (1684–1751), a Wittenberg anatomist and botanist.
> †Henri Hartmann (1860–1952), a professor of surgery in Paris.
>
> LIST 14.10

Detecting an expansile impulse.

a   b   c

A=no impulse; B=transmitted pulsation from a neighbouring artery; C=expansile impulse, the sign of an aneurysm

(ain A, ed. *Hamilton Bailey's physical signs in clinical surgery*, 17th edn. Bristol: John Wright & Sons, 1986.)

with intra-abdominal lumps. To determine whether a mass is in the abdominal wall, ask the patient to fold the arms across the upper chest and sit halfway up. An intra-abdominal mass disappears or decreases in size, but one within the layers of the abdominal wall will remain unchanged. A *divarication* of the rectus sheath will be obvious when a patient sits up (see Fig. 14.42). This weakness in the abdominal wall aponeurosis is very common and causes bulging of the central part of the abdomen when intra-abdominal pressure increases.

Pain can arise from the abdominal wall; this can cause confusion with intra-abdominal causes of pain. To test for *abdominal wall pain*, feel for an area of localised tenderness that reproduces the pain while the patient is supine. If this is found, ask the patient to fold the arms across the upper chest and sit halfway up, then palpate again.[y] If the tenderness disappears, this suggests that the pain is in the abdominal cavity (as tensed abdominal muscles are protecting the viscera), but if the tenderness persists or is greater, this suggests that the pain is arising from the abdominal wall (e.g. muscle strain, nerve entrapment, myositis).[8–10] However, Carnett's test may occasionally be positive when there is visceral disease with involvement of the parietal peritoneum producing inflammation of the overlying muscle (e.g. appendicitis).

Percussion

Percussion is used to define the size and nature of organs and masses, but is most useful for detecting fluid in the peritoneal cavity, and for eliciting tenderness in patients with peritonitis.

Liver

The liver borders should be percussed routinely to determine the liver span. If the liver edge is not palpable and there is no ascites, the right side of the abdomen should be percussed in the midclavicular line up to the right costal margin until dullness is encountered. This defines the liver's lower border even when it is

---

[y] Carnett's test: described by JB Carnett in 1926.

> **SOME CAUSES OF ANTERIOR ABDOMINAL WALL MASSES**
>
> Lipoma
> Sebaceous cyst
> Dermal fibroma
> Malignant deposits (e.g. melanoma, carcinoma)
> Epigastric hernia
> Umbilical or paraumbilical hernia
> Incisional hernia
> Rectus sheath divarication (see Fig. 14.42)
> Rectus sheath haematoma
>
> LIST 14.11

Rectus sheath divarication.

(a) At rest. (b) 'Lift your head off the pillow'

FIGURE 14.42

Percussion of the spleen

FIGURE 14.43

GOOD SIGNS GUIDE 14.2
Ascites

Sign	LR+	LR−
INSPECTION		
Bulging flanks	2.4	0.3
Oedema of ankles	2.8	0.1
PALPATION AND PERCUSSION		
Flank dullness	2.6	0.3
Shifting dullness	5.8	0.5
Fluid thrill	9.6	0.6

not palpable. The upper border of the liver must always be defined by percussing down the midclavicular line. Loss of normal liver dullness may occur in massive hepatic necrosis, or with free gas in the peritoneal cavity (e.g. perforated bowel).

Spleen

Percussion over the left costal margin is more sensitive than palpation for detection of enlargement of the spleen. Percuss over the lowest intercostal space in the left anterior axillary line in both inspiration and expiration with the patient supine (see Fig. 14.43). Splenomegaly should be suspected if the percussion note is dull or becomes dull on complete inspiration. If the percussion note is dull, palpation should be repeated (see also Ch 21 for another method for detecting splenomegaly).

Kidneys

Percussion over a right or left subcostal mass can help distinguish hepatic or splenic from renal masses: in the latter case there will usually be a resonant area because of overlying bowel (be warned, however, that sometimes a very large renal mass may displace overlying bowel).

Bladder

An area of suprapubic dullness indicates the upper border of an enlarged bladder or pelvic mass.

Ascites

The percussion note over most of the abdomen is resonant, due to air in the intestines.[11] The resonance is detectable out to the flanks. When peritoneal fluid (ascites) collects, the influence of gravity causes this to accumulate first in the flanks in a supine patient. Thus, a relatively early sign of ascites (when at least 2 litres of fluid have accumulated) is a dull percussion note in the flanks (see Good signs guide 14.2). When ascites is gross, the abdomen distends, the flanks bulge, umbilical eversion occurs (see Fig. 14.29) and dullness is detectable closer to the midline. However, an area of central resonance will always persist. Routine abdominal examination should include percussion starting in the midline with the finger pointing towards the feet; the percussion note is tested out towards the flanks on each side.

If (and only if) dullness is detected in the flanks, the sign of **shifting dullness** (see Fig. 14.44) should be sought.[11] To detect this sign, while standing on the right side of the bed percuss out to the left flank until dullness is reached (see Fig. 14.45(a)). This point should be marked (usually by leaving a finger over the spot) and the patient rolled towards you. Ideally 30 seconds to 1 minute should then pass so that fluid can move inside the abdominal cavity and then percussion is repeated over the marked point (see Fig. 14.45(b)).

Shifting dullness is present if the area of dullness has changed to become resonant. This is because peritoneal fluid moves under the influence of gravity to the right side of the abdomen when this is the lowermost point. Very occasionally, fluid and air in

CHAPTER 14 THE GASTROINTESTINAL EXAMINATION

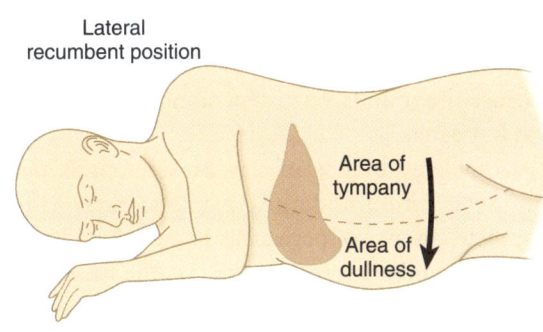

Anatomy of shifting dullness

FIGURE 14.44

Shifting dullness.

(a) Percuss out to the left flank until the percussion note becomes dull. Mark this spot with your finger.

(b) Roll the patient towards you, wait 30 seconds. Shifting dullness is present if the left lateral dull area is now resonant

FIGURE 14.45

dilated small bowel in small-intestinal obstruction, or a massive ovarian cyst filling the whole abdomen, can cause confusion.

To detect a **fluid thrill** (or wave), ask an assistant (or the patient) to place the medial edges of both palms firmly on the centre of the abdomen with the fingers pointing towards each other. Flick the side of the abdominal wall; a pulsation (thrill) is felt by the hand placed on the other abdominal wall. A fluid thrill is of more value when there is massive ascites. Interestingly, it may also occur when there is a massive ovarian cyst or a pregnancy with hydramnios.

The presence of bulging in the flanks has good sensitivity and specificity for the detection of ascites.

Shifting dullness has both good sensitivity and good specificity. The presence of ankle oedema increases the likelihood of ascites. (See Good signs guide 14.2.)

The causes of ascites are outlined in List 14.12.

When significant ascites is present, abdominal masses may be difficult to feel by direct palpation. Here is the opportunity to practise *dipping*. Using the hand placed flat on the abdomen, the fingers are flexed at the metacarpophalangeal joints rapidly so as to displace

CLASSIFICATION OF ASCITES BY THE SERUM ASCITES TO ALBUMIN CONCENTRATION GRADIENT

High gradient (>11 g/L)
- Cirrhosis*
- Alcoholic hepatitis
- Budd–Chiari syndrome (hepatic vein thrombosis) or veno-occlusive disease
- Fulminant hepatic failure
- Congestive heart failure, constrictive pericarditis (cardiac ascites)

Low gradient (<11 g/L)
- Peritoneal carcinomatosis
- Tuberculosis
- Pancreatic ascites
- Nephrotic syndrome

*Patients with a high serum-to-ascites albumin gradient most often have portal hypertension (97% accuracy).

LIST 14.12

Auscultation of the abdomen

FIGURE 14.46

the underlying fluid. This enables the fingers to reach a mass covered in ascitic fluid. In particular, this should be attempted to palpate an enlarged liver or spleen. The liver and spleen may become ballottable when gross ascites is present.

Auscultation

While some cardiologists believe that the sounds produced in the abdominal cavity are not as varied or as interesting as those one hears in the chest, they have some value.

Bowel sounds

Place the diaphragm of the stethoscope just below the umbilicus. Bowel sounds can be heard over all parts of the abdomen in healthy people (see Fig. 14.46). They are poorly localised and there is little point in listening for them in more than one place. Most bowel sounds originate in the stomach, some from the large bowel and the rest from the small bowel. They have a soft gurgling character and occur only intermittently. Bowel sounds should be described as either present or absent; the terms 'decreased' or 'increased' are meaningless because the sounds vary, depending on when a meal was last eaten.

Complete absence of any bowel sounds over a 4-minute period indicates paralytic ileus (this is complete absence of peristalsis in a paralysed bowel). As only liquid is present in the gut, the heart sounds may be audible over the abdomen, transmitted by the dilated bowel.

The bowel that is obstructed produces a louder and higher-pitched sound with a tinkling quality due to the presence of air and liquid ('obstructed bowel sounds'). The presence of normal bowel sounds makes obstruction unlikely. Intestinal hurry or rush, which occurs in diarrhoeal states, causes loud gurgling sounds, often audible without the stethoscope. These bowel sounds are called *borborygmi*.

Friction rubs

These indicate an abnormality of the parietal and visceral peritoneum due to inflammation, but are very rare and non-specific.

They may be audible over the liver or spleen. A rough creaking or grating noise is heard as the patient breathes. Hepatic causes include a tumour within the liver (hepatocellular cancer or metastases), a liver abscess, a recent liver biopsy, a liver infarct, or gonococcal or chlamydial perihepatitis due to inflammation of the liver capsule (Fitz-Hugh–Curtis syndrome[z]). A splenic rub indicates a splenic infarct.

Venous hums

A venous hum is a continuous, low-pitched, soft murmur that may become louder with inspiration and diminish when more pressure is applied to the stethoscope. Typically it is heard between the xiphisternum and the umbilicus in cases of portal hypertension, but is rare. It may radiate to the chest or over to the liver. Large volumes of blood flowing in the umbilical or paraumbilical veins in the falciform ligament are responsible. These channel blood from the left portal vein to the epigastric or internal mammary veins in the abdominal wall. A venous hum may occasionally be heard over the large vessels such as the inferior mesenteric vein or after portacaval shunting. Sometimes a thrill is detectable over the site of maximum intensity of the hum. The Cruveilhier–Baumgarten syndrome[aa] is the association of a venous hum at the umbilicus and dilated abdominal wall veins. It is almost always due to cirrhosis of the liver. It occurs when patients have a patent umbilical vein, which allows portal-to-systemic shunting at this site. The presence of a venous hum or of prominent central abdominal veins suggests that the site of portal obstruction is intrahepatic rather than in the portal vein itself.

Bruits

Uncommonly, an arterial systolic bruit can be heard over the liver. This sound is higher pitched than a venous hum, is not continuous and is well localised. This is usually due to a hepatocellular cancer but may occur in acute alcoholic hepatitis, with an arteriovenous malformation or transiently after a liver biopsy. Auscultation for renal bruits on either side of the midline above the umbilicus is indicated if renal artery stenosis is suspected. A bruit in the epigastrium may be heard in patients with chronic intestinal ischaemia from mesenteric arterial stenosis, but may also occur in the absence of pathology. A bruit may occasionally be audible over the spleen when there is a tumour of the body of the pancreas or a splenic arteriovenous fistula.

Scratch test

The scratch test can help to identify the inferior liver border if the abdomen is very tender, tense or distended. Place the diaphragm of the stethoscope below the xiphoid and lightly but briskly stroke the skin in a direction at right angles to the expected liver edge, starting at the right lower quadrant and working slowly up to the right costal margin along the midclavicular line. When the liver edge is reached, the sound of the scratch is transmitted to the stethoscope. The point of initial (not maximal) sound transmission is most helpful in identifying the liver edge. This test has been controversial but is reliable with moderate accuracy (versus abdominal ultrasound).[12,13]

HERNIAS

Hernias are of surgical importance and should not be missed during an abdominal examination. They are very frequently the focus of student assessment examinations.

Examination anatomy

You need to know the anatomy of the inguinal and femoral canal. A key anatomical landmark is the pubic tubercle (or pubic spine), a palpable round nodule (tubercle) on the upper border of the medial portion of the superior ramus of the pubis (a midline cartilaginous joint uniting the superior rami of the left and right pubic bones). The inguinal ligament attaches to the pubic tubercle (see Fig. 14.47). Find the femoral artery pulsation and go medially to identify the tubercle. The pubic tubercle can usually easily be felt lateral to the symphysis pubis (2–3 centimetres from the midline). In the obese individual, it may be difficult to locate the pubic tubercle; in such situations, if the thigh is flexed and abducted, the adductor longus muscle can be traced proximally, leading you to the pubic tubercle.

From the pubic tubercle to the anterior superior iliac spine lies the inguinal canal. At the mid-inguinal point (midway between the pubic symphysis and the anterior superior iliac spine) is an internal ring. At the pubic tubercle lies an external ring, in men the gateway to the scrotum. Remember that the femoral

---

[z] AH Curtis described hepatic adhesions associated with pelvic inflammatory disease in 1930, while T Fitz-Hugh described right upper abdominal acute gonococcal peritonitis in 1934. However, this syndrome was actually first described by C Stajano in 1920.

[aa] Jean Cruveilhier (1791–1874), a professor of pathological anatomy in Paris, who had been Dupuytren's registrar, and Paul von Baumgarten (1848–1928), a German pathologist.

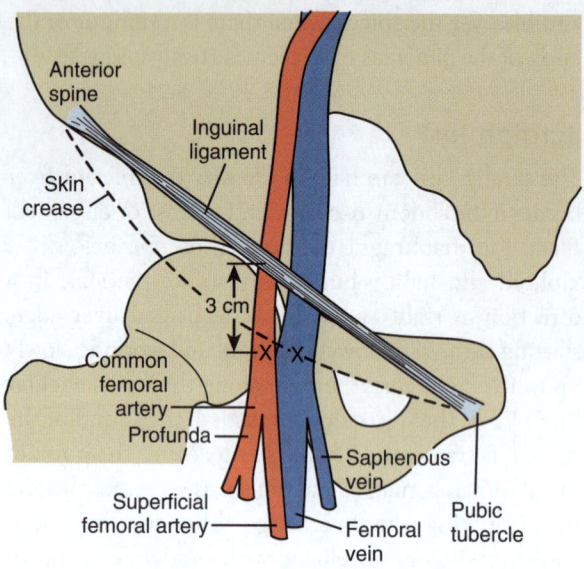

Anatomy of the pubic tubercle and inguinal ligament

(From Kaplan J et al. *Kaplan's cardiac anesthesia*, 6th edn. Philadelphia: Saunders 2011.)

FIGURE 14.47

DIFFERENTIAL DIAGNOSIS OF A SOLITARY GROIN LUMP

Above the inguinal ligament
Inguinal hernia
Undescended testis
Cyst of the canal of Nuck
Encysted hydrocele or lipoma of the cord
Iliac node

Below the inguinal ligament
Femoral hernia
Lymph node
Saphena varix (sensation of a 'jet of water' on palpation, disappears when supine)
Femoral aneurysm (pulsatile)
Psoas abscess (associated with fever, flank pain and flexion deformity)

LIST 14.13

canal is situated lateral to the pubic tubercle, below the inguinal ligament.

Hernias in the groin

The principal sign of a hernia is a lump in the groin. Naturally, not all lumps in the region are hernias (see List 14.13).

A groin lump that is present on standing or during manoeuvres that raise intra-abdominal pressure (such as coughing or straining), and that disappears (or reduces) on recumbency, is easily identified as a hernia.

Some hernias are irreducible. Another term used for irreducible is incarcerated, but this term is best avoided. Some irreducible hernias contain bowel, which may become obstructed, giving rise to symptoms of small-bowel obstruction in addition to the irreducible lump. Sometimes the bowel contents' blood supply becomes jeopardised, and these are known as *strangulated hernias*; they are usually painful, red, tense and tender.

Inguinal hernias typically bulge above the crease of the groin. The lump is found medial to the pubic tubercle, above the inguinal ligament (remember, inguinal=medial and above). Inguinal hernias may be indirect or direct. Indirect inguinal hernias are by far the most common groin hernia. The bowel follows the inguinal canal, bulging through the internal ring and sometimes out through the external ring. Direct inguinal hernias are usually the result of a muscular defect of the inguinal canal (an area known as Hesselbach's triangle,[bb] bounded inferiorly by the inguinal ligament, laterally by the inferior epigastric vessels and medially by the lateral border of the rectus sheath). Usually the hernia does not reach the scrotum. However, differentiating a direct from an indirect hernia is difficult based on clinical signs alone.

A *femoral hernia* bulges through the femoral ring into the femoral canal. Femoral hernias bulge into the groin crease at its medial end. The lump is found lateral to the pubic tubercle, below the inguinal ligament (remember, femoral=lateral and below).

Examination technique

1. Wash your hands and glove up.
2. *Position the patient.* A thorough examination for a hernia should be commenced with the patient

---

[bb] Franz Hesselbach (1759–1816), a professor of surgery in Würzburg, described this triangle bounded by the inguinal ligament, the inferior epigastric artery and the rectus abdominis.

Note the elliptical swelling of an indirect inguinal hernia descending into the scrotum on the right side. Also note the globular swelling of a direct inguinal hernia on the left side

FIGURE 14.48

standing if possible. The patient should be asked to stand with full exposure from the thigh to the upper abdomen.
3. *Point sign.* Ask the patient to point where the lump has been seen or felt.
4. *Inspect.* Pay careful attention to scars from previous surgery, which may be difficult to see. Look for obvious lumps and swellings on both sides.
5. *Cough impulse.* Before palpation, ask the patient to turn his or her head away from you and cough. Fix your eyes in the region of the pubic tubercle and note the presence of a visible cough impulse. Ask the patient to cough again while you inspect the opposite side.
6. *Palpation.* Place your fingers over the region of the pubic tubercle. Once again the patient is asked to cough and a palpable expansile impulse is sought. If a hernia is present, attempts at reduction should not be performed while the patient is erect, as it is more difficult and painful than when the patient is placed supine.
7. *Lay the patient supine.* Ask the patient to lie supine on the examination couch. Perform the procedure of inspection and palpation in the same manner again. The exact position of any hernia is usually easier to define with the patient lying supine.

8. *Identify the hernia type.* If a lump is present, it must be determined whether this is a hernia and, if so, what sort of hernia. Identify the pubic tubercle. Remember, one cannot get above a hernia, but one can get above a hydrocele in the inguinal canal. Try to determine whether the hernia is inguinal (see Fig. 14.48) or femoral based on the position in relation to the pubic tubercle and inguinal ligament (see above).
   Remember, femoral hernias are more dangerous: they are usually smaller and firmer than inguinal hernias and commonly do not exhibit a cough impulse. Because they are frequently irreducible they are commonly mistaken for an enlarged inguinal lymph node. A cough impulse is rare from a femoral hernia and needs to be distinguished from the thrill produced by a saphena varix when a patient coughs.
9. In a male, examine the testes and scrotum. A large inguinal hernia may descend through the external ring immediately above the pubic tubercle into the scrotum. Gentle invagination of the scrotum with the tip of the gloved finger in the external ring may be performed to confirm an indirect hernia in men, but this can be difficult to interpret without substantial experience (see Fig. 14.49). A maldescended testis can be confused with an inguinal hernia;

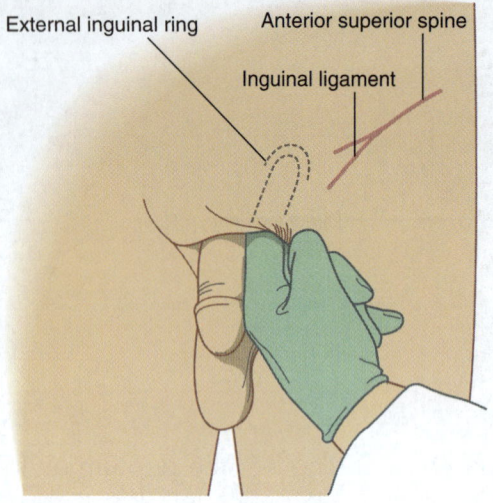

To examine the inguinal canal in a male, the scrotum can be invaginated as shown (always wear gloves)

FIGURE 14.49

always confirm that there is a testis in each scrotum. A large inguinal hernia may present as a lump in the scrotum. It is important to ascertain whether one can get above the lump. If you can get above the lump, the lump is of primary intrascrotal pathology and is not a hernia.

Epigastric hernia

A hernia in the epigastric region is common in older patients. This can be identified by asking the patient to do half a sit-up from the supine position and looking for an obvious bulge. Identify scars that may explain the abdominal wall weakness. Ask the patient whether the lump is painful and palpate it. Feel for a cough impulse. Asymptomatic epigastric hernias are usually best left alone!

Incisional hernias

Any abdominal scar may be the site of a hernia because of abdominal wall weakness. Assess this by asking the patient to cough while you look for abnormal bulges. Next have the patient lift the head and shoulders off the bed while you rest your hand on the patient's forehead and resist this movement. If a bulge is seen, use your other hand to palpate for a fascial layer defect in the muscle, and test the cough impulse.

RECTAL EXAMINATION

The examining physician often hesitates to make the necessary examination because it involves soiling the finger.
    William Mayo (1861–1939)

The abdominal examination is not complete without the performance of a rectal examination (with the aid of gloves; see Fig. 14.50).[14,15] It should be considered in all patients with bowel symptoms admitted to hospital and who are aged 40 or older, unless the examiner has no fingers, the patient no anus or acute illness such as myocardial infarction presents a temporary contraindication.

The patient's permission must be obtained and, if indicated, a chaperone introduced to the patient. Privacy must be ensured for the patient throughout the examination. Following an explanation as to what is to happen and why, the patient lies on his or her left side with the knees drawn up and back to the examiner. This is called the left lateral position. The examination can be performed with the patient standing and in the bent-over position; this may help provide good information about the prostate, but makes assessment of rectal function more difficult.

Don a pair of gloves and begin the inspection of the anus and perianal area by separating the buttocks. The following must be looked for:

1. **Thrombosed external haemorrhoids (piles).** Small (less than 1 centimetre), tense bluish swellings may be seen on one side of the anal margin. They are painful and are due to rupture of a vein in the external haemorrhoidal plexus. They are also called perianal haematomas.
2. **Skin tags.** These look like tags elsewhere on the body and can be an incidental finding or occur with haemorrhoids or Crohn's disease.
3. **Rectal prolapse.** Circumferential folds of red mucosa are visible protruding from the anus. These may become apparent only when the patient is asked to strain as if to pass stool. If there is rectal prolapse, straining may cause a dark red mass to appear at the anal verge;

The rectal examination: regional anatomy
(From Talley NJ. How to do and interpret a rectal examination in gastroenterology. *American Journal of Gastroenterology* 2008; 108:802–803.)

FIGURE 14.50

mucosal prolapse causes the appearance of radial folds, while concentric folds are a sign of complete prolapse. This mass is continuous with the perianal skin and is usually painless. In cases of mucosal rectal prolapse, the prolapsed mucosa can be felt between the examiner's thumb and forefinger. A gaping anus suggests loss of internal and external sphincter tone. This may coexist with prolapse.

4. **Anal fissure (fissure-in-ano).** This is a crack in the anal wall that may be painful enough to prevent rectal examination with the finger. Fissures-in-ano usually occur directly posteriorly and in the midline. A tag of skin may be present at the base: this is called a sentinel pile and indicates that the fissure is chronic. It may be necessary to get the patient to bear down for a fissure to become visible. Multiple or broad-based fissures may be present in patients with inflammatory bowel disease, malignancy or sexually transmitted disease.

5. **Fistula-in-ano.** The entrance of this tract may be visible, usually within 4 centimetres of the anus. The mouth has a red pouting appearance caused by granulation tissue. This may occur with Crohn's disease or perianal abscess.

6. **Condylomata acuminata (anal warts).** Condylomata (see Fig. 14.51) may be confused with skin tags, but are in fact pedunculated papillomas with a white surface and red base. They may surround the anus.

7. **Carcinoma of the anus.** This may be visible as a fungating mass at the anal verge.

8. **Pruritus ani.** The appearance of this irritating anal condition varies from weeping red dermatitis to a thickened white skin. It is usually caused by faecal soiling.

Condylomata (anal warts)

(From Venkatesan A. Pigmented lesions of the vulva. *Dermatology Clinics* 2010; 28(4):795–805.)

FIGURE 14.51

Next ask the patient to strain and watch the perineum: look for incontinence and leakage of faeces or mucus, abnormal descent of the perineum (>4 centimetres) or the presence of a patulous anus. The presence of a gaping anus often correlates with lower resting pressures on anorectal manometry. Internal haemorrhoids can prolapse in the right anterior, right posterior and left lateral positions.

Now test the anal wink. Stroke a cotton pad in all four quadrants around the anus. Usually you will see a brisk anal contraction that indicates the sacral nerve pathways are intact. Sometimes the response is weak in healthy people. However, the complete absence of an anal wink, particularly in the setting of faecal incontinence, suggests that there is a spinal cord problem and indicates the need to perform a more detailed neurological examination and consider further investigations accordingly.

Now the time for action has come. Lubricate the tip of your gloved right index finger and place it over the patient's anus. Ask the patient to breathe in and out quietly through the mouth, as a distraction and to aid relaxation.

If the patient feels excruciating pain at the start of the examination, this strongly suggests that there is an anal fissure and the remainder of the rectal examination should be abandoned. Often the fissure can be seen on inspection. An anal fissure can precipitate constipation but may be secondary to constipation itself. By liberally lubricating the rectum with lignocaine jelly, it may still be possible to complete the rest of the examination, but usually it is better to perform anoscopy under appropriate sedation for these patients. Other causes of significant anal pain during palpation include recently thrombosed external haemorrhoids, an ischiorectal abscess, active proctitis or anal ulceration from another cause.

Unless the patient feels pain, slowly increase the pressure applied with the pulp of your finger until the sphincter is felt to relax slightly. At this stage advance your finger into the rectum slowly. During entry, sphincter tone should be assessed as normal or reduced. The accuracy of this assessment has been questioned in the past, but more recently it has been shown to correlate well with anorectal manometry measurements.[16] This resting tone is predominantly (70%–80%) attributable to the internal anal sphincter muscle. Reduced sphincter tone may indicate a sphincter tear. A high anal resting tone may contribute to difficulties with evacuation.

Palpation of the anterior wall of the rectum for the *prostate gland* in the male and for the *cervix* in the female is performed first. The normal prostate is a firm, rubbery bilobed mass with a central furrow. It becomes firmer with age. With prostatic enlargement, the sulcus becomes obliterated and the gland is often asymmetrical. A very hard nodule is apparent when a carcinoma of the prostate is present. The prostate is boggy and tender in prostatitis. A mass above the prostate or cervix may indicate a metastatic deposit on Blumer's shelf.[cc]

Rotate your finger clockwise so that the left lateral wall, posterior wall and right lateral wall of the rectum can be palpated in turn. Then advance your finger as high as possible into the rectum and slowly withdraw along the rectal wall. A soft lesion, such as a small

---

[cc] George Blumer (1858–1940), a professor of medicine at Yale, in 1909 described cancer in the pouch of Douglas forming a shelf-like structure.

> **CAUSES OF A PALPABLE MASS IN THE RECTUM**
>
> Rectal carcinoma
> Rectal polyp
> Hypertrophied anal papilla
> Diverticular phlegmon (recent or old)
> Sigmoid colon carcinoma (prolapsing into the pouch of Douglas*)
> Metastatic deposits in the pelvis (Blumer's shelf)
> Uterine or ovarian malignancy
> Prostatic or cervical malignancy (direct extension)
> Endometriosis
> Pelvic abscess or sarcoma
> Amoebic granuloma
> Foreign body
>
> *Note:* Faeces, while palpable, also indent.
> *James Douglas (1675–1742), a Scottish anatomist and male midwife, physician to Queen Caroline (wife of George II) in London.
>
> LIST 14.14

rectal carcinoma or polyp, is more likely to be felt in this way (see List 14.14).[dd]

The pelvic floor—special tests for pelvic floor dysfunction

The first test is simple: ask the patient to strain and try to push out your finger. Normally, the anal sphincter and puborectalis should relax and the perineum should descend by 1–3.5 centimetres. If the muscles seem to tighten, particularly when there is no perineal descent, this suggests paradoxical external anal sphincter and puborectalis contraction, which in fact are blocking normal defecation (called pelvic floor dyssynergia or anismus). Ask the patient to strain again when your finger is rotated anteriorly. In this position a *rectocele* (a defect in the anterior wall of the rectum) may be palpable.

Second, press on the posterior rectal wall and ask if this causes pain; this suggests puborectalis muscle tenderness, which can also occur in pelvic floor dyssynergia.

Third, assess whether the anal sphincter and the puborectalis contract when you ask the patient to contract or squeeze the pelvic floor muscles. Puborectalis contraction is perceived as a 'lift'—that is, the muscle lifts the examining finger towards the umbilicus. Many patients with faecal incontinence cannot augment anal pressure when asked to squeeze.

Finally, place your other hand on the anterior abdominal wall while asking the patient to strain again. This provides some information on whether the patient is excessively contracting the abdominal wall (e.g. by performing an inappropriate Valsalva manoeuvre) and perhaps also the pelvic floor muscles while attempting to defecate, which may impede evacuation. However, the exact value of this test is unclear.

Constipation that is due to pelvic floor dysfunction responds to biofeedback in about 70% of cases, and this treatment can result in a laxative-free existence for patients with troubling outlet constipation; the diagnosis should be entertained in all patients with chronic constipation, and a good rectal examination can help guide you as to whether anorectal manometry testing is warranted.

Ending the rectal exam

After your finger has been withdrawn, inspect the glove for bright blood or melaena, mucus or pus, and note the colour of the faeces. Haemorrhoids are not palpable unless thrombosed. Persistent gaping of the anal canal after withdrawal of the examining finger may indicate external anal sphincter denervation.

Testing of the stools for blood

Testing of the stools for blood may be considered in the assessment of anaemia, iron deficiency, gastrointestinal bleeding or symptoms suggesting colonic cancer, or for colon cancer screening in asymptomatic people. In the guaiac test, stool is placed on a guaiac-impregnated paper; blood results in phenolytic oxidation, causing a blue colour.

[dd] It can be useful to perform the rectal examination with the patient supine and the head of the bed elevated; this allows the intra-abdominal contents to descend and a bimanual examination (using the opposite hand to compress the lower abdomen) is possible.

Unfortunately, both false-positive and false-negative results occur with the occult blood tests. Peroxidase and catalase, present in various foods (e.g. fresh fruit, uncooked vegetables), and haem in red meat can cause false-positive results, as can aspirin, anticoagulants and oral iron. Vitamin C can reduce the sensitivity of guaiac results and should not be taken before testing. False-negative results are not uncommon with colorectal neoplasms because they bleed intermittently. Hence testing for faecal occult blood from the glove after a rectal examination is of little value,[17] and more sensitive and specific testing (e.g. colonoscopy) is required, depending on the clinical setting.

OTHER

Examine the legs for bruising or oedema, which may be the result of liver disease. Neurological signs of alcoholism (e.g. a coarse tremor) or evidence of thiamine deficiency (peripheral neuropathy or memory loss) may also be present.

Examination of the cardiovascular system may be helpful in patients with hepatomegaly. Cardiac failure is a common cause of liver enlargement and can even cause cirrhosis. Measurement of the patient's temperature is important, especially in an acute abdominal case or if there is any suggestion of infection.

Examine with particular care all lymph node groups, the breasts and chest if there is any evidence of malignant disease such as firm, irregular hepatomegaly.

EXAMINATION OF THE GASTROINTESTINAL CONTENTS

Faeces

Never miss an opportunity to inspect a patient's faeces, because considerable information about the gastrointestinal tract can be obtained in this way.

Melaena

Melaena stools are poorly formed, black and have a tarry appearance. They have a very characteristic and offensive smell. The cause is the presence of blood digested by gastric acid and colonic bacteria. Melaena usually indicates bleeding from the oesophagus, stomach or duodenum. The most common cause is acute or chronic peptic ulceration. Less often, right-sided colonic bleeding and (rarely) small-bowel bleeding can cause melaena. The differential diagnosis of dark stools includes ingestion of iron tablets, bismuth, liquorice or charcoal. However, these tend to result in small well-formed non-tarry stools and the offensive smell is absent.

Bright-red blood (haematochezia)

This appearance usually results from haemorrhage from the rectum or left colon. Beetroot ingestion can sometimes cause confusion. Blood loss may result from a carcinoma or polyp, an arteriovenous malformation, inflammatory bowel disease or diverticular disease. It can occasionally occur with massive upper gastrointestinal bleeding. The blood is usually mixed in with the bowel motion if it comes from above the anorectum, but if blood appears on the surface of the stool or only on the toilet paper this suggests, but does not guarantee, that bleeding is from a local rectal cause, such as internal haemorrhoids or a fissure. Dark-red jelly-like stools may be seen with ischaemic bowel.

Steatorrhoea

The stools are usually very pale, offensive, smelly and bulky. They float and are difficult to flush away. However, the most common cause of floating stools is gas and water rather than fat.

Steatorrhoea results from malabsorption of fat. In severe pancreatic disease, oil (triglycerides) may be passed per rectum and this is virtually pathognomonic of pancreatic steatorrhoea (lipase deficiency). Oil may also be seen when the patient has used a weight-loss drug that induces fat malabsorption (orlistat).

'Toothpaste' stools

Here the faeces are expressed like toothpaste from a tube: the condition is usually due to severe constipation with overflow diarrhoea. It may, however, also occur in the irritable bowel syndrome, with a stricture or in Hirschsprung's disease.

Rice-water stools

Cholera causes massive excretion of fluid and electrolytes from the bowel, which results in a severe secretory diarrhoea. The pale watery stools are of enormous volume and contain mucous debris.

Vomitus

The clinician who is fortunate enough to have vomitus available for inspection (ill-informed staff may throw out this valuable substance) should not lose the opportunity of a detailed examination. There are a number of interesting types of vomitus.

'Coffee grounds'

An old blood clot in vomitus has the appearance of the dregs of a good cup of espresso coffee. Unfortunately, darker vomitus is often described as having this appearance. This emphasises the need for personal inspection. Iron tablets and red wine, not to mention coffee ingestion, can have the same effect on the vomitus.

Bright-red blood (haematemesis)

Look for the presence of fresh clot. It usually indicates fresh bleeding from the upper gastrointestinal tract.

Yellow-green vomitus

This results from the vomiting of bile and upper small-bowel contents, often when there is obstruction.

Faeculent vomiting

Here brown offensive material from the small bowel is vomited. It is a late sign of small-intestinal obstruction. Recently ingested tea can have the same appearance but lacks the smell.

Brownish-black fluid in large volumes may be vomited in cases of acute dilation of the stomach. A succussion splash will usually be present. Acute dilation may occur in association with diabetic ketoacidosis or following abdominal surgery. It represents a medical emergency because of the risk of aspiration; there is a need for urgent placement of a nasogastric tube.

Projectile vomiting

This term describes the act of vomiting itself and may indicate pyloric stenosis. It may also occur with raised intracranial pressure.

URINALYSIS

Note that testing of the urine can be very helpful in diagnosing liver disease.

Strip colour tests can detect the presence of bilirubin and urobilinogen in the urine. False-positive or false-negative results can occur with vitamin C or even exposure to sunlight. An understanding of the reasons for the presence of bilirubin or urobilinogen in the urine necessitates an explanation of the metabolism of these substances (see Fig. 14.52).

Red blood cells are broken down by the reticuloendothelial system, causing the release of haem, which is converted to biliverdin and then *unconjugated bilirubin*, a water-insoluble compound. For this reason, unconjugated bilirubin released with haemolytic anaemia will not appear in the urine (termed *acholuric jaundice*).

Unconjugated bilirubin is transported in the blood bound largely to albumin but also to other plasma proteins. Unconjugated bilirubin is then taken up by the liver cells and transported to the endoplasmic reticulum, where glucuronyl transferases conjugate bilirubin with glucuronide. This results in the formation of *conjugated bilirubin*, which is water soluble. Conjugated bilirubin is then concentrated and excreted by the liver cells into the canaliculus.

Conjugated bilirubin is virtually all excreted into the small bowel; it is converted in the terminal ileum and colon to *urobilinogen*, and then to *stercobilin*. Stercobilin is responsible for the normal colour of the stools with other non-bilirubinoid dietary pigments. Up to 20% of urobilinogen is reabsorbed by the bowel, and small amounts are excreted in the urine as urinary urobilinogen. This can often be normally detected by reagent strips.

Total biliary obstruction, from whatever cause, results in absence of urinary urobilinogen, as no conjugated bilirubin reaches the bowel, resulting in pale stools (absence of stercobilin). The conjugated bilirubin, unable to be excreted (the rate-limiting step), leaks from the hepatocytes into the blood and from there is excreted into the urine (normally there is no bilirubin detected in urine). This results in dark urine (excess conjugated bilirubin). Acute liver damage, as in viral hepatitis, may sometimes initially result in excessive urinary urobilinogen, because the liver is unable to re-excrete the urobilinogen reabsorbed from the bowel. These changes are summarised in Table 14.2.

Schematic representation of the bilirubin pathway.

Increased haemolysis (1) overwhelms the hepatocytes' ability to conjugate bilirubin and excrete the conjugated form, leading to increased serum levels of unconjugated bilirubin. Low levels of glucuronyl transferase (2) (e.g. Gilbert's disease) cause decreased conjugation. Hepatocellular dysfunction (3) causes decreased uptake, conjugation and excretion with increases of unconjugated bilirubin and conjugated bilirubin. Posthepatic obstruction (4) from stones or tumour prevents passage of bilirubin through the bile ducts into the bowel, leading to increased serum levels of conjugated bilirubin

FIGURE 14.52

Changes in urine and faeces with jaundice

	Causes of jaundice		
Substance and site	**Haemolysis**	**Obstruction or cholestasis**	**Hepatocellular liver disease**
Urine			
Bilirubin (conjugated)	Normal*	Raised	Normal or raised
Urobilinogen	Raised	Absent or decreased	Normal or raised
Faeces			
Stercobilinogen	Raised	Absent or decreased	Normal
Causes	Haemologytic anaemia	Extrahepatic biliary obstruction (e.g. gallstones, carcinoma of pancreas or bile duct, strictures of the bile duct), intrahepatic cholestasis (e.g. drugs, recurrent jaundice of pregnancy)	Hepatitis, cirrhosis, drugs, venous obstruction

*Unconjugated bilirubin levels are elevated in the serum.

TABLE 14.2

T&O'C ESSENTIALS

1. When examining the abdomen, it is important to position the patient flat. While palpating, consider the underlying organs that are present when abnormalities are detected.
2. If an abdominal mass is found, characterise it, then pay special attention to the liver, rectal examination and supraclavicular nodes.
3. A left upper quadrant mass may be a spleen or a kidney. Remember that one cannot get above the spleen and that the spleen is not ballottable.
4. If the liver and spleen are enlarged, examine for other signs of chronic liver disease.
5. If you feel the liver, it may not be enlarged (check the upper border). You may feel an enlarged left lobe only in the epigastrium.
6. An inguinal hernia bulges above the crease of the groin, whereas a femoral hernia bulges into the medial end of the groin crease.
7. Draining lymph node groups must be examined carefully.
8. A gastrointestinal system examination is incomplete without a rectal examination.
9. Examination of the urine is an important extension of the physical examination.

OSCE REVISION TOPICS (see the OCSE video The GI examination [no. 4] at Student CONSULT) – THE GASTROINTESTINAL EXAMINATION

Use these topics, which commonly occur in the OSCE, to help with revision.

1. Please examine this man for signs of chronic liver disease. (pp 230, 274)
2. This woman has had abdominal distension. Please examine her for ascites. (p 258)
3. Please examine this man with chronic liver disease and decide whether there are signs of portal hypertension. (p 274)
4. This man has found a lump in his groin. Please examine him. (p 262)
5. Explain how you would perform a rectal examination. (p 264)

References

1. Sibarte V, Shanahan F. Clinical examination of the gastrointestinal system in the 21st century—is the emphasis right? *Am J Gastroenterol* 2004; 99:1874–1875.
2. Walton S, Bennett JR. Skin and gullet. *Gut* 1991; 32:694–697. An excellent review of skin signs in gastroenterology.
3. Beitman RG, Rost SS, Roth JL. Oral manifestations of gastrointestinal disease. *Dig Dis Sci* 1981; 26:741–747. A detailed review.
4. Naylor CD. The rational clinical examination. Physical examination of the liver. *JAMA* 1994; 271:1859–1865. A valuable review of technique. Palpation is probably superior to percussion (in part because the midclavicular line is a 'wandering landmark'). Auscultation is usually of minimal value.
5. McGee S, *Evidence-based physical diagnosis*, 3rd edn. St Louis: Saunders, 2012.
6. Fink HA, Lederle FA, Roth CS et al. The accuracy of physical examination to detect abdominal aortic aneurysm. *Arch Intern Med* 2000; 160:833–836.
7. Chervu A, Clagett GP, Valentine RJ et al. Role of physical examination in detection of abdominal aortic aneurysms. *Surgery* 1995; 117:454–457.
8. Thomson WH, Francis DM. Abdominal wall tenderness: a useful sign in the acute abdomen. *Lancet* 1977; 2:1053–1054. Although abdominal wall pain can be recognised when the patient tenses the abdominal wall muscles, intraperitoneal inflammation can cause a false-positive sign.
9. Srinivasan R, Greenbaum DS. Chronic abdominal wall pain: a frequently overlooked problem. Practical approach to diagnosis and management. *Am J Gastroenterol* 2002; 97:824–830.
10. Editorial. Abdominal wall tenderness test: could Carnett cut costs? *Lancet* 1991; 337:1134.
11. Williams JW Jr, Simel DL. The rational clinical examination. Does this patient have ascites? How to divine fluid in the abdomen. *JAMA* 1992; 267:2645–2648. This review provides information on the discriminant value of signs. Bulging flanks, shifting dullness and a fluid wave are each reasonably sensitive and specific. The presence of ascites is more easily predicted than its absence.
12. Gupta K, Dhawan A, Abel C et al. A re-evaluation of the scratch test for locating the liver edge. *BMC Gastroenterol* 2013; 13:35.
13. Goodsall TM, Flynn P, Attia JR. The scratch test for determining the inferior hepatic margin. *MJA* 2017; 206:386–387. Excellent description of this test (and a linked video).
14. Muris JW, Starmans R, Wolfs GG et al. The diagnostic value of rectal examination. *Fam Pract* 1993; 10:34–37. A useful procedure in patients with rectal or prostatic symptoms. Based on a literature review but studies in general practice are lacking.
15. Talley NJ. How to do and interpret a rectal examination in gastroenterology. *Am J Gastroenterol* 2008; 108:802–803.
16. Dobben AC, Terra MP, Deutekom M et al. Anal inspection and digital rectal examination compared to anorectal physiology tests and endoanal ultrasonography in evaluating faecal incontinence. *Int J Colorectal Dis* 2007; 22:783–790.
17. Longstreth GF. Checking for 'the occult' with a finger: a procedure of little value. *J Clin Gastroenterol* 1988; 10:133–134. A faecal occult blood test from the glove after rectal examination has too many false-positive and false-negative results to be of value.

CHAPTER 15

Correlation of physical signs and gastrointestinal disease

Bellyache; the colic or pain in the bowels. SAMUEL JOHNSON, A Dictionary of the English Language (1775)

EXAMINATION OF THE ACUTE ABDOMEN

It is very important to try to determine whether a patient who presents with acute abdominal pain requires an urgent operation or whether careful observation with reassessment is the best course of action.[1] Note whether the patient has received pain relief (usually with an opiate)—pain relief should not usually be withheld and does not alter the signs sufficiently to lead to misdiagnosis.[2]

First, take note of the *general appearance* of the patient. The patient who is obviously distressed with pain or who looks unwell often is, and conversely some reassurance can be gained if a patient does not look sick and appears comfortable.

Assess the patient's *vital signs* immediately and recheck these at frequent intervals. Signs of reduced circulating blood volume and dehydration—including:

- tachycardia
- postural hypotension
- tachypnoea
- vasoconstriction
- sweating

are of great concern. These signs, when associated with abdominal pain, are usually an indication of substantial intra-abdominal blood loss (such as a ruptured aortic aneurysm), substantial fluid losses (e.g. due to acute pancreatitis) or septic shock (as with a perforated viscus or abscess).

Take the patient's temperature.

Inspect the abdomen (see Fig. 15.1). Look particularly for lack of movement with respiration, with splinting of the abdominal wall muscles. If there is a history of possible blunt abdominal trauma look for a seatbelt sign (bruising in the distribution of a seatbelt).[3]

Note any abdominal distension, visible peristalsis or other lumps and masses, without forgetting the groin region and hernias. Note also any abdominal scars and enquire as to their nature and age.

Palpate very gently. The presence or absence of peritonism is first assessed. Peritonism is an inflammation that causes pain when peritoneal surfaces are moved relative to each other (see Good signs guide 15.1). Traditionally, rebound tenderness is used to assess whether peritonism is present or not. However, if peritonism is present, this test is far more uncomfortable (and cruel) than eliciting tenderness to light percussion. If the patient is extremely apprehensive, ask him or her first to cough; the reaction will be a guide to the degree of peritonism and also its location. Palpation is then continued slowly, but more deeply if possible and if masses are sought. Do

GOOD SIGNS GUIDE 15.1
Peritonitis

Sign	LR+	LR−
ABDOMINAL EXAMINATION		
Guarding	2.3	0.54
Rigidity	4.4	0.84
Rebound tenderness	2.0	0.42
Abnormal bowel sounds	1.4	0.89
RECTAL EXAMINATION		
Rectal tenderness	1.2	0.91
OTHER TESTS		
Positive abdominal wall tenderness	0.08	1.9

CHAPTER 15 CORRELATION OF PHYSICAL SIGNS AND GASTROINTESTINAL DISEASE

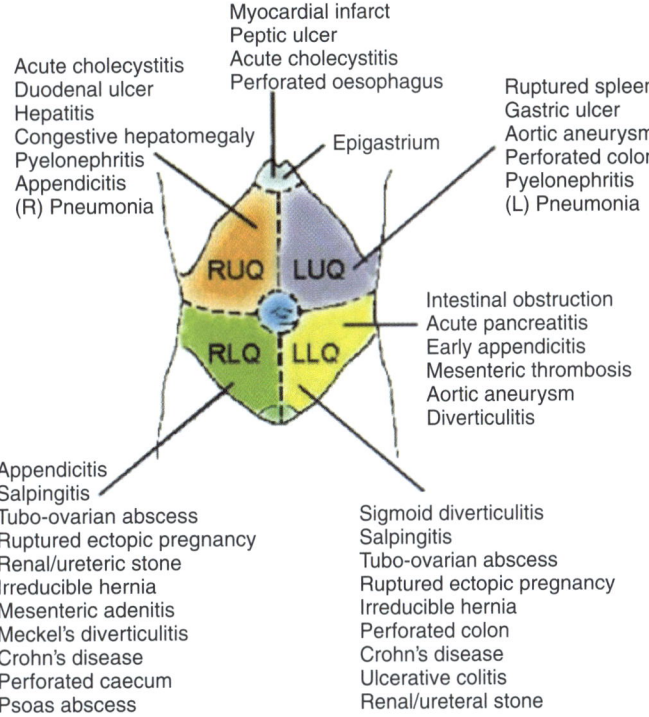

Differential diagnosis of the acute abdomen

FIGURE 15.1

not forget to palpate for the pulsatile mass of a ruptured aneurysm. This may be quite indistinct.

> **T&O'C ESSENTIAL**
>
> *Look repeatedly at the patient's face during palpation to ensure the examination is not causing distress.*

Then perform light *percussion* over areas of tenderness. If generalised peritonitis is present, this almost invariably necessitates a surgical approach, with the notable exception of acute pancreatitis.

Examine for hernias. The presence of a hernia does not necessarily mean that this is the cause of pathology, as they are quite common. However, a tender or irreducible hernia is more likely to be of significance, particularly if this has only very recently been noticed by the patient or has recently become tender.

Auscultation is now performed. In the presence of a bowel obstruction, bowel sounds (see Good signs guide 15.2) will be louder, more frequent and high-pitched.

GOOD SIGNS GUIDE 15.2
Acute bowel obstruction

Sign	LR+	LR−
INSPECTION OF THE ABDOMEN		
Visible peristalsis	18.8	0.94
Abdominal distension	9.7	0.40
ABDOMINAL EXAMINATION		
Guarding	1.0	0.98
Rigidity	1.2	1.0
Rebound tenderness	0.86	1.1
AUSCULTATION		
Increased (obstructed) bowel sounds	5.8	0.61
Abnormal bowel sounds	2.7	0.54
RECTAL EXAMINATION		
Rectal tenderness	0.75	1.0

In an ileus from any cause, bowel sounds are usually reduced or absent.

Rectal and vaginal examinations may be important but the findings are not very helpful for the diagnosis of appendicitis or obstruction; note any tenderness (and its location), masses or blood loss. Clinical findings that increase the likelihood of an ectopic pregnancy include tenderness (cervical motion tenderness [LR, 4.9] and adnexal tenderness [LR, 1.9]) and a mass (adnexal mass [LR, 2.4]).[4]

Per rectal blood should make the examiner think of acute colitis (e.g. Crohn's disease, ulcerative colitis, ischaemic colitis or infectious colitis) or of mesenteric ischaemia. A purulent vaginal discharge suggests salpingitis.

Urinalysis may show glycosuria and ketonuria in diabetic ketoacidosis (which can cause acute abdominal pain), haematuria in renal colic, bilirubinuria in cholangitis or proteinuria in pyelonephritis.

Examine the *respiratory system* for signs of consolidation, a pleural rub or pleural effusion, and examine the *cardiovascular system* for atrial fibrillation (a major cause of embolism to a mesenteric artery). Examine the *back* for evidence of spinal disease that may radiate to the abdomen. Remember that herpes zoster may cause abdominal pain before the typical vesicles erupt.

Consider the symptoms and signs of appendicitis[1] (see Good signs guide 15.3). Malaise and fever are usually associated with abdominal pain, which is at first worst in the hypogastrium and then moves to the right iliac fossa. The examination will often reveal tenderness and guarding in the right iliac fossa. The pain and tenderness are usually maximal over *McBurney's*[a] *point*. McBurney described this point as 3.8 to 5 centimetres along a line from the anterior superior iliac spine to the umbilicus. *Rovsing's*[b] *sign* is another way of testing rebound tenderness. Press over the patient's left lower quadrant, then release quickly; this causes pain in the right iliac fossa. The *psoas sign* is positive when the patient lies on the left side and the clinician attempts to extend the right hip. If this is painful and resisted, the sign is positive. When the appendix causes pelvic inflammation, rectal examination evokes tenderness on the right side. These signs are of variable usefulness.

Remember that in elderly patients these signs may be reduced or absent.

Acute abdomen after blunt trauma

You must assess for intra-abdominal injuries after blunt trauma to the abdomen, such as is common after a motor vehicle accident. A careful clinical assessment to look for shock and abdominal signs should be followed by targeted investigations, most notably an emergency abdominal ultrasound.[3]

Take the patient's pulse and blood pressure. Hypotension is an indicator of intra-abdominal injury (+ve LR, 5.2). Look for bruising. Note the presence of the seatbelt sign from trauma with bruising over the area of impact (LR range for injury, 5.6–9.9). Also look for abdominal distension (LR, 3.8). Palpate for rebound tenderness (LR, 6.5) and guarding (LR, 3.7). Note that no abdominal tenderness on palpation is insufficient to exclude intra-abdominal injury (summary LR, 0.61).

Do an emergency ultrasound as this is more accurate than physical examination. The presence of intraperitoneal fluid or organ injury on bedside ultrasound assessment indicates the need for urgent surgical consultation (LR, 30). A normal ultrasound result is strongly reassuring (LR, 0.26).[3]

LIVER DISEASE

There are many signs that point to chronic liver disease.

GOOD SIGNS GUIDE 15.3
Appendicitis

Sign	LR+	LR−
VITAL SIGNS		
Fever	1.9	0.58
ABDOMINAL EXAMINATION		
Severe right lower quadrant pain	7.3	0.2
McBurney's point tenderness	3.4	0.4
Rovsing's sign	1.1–6.3	0–0.86
RECTAL EXAMINATION		
Rectal tenderness	0.83–5.3	0.36–1.1
OTHER		
Psoas sign	2.4	0.9

(Adapted from Simel DL, Rennie D. *The rational clinical examination: evidence-based diagnosis*. New York: McGraw-Hill, 2009, Table 5.3.)

---

[a] Charles McBurney (1845–1913), a New York surgeon, described this sign to the New York Surgical Society in 1889.
[b] Thorkild Rovsing (1862–1937), a professor of surgery in Copenhagen.

Signs

- **Hands:** leuconychia, clubbing, palmar erythema, bruising, asterixis.
- **Face:** jaundice, scratch marks, spider naevi, fetor hepaticus.
- **Chest:** gynaecomastia, loss of body hair, spider naevi, bruising, pectoral muscle wasting.
- **Abdomen:** hepatosplenomegaly, ascites, signs of portal hypertension, testicular atrophy.
- **Legs:** oedema, muscle wasting, bruising.
- **Fever:** may occur in up to one-third of patients with advanced cirrhosis (particularly when this is secondary to alcohol) or if there is infected ascites.

Physical findings including spider naevi (LR, 4.3), and the presence of ascites (LR, 7.2), and selected screening tests, most notably a low platelet count (<160×10(3)/μL, LR, 6.3), are useful as indicators of cirrhosis in suspected liver disease cases.[5] The presence of two or more of the following signs strongly suggests cirrhosis: (1) spider naevi, (2) palmar erythema, (3) ascites, (4) hepatomegaly (firm liver), (5) abnormal collateral veins on the abdomen, and (6) hepatic encephalopathy. The absence of hepatomegaly suggests cirrhosis is less likely (LR, 0.37). The likelihood ratios are summarised in Good signs guide 15.4.

PORTAL HYPERTENSION

Signs

- **Splenomegaly:** correlates poorly with the degree of portal hypertension.
- **Collateral veins:** haematemesis (from oesophageal or gastric varices).
- **Ascites.**

Causes

1. Cirrhosis of the liver.
2. Other causes:
   a. *Presinusoidal:* (i) portal vein compression (e.g. lymphoma, carcinoma); (ii) intravascular clotting (e.g. in polycythaemia); (iii) umbilical vein phlebitis.
   b. *Intrahepatic:* (i) sarcoid, lymphoma or leukaemic infiltrates; (ii) congenital hepatic fibrosis.
   c. *Postsinusoidal:* (i) hepatic vein outflow obstruction (Budd–Chiari syndrome) may be idiopathic, or caused by myeloproliferative disease, cancer (kidney, pancreas, liver), the contraceptive pill or pregnancy, paroxysmal nocturnal haemoglobinuria (PNH), fibrous membrane, trauma, schistosomiasis; (ii) veno-occlusive disease; (iii) constrictive pericarditis; (iv) chronic cardiac failure.

HEPATIC ENCEPHALOPATHY

Grading

Grade 0	Normal mental state.
Grade 1	Mental changes (lack of awareness, anxiety, euphoria, reduced attention span, impaired ability to add and subtract).
Grade 2	Lethargy, disorientation (for time), personality changes, inappropriate behaviour.
Grade 3	Stupor, but responsive to stimuli; gross disorientation, confusion.
Grade 4	Coma.

Causes

These include:

- acute liver failure (e.g. postviral hepatitis, alcoholic hepatitis)
- cirrhosis
- chronic portosystemic encephalopathy (e.g. from a portacaval shunt).

GOOD SIGNS GUIDE 15.4
Cirrhosis

Sign	LR+	LR−
Spider naevi	4.3*	0.61
Palmar erythema	5.0	0.59
Hepatomegaly (hard)	3.3	0.37*
Encephalopathy	10.0*	0.86
Ascites	7.2*	0.69
Prominent abdominal veins	11.0*	0.72

*Most useful.
(Adapted from Udell JA, Wang CS, Tinmouth J et al. Does this patient with liver disease have cirrhosis? *JAMA* 2012; 307:832–842.)

Encephalopathy may be precipitated by:

- diarrhoea, diuretics or vomiting (resulting in hypokalaemia, which may increase renal ammonia and other toxin production, or alkalosis, which may increase the amount of ammonia and other toxins that cross the blood–brain barrier)
- gastrointestinal bleeding or a relatively high-protein diet (causing an acute increase in nitrogenous contents in the bowel)
- infection (e.g. urinary tract, chest or spontaneous bacterial peritonitis)
- acute liver cell decompensation (e.g. from an alcoholic binge or a hepatoma)
- sedatives
- metabolic disturbances such as hypoglycaemia.

DYSPHAGIA

Dysphagia (difficulty in swallowing) and odynophagia (pain on swallowing) are important symptoms of underlying organic disease. It is important to examine such patients carefully for likely causes, particularly cancer (see List 13.2, p 221).

Signs

- **General inspection.** Note weight loss, due to decreased food intake or oesophageal cancer per se.
- **The hands.** Inspect the nails for koilonychia and the palmar creases for pallor indicative of anaemia. Iron deficiency anaemia can be associated with an upper oesophageal web, which is a thin structure consisting of mucosa and submucosa but not muscle. Iron deficiency anaemia and dysphagia due to an upper oesophageal web is called the Plummer–Vinson[c] (or sometimes the Paterson–Brown–Kelly[d]) syndrome. Also examine the hands for signs of scleroderma.
- **The mouth.** Inspect the mucosa for ulceration or infection (e.g. candidiasis), which can cause odynophagia. Examine the lower cranial nerves for evidence of bulbar or pseudobulbar palsy.
- **The neck.** Palpate the supraclavicular nodes, which may occasionally be involved with oesophageal cancer; examine for evidence of retrosternal thyroid enlargement. A mass on the left side of the neck that is accompanied by gurgling sounds may rarely be caused by a Zenker's[e] diverticulum, an outpouching of the posterior hypopharyngeal wall.
- **The lungs.** Examine for evidence of aspiration into the lungs (due to overflow of retained material, gastro-oesophageal reflux or, rarely, the development of a tracheo-oesophageal reflux from oesophageal cancer).
- **The abdomen.** Feel for hepatomegaly due to secondary deposits from oesophageal cancer and for an epigastric mass from a gastric cancer; perform a rectal examination to exclude melaena (albeit uncommon with oesophageal disease).

GASTROINTESTINAL BLEEDING

Haematemesis, melaena or massive rectal bleeding are dramatic signs of gastrointestinal haemorrhage.[6] It is important in such a case to assess the amount of blood loss and attempt to determine the likely site of bleeding. Haematemesis indicates bleeding from a site proximal to, or in, the duodenum.

Assessing degree of blood loss

First take the pulse rate and the blood pressure with the patient lying and sitting. As a general rule, loss of 1.5 litres or more of blood volume over a few hours results in a fall in cardiac output, causing hypotension and tachycardia. A pulse rate of more than 100 beats per minute, a systolic blood pressure of less than 100 mmHg or a 15 mmHg postural fall in systolic blood pressure suggests severe recent blood loss. The signs depend to some extent on the state of the patient's cardiovascular system. Those who have pre-existing cardiovascular disease will become shocked much earlier than young, fit patients with a normal cardiovascular system.

---

[c] Henry Plummer (1874–1936), a physician at the Mayo Clinic, described the syndrome in 1912; Porter Vinson (1890–1959), a physician at Medical College Virginia, described the syndrome in 1919.

[d] Donald Paterson (1863–1939), a Cardiff otolaryngologist, and Adam Brown-Kelly (1865–1941), a Glasgow otolaryngologist, described this syndrome in 1919.

[e] Friedrich Albert Zenker (1825–1898), a Munich pathologist.

Once signs of shock are present, massive blood loss has occurred. These signs include:
- peripheral cyanosis with cold extremities
- clammy skin
- dyspnoea and air hunger
- anxiety.

The blood pressure is low, with a compensating tachycardia, and urine output is reduced or absent. These are ominous signs in patients with gastrointestinal haemorrhage. Urgent resuscitative measures must be instituted.

Determining the possible bleeding site

The causes of acute gastrointestinal haemorrhage are listed in Table 13.1 (see p 225).

Examine the patient with *acute upper gastrointestinal bleeding* for signs of chronic liver disease and portal hypertension. Part of the assessment should include inspection of the vomitus and stools and a rectal examination (critical). Melaena on rectal examination definitely increases the likelihood that a patient has an upper gastrointestinal bleed (LR, 25).[6]

Remember that, of patients with chronic liver disease and upper gastrointestinal bleeding, only about half are bleeding from varices. The others are usually bleeding from peptic ulceration (either acute or chronic). Examine also for evidence of a bleeding diathesis (generalised bruising or petechiae).

Finally, examine the patient for any evidence of skin lesions that can be associated with vascular anomalies in the gastrointestinal tract, although these are rare (see Table 13.1 on p 225 and Table 14.1 on p 233). For example, pseudoxanthoma elasticum is an autosomal recessive disorder of elastic fibres that results in xanthoma-like yellowish nodules, particularly in the axillae or neck (see Fig. 15.2). These patients may also have angioid streaks of the optic fundus and angiomatous malformations of blood vessels that can bleed into the gastrointestinal tract. Ehlers–Danlos syndrome is a group of connective tissue disorders resulting in fragile and hyperextensible skin (see Fig. 15.3). In a number of types, blood vessels are involved. Type IV is characterised by gastrointestinal tract bleeding, spontaneous bowel perforation, but minimal skin hyperelasticity and minimal joint hyperextension.

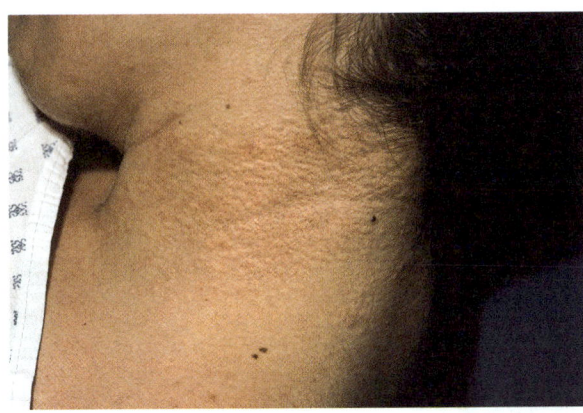

Pseudoxanthoma elasticum (axillae or neck)
(From Paller AS, Mancini AJ. *Hurwitz clinical pediatric dermatology*, 4th edn. Philadelphia: Saunders 2011.)

FIGURE 15.2

Examine the patient with *acute lower gastrointestinal bleeding* as described above, paying close attention to the abdominal examination and the rectal examination. Inspect the stools and test them for blood. Note that the finding of blood clots in the stool (LR, 0.05) decreases the likelihood of bleeding from the upper gut[6] and directs you to the colon (but this is not an absolute rule).

INFLAMMATORY BOWEL DISEASE

Inflammatory bowel disease refers to two chronic idiopathic diseases of the gastrointestinal tract: ulcerative colitis and Crohn's disease.

Ulcerative colitis

In the gastrointestinal tract only the large bowel is affected. Occasionally the terminal ileum can be secondarily involved (backwash ileitis). The disease almost always involves the rectum and may extend, without skip areas, to involve a variable part of the colon.

- **Abdominal signs:** if there is proctitis only, there are usually no abnormal external findings (except at colonoscopy and biopsy). Occasionally, anal fissures are present; with colitis, in the uncomplicated case the abdominal examination

Ehlers–Danlos syndrome: (a) arms; (b) hands. Abnormal elasticity of the skin is typical of the Ehlers–Danlos syndrome. The skin may be greatly stretched and takes much longer than normal to return to its normal position. It is also more fragile than normal. Joint hypermobility occurs in type III Ehlers–Danlos syndrome

FIGURE 15.3

Erythema nodosum

(From McDonald FS, ed. *Mayo Clinic images in internal medicine*, with permission. © Mayo Clinic Scientific Press and CRC Press. Reproduced by permission of Taylor and Francis Group, LLC, a division of Informa plc.)

FIGURE 15.4

may be normal or there may be tenderness and guarding over the affected colon.

- **Signs of complications:** local signs include the following:
  - *toxic dilation (megacolon)*—one of the most feared complications in which there are signs of distension, generalised guarding and rigidity (peritonism), pyrexia and tachycardia
  - *massive bleeding or perforation*
  - *carcinoma*—there is an increased incidence of colonic cancer in extensive, long-standing ulcerative colitis.
- Systemic signs include:
  - *chronic liver disease*—primary sclerosing cholangitis or cirrhosis
  - *anaemia*—due to chronic disease per se, or blood loss, or autoimmune haemolysis
  - *arthritis*—there may be a peripheral non-deforming arthropathy affecting particularly the knees, ankles and wrists (10%), and there may be signs of ankylosing spondylitis in 3% of affected patients
  - *skin manifestations:* erythema nodosum (2%) consists of tender red nodules usually on the shins (see Fig. 15.4); pyoderma gangrenosum (rare) starts as a tender, red raised area that becomes bullous and ulcerates (see Fig. 15.5)—it may occur anywhere but is often on the anterior aspects of the legs; mouth ulcers are common and are due to aphthous ulceration (5%); finger clubbing may be present
  - *ocular changes* include conjunctivitis, iritis and episcleritis (see Fig. 15.6), which are strongly associated with arthritis and skin rash. (*Conjunctivitis* is an inflammation of the conjunctiva, which then appears red and swollen; the eye itself is not tender. *Iritis* is an inflammation of the iris with central scleral

CHAPTER 15 CORRELATION OF PHYSICAL SIGNS AND GASTROINTESTINAL DISEASE

Pyoderma gangrenosum

(From Misiewicz JJ, Bantrum CI, Cotton PB et al. *Slide atlas of gastroenterology*. London: Gower Medical Publishing, 1985.)

FIGURE 15.5

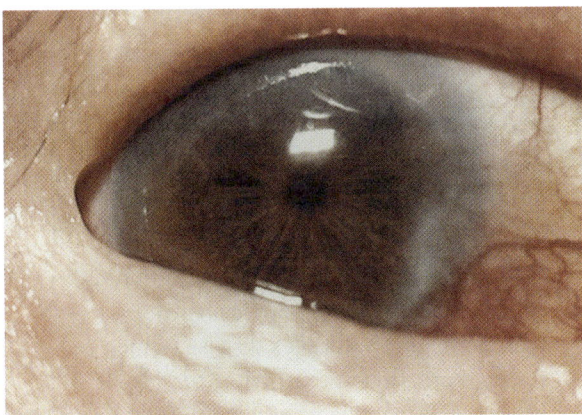

Iritis and episcleritis

(From Guerrant DL. *Tropical infectious diseases: principles, pathogens and practice*, 3rd edn. Philadelphia: Saunders, 2011.)

FIGURE 15.6

injection, which radiates out from the pupil; the eye is tender. *Episcleritis* is a nodule of inflammation on the scleral surface.)

Crohn's disease

The whole of the gastrointestinal tract may be affected from the mouth to the anus. However, most commonly the terminal ileum, with or without the colon, is involved.

- **Abdominal signs:** if the condition affects only the terminal ileum there are often no abnormal findings, although tenderness, fullness or a mass (either soft or firm) in the right iliac fossa may be present. Occasionally, there may be signs of an abdominal abscess; these patients may have a high swinging fever, localised tenderness, a palpable mass and evidence of bowel obstruction (pain, vomiting and constipation with dehydration, abdominal distension and tenderness, and an empty rectum). Anal disease is common, including skin tags, fissures, fistulae and abscesses. Colonic involvement produces the same signs as ulcerative colitis.
- **Signs of complications:** these are similar to those of ulcerative colitis with the following exceptions:
  - *liver disease*—primary sclerosing cholangitis is less common
  - *osteomalacia* and *osteoporosis*, which may occur in patients with extensive terminal ileal involvement, results in bone tenderness and fracture
  - *signs of malabsorption* may be present
  - *finger clubbing* is more common
  - *signs of gastrointestinal malignancy* (colonic carcinoma); the incidence is increased if the colon is inflamed
  - the incidence of *gallstones and renal stones* is increased
  - *renal disease* due to pyelonephritis, hydronephrosis or very rarely secondary amyloidosis may occur.

MALABSORPTION AND NUTRITIONAL STATUS

Numerous diseases can cause maldigestion or malabsorption of food. Fat, protein and/or carbohydrate absorption may be affected.

Signs

- **General:** wasting (protein and fat malabsorption), folds of loose skin (recent weight loss), pallor (anaemia) or pigmentation (e.g. as in Whipple's[f] disease).
- **Stools:** steatorrhoea (pale, bulky and offensive stools).
- **Mouth:** glossitis and angular stomatitis (deficiency in vitamin B_2, vitamin B_6, vitamin B_{12}, folate or niacin) or intraoral purpura (vitamin K deficiency).
- **Limbs:** bruising (vitamin K deficiency), oedema (protein deficiency), peripheral neuropathy (vitamin B_{12} or thiamine deficiency), bone pain (vitamin D deficiency).
- **Signs suggesting the underlying cause:** in the abdomen these include scars from previous surgery, such as a gastrectomy, operations for Crohn's disease or massive small-bowel resection; on the skin may be found dermatitis herpetiformis (itchy red lumps on the extensor surfaces; see Fig. 15.7)—this condition is strongly associated with coeliac disease and the histocompatibility antigen HLA-DQ2 or DQ8; there may be signs of chronic liver disease, or signs of inflammatory bowel disease.

Causes

Common causes include coeliac disease, chronic pancreatitis and a previous gastrectomy.

Classification of malabsorption

- **Lipolytic phase defects** (pancreatic enzyme deficiency): (1) chronic pancreatitis; (2) cystic fibrosis.
- **Micellar phase defects** (bile salt deficiency): (1) extrahepatic biliary obstruction; (2) chronic liver disease; (3) bacterial overgrowth; (4) terminal ileal disease, such as Crohn's disease or resection.

Dermatitis herpetiformis: pruritic papulovesicles over extensor surfaces in coeliac disease

(From Fitzpatrick JE, Morelli JG. *Dermatology secrets plus*, 4th edn. Maryland Heights, MO: Mosby 2010.)

FIGURE 15.7

- **Mucosal defects** (diseased epithelial lining): (1) coeliac disease; (2) tropical sprue; (3) lymphoma; (4) Whipple's disease (which causes pigmentation and arthritis; see Fig. 15.8); (5) bowel ischaemia or resection; (6) amyloidosis; (7) hypogammaglobulinaemia; (8) HIV infection.
- **Delivery phase defects** (inability to transport fat out of cells to lymphatics): (1) intestinal lymphangiectasia; (2) abetalipoproteinaemia; (3) carcinomatous infiltration of lymphatics.

---

[f] George Hoyt Whipple (1878–1976), a Baltimore pathologist, described this rare disease characterised by diarrhoea, arthralgia, central nervous system signs and pigmentation. He shared the 1934 Nobel Prize for work on liver treatment in anaemia and coined the word *thalassaemia*.

CHAPTER 15 CORRELATION OF PHYSICAL SIGNS AND GASTROINTESTINAL DISEASE 281

Pigmentation in Whipple's disease

(From Schaller J, Carlson JA. Erythema nodosum-like lesions in treated whipple's disease. *Journal of the American Academy of Dermatology* Copyright © 2008, American Academy of Dermatology, Inc.)

FIGURE 15.8

T&O'C ESSENTIALS

1. In assessing for an acute abdomen percuss before palpation for peritonism.
2. Know the signs for chronic liver disease. Dupuytren's contracture is a sign of alcohol use or trauma, not chronic liver disease.
3. Look for signs of nutritional deficiency when assessing for gastrointestinal or liver disease.
4. Erythema nodosum or pyoderma gangrenosum may occur in ulcerative colitis or Crohn's disease.

References

1. Wagner JM, Mckinney WP, Carpenter JL. Does this patient have appendicitis? *JAMA* 1996; 276:1589–1594. A 'must read' that discusses the key symptoms and signs that help make the correct diagnosis.
2. Ranji SR, Goldman LE, Simel DL, Shojania KG. Do opiates affect the clinical evaluation of patients with acute abdominal pain? *JAMA* 2006; 296(14):1764–1774. The answer is no, not enough to withhold pain relief.
3. Nishijima DK, Simel DL, Wisner DH, Holmes JF. Does this adult patient have a blunt intra-abdominal injury? *JAMA* 2012; 307(14):1517–1527.
4. Crochet JR, Bastian LA, Chireau MV. Does this woman have an ectopic pregnancy?: the rational clinical examination systematic review. *JAMA* 2013; 309(16):1722–1729.
5. Udell JA, Wang CS, Tinmouth J et al. Does this patient with liver disease have cirrhosis? *JAMA* 2012; 307(8):832–842.
6. Srygley FD, Gerardo CJ, Tran T, Fisher DA. Does this patient have a severe upper gastrointestinal bleed? *JAMA* 2012; 307(10):1072–1079. Malaena on rectal examination suggests an upper gut bleed, but blood clots in stool are against an upper GI bleed. Do a rectal exam!

CHAPTER 16

A summary of the gastrointestinal examination and extending the gastrointestinal examination

Jaundice is a disease your friends diagnose. SIR WILLIAM OSLER (1849–1919)

The gastrointestinal examination: a suggested method

Gastrointestinal system examination

FIGURE 16.1

Lying flat (1 pillow)
1. General inspection
   Jaundice (liver disease)
   Pigmentation (haemochromatosis, Whipple's disease)
   Xanthomata (chronic cholestasis)
   Mental state (encephalopathy)
2. Nails
   Clubbing
   Leuconychia
   Palmar erythema
   Dupuytren's contractures (alcohol)
   Arthropathy
   Hepatic flap
3. Arms
   Spider naevi
   Bruising
   Wasting
   Scratch marks (chronic cholestasis)
4. Face
   Eyes
   Sclerae: jaundice, anaemia, iritis

TEXT BOX 16.1

The gastrointestinal examination: a suggested method *continued*

    Cornea: Kayser–Fleischer rings (Wilson's disease)
    Parotids (alcohol)
    Mouth
    Breath: fetor hepaticus
    Lips: stomatitis, leucoplakia, ulceration, localised pigmentation (Peutz–Jeghers syndrome), telangiectasia (hereditary haemorrhagic telangiectasia)
    Gums: gingivitis, bleeding, hypertrophy, pigmentation, monilia
    Tongue: atrophic glossitis, leucoplakia, ulceration
5. Cervical / axillary lymph nodes
6. Chest
    Gynaecomastia
    Spider naevi
    Body hair
7. Abdomen
    Inspect
    Scars
    Distension
    Prominent veins—determine direction of flow (caput Medusae; inferior vena cava obstruction)
    Striae
    Bruising
    Pigmentation
    Localised masses
    Visible peristalsis
    Palpate
    Superficial palpation—tenderness, rigidity, outline of any mass
    Deep palpation—organomegaly (liver, spleen, kidney), abnormal masses
    Roll onto right side (spleen)
    Percuss
    Liver, spleen
    Ascites—shifting dullness (if dull in flanks)
    Auscultate
    Bowel sounds
    Bruits, hums, rubs
8. Groin
    Testes
    Lymph nodes
    Hernial orifices (standing up)
9. Legs
    Bruising
    Oedema
    Neurological signs (alcohol)
10. Other
    Rectal examination—inspect (fistulae, tags, blood, mucus), palpate (masses)
    Urine analysis (bile)
    Cardiovascular system (cardiomyopathy, cardiac failure, constrictivepericarditis)
    Temperature chart (infection)

As with the other systems this examination will usually be targeted. However, it cannot be performed properly, even in a busy clinic, unless the patient lies down and removes sufficient clothing—if necessary in stages and with a chaperone.

Position the patient correctly with one pillow for the head and complete exposure of the abdomen. Look briefly at the **general appearance** and inspect particularly for signs of chronic liver disease.

Examine the patient's **hands**. Ask the patient to extend his or her arms and hands and look for the hepatic flap. Look also at the nails for clubbing and for white nails (leuconychia), and note any palmar erythema or Dupuytren's contractures. The arthropathy of haemochromatosis may also be present. Look now at the patient's **arms** for bruising, scratch marks and spider naevi.

Then go to the patient's **face**. Note any scleral abnormality (jaundice, anaemia or iritis). Look at the corneas for Kayser–Fleischer rings. Feel for parotid enlargement, then inspect the mouth with a torch and spatula for angular stomatitis, ulceration, telangiectasias and atrophic glossitis. Smell the breath for fetor hepaticus. Now look at the chest for spider naevi and in men for gynaecomastia and loss of body hair.

Inspect the patient's **abdomen** from the side, squatting to the patient's level. Large masses may be visible. Ask the patient to take slow, deep breaths and look especially for the hepatic, splenic and gallbladder outlines. Now stand up and look for scars, distension, prominent veins, striae, hernia, bruising and pigmentation.

Palpate lightly in each region for masses, having asked first whether any area is particularly tender. This will avoid causing the patient pain and may also provide a clue to a site of possible pathology. Next palpate each region more deeply; then feel specifically for hepatomegaly and splenomegaly. If there is hepatomegaly, confirm this with percussion and estimate the

TEXT BOX 16.1

Continued

The gastrointestinal examination: a suggested method *continued*

span. If no spleen is felt, percuss over the left costal margin in the left anterior axillary line during complete inspiration (dullness suggests splenomegaly). Always **roll** the patient onto the right side and palpate again if the spleen is not felt initially. Attempt now to feel the kidneys bimanually. Remember the important distinguishing features of a spleen as opposed to a kidney.

Percuss for ascites only if there is dullness in the flanks (and usually this will be obvious). If the abdomen is resonant right out to the flanks, do not roll the patient over. Otherwise test for shifting dullness. This is performed by percussing away from your side of the bed until you reach a dull note. Then **roll** the patient towards you and, after waiting a minute or so, begin percussing again for resonance.

By **auscultation** note the presence of bowel sounds. Next auscultate briefly over the liver, spleen and renal areas, listening for bruits, hums and rubs.

Examine the patient's **groin** next. Palpate for inguinal lymphadenopathy. Examine for hernias by asking the patient to stand and then cough. The testes should be palpated. Now look at the legs for oedema and bruising. Neurological examination of the **legs** may be indicated if there are signs of chronic liver disease.

If the **liver** is enlarged or cirrhosis is suspected ask the patient to sit up to 45° and estimate the jugular venous pressure. This will avoid missing constrictive pericarditis or chronic cardiac failure as a cause of liver disease. While the patient is sitting up, palpate in the supraclavicular fossae for **lymph nodes** and feel at the back for **sacral oedema**. If ascites is present, it is necessary to examine the chest for a pleural effusion.

If malignant disease is suspected, examine all lymph node groups, the breasts and the lungs.

A **rectal** examination should always be considered and specimens of the patient's vomitus or faeces should be inspected, if available and symptoms point to abnormalities. Perform a **urinalysis** (for bilirubin and urobilinogen, and glucose) and check the patient's **temperature**.

TEXT BOX 16.1

EXTENDING THE GASTROINTESTINAL EXAMINATION

Radiology, endoscopy, biochemical and special tests of function provide important diagnostic and prognostic information in gastrointestinal and liver diseases. An introduction to testing is provided here.

Endoscopy

Endoscopy allows the clinician to extend the physical examination directly into the gastrointestinal tract. The oesophagus, stomach and duodenum (second part) are usually easily reached by a standard gastroscope, while a colonoscope can reach into the terminal ileum. Small-bowel enteroscopy allows visualisation of the entire small intestine, although this remains technically challenging, but a small-bowel capsule is easily swallowed and provides images of the small intestine (e.g. to determine the cause of obscure gastrointestinal bleeding). An endoscopic ultrasound (where an ultrasound probe is passed through the endoscope biopsy channel) allows excellent imaging of the pancreas and biliary ducts.

Inspection is a critical endoscopy skill and a systematic approach is key to ensuring that pathology is identified correctly.

Indications for upper endoscopy include dysphagia (although a barium swallow may be considered first to help guide endoscopic management), odynophagia, gastrointestinal bleeding, recurrent vomiting, weight loss and heartburn or dyspepsia resistant to treatment. The procedure is also used to determine whether oesophageal varices are present so that prophylactic treatment can be considered. Colonoscopy is used to screen for colon cancer and investigate unexplained lower gastrointestinal symptoms.

Informed consent is always required prior to the procedure as there are well-defined risks (most notably perforation, bleeding and anaesthetic risks).

Relative contraindications to endoscopy include intestinal perforation, severe cardiorespiratory disease or obstructive sleep apnoea (as the sedation risk is increased), a recent myocardial infarction (last 6 months) and anticoagulation (because of the bleeding risk, especially if biopsies are required).

Biochemistry

Blood testing for liver enzymes provides some useful guidance when approaching possible liver disease. As a simple rule (although no rule is absolute in medicine), always confirm an isolated abnormal blood test value before marching on to do more intensive investigations.

With liver inflammation (e.g. hepatitis), the liver transaminase enzymes alanine transaminase (ALT [SGPT]) and aspartate aminotransferase (AST [SGOT]) both increase. ALT is more liver specific (ALT-Liver) and is usually higher than AST in acute viral hepatitis. In alcoholic liver disease, AST is higher than ALT (the ratio is about 3:1 because alcohol specifically injures mitochondria and AST comes from mitochondria).

Another indicator of liver dysfunction is the serum alkaline phosphatase (SAP), but this enzyme may arise from the liver (e.g. bile duct obstruction) or bone (e.g. metastases). If the gamma glutamyl transpeptidase (GGT) is also increased, this suggests a liver origin, as this enzyme rises in parallel with SAP. An ultrasound is usually indicated to rule out dilated bile ducts (e.g. from cancer).

A low albumin level may indicate that the liver is not synthesising this protein. An elevated international normalised ratio (INR) occurs if there is vitamin K deficiency (e.g. because the liver is not synthesising clotting factors II, VII, IX and X).

If the liver transaminases are increased, the cause needs to be identified. Review the alcohol history. Check the body mass index (e.g. fatty liver causing inflammation: non-alcoholic steatohepatitis). Testing for hepatitis A, B or C and searching for diseases that cause infiltration of the liver (e.g. iron overload in haemochromatosis, by testing the serum ferritin and iron studies) are further steps to consider based on the clinical picture.

IMAGING THE GASTROINTESTINAL SYSTEM

The three modalities most commonly used in abdominal imaging are abdominal X-rays Figs 16.2–16.7), computed tomography (CT) scans (Figs 16.8–16.9) and ultrasound (Figs 16.9–16.10).

Abdominal X-rays (see the OCSE X-ray library at Student CONSULT)

Indications

Plain film radiographs of the abdomen are indicated initially to identify three conditions: bowel obstruction, intraperitoneal free gas and radio-opaque calculi. Up to 50% of abdominal aortic aneurysms, 90% of renal calculi and at least 10% of gallstones have enough calcium to be detectable on plain films. Occasionally, the degree of faecal loading may also be assessed with an abdominal X-ray. Non-specific abdominal pain should not be an indication for an abdominal X-ray examination.

Technique of examination

The routine radiographic assessment of the abdomen includes supine AP, erect AP and PA erect chest X-rays. If the patient is unable to be placed upright, a left lateral decubitus is substituted. The term **KUB** is occasionally applied to an abdominal X-ray, denoting Kidneys, Ureters and Bladder. All three images should be interpreted systematically.

Principles of interpretation

Interpretation of the plain radiograph requires knowledge of basic anatomy and pathological processes. The soft-tissue density of the abdominal organs is similar to that of water. Therefore, they are not usually visible unless outlined by fat or adjacent gas. For example, fluid-filled bowel is not visible, but the bowel walls are outlined by the contained gas.

The five fundamental radiographic densities that need to be interpreted are gas, fat, solid organ, calcification and metal (see Table 16.1). Because of the intrinsic lack of contrast in the abdomen, radio-opaque contrast media are used to highlight various organs. Barium meals, barium enemas, intravenous urograms and arteriograms are contrast studies.

Reading an abdominal X-ray

As with chest X-rays, the name and date should be checked. The left and right sides should be easily distinguished by the stomach gas on the left and the

Fundamental plain abdominal X-ray densities	
Content	**Density**
Gas	Very black
Fat	Black
Solid organ	Grey
Calcification	White
Metal	Very white

TABLE 16.1

Free peritoneal gas.

The erect chest X-ray is superior to an erect abdominal film for the demonstration of free gas. On the erect chest X-ray, free peritoneal gas is seen below the hemidiaphragm (black arrows). The free gas on the left must be distinguished from gas in the gastric fundus (open arrow). This free gas (black arrow) on the left is crescentic in shape because it outlines the spleen and lies at the apex of the hemidiaphragm. It indicates a perforation of a hollow abdominal viscus unless there has been recent surgery or penetrating trauma

(From Leal RF. Free peritoneal perforation in a patient with Crohn's disease. Report of a case. *International Journal of Surgery Case Reports* 2013; 4(3):322–324.)

FIGURE 16.2

triangular bulky soft tissue of the liver seen in the right hypochondrium.

Review the following:
- **Boundaries:** diaphragm, psoas muscles, extraperitoneal fat ('flank lines').
- **Bones:** lower ribs and costal cartilages, lumbar spine, pelvis.
- **Hollow viscera gas:** gas outlining the stomach, small bowel and large bowel.
- **Solid organs:** size of liver, spleen and kidneys.
- **Pelvic organs:** bladder size.
- **Vascular:** aortic calcification.
- **Abnormalities:** renal or biliary calculi, dilated bowel, free peritoneal gas (see Fig. 16.2).
- **Bowel gas pattern:** supine films are taken in most conditions to show the distribution of the bowel gas. In patients with an acute abdomen, a horizontal beam film, usually an erect view, is also taken to show air–fluid levels. With obstruction, there is an accumulation of fluid and gas proximally. In inflammatory or ischaemic colitis, the swollen bowel mucosa will be outlined by gas ('thumb-printing').
- **Bowel dilation:** when an ileus (see Fig. 16.3) or obstruction (see Figs 16.4 and 16.5) is present, it is possible to distinguish small- from large-bowel dilation. The *large-bowel loops* are peripheral, few in number, have diameters greater than 5 centimetres, contain faeces and have haustral margins that do not extend across the bowel lumen. In contrast, the *small-bowel loops* are central, multiple, between 3 and 5 centimetres in diameter and do not contain faeces. Valvulae conniventes that extend completely across the bowel lumen are seen in the jejunal loops. With gastric dilation, the stomach may be massively enlarged and distended with air (see Fig. 16.6).
- **Calcification:** calcification shows up well against the grey, soft-tissue densities. About 90% of renal stones are calcified, whereas only 10% of gallstones are calcified. To identify radiolucent gallstones, an ultrasound examination is the test of choice. Calcification may be seen in the pancreas in chronic pancreatitis (see Fig. 16.7). Costal cartilage calcification is commonly seen in

Generalised ileus.

The large bowel is filled with gas and is dilated, except in the descending colon. Dilated small bowel is also seen in the right hypochondrium (upper arrow). As gas is seen around the rectum (lower arrow), mechanical obstruction is excluded

(From Herring W. *Learning radiology: recognizing the basics*. St Louis, MO: Mosby, 2012.)

FIGURE 16.3

Large-bowel obstruction.

The large bowel is markedly distended around the sigmoid colon, where it abruptly stops (arrow). The common causes of obstruction are carcinoma or diverticular stricture. The increased peristalsis occurring at the onset of obstruction can remove the gas and faeces distal to the obstruction. Therefore, no gas is seen in this patient

(From Keighley M. *Surgery of the anus, rectum and colon*. Philadelphia: Elsevier, 2008.)

FIGURE 16.4

---

elderly patients, projected over the hypochondrial regions. Calcification in the walls of an abdominal aortic aneurysm may be seen on a lateral abdominal film. Splenic and renal artery aneurysms are also often calcified. Vascular calcification may frequently be seen in the elderly.

- **Ascites:** with accumulation of peritoneal fluid within the peritoneal cavity, the film looks generally grey and lacks detail. On the supine film, the bowel loops float towards the middle of the abdomen. Ascites is best identified by ultrasound.

Abdominal ultrasound

Diagnostic ultrasound is a safe and rapid imaging technique. It is non-invasive, usually painless, requires no contrast medium and involves limited or no patient preparation.

Ultrasound is unsuitable for patients who are obese or extremely muscular, have large amounts of gas, cannot follow instructions, are in severe pain or have large open wounds and surgical dressings.

Indications

Ultrasound is the abdominal imaging technique of choice in the initial investigation of hepatobiliary disease including splenomegaly, renal and bladder disease,

Small-bowel obstruction.

There is gross dilation of the small bowel. It is recognised as small bowel from its central position and its transverse mucosal bands—the valvulae conniventes (black arrow). Air–fluid levels are seen on the erect view (a). The supine view (b) gives a better view of the distribution of the dilated loops. From the number and position of the displayed dilated loops, the obstruction would be at the level of the mid small bowel. The round radio-opaque shadow in the left hypochondrium is a tablet (open arrow)

(From Koch MR. *Abdominal imaging*. Philadelphia: Saunders, 2011.)

FIGURE 16.5

Gastric dilation.

The stomach is massively enlarged and distended with air. When this occurs acutely, prompt nasogastric aspiration is necessary. Mechanical obstruction due to a pyloric ulcer or carcinoma needs exclusion. Atonic dilation is usually a postoperative complication, but may occur with diabetic coma, trauma, pancreatitis or hypokalaemia

(From Gore R. *High-yield imaging: gastrointestinal*. Philadelphia: Saunders, 2010.)

FIGURE 16.6

appendicitis, ascites and aortic aneurysm. Where acute abdominal trauma has occurred, rapid assessment for free fluid by five-location ultrasound is commonly used (a **FAST** scan: Focused Assessment with Sonography in Trauma). Ultrasound is especially suited in paediatrics and obstetrics given the absence of the harmful effects of ionising radiation.

Technique of examination

Ultrasound images are formed when high-frequency sound waves ranging from 2 to 15 megahertz are transmitted through the body originating from a hand-placed transducer (probe) on the skin. The generated sonographic waves pass through the underlying body tissues and are reflected back as returning echoes. The time taken for a generated wave to enter and then return is converted to a depth, while

Pancreatic calcification.

Stippled calcification is seen in the region of the pancreas (arrow), indicating chronic calcific pancreatitis. The most likely cause is alcohol excess

(From Miller FH. *Textbook of gastrointestinal radiology*. Philadelphia: Saunders, 2008.)

FIGURE 16.7

Fundamental ultrasound terminology		
Ultrasound term	**Definition**	**Correlation**
Anechoic	Absence of echo, very black	Gallbladder, cyst
Hypoechoic	Decreased echo, black to dark grey	Kidney medulla, solid tumour
Hyperechoic	Increased echo, white to light grey	Renal sinus fat, acute haemorrhage
Echogenic	Increased echo, white to light grey	Fat, haemorrhage
Isoechoic	Same density as surrounding tissue	Gallbladder, cyst
Acoustic enhancement	Increased density behind a structure	Gallbladder, cyst
Acoustic shadowing	Decreased density behind a structure	Rib, bowel, calculus
Doppler	Technique to assess vascular flow	Portal vein, aorta

TABLE 16.2

Fundamental abdominal ultrasound densities	
Content	**Density**
Air	Hyperechoic interface with posterior acoustic shadowing
Fat	Echogenic
Hollow organ	Hypoechoic interface with posterior acoustic enhancement
Solid organ	Echogenic
Calcification	Hyperechoic interface with posterior acoustic shadowing

TABLE 16.3

the number of returning echoes is converted to a density ('echogenicity')—be it black, white or many shades of grey. Tissues that allow through transmission with few echoes are displayed black (hypoechoic, anechoic), whereas high numbers of returning echoes are displayed white (hyperechoic, echogenic; see Tables 16.2 and 16.3).

Principles of interpretation

Each organ is first identified and scanned in real time in its entirety. Selected images of each organ are then made systematically in longitudinal and transverse section. Doppler examination is applied to identify vascular flow in the portal vein, aorta, renal arteries, hepatic veins and inferior vena cava. Any pathological condition, such as a mass, is also scrutinised with Doppler to characterise its vascular flow. Each organ is assessed as to its size, shape, margins, internal architecture, echogenicity and vascularity. Any abnormality detected is targeted to determine its characteristics, including its exact anatomical location, size, internal structure and margin features, as well as its vascularity (see Figs 16.9–16.10).

CT of the abdomen
Indications

CT scanning of the abdomen has become the imaging technique of choice for the investigation of many

Pancreatic pseudo-cyst

FIGURE 16.8

abdominal diseases. The main advantages of CT are the short time required for image acquisition, the exquisite anatomical detail provided, the wide limits of body coverage and the ability to assess blood vessels and perfusion characteristics of organs and lesions. Patient morbidity is mainly related to the radiation dose incurred and to complications from the intravenous iodinated contrast such as renal failure and allergic reactions.

Technique of examination

Images are obtained in a transverse plane (axial) in a continuous spiral as the patient is moved through the imaging beam. As the X-ray passes through the patient it decreases in energy (is attenuated) according to the tissue density and is registered on a row of detectors and converted into a density. Once a body area has been scanned the data can be recalculated into any density or plane including three-dimensional renditions. Multi-row CT scanners allow more rapid acquisition with thinner slices. This allows the detection of more detail and smaller abnormalities.

Intravenous contrast containing iodine is injected to improve organ depiction, identify blood vessels and show vascularity. Oral contrast is given to show intestinal details.

Many variations in CT technique can be obtained to optimise the depiction of abnormalities (see Table 16.4, Figs 16.8, 16.9a, 16.11).

Principles of interpretation

First, the initial scanogram of the abdomen should be reviewed, because in up to 10% of cases the diagnosis can be made or modified by the findings. Second, an overview of the entire scan is performed slice by slice, to identify any major abnormalities such as bowel loop dilation, ascites, organomegaly, aortic aneurysm or mass. Third, an organ-by-organ analysis is completed to check its size, margins, enhancement characteristics and any mass lesion. At the periphery of each normal organ the transition from the surface to the adjacent fat should be sharp and distinct—a feature that if absent frequently denotes inflammatory change, haemorrhage or tumour infiltration. Fourth, free fluid and free gas are identified by surveying the subdiaphragmatic spaces, paracolic gutters, renal recesses and the pelvis. Finally, change the image setting to the *lung window* to view basal pathology such as pleural effusion, hiatus hernia and tumours or to the *bone window* to view the spine, ribs and bony pelvis optimally.

Liver cyst.

(a) CT, (b) ultrasound and (c) MRI. The cyst displays no internal echoes but distinct posterior acoustic enhancement on ultrasound. There is an internal septum present, which is thin. Features are that of a septated hepatic cyst

(From Shaked O. Biologic and clinical features of benign solid and cystic lesions of the liver. *Clinical Gastroenterology and Hepatology* 2011; 9(7):547–562. AGA Institute, ©2011.)

FIGURE 16.9

Ultrasound of liver metastasis.

Multiple echogenic round lesions are demonstrated in the liver from metastatic colon carcinoma. Note also that the liver margin is lobulated owing to macronodular cirrhosis

(From Jarnagin WR. *Blumgart's surgery of the liver, biliary tract and pancreas.* Philadelphia: Elsevier, 2012.)

FIGURE 16.10

CT of gallbladder (GB) and liver.

Ultrasound is superior for identifying gallstones

(From Gore R. *High-yield imaging*. Philadelphia: Saunders, 2010.)

FIGURE 16.11

Summary of common CT techniques of the abdomen

Technique	Contrast	Applications	Example
Non-contrast (CT —helical or CT KUB non-helical)	None given	Calcifications, gas	Renal calculus, calcified lymph nodes, calcification within tumours Foreign body Gas—pneumoperitoneum, intrahepatic gas, gas within the bowel wall
Arterial (CTA)	IVI 20-second delay	Vessel disease (aneurysm) Acute haemorrhage Organ viability Lesion perfusion	Aortic aneurysm, arterial occlusion or dissection Angiodysplasia Necrotic pancreatitis Metastasis
Portal venous	IVI 70-second delay	Routine assessment Organ perfusion	All diseases, e.g. solid organ disease, duct obstruction
Triple phase	Non-contrast Arterial Portal venous	Organ perfusion	Necrotic pancreatitis Infarction, haemorrhage, lesion characterisation
Delayed	IVI 2–10-minute delay	Vessel leak Acute haemorrhage Renal pelvis–ureter tear / tumour Bladder	Gastrointestinal bleed Leaking aneurysm Torn ureter or tumour Bladder tumour, liver lesions
CT cholangiogram	IVI bilirubin analogue	Biliary tree disease	Stone Stricture Tumour Leak
CT colonography	PR carbon dioxide	Colon disease	Tumour Stenosis

CTA = computer tomography angiography; IVI = intravenous infusion; KUB = kidneys, ureters and bladder; PR = per rectal.

TABLE 16.4

T&O'C ESSENTIALS
ABDOMINAL CT INTERPRETATION

1. Check patient's name and date of scan.
2. Type of scan:
   - non-contrast
   - contrast
   - phase, e.g. kidneys, ureters and bladder (KUB), triple phase, portal phase.
3. General review:
   - look at the topogram (this image shows the abdomen as a frontal X-ray with a wider coverage than the CT scans)
   - find the axial and the coronal images
   - find the top—lung bases and bottom—pelvis images
   - look for obvious abnormalities.
4. Review important areas:
   - symphysis pubis (bottom scan)
   - pelvis
   - iliac crest
   - kidneys
   - liver
   - lung bases (top scan).
5. Look everywhere systematically:
   - organ by organ
   - slice by slice.
6. Specific search:
   - skeleton
   - lung bases
   - inguinal area
   - lymph node groups
   - air in peritoneum.
7. Compare with previous studies and clinical findings.

REVISION OSCES

1. Outline the indications for abdominal ultrasonography. Explain what important abnormalities may be picked up. (p 289)
2. Look at this abdominal CT scan and point out the main anatomical features. (p 290)
3. Outline the main indications for upper and lower bowel endoscopy. What are some of the limitations of the procedure? (p 284)
4. Explain how you would investigate this patient who has iron deficiency anaemia. (pp 279, 284, 331, 350)

SECTION 5
The genitourinary system

CHAPTER 17

The genitourinary history

CHAPTER 18

The genitourinary examination

CHAPTER 19

The genitourinary tests and scans, summary of the renal examination

CHAPTER 17

The genitourinary history

Falstaff: 'What says the doctor to my water?'

Page: 'He said, sir, the water itself was a good healthy water: but for the party that owed it, he might have more diseases than he knew for.'   WILLIAM SHAKESPEARE, Henry IV, Part 1

Despite their very different functions the male and female genital and urinary systems are intimately associated anatomically and are usually assessed together.

PRESENTING SYMPTOMS

Presenting symptoms may include a change in the appearance of the urine, abnormalities of micturition, suprapubic or flank pain or the systemic symptoms of renal failure (see List 17.1). Some patients have no symptoms but are found to be hypertensive or to have abnormalities on routine urinalysis or serum biochemistry. Investigations of relatives of patients with inherited renal disease may have led to the diagnosis (e.g. polycystic kidney disease; see List 17.2). Others may feel unwell but not have localising symptoms (see Questions box 17.1). The major renal syndromes are set out in Table 17.1.

Basic male and female reproductive anatomy is shown in Figs 18.8 (p 313) and 40.3 (p 754).

GENITOURINARY HISTORY

Major symptoms

Change in appearance of urine (e.g. haematuria)

Change in urine volume or stream:
- Polyuria
- Nocturia
- Anuria
- Decrease in stream size
- Hesitancy
- Dribbling
- Urine retention
- Strangury
- *Pis-en-deux*—double-voiding (incomplete bladder emptying)
- Incontinence of urine

Dysuria (painful micturition)

Frequency, urgency

Fever, loin pain

Renal colic

Urethral discharge

Symptoms suggestive of chronic kidney disease (uraemia):
- Oliguria, nocturia, polyuria
- Anorexia, a metallic taste, vomiting, fatigue, hiccup, insomnia
- Itch, bruising, oedema

Menses:
- Age of onset
- Regularity
- Last period (date)
- Dysmenorrhoea, menorrhagia

Erectile dysfunction

Loss of libido

Infertility

Pregnancies: number and any complications

Urethral or vaginal discharge

Genital rash

LIST 17.1

Change in appearance of the urine

Some patients present with discoloured urine. A red discoloration suggests haematuria (blood in the urine).[1] Urethral inflammation or trauma, or prostatic disease, can cause haematuria at the beginning of micturition which then clears, or haematuria only at the end of micturition (see List 17.3). Patients with porphyria can have urine that changes colour on standing. Consumption of certain drugs (e.g. rifampicin) or large amounts of beetroot and, rarely, haemoglobinuria (due to destruction of red blood cells and release of free haemoglobin) or myoglobinuria (due to muscle trauma and breakdown) can cause red discoloration of the urine. Foamy, tea-coloured or brown urine may be a presenting sign of nephrosis or kidney failure. It is worth noting that the colour of the urine is not a reliable guide to its concentration.

> **HISTORY SUGGESTING POLYCYSTIC KIDNEY DISEASE**
>
> Family history (20% have no family history)
> Flank pain
> Back pain
> Haematuria
> History of hypertension
> Abdominal enlargement
>
> LIST 17.2

Urinary tract infection

Urinary tract infection (UTI) includes both upper UTI (renal) and lower UTI (mostly the bladder—cystitis).

> **QUESTIONS TO ASK THE PATIENT WITH SUSPECTED RENAL DISEASE**
>
> ! denotes symptoms for the possible diagnosis of an urgent or dangerous problem.
>
> 1. How did your kidney problems begin? Have you had tiredness, the need to pass urine at night (nocturia) or loss of appetite?
> 2. Was the kidney trouble thought to be brought on by any medications you were taking (e.g. non-steroidal anti-inflammatory drugs, ACE inhibitors/angiotensin receptor blockers or contrast used for an X-ray procedure)?
> 3. Were you told there was inflammation of the kidneys (glomerulonephritis) or protein in the urine?
> 4. Have you had kidney infections recently or as a child?
> 5. Have you had kidney stones or urinary obstruction?
> ! 6. Have you passed blood in the urine? (Urinary tract malignancy)
> 7. Have you had a biopsy of your kidney? Do you know the result?
> 8. Have you had diabetes or high blood pressure?
> 9. Have you had cardiovascular disease or peripheral vascular disease?
> 10. Have you had kidney surgery or removal of a kidney, or have you been told you have only one functioning kidney?
> 11. Is there a history in the family of enlarged kidneys and high blood pressure? (Polycystic kidneys)
> 12. Have you had problems with rashes or arthritis? (Systemic lupus erythematosus, scleroderma)
> 13. Have you had problems with swelling or shortness of breath? (Fluid retention)
> 14. Have you been told how bad your kidney function is and whether you may need dialysis one day?
> 15. Are you taking medications to help the kidney function?
> 16. What tablets and medications (including over-the-counter products, herbal remedies, etc.) are you taking?
>
> QUESTIONS BOX 17.1

The major renal syndromes

Name	Definition	Example
Nephrotic	Massive proteinuria	Minimal change disease
Nephritic	Haematuria, renal failure	Poststreptococcal glomerulonephritis
Tubulointerstitial nephropathy	Renal failure, mild proteinuria	Analgesic nephropathy
Acute kidney injury (AKI)*	Sudden fall in function, rise in creatinine	Acute tubular necrosis
Rapidly progressive renal failure	Fall in renal function, over weeks	Malignant hypertension or 'crescentic' glomerulonephritis
Asymptomatic urinary abnormality	Isolated haematuria, or mild proteinuria	Immunoglobulin A nephropathy

*Previously called acute renal failure.

(Levin A, Warnock D, Mehta R, Kellum J, Shah S, Melitoris B, Ronco C. Improving outcome for AKI. *Am J Kidney Dis* 2007; 50(1):1–4.)

TABLE 17.1

HAEMATURIA

Favours urinary tract infection (UTI)
Dysuria
Fever (prostatitis, pyelonephritis)
Suprapubic pain (cystitis)
Moderate flank or back pain (pyelonephritis)

Favours renal calculi
Severe loin pain

Favours source that is not glomerular
Clots in urine

Favours blood not in urine
Menstruation

Favours immunoglobulin A (IgA) nephropathy
Multiple episodes over months

Favours trauma
Recent indwelling urinary catheter or procedure
Recent back or abdominal injury

Favours bleeding disorder
Use of anticoagulant drugs

LIST 17.3

RISK FACTORS FOR URINARY TRACT INFECTION (UTI)

Female sex
Coitus
Pregnancy
Diabetes
Indwelling urinary catheter
Previous UTI
Lower urinary tract symptoms of obstruction

LIST 17.4

UTI is much more common in women than in men, but there are a number of risk factors for the disease (see List 17.4). It can be strongly suspected on the basis of the patient's symptoms.[2] These include:

- dysuria (pain or stinging during urination)
- frequency (need to pass small amounts of urine frequently)
- haematuria
- loin pain (more suggestive of upper UTI)
- back pain.

Women who believe they have a UTI are usually right. The positive predictive value has been reported as 84%[3] (see Good symptoms and signs guide 17.1). Ask about fever, rigors and lower abdominal discomfort. Physical examination may reveal loin tenderness when the renal angle is ballotted posteriorly.

The latter findings are more suggestive of complicated UTI or pyelonephritis. The presence of a

Possibly as much as 50% of lower UTIs also involve the kidneys. Renal infection may be difficult to distinguish clinically from lower UTI, but is a more serious condition and more likely to involve systemic complications such as septicaemia.

> **GOOD SYMPTOMS AND SIGNS GUIDE 17.1**
> **Urinary tract infection**
>
> | Symptom or sign | LR+ | LR− |
> |---|---|---|
> | Dysuria | 1.5 | 0.48 |
> | Frequency | 1.8 | 0.59 |
> | Haematuria | 2.0 | 0.92 |
> | Fever | 1.6 | 0.9 |
> | Flank pain | 1.1 | 0.84 |
> | Lower abdominal pain | 1.1 | 0.89 |
> | Patient says | 4.0 | 0 |
> | Vaginal discharge | 0.3 | 3.1 |
>
> (Adapted from Simel DL, Rennie D. *The rational clinical examination: evidence-based diagnosis.* New York: McGraw-Hill, 2009, Table 51-2.)

vaginal discharge or irritation is against the diagnosis. Elderly patients with a UTI often present with confusion and few other symptoms or signs. A UTI in a male or frequent, relapsing or recurrent UTI in a female suggests an anatomical abnormality and requires urological evaluation.

Urinary obstruction

Urinary obstruction is common in elderly men and causes lower urinary tract symptoms—(LUTS; formerly known as prostatism) or bladder outflow obstruction. The patient may have noticed hesitancy (difficulty starting micturition—urination), followed by a decrease in the size of the stream of urine and terminal dribbling of urine. Strangury (recurrently, a small volume of bloody urine is passed with a painful desire to urinate each time) and *pis-en-deux*/double-voiding (the desire to urinate despite having just done so) may occur.[4] When obstruction is complete there may be overflow incontinence of urine. Obstruction is associated with an increased risk of urinary infection.

Renal calculi can cause ureteric obstruction (see Fig. 19.2 on p 322). The presenting symptom here, however, is usually severe colicky or constant loin or lower quadrant pain that may radiate down towards the symphysis pubis or perineum or testis (renal colic). Sometimes the main symptoms are abdominal pain and nausea and the condition must be distinguished from an acute abdomen. Urinary obstruction can be a cause of acute kidney injury (AKI, or renal failure; see List 17.5).

Urinary incontinence

This is the inability to hold urine in the bladder voluntarily. It is not a consequence of normal ageing alone. The problem can occur transiently with UTIs, delirium, excess urine output (e.g. from the use of diuretics), immobility (because patients are unable to reach the toilet), urethritis or vaginitis, or stool impaction.

Causes of established urinary incontinence include:

1. *Stress incontinence* (instantaneous leakage after the stress of coughing or after a sudden rise in intra-abdominal pressure of any cause)—this problem is more common in women owing to vaginal deliveries or an atrophic vaginal wall postmenopause causing a hypermobile urethra.
2. *Urge incontinence* (*overactivity of the detrusor muscle*), which is characterised by an intense urge to urinate and then leakage of urine in the absence of cough or other stressors—this occurs in both men and women.
3. *Detrusor underactivity*—this is rare and is characterised by urinary frequency, nocturia and the frequent leaking of small amounts of urine from neurological disease.
4. *Overflow incontinence* (*urethral obstruction*)—this occurs typically in men with disease of the prostate and is characterised by dribbling incontinence after incomplete urination.
5. A *vesico/urethral fistula*—a complication of obstructed labour.

Chronic kidney disease

The clinical features of chronic kidney disease (CKD; chronic renal failure) can be deduced in part by considering the normal functions of the kidneys.

1. Failure of excretory function leads to accumulation of numerous 'uraemic' toxins, hence the widely used term *uraemia*. This frequently leads to malaise, lethargy, anorexia, malnutrition and hiccups.[a]

---

[a] We prefer not to spell this as 'hiccoughs'. But then we still argue over the merits of US or English spelling in medicine!

CAUSES OF ACUTE KIDNEY INJURY

Onset over days

This is defined as a rapid deterioration in renal function severe enough to cause accumulation of waste products, especially nitrogenous wastes, in the body. Usually the urine flow rate is less than 20 mL/hour or 400 mL/day, but occasionally it is normal or increased (high-output renal failure).

PRERENAL

Fluid loss: blood (haemorrhage), plasma or water and electrolytes (diarrhoea and vomiting, fluid volume depletion)

Hypotension: myocardial infarction, septicaemic shock, drugs

Renovascular disease: embolus, dissection or atheroma

Increased renal vascular resistance: hepatorenal syndrome

RENAL

Acute-on-chronic kidney failure (precipitated by infection, fluid volume depletion, obstruction or nephrotoxic drugs)—see List 17.1

Acute renal disease:
- e.g. primary or secondary glomerulonephritis, connective tissue diseases

Acute tubular necrosis secondary to:
- ischaemia (hypovolaemia)
- toxins and drugs (such as aminoglycoside antibiotics, radiocontrast material, heavy metals)
- rhabdomyolysis, haemoglobinuria

Tubulointerstitial disease:
- e.g. drugs (such as proton pump inhibitors, sulfonamides, cyclosporin A), urate or calcium deposits, phosphate, oxalate, crystal nephropathy

Vascular disease:
- e.g. vasculitis, scleroderma

Myeloma

Acute pyelonephritis (rare)

POSTRENAL (COMPLETE URINARY TRACT OBSTRUCTION)

Urethral obstruction:
- e.g. calculus or blood clot, sloughed papillae, trauma, phimosis or paraphimosis (a tight narrowing of the foreskin that prevents it being retracted and that can obstruct the urinary meatus)

At the bladder neck:
- e.g. calculus or blood clot, prostatic hypertrophy or cancer

Bilateral ureteric obstruction:
- intraureteric, e.g. blood clot, pyogenic debris, calculi
- extraureteric, e.g. retroperitoneal fibrosis (due to radiation, methysergide or idiopathic), retroperitoneal/pelvic tumour or surgery, uterine prolapse

Causes of rapidly progressive kidney failure (onset over weeks to months)

Urinary tract obstruction

Rapidly progressive glomerulonephritis

Bilateral renal artery stenosis (may be precipitated by angiotensin-converting enzyme [ACE] inhibitor or angiotensin receptor blocker use)

Multiple myeloma

Scleroderma renal crisis

Malignant hypertension

Haemolytic uraemic syndrome

Note: Anuria may be due to urinary obstruction, bilateral renal artery occlusion, rapidly progressive (crescentic) glomerulonephritis, renal cortical necrosis or a renal stone in a solitary kidney.
(Levin A, Warnock D, Mehta R et al. Improving outcome for AKI. *Am J Kidney Dis* 2007; 50(1):1–4.)

LIST 17.5

---

2. Urinary concentrating ability may be lost early, leading to the risk of dehydration; nocturia can be an early symptom.
3. Various factors such as the failure to excrete sodium may lead to hypertension.
4. Damage to the renal tubules may lead to sodium loss and hypotension.
5. Excretion of potassium depends in part on urine volume. Hyperkalaemia usually becomes a problem when a patient is oliguric (passes less than 400 mL urine/day) and may occur when taking potassium-sparing diuretics or agents that promote potassium retention (ACE inhibitors, angiotensin receptor blockers,

Classification of chronic kidney disease by glomerular filtration rate (GFR)

Stage	Description	GFR (mL/min/1.73 m²)
—	Increased risk for CKD (e.g. diabetes, hypertension)	>90
1	Kidney damage but normal GFR	>90
2	Kidney damage and mild GFR reduction	60–89
3	Moderate reduction in GFR	30–59
4	Severe reduction in GFR	15–29
5	Kidney failure	<15

TABLE 17.2

non-steroidal anti-inflammatory drugs [NSAIDs]).
6. Failure of acid excretion leads to metabolic acidosis.
7. Disordered mineral and bone metabolism (abnormal levels of calcium, phosphorus, parathyroid hormone [PTH] and vitamin D) may lead to abnormalities in bone and blood vessels or soft-tissue calcification.[5]
8. Failure to secrete erythropoietin leads to normochromic normocytic anaemia.
9. Alterations in the metabolism of those medications that are excreted by the kidneys.
10. Adequacy of renal function is defined by the glomerular filtration rate (GFR). This is the volume of blood filtered by the kidneys per unit of time. The normal range is 90–120 mL/min. The GFR is estimated by calculating the clearance of creatinine (a normal breakdown product of muscle) from the blood. The serum creatinine and urea levels also provide a measure of accumulation of uraemic toxins and therefore of renal function. Most laboratories now provide an estimated GFR (eGFR) measurement calculated from the serum creatinine and the patient's age and sex.

CKD is defined as kidney damage or GFR <60 mL/min/1.73 m² for 3 months or more, irrespective of cause.[6] Further, kidney disease has been divided into six groups according to GFR (see Table 17.2). These allow planning of investigations and treatment that might slow progression of the disease.

A uraemic patient may present with:
- anuria (defined as failure to pass more than 50 mL urine daily)
- oliguria (less than 400 mL urine daily)
- nocturia (the need to get up during the night to pass urine), or
- polyuria (the passing of abnormally large volumes of urine).

Nocturia may be an indication of failure of the kidneys to concentrate urine normally, and polyuria may indicate complete inability to concentrate the urine (or a large intake of fluids[b]).

The more general symptoms of renal failure include anorexia, vomiting, fatigue, hiccups and insomnia. Pruritus (a general itchiness of the skin), easy bruising and oedema due to fluid retention may also be present. Other symptoms indicating complications include bone pain, fractures because of renal bone disease, and the symptoms of hypercalcaemia (including anorexia, nausea, vomiting, constipation, increased urination, mental confusion) because of tertiary (or primary) hyperparathyroidism.[c] Patients may also present with the features of pericarditis, hypertension, cardiac failure, ischaemic heart disease, neuropathy or peptic ulceration.

Find out whether the patient is undergoing dialysis and whether this is haemodialysis or peritoneal dialysis. There are a number of important questions that must be asked of dialysis patients (see Questions box 17.2).

Ask about any complications that have occurred, including recurrent peritonitis with peritoneal dialysis or problems with vascular access for haemodialysis.

Renal transplantation is a common treatment for renal failure. A patient may know how well the graft is functioning and what the most recent renal function tests have shown. Find out whether the patient knows of rejection episodes, how these were treated and whether there has been more than one renal transplant. It is

---
[b] Many people deliberately and proudly drink 8–10 glasses of water per day.
[c] In secondary hyperparathyroidism, serum calcium is low and phosphate is high. In tertiary hyperparathyroidism, where parathyroid function has become autonomous, serum calcium and phosphate levels are both high.

> **QUESTIONS TO ASK THE DIALYSIS PATIENT**
>
> ! denotes symptoms for the possible diagnosis of an urgent or dangerous problem.
>
> 1. What fluid restriction have you been recommended?
> 2. Have phosphate-binding drugs been prescribed? When do you take these relative to meals?
> 3. Do you use haemodialysis or peritoneal dialysis? Do you do this at home? How many times a week?
> ! 4. Have you had abdominal pain or fever recently? (Peritonitis related to peritoneal dialysis)
> 5. Have you had any problems with haemodialysis, such as low blood pressure, or with the fistula used for haemodialysis? Have you had any problems with peritonitis with peritoneal dialysis?
> 6. How much weight do you gain between each haemodialysis?
> 7. Do you still pass any urine? If so, how much?
> 8. Are you on a renal transplant list or have you previously had a transplant?
> 9. Do you follow recommended dietary restrictions?
> 10. What other medications do you take?
> 11. Have you had heart or blood vessel problems?
> 12. Have you had overactive parathyroid glands or parathyroid surgery?
>
> QUESTIONS BOX 17.2

necessary to ascertain whether there have been any problems with recurrent infection, urine leaks or side effects of treatment. Long-term problems with immunosuppression may have occurred, including the development of cancers, chronic nephrotoxicity (e.g. from cyclosporin or tacrolimus), obesity and hypertension from steroids, or recurrent infections. The patient should be aware of the need to avoid skin exposure to the sun and women should know that they need regular Papanicolaou[d] (Pap) smears for cancer surveillance.

Ask if the kidney was a cadaveric transplant or from a live donor—often a relative. The source of the kidney may affect the patient and family psychologically (e.g. early failure of a graft donated by a relative).

MENSTRUAL AND SEXUAL HISTORY

Sexual history taking can be embarrassing for the patient (and student); unless it is very relevant to the presenting problem, it should probably be left to a second or later interview. By this time the patient and clinician will have become more used to each other and the questions are likely to seem less intrusive.

For the menstrual history, the menarche or date of the first period is important. The regularity of the periods over the preceding months or years and the date of the last period are also both relevant. The patient may complain of dysmenorrhoea (painful menstruation) or menorrhagia (an abnormally heavy period or series of periods).

Vaginal discharge can occur in patients with infections of the genital tract. Sometimes the type of discharge is an indication of the type of infection present. The history of the number of pregnancies and births is relevant: *gravidity* refers to the number of times a woman has conceived, while *parity* refers to the number of babies delivered (live births or stillbirths). Also ask about any complications that occurred during pregnancy (e.g. hypertension).

The sexual history is also relevant.[7] Ask about contraceptive methods and the possibility of pregnancy.[8] Ask men about erectile dysfunction (impotence). Erectile dysfunction is defined as inability to achieve or maintain a satisfactory erection during a 3-month period. Most causes are organic (neurogenic [e.g. diabetes], vascular [related to endothelial dysfunction] or drug related [e.g. beta-blockers, thiazide diuretics]). The onset is gradual and often begins with the loss of morning erections in older men.

---

[d] Georgios N Papanicolaou (1884–1962). After studying at the University of Athens he worked in the pathology department at New York Hospital.

TREATMENT

A detailed drug history must be taken. Note all the drugs, including steroids and immunosuppressants, and their dosages. In patients with decreased renal function, the dosages of many drugs that are cleared by the kidneys must be adjusted. The patient with CKD should be well informed about the need for protein, phosphate, potassium, fluid or salt restriction. Patients with UTIs may have had a number of courses of antibiotics. Contrast agents used for angiography CT scans and MRI scans can be nephrotoxic. Has the patient had exposure to these recently? Treatment of hypertension should be documented. Certain drugs should be used with caution. For example, NSAIDs can worsen renal function or cause CKD.

PAST HISTORY

Find out whether there have been previous or recurrent UTIs or renal calculi. There may have been operations to remove urinary tract stones, or pelvic surgery may have been performed because of urinary incontinence in women or prostatism in men. The patient may know about the previous detection of proteinuria or microscopic haematuria at a routine examination. Glomerulonephritis will usually have been diagnosed by renal biopsy, a procedure that is often a memorable event. Histories of diabetes mellitus or gout are relevant, as these diseases may lead to renal complications. It is most important to find out about hypertension, because this may not only cause renal impairment but is also a common complication of renal disease. Similarly, a history of episodes of AKI, a history of cancer treated with chemotherapy or radiotherapy, severe allergic reactions and exposure to nephrotoxic substances are all relevant. A history of childhood enuresis (bedwetting) beyond the age of 3 years old can be associated with vesicoureteric reflux and subsequent renal scarring.

Renovascular disease is more likely if there is a history of vascular disease elsewhere, such as myocardial ischaemia or cerebrovascular disease. In elderly patients, specific questions relating to ingestion of Bex or Vincent's powders may suggest a diagnosis of analgesic nephropathy. This is particularly important as these patients require surveillance for urothelial malignancy in addition to managing their renal impairment.

SOCIAL HISTORY

Patients with CKD may have many social problems. There may be a need for access to equipment at home for dialysis. Who does the patient contact if there is a problem with home dialysis? You must ask detailed questions to find out how the patient and his or her family are coping with the chronic illness and its complications. Has the patient been able to work? Find out how well informed the patient is about the transplant, if this has been the treatment. Also find out what sort of support the patient has obtained from relatives and friends. Can dialysis be organised at other centres so that the patient can go on holidays?

FAMILY HISTORY

Some forms of renal disease are inherited. Polycystic kidney disease, for example, is an autosomal-dominant condition. Ask about diabetes and hypertension in the family. A family history of deafness and renal impairment suggests Alport's[e] syndrome, a hereditary form of nephritis. A family history of kidney disease of any type is a risk factor for the development of CKD.

> **T&O'C ESSENTIALS**
>
> 1. Patients with early renal disease are often asymptomatic.
> 2. A routine urine or blood test may lead to the need to take a renal history.
> 3. Many drugs are nephrotoxic. A change of medications may explain deterioration in renal function.
> 4. Patients with chronic kidney disease are at increased risk of cardiovascular and bone disease.
> 5. Chronic kidney disease can have a profound effect on a patient's life. Questions about coping and support should be routine.

---

[e] Cecil Alport, 1880–1959, a South African physician who worked in London and Egypt, described this syndrome in 1927 while working at St Mary's Hospital, London.

> **OSCE REVISION TOPICS – GENITOURINARY HISTORY**
>
> *Use these topics, which commonly occur in the OSCE, to help with revision.*
>
> 1. Please take a detailed history from this man who had a renal transplant 6 years ago. (p 302)
> 2. Ask this patient about her dialysis regimen and how she copes. (p 303)
> 3. Please take a history from this woman who has had recurrent urinary tract infections. (p 298)
> 4. This man has hypertension and has been told he has stage 4 kidney disease. Please take a history from him. (pp 124, 298)

References

1. Marazzi P, Gabriel R. The haematuria clinic. *BMJ* 1994; 308:356.
2. Bent S, Nallamothu BK, Simel DL et al. Does this woman have an acute uncomplicated urinary tract infection? *JAMA* 2002, 287; 20:2701–2710. Dysuria, frequency, haematuria, back pain and costovertebral tenderness increase the likelihood of UTI (positive LRs between 1.5 and 2.0). No vaginal discharge or irritation decreases the likelihood.
3. Scoles D, Hooton TM, Roberts PL et al. Risk factors for recurrent urinary tract infection in young women. *J Infect Dis* 2000; 182(4):1177–1182.
4. Dawson C, Whitfield H. Urological evaluation (ABC of urology). *BMJ* 1996; 312:695–698. This article provides useful definitions and interpretation of symptoms.
5. Moe S, Cunningham J, Goodman W et al. Definition, evaluation, and classification of renal osteodystrophy: a position statement of the Kidney Disease: Improving Global Outcomes (KDIGO). *Kidney Int* 2006; 69: 1945–1953.
6. Levey A, Eckarrdt K, Tsukanoto Y et al. Definition and classification of CKD: a position statement of KDIGO. *Kidney Int* 2005; 67:2089–2100.
7. Dean J. ABC of sexual health: examination of patient with sexual problems. *BMJ* 1998; 317:1641–1643.
8. Bastian LA, Pistcitelli JT. Is this patient pregnant? Can you reliably rule in or rule out early pregnancy by clinical examination? *JAMA* 1997; 278:586–591. Clinical features (amenorrhoea, morning sickness, tender breasts, enlarged uterus after 8 weeks with a soft cervix) cannot reliably diagnose early pregnancy—a pregnancy test, however, can.

CHAPTER 18

The genitourinary examination

Don't touch the patient—state first what you see, cultivate your powers of observation

SIR WILLIAM OSLER (1849–1919)

EXAMINATION ANATOMY

Fig. 18.1 shows an outline of the anatomy of the urinary tract. Fig. 18.2 shows the arterial supply of the kidneys as demonstrated on a CT renal angiogram and Fig. 18.3 shows the outline of the renal collecting system. Problems with function can arise in any part, from the arterial blood supply of the kidneys, the renal parenchyma, the ureters and bladder (including their innervation) to the urethra.

THE EXAMINATION

A set examination of the genitourinary system is not routinely performed. However, if renal disease is suspected or known to be present, then certain signs must be sought. These are mostly the signs of chronic kidney disease (CKD) (uraemia) and its causes (see List 18.1). However, examination of the male genitalia or female pelvis (see Ch 40) is part of the routine general examination.

GENERAL APPEARANCE

The general inspection remains crucial. Look for *hyperventilation*, which may indicate an underlying metabolic acidosis. *Hiccupping* may be present and can be an ominous sign of advanced uraemia. There may be the ammoniacal fish breath (*uraemic fetor*) of kidney failure. This musty smell is not easy to describe but once detected is easily remembered. Patients with CKD commonly have a sallow complexion (a dirty brown appearance or *uraemic tinge*). This may be due to impaired excretion of urinary pigments (urochromes) combined with anaemia. The skin colour may be from slate grey to bronze, caused by iron deposition in dialysis patients who have received multiple blood transfusions, but these signs are becoming less frequent with the use of exogenous erythropoietin. In terminal renal failure, patients become drowsy and finally sink into a coma owing to nitrogen or toxin retention. Twitching due to myoclonic jerks, and tetany and epileptic seizures due to neuromuscular irritability or a low serum calcium level, occur late in renal failure. Overvigorous correction of acidosis (e.g. with bicarbonate infusions) may also precipitate seizures and coma. There may be typical skin nodules related to calcium phosphate deposition.

The state of fluid balance should be assessed in all patients with renal disease. Severe fluid-volume depletion can be a cause of acute kidney injury (AKI) and can cause precipitous decompensation in patients with CKD. Conversely, volume excess can result from intravenous infusions of fluid used in an attempt to correct AKI and cause pulmonary oedema. Patients should be weighed regularly as an objective measure of their fluid status.

The distinctive ketone-like smell of a urinary tract infection (UTI) may be apparent. There may be evidence of urinary incontinence on the patient's clothing.

HANDS

Inspect the patient's *nails*. Look for leuconychia. Muehrcke's nails[a] refer to paired white transverse lines near the end of the nails; these occur in hypoalbuminaemia (e.g. nephrotic syndrome).[1] A single transverse white band (Mees' lines[b]; see Fig. 18.4) may occur in arsenic poisoning, as well as in chronic kidney disease. Half-and-half nails (distal nail brown or red, proximal nail pink or white) are also seen in CKD.

---

[a] RC Meuhrcke reported this sign in the *British Medical Journal* in 1956.
[b] RA Mees, a Dutch physician, reported this sign in 1919. It had previously been reported (1901) in the *Lancet* by E Reynolds among drinkers of beer contaminated by arsenic in the north of England.

CHAPTER 18 **THE GENITOURINARY EXAMINATION** 307

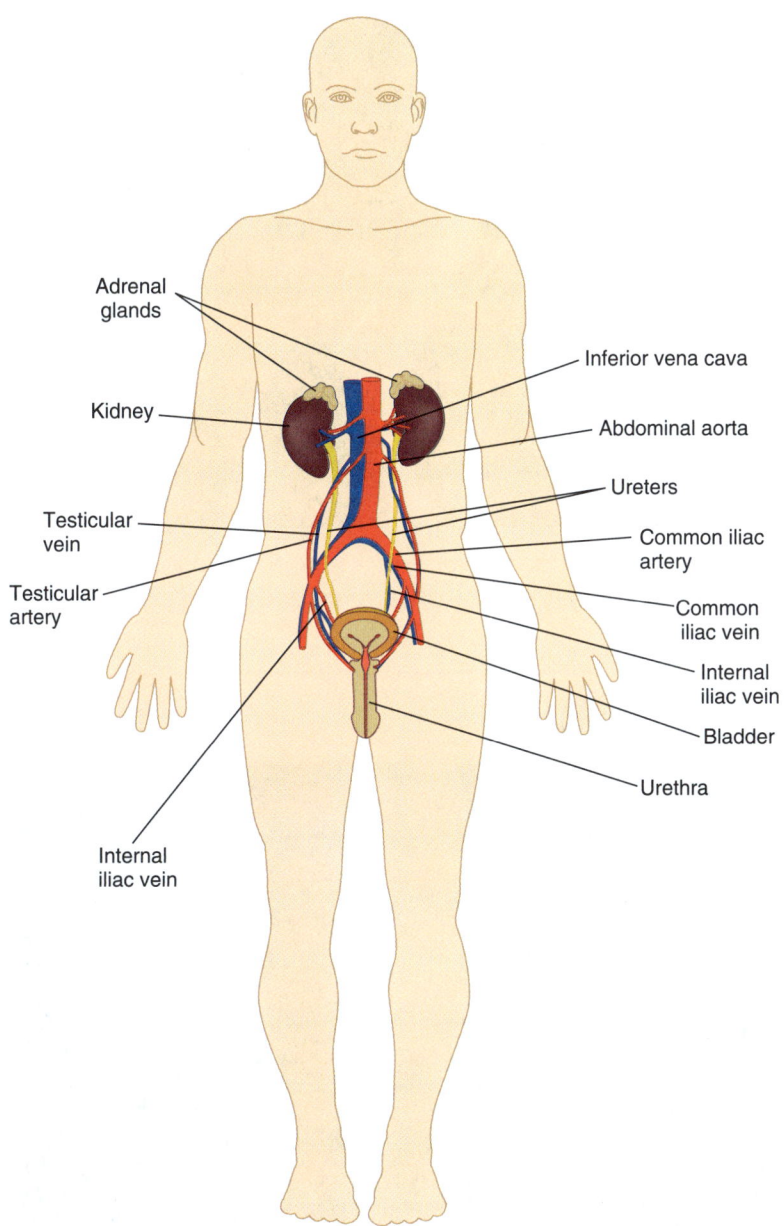

The anatomy of the kidneys and the urinary tract

FIGURE 18.1

Anaemia is common and causes palmar crease pallor. There are a number of causes of anaemia in patients with CKD, including poor nutrition (especially folate deficiency), blood loss, erythropoietin deficiency, haemolysis, bone marrow depression and the chronic disease state.

Asterixis (p 236) may be present in terminal CKD.

ARMS

Inspect the patient's wrists and forearms for scars and palpate for surgically created arteriovenous fistulae or shunts, used for haemodialysis access. There is a longitudinal swelling and a palpable continuous thrill—a characteristic buzzing feel—present over the

CT angiogram showing the origins and course of the renal arteries (large arrows) from the abdominal aorta; the left and right inferior phrenic arteries are visible arising superiorly

FIGURE 18.2

Outline of the renal collecting system.

This intravenous pyelogram shows the outline of the kidneys (1), the renal pelves (2) and the calyces (3) and ureters (4)

FIGURE 18.3

fistula (see Fig. 18.5). There may be scars from previous thrombosed shunts or carpal tunnel syndrome surgery present on either side. Look for signs of the carpal tunnel syndrome.

Bruising occurs because of nitrogen retention, which causes impaired prothrombin consumption, a defect in platelet factor III and abnormal platelet aggregation in CKD. *Skin pigmentation* is common, reflecting a failure to excrete urinary pigments. *Scratch marks and excoriations*, due to uraemic pruritus, often associated with hyperphosphataemia, may be present. This occurs commonly and can be extremely debilitating. *Uraemic*

CAUSES OF CHRONIC KIDNEY DISEASE (CKD)

This is defined as a severe reduction in nephron mass over a variable period of time resulting in uraemia.*

1. Glomerulonephritis
2. Diabetes mellitus
3. Systemic vascular disease
4. Analgesic nephropathy
5. Reflux nephropathy
6. Hypertensive nephrosclerosis
7. Polycystic kidney disease
8. Obstructive nephropathy
9. Amyloidosis
10. Renovascular disease
11. Atheroembolic disease
12. Hypercalcaemia, hyperuricaemia, hyperoxaluria
13. Autoimmune diseases
14. Haematological diseases
15. Toxic nephropathies
16. Granulomatous diseases
17. Chronic tubulointerstitial nephritis

Clinical features suggesting that renal failure is chronic rather than acute

Small kidney size (except with polycystic kidneys, diabetes, amyloidosis and myeloma)

Renal bone disease

Anaemia (with normal red blood cell indices)

Peripheral neuropathy

*Note that this list is not all-inclusive.
(Levey A, Eckarrdt K, Tsukanoto Y et al. Definition and classification of CKD: a position statement of KDIGO. *Kidney Int* 2005; 67:2089–2100.)

LIST 18.1

Mees' lines

(From McDonald FS, ed. *Mayo Clinic images in internal medicine*, with permission. © Mayo Clinic Scientific Press and CRC Press. Reproduced by permission of Taylor and Francis Group, LLC, a division of Informa plc.)

FIGURE 18.4

Arteriovenous fistula in the forearm of a haemodialysis patient

FIGURE 18.5

frost is a fine white powder present on the skin where very high concentrations of urea have precipitated out of the sweat in terminal CKD; it is very rare. Evidence of *vasculitis*, which can cause renal disease, should also be sought.

Look for signs of *peripheral neuropathy* (p 583) in the limbs. Sensory impairment is more marked than motor impairment initially. Myopathy and bone tenderness can also occur.

FACE

The presence of a *rash* or skin tethering may indicate an underlying connective tissue disease such as systemic lupus erythematosus or systemic sclerosis.

The presence of hearing aids may be consistent with Alport's syndrome (hereditary nephritis, often with sensorineural hearing loss and eye disease of the retina or cornea).

Inspect the patient's eyes and look for signs of *anaemia* and, rarely, *jaundice* (retention of nitrogenous wastes can cause haemolysis). *Band keratopathy* is a calcium deposition beneath the corneal epithelium in line with the interpalpebral fissure—it is due to secondary or tertiary hyperparathyroidism, or excessive replacement of calcium in patients with CKD.

A uraemic *fetor* may be present in the patient's mouth. This is an ammoniacal, musty odour that results from the breakdown of urea to ammonia in the saliva. Mucosal *ulcers* can occur as there is a decrease in saliva flow, and patients with CKD are prone to infection (e.g. thrush), owing to decreased acute inflammatory responses as a result of nitrogen retention. Transplant patients treated with calcineurin inhibitors (cyclosporin and tacrolimus) frequently develop *gingival hyperplasia* (thickening of the gums).

NECK

Carefully check the *jugular venous pressure* (see Fig. 5.6, p 77) to help assess the intravascular volume status. Auscultate for *carotid artery bruits*; these provide a (rather unreliable) clue that there may be generalised atherosclerotic disease (which can cause renal artery stenosis or complicate CKD). Look for signs of previous *jugular vein puncture* due to previous vascular access insertion ('vascath') for haemodialysis. Surgical scars from previous *parathyroidectomy* performed for management of tertiary hyperparathyroidism may be present.

CHEST

Examine the heart and lungs. In CKD there may be *congestive cardiac failure* due to fluid retention, and *hypertension* as a result of sodium and water retention or excess vasoconstrictor activity, or both. Signs of *pulmonary oedema* may also be present owing to uraemic lung disease (a type of non-cardiogenic pulmonary oedema associated with a typical 'bat's wing' pattern on chest X-ray; see Fig. 8.5, p 152), volume overload or uraemic cardiomyopathy.

Pericarditis, which can be fibrinous or haemorrhagic in CKD, is secondary to retained metabolic toxins and can cause a pericardial effusion; there may be a pericardial rub or signs of cardiac tamponade. Lung infection is also common as a result of the immunosuppression present from the CKD itself or of treatment.

THE ABDOMINAL EXAMINATION

Abdominal examination is performed as described on page 244. However, particular attention must be paid to the following.

Inspection

The presence of a Tenckhoff catheter (peritoneal dialysis catheter) should be noted. It is important to look for nephrectomy *scars* (see Fig. 14.28, p 245). These are often more posterior than one might expect. It may be necessary to roll the patient over and look in the region of the loins. Renal transplant scars are usually found in the right or left iliac fossae. A *transplanted kidney* may be visible as a bulge under the scar, as it is placed in a relatively superficial plane. Peritoneal dialysis results in small scars from catheter placement in the peritoneal cavity; these are situated on the lower abdomen, at or near the midline.

The abdomen may be distended because of large polycystic kidneys or *ascites* (as a result of the nephrotic syndrome, or peritoneal dialysis fluid).

Inspect the scrotum for masses and genital oedema.

Palpation

Particular care is required here so that renal masses (see List 18.2) are not missed. Remember that an enlarged kidney usually bulges forwards, while perinephric abscesses or collections tend to bulge backwards. Transplanted kidneys in the right or left iliac fossa may be palpable as well. Tenderness over the transplant can be a sign of rejection. Patients with polycystic kidneys may also have a polycystic liver and there may be hepatomegaly as a result of hepatic cysts (see List 18.3). Feel for the presence of an enlarged bladder.[2] Also palpate for an abdominal aortic aneurysm. In the patient with abdominal pain, renal colic should be suspected if there is renal tenderness (LR+, 3.6) or loin tenderness (LR+, 27.7).[3]

> ### RENAL MASSES
>
> **Unilateral palpable kidney**
> Renal cell carcinoma
> Hydronephrosis or pyonephrosis
> Xanthogranulomatous pyelonephritis
> Polycystic kidneys (with asymmetrical enlargement)
> Normal right kidney or solitary kidney
> Acute renal vein thrombosis (unilateral)
> Acute pyelonephritis
> Renal abscess
> Compensatory hypertrophy of single functioning kidney
>
> **Bilateral palpable kidneys**
> Polycystic kidneys
> Hydronephrosis or pyonephrosis bilaterally
> Renal cell carcinoma bilaterally
> Diabetic nephropathy (early)
> Nephrotic syndrome (see List 19.2, p 321)
> Infiltrative disease, e.g. amyloid, lymphoma
> Acromegaly
> Bilateral renal vein thrombosis
>
> LIST 18.2

> ### ADULT POLYCYSTIC KIDNEY DISEASE
>
> If you find polycystic kidneys, remember these very important points.
>
> 1. Take the blood pressure (75% of affected patients have hypertension).
> 2. Examine the urine for haematuria (due to haemorrhage into a cyst) and proteinuria (usually less than 2 g/day).
> 3. Look for evidence of anaemia (due to CKD) or polycythaemia (due to high erythropoietin levels). Note that the haemoglobin level is higher than expected for the degree of renal failure.
> 4. Note the presence of hepatomegaly or splenomegaly (due to cysts). These may cause confusion when one is examining the abdomen.
> 5. Tenderness on palpation may indicate an infected cyst.
>
> *Note:* Subarachnoid haemorrhage occurs in 3% of patients with polycystic kidney disease due to rupture of an associated intracranial aneurysm. As polycystic kidney disease is an autosomal dominant condition, all family members should also be assessed.
>
> LIST 18.3

Ballotting

From the French word meaning *to shake about*, ballotting is an examination technique for palpating the kidney by attempting to flick it forwards. Place one hand under the renal angle and flick your fingers upwards while your other hand—placed anteriorly in the right or left upper quadrant—waits to feel the kidney move upwards and then float down again (see Fig. 18.6).

Percussion

This is necessary to confirm the presence of ascites by examining for shifting dullness. Also percuss for an enlarged bladder.[4] Obesity and ascites make direct percussion of the bladder difficult. This is an opportunity to attempt *auscultatory percussion*.[2] Place the diaphragm of the stethoscope just above the border of the symphysis pubis and perform direct percussion of the abdominal wall, starting at the subcostal margin in the middle

Ballotting the kidneys

FIGURE 18.6

line. There is a sudden increase in loudness when the upper border of the bladder is reached. It is even possible to estimate the volume of urine in the bladder by this method. An upper border less than 2 centimetres from the stethoscope suggests a fairly empty bladder, while an upper border more than 8 centimetres higher corresponds to a urine volume of between 750 mL and 1 L.

Auscultation

The important sign here is the presence of a *renal bruit*. Renal bruits are best heard above the umbilicus, about 2 centimetres to the left or right of the midline. Listen with the diaphragm of the stethoscope over both these areas. Next ask the patient to sit up, and listen in both flanks. The presence of a systolic and diastolic bruit is important. A diastolic component makes the bruit more likely to be haemodynamically significant. Its presence suggests renal artery stenosis due to fibromuscular dysplasia or atherosclerosis. Approximately 50% of patients with renal artery stenosis will have a bruit. In a patient with hypertension that is difficult to control, the presence of a systolic/diastolic abdominal bruit has a positive LR for renal artery stenosis of over 40.[3] On the other hand, if only a soft systolic bruit is audible, at least half these patients do not have any significant renal artery stenosis. In such cases the aorta or splenic artery may be the source of the sound. The absence of hypertension makes the diagnosis of renal artery stenosis less likely. The occurrence of unexplained pulmonary oedema of sudden onset ('flash' pulmonary oedema) in a patient with renal impairment and hypertension makes a diagnosis of renal artery stenosis more likely.

Rectal and pelvic examination

Here the presence of prostatomegaly[5,6] in men and a frozen pelvis from cervical cancer in women is important, as this may be a cause of urinary tract obstruction and secondary renal failure. (For female pelvic examination, see Ch 40, p 752.)

THE BACK

Strike the patient's vertebral column gently with the base of your fist to elicit bony tenderness. This may be

Murphy's kidney punch (not too hard)

FIGURE 18.7

due to renal osteodystrophy from osteomalacia, secondary hyperparathyroidism or multiple myeloma. Back pain in the context of renal failure should always raise the possibility of an underlying paraproteinaemia.

Gentle use of the clenched fist to strike the patient in the renal angle is known as Murphy's kidney punch (see Fig. 18.7) and is designed to elicit renal tenderness in patients with renal infection. Similar information may be gained from more gentle ballotting of the renal angle when the patient lies supine. Look also for sacral oedema in a patient confined to bed, particularly if the nephrotic syndrome or congestive cardiac failure is suspected. The presence of ulcerations of the toes suggests atheroembolic disease.

LEGS

The important signs here are oedema, purpura (p 346), livedo reticularis (a red–blue reticular[c] pattern from vasculitis or atheroembolic disease), pigmentation, scratch marks and signs of peripheral vascular disease. Examination for peripheral neuropathy and myopathy is indicated, as in the arms. Gouty tophi or the presence of gouty arthropathy may very occasionally provide an explanation for the patient's renal failure (although secondary uric acid retention is common with CKD, it rarely causes clinical gout).

---

[c] *Reticulum* is the Latin word for a 'little net'.

BLOOD PRESSURE

It is of the utmost importance to take the blood pressure in every patient with renal disease. This is because hypertension can be the cause of renal disease or one of its complications. Test for postural hypotension, as hypovolaemia may precipitate AKI.

FUNDI

Examination of the fundi is important. Look especially for hypertensive changes and diabetic changes. Diabetes can be a cause of CKD.

MALE GENITALIA

Inspect the genitals (see Figs 18.8 and 18.9) for evidence of mucosal ulceration. This can occur in a number of systemic diseases, including Reiter's syndrome (reactive arthritis) and the rare Behçet's syndrome. For aesthetic and protective reasons, it is essential to wear gloves for this examination. Retract the foreskin to expose the glans penis. This mucosal surface is prone to inflammation or ulceration in both infective and connective tissue diseases (see List 18.4). Look also for urethral discharge. If there is a history of discharge, attempt to express fluid by compressing or 'milking'

the shaft. Any fluid obtained must be sent for microscopic examination and culture.

Inspect the scrotum with the patient standing. Usually the left testis hangs lower than the right. This is the only part of the body that consistently does not appear bilaterally symmetrical on inspection. Torsion

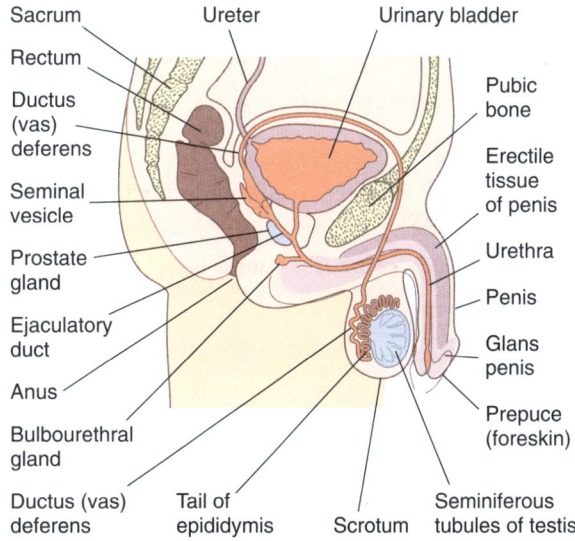

Male reproductive anatomy

FIGURE 18.8

(a) To palpate the epididymis, feel along the posterior pole of the testis

(b) Scrotal swelling—fingers can 'get above' mass

(c) Inguinal hernia with descent into the scrotum—fingers cannot 'get above' mass

Examination of scrotum

(From Douglas G, Nicol F, Robertson C. *Macleod's clinical examination*, 12th edn. Edinburgh: Churchill Livingstone, 2009.)

FIGURE 18.9

> **CAUSES OF GENITAL LESIONS**
>
> **Ulcerative**
> Herpes simplex (vesicles followed by ulcers: tender)
> Syphilis (non-tender)
> Malignancy (squamous cell carcinoma: non-tender)
> Chancroid (*Haemophilus ducreyi* infection: tender)
> Behçet's syndrome
>
> **Non-ulcerative**
> Balanitis, due to Reiter's syndrome or poor hygiene
> Venereal warts
> Primary skin disease (e.g. psoriasis)
>
> *Note:* Always consider HIV infection.
>
> LIST 18.4

of the testis may cause the involved testis to appear higher and to lie more transversely than normal. Inspect for oedema of the skin, sebaceous cysts, tinea cruris (an erythematous rash caused by a fungal infection of the moist skin of the groin) or scabies. Scrotal oedema is common in severe cardiac failure and may occur with the nephrotic syndrome and ascites.

Palpate each testis gently using the fingers and thumb of the (gloved) right hand or cradle the testis between the middle and index fingers of the right hand and palpate it with the ipsilateral thumb.[7] The testes are normally equal in size, smooth and relatively firm. Absence of one or both testes may be due to previous excision, failure of the testis to descend or to a retractile testis. In children the testes may retract as examination of the scrotum begins because of a marked cremasteric reflex. A maldescended testis (one that lies permanently in the inguinal canal or higher) has a high chance of developing malignancy. An exquisitely tender, indurated testis suggests orchitis.[8] This is often due to mumps in postpubertal patients and occurs about 5 days after the parotitis. An undescended testis may be palpable in the inguinal canal, usually at or above the external inguinal ring. The presence of small firm testes suggests an endocrine disease (hypogonadism) or testicular atrophy due to alcohol or drug ingestion.

Feel posteriorly for the epididymis and then upwards for the vas deferens and the spermatic cord. It should be possible to differentiate the vas from the testis.

A varicocele feels like a bag of worms in the scrotum. The testis on the side of the varicocele often lies horizontally. It is unclear whether this is a cause or effect of the varicocele. A left varicocele is sometimes found when there is an underlying left renal tumour or left renal vein thrombosis. The significance of the rarer right varicocele is disputed.[9]

Differential diagnosis of a scrotal mass

If a mass is palpable in the scrotum, decide first whether it is possible to get above it. Have the patient stand up. If no upper border is palpable, it must be descending down the inguinal canal from the abdomen and is therefore an inguinoscrotal hernia (see Fig. 18.10). If it is possible to get above the mass, it is necessary to decide whether it is separate from or part of the testis, and to test for translucency. This is performed using a transilluminoscope (a torch; see Fig. 18.11). With the patient in a darkened room, a small torch is applied to the side of the swelling by invaginating the scrotal wall. A cystic mass will light up, whereas a solid mass remains dark.

A mass that is part of the testis and that is solid (non-translucent) is likely to be a tumour or, rarely, a syphilitic gumma. The testes may be enlarged and hard in men with leukaemia. A mass that is cystic (translucent) with the testis within it is a hydrocele (a collection of fluid in the tunica vaginalis of the testis). A mass that appears separate from the testis and transilluminates is probably a cyst of the epididymis, whereas a similar mass that fails to transilluminate is probably the result of chronic epididymitis. By feeling along the testicular–epididymal groove it is usually possible to separate an epididymal mass from the testis itself.

CHAPTER 18 THE GENITOURINARY EXAMINATION 315

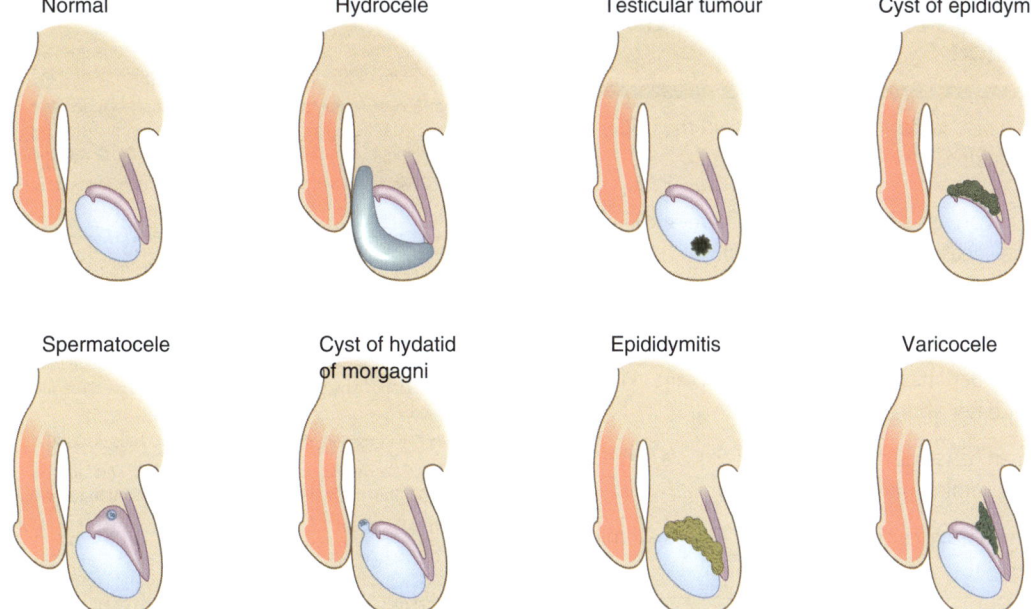

Differential diagnosis of a scrotal mass

(Adapted from Dunphy JE, Botsford TW. *Physical examination of the surgical patient. An introduction to clinical surgery*, 4th edn. Philadelphia: WB Saunders, 1975.)

FIGURE 18.10

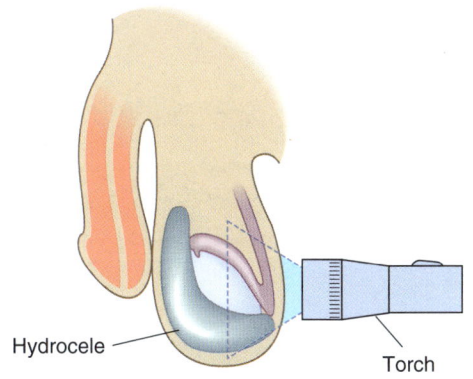

Transillumination of the scrotum

FIGURE 18.11

T&O'C ESSENTIALS

1. There may be no signs in a patient with renal disease.
2. The kidneys (unless transplanted) are retroperitoneal structures and are best palpated by ballotting.
3. Transplanted kidneys are easily felt on abdominal palpation and are superficial.
4. Polycystic kidneys may be very large but can be confused with an enlarged liver and spleen.
5. Examination of the urine is an extension of the renal examination.
6. A systematic approach is required for the male (and female) genital examination.

OSCE REVISION TOPICS – GENITOURINARY EXAMINATION

Use these topics, which commonly occur in the OSCE, to help with revision.

1. This woman has a family history of polycystic kidney disease. Please examine her. (p 310)
2. This man is undergoing haemodialysis. Please examine him. (p 306)
3. This woman has had a renal transplant. Please examine her abdomen. (p 310)
4. This man has stage 4 kidney disease and is a diabetic. Please examine him. (p 306)
5. This man has noticed a scrotal mass. Please examine him. (p 313)

References

1. Muehrcke RC. The fingernails in chronic hypoalbuminaemia: a new physical sign. *BMJ* 1956; 1:1327–1328. The classic description of this sign.
2. Guarino JR. Auscultatory percussion of the urinary bladder. *Arch Intern Med* 1985; 145:1823–1825. This careful study makes a convincing case for the use of this technique, especially in obese patients or those with ascites.
3. McGee S. *Evidence-based physical diagnosis*, 3rd edn. St Louis: Saunders, 2012.
4. D'Silva KA, Dahm P, Wong CL. Does this man with lower urinary tract symptoms have bladder outlet obstruction?: The Rational Clinical Examination: a systematic review. *JAMA* 2014; 312(5):535–542.
5. Guinan P, Bush I, Ray V et al. The accuracy of the rectal examination in the diagnosis of prostate carcinoma. *N Engl J Med* 1980; 303:499–503. This article suggests that rectal examination is an excellent technique for distinguishing benign prostatic hyperplasia and cancer, but this has subsequently been questioned.
6. Schroder FH. Detection of prostate cancer. *BMJ* 1995; 310:140–141.
7. Zornow DH, Landes RR. Scrotal palpation. *Am Fam Physician* 1981; 23:150–154. This article describes standard examination techniques.
8. Rabinowitz R, Hulbert WC Jr. Acute scrotal swelling. *Urol Clin North Am* 1995; 22:101–105.
9. Roy CR, Wilson T, Raife M, Horne D. Varicocele as the presenting sign of an abdominal mass. *J Urol* 1989; 141:597–599. A sign of late-stage renal cell carcinoma, due to testicular vein compression, but can be on the left or right side!

CHAPTER 19

A summary of the examination of chronic kidney disease and extending the genitourinary examination

The ghosts of dead patients that haunt us do not ask why we did not employ the latest fad of clinical investigation; they ask why did you not test my urine? SIR ROBERT HUTCHISON (1871–1960)

Examination of the patient with chronic kidney disease: a suggested method

Chronic kidney disease examination

FIGURE 19.1

1. General inspection
   Mental state
   Hyperventilation (acidosis), hiccups
   Sallow complexion ('uraemic tinge')
   Hydration
   Subcutaneous nodules (calcium phosphate deposits)
2. Hands
   Nails—leuconychia; white lines; distal brown arc
   Arteriovenous fistulae
   Asterixis
   Neuropathy
3. Arms
   Bruising
   Pigmentation
   Scratch marks/excoriations
   Myopathy
4. Face
   Eyes—anaemia, jaundice, band keratopathy
   Mouth—dryness, ulcers, fetor, gingival hypertrophy
   Rash (lupus, vasculitis, etc.)
5. Neck
   Jugular venous pressure
   Carotid bruits
   Scars from previous vascath insertion
   Parathyroidectomy scars
6. Abdomen
   Tenckhoff catheter
   Scars—dialysis, operations
   Kidneys—transplant kidney
   Bladder

TEXT BOX 19.1

Continued

Examination of the patient with chronic kidney disease: a suggested method *continued*

- Liver
- Lymph nodes
- Ascites
- Bruits
- Rectal and pelvic examination (prostatomegaly, frozen pelvis, bleeding)
7. Back
   - Nephrectomy scar
   - Tenderness
   - Oedema
8. Chest
   - Heart—heaving apex, pericarditis, failure
   - Lungs—infection, pulmonary oedema
9. Legs
   - Oedema—nephrotic syndrome, cardiac failure
   - Bruising
   - Pigmentation
   - Scratch marks/excoriation
   - Neuropathy
   - Vascular access
10. Urine analysis
    - Specific gravity, pH
    - Glucose—diabetes mellitus
    - Blood—'nephritis', infection, stone
    - Protein—'nephritis', etc.
11. Other
    - Blood pressure—lying and standing
    - Fundoscopy—hypertensive and diabetic changes, etc.
    - Rash, livedo reticularis
    - Genital examination, where indicated

Lay the patient flat in bed while performing the usual **general inspection**. Some patients with kidney failure may have fluid overload or a problem with heart failure and be unable to lie flat comfortably. Always ask whether the patient will be comfortable lying flat before dropping the head of the bed.* Note particularly the patient's mental state and the presence of a sallow complexion, whether the patient appears properly hydrated and whether there is any hyperventilation or hiccupping.

The detailed examination begins with the **hands** and inspection of the nails, which may reveal leuconychia, white transverse lines (Muehrcke's nails), a single white band (Mees' lines) or a distal brown arc (half-and-half nails). Examine the wrists and arms for a vascular access fistula.

Get the patient to hold out his or her hands and look for asterixis. Then inspect the **arms** for bruising, subcutaneous nodules (calcium phosphate deposits), pigmentation, scratch marks and gouty tophi.

Go now to the patient's **face** and begin by examining the eyes for anaemia, jaundice or band keratopathy. Examine the mouth for dryness, ulcers or fetor, and note the presence of any vasculitic rash on the face.

Check the **neck** for surgical scars, and listen for carotid bruits. Look at the jugular venous pressure with the patient at 45°.

The patient should then lie flat while you examine the **abdomen** for scars indicating peritoneal dialysis or operations, including renal transplants. Palpate for the kidneys, including transplanted kidneys, and then examine the liver and spleen. Feel for an abdominal aortic aneurysm. Percuss over the bladder, determine whether there is ascites, and listen for renal bruits. Rectal examination is indicated to detect prostatomegaly or bleeding.

Sit the patient up and palpate the **back** for tenderness and sacral oedema.

Examine the **heart** for signs of pericarditis or cardiac failure and the **lungs** for pulmonary oedema.

Lay the patient down again. Look at the **legs** for oedema (due to the nephrotic syndrome or cardiac failure), bruising, pigmentation, scratch marks or the presence of gout. Examine for peripheral neuropathy (decreased sensation, loss of the more distal reflexes).

Urinalysis is performed, testing for specific gravity, pH, glucose, blood, protein or leucocytes. The examination ends with measurement of the **blood pressure**, lying and standing (for orthostatic hypotension), and **fundoscopy** to look for hypertensive and diabetic changes.

---

*Some patients with vertigo are also very uncomfortable when lying flat.

TEXT BOX 19.1

EXTENDING THE GENITOURINARY EXAMINATION

Investigations

Kidney disease is investigated by the following:

1. Examination of the urine (e.g. dipstick testing, urine culture for infection) and urinary sediment.
2. Tests of renal function—for example, glomerular function by serum creatinine and estimated glomerular filtration rate (e-GFR, which is derived from the serum creatinine level), and tubular function by measuring electrolytes and urine (pH, specific gravity, glucose, protein excretion).
3. Blood tests to search for the causes of renal dysfunction—for example, looking for renal disease: hepatitis B or C, HIV, complement and immune complexes, tests for autoimmune disease, immunoelectrophoresis.
4. Blood tests to assess the effects of renal disease—for example, electrolyte changes; blood count (for anaemia); serum glucose (diabetes mellitus); calcium, phosphate and parathyroid hormone; uric acid.
5. Ultrasound and other scans (see Figs 19.4–19.7) to look at renal size and for any renal mass or urinary obstruction (ureters and bladder), and arterial Doppler to measure renal blood supply. Ultrasound of the scrotum is used to identify scrotal masses (see Fig. 19.8). Note the kidneys are usually both small on ultrasound in chronic kidney disease (CKD), but the exceptions include diabetes mellitus and amyloid or polycystic kidneys.
6. Renal biopsy—for example, to diagnose glomerulonephritis.

The urine

This valuable fluid must not be discarded in any patient in whom a renal, diabetic, gastrointestinal or other major system disease is suspected.

Colour

Look at the colour of the urine (see Table 19.1).

Some causes of urine colour changes

Colour	Underlying causes
Very pale or colourless	Dilute urine (e.g. overhydration, recent excessive beer consumption, diabetes insipidus,* post-obstructive diuresis)
Yellow-orange	Concentrated urine (e.g. dehydration) Bilirubin Tetracycline, anthracene, sulfasalazine, riboflavin, rifampacin
Brown	Bilirubin Nitrofurantoin, phenothiazines; chloroquine, senna, rhubarb (yellow to brown or red)
Pink	Beetroot consumption Phenindione, phenolphthalein (laxatives), uric acid crystalluria (massive)
Red	Haematuria, haemoglobinuria, myoglobinuria (may also be pink, brown or black) Porphyrins, rifampicin, phenazopyridine, phenytoin, beetroot
Green	Methylene blue, triamterene, myoglobinuria when mild
Black	Severe haemoglobinuria Methyldopa, metronidazole, unipenem Melanoma, ochronosis; porphyrins, alkaptonuria (red to black on standing)
White / milky	Chyluria

*Diabetes *comes from a Greek word meaning 'passing through' and refers to the large amount of urine passed by people with uncontrolled diabetes mellitus or with diabetes insipidus.* Mellitus *means 'sweet' and* insipidus *means 'tasteless'. We should be grateful that taste testing is no longer a part of the urinary examination.*

TABLE 19.1

Transparency

Phosphate or urate deposits can occur normally and produce white (phosphate) or pink (urate) cloudiness. Fainter cloudiness may be due to bacteria. Pus, chyle (lymphatic fluid) or blood can cause a more turbid appearance.

Smell

A mild ammoniacal smell is normal. A urinary tract infection (UTI) causes a fishy smell, and antibiotics can sometimes be smelt in the urine, as can asparagus.

Specific gravity

A urinometer, which is a weighted float with a scale, is used to measure specific gravity. The depth to which the float sinks in the urine indicates the specific gravity, which is read off the scale on the side. The specific gravity can also be estimated by dipstick methods.

Water has a specific gravity of 1, and the presence of solutes (especially heavy solutes such as glucose or an iodine contrast medium) in urine increases the specific gravity. The normal range is 1.002–1.025. A consistently low specific gravity suggests CKD (as there is failure of the kidneys to concentrate the urine) or diabetes insipidus (where there is a deficiency of antidiuretic hormone resulting in passage of a large volume of dilute urine). A high specific gravity suggests fluid volume depletion or diabetes mellitus with the presence of large amounts of glucose in the urine.

There is a rough correlation between the specific gravity of the urine and its osmolarity. For example, a specific gravity of 1.002 corresponds to an osmolarity of 100 mOsm/kg, and a specific gravity of 1.030 corresponds to 1200 mOsm/kg.

Chemical analysis

A chemical reagent colour strip allows simultaneous multiple analyses of pH, protein, glucose, ketones, blood, nitrite, specific gravity, the presence of leucocytes, bile and urobilinogen. The strip is dipped in the urine and colour changes are measured after a set period. The colours are compared with a chart provided. It should be noted that the specific gravity by dipstick is pH dependent and insensitive to non-ionised molecules, and therefore correlates poorly with urine osmolality.

pH

Normal urine is acidic, except after meals when for a short time it becomes alkaline (the alkaline tide). Measuring the pH of urine is helpful in a number of critical circumstances. Sometimes the urine has to be made alkaline for therapeutic purposes, such as treating myoglobinuria or recurrent urinary calculi due to uric acid or cystine. Distal renal tubular acidosis should be suspected if the early-morning urine is consistently alkaline and cannot be acidified. Urinary tract infections (UTIs) with urea-splitting organisms, such as *Proteus mirabilis*, can also cause an alkaline urine which, in turn, favours renal struvite stone formation.

Protein

The colours are compared with a chart provided. The strip tests give only a semiquantitative measure of urinary protein (+ to ++++) and, if positive, must be confirmed by other tests. It is very important to note that the dipstick is sensitive to albumin but not to other

---

CAUSES OF PROTEINURIA

Persistent proteinuria

1. Renal disease

Almost any renal disease may cause a trace of proteinuria. Moderate or large amounts tend to occur with glomerular disease (see List 19.2).

2. No renal disease (functional)

Exercise
Fever
Hypertension (severe)
Congestive cardiac failure
Burns
Blood transfusion
Postoperative
Acute alcohol abuse

Orthostatic proteinuria

Proteinuria that occurs when a patient is standing but not when recumbent is called orthostatic proteinuria. In the absence of abnormalities of the urine sediment, diabetes mellitus, hypertension or reduced renal function, it probably has a benign prognosis.

LIST 19.1

---

proteins. A reading of + of proteinuria may be normal, as up to 150 mg of protein a day is lost in the urine. Causes of abnormal amounts of protein in the urine are outlined in Lists 19.1 and 19.2. Chemical dipsticks do not detect the presence of Bence Jones proteinuria[a] (immunoglobulin light chains).

If proteinuria is detected on dipstick testing, this should be quantified and careful urine (phase-contrast) microscopy should be carried out to look for evidence of active renal disease.

Glucose and ketones

A semiquantitative measurement of glucose and ketones is available. Glycosuria usually indicates diabetes mellitus, but can occur with other diseases (see List 19.3).

Ketones in the urine of patients with diabetes mellitus are an important indication of the presence of diabetic ketoacidosis (see List 19.3). The three ketone bodies are acetone, beta-hydroxybutyric acid and acetoacetic acid. Lack of glucose (starvation) or lack of glucose availability for the cells (diabetes mellitus)

---

[a] Henry Bence Jones (1818–73), physician at St George's Hospital, London, described this in 1848.

NEPHROTIC SYNDROME

Definition
1. Proteinuria (>3.5 g per 24 hours) (*Note:* the other features can all be explained by loss of protein)
2. Hypoalbuminaemia (serum albumin <30 g/L, due to proteinuria)
3. Oedema (due to hypoalbuminaemia)
4. Hyperlipidaemia (due to increased LDL and cholesterol, possibly from loss of plasma factors that regulate lipoprotein synthesis)

Causes
PRIMARY RENAL PATHOLOGY
1. Membranous glomerulonephritis
2. Minimal change glomerulonephritis
3. Focal and segmental glomerulosclerosis

SECONDARY RENAL PATHOLOGY
1. Drugs (e.g. penicillamine, lithium, ampicillin, bisphosphonates, non-steroidal anti-inflammatory drugs)
2. Systemic disease (e.g. SLE, diabetes mellitus, amyloidosis)
3. Malignancy (e.g. carcinoma, lymphoma, multiple myeloma)
4. Infections (e.g. hepatitis B, hepatitis C, infective endocarditis, malaria, HIV)

LDL = low-density lipoprotein; SLE = systemic lupus erythematosus; HIV = human immunodeficiency virus.

LIST 19.2

CAUSES OF GLYCOSURIA AND KETONURIA

Glycosuria
Diabetes mellitus

Other reducing substances (false positives): metabolites of salicylates, ascorbic acid, galactose, fructose

Impaired renal tubular ability to absorb glucose (renal glycosuria) e.g. Fanconi's* syndrome (proximal renal tubular disease)

Ketonuria
Diabetic ketoacidosis
Starvation

*Guido Fanconi (1892–1972), a Zürich paediatrician. Considered a founder of modern paediatrics, he described this in 1936. It had previously been described by Guido De-Toni in 1933 and is sometimes called the De-Toni–Fanconi syndrome.

LIST 19.3

---

causes activation of carnitine acetyltransferase, which accelerates fatty acid oxidation in the liver. However, the pathway for the conversion of fatty acids becomes saturated, leading to ketone body formation. The strip tests react only to acetoacetic acid. Ketonuria may also be seen associated with fasting, vomiting and strenuous exercise.

Blood
Blood in the urine (haematuria) is abnormal and can be seen with the naked eye if 0.5 mL is present per litre of urine (see List 19.4). Blood may be a contaminant of the urine when women are menstruating. A positive dipstick test is abnormal and suggests haematuria, haemoglobinuria (uncommon) or myoglobinuria (also uncommon). The presence of more than a trace of protein in the urine in addition suggests that the blood is of renal origin. False-positives may occur when there is a high concentration of certain bacteria and false-negative results can occur if vitamin C is being taken.

Nitrite
If positive, this usually indicates infection with bacteria that produce nitrite. More-specific dipstick tests for white cells are now available; a positive test has an LR of 4.2 for a urinary infection and a negative test has an LR of 0.3.[1]

The urine sediment
Every patient with suspected renal disease should have a midstream urine sample examined (see Good signs guide 19.1). Centrifuge 10 mL of the urine at 2000 r.p.m. for 4 minutes. Remove the supernatant, leaving 0.5 mL; shake well to resuspend, then place one drop on a slide with a coverslip. Look at the slide using a low-power microscope and at specific formed elements under the high-power field (HPF) for identification. There is a significant false-negative rate when there are low numbers of formed elements in the urine. Look for red blood cells (RBCs), white blood cells (WBCs) and casts.

Red blood cells
These appear as small circular objects without a nucleus. Usually none are seen, although up to 5 RBCs/low-power

CAUSES OF POSITIVE DIPSTICK TEST FOR BLOOD IN THE URINE

Haematuria

RENAL
Glomerulonephritis
Polycystic kidney disease
Pyelonephritis
Renal cell carcinoma
Analgesic nephropathy
Malignant hypertension
Renal infarction (e.g. infective endocarditis, vasculitis)
Bleeding disorders

RENAL TRACT
Cystitis
Calculi (see Fig. 19.2)
Bladder or ureteric tumour
Prostatic disease (e.g. cancer, benign prostatic hypertrophy)
Urethritis

Haemoglobinuria

Intravascular haemolysis, e.g. microangiopathic haemolytic anaemia, march haemoglobinuria, prosthetic heart valve, paroxysmal nocturnal haemoglobinuria, chronic cold agglutinin disease

Myoglobinuria

This is due to rhabdomyolysis (muscle destruction):
- muscle infarction (e.g. trauma)
- excessive muscle contraction (e.g. convulsions, hyperthermia, marathon running)
- viral myositis (e.g. influenza, Legionnaires' disease)
- drugs or toxins (e.g. alcohol, snake venom, statins)
- idiopathic.

LIST 19.4

Renal calculus.

The large staghorn calculus shown here is occupying the calyces of the left renal pelvis. This type of calculus is almost always radio-opaque. Phleboliths (calcifications related to blood vessels) are rounded opacities seen in the pelvis below the level of the ischial spines, whereas ureteric calculi lie above this level, in the line of the ureters. An abdominal ultrasound examination (intravenous pyelograms [IVPs] are almost never performed in this context today) is necessary to check whether there is an obstruction at the pelviureteric junction. In general, 90% of renal calculi are radio-opaque and visible on plain X-ray films. A significant proportion of patients presenting with renal colic due to calcium calculi have hyperparathyroidism

FIGURE 19.2

GOOD SIGNS GUIDE 19.1
Urinalysis and chronic kidney disease

Sign	LR+	LR−
Blood on urine dipstick	1.55	0.89
Protein on urine dipstick	3.0	0.61
Blood or protein on urine dipstick	1.4	0.56
Red blood cells on urine microscopy	1.3	0.78
Casts on urine microscopy	4.1	0.22
Microalbuminuria	3.4	0.76

field (LPF) may be normal in very concentrated urine. If their numbers are increased, try to determine whether the RBCs originate from the glomeruli (more than 80% of the RBCs are dysmorphic—irregular in size and shape) or the renal tract (the RBCs are typically uniform).

White blood cells

These cells have lobulated nuclei. Usually fewer than 6 WBCs/HPF are present, although up to 10 may be normal in very concentrated urine. Tubular epithelial cells have a compact nucleus and are larger. Pyuria indicates urinary tract inflammation. Bacteria may also be seen if there is infection, but bacterial contamination is more likely if squamous epithelial cells (which are larger and have single nuclei) are prominent. Sterile pyuria is characteristic of renal tuberculosis but may also occur in acute or chronic tubulointerstitial disease. Multistix test strips will often test for the presence of WBCs.

Casts

Casts are cylindrical moulds formed in the lumen of the renal tubules or collecting ducts (see Fig. 19.3). They are signs of a damaged glomerular basement membrane or damaged tubules. The size of a cast is determined by the dimension of the lumen of the nephron in which it forms. The presence of casts is a very important abnormality and indicates renal disease.

Hyaline casts are long cylindrical structures. One or two RBCs or WBCs may be present in the cast. Normally there are fewer than 1 per LPF. They consist largely of Tamm–Horsfall mucoprotein secreted by the renal tubules.

Granular casts are abnormal cylindrical granular structures that arise from the tubules, usually in patients with proteinuria. They consist of hyaline material containing fragments of serum proteins.

Red cell casts are always abnormal and indicate primary glomerular disease (haematuria of glomerular origin or vasculitis). They contain 10 to 50 red cells, which are well defined.

With **white cell casts** many WBCs adhere to or inside the cast. These are abnormal, indicating bacterial pyelonephritis or less commonly glomerulonephritis, kidney infarction or vasculitis.

Fatty casts (i.e. the presence of fat in casts) are suggestive of the nephrotic syndrome.

Electrolyte abnormalities

The kidneys play an important role in maintaining fluid and electrolyte balance within the body. The most common electrolyte abnormalities are:

- hyperkalaemia (increased potassium concentration in the blood)
- hypokalaemia (reduced potassium concentration)
- hypernatraemia (increased sodium concentration)
- hyponatraemia (reduced sodium concentration).

Hyperkalaemia
Causes:

- Severe CKD—can be an indication for dialysis.
- Renal tubular acidosis (type 4)—often seen in diabetics mellitus.
- Addison's disease (low mineralocorticoid levels).
- Drugs—angiotensin-converting enzyme (ACE) inhibitors and angiotensin II receptor (AR) blockers, spironolactone.

Ask the patient about muscle weakness, medications and kidney or endocrine disease. Palpitations or syncope may indicate cardiac arrhythmias (see the OCSE ECG library, Cardiac arrrythmia at Student CONSULT).

A red cell cast of urine.

Red cell casts are the deposition of red cells in Tamm-Horsfall protein excreted within renal tubules, and acting as a matrix of urinary casts. These occur only in glomerular inflammation, and are quantitatively linked to severity (number of casts per high-power field)

(Henry JB. *Clinical diagnosis and management by laboratory methods*, 20th edn. Figure 28.21, Saunders, 2001, 445–479pp.)

FIGURE 19.3

Hypokalaemia

Causes:
- Loss of fluid, e.g. diarrhoea and vomiting.
- Hyperaldosteronism leading to hypertension.
- Drugs, e.g. diuretics.
- Some forms of renal tubular acidosis.
- Anorexia nervosa.

Ask about muscle weakness and palpitations (e.g. from ectopic beats or ventricular tachycardia; see the OCSE ECG library, Ventricular tachycardia at Student CONSULT). Ask about diuretic or laxative use, diarrhoea and vomiting.

Look for underweight and ask about diet—anorexia nervosa.

Hypernatraemia

Remember that the problem is not too much sodium but rather not enough water.

Cause:
- Dehydration—more sodium is conserved (aldosterone) than water (vasopressin)

This may be due to:
- loss of water from the kidneys
  - glycosuria (diabetes)
  - reduced vasopressin release (diabetes insipidus)
  - use of osmotic diuretics, e.g. mannitol
  - age-related reduced renal concentrating ability
- loss of water from other places
  - sweating, burns
  - very severe diarrhoea
  - severe vomiting.

Ask about diarrhoea and vomiting, diabetes and recent blood sugar levels, extreme exercise and sweating, muscle weakness, seizures.

Look for signs of dehydration (p 44), muscular and cerebral irritability, and seizures and coma.

Hyponatraemia

Hyponatraemia is quite common. The problem is usually too much water rather than not enough salt. Patients may be euvolaemic, hypervolaemic or hypovolaemic.

Causes:
- *Euvolaemia:* syndrome of inappropriate antidiuretic hormone (SIADH)—(see List 19.5), serious illnesses, pain, polydipsia.
- *Hypervolaemic:* liver failure, cardiac failure, CKD.
- *Hypovolaemic:* fluid loss—vomiting, diarrhoea and diuretic use.

Ask (if the patient is able to answer) in detail about drug use (diuretics and drugs that can cause SIADH), water drinking, liver, heart or kidney disease.

Look for signs of confusion and serious illnesses (e.g. pneumonia, head injury).

CAUSES OF SYNDROME OF INAPPROPRIATE ANTIDIURETIC HORMONE (SIADH)

1. Drugs—anticonvulsants, psychotropics, antidepressants, cytotoxics, opiates, oral hypoglycaemic agents
2. Tumours, e.g. small cell carcinoma of the lung
3. Stroke, head injury, cerebral abscess
4. Pneumonia, tuberculosis
5. Postoperative state, pain

LIST 19.5

CHAPTER 19 **A SUMMARY OF THE EXAMINATION OF CHRONIC KIDNEY DISEASE** 325

Imaging the kidneys and scrotum

Some common scan findings are presented in Figs 19.4–19.8.

Ultrasound of polycystic kidneys. There are multiple discrete cysts, the largest being 1.2×1.2 centimetres

(From Kaplan BS, Meyers K. *Paediatric nephrology and urology: requisites*, 1st edn. St Louis, MO: Mosby, 2004.)

FIGURE 19.5

Ultrasound of (a) normal kidneys and (b) hydronephrosis with cortical atrophy

(From Adam A, Dixon A, Gillard J et al. *Grainger & Allison's diagnostic radiology*, 5th edn. Edinburgh: Churchill Livingstone, 2008.)

FIGURE 19.4

Nuclear scan of small scarred left kidney in a patient with hypertension. There is an area of infarction in the upper pole of the right kidney

(From Mason J, Pusey C. *The kidney in systemic autoimmune diseases. Volume 7, Handbook of systemic autoimmune diseases.* London: Elsevier, 2007.)

FIGURE 19.6

CT scan of renal tumour showing needles used for ablation treatment

(From Allan PL, Baxter GM, Weston M. *Clinical ultrasound*, 3rd edn. Edinburgh: Churchill Livingstone, 2011.)

FIGURE 19.7

Ultrasound of scrotal mass; sagittal and transverse scans of a seminoma. There is a lobulated heterogeneous mass with a thin rim of normal testis

(From Rumack CM, Wilson S, Charboneau JW, Levine D. *Diagnostic ultrasound*, 4th edn. St Louis, MO: Mosby, 2010.)

FIGURE 19.8

T&O'C ESSENTIALS

1. Assessment of kidney disease and its severity depend on blood tests that provide data about renal function.
2. Analysis of the urine is important, especially as a screening test—for example, by the detection of blood or excess protein.
3. Renal ultrasound can help distinguish CKD (usually, small kidneys) from acute kidney disease (usually, normal-sized kidneys).
4. Renal biopsy may be needed for the accurate diagnosis of renal pathology, especially for the identification of glomerulonephritis.

OSCE REVISION TOPICS

1. Perform dipstick testing on this urine sample. Explain the significance of the findings. (p 319)
2. Discuss the significance of this urinalysis, which shows ++++ proteinuria. What physical examination would you perform for the patient? (p 320)
3. This woman has large kidneys on examination. Discuss the appropriate investigations for her. (p 325)

Reference

1. McGee S. *Evidence-based physical diagnosis*, 3rd edn. St Louis: Saunders, 2012.

SECTION 6
The haematological system

CHAPTER 20

The haematological history

CHAPTER 21

The haematological examination

CHAPTER 22

A summary of the haematological examination and extending the haematological examination

CHAPTER 20
The haematological history

The blood is the generative part, the fountain of life, the first to live, the last to die and the primary seat to the soul. WILLIAM HARVEY (1578–1657)

HAEMATOLOGICAL DISORDERS

The range of haematological disorders includes the following:

- Abnormalities of red cells—for example, anaemia (too few red cells), polycythaemia (too many red cells) and haemoglobinopathies (abnormal haemoglobin molecules). Small red cells (microcytosis) and anaemia are usually a result of iron deficiency. Large red cells (macrocytosis) and anaemia can be secondary to vitamin B_{12} or folate deficiency (oval macrocytosis), recent blood loss (new red cells are large) or excessive alcohol consumption and liver disease of any cause (round macrocytosis). Chronic kidney disease is usually associated with anaemia partly as a result of reduced erythropoietin production by the kidneys.
- Abnormalities of platelets—for example, thrombocytopenia (reduced platelet numbers), thrombocytosis (increased platelet numbers) and reduced platelet function, for example as a result of the use of antiplatelet drugs (aspirin being the commonest).
- Abnormalities of clotting factors—for example, haemophilia (clotting factor VIII or IX deficiency) and increased tendency to clotting (e.g. presence of factor V Leiden mutation).
- Abnormalities of white cells—for example, neutropenia (reduced neutrophil numbers) and leukaemia (increased numbers of white cells, mature, immature or both).
- Reductions in bone marrow production of white or red cells, or both (e.g. myelodysplastic syndrome [MDS], myelofibrosis, bone marrow infiltration and drug- or immune-induced aplasia).
- Cancers of lymph nodes (Hodgkin's lymphoma and non-Hodgkin's lymphoma [NHL]).
- Abnormalities of immunoglobulin-producing cells—for example, multiple myeloma (monoclonal overproduction) and immunoglobulin deficiencies.

PRESENTING SYMPTOMS

Major presenting symptoms are outlined in List 20.1.

Red cell abnormalities

The numerous causes of anaemia make a careful history important in helping to work out the aetiology (see Questions box 20.1).

Patients with anaemia may present with weakness, tiredness, dyspnoea, fatigue or postural dizziness. Angina and heart failure may be precipitated by anaemia. Anaemia due to iron deficiency is often the result of gastrointestinal blood loss, or sometimes recurrent heavy menstrual blood loss, so these symptoms should be sought. The anaemia of chronic disease (red cells are normal in size—normochromic) occurs as a result of bone marrow suppression associated with chronic illness such as rheumatoid arthritis, infective endocarditis and chronic kidney disease.

Ask about other illnesses and travel. In much of the world chronic malarial infection or intestinal parasitic infection is the cause of chronic anaemia.

Ask about alcohol intake, diet and possible vitamin B_{12} deficiency if the patient is known to have macrocytic anaemia. Some vegan diets can lead to B_{12} deficiency.

HAEMATOLOGICAL HISTORY

Major symptoms

SYMPTOMS OF ANAEMIA
- Weakness
- Tiredness
- Dyspnoea
- Fatigue
- Postural dizziness

The patient may be aware of a problem that is associated with anaemia:
- bleeding (menstrual, gastrointestinal, after dental extractions)
- dietary iron (microcytic anaemia; p 353) and vitamin B_{12} or folate deficiency (macrocytic anaemias; p 353)
- bone pain due to marrow abnormalities (e.g. infiltration, multiple myeloma, leukaemia)
- chronic disease (e.g. rheumatoid arthritis)
- haemoglobinopathy (family history of thalassaemia)
- malaria.

SYMPTOMS OF BLEEDING AND CLOTTING ABNORMALITIES
- Easy bruising
- Petechiae (pinhead red, non-bleeding flat spots)
- Purpura (>5 mm)
- Bleeding into joints (haemophilia)
- Thrombotic tendency

The patient may know of previous problems with:
- coagulation (e.g. haemophilia)
- platelets (e.g. ITP [a low platelet count], antiplatelet drugs)
- an increased risk of clotting, thrombophilia (e.g. previous deep vein thrombosis [DVT], inherited clotting abnormality).

SYMPTOMS OF ABNORMALITIES OF WHITE CELLS
- Recurrent infections (e.g. neutropenia, multiple myeloma, bone marrow suppression)
- Fever or jaundice
- Mouth ulcers

SYMPTOMS OF LYMPHOMA
- Lymph gland enlargement
- Loss of weight, fever, sweats, tiredness

SYMPTOMS OF MYELOMA
- CRAB:
  - **C**alcium, hypercalcaemia symptoms
  - **R**enal impairment, fatigue
  - **A**naemia, dyspnoea and palpitations
  - **B**one pain, or fractures

OTHER
- Recurrent infections (e.g. pneumonia)
- Enlargement of the tongue from secondary amyloidosis

LIST 20.1

Previous resection of the stomach or terminal ileum (intrinsic factor not produced—stomach; or B_{12} not absorbed—ileal resection) can also lead to B_{12} deficiency. Serious gastrointestinal disease can cause folate and iron deficiency because of malabsorption.

Polycythaemia may be associated with pruritus and headache. Ask about smoking and chronic lung disease (hypoxia), which can be a cause.

Clotting and bleeding

Consider the important causes of abnormal bleeding.

Platelets

Disorders of platelet function may present with petechiae (flat red pinhead-sized spots), easy bruising or bleeding problems (Table 20.1). Ask about drug treatment; antiplatelet drugs are commonly prescribed for vascular disease. Reduced platelet numbers (thrombocytopenia), sometimes associated with increased bleeding risk, can occur as a result of autoimmune disorders (idiopathic thrombocytopenic purpura [ITP]). Ask about previous traumatic or surgical splenectomy, which can result in increased platelet numbers (thrombocytosis).

QUESTIONS TO ASK THE PATIENT WITH ANAEMIA

1. How was the problem diagnosed? (Routine tests or symptoms)
2. What symptoms have you had (e.g. tiredness, dyspnoea, angina)?
3. Have you noticed any bleeding from the bowel, or vomited any blood?
4. Have you noticed black bowel motions?
5. Have you had problems with stomach ulcers or inflammation of the bowel (colitis) or previous bowel operations?
6. Have you been taking arthritis tablets or blood-thinning tablets?
7. Have you had a recent operation or procedure? (Blood loss)
8. Have you had heavy periods?
9. What is your diet like? Are you a vegetarian or vegan? Do you drink much alcohol?
10. Do you take iron or vitamin supplements?
11. Have you had problems with your kidneys or a chronic severe arthritis? (Anaemia of chronic disease)
12. Have you ever needed a blood transfusion?
13. Have you been generally unwell or had problems with recurrent infections or ulcers?
14. Is there a history of anaemia in the family? Do you know what the cause was? (Haemoglobinopathy)

QUESTIONS BOX 20.1

Features of bleeding abnormalities

	Platelet abnormalities	Coagulation abnormalities
Family or medication history	Sometimes	Often
Sex	Females > males	Males > females
Petechiae	Usual	Unusual
Superficial ecchymoses (bruises)	Small, numerous	Large, single
Bleeding into joints (haemarthrosis)	Rare	Common
Delayed bleeding after trauma	Rare	Common
Haematoma (deeper bruises)	Rare	Common

TABLE 20.1

Coagulation abnormalities

Haemophilia

Deficiency of factor VIII causes haemophilia A and of factor IX, haemophilia B. These are X-linked recessive disorders.

The clinical picture depends on the severity of the reduction of the clotting factor in the blood. Severe reduction in levels is associated with spontaneous bleeding, particularly into load-bearing joints, especially the knees (haemarthroses). Recurrent joint bleeds lead to arthropathy. Bleeding into large muscles—thigh, iliopsoas, calf and abdominal wall—is common. Spontaneous cerebral bleeding is uncommon but can occur after minor trauma.

The patient with severe haemophilia will often be well informed about this lifelong condition but less severe disease may have been diagnosed only after testing because of unusual bleeding following surgery. Questions box 20.2 outlines important questions to ask a patient with haemophilia.

Von Willebrand's disease[a]

Von Willebrand factor, which is encoded on chromosome 12, binds to collagen at the site of vascular injury and attracts platelets to these sites. It also protects factor VIII from degradation.

Venous thrombosis and embolism

Ask about abnormal clotting anywhere in the body. Deep vein thrombosis (DVT) may present with pain and swelling in the calves and thrombosis in the proximal leg veins may be complicated by pulmonary embolism. This may have been diagnosed as a result of breathlessness and chest pain and when the embolus was very large by hypoxia and shock. The patient may remember having had a CT pulmonary angiogram or

---

[a] EA von Willebrand (1870–1949), a Swedish physician, described this in 1926.

> **HAEMOPHILIA**
>
> 1. Do you know whether you have haemophilia A or B?
> 2. Has anyone in the family been affected?
> 3. How old were you when it was diagnosed?
> 4. Do you know how low your factor VIII or IX level is?
> 5. What bleeding problems have you had?
> 6. Have you had damage to your joints? Which ones?
> 7. How does this affect your ability to exercise or work?
> 8. What precautions do you take to protect yourself from bleeding?
> 9. How do you get factor VIII injections when you need them?
> 10. What do you do if you hurt yourself or need dental work or an operation?
>
> QUESTIONS BOX 20.2

> **RISK FACTORS FOR THROMBOSIS**
>
> **Patient:**
> - Obesity
> - Advanced age
> - Smoking
> - Oral contraceptive or hormone replacement treatment
> - Pregnancy
> - Prolonged immobilisation—bedbound, long-distance travel
>
> **Surgery**
> - Lower limb orthopaedic surgery
> - Trauma and immobilisation
> - Pelvic or abdominal surgery especially for malignancy
> - Lower limb immobilisation after surgery or trauma—splints, etc.
>
> **Medical illnesses**
> - Malignancy
> - Cardiac failure
> - Vasculitis
> - Inflammatory bowel disease
>
> **Haematological prothrombotic abnormalities**
> - Prothrombin gene mutation
> - Factor V Leiden mutation
> - Antiphospholipid syndrome
> - Deficiency of endogenous anticoagulants, e.g. protein C, protein S, antithrombin 3
>
> These factors interact with each other. For example, factor V Leiden mutation and oral contraceptive use together increase thrombotic risk 100 fold.
>
> LIST 20.2

V/Q lung scan. The number of lung segments involved may be known. The patient may know about late complications including:
- chronic venous insufficiency in the legs
- the development of pulmonary hypertension
- recurrent episodes.

Venous thrombosis can also occur in other veins, for example the axillary vein,[b] vena cava (extension from leg veins or associated with renal cell carcinoma).

Find out whether the patient has any prothrombotic risk factors (List 20.2).

Finally ask what the patient knows about the longer-term prognosis and measures recommended to prevent further episodes. How has this life-threatening disease affected his or her life and family?

Arterial thrombosis and embolism

Arterial thrombosis and embolism may present as stroke, limb ischaemia, or mesenteric or renal ischaemia. Although the majority of cases are due to atherosclerosis or cardiac causes (e.g. atrial fibrillation), there are a number of haematological causes to consider:
- polycythaemia
- sickle cell anaemia
- heparin-induced thrombocytopenia and thrombosis (HITT)
- systemic lupus erythematosus (SLE)
- antiphospholipid syndrome
- inherited causes (e.g. protein C or S deficiency).

---

[b] Traditionally caused by the patient's having drunk too much alcohol and falling asleep with his arm draped over a bar stool.

> **DIFFERENTIAL DIAGNOSIS OF SUSPECTED LYMPHADENOPATHY**
>
> 1. Lipoma—usually large and soft; may not be in lymph node area
> 2. Abscess—tender and erythematous, may be fluctuant
> 3. Sebaceous cyst—intradermal location
> 4. Thyroid nodule—forms part of thyroid gland
> 5. Secondary to recent immunisation, or cellulitis
>
> LIST 20.3

Recurrent infection

Recurrent infection such as pneumonia may be the first symptom of a disorder of the immune system, including leukaemia (due to low neutrophils), multiple myeloma (due to low-normal immunoglobulin levels), HIV infection (lymphopenia) or inherited or acquired immunoglobulin deficiency. The patient may have noticed lymph node enlargement, which can occur with lymphoma or leukaemia. Not all lumps are lymph nodes: consider the differential diagnosis (see List 20.3). Ask about fever, its duration and pattern. Lymphomas can be a cause of chronic fever, and viral infections such as cytomegalovirus and infectious mononucleosis are associated with haematological abnormalities and fever.

Immunoglobulin deficiency is associated with recurrent severe respiratory tract infections and sinusitis. Ask about symptoms of sinusitis and bronchiectasis.

TREATMENT HISTORY TO ASK ABOUT

- Anaemia may have been treated with iron supplements or vitamin B_{12} injections.
- Anti-inflammatory drugs or anticoagulants may be the cause of bleeding.
- Supportive treatment for anaemia due to myelodysplastic syndrome (MDS), myelofibrosis or bone marrow failure may have included regular blood transfusions.
- Patients with chronic kidney disease may be taking erythropoietin.
- Polycythaemia or haemochromatosis may have been treated with regular venesections.
- Treatment for leukaemia, myeloma or lymphoma may have involved chemotherapy, radiotherapy, or both, or bone marrow transplant. Ask about the effects these complicated treatments have had on the patient's life.
- Splenectomy may have been performed for thrombocytopenia or lymphoma.
- Corticosteroids and sometimes immunosuppressive drugs are also used for idiopathic thrombocytopenia.
- Regular immunoglobulin infusions are used for patients with immunoglobulin deficiency. Ask whether these have been effective at reducing infections.
- Factor VIII will have been used to treat factor-VIII-deficient haemophiliacs. This may be derived from blood donors of a recombinant product. Older patients may have been exposed to hepatitis and human immune deficiency viruses. Ask whether the patient knows his or her hepatitis and HIV status.
- Recombinant and donor-obtained factor IX concentrate is available for patients with haemophilia B.

What treatment has been recommended for the patient with a history of thrombosis and for what period? Ask about:

- intravenous or subcutaneous heparin
- oral anticoagulation—e.g. with warfarin or direct oral anticoagulant (DOAC), e.g. apixaban, rivaroxaban or dabigatran
- if warfarin is being taken, the monitoring of this drug (INR testing) and the recommended INR range
- whether there have been problems with drug treatment—especially bleeding
- aspirin—used for prophylaxis against DVT after treatment with an anticoagulant
- whether other treatment has been needed, e.g. surgery to remove clots, a vena caval filter to prevent more pulmonary emboli.

PAST HISTORY

A history of colonoscopy for polyps or bowel cancer, or malabsorption may give a clue regarding the underlying cause of anaemia. Anaemia in patients with systemic disease such as rheumatoid arthritis or chronic kidney disease can be multifactorial.

SOCIAL HISTORY

A patient's racial origin is relevant. Thalassaemia is common in people of Mediterranean or southern Asian origin and sickle cell disease in Africans. Find out the patient's occupation and whether he or she has had very heavy work exposure to toxins such as benzene (risk of leukaemia). Ask whether the patient has had previous chemotherapy for a malignancy (drug-related development of leukaemia or MDS). Find out whether the patient drinks alcohol and how much.

FAMILY HISTORY

There may be a history of thalassaemia or sickle cell anaemia in the family. Haemophilia is a sex-linked recessive disease, whereas von Willebrand's[a] disease is autosomal dominant with incomplete penetrance.

OSCE REVISION TOPICS

1. This man has haemophilia A. Take a history from him. (p 330)

2. This woman has iron deficiency anaemia. Take a history from her and outline the possible causes. (pp 331, 353)

3. This woman has been bruising easily. Take a history from her and give a possible differential diagnosis. (p 330)

T&O'C ESSENTIALS

1. Haematological symptoms are often not specific: many haematological and other diseases cause tiredness and malaise.

2. Anaemia and chronic leukaemias are most often diagnosed on a routine blood test, not physical examination, but taking a careful history from patients can often give clues about its aetiology and help direct further tests.

3. Many medications can cause haematological problems and patients do not always appreciate these medications as being relevant (e.g. over-the-counter aspirin). Careful questioning is important to identify possible drug side effects as a cause of haematological disease.

4. Recurrent infection should arouse suspicions about underlying acute or chronic haematological disease.

CHAPTER 21
The haematological examination

Blood; the red liquor that circulates in the bodies of animals. SAMUEL JOHNSON, A dictionary of the English language *(1775)*

Haematological assessment does not depend only on the microscopic examination of the blood constituents. Physical signs, followed by examination of the blood film, can give vital clues about underlying disease. Haematological disease can affect the red blood cells (RBCs), the white blood cells (WBCs), the platelets and other haemostatic mechanisms, as well as the mononuclear–phagocyte (reticuloendothelial) system.

EXAMINATION ANATOMY

An important part of the examination involves assessment of all the palpable groups of lymph nodes. As each group is examined its usual drainage area must be kept in mind (see Fig. 21.1). It follows that whenever an abnormality is discovered anywhere that might be due to infection or malignancy its **draining lymph nodes must be examined**. A decision about the size of the spleen is one of the most important aspects of the haematological examination. The normal spleen lies almost completely under the ribs and is not palpable. An enlarging spleen cannot displace the spine, kidney (it is retroperitoneal) or the diaphragm and so moves downwards and displaces the stomach. Its anterior pole follows a course in line with the bony part of the tenth rib and as it descends below the rib cage moves across the abdomen towards the right iliac fossa.

Ludwig Traube described a space defined superiorly by the sixth rib, laterally by the midaxillary line and inferiorly by the left costal margin that is normally resonant to percussion. He noted that it became dull in the presence of a pleural effusion but did not realise that enlargement of the spleen also caused this resonance to disappear (p 258).

GENERAL APPEARANCE

Position the patient as for the gastrointestinal examination—lying on the bed with one pillow (see Fig. 14.2, p 230). Look for signs of wasting and for *pallor* (which may be an indication of anaemia).[1-3] Note the patient's racial origin (e.g. thalassaemia and sickle cell disease). If there is any *bruising*, look at its distribution and extent. *Jaundice* may be present and can indicate haemolytic anaemia. *Scratch marks* (following pruritus, which sometimes occurs with lymphoma and myeloproliferative disease) should be noted.

HANDS

The detailed examination begins in the usual way with assessment of the hands. Look at the nails for *koilonychia*—these are dry, brittle, ridged, spoon-shaped nails, which are rarely seen today. They can be due to severe iron deficiency anaemia, although the mechanism is unknown. Occasionally koilonychia may be due to fungal infection. They may also be seen in Raynaud's phenomenon (see Fig. 21.2). Digital infarction (see Fig. 21.3) may be a sign of abnormal globulins (e.g. cryoglobulinaemia). Pallor of the nail beds may occur in anaemia but is an unreliable sign. Pallor of the *palmar creases* suggests that the haemoglobin level is less than 70 g/L, but this is also a rather unreliable sign.[1]

Note any changes of rheumatoid or gouty *arthritis*, or connective tissue disease (see Ch 25). Rheumatoid arthritis, when associated with splenomegaly and neutropenia, is called Felty's syndrome:[a] the mechanism

---
[a] Augustus Roi Felty (1895–1963), a physician at Hartford Hospital, Connecticut, described this in 1924.

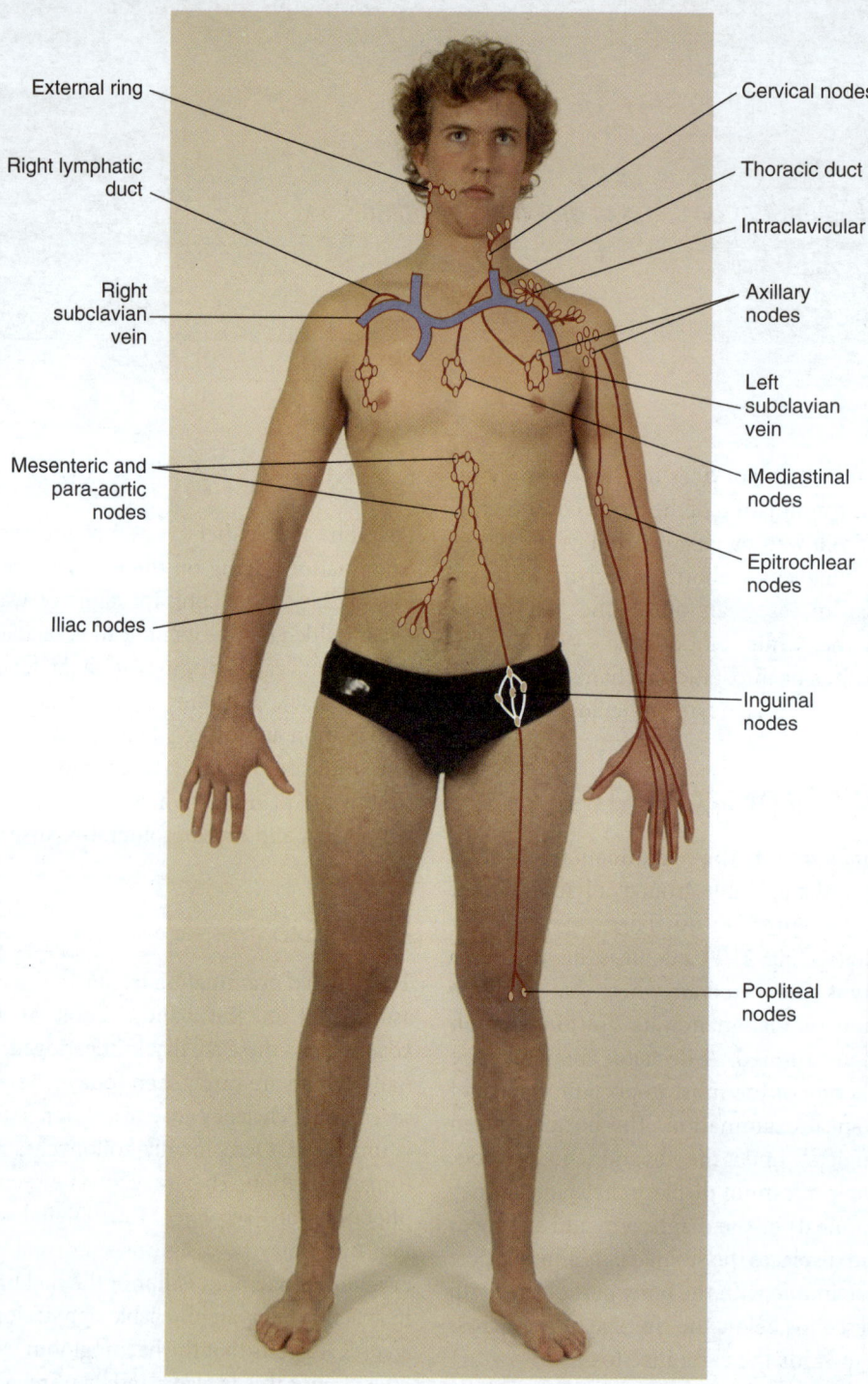

Usual drainage areas of lymph nodes

(Adapted from Epstein O, Perkin G, Cookson J et al. *Clinical examination*, 4th edn. Edinburgh: Mosby, 2008.)

FIGURE 21.1

Raynaud's phenomenon

FIGURE 21.2

Thrombocytopenic purpura (petechiae)

FIGURE 21.4

Digital infarction

FIGURE 21.3

Ecchymoses

(From Vidimos A, Ammirati C, Poblete-Lopez C. *Dermatologic surgery*, 1st edn. Philadelphia: Saunders, 2008.)

FIGURE 21.5

of the neutropenia is likely to be autoimmune and is often associated with large granular lymphocytes, but it can result in severe infection. Felty's syndrome may also be associated with thrombocytopenia (see Fig. 21.4), haemolytic anaemia, skin pigmentation and leg ulceration. Gouty tophi and arthropathy may be present in the hands. Gout may be a manifestation of a myeloproliferative disease. Connective tissue diseases can cause anaemia because of the associated chronic inflammation.

Now take the patient's *pulse*. A tachycardia may be present. Anaemic patients have an increased cardiac output and compensating tachycardia because of the reduced oxygen-carrying capacity of their blood.

Look for *purpura* (see Fig. 21.4), which is really any sort of bruising, due to haemorrhage into the skin. The lesions can vary in size from pinheads called petechiae (from Latin *petechia* 'a spot'; see List 21.1) to large bruises (>5 mm) called *ecchymoses* (see Fig. 21.5 and List 21.2).

If the petechiae are raised (*palpable purpura*) they are not due to thrombocytopenia, but rather this suggests an underlying systemic vasculitis, where the lesions are painful, or bacteraemia.

CAUSES OF PETECHIAE

Thrombocytopenia
Platelet count $<100 \times 10^9/\text{L}$

INCREASED DESTRUCTION
Immunological:
- immune thrombocytopenic purpura (ITP)
- systemic lupus erythematosus (SLE)
- drugs (e.g. quinine, sulfonamides, methyldopa)

Non-immunological:
- damage (e.g. prosthetic heart valve)
- consumption (e.g. disseminated intravascular coagulation [DIC] loss, e.g. haemorrhage)

REDUCED PRODUCTION
Marrow aplasia (e.g. drugs, chemicals, radiation)
Marrow malignancy (e.g. myelodysplastic syndrome [MDS], carcinoma, multiple myeloma, acute leukaemia, myelofibrosis)

SEQUESTRATION
Hypersplenism

Platelet dysfunction
Congenital or familial

Acquired:
- myeloproliferative disease
- dysproteinaemia
- chronic kidney disease, chronic liver disease
- drugs (e.g. aspirin)

Bleeding due to small vessel disease
Infection:
- infective endocarditis
- septicaemia (e.g. meningococcal)
- viral exanthemata (e.g. measles)

Drugs (e.g. steroids)

Scurvy (vitamin C deficiency)—classically perifollicular purpura on the lower limbs, which is almost diagnostic of this condition

Cushing's syndrome

Vasculitis:
- polyarteritis nodosa
- Henoch–Schönlein purpura*

Fat embolism

Dysproteinaemia

*Eduard Henoch (1820–1910), professor of paediatrics, Berlin, described this in 1865, and Johannes Schönlein (1793–1864), Berlin physician, described it in 1868.

LIST 21.1

CAUSES OF PURPURA AND BRUISING/BLEEDING

Trauma

Thrombocytopenia or platelet dysfunction

Coagulation disorders
ACQUIRED
Vitamin K deficiency (leading to factor II, VII, IX and X deficiency)
Liver disease (impaired synthesis of clotting factors)
Anticoagulants (e.g. heparin, warfarin, novel (direct) oral anticoagulants [NOACs])
Disseminated intravascular coagulation

CONGENITAL (RARELY CAUSE ECCHYMOSES AND USUALLY PRESENT WITH HAEMORRHAGE)
Haemophilia A (factor VIII deficiency)
Haemophilia B (factor IX deficiency, Christmas disease)
Von Willebrand's disease (an inherited abnormality of the von Willebrand protein, which is part of the factor VIII complex and causes a defect in platelet adhesion)

Senile ecchymoses (due to loss of skin elasticity, or chronic corticosteroid use)

LIST 21.2

Feeling for the epitrochlear lymph node

FIGURE 21.6

FOREARMS

If thrombocytopenia or capillary fragility is suspected, the Hess[b] test can be performed.[c]

EPITROCHLEAR NODES

Now feel for enlarged epitrochlear nodes. The best method is to flex the patient's elbow to 90°, abduct the upper arm a little and place the palm of your right hand under the patient's right elbow (see Fig. 21.6). Your thumb can then be placed over the appropriate area, which is proximal and slightly anterior to the medial epicondyle. This is repeated with the left hand for the other side. An enlarged epitrochlear node is usually pathological. It occurs with local infection, non-Hodgkin's lymphoma[d] or, rarely, syphilis. Note the features and different causes as outlined in Lists 21.3 and 21.4. Certain symptoms and signs suggest lymphadenopathy may be the result of a significant disease (see Good signs guide 21.1).

---

[b] Alfred Hess (1875–1933), a professor of paediatrics in New York, described this in 1914.
[c] This test is only of historical interest these days, as a platelet count can be obtained almost as quickly in most hospitals and clinics. A blood pressure cuff, placed over the upper arm, is inflated to a point 10 mmHg above the diastolic blood pressure. Wait for 5 minutes, then deflate the cuff and wait for another 5 minutes before inspecting the arm. Look for petechiae, which are usually most prominent in the cubital fossa and near the wrist, where the skin is most lax. Fewer than 5 petechiae per cm^2 is normal, whereas more than 20 is definitely abnormal, suggesting thrombocytopenia, abnormal platelet function or capillary fragility.
[d] Thomas Hodgkin (1798–1866), a famous student at Guy's Hospital, London, described his disease in 1832. The first case he described was a patient of Richard Bright's. Hodgkin was one of the first to use the stethoscope in England. On failing to be appointed a physician, he gave up medicine and became a missionary.

CHARACTERISTICS OF LYMPH NODES

During palpation of lymph nodes the following features must be considered.

Site

Palpable nodes may be localised to one region (e.g. local infection, early lymphoma) or generalised (e.g. late lymphoma).

The palpable lymph node areas are:
- epitrochlear
- axillary
- cervical and occipital
- supraclavicular
- para-aortic (rarely palpable)
- inguinal
- popliteal.

Size

Large nodes are usually abnormal (greater than 1 centimetre).

Consistency

Hard nodes suggest carcinoma deposits, soft nodes may be normal, and rubbery nodes may be due to lymphoma.

Tenderness

This implies infection or acute inflammation.

Fixation

Nodes that are fixed to underlying structures are more likely than mobile nodes to be infiltrated by carcinoma.

Overlying skin

Inflammation of the overlying skin suggests infection, and tethering to the overlying skin suggests carcinoma.

LIST 21.3

AXILLARY NODES

Now feel for enlarged axillary nodes (see Fig. 21.7). To palpate for these, raise the patient's arm and, using your left hand for the right side, push your fingers as high as possible into the axilla (see Fig. 21.8a). Then bring the patient's arm down to rest on your forearm and ask him or her to relax and allow you to take the

> **CAUSES OF LOCALISED LYMPHADENOPATHY**
>
> 1. Inguinal nodes: infection of lower limb, sexually transmitted disease, abdominal or pelvic malignancy, immunisations
> 2. Axillary nodes: infections of the upper limb, carcinoma of the breast, disseminated malignancy, immunisations
> 3. Epitrochlear nodes: infection of the arm, lymphoma, sarcoidosis
> 4. Left supraclavicular nodes: metastatic malignancy from the chest, abdomen (especially stomach—Troisier's sign) or pelvis
> 5. Right supraclavicular nodes: malignancy from the chest or oesophagus
> 6. Cervical nodes: cancers of the oropharynx and head and neck
>
> LIST 21.4

Enlarged axillary nodes

(Courtesy of Dr A Watson, Infectious Diseases Department, The Canberra Hospital.)

FIGURE 21.7

GOOD SIGNS GUIDE 21.1
Factors suggesting lymphadenopathy is associated with significant disease (particularly lymphoma)

Sign	LR+	LR−
Age >40	2.25	0.41
Weight loss	2.3	0.85
Fever	0.71	1.1
Head and neck but not supraclavicular	0.84	1.2
Supraclavicular	3.1	0.76
Axillary	0.86	1.0
Inguinal	0.76	1.0
Size		
<4 cm^2	0.44	3.6
4–9 cm^2	2.0	0.87
>9 cm^2	8.4	0.65
Hard texture	3.3	0.64
Tender	0.61	1.2
Fixed node	13.0	0.73

weight. The opposite is done for the left side (see Fig. 21.8b).

There are five main groups of axillary nodes (see Fig. 21.9):

1. central
2. lateral (above and lateral)
3. pectoral (medial)
4. infraclavicular, and
5. subscapular (most inferior).

An effort should be made to feel for nodes in each of these areas of the axilla.

FACE

The patient's *eyes* should be examined for the presence of scleral jaundice, haemorrhage or injection (due to increased prominence of scleral blood vessels, as in polycythaemia; see Fig. 21.10). Conjunctival pallor may suggest severe anaemia and is more reliable than examination of the nail beds or palmar creases (pp 49, 776).[3] In northern Europeans the combination of prematurely grey hair and blue eyes may indicate a predisposition to the autoimmune disease *pernicious anaemia*, where there is a vitamin B_{12} deficiency due to lack of intrinsic factor secretion by an atrophic gastric mucosa.

The *mouth* should be examined for hypertrophy of the gums, which may occur with infiltration by leukaemic cells, especially in acute monocytic leukaemia, or with swelling in scurvy (rare). Gum bleeding must also be looked for, and ulceration, infection and haemorrhage of the buccal and pharyngeal mucosa noted. Atrophic glossitis occurs with megaloblastic anaemia or iron

CHAPTER 21 THE HAEMATOLOGICAL EXAMINATION 341

The main groups of axillary lymph nodes.

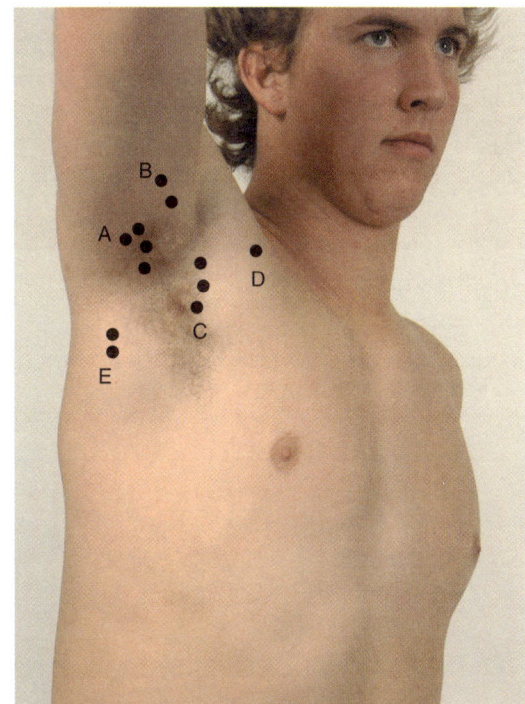

A=central; B=lateral; C=pectoral;
D=infraclavicular; E=subscapular

FIGURE 21.9

(a) Feeling for the axillary lymph nodes, right side. (b) Left side: patient's arm rests on the examiner's arm to relax the shoulder

FIGURE 21.8

deficiency anaemia. Multiple telangiectasias may appear around or in the mouth of patients with *hereditary haemorrhagic telangiectasia*. Look to see whether the tonsils are enlarged. *Waldeyer's ring*[e] is a circle of lymphatic tissue in the posterior part of the oropharynx and nasopharynx, and includes the tonsils and adenoids. Sometimes non-Hodgkin's lymphoma will involve Waldeyer's tonsillar ring, but Hodgkin's disease rarely does.

---

[e] Heinrich Wilhelm Gottfried von Waldeyer-Hartz (1836–1921), Berlin anatomist.

CERVICAL AND SUPRACLAVICULAR NODES

Sit the patient up and examine the cervical nodes from behind. There are eight groups. Attempt to identify each of the groups of nodes with your fingers (see Fig. 21.11). First palpate the *submental node* (see Fig. 21.12), which lies directly under the chin, and then the *submandibular nodes*, which are below the angle of the jaw. Next palpate the *jugular chain* (see Fig. 21.13), which lies anterior to the sternomastoid muscle, and then the *posterior triangle nodes*, which are posterior to the sternomastoid muscle. Palpate the occipital region for *occipital nodes* and then move to the *postauricular node* (see Fig. 21.14) behind the ear and the *preauricular node* in front of the ear. Finally from the front, with the patient's shoulders slightly shrugged, feel in the supraclavicular fossa and at the base of the sternomastoid muscle for the *supraclavicular nodes* (see Fig. 21.15).

Polycythaemia rubra vera—prominent scleral blood vessels

(From Marx J, Hockberger R, Walls R. *Rosen's emergency medicine.* St Louis, MO: Mosby, 2009.)

FIGURE 21.10

Causes of lymphadenopathy, localised and generalised, are given in List 21.5. Note that small cervical nodes are often palpable in healthy young people.[4,5]

The detection of lymphadenopathy should lead to a search of the area drained by the enlarged nodes. This may reveal the likely cause (see List 21.5). Lymphangitis (see Fig. 21.16), which is inflammation of the lymphatic vessels, may be visible in the drainage area of the abnormal nodes, especially if the enlargement is caused by infection.

BONE TENDERNESS

While the patient is sitting up, gently but firmly tap over the spine with your fist for bony tenderness. This

(a) Cervical and supraclavicular lymph nodes. 1=submental; 2=submandibular; 3=jugular chain (posterior cervical and anterior or deep cervical); 4=supraclavicular; 5=posterior triangle; 6=postauricular; 7=preauricular; 8=occipital. (b) Cervical lymphadenopathy. (c) Submandibular lymphadenopathy

((b) and (c) Courtesy of Dr A Watson, Infectious Diseases Department, The Canberra Hospital.)

FIGURE 21.11

Feeling for the submental node

FIGURE 21.12

Feeling for enlarged postauricular nodes

FIGURE 21.14

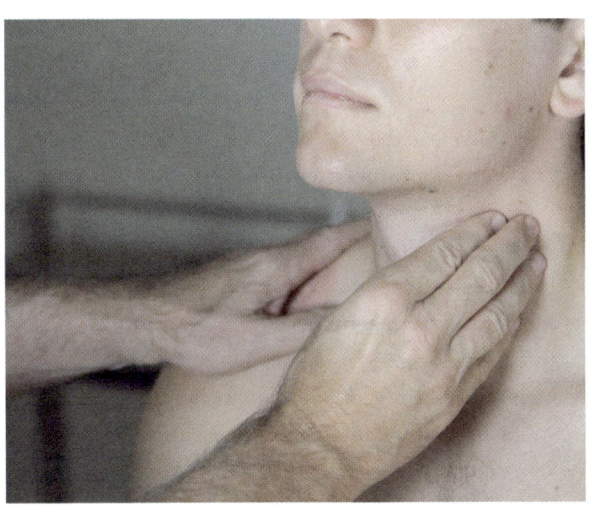

Palpating the jugular chain of lymph node

FIGURE 21.13

'Shrug your shoulders for me'—feeling for the supraclavicular lymph nodes

FIGURE 21.15

may be caused by an enlarging marrow due to infiltration by multiple myeloma, lymphoma or carcinoma, or due to malignant disease of the bony skeleton. Also gently press the sternum and both clavicles with the heel of your hand and then test both shoulders by pushing them towards each other with your hands.

THE ABDOMINAL EXAMINATION

Lay the patient flat again. Examine the abdomen carefully, especially for splenomegaly[6] (see List 21.6 and Good signs guide 21.2), hepatomegaly, para-aortic nodes (rarely palpable unless very enlarged), inguinal nodes and testicular masses. Remember that a central deep abdominal mass may occasionally be due to enlarged para-aortic nodes. Para-aortic adenopathy strongly suggests lymphoma or lymphatic leukaemia. The rectal examination may reveal evidence of bleeding or a carcinoma.

Two further methods of assessing for splenomegaly are described here:

1. *Percussion of the Traube space:* with the patient supine, abduct the patient's left arm slightly, ask the patient to breathe normally and percuss across the space from its medial to lateral

CAUSES OF LYMPHADENOPATHY

Generalised lymphadenopathy

Lymphoma (rubbery and firm)

Leukaemia (e.g. chronic lymphocytic leukaemia, acute lymphocytic leukaemia)

Infections:
- viral (e.g. infectious mononucleosis, cytomegalovirus, human immunodeficiency virus)
- bacterial (e.g. tuberculosis, brucellosis, syphilis)
- protozoal (e.g. toxoplasmosis)

Connective tissue diseases (e.g. rheumatoid arthritis, systemic lupus erythematosus)

Infiltration (e.g. sarcoid)

Drugs (e.g. phenytoin [pseudolymphoma])

Localised lymphadenopathy

Local acute or chronic infection

Metastases from carcinoma or other solid tumour

Lymphoma, especially Hodgkin's disease

LIST 21.5

Lymphangitis in the groin

FIGURE 21.16

CAUSES OF SPLENOMEGALY

Massive

COMMON

Chronic myeloid leukaemia

Idiopathic myelofibrosis

Chronic lymphocytic leukaemia

RARE

Malaria

Kala azar

Primary lymphoma of spleen

Moderate

The above causes

Portal hypertension

Non-Hodgkin's lymphoma (NHL)

Leukaemia (acute or chronic)

Thalassaemia

Storage diseases (e.g. Gaucher's disease*)

Small

The above causes

Other myeloproliferative disorders:
- polycythaemia rubra vera
- essential thrombocythaemia

Haemolytic anaemia

Megaloblastic anaemia (rarely)

Infection:
- viral (e.g. infectious mononucleosis, hepatitis)
- bacterial (e.g. infective endocarditis)
- protozoal (e.g. malaria)

Connective tissue diseases:
- rheumatoid arthritis
- systemic lupus erythematosus
- polyarteritis nodosa

Infiltrations (e.g. amyloid, sarcoid)

Splenomegaly may be found in 3%–12% of the normal population.

Note: Secondary carcinomatosis is a very rare cause of splenomegaly.

*Phillipe Charles Ernest Gaucher (1854–1918), who described this in 1882, was a physician and dermatologist at the Hôpital St-Louis, Paris.

LIST 21.6

margins at a couple of levels. The note should remain resonant unless the spleen is enlarged.[6,7]

2. *Percussion by the Castell method:* with the patient still supine, percuss over the *Castell spot* (see Fig. 21.17)—the lowest left intercostal space in the anterior axillary line—with the patient in full inspiration and expiration. The note will become

GOOD SIGNS GUIDE 21.2
Splenomegaly

Finding	LR+	LR−
Spleen palpable	8.2	0.4
Spleen percussion positive (Traube space)	2.3	0.48
Spleen percussion (Castell spot)	1.2	0.45

(Adapted from Simel DL, Rennie D. *The rational clinical examination: evidence-based clinical diagnosis*, 1st edn. Chicago, IL: American Medical Association, 2008.)

ASSESSING THE PATIENT WITH SUSPECTED MALIGNANCY

1. Palpate all draining lymph nodes.
2. Examine all remaining lymph node groups.
3. Examine the abdomen, particularly for hepatomegaly and ascites.
4. Feel the testes.
5. Perform a rectal examination and pelvic examination.
6. Examine the lungs.
7. Examine the breasts.
8. Examine all the skin and nails for melanoma.

LIST 21.7

Castell spot

(From Mangione S. *Physical diagnosis secrets*, 2nd edn. St Louis, MO: Mosby, 2007.)

FIGURE 21.17

The groups of inguinal lymph nodes and their drainage areas

(Adapted from Epstein O, Perkin G, Cookson J et al. *Clinical examination*, 4th edn. Edinburgh: Mosby, 2008.)

FIGURE 21.18

dull during inspiration if the spleen is enlarged. The sensitivity and specificity of this test have been recorded as high as 82% and 83%, respectively.[6]

Assessment of the patient with suspected malignancy is presented in List 21.7.

INGUINAL NODES

There are two groups of inguinal nodes: one along the inguinal ligament and the other along the femoral vessels (see Fig. 21.18). Small, firm mobile nodes are commonly found in thin normal subjects.

LEGS

Inspect for any petechiae, bruising, pigmentation or scratch marks. Palpable purpura over the buttocks and legs are present in Henoch–Schönlein purpura[f] (see Fig. 21.19). Drug reactions may cause petechiae or purpura on the legs or elsewhere (see Fig. 21.20). Leg

---

[f] Henoch–Schönlein purpura is also characterised by glomerulonephritis (manifested by haematuria and proteinuria), arthralgias and abdominal pain.

Henoch–Schönlein purpura

(From McDonald FS, ed. *Mayo Clinic images in internal medicine*, with permission. © Mayo Clinic Scientific Press and CRC Press. Reproduced by permission of Taylor and Francis Group, LLC, a division of Informa plc.)

FIGURE 21.19

ulcers may occur above the medial or lateral malleolus in association with haemolytic anaemia (including sickle cell anaemia and hereditary spherocytosis), probably as a result of tissue infarction due to abnormal blood viscosity. Leg ulcers can also occur with thalassaemia, macroglobulinaemia, thrombotic thrombocytopenic purpura and polycythaemia, as well as in Felty's syndrome. Chronic use of hydroxyurea for myeloproliferative disorders can cause malar ulcers.

Occasionally, popliteal nodes may be felt in the popliteal fossa.

The legs should also be examined for evidence of the neurological abnormalities caused by vitamin B_{12} deficiency: peripheral neuropathy and subacute combined degeneration of the spinal cord. Vitamin B_{12} is an essential cofactor in the conversion of homocysteine to methionine; in B_{12} deficiency, the lack of methionine impairs methylation of myelin basic protein. Deficiency of vitamin B_{12} can also result in optic atrophy and mental changes. Lead poisoning causes anaemia and foot (or wrist) drop.

Signs of venous disease in the legs may indicate previous venous thromboses and damage to the venous valves between the superficial and deep veins. Look for signs of current venous thrombosis.

Examine the weight-bearing joints of the lower limbs for signs of deformity and chronic arthritis resulting from haemarthroses in the patient with haemophilia (see Fig. 26.12 on p 435).

FUNDI

Examine the fundi. An increase in blood viscosity, which occurs in diseases such as macroglobulinaemia, myeloproliferative disease or chronic granulocytic leukaemia, can cause engorged retinal vessels and later papilloedema. Haemorrhages may occur because of a haemostatic disorder. Retinal lesions (multiple yellow–white patches) may be present in toxoplasmosis (see Fig. 45.5 on p 840) and cytomegalovirus infections (see Fig. 45.6 on p 840).

Drug purpura

FIGURE 21.20

T&O'C ESSENTIALS

1. The whole body must be examined for signs of haematological disease.
2. Accurate assessment of lymph node size and character requires practice.
3. Palpation of the spleen can be difficult. Students should practise a number of techniques.
4. The causes of splenomegaly are very varied and the size of the spleen, the presence of associated lymphadenopathy and the patient's history all need to be taken into account when considering the differential diagnosis.

References

1. Strobach RS, Anderson SK, Doll DC, Ringenberg QS. The value of the physical examination in the diagnosis of anaemia: correlation of the physical findings and the haemoglobin concentrations. *Arch Intern Med* 1988; 148:831–832. Palmar crease pallor can occur above a haemoglobin value of 70 g/L.
2. Nardone DA, Roth KM, Mazur DJ, McAfee JH. Usefulness of physical examination in detecting the presence or absence of anemia. *Arch Intern Med* 1990; 150:201–204.
3. Sheth TN, Choudray NK, Bowes M, Detsky AS. The relation of conjunctival pallor to the presence of anemia. *J Gen Intern Med* 1997; 12:102–106. The presence of conjunctival pallor is a useful indicator of anaemia, but its absence is unhelpful. It is also a reliable sign.
4. Linet OI, Metzler C. Practical ENT: incidence of palpable cervical nodes in adults. *Postgrad Med* 1977; 62:210–211, 213. In young adults without chronic disease, palpable cervical lymph nodes are often detected but are not clinically important. Remember, posterior cervical nodes are almost never normal.
5. Habermann TM, Steensma DP. Lymphadenopathy. *Mayo Clin Proc* 2000; 75(7):723–732.
6. Grover SA, Barkun AN, Sackett DL. Does this patient have splenomegaly? *JAMA* 1993; 270:2218–2221. A valuable guide to assessment of splenomegaly, although the recommendations are controversial. A combination of percussion and palpation may best identify splenomegaly but, in contrast to hepatomegaly, percussion may be modestly more sensitive, according to the few available studies. Our conclusion is that this needs to be better established; in practice, splenomegaly is often missed by percussion alone.
7. Barkun AN, Camus M, Meagher T et al. Splenic enlargement and Traube's space; how useful is percussion? *Am J Med* 1989; 87:562–566.

CHAPTER 22
A summary of the haematological examination and extending the haematological examination

Acquire the art of detachment, the virtue of method, and the quality of thoroughness but above all the grace of humility. SIR WILLIAM OSLER (1849–1919)

The haematological examination: a suggested method

Haematological system examination
FIGURE 22.1

Lying flat (1 pillow)
1. General inspection
   Weight (normal, reduced, increased)
   Bruising (thrombocytopenia, scurvy, etc.)
   - Petechiae (pinhead bleeding)
   - Ecchymoses (large bruises)
   Pigmentation (lymphoma)
   Rashes and infiltrative lesions (lymphoma)
   Ulceration (neutropenia)
   Cyanosis (polycythaemia)
   Plethora (polycythaemia)
   Jaundice (haemolysis)
   Scratch marks (myeloproliferative diseases, lymphoma)
   Racial origin
2. Hands
   Nails—koilonychia, pallor
   Palmar crease pallor (anaemia)
   Arthropathy (haemophilia, secondary gout, drug treatment, etc.)
   Pulse
3. Epitrochlear and axillary nodes
4. Face
   Sclera—jaundice, pallor, conjunctival suffusion (polycythaemia)
   Mouth—gum hypertrophy (monocytic leukaemia, etc.), ulceration, infection, haemorrhage (marrow aplasia, etc.); atrophic glossitis, angular stomatitis (iron, vitamin deficiencies)
   Tongue—amyloidosis
5. Cervical nodes (sitting up)
   Palpate from behind
6. Bony tenderness
   Spine
   Sternum

TEXT BOX 22.1

The haematological examination: a suggested method *continued*

    Clavicles
    Shoulders
7. Abdomen (lying flat) and genitalia
    Inguinal nodes
    Detailed examination
8. Legs
    Vasculitis (Henoch–Schönlein purpura—buttocks, thighs)
    Bruising

    Pigmentation
    Ulceration (e.g. haemoglobinopathies)
    Neurological signs (subacute combined degeneration, peripheral neuropathy)
9. Other
    Fundi (haemorrhages, infection, etc.)
    Temperature chart (infection)
    Urine analysis (haematuria, bile, etc.)
    Rectal and pelvic examination (blood loss)

This will be a targeted examination during follow-up consultations but should be completed in full for the first visit if haematological disease is suspected or known.

Position the patient as for a gastrointestinal examination. Make sure he or she is fully undressed, in stages and with a gown for women. Look for **bruising**, **pigmentation**, **cyanosis**, **jaundice** and **scratch marks** (due to myeloproliferative disease or lymphoma). Also note the racial origin of the patient.

Pick up the patient's **hands**. Look at the nails for koilonychia (spoon-shaped nails, which are rarely seen today and indicate iron deficiency) and the changes of vasculitis. Pale palmar creases may indicate anaemia (typically the haemoglobin level has to be lower than 70 g/L). Evidence of arthropathy may be important (e.g. rheumatoid arthritis and Felty's syndrome, recurrent haemarthroses in bleeding disorders, secondary gout in myeloproliferative disorders).

Examine the **epitrochlear nodes**. Note any bruising. Remember, petechiae are pinhead haemorrhages, whereas ecchymoses are larger bruises.

Go to the **axillae** and palpate the axillary nodes. There are five main areas: central, lateral (above and lateral), pectoral (most medial), infraclavicular and subscapular (most inferior).

Look at the **face**. Inspect the eyes, noting jaundice, pallor or haemorrhage of the sclerae, and the injected sclerae of polycythaemia. Examine the mouth. Look for perioral telangiectasias. Note gum hypertrophy (e.g. from acute monocytic leukaemia or scurvy), ulceration, infection, haemorrhage, atrophic glossitis (e.g. from iron deficiency, or vitamin B_{12} or folate deficiency) and angular stomatitis. Look for tonsillar and adenoid enlargement (Waldeyer's ring).

Sit the patient up. Examine the **cervical nodes** from behind. There are eight groups: submental, submandibular, jugular chain, supraclavicular, posterior triangle, postauricular, preauricular and occipital. Then feel the supraclavicular area from the front. Tap the spine with your fist for **bony tenderness** (caused by an enlarging marrow—e.g. in myeloma or carcinoma). Also gently press the sternum, clavicles and shoulders for bony tenderness.

Lay the patient flat again. Examine the **abdomen**. Focus on the liver and spleen. Feel for para-aortic nodes. Do not forget to feel the testes in males and to perform a rectal and pelvic examination (for tumour or bleeding). Spring the hips for pelvic tenderness. Palpate the inguinal nodes. There are two groups: along the inguinal ligament and along the femoral vessels.

Examine the **legs**. Note particularly leg ulcers. Examine the legs from a neurological aspect, for evidence of vitamin B_{12} deficiency or peripheral neuropathy from other causes. Remember, hypothyroidism can cause anaemia and neurological disease.

Finally, examine the **fundi**, look at the **temperature** chart and test the **urine**.

TEXT BOX 22.1

EXTENDING THE HAEMATOLOGICAL PHYSICAL EXAMINATION

Haematology tests

Diagnosis of haematological disease depends on the history, physical examination and thoughtful testing. Although haematology is a test-heavy specialty, the ultimate diagnosis is still guided by the clinical setting.

Key tests to consider include:

- *Complete blood count (CBC) or full blood count (FBC)*—starts with the automated indices to identify anaemia and the likely cause (which must be confirmed by more specific testing), or to identify white cell disorders (e.g. leukaemia) or platelet disorders (low: thrombocytopenia, or high: thrombocytosis).
- *Peripheral blood smear*—an extension of the physical examination to identify disease (e.g. target cells in liver disease, spherocytes (round red blood cells [RBCs]) and polychromasia (the presence of large greyish-stained cells—reticulocytes) in immune haemolysis, burr cells in renal disease, teardrop cells in bone marrow infiltration—see below).
- *Reticulocyte count*—low if there are red cell production or maturation defects, or high if red cell survival is short and red cell production is increased (as occurs with blood loss, or haemolysis) and is correlated with polychromasia (reticulocytes are immature red cells released from the bone marrow).
- *Tests for excess bleeding*—for example, the prothrombin time (international normalised ratio [INR]) is increased with liver disease and vitamin K deficiency or warfarin therapy. The activated partial thromboplastin time (APTT) is prolonged in haemophilia or heparin therapy. Factor VIII and IX levels can be measured and used to predict bleeding risk and treatment requirements for patients with haemophilia.
- *Tests for excess clotting propensity (thrombophilia)* (such as a history of multiple deep venous thromboses)—for example, factor V Leiden mutation, antithrombin deficiency, protein C or S deficiency, antiphospholipid antibodies.
- *Special tests*—for example, *JAK2* mutation in polycythaemia rubra vera and other myeloproliferative neoplasms, *BCR-ABL* oncogene mutation (correlates with Philadelphia chromosome) in chronic myelogenous leukaemia, immunoelectrophoresis of serum and urine and serum free light chains for multiple myeloma, tests for haemolysis (including direct antiglobulin test [DAT], previously called direct Coombs test, for antibody-mediated red cell damage), immunophenotyping of peripheral blood lymphocytes for chronic lymphocytic leukaemia.
- *Bone marrow*—e.g. to identify the type of myelodysplastic syndrome (MDS) or leukaemia, or excess plasma cells (multiple myeloma).

Examination of the peripheral blood film

This is a simple and useful clinical investigation. After interpretation of the automated red cell, white cell and platelet indices, a properly made peripheral blood film is one of the simplest, least invasive and most readily accessible forms of 'tissue biopsy' and can be a very useful diagnostic tool in clinical medicine. An examination of the patient's blood film can: (1) assess whether the morphology of RBCs, white blood cells (WBCs) and platelets is normal, (2) help characterise the type of anaemia, (3) detect the presence of abnormal cells and provide clues about quantitative changes in plasma proteins (e.g. paraproteinaemia), and (4) help make the diagnosis of an underlying infection, malignant infiltration of the bone marrow or primary proliferative haematological disorder.

The following pages present illustrated examples of some clinical problems diagnosed by examination of the blood film (see Figs 22.2 to 22.14).

Anaemia

Anaemia is a reduction in the concentration of haemoglobin below 135 g/L in an adult man and 115 g/L in an adult woman. Anaemia is not a disease itself but results from an underlying pathological process (see List 22.1). It can be classified according to the blood film. RBCs with a low mean cell volume (MCV) appear small (microcytic) and pale (low mean

Spherocytic anaemia.

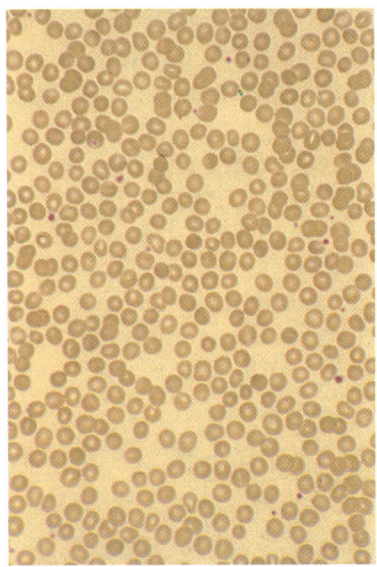

Hereditary spherocytosis or autoimmune haemolytic anaemia. The numerous RBCs that are small, round and lack central pallor are spherocytes (the big RBCs are probably reticulocytes)

FIGURE 22.2

Autoagglutination.

Cold haemagglutinin disease. Film shows clumping of red cells (low power)

FIGURE 22.3

Microangiopathic haemolysis (e.g. disseminated intravascular coagulation).

Frequent fragmented (bitten) red cells

FIGURE 22.4

Sickle cell anaemia.

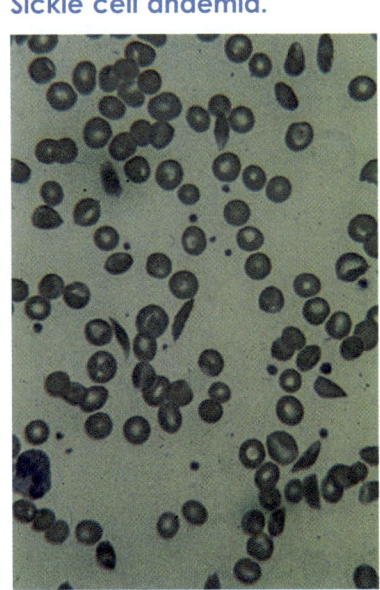

Film shows several sickle-shaped cells with target cells probably secondary to the 'autosplenectomy' that occurs in this disease

FIGURE 22.5

Leucoerythroblastic film.

Film indicative of bone marrow infiltration. Shows circulating nucleated RBCs and immature WBCs

FIGURE 22.6

Postsplenectomy picture.

Film shows several Howell–Jolly bodies, target cells and crenated cells

FIGURE 22.7

Myelofibrosis.

Film shows a dysplastic nucleated RBC, frequent teardrop poikilocytes and a primitive granulocyte

FIGURE 22.8

Malaria.

The two RBCs in the centre show the trophozoite

FIGURE 22.9

Viral illness (e.g. infectious mononucleosis).

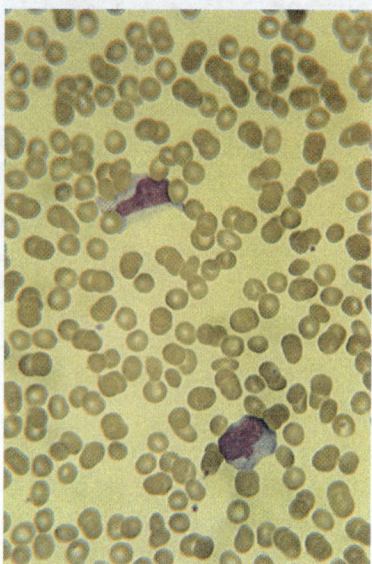

Film shows two atypical or 'switched-on' lymphocytes

FIGURE 22.10

Bacterial infection (e.g. pneumonia, infective endocarditis).

The WBC in the centre is a band form with prominent 'toxic' granules

FIGURE 22.11

Acute leukaemia.

The film shows two very primitive WBCs with prominent nucleoli

FIGURE 22.12

Iron-deficiency anaemia.

RBCs show varying shape and size; they are generally hypochromic

FIGURE 22.13

CAUSES OF ANAEMIA

Microcytic anaemia

- Iron-deficiency anaemia (iron is essential for haem production)
  - Chronic bleeding (most common cause, usually from gastrointestinal or menstrual loss)
  - Malabsorption (e.g. coeliac disease)
  - Hookworm (blood loss)
  - Pregnancy (increased demand)

  Note: Dietary inadequacy alone is rarely the sole cause.
- Thalassaemia minor (an abnormal haemoglobin)
- Sideroblastic anaemia of MDS (iron incorporation into haem is abnormal)
- Long-standing anaemia of chronic disease

Macrocytic anaemia

- Megaloblastic bone marrow (oval macrocytes on the blood film)
  - Vitamin B_{12} deficiency due to:
    pernicious anaemia
    tropical sprue or bacterial overgrowth
    ileal disease (e.g. Crohn's disease, ileal resection >60 cm)
    fish tapeworm (*Diphyllobothrium latum*) in Scandinavia especially
    poor diet (vegans, rare)
  - Folate deficiency due to:
    dietary deficiency, especially alcoholics
    malabsorption, especially coeliac disease
    increased cell turnover, e.g. pregnancy, leukaemia, chronic haemolysis, chronic inflammation
    antifolate drugs, e.g. phenytoin, methotrexate, sulfasalazine
- Non-megaloblastic bone marrow (round macrocytes on the blood film)
  - Alcohol
  - Cirrhosis of the liver
  - Reticulocytosis (e.g. haemolysis, haemorrhage)
  - Hypothyroidism
  - Marrow infiltration
  - MDS
  - Myeloproliferative disease

Normocytic anaemia

- Bone marrow failure
  - Aplastic anaemia (bone marrow fatty or empty) (e.g. drugs [such as chloramphenicol, indometacin, phenytoin, sulfonamides, antineoplastics], radiation, systemic lupus erythematosus, viral hepatitis, pregnancy, Fanconi syndrome, idiopathic)
  - Ineffective haematopoiesis (normal or increased bone marrow cellularity) (e.g. myelodysplastic syndrome, PNH)
  - Infiltration (e.g. leukaemia, lymphoma, myeloma, granuloma, myelofibrosis)
- Anaemia of chronic disease
  - Chronic inflammation (e.g. infection [abscess, tuberculosis], connective tissue disease)
  - Malignancy
  - Endocrine deficiencies (e.g. hypothyroidism, hypopituitarism, Addison's disease)
  - Liver disease
  - Chronic kidney disease
  - Malnutrition
- Haemolytic anaemia
  - Intracorpuscular defects (e.g. hereditary spherocytosis, elliptocytosis; haemoglobinopathies—sickle cell anaemia, thalassaemia; paroxysmal nocturnal haemoglobinuria)
  - Extracorpuscular defects (e.g. immune-autoimmune [warm or cold antibody] or incompatible blood transfusion; hypersplenism; trauma [marathon runners, prosthetic heart valves]; microangiopathic—disseminated intravascular coagulation; toxic—malaria)

MDS=myelodysplastic syndrome; PNH=paroxysmal nocturnal haemoglobinuria.

LIST 22.1

Megaloblastic anaemia.

RBCs are macrocytic with many oval forms and the neutrophil is hypersegmented

FIGURE 22.14

cell haemoglobin—MCH, hypochromic). Those with a high MCV appear large and round or oval-shaped (macrocytic). Alternatively, the RBCs may be normal in shape and size (normochromic, normocytic) but reduced in number. Spherocytosis occurs in autoimmune haemolytic anaemia and hereditary spherocytosis. If there is a mixture of small and large red cells the MCV may be normal, but the red cell distribution width (RDW) will be increased.

Signs of a severe anaemia of any cause include pallor, tachycardia, wide pulse pressure, systolic ejection murmurs due to a compensatory rise in cardiac output and cardiac failure if myocardial reserve is reduced. There may be signs of the underlying cause.

Pancytopenia

Signs

There may be clinical evidence of anaemia, leucopenia (reduced numbers of WBCs resulting in susceptibility to infection, mainly with neutropenia) and thrombocytopenia (petechiae and bleeding)—a deficiency in all three bone marrow cell lines. If confirmed on a blood count, this condition is called pancytopenia.

Causes

- **Aplastic anaemia:** severe hypoplasia of the erythroid, myeloid and platelet precursor cell lines in the bone marrow, resulting in a bone marrow that is fatty and empty of cells. The causes are listed in List 22.1; 50% have no cause identified.
- **Marrow infiltration** by MDS, leukaemia, lymphoma, carcinoma, multiple myeloma, myelofibrosis or granulomata.
- **Other:** pernicious anaemia, hypersplenism, systemic lupus erythematosus, folate deficiency, paroxysmal nocturnal haemoglobinuria (PNH).

Acute leukaemia

Leukaemia is a neoplastic proliferation of one of the blood-forming cells. Acute leukaemia presents with marrow failure from progressive infiltration of the marrow with immature cells. The course is rapidly fatal without treatment. Acute leukaemia can be divided into two main types: acute lymphoblastic leukaemia and acute myeloid leukaemia, both of which are subdivided further on special testing, which then determines optimal therapy.

General signs of acute leukaemia

Pallor (anaemia), fever (which usually indicates infection secondary to neutropenia) and petechiae (thrombocytopenia) are all due to bone marrow failure. Weight loss, muscle wasting (hypercatabolic state) and localised infections (e.g. mouth ulcers, the tonsils or perirectal region, due to neutropenia) also occur.

Signs of infiltration of the haematopoietic system

These include: (1) bony tenderness, due to infiltration or infarction; (2) lymphadenopathy (slight to moderate, especially in acute lymphoblastic leukaemia); (3) splenomegaly (slight to moderate, occurs especially in acute lymphoblastic leukaemia; the spleen may be tender owing to splenic infarction); and (4) hepatomegaly (slight to moderate).

Signs of infiltration of other areas

There may be: (1) tonsillar enlargement (especially in acute lymphoblastic leukaemia); (2) swelling or bleeding of the gums, especially in monocytic leukaemia; (3) pleural effusions; (4) nerve palsies, involving the spinal nerve roots or the cranial nerves; or (5) meningism due to infiltration of the meninges, especially in acute lymphoblastic leukaemia.

Chronic leukaemia

This is a haematological malignancy in which the leukaemic cell is at first well differentiated. These have a better prognosis untreated than acute leukaemia. Most patients are asymptomatic at diagnosis, which is usually made when a blood count is being performed for an unrelated reason. There are two main types: chronic myeloid leukaemia and chronic lymphocytic leukaemia. Chronic lymphocytic leukaemia is usually a low-grade condition and treatment is often not necessary for many years; some patients never require therapy. However, chronic myeloid leukaemia will undergo transformation to acute leukaemia and death in a median 3.5 years and therefore detection and treatment early in the chronic phase are essential.

Signs of chronic myeloid leukaemia

Chronic myeloid leukaemia is one of the myeloproliferative disorders and diagnosis is made by detection of the *BCR-ABL* oncogene (the molecular counterpart of the Philadelphia chromosome). There is an expanded granulocytic mass in the bone marrow, liver and spleen.

- **General signs** may include pallor (anaemia due to bone marrow infiltration) and secondary gout (common).
- **Haematopoietic system signs** include massive splenomegaly and moderate hepatomegaly. (*Note:* lymphadenopathy is usually a sign of blast transformation.)

Signs of chronic lymphocytic leukaemia

Chronic lymphocytic leukaemia is a lymphoproliferative disorder (related to non-Hodgkin's lymphoma) and diagnosed on immunophenotyping of the peripheral blood lymphocytes. There may be tiredness and pallor. Recurrent acute infections may occur.

Haematopoietic system signs include marked or moderate lymphadenopathy and moderate hepatosplenomegaly.

Other abnormalities may include a DAT (Coombs'[a] test)—positive haemolytic anaemia, herpes zoster skin infections and nodular infiltrates. Patients may note a hypersensitivity to insect bites before the diagnosis is made.

Myeloproliferative disease

This is a group of disorders of the haematopoietic stem cell. These include polycythaemia vera, primary myelofibrosis, chronic myeloid leukaemia and essential thrombocythaemia. Overlapping clinical and pathological features occur in these disorders. Therefore, patients may have signs of one or more of the conditions. Any of them may progress to acute myeloid leukaemia.

Polycythaemia

This is an elevated haemoglobin concentration and can result from an increased RBC mass or a decreased plasma volume. Polycythaemia vera results from an autonomous increase in the RBC production. Patients with polycythaemia often have a striking ruddy, plethoric appearance. To examine a patient with suspected polycythaemia, assess for both the manifestations of polycythaemia vera and other possible underlying causes of polycythaemia (see List 22.2).

Look at the patient and estimate the state of hydration (dehydration alone can cause an elevated haemoglobin due to haemoconcentration). Note whether there is a Cushingoid (p 459) or virilised (p 475) appearance. Cyanosis may be present because of an underlying condition such as cyanotic congenital heart disease or chronic lung disease. Look for nicotine staining (smoking). All these diseases can result in secondary polycythaemia.

Inspect the patient's arms for scratch marks; post-bathing pruritus occurs in polycythaemia vera, possibly owing to basophil histamine release. Take the blood pressure: very rarely a phaeochromocytoma will cause secondary polycythaemia and hypertension.

Examine the patient's eyes. Look for injected conjunctivae. Fundal hyperviscosity changes—including engorged, dilated retinal veins and haemorrhages—may be present. Inspect the tongue for central cyanosis.

---

[a] Robin Coombs (1921–2006), Quick professor of biology, Cambridge.

POLYCYTHAEMIA

Signs of polycythaemia vera

Plethoric appearance including engorged conjunctival and retinal vessels (not specific)

Scratch marks (generalised pruritus)

Splenomegaly (80%)

Bleeding tendency (platelet dysfunction)

Peripheral vascular and ischaemic heart disease (thrombosis, slow circulation)

Gout

Mild hypertension

Causes of polycythaemia

ABSOLUTE POLYCYTHAEMIA (INCREASED RBC MASS)

Idiopathic: polycythaemia vera

Secondary polycythaemia

- Increased erythropoietin:
    - Renal disease—polycystic disease, hydronephrosis, tumour; after renal transplantation
    - Hepatocellular carcinoma
    - Cerebellar haemangioblastoma
    - Uterine fibroma
    - Virilising syndromes
    - Cushing's syndrome
    - Phaeochromocytoma
- Hypoxic states (erythropoietin secondarily increased):
    - Chronic lung disease
    - Sleep apnoea
    - Living at high altitude
    - Cyanotic congenital heart disease
    - Abnormal haemoglobins
    - Carbon monoxide poisoning

RELATIVE POLYCYTHAEMIA (DECREASED PLASMA VOLUME)

Dehydration

Stress polycythaemia: Gaisböck's* disease

*Felix Gaisböck (1868–1955), a German physician, described this in 1905.

LIST 22.2

Examine the cardiovascular system for signs of cyanotic congenital heart disease and the respiratory system for signs of chronic lung disease. Assess the abdomen carefully for splenomegaly, which occurs in 80% of cases of polycythaemia vera but does not usually occur with the other forms of polycythaemia. There may be evidence of chronic liver disease or hepatocellular carcinoma, which may cause secondary polycythaemia. Palpate for the kidneys and perform a urinalysis. In women palpate the uterus. Polycystic kidney disease, hydronephrosis, renal carcinoma and uterine fibromas can all rarely cause secondary polycythaemia.

Inspect the patient's legs for scratch marks, gouty tophi (see Fig. 25.6 on p 412) and arthropathy, as well as for signs of peripheral vascular disease. In polycythaemia rubra vera, secondary gout occurs owing to the increased cellular turnover resulting in hyperuricaemia. Peripheral vascular disease occurs in polycythaemia vera because of thrombosis (as there is increased platelet adhesiveness and accelerated atherosclerosis) and slowed circulation due to hyperviscosity.

Look for cerebellar signs, which may be due to the presence of a cerebellar haemangioblastoma, a very rare cause of secondary polycythaemia. Examine the central nervous system for signs of a stroke due to thrombosis.

Primary myelofibrosis

This is a clonal haematopoietic stem cell disorder with fibrosis as a secondary phenomenon. Gradual replacement of the marrow by fibrosis and progressive splenomegaly characterise the disease.

- **General signs** include pallor (anaemia occurs in most patients eventually) and petechiae (in 20% of patients, due to thrombocytopenia).
- **Haematopoietic system signs** include splenomegaly (in almost all cases, and often to a massive degree—there may also be a splenic rub due to splenic infarction), hepatomegaly (occurs in 50% of patients and can be massive) and lymphadenopathy (very uncommon).
- **Other signs** are bony tenderness (uncommon) and gout (occurs in 5% of patients).

Chronic myeloid leukaemia

(See p 355.)

Essential thrombocythaemia

This is a sustained elevation of the platelet count above normal without any primary cause, and requires exclusion of iron deficiency, which may be masking polycythaemia vera.

- **General signs** include spontaneous bleeding and thrombosis.
- **Haematopoietic system signs** include splenomegaly.

Causes of thrombocytosis (platelet count more than $450 \times 10^9/L$) include: (1) following haemorrhage or surgery, (2) postsplenectomy, (3) iron deficiency, (4) chronic inflammatory disease, and (5) malignancy.

Causes of thrombocytosis (platelet count more than $800 \times 10^9/L$) include: (1) myeloproliferative disease and (2) secondary to recent splenectomy, malignancy or marked inflammation occasionally.

Lymphoma

Lymphoma is a malignant disease of the lymphoid system. There are two main clinicopathological types: Hodgkin's lymphoma (HL, with the characteristic Reed–Sternberg[b] cell in most cases) and non-Hodgkin's lymphoma (NHL). NHL refers to an extensive range of clinically and histopathologically distinct subtypes that range from indolent (only requiring observation without treatment) to highly aggressive, which have a poor prognosis if not treated urgently. Signs of lymphoma depend on the stages of the disease. Hodgkin's lymphoma often presents in stage I or II, whereas NHL usually presents in stage III or IV.

Staging of lymphoma using Ann Arbor classification:

Stage I   Disease confined to a single lymph node region or a single extralymphatic site (IE)

Stage II Disease confined to two or more lymph node regions on one side of the diaphragm

ECOG performance status

Grade	ECOG performance status
0	Fully active; no restriction on activities compared with before the disease
1	Restricted, but only from strenuous activity. Able to perform light or sedentary work
2	Able to look after self. Mobile but not able to work
3	Only partly able to look after self. In bed or chair more than 50% of waking hours
4	Completely confined to bed or chair. Unable to look after self at all

ECOG = Eastern Cooperative Oncology Group.

TABLE 22.1

Stage III Disease confined to lymph nodes on both sides of the diaphragm with or without localised involvement of the spleen (IIIS), other extralymphatic organ or site (IIIE), or both (IIIES)

Stage IV Diffuse disease of one or more extralymphatic organs (with or without lymph node disease)

For any stage, a = no symptoms and b = fever, weight loss greater than 10% in 6 months or night sweats.

An assessment of the patient's general state helps in determining prognosis and practicality of further treatment for haematological malignancies. This is called the ECOG (Eastern Cooperative Oncology Group) performance status (Table 22.1).

Signs of Hodgkin's lymphoma

1. Lymph node enlargement (see Fig. 22.15): discrete, rubbery, painless, large and superficial nodes, often confined to one side and one lymph node group.
2. Splenomegaly and hepatomegaly. Splenomegaly does not always indicate extensive disease.
3. Organ infiltration occurs seldom and with advanced stage disease. Look especially for signs of: (a) lung disease, such as a pleural effusion, (b) bone pain or pathological fractures (rare), (c) spinal cord or nerve compression (rare), and (d) nodular skin infiltrates (rare).
4. Profuse night sweats, weight loss and fever with or without infection (reduced cell-mediated

---

[b] Dorothy Reed (1874–1964), a pathologist at Johns Hopkins Hospital, Baltimore, described these cells in 1906 and Karl Sternberg (1872–1935), a pathologist, described giant cells in 1898.

Cervical lymph node enlargement in a patient with lymphoma

(From Mir MA. *Atlas of clinical diagnosis*, 2nd edn. Edinburgh: Saunders, 2003.)

FIGURE 22.15

CT scan of the abdomen.

A normal-sized spleen is visible (arrow)

(From Halpert RD. *Gastrointestinal imaging: the requisites*, 3rd edn. Maryland Heights: Mosby, 2006.)

FIGURE 22.16

immunity) suggest a poorer prognosis, or more advanced disease.

Signs of non-Hodgkin's lymphoma

1. Lymph node enlargement: often more than one site is involved and Waldeyer's ring is more commonly affected than in HL.
2. Hepatosplenomegaly may occur.
3. Systemic 'B' signs (e.g. profuse night sweats, weight loss or fever)
4. Signs of extranodal spread are more common than in HL.
5. The disease may sometimes arise at an extranodal site (e.g. the gastrointestinal tract).

Multiple myeloma

This is a disseminated malignant disease of plasma cells. Remember the 'CRAB' features (Calcium high, Renal function abnormal, Anaemia, Bone disease), which differentiate myeloma from the benign, premalignant prodromal disease monoclonal gammopathy of undetermined significance (MGUS).

General signs

There may be signs of anaemia (due to bone marrow infiltration or as a result of chronic kidney disease), purpura (due to bone marrow infiltration and thrombocytopenia) or infection (particularly pneumonia).

Bony tenderness and pathological fractures may be present. Weight loss may be a feature.

Skin changes include hypertrichosis, erythema annulare, yellow skin and secondary amyloid deposits.

There may be signs of spinal cord compression, or mental changes (due to hypercalcaemia).

Look for signs of chronic kidney disease (which may be due to tubular damage from filtered light chains, uric acid nephropathy, hypercalcaemia, urinary tract infection, secondary amyloidosis or plasma cell infiltration).

Haematological imaging

CT and ultrasound are often used to help determine the presence of splenomegaly or lymphadenopathy (see Figs 22.16 and 22.17). A PET (positron emission tomography) scan is now a routine staging investigation in lymphoma. Multiple myeloma requires a plain X-ray skeletal survey looking for osteolytic bone lesions (e.g. 'pepper-pot' skull), and usually MRI of the whole spine to exclude plasmacytomas threatening spinal cord compression.

CT scans of the chest revealing extensive lymphadenopathy, typical of a lymphoma. There are numerous lymph nodes in the anterior mediastinum displacing the thymus.

(From Schaaf HS, Zumla A. *Tuberculosis*, 1st edn. Edinburgh: Saunders, 2009.)

FIGURE 22.17

T&O'C ESSENTIALS

1. Systemic symptoms may be the clue to a haematological problem.
2. Many haematological abnormalities are detected on a routine blood film.
3. Easy bruising may be the first indication of a bleeding abnormality.
4. Anaemia is common and its symptoms tend to be generalised. The history can be of great assistance in working out the cause.
5. A thorough lymph node examination is a routine part of the haematological examination.
6. You should be able to detect moderate to massive splenomegaly on physical examination.
7. Painless firm, rubbery lymphadenopathy is very suggestive of lymphoma. Lymph nodes of secondary malignant spread are usually hard and irregular. Tender nodes usually indicate an infective cause.

OSCE REVISION TOPICS – THE HAEMATOLOGICAL SYSTEM

Use these topics, which commonly occur in the OSCE, to help with revision.

1. This man has been treated for lymphoma. Take a history from him. (p 357)
2. This man has had a diagnosis of myeloma. Please take a history from him. (p 358)
3. This man has noticed some lymph node enlargement. Please take a history from him. (pp 340, 344)
4. This woman has noticed enlarged lymph nodes. Please examine her. (p 348)
5. This woman has been found to have a mass in the left upper quadrant. Please examine her for splenomegaly. (pp 251, 343)

SECTION 7
The rheumatological system

CHAPTER 23

The rheumatological history

CHAPTER 24

The rheumatological examination

CHAPTER 25

Correlation of physical signs and rheumatological disease

CHAPTER 26

A summary of the rheumatological examination and extending the rheumatological examination

CHAPTER 23

The rheumatological history

The rheumatism is a common name for many aches and pains which have yet got no peculiar appellation, though owing to very different causes. WILLIAM HEBERDEN (1710–1801)

PRESENTING SYMPTOMS

The major presenting symptoms of the rheumatological history are shown in List 23.1.

Peripheral joints
Pain and swelling

The underlying aetiology of joint pain can often be worked out by asking about the distribution, duration and characteristics of joint involvement (see Questions box 23.1).

It is often useful to ask the patient to point to the painful place or area. For example, pain said to affect the knee may be in the popliteal fossa, the knee joint itself or the supra- or infrapatellar bursa. Remember also that pain in the knee or lower thigh may be referred from the hip (see Fig. 23.1).

Patterns of presentation with rheumatological disease that can help establish the differential diagnosis include the following:

- articular vs non-articular (joint itself or surrounding structures such as tendons)

RHEUMATOLOGICAL HISTORY

Major symptoms
JOINTS
Pain
Swelling
Morning stiffness
Stiffness after inactivity
Loss of motion
Loss of function
Deformity
Weakness
Instability
Changes in sensation

EYES
Dry eyes and mouth
Red eyes

SYSTEMIC
Raynaud's phenomenon
Rash, fever, fatigue, weight loss, diarrhoea, mucosal ulcers

LIST 23.1

QUESTIONS TO ASK THE PATIENT WITH JOINT PAIN

❗ denotes symptoms for the possible diagnosis of an urgent or dangerous problem.

1. Which joints are sore?
2. Is it only one joint (monoarthritis) or several joints (polyarthritis)? Show me where. (See Lists 23.2, 23.3 and 23.4.)
3. Are the joints swollen or red (arthritis), or not (arthralgia)?
4. Are they getting better or worse?
5. Is the pain worse in the morning (morning stiffness: rheumatoid arthritis) or after exercise (osteoarthritis)?
6. Have you injured the joint?
❗ 7. Is the back pain worse at night? (Possible ankylosing spondylitis or malignancy)
8. Did back pain start suddenly? (Crush fracture)

QUESTIONS BOX 23.1

364 SECTION 7 THE RHEUMATOLOGICAL SYSTEM

Map of referral patterns for different joints.

(a) Acromioclavicular and sternoclavicular joints; (b) scapulohumeral joint; (c) hip; (d) knee

(Adapted from Epstein O, Perkin G, Cookson J et al. *Clinical examination*, 4th edn. Edinburgh: Mosby, 2008.)

FIGURE 23.1

CAUSES OF MONOARTHRITIS

A single hot, red swollen joint (acute monoarthritis)

Septic arthritis
- Haematogenous (e.g. staphylococcal or gonococcal—latter may be polyarticular)
- Secondary to penetrating injury

Traumatic

Gout, pseudogout or hydroxyapatite arthritis

Haemarthrosis (e.g. haemophilia; see Fig. 26.5 on p 433)

Seronegative spondyloarthritis (occasionally)

A single painful but not inflamed joint

Osteoarthritis

A single chronic inflamed joint (chronic monoarthritis)

Chronic infection (e.g. atypical mycobacterial infection)

Seronegative spondyloarthritis

Pigmented villonodular synovitis

Synovial (osteo)chondromatosis

LIST 23.2

- inflammatory vs non-inflammatory (e.g. rheumatoid vs osteoarthritis)
- acute vs chronic
- peripheral vs axial (i.e. spinal or sacroiliac [SI])
- additive vs migratory (joints improve and new ones become involved) vs palindromic (recurrences and relapses)
- inflammatory monoarthritis vs oligoarthritis (2–5 joints) vs polyarthritis (>5 joints).

The causes of monoarthritis (single joint) and polyarthritis (more than one joint) are outlined in Lists 23.2 and 23.3, and the patterns of polyarthritis in various diseases are outlined in List 23.4.

Mode of onset

This may be sudden or gradual or insidious. When the onset is sudden, ascertain whether there is an obvious cause:

- Is it injury?
- Is it high alcohol intake (gout)?
- Is it joint infection, or reactive—e.g. urinary tract or gastrointestinal infection?

> **CAUSES OF POLYARTHRITIS**
>
> **Acute polyarthritis**
> Infection—viral, bacterial
> Onset of chronic polyarthritis
>
> **Chronic polyarthritis**
> Rheumatoid arthritis
> Seronegative spondyloarthritis
> Osteoarthritis
> Gout, pseudogout or hydroxyapatite arthritis
> Connective tissue disease (e.g. systemic lupus erythematosus)
> Infection (e.g. spirochaetal infection—rare)
> - TB—infectious monoarthritis
>   - Inflammatory (Poncet[a] disease): large and small joints
> - Hepatitis C
> - Looks like RA
>
> RA = rheumatoid arthritis; TB = tuberculosis.
>
> LIST 23.3

> **T&O'C ESSENTIAL**
>
> 1. If a patient with well-controlled rheumatoid arthritis (RA) presents with a single hot joint, it must be presumed septic. NB. Immunosuppressants mask the signs of sepsis.
> 2. Aspirate a suspected septic joint; it is an emergency.

No apparent cause (spontaneous onset) suggests inflammation:
- Is it a flare-up of chronic arthritis?
- Is it migratory arthritis?

Morning stiffness vs mechanical pain

Ask about the presence of early-morning stiffness and the length of time that this stiffness lasts (typically it lasts for at least an hour). Morning stiffness classically occurs in rheumatoid arthritis and other inflammatory arthropathies, and the duration of stiffness is a guide to its severity. Stiffness after inactivity, such as sitting, is characteristic of osteoarthritis of the hip or knee. The mechanical pain of osteoarthritis is better with rest and worse with activity.

Deformity

The patient may have noticed deformity of a joint or bone. If there has been progressive change in the shape of the area, this is more likely to be significant.

Instability

Joint instability may be described by the patient as a 'giving way', or occasionally 'coming out', of the joint in certain conditions. This may be due to true dislocation (e.g. with the shoulder or the patella) or alternatively to muscle weakness or a ligamentous problem.

Change in sensation

This may occur as a result of nerve entrapment or injury, and sometimes as a result of ischaemia. Ask about numbness or paraesthesias (pins and needles). The distribution of the change of sensation should help distinguish nerve damage or entrapment (a specific distribution) from ischaemia.

Up to 50% of type 1 and some type 2 diabetics develop diabetic *cheiroarthritis*.[b] The small and then larger joints of the hands are involved. There is pain and restriction of movement, especially of extension of the fingers. The skin becomes thickened and tight. The cause is probably diabetic microangiopathy, which leads to damage to the skin and connective tissue.

Back pain

This is a very common symptom. It is most often a consequence of local musculoskeletal disease.

Ask where the pain is situated, whether it began suddenly or gradually, whether it is localised or diffuse, whether it radiates to the limbs or elsewhere, and whether the pain is aggravated by movement, coughing or straining. Musculoskeletal pain is characteristically well localised and is aggravated by movement. If there is a spinal nerve root irritation there may be pain that occurs in a dermatomal distribution. This helps to localise the level of the lesion. Diseases such as osteoporosis (with crush fractures), infiltration of carcinoma, leukaemia

---

[a] Antonin Poncet (1849–1913), a French surgeon in Lyon.

[b] From the Greek word χειρ (keir) meaning 'hand'.

PATTERNS OF POLYARTHRITIS

Rheumatoid arthritis

This is usually a symmetrical polyarthritis.

Hands: proximal interphalangeal, metacarpophalangeal and wrist joints

Elbows

Small joints of the upper cervical spine

Knees

Ankles

Feet: tarsal and metatarsophalangeal joints

Cervical spine and temporomandibular joints may also be affected.

Spondyloarthritis

ANKYLOSING SPONDYLITIS

Sacroiliac joints and spine

Hips, knees and shoulders

PSORIATIC ARTHRITIS

Asymmetrical oligoarthritis (2–5 joints)

Sausage digits

Terminal interphalangeal joints

Sacroiliac joints

Rheumatoid pattern

Clues:
- Family history of psoriasis
- Psoriasis—in addition to the usual skin surfaces, hairline, umbilicus, and natal cleft
- Pitting of the nails

REACTIVE ARTHRITIS (REITER'S SYNDROME)

Sacroiliac joints and spine

Hips

Knees

Ankles and joints of the feet

Primary osteoarthritis

This is usually symmetrical and can affect many joints.

Fingers: distal (Heberden's nodes) and proximal (Bouchard's nodes) interphalangeal joints, and metacarpophalangeal joints of the thumbs

Acromioclavicular joints

Small joints of the spine (lower cervical and lumbar)

Knees

Metatarsophalangeal joints of the great toes

Secondary osteoarthritis

This is:
- asymmetrical and affects previously injured, inflamed or infected weight-bearing joints, particularly the hip and knee
- a result of metabolic conditions (e.g. haemochromatosis); symptoms and findings are generalised.

LIST 23.4

---

or myeloma may cause progressive and unremitting back pain, which is often worse at night. The pain may be of sudden onset but is usually self-limiting if it results from the crush fracture of a vertebral body. In ankylosing spondylitis the pain is usually situated over the sacroiliac joints and lumbar spine. There may be buttock pain that radiates to posterior thigh and mimics S1 nerve root pain and hamstring strains. It is also worse at night and is associated with morning stiffness. The pain of ankylosing spondylitis is typically better with activity, which helps distinguish it from mechanical back pain.[1–3] Pain from diseases of the abdomen and chest (e.g. dissecting abdominal or thoracic aortic aneurysm) can also be referred to the back.

The sudden onset of back pain without obvious cause or with minimal trauma suggests an osteoporotic crush fracture. Ask about the factors that increase the risk of osteoporosis:
- menopause
- alcohol
- cigarettes
- endocrine abnormalities—thyroid
- chronic kidney disease
- chronic liver disease.

Limb pain

This can occur from disease of the musculoskeletal system, the skin, the vascular system or the nervous system.

Musculoskeletal pain may be due to trauma or inflammation. Muscle disease such as *polymyositis* can present with an aching pain in the proximal muscles around the shoulders and hips, associated with weakness. Pain and stiffness in the shoulders and hips in patients over the age of 50 years may be due to *polymyalgia rheumatica*. The acute or subacute onset of symptoms in multiple locations suggests an inflammatory process. Bone disease such as osteomyelitis, osteomalacia, osteoporosis or tumours can cause limb pain. Inflammation of tendons (*tenosynovitis*) can produce local pain over the affected area.

Vascular disease may also produce pain in the limbs. Acute arterial occlusion causes severe pain of sudden onset, often with coolness or pallor. Chronic peripheral vascular disease can cause intermittent claudication (p 113). Venous thrombosis can also cause diffuse aching pain in the legs associated with swelling.

Spinal stenosis can cause pseudoclaudication—pain on walking that, unlike the pain of peripheral arterial disease, is relieved by leaning forwards, and the peripheral pulses are present.

Nerve entrapment and *neuropathy* can both cause limb pain that is often associated with paraesthesias or weakness. The usual cause is synovial thickening or joint subluxation, especially for patients with rheumatoid arthritis. The vasculitis associated with the inflammatory arthropathies can also cause neuropathy leading to diffuse peripheral neuropathy or mononeuritis multiplex.

Patients with chronic rheumatoid arthritis often develop subluxation of the cervical spine at the atlanto-axial joint. This is caused by erosion of the transverse ligament around the posterior aspect of the odontoid process (dens). The patient may describe shooting paraesthesias down the arms and an occipital headache. Neck flexion leads to indentation of the cord by the dens and can cause tetraplegia or sudden death. The abnormality may be obvious on lateral X-rays of the cervical spine (see Fig. 26.3, p 431).

Injury to peripheral nerves can result in vasomotor changes and severe limb pain. This is called *causalgia*. Even following amputation of a limb, phantom limb pain may develop and persist as a chronic problem.

Raynaud's phenomenon

Raynaud's[c] phenomenon is an abnormal response of the fingers and toes to cold. Classically, the fingers first turn white, then blue and finally red after exposure to cold.

It may be painful. Patients with Raynaud's disease have Raynaud's phenomenon without an obvious underlying cause. The disease tends to be familial and females are more likely to be affected. This is a benign condition. However, Raynaud's phenomenon in patients with connective tissue diseases, especially systemic sclerosis, can lead to the formation of digital ulcers (see List 23.5). It may be the first sign of this condition (see Fig. 21.2 on p 337).

Dry eyes and mouth

Dry eyes and dry mouth are characteristic of Sjögren's syndrome (see List 23.6). This syndrome may occur

---

CAUSES OF RAYNAUD'S PHENOMENON (WHITE-BLUE-RED FINGERS AND TOES IN RESPONSE TO COLD)

Reflex
Raynaud's disease (idiopathic)
Vibrating machinery injury
Cervical spondylosis

Connective tissue disease
Systemic sclerosis, diffuse or limited type
Mixed connective tissue disease
Systemic lupus erythematosus
Polyarteritis nodosa
Rheumatoid arthritis
Polymyositis
Vasculitis

Arterial disease
Embolism or thrombosis
Buerger's disease (thromboangiitis obliterans)—smokers
Trauma

Haematological
Polycythaemia
Leukaemia
Dysproteinaemia
Cold agglutinin disease

Poisons
Drugs: beta-blockers, ergotamine
Vinyl chloride

LIST 23.5

---

[c] Maurice Raynaud (1834–81) described this in his first work, published in Paris in 1862.

> **CLINICAL FEATURES OF SJÖGREN'S SYNDROME**
>
> In this syndrome, mucus-secreting glands are infiltrated by lymphocytes and plasma cells, which cause atrophy and fibrosis of glandular tissue.
>
> 1. Dry eyes: conjunctivitis, keratitis, corneal ulcers (rarely vascularisation of the cornea)
> 2. Dry mouth
> 3. Chest: infection secondary to reduced mucus secretion, and IgA subclass deficiencies or interstitial pneumonitis
> 4. Kidneys: renal tubular acidosis or nephrogenic diabetes insipidus
> 5. Genital tract: atrophic vaginitis
> 6. Pseudolymphoma: sublingual lymphadenopathy and splenomegaly, which may rarely progress to a true (usually non-Hodgkin's) lymphoma
>
> *Note:* This syndrome occurs in rheumatoid arthritis and with the connective tissue diseases.
> IgA = immunoglobulin A.
>
> **LIST 23.6**

in isolation (primary Sjögren's) and is very common in association with rheumatoid arthritis and other connective tissue disease. Mucus-secreting glands become infiltrated with lymphocytes and plasma cells, which cause atrophy and fibrosis. The dry eyes can result in conjunctivitis, keratitis and corneal ulcers. Sjögren's syndrome can also have an effect on other organs such as the lungs or kidneys.

Red eyes

The spondyloarthritides and Behçet's[d] syndrome, but not rheumatoid arthritis, may be complicated by iritis (eye pain with central scleral injection—a 'red eye'—radiating out from the pupil; see Fig. 25.3 on p 411). In other diseases, such as Sjögren's, red eyes may be due to dryness, episcleritis or scleritis.

Systemic symptoms

Fatigue is common with connective tissue disease. *Weight loss* and *diarrhoea* may occur with systemic sclerosis, because of small-bowel bacterial over-growth. Mucosal ulcers and rashes are common in some connective tissue diseases such as systemic lupus erythematosus (SLE). *Generalised stiffness* can be due to rheumatoid arthritis or systemic sclerosis, but other causes include systemic infection (e.g. influenza), excessive exercise, polymyalgia rheumatica, neuromuscular disease (e.g. extrapyramidal disease, tetanus, myotonia, dermatomyositis) and hypothyroidism. Finally, on occasion *fever* may be associated with the connective tissue diseases, especially SLE, but infection should always be excluded.

TREATMENT HISTORY

Document current and previous antiarthritic medications (e.g. non-steroidal anti-inflammatory drugs [NSAIDs], sulfasalazine, lefunomide, hydroxychloroquine, gold, methotrexate, steroids, tumour necrosis factor inhibitors and other biological agents). Any side effects of these drugs (e.g. gastric ulceration or haemorrhage—NSAIDs), steroid side effects or serious infections (biological agents) also need to be identified. Patients commenced on biological agents have usually had screening tests performed to exclude infection with tuberculosis (e.g. chest X-ray, Mantoux test). Biological agents may allow reactivation of TB.

Ask also about physiotherapy and whether that has been helpful.

PAST HISTORY

It is important to enquire about any history of trauma, joint or tendon surgery (perhaps just another type of trauma) in the past. Similarly, a history of recent infection—including hepatitis, streptococcal pharyngitis, rubella, dysentery, gonorrhoea or tuberculosis—may be relevant to the onset of arthralgia or arthritis.

A history of tick bite may indicate that the patient has tick-bite arthritis. Other possible causes include:

- Ross river fever (Australia—usually rural)
- Barmah fever virus (Northern Australia)
- epidemic chikungunga (if the patient has travelled to the tropics)
- parvovirus infection
- Q fever and TB, which can cause a monoarthritis or osteomyelitis
- reactive arthritis, which may occur after recent sexually transmitted infections such as

---
[d] Halushi Behçet (1889–1948), a Turkish dermatologist.

Functional assessment in rheumatoid arthritis	
Class	**Assessment**
Class 1	Normal functional ability
Class 2	Ability to carry out normal activities, despite discomfort or limited mobility of one or more joints
Class 3	Ability to perform only a few of the tasks of the normal occupation or of self-care
Class 4	Complete or almost complete incapacity, with the patient confined to a wheelchair or to bed

TABLE 23.1

gonorrhoea and chlamydia and after episodes of dysentery
- a mono- or polyarthritis or tenosynovitis and acute rheumatic fever in children
- Lyme disease[e] (usually large joints).

A history of psoriasis may indicate that the arthritis is due to psoriatic arthritis. Joint disease may precede the rash in patients with psoriatic arthritis, so a family history of psoriasis (first-degree relative) may be a clue to this condition. It is also important to enquire about any history of arthritis in childhood. The smoking history is important: RA is more common in smokers, and smoking adds to their already increased risk of cardiovascular disease.

SOCIAL HISTORY

Determine the patient's ability to function (see Table 23.1). Ask about the domestic set-up, occupation, hobbies and sporting interests. This is particularly relevant if a chronic disabling arthritis has developed. Any history of sexually transmitted infection in the past is important, but non-specific urethritis and gonorrhoea are especially relevant.

FAMILY HISTORY

Some diseases associated with chronic arthritis run in families. These include RA, gout and primary osteoarthritis (OA), haemochromatosis, the spondyloarthritides, psoriasis and inflammatory bowel disease. A family history of bleeding disorder may explain an acutely swollen tender joint (haemophilia) in a boy.

T&O'C ESSENTIALS

1. Many rheumatological diseases have associated systemic abnormalities. Asking about extra-joint symptoms must be part of the history taking.
2. Back pain that wakes a patient from sleep may be associated with malignancy.
3. Chronic rheumatological disease can have a profound effect on a patient's life and work. It is essential to take a detailed history of the effects of the disease on the patient.
4. A history of morning stiffness (usually lasting for an hour or more) is characteristic of RA and helps distinguish it from OA; its duration is a guide to disease severity.

OSCE REVISION TOPICS – THE RHEUMATOLOGICAL HISTORY

Use these topics, which commonly occur in the OSCE, to help with revision.

1. Take a history from this woman with joint pains. (p 363)
2. This man has a long history of back pain and skin rash. Please take a history from him. (pp 365, 366)
3. This woman has stiffness in her joints in the morning. Please take a history from her. (p 363)
4. This man has the recent onset of severe back pain and fever. Please take a history from him. (p 366)

References

1. Van den Hoogen HMM, Koes BW, Van Eijk JTM, Bouter LM. On the accuracy of history, physical, and the erythrocyte sedimentation rate in diagnosing low back pain in general practice: a criteria based review of the literature. *Spine* 1995; 20:318–327. Unfortunately, distinguishing mechanical from non-mechanical causes of low back pain such as ankylosing spondylitis is clinically difficult. However, tenderness to pressure over the anterior superior iliac spines and over the lower sacrum may, based on other studies, be somewhat helpful for the positive diagnosis of ankylosing spondylitis.
2. Deyo RA, Rainville J, Kent DL. What can the history and physical examination tell us about low back pain? *JAMA* 1992; 268:760–765.
3. Chou R. In the clinic. Low back pain. *Ann Intern Med* 2014; 160:ITC 6-1.

---
[e] Lyme disease cannot be acquired in Australia, but frequent false-positive tests for Lyme disease occur particularly in patients with autoimmune disease owing to cross-reaction with rheumatoid factors and antinuclear antibody.

CHAPTER 24
The rheumatological examination

How dare thy joints forget to pay their awful duty to our presence. WILLIAM SHAKESPEARE, Richard II

EXAMINATION ANATOMY

Rheumatoid arthritis first inflames the joint synovium. Thickening of this may be palpable and is called *pannus*. Later, destruction of surrounding structures including tendons, articular cartilages and the bone itself occurs.

Joint pain may be well localised if there is inflammation close to the skin, but deeper joint abnormalities may cause pain to be referred. The areas where joint pain is felt correspond to the innervation of the muscle attached to that joint—the myotome. For example, the glenohumeral joint of the shoulder and the posterior scapular muscles are supplied from C5 and C6, so pain over the shoulder or scapula may arise from any structure supplied from these nerve roots—including the shoulder muscles and joints but also the C5 and C6 segments of the spine. The pattern of joint involvement may help in working out the type of arthritis. Remember though that more than one type of arthritis may be present. Fig. 24.1a shows typical synovial joints affected in rheumatoid arthritis, 24.1b thoracic joint involvement in spondyloarthropathies, 24.1c the pattern of involvement in psoriatic arthritis and 24.1d knee joint involvement in osteoarthritis. There are certain risk factors for osteoarthritis (see List 24.1).

The extra-articular structures that surround a joint (Fig. 24.2)—the ligaments, tendons and nerves—may also be the source of joint pain. Disease of the joint itself tends to limit movement of the joint in all directions, both active movement (moved by the patient) and passive movement (moved by the examiner). Extra-articular disease causes variable limitation of movement in different directions and tends to cause more limitation of active movement than of passive movement.

> **RISK FACTORS FOR OSTEOARTHRITIS**
> - Age
> - Female sex
> - Obesity (especially knee)
> - Genetic factors
> - Trauma
> - Manual labour (hand)
> - Occupational or recreational usage (e.g. farmer's hip, footballer's knee)
> - Race (e.g. Caucasians—hip and hand)
>
> Note: lifetime risk of symptomatic OA of knee is 27% and of hip 45%
>
> LIST 24.1

General inspection

There are certain established ways of examining the joints and related structures[1] and it is important to be aware of the numerous systemic complications of rheumatological diseases. The actual system of examination depends on the patient's history and sometimes on the examiner's noticing an abnormality on general inspection. Formal examination of all the joints is rarely part of the routine physical examination, but students should learn how to handle each joint properly and a formal examination is an important part of the evaluation of patients who present with joint symptoms or who have an established diagnosis and active symptoms. Diseases of the extra-articular soft tissues are particularly common.

General inspection is important for two reasons: first, it gives an indication of the patient's functional disability, which is essential in all rheumatological

CHAPTER 24 THE RHEUMATOLOGICAL EXAMINATION 371

(a) Typical synovial joints affected in rheumatoid arthritis (symmetrical, arms and legs, large and small joints); (b) Courtesy of MA Mir, from Atlas of Clinical Diagnosis, Saunders 2003—fig. A; RT Emond, PD Welsby and HA Rowland, from Colour Atlas of Infectious Diseases, Mosby 2003—fig. C); (c) Clinical Dermatology, Psoriasis and Other Papulosquamous Diseases, Figure 8.25, 2010; (d) Manual of Clinical and Practical Medicine, Musculoskeletal system, Figure 9.57, 2010, 277–302pp

FIGURE 24.1

Hand bones and finger joint—a typical synovial joint

FIGURE 24.2

assessments, and second, certain conditions can be diagnosed by careful inspection. Look at the patient as he or she walks into the room. Does walking appear to be painful and difficult? What posture is taken? Does the patient require assistance such as a stick or walking frame? Is there obvious deformity, and what joints does it involve? Note the pattern of joint involvement, which gives a clue about the likely underlying disease (see Lists 23.2 and 23.4 on pp 364 and 366).

For a more detailed examination the patient should be undressed as far as practical, usually to the underclothes. Depending on the patient's condition and the parts of the body to be examined, the examination may best be begun with the patient in bed, or sitting over the side of the bed or in a chair, or standing. The opportunity of watching the patient remove the clothes should not be lost because arthritis can interfere with this essential daily task.

Consider the characteristic changes of osteoarthritis (see List 24.2).

PRINCIPLES OF JOINT EXAMINATION

Certain general rules apply to the examination of all the joints and they can be summarised as: *look, feel, move, measure* and *compare with the opposite side*.

> **TYPICAL FINDINGS IN OSTEOARTHRITIC JOINTS**
>
> - Osteophytes (bony swellings) around the joint margins (e.g. Heberden's nodes)
> - Little or no synovitis
> - Deformity with little instability
> - Reduced movement—passive and active
> - Crepitus on joint movement
> - Tenderness over the joint
> - Wasting and weakness of muscles
>
> LIST 24.2

Look

The first principle is always to compare right with left. Remember that joints are three-dimensional structures and need to be inspected from the front, the back and the sides. Inspect the skin for *erythema* indicating underlying inflammation and suggesting active, intense arthritis or infection, *atrophy* suggesting chronic underlying disease, *scars* indicating previous operations such as tendon repairs or joint replacements, and *rashes*. For example, psoriasis is associated with a rash and polyarthritis (inflammation of more than one joint). The psoriatic rash consists of scaling erythematous plaques on extensor surfaces. The nails are often also affected (see Fig. 24.6). Also look for a vasculitic skin rash (inflammation of the blood vessels of the skin), which can range in appearance from palpable purpura or livedo reticularis (bluish-purple streaks in a net-like pattern) to skin necrosis.

A small, firm, painless swelling over the back (dorsal surface) of the wrist is usually a synovial cyst—a ganglion.[a] A larger, localised, soft area of swelling of the dorsum of the wrist generally indicates tenosynovitis.

Note any *swelling* over the joint. There are a number of possible causes; these include effusion into the joint space, hypertrophy and inflammation of the synovium (e.g. rheumatoid arthritis), or bony overgrowths at the joint margins (e.g. osteoarthritis). It may also occur when tissues around the joints become involved, as with the tendinitis or bursitis of rheumatoid arthritis. Swelling of the lower legs may be due to fluid retention, which is painless and can occur in association with inflammation anywhere in the leg. Painful swelling may result from inflammation of the ankle joints or tendons, or of the fascia, or from inflammatory oedema of the skin and subcutaneous tissue.

Deformity is the sign of a chronic, usually destructive, arthritis and ranges from mild ulnar deviation of the metacarpophalangeal joints in early rheumatoid arthritis to the gross destruction and disorganisation of a denervated (Charcot's[b]) joint (see Fig. 29.4 on p 466). Deviation of the part of the body away from the midline is called *valgus* deformity, and that towards the midline it is called *varus* deformity. For example, *genu valgum* means knock-kneed and *genu varum* means bow-legged.

Look for abnormal bone alignment. *Subluxation* is said to be present when displaced parts of the joint surfaces remain partly in contact. *Dislocation* is used to describe displacement where there is loss of contact between the joint surfaces.

Muscle wasting results from a combination of disuse of the joint, inflammation of the surrounding tissues and sometimes nerve entrapment. It tends to affect muscle groups adjacent to the diseased joint (e.g. quadriceps wasting with active arthritis of the knee) and is a sign of chronicity.

Feel

Palpate for skin *warmth*. This is done traditionally with the backs of the fingers where temperature appreciation is said to be better. A cool joint is unlikely to be involved in an acute inflammatory process. A swollen and slightly warm joint may be affected by active synovitis (see below), infection (very warm, e.g. *Staphylococcus*) or crystal arthritis (e.g. gout).

Tenderness is a guide to the acuteness of the inflammation, but may be present over the muscles of patients with fibromyalgia. Tenderness elicited over the margins of a joint indicates inflammation. Where the joint cannot be examined directly (e.g. hips, midtarsal joints), passive movement that causes pain is a surrogate for this. Tell the patient to state if the examination is becoming uncomfortable. Tenderness can be graded as follows:

Grade I	Patient complains of pain
Grade II	Patient complains of pain and winces
Grade III	Patient complains of pain, winces and withdraws the joint
Grade IV	Patient does not allow palpation.

This may result from joint inflammation or from lesions outside the joints (periarticular tissues), including inflamed tendons, bursae or attachments (entheses). Infected joints are extremely tender and patients will often not let the examiner move the joint at all. Palpation of a joint or area for tenderness must be performed gently, and the patient's face rather than the joint itself should be watched for signs that the examination is uncomfortable.

Palpate the joint deliberately now, if possible, for evidence of *synovitis*, which is a soft and spongy (boggy) swelling. This must be distinguished from an *effusion*, which tends to affect large joints but can occur in any joint. Here the swelling is fluctuant and can be made to shift within the joint. *Bony swelling* feels hard and immobile, and suggests osteophyte formation or subchondral bone thickening.

Move

Much information about certain joints is gained by testing the range of *passive* movement. (Passive movement is obviously contraindicated in cases of recent injury to the limb or joint, such as a suspected fracture.) Ask the patient to relax and let you move

---

[a] The traditional treatment, striking the lesion very hard with the family Bible, is not effective.
[b] Jean Martin Charcot (1825–1893), a Parisian physician and neurologist. He became professor of nervous diseases, holding the first Chair of Neurology in the world. His pupils included Babinski, Marie and Freud.

the joint. This must be attempted gently and will be limited if the joint is painful (secondary to muscle spasm), if a tense effusion is present, if there is capsular contraction or if there is a fixed deformity. The joints may have limited extension (called fixed flexion deformity) or limited flexion (fixed extension deformity). Passive movement of the spine is not a practical manoeuvre (unless the examiner is very strong), and active movement is tested here. *Active* movement is more helpful in assessing integrated joint function. Hand function and gait are usually applied as tests of *function*. *Pain on motion* indicates a joint or periarticular problem.

> **HINT BOX**
>
> 1. When pain is present with both active and passive joint movement there is likely to be an intrinsic joint (articular) problem.
> 2. When pain is present only on active movement—consider a periarticular abnormality.
> 3. If active is impaired, but passive is normal—consider soft-tissue injury or neurological disease.

Stability of the joint is important and depends largely on the surrounding ligaments. This is tested by attempting to move the joint gently in abnormal directions to its usual limits, set by ligaments and muscular tone.

Joint crepitus, which is a grating sensation or noise from the joint, indicates irregularity of the articular surfaces. Its presence suggests chronicity.

Measure

Accurate measurement of the range of movement of a joint is possible with a goniometer, which is a hinged rod with a protractor in the centre. Open the instrument's jaws and line them up with the joint. Measurement of joint movements is performed from the zero starting position. For most joints this is the anatomical position in extension (e.g. the straightened knee). Movement is then recorded as the number of degrees of flexion from this position. A knee with a fixed flexion deformity may be recorded as '30° to 60°', which indicates that there is 30° of fixed flexion deformity

and that flexion is limited to 60°. At some joints both flexion and extension from the anatomical position can be measured, as at the wrists. The goniometer is not routinely used by non-rheumatologists and there is a wide range of normal values for joint movement. Most clinicians estimate the approximate joint angles.

A tape measure is useful for measuring and following serially the quadriceps muscle bulk and in examination of spinal movements.

ASSESSMENT OF INDIVIDUAL JOINTS

Hands and wrists

(See Figs 24.3 to 24.8.)

Examination anatomy

The articulations between the phalanges are synovial hinge joints. The eight bones of the wrist (carpal bones) form gliding joints that allow wrist movements—flexion / extension and abduction / adduction as they slide over each other.

X-ray of normal hand

(Courtesy of M Thomson, National Capital Diagnostic Imaging, Canberra.)

FIGURE 24.3

History

Pain may be present in some or all of the joints. It is more likely to be vague or diffuse if it has radiated from the shoulder or neck or is due to carpal tunnel syndrome, and to be localised if it is due to arthritis. *Stiffness* is typically worse in the mornings in rheumatoid arthritis. *Swelling* of the wrist may indicate arthritis or tendon sheath inflammation. Swelling of individual joints suggests arthritis. *Deformity* of the fingers and hand due to rheumatoid arthritis or of the fingers as a result of arthritis or gouty tophi may be the presenting complaint. The sudden onset of deformity suggests tendon rupture. *Locking or snapping* of a finger (trigger finger) is typical of inflammation of a flexor tendon sheath (tenovaginitis). *Loss of function* is a serious problem when it involves the numerous functions of the hand and wrist. Ask what problems this has caused. *Neurological symptoms* as a result of nerve compression may cause paraesthesias, numbness or sometimes hyperaesthesia or limitation of strength or of complicated hand functions.

Examination

First sit the patient over the side of the bed and place the patient's hands on the pillow with palms down. Often examination (Text box 24.1) or even inspection of the hands alone will give enough information for the examiner to make a diagnosis. As a result this is quite a popular test in the OSCE.

> **T&O'C ESSENTIALS**
>
> In the setting of polyarthritis of the hands, if the distal interphalangeal (DIP) joints are spared the diagnosis is likely to be rheumatoid arthritis or systemic lupus erythematosus. If the DIP joints are involved consider: osteoarthritis, gouty arthritis or psoriatic arthritis.

Look

Start the examination at the *wrists and forearms*. Inspect the skin for erythema, scleroderma, atrophy, scars and rashes. Look for swelling and its distribution. Next, look at the wrist for swelling, deformity, ulnar and styloid prominence. Then look for muscle wasting of the intrinsic muscles of the hand. This results in the appearance of hollow ridges between the metacarpal bones. It is especially obvious on the dorsum of the hand.

Go on to the *metacarpophalangeal (MCP) joints*. Again note any skin abnormalities, swelling or deformity. Look especially for ulnar deviation and volar (palmar) subluxation of the fingers. Ulnar deviation is deviation of the phalanges at the metacarpophalangeal joints towards the medial (ulnar) side of the hand. It is usually associated with anterior (Volar) subluxation of the fingers (see Fig. 24.4). These deformities are characteristic but not pathognomonic of rheumatoid arthritis (see List 24.3).

Next inspect the *proximal interphalangeal (PIP)* and *distal interphalangeal* joints. Again note any skin changes and joint swelling. Look for the characteristic deformities of *rheumatoid arthritis* (see Fig. 24.4). These include *swan neck* and *boutonnière* deformity of the fingers and *Z deformity* of the thumb. They are due to joint destruction and tendon dysfunction. The swan neck deformity is hyperextension at the proximal interphalangeal joint and fixed flexion deformity at the distal interphalangeal joint. It is due to subluxation at the proximal interphalangeal joint and tendon shortening at the distal interphalangeal joint. The boutonnière (buttonhole) deformity consists of fixed flexion of the proximal interphalangeal joint and extension of the distal interphalangeal joints. This is due to protrusion of the proximal interphalangeal joint through its ruptured extensor tendon. The Z deformity of the thumb consists of hyperextension of the interphalangeal joint and fixed

> **DIFFERENTIAL DIAGNOSIS OF A DEFORMING POLYARTHROPATHY**
>
> Rheumatoid arthritis
> Seronegative spondyloarthritis, particularly psoriatic arthritis, ankylosing spondylitis or Reiter's disease
> Chronic tophaceous gout (rarely symmetrical)
> Primary generalised osteoarthritis
> Erosive or inflammatory osteoarthritis
> Jaccoud's* arthritis (rheumatic fever)
>
> *François Jaccoud (1830–1913), a professor of medicine in Geneva.
>
> LIST 24.3

Examination of the hands and wrists

Sitting up (hands on a pillow)

1. General inspection
   Cushingoid
   Weight
   Iritis, scleritis, etc.
   Obvious other joint disease
2. Look
   Dorsal aspect
   - Wrists
     Skin—scars, redness, atrophy, rash
     Swelling—distribution
     Deformity
     Muscle wasting
   - Metacarpophalangeal joints
     Skin
     Swelling—distribution
     Deformity—ulnar deviation, volar
       subluxation, etc.
   - Proximal and distal interphalangeal joints
     Skin
     Swelling—distribution
     Deformity—swan necking, boutonnière, Z, etc.
   - Nails
     Psoriatic changes—pitting, ridging, onycholysis, hyperkeratosis, discoloration
3. Feel and move passively
   Wrists
   - Synovitis
   - Effusions
   - Range of movement
   - Crepitus
   - Ulnar styloid tenderness
   Metacarpophalangeal joints
   - Synovitis
   - Effusions
   - Range of movement
   - Crepitus
   - Subluxation
   Proximal and distal interphalangeal joints
   - As above
   Palmar tendon crepitus
   Carpal tunnel syndrome tests
   Palmar aspect
   - Skin—scars, palmar erythema, palmar creases (anaemia)
   - Muscle wasting
4. Hand function
   Grip strength
   Key grip
   Opposition strength
   Practical ability
5. Other
   Elbows—subcutaneous nodules—psoriatic rash
   Other joints
   Signs of systemic disease

TEXT BOX 24.1

---

flexion and subluxation of the metacarpophalangeal joint.

Now look for the characteristic changes of *osteoarthritis* (see Fig. 24.5). Here the distal interphalangeal and first carpometacarpal joints are usually involved. *Heberden's nodes*[c] are a common deformity caused by marginal osteophytes that lie at the base of the distal phalanx. Less commonly, the proximal interphalangeal joints may be involved and osteophytes here are called *Bouchard's*[d] nodes.

Look also to see whether the phalanges appear *sausage-shaped (dactylitis)*. This is characteristic of psoriatic arthropathy, but can also occur in patients with reactive arthritis. It is due to interphalangeal arthritis and flexor tendon sheath oedema. Finger shortening due to severe destructive arthritis also occurs in psoriatic disease and is called *arthritis mutilans*. The hand may take up a *main en lorgnette* ('hand holding long-handled opera glasses') appearance owing to a combination of shortening and telescoping of the digits. This is very rare now as a result of improved treatment of rheumatoid arthritis.

Look at the finger pulps for atrophy and digital ulcers, which suggest systemic sclerosis.

Now examine the *nails*. Characteristic *psoriatic* nail changes may be visible: these include onycholysis, pitting (small depressions in the nail), onycholysis (see Fig. 24.6) and, less commonly, hyperkeratosis (thickening of the nail), ridging (a non-specific sign) and discoloration.

---

[c] William Heberden (1710–1801), a London physician, and doctor to George III and Samuel Johnson, described these in 1802. He was the first person to describe angina.
[d] Charles Jacques Bouchard (1837–1915), a Parisian physician.

(a) The hands in rheumatoid arthritis showing ulnar deviation and Z deformity. (b) Rheumatoid hands showing swan neck deformity and DIP. (c) A swan's neck as it feeds (neck extended at body, head flexed). (d) Boutonnière deformity of the PIP and DIP joints

FIGURE 24.4

The presence of *vasculitic* changes around the nail folds implies active disease. These consist of black to brown 1–2 millimetre lesions due to skin infarction and occur typically in rheumatoid arthritis (see Fig. 24.7). Splinter haemorrhages may be present in patients with systemic lupus erythematosus (and infective endocarditis) and are due to vasculitis. Unlike nail-fold infarcts they are located under the nails in the nail beds. Periungual telangiectasias occur in systemic lupus erythematosus, scleroderma or dermatomyositis.

Now turn the patient's hands over and reveal the *palmar surfaces*. Look at the palms for scars (from tendon repairs or transfers), palmar erythema and muscle wasting of the thenar or hypothenar eminences (due to disuse, vasculitis or peripheral nerve entrapment). A Dupuytren's contracture may be visible (p 236). Telangiectasia here would support the diagnosis of scleroderma.

> **HINT BOX**
>
> Even when asked to examine hands, look at the extensor surfaces at the elbows for:
>
> - rheumatoid nodules
> - gouty tophi
> - psoriasis.

Feel and move

Turn the hands back again to the palm-down position. Palpate the *wrists* with both thumbs placed on the dorsal surface by the wrists, supported underneath by the index fingers (see Fig. 24.8). Feel gently for synovitis (boggy swelling) and effusions. The wrist should be gently dorsiflexed (normally possible to 75°) and palmar

Hand of a patient with osteoarthritis showing Heberden's nodes (distal interphalangeal joints) and Bouchard's nodes (proximal interphalangeal joints)

FIGURE 24.5

Rheumatoid vasculitis (arrows)

FIGURE 24.7

Psoriatic nails, showing onycholysis and discoloration, with typical pitting and ridging

FIGURE 24.6

Palpating the wrist joint—approved method

FIGURE 24.8

flexed (also possible to 75°) with your thumbs. Then radial and ulnar deviation (20°) is tested (see Fig. 24.9). Note any tenderness or limitation of movement or joint crepitus. Palpate the ulnar styloid for tenderness, which can occur in rheumatoid arthritis.

Test for tenderness at the tip of the radial styloid. This suggests de Quervain's[e] tenosynovitis. Boggy swelling distal to the styloid suggests synovitis.

Feel for tenderness in the anatomical snuff box (see Fig. 24.9), which can be the result of first carpometacarpal joint arthritis or of scaphoid injury. Test for tenderness distal to the head of the ulna for extensor carpi ulnaris tendinitis.

Go on now to the *metacarpophalangeal joints*, which are palpated in a similar way with the two thumbs. Again passive movement is tested. The joints are best examined in 90° flexion, which opens the joint margins. Volar subluxation can be demonstrated by flexing the

[e] Fritz de Quervain (1868–1940), a professor of surgery in Berne, Switzerland.

Movements of the wrist joint.

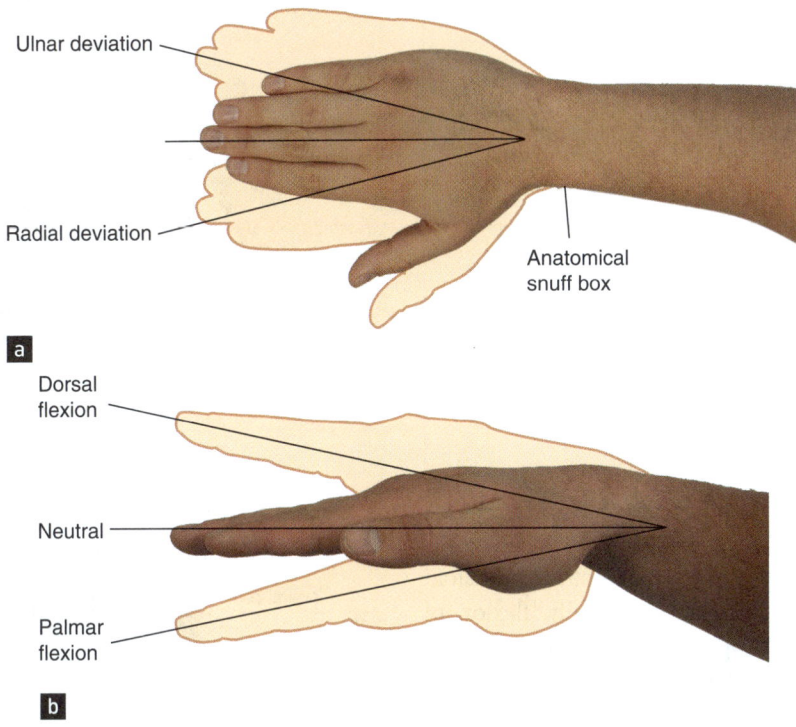

(a) Ulnar and radial deviation; (b) dorsal and palmar flexion

FIGURE 24.9

metacarpophalangeal joint with the proximal phalanx held between the thumb and forefinger; the joint is then rocked backwards and forwards (see Fig. 24.10). Very little movement occurs with this manoeuvre at a normal joint. Considerable movement may be present when ligamentous laxity or subluxation is present.

Palpate the *proximal* and *distal interphalangeal* joints for tenderness, swelling and osteophytes. Use the thumb and forefinger of each hand and examine in two planes.

Next test for *palmar tendon crepitus*. Place the palmar aspects of your fingers against the palm of the patient's hand while he or she flexes and extends the metacarpophalangeal joints. Inflamed palmar tendons can be felt creaking in their thickened sheaths and nodules can be palpated. This indicates tenosynovitis.

A *trigger finger* may also be detected by this manoeuvre. Here, the thickening of a section of digital flexor tendon is such that it tends to jam when passing

Examination for volar subluxation at the metacarpophalangeal joints

FIGURE 24.10

> **CAUSES OF CARPAL TUNNEL SYNDROME**
>
> Occupation-related: working with wrists and hands flexed
> Rheumatoid arthritis
> Hypothyroidism
> Acromegaly
> Pregnancy
> Gout
> Obesity
> Amyloidosis
> Diabetes mellitus
> Idiopathic
> Carpal bone osteomyelitis
>
> LIST 24.4

(a) Active wrist extension; (b) active wrist flexion

FIGURE 24.11

through a narrowed part of its tendon sheath. Rheumatoid arthritis is an important cause. Typically, flexion of the finger occurs freely up to a certain point where it sticks and cannot be extended (as flexors are more powerful than extensors). The application of greater force overcomes the resistance with a snap.

If the carpal tunnel syndrome is suspected, ask the patient to flex both wrists for 30 seconds—paraesthesias will often be precipitated in the affected hand if the syndrome is present (*Phalen's*[f] wrist flexion test). The paraesthesias (pins and needles) are in the distribution of the median nerve (p 559), when thickening of the flexor retinaculum has entrapped the nerve in the carpal tunnel (see List 24.4). This test is more reliable than *Tinel's*[g] *sign*, in which tapping over the flexor retinaculum (which lies at the proximal part of the palm) may cause similar paraesthesias.[2]

Now test active movements. First assess *wrist flexion and extension* as shown in Fig. 24.11. Compare the two sides. Now go on to *thumb movements* (see Fig. 24.12). The patient holds the hand flat, palm upwards, and your hand holds the patient's fingers. Test *extension* by asking the patient to stretch the thumb outwards; *abduction* by asking for the thumb to be pointed straight upwards; *adduction* by asking the patient to squeeze your finger and *opposition* by getting the patient to touch the little finger with the thumb. Look for limitation of these movements and discomfort caused by them. Next test *metacarpophalangeal and interphalangeal movements*. As a screening test, ask the patient to make a fist then to straighten out the fingers (see Fig. 24.13). Then test the fingers individually. If active flexion of one or more fingers is reduced, test the superficial and profundus flexor tendons (see Fig. 24.14). Hold the proximal finger joint extended and instruct the patient to bend the tip of the finger; the distal fingertip will only flex if the flexor profundus is intact. Then hold the other fingers extended (to inactivate the profundus) with the finger to be tested resting above your fingers and instruct the patient to bend the whole finger (inability indicates the superficialis is unable to work). The most common tendon ruptures are of the extensors of the fourth and fifth fingers.

---

[f] George Phalen, an orthopaedic surgeon at the Cleveland Clinic.
[g] Jules Tinel (1879–1952), a physician and neurologist in Paris. In 1915 he described tingling in the distribution of a nerve that had been severed and was regrowing when it was percussed.

Thumb movements.

(a) Extension; (b) abduction; (c) adduction; (d) opposition

FIGURE 24.12

Function

It is important to test the function of the hand. *Grip strength* is tested by getting the patient to squeeze two of your fingers. Even an angry patient will rarely cause pain if given only two fingers. Serial measurements of grip strength can be made by asking the patient to squeeze a partly inflated sphygmomanometer cuff and noting the pressure reached. *Key grip* (see Fig. 24.15) is the grip with which a key is held between the pulps of the thumb and forefinger. Ask the patient to hold this grip tightly and try to open up his or her fingers. *Opposition strength* (see Fig. 24.16) is where the patient opposes the thumb and individual fingers. The difficulty with which these can be forced apart is assessed. Finally, *a practical test*, such as asking the patient to undo a button or write with a pen, should be performed.

Tests of hand function should be completed by formally assessing for neurological changes (see Ch 34).

Examination of the hands is not complete without feeling for the *subcutaneous nodules* of rheumatoid arthritis near the elbows (see Fig. 24.17). These are 0.5–3 centimetre firm, shotty,[h] non-tender lumps that occur typically over the olecranon. They may be attached to bone. They are found in rheumatoid-factor-positive

---

[h] They feel like the pellets emitted by a shot-gun.

Screening metacarpophalangeal and interphalangeal movements.

(a) Flexion—'Make a fist'; (b) extension—'Now open your hand up'

FIGURE 24.13

Testing the superficial and profundus flexor tendons.

(a) Flexor profundus; (b) flexor superficialis

FIGURE 24.14

The key grip

FIGURE 24.15

Testing opposition strength

FIGURE 24.16

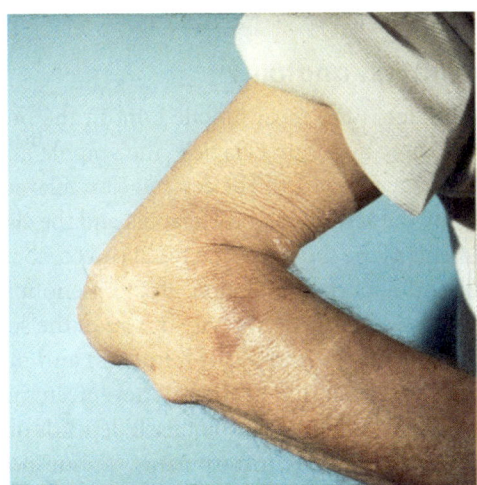

Subcutaneous nodules in rheumatoid arthritis

FIGURE 24.17

rheumatoid arthritis. Rheumatoid nodules are areas of fibrinoid necrosis with a characteristic histological appearance and are probably initiated by a small-vessel vasculitis. They are localised by trauma but can occur elsewhere, especially attached to tendons, over pressure areas in the hands or feet, in the lung, pleura, myocardium or vocal cords. They are most commonly found firmly attached over the proximal ulna, just distal to the elbow. Occasionally they are within the olecranon bursa and can be moved freely within it. The combination of arthritis and nodules suggests the diagnostic possibilities outlined in List 24.5.

If the patient has diabetes mellitus, look for the features of diabetic cheiroarthropathy and then test function. The skin appears thick and tight and the patient may be unable to extend *all* digits fully. This is different to Dupuytren's contractures, which usually affect only the fourth and fifth digits. Two simple tests can be helpful:

- To recognise contractures in the metacarpophalangeal, proximal interphalangeal and distal interphalangeal joints, ask the patient to bring the flat of the hands together as if praying (**prayer sign**).
- To recognise contractures in the metacarpophalangeal joints, ask the patient to flatten the palm against the surface of a table (**table-top test**).

CAUSES OF ARTHRITIS PLUS NODULES*

Rheumatoid arthritis
Systemic lupus erythematosus (rare)
Rheumatic fever (Jaccoud's arthritis) (very rare)
Granulomas (e.g. sarcoidosis) (very rare)

*Gouty tophi and xanthomata from hyperlipidaemia may cause confusion.

LIST 24.5

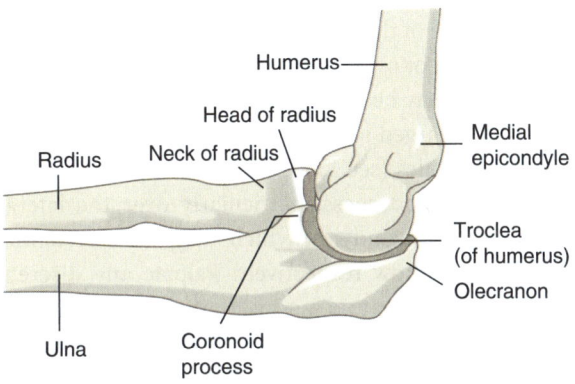

Anatomy of the elbow

FIGURE 24.18

Elbows
Examination anatomy

The humerus, radius and ulna meet at the elbow, which is both a hinge and a pivot joint (see Fig. 24.18). Pivoting occurs between the radius and ulna, and the articulation between all three bones forms a hinge joint.

History

Pain from the elbow is usually diffuse and may radiate down the forearm. It may occur over the lateral or medial epicondyle if the patient has tendinitis (tennis or golfer's elbow). The patient may have noticed some swelling as a result of inflammation. *Swelling* over the back suggests olecranon bursitis. *Stiffness* may interfere with elbow movements and the patient may complain of difficulty combing the hair. When supination and pronation are affected the patient may complain of difficulty with carrying and holding. If the patient is aware of the elbow moving abnormally this suggests *instability* of the joint and may be a result of rheumatoid arthritis or trauma. Ulnar nerve trauma at the elbow may lead to a complaint of *numbness* or *paraesthesias* in the distribution of that nerve.

Examination

Watch as the patient undresses, for difficulty disentangling the arms from clothing. The upper arms should be exposed completely. Note any deformity or difference in the normal 5–10° valgus position (carrying angle[i]) as the patient stands with the palms facing forwards.

Look for a joint effusion, which appears as a swelling on either side of the olecranon. Discrete swellings over the olecranon or over the proximal subcutaneous border of the ulna may be due to rheumatoid nodules, gouty tophi, an enlarged olecranon bursa or, rarely, to other types of nodules (see List 24.5).

Feel for tenderness, particularly over the lateral and medial epicondyles, which may indicate tennis and golfer's elbow respectively. Palpate any discrete swellings. Rheumatoid nodules are quite hard, may be tender and are attached to underlying structures. Gouty tophi have a firm feeling and often appear yellow under the skin, but are sometimes difficult to distinguish from rheumatoid nodules. A fluid collection in the olecranon bursa is softly fluctuant and may be tender if inflammation is present. These collections are associated with rheumatoid arthritis and gout, but often occur independently of these diseases.

Small amounts of fluid or synovitis of the elbow joint may be detected by the examiner, facing the patient, placing the thumb of the opposite hand along the edge of the ulnar shaft just distal to the olecranon where the synovium is closest to the surface. Full extension of the elbow joint will cause a palpable bulge in this area if fluid is present.

Move the elbow joints passively. The elbow is a hinge joint. The zero position is when the arm is fully extended (0°). Normal flexion is possible to 150°. Limitation of extension is an early sign of synovitis.

If lateral epicondylitis is suspected, ask the patient to extend and supinate the wrist actively against resistance. Test the range of active movements by standing in front of the patient and demonstrating. If there is any deformity or complaint of numbness, a neurological examination of the hand and arm is indicated for ulnar nerve entrapment.

Shoulders

Examination anatomy

The shoulder is the most mobile joint in the body. It involves three bones: the clavicle, the scapula and the humerus (see Fig. 24.19). The acromioclavicular joint is formed by the acromion of the scapula and the clavicle. Movements of the shoulder are a result of a combination of ball-and-socket articulation at the glenohumeral joint (between the glenoid cavity [fossa] of the scapula and the ball-shaped end of the humerus) and motion between the scapula and the thorax. Seventeen muscles are involved. Stability of the joint itself depends on four muscles: supraspinatus, infraspinatus, teres minor and subscapularis—the rotator cuff muscles. The shallow glenoid fossa is extended by a cartilage rim (the glenoid labrum). This cushions the humeral head and increases the depth and surface area of articulation. Instability of the joint can result from abnormality of, or injury to, any of these structures.

The joint is encased in a capsule and is lined with synovium.

This complicated joint is frequently affected by a number of non-arthritic conditions involving its bursa, capsule and surrounding tendons—for example, 'frozen (stiff) shoulder' (adhesive capsulitis), tendinitis and bursitis. All of these disorders affect movement of the shoulder.

Instability of the joint can result in dislocation (all contact between the articular surfaces is lost) or subluxation (partial contact remains). Anterior dislocation or subluxation tends to occur after a fall onto an outstretched arm. More chronic instability is associated with gradual stretching of the supporting structures by sporting or work activities that involve use of the arm above the head. Patients with ligamentous laxity may have multidirectional instability and some are able to dislocate their shoulders voluntarily (e.g. at parties).

History

Pain is the most common symptom of a patient with shoulder problems.[3] Typically it is felt over the front and lateral part of the joint. It may radiate to the insertion of the deltoid or even further. Pain felt over the top of the shoulder is more likely to come from the acromioclavicular joint or from the neck. *Deformity* has to be severe before it becomes obvious. *Pain and stiffness* may severely limit shoulder movement. *Instability* may

---

[i] This is wider in women so that their larger hips are accommodated.

Examination of the shoulders.

(a) Anatomy of the shoulder. (b) X-ray of left shoulder in the neutral position; the relative positions of the humeral head, clavicle and scapulae can be seen. (c) X-ray of left shoulder in abduction; abduction of the arm rotates the head of the humerus and the clavicle moves upwards

(X-rays courtesy of M Thomson, National Capital Diagnostic Imaging, Canberra.)

FIGURE 24.19

cause the alarming feeling that the shoulder is jumping out of its socket. This is most likely to occur during abduction and external rotation (e.g. while attempting to serve a tennis ball). *Loss of function* may result in difficulty using the arms at above shoulder height or reaching around to the back. A clinical clue is that rotator cuff tears tend to occur in older patients (>50 years) whereas tendinits and impingement affect younger patients.[4]

Examination

Watch the patient undressing and note forward, backward and upward movements of the shoulders and whether these seem limited or cause the patient pain. Stand back and compare the two sides. The arms should be held at the same level and the outlines of the acromioclavicular joints should be the same. There may be wasting of one of the deltoid muscles that will not be obvious unless the two are compared.

Deltoid wasting is characteristic of shoulder problems, whereas trapezius muscle wasting suggests cervical spine problems.

Look at the joint. A swelling may be visible anteriorly, but unless effusions are large and the patient is thin these are difficult to detect. Look for asymmetry and for scars as a result of injury or previous surgery.

Feel for tenderness and swelling. Stand beside the patient, rest one hand on the patient's shoulder and move the arm into different positions (see below). As the shoulder moves, feel the acromioclavicular joint and then move your hand along the clavicle to the sternoclavicular joint.

Move the joint (see Figs 24.20 and 24.21). The zero position is with the arm hanging by the side of the body so that the palm faces forwards. *Abduction* tests glenohumeral abduction, which is normally possible to 90°. For the right shoulder, stand behind the patient resting your left hand on the patient's shoulder, while your right hand abducts the elbow from the shoulder. *Elevation* is usually possible to 180° when it is performed actively, as movement of the scapula is then included. *Adduction* is possible to 50°; the arm is carried forwards across the front of the chest. *External rotation* is possible to 65°; with the elbow bent to 90° the arm is turned laterally as far as possible. *Internal rotation* is usually possible to 90°; it is tested actively by asking the patient to place his or her hand behind the back and then to try to scratch the back as high up as possible with the thumb. Patients with rotator cuff problems complain of pain when they perform this manoeuvre. *Flexion* is possible to 180°, of which the glenohumeral joint contributes about 90°. *Extension* is possible to 65°; the arm is swung backwards as in marching. During all these manoeuvres, limitation with or without pain and joint crepitus are assessed.

Rapid assessment of shoulder movement is possible using the three-step Apley[j] scratch test (see Fig. 24.22). Stand behind and ask the patient to scratch an imaginary itch over the opposite scapula, first by reaching over the opposite shoulder, next by reaching behind the neck and finally by reaching behind the back. If this test is normal there is usually no need to test passive shoulder movements.

The anterior stability of the shoulder joint is traditionally assessed by the *apprehension test*; stand behind the patient, abduct, extend and externally rotate the shoulder (see Fig. 24.21c) while pushing the head of the humerus forwards with the thumb. The patient will strongly resist this manoeuvre if there is impending dislocation (LR+ 1.8; LR− 0.23). There will be a similar response if the arm is adducted and internally rotated and posterior dislocation is about to occur. The *clunk test* is probably kinder to the patient and more accurate. The patient lies supine with the arm fully abducted. It is then put into full external rotation and the head of the humerus is pushed a little anteriorly. Rather than looking for signs of distress, the examiner listens and feels for a grinding sensation from the shoulder (LR+ 16; LR− 0.67).

This is also the time to test biceps function. The patient flexes the elbow against resistance. A ruptured biceps tendon causes the biceps muscle to roll up into a ball.

As a general rule, intra-articular disease produces *painful* limitation of movement in *all* directions, whereas tendinitis produces *painful* limitation of movement in *one* plane only and tendon rupture or neurological lesions produce *painless* weakness. For example, if the abnormal sign is limited shoulder abduction in the middle range (45–135°), this suggests rotator cuff problems (i.e. the supraspinatus, infraspinatus, subscapularis and teres minor muscles) rather than arthritis.

The *drop-arm test* can help diagnose a supraspinatus tear. Abduct the patient's arm to 90° and ask him or her to let the arm down slowly to the waist. A positive test (the arm drops suddenly) indicates a supraspinatus tear.

Bicipital tendinitis causes localised tenderness over the groove. The supraspinatus tendon is a little higher, just under the anterior surface of the acromion. Supraspinatus tendinitis is common. Testing for it involves placing a finger over the head of the tendon while the shoulder is in extension. As this pushes the tendon forwards against your finger, the movement is painful. When the shoulder is then flexed the tendon moves away and the pain disappears.

Do not forget that arthritis affecting the acromioclavicular joint can be confused with glenohumeral disorders. The *cross-arm test* can help. Ask the patient to abduct the arm to 90° and then adduct the arm across the body. The test is positive if pain is felt in the acromioclavicular joint region.

---

[j] Alan Apley, an orthopaedic surgeon at St Thomas's Hospital, London.

Movements of the shoulder joint.

(a) Abduction using the glenohumeral joint; (b) abduction using the glenohumeral joint and the scapula; (c) extension; (d) adduction

FIGURE 24.20

Examining the shoulder joint.

(a) Extension; (b) flexion; (c) apprehension test; (d) internal rotation and abduction

FIGURE 24.21

Also remember to examine the neck and axillae in patients with shoulder pain.

Temporomandibular joints
History
The usual symptoms of temporomandibular joint (TMJ) dysfunction include clicking and pain on opening the mouth. The jaw may sometimes lock in the open position.

Examination
Look in front of the ear for swelling. **Feel** by placing a finger just in front of the ear while the patient opens and shuts the mouth (see Fig. 24.23). The head of the mandible is palpable as it slides forwards when the jaw is opened. Clicking and grating may be felt. This is sometimes associated with tenderness if the joint is involved in an inflammatory arthritis. Rheumatoid arthritis may affect the temporomandibular joint.

Neck
Examination anatomy—the spine
The spinal column (see Fig. 24.24) is like a tower of bones that protects the spinal cord and houses its blood supply and efferent and afferent nerves. It provides

(a) to (c) Apley scratch test to assess shoulder movement

FIGURE 24.22

Examining the temporomandibular joints—'Open and shut your mouth for me'

FIGURE 24.23

mechanical support for the body and is flexible enough to allow bending and twisting movements. There are diarthrodial joints between the articular processes of the vertebral bodies, and the vertebral bodies are separated by the vertebral discs. These pads of cartilage are flexible enough to allow movement between the vertebrae. In the cervical spine from C3 to C7, the uncovertebral joints of Luschka[k] are present. These are formed between a lateral bony extension (uncinate process) from the margin of the more inferior vertebral body and the one above. Osteoarthritic hypertrophy of these joints may result in pain or nerve root irritation.

History

Pain is the most common neck symptom. Musculoskeletal neck pain usually arises in the structures at the back of the neck—the cervical spine, the splenius, semispinalis and trapezius muscles—or in the cervical nerves or nerve roots. Pain in the front of the neck may come from the oesophagus, trachea, thyroid gland or anterior neck muscles (e.g. sternomastoid and platysma). Pain may be referred to the front of the neck from the heart.

There may be a history of trauma from direct injury or a sudden deceleration causing hyperextension of the neck: 'whiplash' injury. Injury can also be caused by attempted therapeutic neck manipulations. The possibility of spinal cord injury must be considered in these patients. Ask about weakness or altered sensation in the arms and legs and any problem with bowel or bladder function.

---

[k] Hubert von Luschka (1820–75), a professor of anatomy in Tübingen.

(a) Structure of the spine; (b) MRI scan of the lumbar spine showing the anatomical features seen in (a)

(MRI scan courtesy of M Thomson, National Capital Diagnostic Imaging, Canberra.)

FIGURE 24.24

The pain may have begun suddenly, suggesting a disc prolapse, or more gradually owing to disc degeneration.

Postural tendon and muscle strains are common causes of temporary neck pain. These are often related to overuse. Ask about the patient's occupation and whether work or recreational activities involve repeated and prolonged extension of the neck (e.g. painters and cyclists). These patients often describe neck stiffness, and pain and muscle spasm are often present. The repeated holding of a telephone between the shoulder and the ear can cause nerve root problems. Neck movement may cause *radicular symptoms* such as paraesthesias in the distribution of a cervical nerve after a hyperextension injury or cervical spine arthritis. Ask about paraesthesias and weakness in the arms and hands.

Rheumatoid arthritis.

Note the head tilt due to right atlantoaxial subluxation, the rheumatoid hands and the subcutaneous rheumatoid nodules

FIGURE 24.25

Movements of the neck.

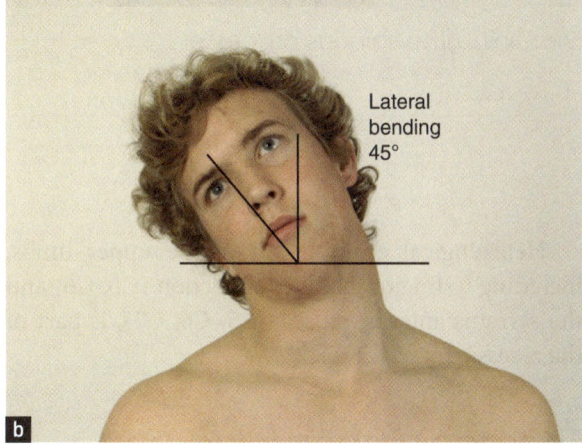

(a) Extension—'Look up and back'; (b) lateral bending—'Now touch your right ear onto your shoulder' (45°); rotation—'Now look over your shoulder to the right and then to the left' (70°)

FIGURE 24.26

Deformity may occur as a result of muscle spasm or sometimes following disc prolapse. *Torticollis* is a chronic and uncontrollable twisting of the neck to one side as a result of a muscle dystonia or cervical nerve root problem.

Examination

The patient should be undressed so as to expose the neck, shoulders and arms (see Fig. 24.25).

Look at the cervical spine while the patient is sitting up, and note particularly his or her posture. **Movement** should be tested actively. Flexion is tested by asking the patient to try to touch his or her chest with the chin (normal flexion is possible to 45°). Extension (see Fig. 24.26(a)) is tested by asking the patient to look up and back (normally possible to 45°). Lateral bending (see Fig. 24.26(b)) is tested by getting the patient to try to touch his or her shoulder with the ear (normally possible to 45°). Rotation is tested by getting the patient to look over the shoulder to the right and then to the left (normally possible to 70°).

Feel the posterior spinous processes. This is often easiest to do when the patient lies prone with the chest supported by a pillow and the neck slightly flexed. Feel for tenderness and uneven spacing of the spinous processes. Tenderness of the facet joints will be elicited by feeling a finger's breadth lateral to the middle line on each side (see Fig. 24.27).

Nerve root symptoms may be reproduced using the *Spurling*[1] test.[5] Extending and rotating the patient's neck towards the affected side worsens the symptoms (over 90% specific for cervical root compression). Then get the patient to lift the affected arm and place it on the head. This will relieve the symptoms—*shoulder abduction relief test.*

---

[1] Roy Spurling 1894–1968, an American neurosurgeon, worked for Harvey Cushing as an intern.

Examining the spinous processes

FIGURE 24.27

Neurological examination of the upper limbs, including testing of shoulder abduction (C5, C6) and the serratus anterior muscle (C5, C6, C7), is part of the assessment of the neck.

Thoracolumbar spine and sacroiliac joints

History

Lower back pain is a very common symptom (see List 24.6). The discomfort is usually worst in the lumbosacral area. Ask whether the onset was sudden and associated with lifting or straining or whether it was gradual.[6,7] Stiffness and pain in the lower back that is worse in the morning is characteristic of an inflammatory spondyloarthritis. Pain that shoots from the buttock and thigh along the sciatic nerve distribution is called *sciatica*. In sciatic nerve compression at a lumbosacral nerve root, the pain is often aggravated by coughing or straining or when the patient leans forwards slightly, for example to brush the teeth. The back pain that patients may call 'lumbago' is often due to referred pain (e.g. from the vertebral joints). There may be other *neurological symptoms* in the legs due to nerve compression or irritation. The distribution of the paraesthesias or weakness may indicate the level of spinal cord or nerve root abnormality. Ask about urinary incontinence and retention as well as numbness in the 'saddle region', erectile dysfunction and bowel incontinence, which can be a result of cauda equina involvement.

Examination

To start the examination, have the patient standing and clothed only in underpants. Look for deformity, inspecting from both the back and the side. Note especially loss of the normal thoracic kyphosis and lumbar lordosis, which is typical of ankylosing spondylitis. Also note any evidence of scoliosis, a lateral curvature of the spine that may be simple ('C' shaped) or compound ('S' shaped) and that can result from trauma, developmental abnormalities, vertebral body disease (e.g. rickets, tuberculosis) or muscle abnormality (e.g. polio).

Feel each vertebral body for tenderness and palpate for muscle spasm.[6]

Movement is assessed actively. Bending movements largely take place at the lumbar spine, whereas rotational movements occur at the thoracic spine. Range of movement is tested by observation (see Fig. 24.28) and the use of Schober's test (see below and Fig. 24.29).

Flexion is tested by asking the patient to touch the toes with the knees straight. The normal range of flexion is very wide. Many people can reach only halfway down the shins when the knees are kept straight. As the patient bends, look at the spine: there is normally a gentle curve along the back from the shoulders to the pelvis. Patients with advanced ankylosing spondylitis have a flat ankylosed spine and all the bending occurs at the hips. Test *extension* by asking the patient to lean backwards. Patients with back pain usually find this less uncomfortable than bending forwards. *Lateral bending* is assessed by getting the patient to slide the right hand down the right leg as far as possible without bending forwards, and then the same for the left side. This movement tends to be restricted early in ankylosing spondylitis. *Rotation* is tested with the patient sitting on a stool (to fix the pelvis) and asking him or her to rotate the head and shoulders as far as possible to each side. This is best viewed from above. It can also be tested while the patient is lying (see Fig. 24.28d).

Measure the lumbar flexion with *Schober's test* (see Fig. 24.29). Make a mark at the level of the posterior iliac spine on the vertebral column (approximately at L5). Place one finger 5 centimetres below and another

> **DIFFERENTIAL DIAGNOSES FOR BACK PAIN**
>
> Remember that serious causes of back pain are rare in otherwise well patients (<1%).
>
> **!** denotes symptoms for the possible diagnosis of an urgent or dangerous problem.
>
> **Suggests non-specific or musculoskeletal cause**
> (Although often said to be due to disc herniation, there is little correlation between MRI-scan-detected disc herniation and pain—it is found in 30% of asymptomatic people)
> Gradual onset
> No neurological symptoms or signs
> Recent minor injury
>
> **Suggests ankylosing spondylitis**
> Systemic symptoms
> Pain at rest
>
> **! Suggests malignant pain**
> Worse at rest, keeps patient awake
> Present for more than 4 weeks
> Weight loss
> Known malignancy
>
> **! Suggests abscess**
> Worse at rest
> Fever
> Immunosuppression
>
> **! Suggests cauda equina syndrome**
> (Compression of sacral nerve roots, usually due to large midline herniation of a disc, but can be caused by infection or malignancy that causes narrowing of the spinal canal)
> Severe pain
> Urinary retention or incontinence
> Faecal incontinence
> Saddle anaesthesia
> Leg weakness
>
> **Suggests fracture of vertebral body**
> Sudden onset of severe pain
> Known osteoporosis
> Steroid use
> Trauma
> Tenderness over vertebral body
>
> **Suggests sciatica**
> (Irritation or compression of L4–S1 nerve roots)
> Pain radiates down leg beyond knee
> Suggests spinal canal stenosis
> Pain worse with walking
> Improved by bending
>
> **Suggests referred pain**
> Abdominal pain (diverticular abscess, pyelonephritis)
> Nausea and vomiting, dysuria (pyelonephritis)
> **!** Sudden-onset tearing pain, hypotension, shock (ruptured abdominal aortic aneurysm)
>
> LIST 24.6

10 centimetres above this mark. Then ask the patient to touch the toes. An increase of less than 5 centimetres in the distance between the two fingers indicates limitation of lumbar flexion. The finger-to-floor distance at full flexion can be measured serially to give an objective indication of disease progression.

Assess *straight leg raising* (Lasègue's[m] test includes passive ankle dorsiflexion). With the patient lying down, lift the straightened leg if sciatica is suspected (normally to 80–90°). Ask the patient to tell you as soon as there is pain and where it occurs. A disc compression of the lumbar or sacral roots will limit leg raising, because of pain in the ipsilateral leg that will be increased by foot dorsiflexion (less than 60°—sensitivity 91%).[8]

Press directly on the anterior superior iliac spine on each side and apply lateral pressure so as to attempt to separate them. This may elicit pain in the sacroiliac joints when patients have sacroiliitis.

Now get the patient to lie in bed on the stomach. Look for gluteal wasting. The sacroiliac joints lie deep

---

[m] Charles E Lasègue (1816–83), a professor of medicine in Paris and pupil of Trousseau.

Movements of the thoracolumbar spine.

(a) Flexion; (b) extension; (c) lateral bending; (d) rotation

FIGURE 24.28

(a–c) Schober's test

(From Douglas G, Nicol F and Robertson C. *Macleod's clinical examination*, 12th edn. Edinburgh: Churchill Livingstone, 2009.)

FIGURE 24.29

to the dimples of Venus.[n] By tradition, firm palpation with both palms overlying each other is used to elicit tenderness in patients with sacroiliitis. Test each side separately.

Now ask the patient to lie on one side. Apply firm pressure to the upper pelvic rim. This will also elicit pain in the sacroiliac joints.

The complete examination of the back also requires neurological assessment of the lower limbs.[9]

Hips
Examination anatomy

The hip is a ball-and-socket synovial joint (see Fig. 24.30). The socket is formed by three bones: the ilium, the ischium and the pubis. The ball is the head of the femur. Surrounding tendons and nerves may cause symptoms that need to be distinguished from hip abnormalities.

History

The word 'hip' is used variably by patients to indicate a number of sites including the buttocks, low back or trochanteric region. Ask the patient to point to the site of pain (see List 24.7). The patient with true hip joint problems will often have pain that is felt anteriorly in the groin or may radiate to the knee. Athletes with 'groin strain' often have adductor tendinitis or osteitis pubis caused by trauma or overuse. Pain over the greater trochanter is more often a result of trochanteric bursitis, gluteus medius tendinitis or tear. It is exacerbated by crossing the legs. Find out what sport the patient plays. The condition is common in sports involving running. Typically the pain is present at the start of exercise and improves as the athlete 'warms up', only to recur later at rest. Take a detailed work history. Overuse syndromes related to work may be worst on Fridays and improve over the weekend. Jumping down off of trucks or platforms may cause repeated trauma to the joint.

A *limp* may be noticed by the patient. When associated with pain it is a compensating mechanism,

---
[n] Roman goddess of love—her ancient Greek equivalent was Aphrodite.

A history of a fall and inability to walk or bear weight on the leg suggests a fracture of the neck of the femur. A history of rheumatoid arthritis and pain that is present at rest suggests rheumatoid arthritis of the hip. Osteoarthritis is more likely to evolve gradually in older people and is associated with obesity and with recurrent trauma.

Ask about systemic symptoms such as fever and weight loss, which might be a sign of septic arthritis.

Pain that is associated with paraesthesias and radiates in the distribution of the lateral cutaneous nerve of the thigh suggests an entrapment syndrome (meralgia paraesthetica).

Examination

Watch the patient walking into the room and note the use of a walking stick, a slow and obviously uncomfortable gait or a limp.

Get the patient to lie down, first on the back.

Looking at the hip joint itself is not possible because so much muscle overlies it. However, you must inspect for scars and deformity. The patient may adopt a position with one leg rotated because of pain.

Feel just distal to the midpoint of the inguinal ligament for joint tenderness. This point lies over the only part of the femoral head that is not intra-acetabular. Now feel for the positions of the greater trochanters. Place your thumbs on the anterior superior iliac spine on each side while moving your fore and middle fingers posteriorly to find the tips of the greater trochanters. These should be at the same level. If one side is higher than the other, the higher side is likely to be the abnormal one.

Move the hip joint passively (see Fig. 24.31). *Flexion* is tested by flexing the patient's knee and moving the thigh towards the chest. Keep the pelvis on the bed by holding the other leg down. A fixed flexion deformity (inability to extend a joint normally) may be masked by the patient's arching the back and tilting the pelvis forwards and increasing lumbar lordosis unless *Thomas's*° test is applied. The legs are fully flexed to straighten the pelvis. One leg is then extended. A fixed flexion deformity (e.g. as result of osteoarthritis) will prevent straightening. *Rotation* is tested with the knee and hip flexed. One hand holds

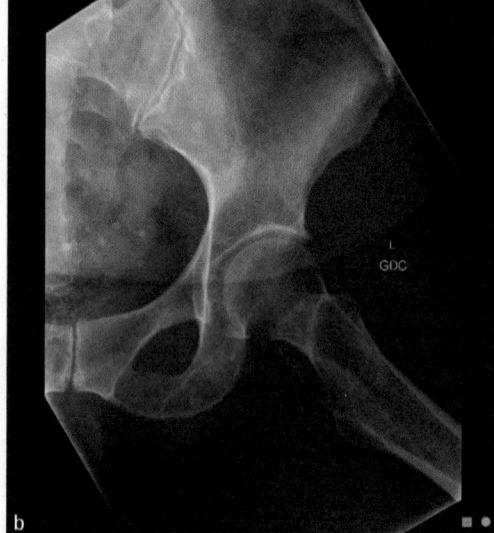

X-rays of: (a) pelvis and hip joints; (b) hip in abduction

(Courtesy of M Thomson, National Capital Diagnostic Imaging, Canberra.)

FIGURE 24.30

but when painless it may be due to differing limb length or instability of the joint. Patients are sometimes aware of *clicking* or *snapping* coming from the region of the hip. This may be due to a psoas bursitis or to slipping of the tendon of the gluteus maximus over the edge of the greater trochanter. *Functional impairment* usually results in difficulty walking and climbing stairs. Sitting down and standing up can become progressively more uncomfortable because of stiffness and pain.

° Hugh Thomas (1834–91), 'the father of orthopaedic surgery', worked in Liverpool as a bone-setter but did not have a hospital appointment.

DIFFERENTIAL DIAGNOSIS OF HIP AND THIGH PAIN

Favours fractured neck of femur
Known osteoporosis
History of a fall
Severe sudden pain
Inability to bear weight

Favours osteoarthritis
Advanced age
Obesity
Gradual onset
Pain when walking
Work involves jumping off trucks or platforms

Favours rheumatoid arthritis
Pain at rest
Pain worse in the morning
Other typical joint involvement
Walking may be severely limited

Favours septic arthritis
Fever
Malaise

Favours aseptic necrosis of the femoral head
Sudden onset of pain
Inability to bear weight on leg
Steroid use
Known fracture
Diabetes mellitus
Sickle cell anaemia

Favours meralgia paraesthetica
(Lateral cutaneous nerve of the thigh entrapment)
Anterior thigh pain with paraesthesias
Occupation involves long periods of sitting
Use of a constricting lumbar support belt

Favours trochanteric bursitis
Pain involves lateral thigh
Worse when:
- climbing stairs
- bending forward
- lying on side

LIST 24.7

---

the knee, the other the foot. The foot is then moved medially (*external rotation of the hip*, normally possible to 45°), then laterally (*internal rotation of the hip*, normal to 45°). *Abduction* is tested by standing on the same side of the bed as the leg to be tested. The right hand grasps the heel of the right leg while the left hand is placed over the anterior superior iliac spine to steady the pelvis. The leg is then moved outwards as far as possible; this is normally possible to 50°. *Adduction* is the opposite: the leg is carried immediately in front of the other limb and this is normally possible to 45°.

The *FABER test* assesses **F**lexion, **AB**duction and External **R**otation of the hip. The patient, lying flat, abducts and externally rotates the hip so as to place the leg across the other thigh in a figure-4 position. Normal hip function will allow the leg to lie parallel to the bed. Pushing on the patient's knee puts pressure on the ipsilateral sacroiliac joint. Pain there suggests sacroiliac disease, and inability to place the leg parallel with the bed suggests hip disease.

Ask the patient to roll over onto the stomach. *Extension* is then tested by placing one hand over the sacroiliac joint while the other elevates each leg. This is normally possible to about 30°. Now ask the patient to stand and perform the Trendelenburg[p] test. The patient stands first on one leg and then on the other. Normally the non-weight-bearing hip rises, but with proximal myopathy or hip joint disease the non-weight-bearing side sags.

Finally, the true *leg length* (from the anterior superior iliac spine to the medial malleolus) and apparent leg length (from the umbilicus to the same lower point) for each leg should be measured. A difference in true leg length indicates hip disease on the shorter side, whereas apparent leg length differences are due to tilting of the pelvis.

In patients with osteoarthritis of the joint, internal rotation, abduction and extension are usually restricted.[10]

---

[p] Friedrich Trendelenburg (1844–1924), a professor of surgery at Rostock, Bonn and Leipzig.

Movements of the hip.

(a) Flexion; (b) extension; (c) flexion, knee bent; (d) internal rotation; (e) external rotation; (f) abduction

FIGURE 24.31

CHAPTER 24 THE RHEUMATOLOGICAL EXAMINATION

Knee anatomy

FIGURE 24.32

Differential diagnosis of knee pain	
Area of pain	**Associated features**
Lateral aspect of knee	
Tear of lateral meniscus	History of trauma Locking or clicking Swelling delayed after injury
Tear of lateral collateral ligament	Knee gives way
Biceps femoris strain	Overuse or injury
Medial aspect of knee	
Tear of medial meniscus	History of trauma Locking or clicking Swelling delayed after injury
Tear or strain of medial collateral ligament	Knee gives way
Hamstring strain	Overuse or injury
Patellofemoral syndrome	Overuse Chronic symptoms
Back of the knee	
Baker's cyst	Sudden pain
Bursitis (e.g. popliteal, semimembranosus)	Localised swelling and tenderness
Hamstring strain	Overuse pattern
Deep venous thrombosis	Chronic pain Injury or overuse
Front of the knee	
Patellar fracture	Injury Sudden pain and tenderness Swelling Separation of fractured segments, visible or palpable
Patellar tendinitis	Overuse
Osteoarthritis	Chronic pain Worse with walking History of old injuries
Prepatellar bursitis (housemaid's knee*)	Occupation
Infrapatellar bursitis (clergyman's knee)	Occupation

*Described by Henry Hamilton Bailey (1894–1961) as 'the most elementary diagnosis in surgery'.

TABLE 24.1

Osteoarthritic joints show loss of joint space, sclerosis (thickening and increased radiodensity) at the joint margins and osteophyte (bony outgrowth) formation on plain X-ray films.

Knees

Examination anatomy

The knee is a complex hinge joint formed by the distal femur, the patella and the proximal end of the tibia (see Fig. 24.32). The bones are enclosed in a joint capsule with an extensive synovial membrane. Lateral stability is provided by the lateral collateral ligaments, and anteroposterior movement is restricted by the cruciate ligaments. There is extensive articular cartilage that acts as a shock absorber and allows smooth gliding movements between the ends of the bones.

History

Pain is a common knee problem (see Table 24.1). If there has been an injury or if the pain is due to a mechanical abnormality, it is often localised. Inflammatory diseases more often cause diffuse pain. Ask the patient to point to the place where the pain is most severe. *Stiffness* is usually of gradual onset and is typical of osteoarthritis. It tends to be worse after inactivity. *Locking* of the knee usually means there is a sudden inability to reach full extension. The knee is often stuck at about 45° of flexion. Unlocking may occur just as suddenly, sometimes following some form of manipulation by the patient. The cause is mechanical: a loose body or torn meniscus has become wedged between the articular surfaces of the joint. *Swelling* that occurs suddenly after an injury is often due to a haemarthrosis from a fracture or ligamentous tear; if swelling occurs after a few hours, a torn meniscus is more likely to be the cause. Arthritis and synovitis cause a chronic swelling. Patients sometimes notice *deformity*, which in later life is usually due to arthritis. Sometimes the patient may complain that the knee is *unstable* or *gives way*. Patellar instability and ruptured ligaments may present this way. Always ask about *loss of function*. There is often a reduced ability to walk distances, climb stairs and get into and out of chairs.

Osteoarthritis of the knee is very common. Older age, previous injury and stiffness lasting less than half an hour are in favour of this diagnosis as the cause of knee pain. Physically active adolescents may present with pain and swelling below the knee at the point of attachment of the patellar tendon to the tibial tuberosity—tibial apophysitis or Osgood–Schlatter's[q] disease. This is the most common *traction apophysitis*.

Ask whether there has been previous knee surgery or arthroscopy.

Take an occupational and sporting history. Injury and overuse syndromes are often related to exercise (particularly competitive sport) and occupations associated with repetitive minor injuries to the knees.

Examination

This is performed with the patient in a number of positions and, of course, walking.[11,12] Even more than with the other joints, it is important to examine the more normal or uninjured knee first. This will help with the interpretation of changes in the other knee and give the patient more confidence that the examination will not be painful.

Look first with the patient lying down on the back with both knees and thighs fully exposed. The affected knee will often be flexed, the most comfortable position. Note any quadriceps wasting. This begins quite soon after knee abnormalities lead to disuse of the muscle. Examine the knees themselves for skin changes, scars (including those from previous surgery or arthroscopy), swelling and deformity. Compare one side with the other. Localised swellings may move about as the knee flexes and extends. They are often cartilaginous loose bodies. Fixed lumps in the line of the joint may be meniscal cysts.

Swelling of the synovium or a knee effusion is usually seen medial to the patella and in the joint's suprapatellar extension. Loss of the peripatellar grooves may be an early sign of an effusion. Assess fixed flexion deformity by squatting down and looking at each knee from the side. A space under the knee will be visible if there is permanent flexion deformity arthritis.

Varus and valgus deformity may be obvious here but are more easily seen when the patient stands. Varus deformity is often related to osteoarthritis and valgus deformity to rheumatoid arthritis.

Now watch as the patient flexes and straightens each knee in turn. As the knee extends the patella glides upwards and remains centred over the femoral condyles. If there is patellar subluxation it will slip laterally during knee flexion and return to the midline during knee extension.

Feel the quadriceps for wasting. Palpate over the knees for warmth and synovial swelling.

Test carefully for a joint effusion. The *patellar tap* is used to confirm the presence of large effusions (see Fig. 24.33a). Rest one hand over the lower part of the quadriceps muscle and compress the suprapatellar extension of the joint space. With your other hand push the patella downwards. The sign is positive if the patella is felt to sink and then comes to rest with a tap as it touches the underlying femur. The *bulge sign* is used to detect small effusions (see Fig. 24.33b). Use your left hand to compress the suprapatellar pouch while you run the fingers of your right hand along the groove beside the patella on one side and then on the other. A bulging along the groove due to a fluid wave,

---

[q] Robert Osgood (1873–1956) worked in France during World War I and then at the Massachusetts General Hospital where he founded the X-ray department and subsequently developed several radiation-induced skin tumours. Carl Schlatter (1864–1934), a professor of surgery in Zurich, pioneered a total gastrectomy operation in 1897.

Testing for patellar effusion.

(a) The patellar tap; (b) the bulge sign: compressing the suprapatellar pouch

FIGURE 24.33

Knee examination.

(a) Testing knee flexion—'Let me bend your knee'; (b) testing the collateral ligaments; (c) testing the cruciate ligaments

FIGURE 24.34

on the side not being compressed, is a sign of a small effusion.

Examine for patellofemoral lesions by sliding the patella sideways across the underlying femoral condyles.

Move the joint passively. Test *flexion* (normally possible to 135°) and *extension* (normal to 5°) by resting one hand on the knee cap while the other moves the leg up and down (see Fig. 24.34(a)). Note the range of movements and the presence of crepitus. While holding the knee flexed, feel for and attempt to localise tenderness. Feel gently for tenderness along the joint line at the patellar ligament and at the sites of attachment of the collateral ligaments.

Test the *ligaments* next (see Good signs guide 24.1).[13–15] The lateral and medial *collateral ligaments*

GOOD SIGNS GUIDE 24.1
Ligament and meniscal injuries

Finding[+]	Sensitivity (%)	Specificity (%)	LR+	LR−
DETECTING ANTERIOR CRUCIATE LIGAMENT TEAR*				
Anterior drawer sign[12]	78	100	37	0.2
Lachman's sign	89	100	42	0.1
DETECTING MENISCAL INJURY*[14]				
McMurray's sign	56	100	8.9	0.5
Joint line tenderness	76	43	1.3	0.6
Joint effusion	35	100	5.7	0.7

NA = not available.
[+]Definition of findings: see text.
*Diagnostic standard: for anterior cruciate tear, tear demonstrated by MRI imaging, arthroscopy or surgery; for meniscal tear, arthroscopy.
(Adapted from Simel DL, Rennie D. *The rational clinical examination: evidence-based diagnosis*. New York: McGraw-Hill, 2009, Table 27.6.)

Baker's cyst of the right knee, viewed from behind

FIGURE 24.35

are assessed by having the knee slightly flexed while holding the leg, with your forearm resting along the length of the tibia; lateral and medial movements of the leg on the knee joint are tested (see Fig. 24.34(b)). Meanwhile steady the thigh with your other hand. Movements of more than 5–10° are abnormal. The *cruciate ligaments* (Fig. 24.34(c)) are tested next. Steady the patient's foot with your elbow or by sitting on it. Flex the patient's knee to 90°. Grasp the tibia and attempt anterior and posterior movements of the leg on the knee joint. Movement may be detected by your thumbs positioned at the joint margins. Again, movement of more than 5–10° is abnormal. Increased anterior movement suggests anterior cruciate ligamentous laxity, and increased posterior movement suggests posterior cruciate ligamentous laxity. The Lachman test may be more accurate (LR+ 42.0; LR− 0.1).[11] Here the knee is flexed 20–30° while the patient is lying supine. Grasp the femur (place your hand above the knee) to steady it, then grab the lower leg below the knee and give it a quick forward tug. It is abnormal when there is exaggerated anterior tibial movement or the knee fails to stop with a thud.

When recurrent dislocation or subluxation of the patella is suspected, the *patellar apprehension test* should be performed. Push the patella firmly in a lateral direction while slowly flexing the knee. The patient's face should be studied for the anxious look that suggests impending dislocation (it is then time to suspend the test).

Ask the patient to roll into the prone position. Look and feel in the popliteal fossa for a Baker's[r] cyst. This is a pressure diverticulum of the synovial membrane that occurs through a hiatus in the knee capsule (see Fig. 24.35). It is best seen with the knee extended and if not obvious when the patient is lying down look again when he or she is standing and with the knee hyperextended. Rupture of this into the calf muscle produces signs that may mimic a deep venous thrombosis. Rupture is often associated with the 'crescent sign'—ecchymoses below the malleoli of the ankle. A Baker's cyst must be distinguished from an aneurysm of the popliteal artery, which will be pulsatile, and a bony tumour (very hard).

This is also the position in which Apley's *grinding test* may be performed (see Fig. 24.36). This is a test of meniscal damage. Flex the patient's leg to 90°, stabilise the thigh by kneeling lightly on it and, while pressing on the foot, rotate the leg backwards and forwards. Pain or clicking makes the test positive. The *distraction test* is the opposite. Here the patient's leg is pulled upwards so as to take the strain off the menisci and stretch

---

[r] William Baker (1839–96), a surgeon at St Bartholomew's Hospital, London, described this in 1877.

Apley's grinding test (push hard)

FIGURE 24.36

McMurray's test of the knee

FIGURE 24.37

the ligaments. If the patient finds the test painful, a ligamentous abnormality may be the cause.

McMurray's[s] test (see Fig. 24.37) is another way of detecting a meniscal tear. With the patient lying on the back, stand on the side to be tested and hold the patient's ankle. Place your other hand on the medial side of the knee and push to apply valgus force. Extend the patient's leg from the flexed position while internally and then externally rotating it. The test is positive if there is a popping sensation, which may be followed by inability to extend the knee.

---

[s] Thomas McMurray (1888–1949), the first professor of orthopaedic surgery in Liverpool.

Stand the patient up. Look particularly for varus (bow-leg) and valgus (knock-knee) deformity.

Finish with a test of function. Get the patient to walk to and fro. Study the gait and the movement of the knees; particularly look for a sideways wobble.

Ankles and feet
Examination anatomy

The ankle is a synovial hinge joint formed between the distal ends of the tibia and the fibula, and the talus bone (see Fig. 24.38). Protrusions from the ends of the tibia and the fibula, which are called malleoli, form a socket that in combination with lateral ligaments stabilises the joint. The proximal part of the foot is called the *tarsus* and contains the seven tarsal bones (talus, calcaneus [heel], navicular, cuboid and the three cuneiform bones) with their supporting ligaments and joint capsules. The joints and ligaments around these bones allow the movements of the foot: inversion and eversion, dorsi- (upward) and plantar (downward) flexion.

History

The usual symptom is pain. If this is present only when the patient wears shoes, the shoes rather than the feet may be the problem. There may be a specific area that is painful and the patient should be asked to point to this. There may be a history of injury or of intensive or unusual exercise. Ankle injuries are common in certain sports that involve twisting of the foot on the leg (e.g. netball, football; see List 24.8). Rupture of the Achilles tendon occurs in squash and tennis players over 50 years of age and following forced dorsiflexion of the foot. Heel pain (both plantar and retrocalcaneal) is often due to plantar fasciitis, Achilles tendinitis or retrocalcaneal bursitis.

Patients with foot pain (see List 24.9) or ankle pain may have a history of rheumatoid arthritis. This can cause pain and deformity and affect the ankle subtalar, midtarsal and metatarsophalangeal joints.

Very severe pain involving the first metatarsophalangeal joint is usually due to gout. Pain right over one of the metatarsals that comes on after unusually vigorous exercise may be due to a stress fracture.

There may be deformity involving the ankle or toes. Patients find this especially troublesome if it makes it difficult to put on shoes. The patient may have noticed

The ankles and feet.

(a) Anatomy of the ankle and foot; (b) X-ray of the ankle; (c) MRI scan of the left foot; (d) MRI scan of the ankle

(X-ray and MRI scans courtesy of M Thomson, National Capital Diagnostic Imaging, Canberra.)

FIGURE 24.38

swelling; ask whether this is painful or not and whether it involves one or both feet. Bilateral swelling is more likely to be due to inflammation. Swelling over the medial aspect of the first metatarsal head (a bunion; Fig. 24.39) occurs commonly as people get older, but may be associated with rheumatoid arthritis.

Paraesthesias in the feet may have been noticed. Try to find out the distribution of the abnormal sensation, which may be a result of peripheral nerve injury or peripheral neuropathy. Coldness of the feet is very common but cyanosis and ulceration are more worrying problems. Chronic foot ulcers mean that diabetes must be excluded.

Examination

This examination includes the ankles, feet and toes.

Look at the skin. Note any swelling, scars, deformity or muscle wasting. Deformities affecting the forefoot

DIFFERENTIAL DIAGNOSES OF ANKLE PAIN

Chronic or persistent pain suggests
Osteoarthritis (worse with walking)
Inflammatory arthritis (often painful at rest)

Pain behind the ankle suggests
Achilles tendinitis (tender lump behind foot, associated with rheumatoid arthritis)
Achilles tendon rupture (pain sudden and severe)

Pain over lateral aspect of ankle suggests
Lateral ligament injury—sprain (history of forced inversion of the ankle)
Lateral malleolus fracture (severe pain, history of trauma)

Pain over medial aspect of ankle suggests
Deltoid ligament injury—sprain (history of forced eversion of the ankle)
Posterior tibial tendinitis
Tarsal tunnel syndrome (posterior tibial nerve entrapment)
Fracture of medial malleolus (severe pain, history of trauma)

LIST 24.8

DIFFERENTIAL DIAGNOSES OF FOOT PAIN

Hindfoot or midfoot pain suggests
Osteoarthritis
Rheumatoid arthritis
Plantar fibromas
Plantar fasciitis (heel pain)
Calcaneal fracture

Forefoot pain suggests
Metatarsalgia
Metatarsal fracture
Interdigital neuroma (interdigital nerve entrapment neuropathy)
Gout (severe pain and swelling, usually of first metatarsophalangeal joint)
Toe problems (bunions, ingrown toenail, claw toes, hammer toes)

LIST 24.9

Bunion

FIGURE 24.39

Sausage-shaped first and second toes in psoriatic arthritis

FIGURE 24.40

include hallux valgus (fixed lateral deviation of the main axis of the big toe), clawing (fixed flexion deformity) and crowding of the toes, as occurs in rheumatoid arthritis. Sausage deformities of the toes occur with psoriatic arthropathy or Reiter's[†] disease (see Fig. 24.40).

Look for the nail changes that suggest psoriasis. Inspect the transverse arch of the foot, which runs underneath the metatarsophalangeal joints, and the longitudinal arch, which runs from the first

---

[†] Hans Reiter (1881–1969), a professor of hygiene in Berlin, described the syndrome in 1916. This was well before he became an enthusiastic Nazi.

Rheumatoid feet showing bilateral hallux valgus and calluses over the metatarsal heads

FIGURE 24.41

Rheumatoid nodule of the Achilles tendon

FIGURE 24.42

metatarsophalangeal joint to the heel. These arches, which bear the weight of the body, may be flattened in arthritic conditions of the foot such as rheumatoid arthritis. Calluses over the metatarsal heads on the plantar surface of the foot occur with subluxation of these joints (see Fig. 24.41).

Feel, starting with the ankle, for swelling around the lateral and medial malleoli. This should not be confused with pitting oedema. If an ankle fracture is suspected because of a history of injury, tenderness over the posterior medial malleolus is a useful sign.[16]

Move the *talar (ankle) joint*, grasping the midfoot with one hand. *Dorsiflexion* is tested by raising the foot towards the knee—normally possible to 20°—and *plantar flexion* by performing the opposite manoeuvre, which is normally possible to 50°.

With the subtalar joint, only *inversion* and *eversion* of the foot on the ankle are tested. Pain on movement is more important than range at this joint. The midtarsal (midfoot) joint allows rotation of the forefoot when the hindfoot is fixed. This is done by steadying the ankle with one hand and rotating (twisting) the forefoot. Again, pain on motion rather than loss of range of movement is noted.

Squeeze the *metatarsophalangeal joints* by compressing the first and fifth metatarsals between your thumb and forefinger. Tenderness suggests inflammation, which is common in early rheumatoid arthritis. Press upwards from the sole of the foot just proximal to the metatarsophalangeal joints of the third and fourth toes. Pain here suggests *Morton's*[u] neuroma. This is due to entrapment and swelling of the digital nerve between the toes. It is associated with pain and numbness of the sides of these toes.

Each *individual interphalangeal joint* is then assessed by feeling and moving. These are typically affected in the seronegative spondyloarthropathies. Extremely tender involvement of the first metatarsophalangeal joint is characteristic of acute gout. In this case the joint also looks red and swollen.

Palpate the *Achilles tendon* for rheumatoid nodules (see Fig. 24.42) and tenderness due to Achilles tendinitis. The achilles tendinitis of spondyloarthritis is diffuse swelling at the attachment on calcaneus (ethesitis). An old Achilles tendon rupture may be detected by squeezing the calf: normally, the foot plantar flexes unless the tendon has previously ruptured (Simmonds[v] test). Also palpate the inferior aspect of the *heel* for tenderness; this may indicate plantar fasciitis, which occurs in seronegative spondyloarthritis and sometimes for no apparent reason.

---

[u] Thomas Morton (1835–1903), a general and eye surgeon at Philadelphia Hospital, performed one of the first appendicectomies.
[v] Franklin Simmonds (1911–83), an orthopaedic surgeon at Rowley Bristow Hospital, Surrey, UK.

T&O'C ESSENTIALS

1. The examination of a patient with arthritis must always be limited by the patient's pain or discomfort. Always compare both sides.
2. Functional assessment is necessary in most joint examinations.
3. Wasting of adjacent muscle groups may be a clue to the presence of arthritis.
4. Look for abnormalities of other adjacent structures such as tendons and skin when examining an arthritic joint.
5. A septic arthritis is a medical emergency.
6. Remember to examine for the systemic manifestations of rheumatic conditions.

OSCE REVISION TOPICS – THE RHEUMATOLOGICAL EXAMINATION

Use these topics, which commonly occur in the OSCE, to help with revision.

1. Please examine this man's back. (p 392)
2. Please examine this woman's hands. (p 374)
3. This woman has noticed tight skin on her hands and chest. Please examine her. (pp 374, 416)
4. This woman has had pain in her left hip. Please examine her. (p 396)
5. This man has had pain with some movements of his shoulders. Please examine him. (p 385)
6. This man has had pain in his left knee. Please examine him. (p 400)
7. This woman has had difficulty walking because of pain in her feet. Please examine her. (p 404)

References

1. Fuchs HA. Joint counts and physical measures. *Rheum Dis Clin North Am* 1995; 21:429–444. Describes useful quantitative methods to evaluate tenderness, pain on motion, swelling, deformity and limitation of movement.
2. Katz JN, Larson ME, Sabra A et al. The carpal syndrome: diagnostic utility of the history and physical examination findings. *Ann Intern Med* 1990; 112:321–327. This study compares the neurophysiological assessment of the carpal tunnel syndrome with the information obtained by examination and history. No single symptom or sign is sufficiently predictive.
3. Glockner SM. Shoulder pain: a diagnostic dilemma. *Am Fam Phys* 1995; 51:1677–1687, 1690–1692. Reviews the utility of symptoms and signs in differential diagnosis.
4. Leech MT, Hall ST. Examination of the shoulder joint. *Med J Aust* 2016; 205(10):444–445.
5. Shabat S, Leitner Y, David R, Folman, Y. The correlation between spurling test and imaging studies in detecting cervical radiculopathy. *J Neuroimaging* 2012; 22(4):375–378.
6. Van den Hoogen HMM, Koes BW, Van Eijk JTM, Bouter LM. On the accuracy of history, physical, and the erythrocyte sedimentation rate in diagnosing low back pain in general practice: a criteria based review of the literature. *Spine* 1995; 20:318–327. Unfortunately, distinguishing mechanical from non-mechanical causes of low back pain such as ankylosing spondylitis is clinically difficult. However, tenderness to pressure over the anterior superior iliac spines and over the lower sacrum may, based on other studies, be somewhat helpful for the positive diagnosis of ankylosing spondylitis.
7. Deyo RA, Rainville J, Kent DL. What can the history and physical examination tell us about low back pain? *JAMA* 1992; 268:760–765.
8. Chou R, Qaseem A, Snow V et al. Diagnosis of low back pain. *Ann Intern Med* 2007; 147:478–491.
9. Katz JN, Dalgas M, Stucki G et al. Degenerative lumbar spinal stenosis. Diagnostic value of the history and physical examination. *Arth Rheum* 1995; 38:1236–1241. Describes symptoms (severe lower limb pain that is absent when the patient is seated) and signs (including a wide-based gait, positive Romberg's sign, thigh pain with lumbar extension) that help predict this rare condition in older patients.
10. Murtagh J. Diagnosis of early osteoarthritis of the hip joint: the four-step stress test. *Aust Fam Phys* 1990; 19:389. Discusses the diagnosis of osteoarthritis of the hip in a systematic way, suggesting a four-step approach.
11. Solomon DH, Simel DL, Bates DW et al. Does this patient have a torn meniscus or ligament of the knee? *JAMA* 2001; 286:1610–1620.
12. Scholten RJ, Opstetten W, van der Plas CG et al. Accuracy of physical diagnostic tests for assessing ruptures of the anterior cruciate ligament: a meta-analysis. *J Fam Pract* 2003; 52:689–694.
13. Lee JK, Yao L, Phelps CT et al. Anterior cruciate ligament tears: MR imaging compared with arthroscopy and clinical tests. *Radiology* 1988; 166(3):861–864.
14. Liu SH, Osti L, Henry M, Bocchi L. The diagnosis of acute complete tears of the anterior cruciate ligament. *J Bone and Joint Surg Br* 1995; 77(4):586–588.
15. Barry OCD, Smith H, McManus F, MacAuley P. Clinical assessment of suspected meniscal tears. *Ir J Med Sci* 1983; 152(4):149–151.
16. McGee S. *Evidence-based clinical diagnosis*, 3rd edn. Philadelphia: Saunders, 2012.

CHAPTER 25
Correlation of physical signs with rheumatological and musculoskeletal disease

The greater the ignorance the greater the dogmatism. SIR WILLIAM OSLER (1849–1919)

RHEUMATOID ARTHRITIS

Rheumatoid arthritis is a chronic systemic inflammatory disease of unknown aetiology that characteristically involves the joints (see Fig. 25.1). In the majority of cases, patients with rheumatoid arthritis have rheumatoid factor present in the serum (seropositive disease). These are heterogeneous antibodies directed against the Fc portion of immunoglobulin G (IgG), but are not specific for rheumatoid arthritis. Anti-cyclic citrullinated peptide (anti-CCP) antibodies occur in 70% of rheumatoid arthritis (mostly the rheumatoid-factor-positive group), and are associated with more aggressive disease and extra-articular manifestations (especially pulmonary and cardiovascular).

To examine the patient with suspected rheumatoid arthritis (see Text box 25.1 and Fig. 25.1), sit him or her up in bed or on a chair.

General inspection

Look to see whether the patient has a Cushingoid appearance due to steroid treatment (p 458), or whether there are signs of weight loss that may indicate active disease.

Hands

Put the patient's hands on a pillow. Look especially for symmetrical small joint synovitis (the distal interphalangeal joints are usually spared). The other abnormalities in advanced disease are ulnar deviation, volar subluxation of the metacarpophalangeal joints, Z deformity of the thumb with swan neck[a] and boutonnière deformity of the fingers (p 375). Examine the fingernails and periungual areas for splinter-like vasculitic changes and look for wasting of the small muscles of the hand. Look at the palms for palmar erythema. Feel the palms for palmar tendon crepitus while the patient extends and flexes the fingers. Look for signs of an ulnar nerve palsy (from ulnar nerve entrapment at the elbow) and a median nerve palsy (carpal tunnel).

Wrists

Look for synovial thickening and perform Phalen's sign (carpal tunnel).

Elbows

Look around the elbows for rheumatoid nodules, which suggest seropositive disease, and examine the elbow joint. Flexion contractures are common.

Shoulders and axillae

Examine for tenderness and limitation of movement. Also palpate the axillary nodes because enlarged nodes may indicate active disease of joints in the area that they drain.

Eyes

Look at the eyes for redness, which may indicate the dryness of Sjögren's syndrome (see List 23.6 on p 368), which occurs in 10%–15% of cases. Note also nodular scleritis—an elevated white or purple-red lesion, which is pathologically a rheumatoid nodule and usually appears surrounded by the intense redness of the injected sclera (see Fig. 25.2). These nodules occur especially in the superior parts of the sclera and

---

[a] The appearance resembles a swan dipping its head into the water.

Examining for rheumatoid arthritis

Rheumatoid arthritis

FIGURE 25.1

1. **General inspection**
   Cushingoid appearance
   Weight
2. **Hands**
3. **Arms**
   Entrapment neuropathy (e.g. carpal tunnel)
   Subcutaneous nodules
   Elbow joint
   Shoulder joint
   Axillary nodes
4. **Face**
   Eyes—dry eyes (Sjögren's), scleritis, episcleritis, scleromalacia perforans, anaemia, cataracts (steroids, chloroquine)
   Fundi—hyperviscosity
   Face—parotids (Sjögren's)
   Mouth—dryness, ulcers, dental caries
   Temporomandibular joint (crepitus)
5. **Neck**
   Cervical spine
   Cervical nodes
6. **Chest**
   Heart—pericarditis, valve lesions
   Lungs—effusion, fibrosis, infarction, infection, nodules (and Caplan's syndrome)
7. **Abdomen**
   Splenomegaly (e.g. Felty's syndrome)
   Inguinal nodes
8. **Hips**
9. **Knees**
10. **Lower limbs**
    Ulceration (vasculitis)
    Calf swelling (ruptured synovial cyst)
    Peripheral neuropathy
    Mononeuritis multiplex
    Cord compression
11. **Feet**
12. **Other**
    Urine: protein, blood (drugs, vasculitis, amyloidosis)
    Rectal examination (blood)

TEXT BOX 25.1

are often bilateral, but affect only 1% of patients. Iritis does *not* occur.

With severe scleritis, scleral thinning may occur, exposing the underlying choroid. This is called *scleromalacia*. Look for cataracts due to steroid treatment. Conjunctival pallor may be present, indicating anaemia due to iron deficiency. This can be a result of blood loss from non-steroidal anti-inflammatory drug use, folate deficiency from a poor diet, hypersplenism or chronic inflammation, or some combination of these.

Parotids

Look for enlargement of the parotid glands, as occurs with Sjögren's syndrome.

Mouth

Look for dryness of the mouth and dental caries (Sjögren's syndrome), and ulcers related to drug treatment (e.g. methotrexate).

Nodular scleritis involving the sclera lateral to the iris

FIGURE 25.2

Temporomandibular joints

Feel the temporomandibular joints for crepitus as the patient opens and shuts the mouth.

Neck

Go on to examine the cervical spine for tenderness, muscle spasm and reduction of rotational movement. Examine for cervical lymphadenopathy.

Chest

Now examine the lungs for signs of pleural effusions or pulmonary fibrosis. Caplan's[b] syndrome is the presence of rheumatoid lung nodules in combination with pneumoconiosis.

Heart

Listen to the heart for a pericardial rub (relatively common) and for murmurs indicating valvular regurgitation (especially the aortic valve), which may occur owing to nodular involvement of a heart valve.

Abdomen

Feel the abdomen for splenomegaly (this occurs in up to 10% of patients and suggests the possibility of Felty's syndrome) and hepatomegaly. Feel the inguinal lymph nodes.

---

[b] Anthony Caplan, a Welsh physician, described this in 1953.

Lower limbs

Examine the hips for limitation of joint movement. The knees, however, are more often affected and here one must note any quadriceps wasting (an important sign of knee arthritis), synovial effusions and flexion contractures. Valgus deformity (a result of lateral arthritic changes—osteoarthritis causes varus deformity) and ligamentous instability may occur as late complications. Look in the popliteal fossae for Baker's cysts. Go on to look at the lower parts of the legs for ulceration; this can occur as a vasculitic complication of Felty's syndrome. Examine for a stocking distribution peripheral neuropathy and for mononeuritis multiplex of the nerves of the lower limbs. There may also be signs of spinal cord compression due to anterior dislocation of the first cervical vertebra or vertical subluxation of the odontoid process.

Ankles and feet

Now look for foot drop (peroneal nerve entrapment or vasculitis) and examine the ankle joint for limitation of movement. Look at the metatarsophalangeal joints for swelling and subluxation. There may also be lateral deviation and clawing of the toes. Remember that the interphalangeal joints are very rarely involved. Finally, feel the Achilles tendon for nodules—a sign of seropositive disease.

An assessment of the activity of the disease is an important way of assessing the adequacy of treatment and is used routinely by rheumatologists. This includes criteria such as the duration of morning stiffness, joint pain, fatigue, joint tenderness, soft-tissue swelling and the presence of extra-articular manifestations. These criteria can be found on the websites of the various rheumatological societies but the core set of parameters includes:

- tender joint count (the number of tender joints)
- swollen joint count
- patient global score
- erythrocyte sedimentation rate (ESR)
- C-reactive protein (CRP).

SERONEGATIVE SPONDYLOARTHRITIDES

Four conditions are generally accepted as belonging to this group: ankylosing spondylitis, Reiter's

CHAPTER 25 CORRELATION OF PHYSICAL SIGNS WITH RHEUMATOLOGICAL AND MUSCULOSKELETAL DISEASE

disease (reactive arthritis), psoriatic arthritis and enteropathic arthritis. These are called the seronegative spondyloarthritides because they were originally distinguished from rheumatoid arthritis by the absence of anti-CCP antibody in the serum. However, up to 30% of patients with otherwise classical rheumatoid arthritis are anti-CCP antibody negative. The seronegative spondyloarthropathies overlap clinically and pathologically, and have an association with HLA-B27.

Ankylosing spondylitis

The following areas should be examined:

- **Back and sacroiliac joints:** may show loss of lumbar lordosis and thoracic kyphosis, severe flexion deformity of the lumbar spine (rare), tenderness of the lumbar vertebrae, reduction of movement of the lumbar spine in all directions, and tenderness of the sacroiliac joints. Measure the occiput to wall distance: serial measurements that show an increasing distance indicate worsening deformity. Perform Schober's test and test for lateral movement of the spine by asking the patient to run a hand straight down the side of each leg in turn. This movement is often severely restricted.
- **Legs:** Achilles tendinitis, plantar fasciitis, and signs of cauda equina compression (rare)—lower limb weakness, loss of sphincter control, saddle sensory loss.
- **Lungs:** decreased chest expansion (less than 5 centimetres); signs of apical fibrosis.
- **Heart:** signs of aortic regurgitation.
- **Eyes:** acute iritis (tends to recur)—painful red eye (10%–15%) (see Fig. 25.3).
- **Rectal and stool examination:** signs of inflammatory bowel disease (either ulcerative colitis or Crohn's disease). *Note:* signs of secondary amyloidosis—e.g. hepatosplenomegaly, renal enlargement, proteinuria—may be present, although this is a very rare complication.

Reactive arthritis[c]

Classically this disease follows urethritis or diarrhoea, with conjunctivitis and arthritis (usually asymmetrical)

Iritis of the right eye

FIGURE 25.3

Circinate balanitis

FIGURE 25.4

of the large weight-bearing joints such as the hip, knee or ankle. The following areas should be examined:

- **Genital region:** urethral discharge; circinate balanitis—scaly, superficial reddened erosions with well-demarcated borders on the glans penis (see Fig. 25.4).
- **Prostate:** prostatitis.
- **Eyes:** conjunctivitis; iritis (rare).
- **Mouth:** painless smooth mucosal lesions, especially of the tongue.
- **Back:** sacroiliac joints (may be unilaterally involved).
- **Lower limbs** (more commonly affected): knees, ankles; metatarsophalangeal joints and toes

---

[c] Reiter's syndrome was recognised by Hans Conrad Reiter (1881–1969), who was convicted for war crimes at Buchenwald.

('sausage toes'); plantar fasciitis, Achilles tendinitis; keratoderma blennorrhagica on the sole (non-tender reddish-brown macules, which become scaling papules)—this is indistinguishable from pustular psoriasis; nails thickened, opaque and brittle.
- **Hands** (less commonly involved): wrists; metacarpophalangeal joints, proximal interphalangeal joints, distal interphalangeal joints; keratoderma blennorrhagica on the palms; nail changes.
- **Cardiovascular system:** aortic regurgitation (rare).

Psoriatic arthritis

Some 10% of patients with psoriasis have arthritis.

Examine as for rheumatoid arthritis, but include the spine and sacroiliac joints. There are five distinct groups of psoriatic arthritis, but overlap is common:
- Monoarticular and asymmetrical oligoarticular arthritis of the hands and feet and other joints (note sausage-shaped digits in Fig. 24.40—see p 405). Most psoriatic arthritis is of this type.
- Symmetrical polyarthritis, similar to rheumatoid arthritis (but seronegative).
- Distal interphalangeal joint involvement with psoriatic nail changes (see Fig. 24.6 on p 378).
- Arthritis mutilans (destructive polyarthritis).
- Sacroiliitis with or without peripheral joint involvement.

Enteropathic arthritis

There are two patterns of involvement of the joints with ulcerative colitis and Crohn's disease:
- *Peripheral joint disease.* This is an asymmetrical oligoarthritis, usually affecting the lower limbs, especially the knees and ankles. It rarely causes deformity.
- *Sacroiliitis.* This is indistinguishable clinically from ankylosing spondylitis.

GOUTY ARTHRITIS

Begin with the feet, as acute gouty arthritis affects the metatarsophalangeal joint of the great toe in 75% of cases (see Fig. 25.5). Next examine the ankles and knees,

Acute gout of first metatarsophalangeal joint

(Hochberg MC. *Rheumatology*, 5th edn. Philadelphia: Elsevier, 2010.)

FIGURE 25.5

Gouty tophi of the fingers

FIGURE 25.6

which tend to be involved after recurrent attacks. The fingers, wrists and elbows are affected late (see Fig. 25.6). Inspect and palpate for gouty tophi[d] (these are urate deposits with inflammatory cells surrounding them). The presence of tophi indicates chronic recurrent gout. They tend to occur over the joint synovia, the olecranon bursa (see Fig. 25.7), the extensor surface of the forearm, the helix of the ear (see Fig. 25.8) and the infrapatellar and Achilles tendons.

---

[d] From the Latin *tophus*, which means 'chalk stone'.

CHAPTER 25 CORRELATION OF PHYSICAL SIGNS WITH RHEUMATOLOGICAL AND MUSCULOSKELETAL DISEASE

Large gouty tophus in the olecranon bursa

FIGURE 25.7

> **HINT BOX**
>
> 1. A common cause of gout in the hospital setting is chronic kidney disease.
> 2. In these patients, gout can look just like RA. There may be symmetrical destructive arthritis of the wrists, MCP joints and lumps on elbows. Aspiration of the joints for crystals and a negative anti-CCP test (p 429) helps make a diagnosis of gout. Remember that there is a negative association between gout and RA.

CALCIUM PYROPHOSPHATE ARTHRITIS (PSEUDOGOUT)

This may present a similar picture to that described above for true gout, but usually large joints (especially the knees) and wrists are involved. In a minority of patients there will be signs of hyperparathyroidism, haemochromatosis or true gout.

CALCIUM HYDROXYAPATITE ARTHRITIS

This causes large-joint arthritis (especially knee and shoulder) and is more common in elderly patients.

OSTEOARTHRITIS

Degenerative arthritis or osteoarthritis (OA) is the most common form of arthritis. It becomes increasingly common with old age. The condition affects synovial joints (see Fig. 24.2 on p 372) and is characterised by a loss of articular cartilage, new bone formation and changes to the shape of the joint. There are certain risk factors for osteoarthritis (see List 24.1 on p 370).

Patients typically give a history of pain and stiffness in the affected joint. If morning stiffness is reported it is usually brief (less than half an hour). Stiffness may improve with use of the joint. Pain is often intermittent but patients usually report a decline in function of the joint over time. Swelling, warmth and joint effusions can occur but are much less prominent than in inflammatory arthritides.

Gouty tophus of the ear

FIGURE 25.8

Finally, examine for signs of the causes of secondary gout: increased purine turnover due to myeloproliferative disease (p 355), lymphoma (p 357) or leukaemia; and decreased renal urate excretion due to renal disease or hypothyroidism. Hypertension, diabetes mellitus and ischaemic heart disease are more common among sufferers of gout.

Any synovial joint can be affected. Osteoarthritis can also occur secondary to a number of other joint and associated abnormalities:

- injury
- inflammatory arthritis (e.g. rheumatoid arthritis, gouty arthritis)
- avascular necrosis
- infective arthritis
- osteopetrosis (congenital condition with increased bone mass)
- haemochromatosis (2nd and 3rd metacarpals)
- Ehlers–Danlos syndrome (genetic disorders of corrective tissue leading to skin hyperextensability and joint hypermobility).

SYSTEMIC LUPUS ERYTHEMATOSUS

Systemic lupus erythematosus (SLE) is a multisystemic chronic inflammatory disease of unknown origin, named because the erosive nature of the condition was likened to the damage caused by a hungry wolf.[e]

General inspection

Look for weight loss (due to chronic inflammation) or a Cushingoid appearance (steroid treatment; see Text box 25.2, Fig. 25.9). While taking the history note any abnormal mental state—psychosis may occur due to the lupus itself or to steroid therapy.

Hands

Note any vasculitic-appearing lesions around the nail bed, or telangiectasia and erythema of the skin of the nail base. A rash may occur—photosensitivity is common. The hand rash of lupus tends to occur over the phalanges, as opposed to that of dermatomyositis, which affects the knuckles.

Raynaud's phenomenon may occur if the weather is cold (see List 23.5 on p 367).

Examine for arthritis: synovitis of the proximal and metacarpophalangeal joints. The arthritis of SLE is not erosive, but if severe may lead to reducible deformities due to damage to supporting structures.

Forearms

Livedo reticularis may occur here (see Fig. 25.10); in Latin this describes skin discoloration in the form of a small net. This is formed by connected bluish-purple streaks without discrete borders. They occur usually on the limbs. Livedo can occur in vasculitis and in the antiphospholipid syndrome[f] or from atheroembolism.[1] Look also for purpura (due to vasculitis[2] or autoimmune thrombocytopenia). Examine for a proximal myopathy (due to the disease itself or to steroid treatment). Subcutaneous nodules very rarely occur in SLE. The axillary nodes may be enlarged but will not be tender. (See also Ch 43, p 802.)

Head and neck

Alopecia (hair loss) is an important diagnostic clue that occurs in about two-thirds of patients and may be associated with scarring. Look especially for lupus hairs, which are short, broken hairs above the forehead. There may be alopecia areata: circular lesions the size of a 20 cent coin with hair loss. Hair typically grows back. The hair as a whole may be coarse and dry, as in hypothyroidism.

Examine the eyes for scleritis and episcleritis (more common as a manifestation of rheumatoid arthritis than SLE). The eyes may be red and dry (Sjögren's syndrome). Pallor of the conjunctivae occurs with anaemia, usually due to chronic disease. Occasionally, jaundice due to autoimmune haemolytic anaemia may be found. Perform a fundoscopy for cytoid bodies, which are hard exudates (white spots) due to aggregates of swollen nerve fibres and are secondary to vasculitis.

A facial rash may be diagnostic (see Fig. 25.11). The classical rash is an erythematous 'butterfly rash' over the cheeks and bridge of the nose and must be distinguished from rosacea. Mouth ulcers on the soft or hard palate may occur and the mouth may be dry (Sjögren's syndrome).

The *rash of discoid lupus* may be found in the same area or affect different parts of the body. Lesions begin as spreading red plaques that have a central area of hyperkeratosis and follicular plugging. An active lesion has an oedematous edge. The appearance

---

[e] From the Latin *lupus*, which means 'wolf'. Lupus has been used as a name for any erosive disease of the skin; for example, lupus vulgaris is tuberculosis of the skin.

[f] Antiphospholipid syndrome refers to venous or arterial thrombosis or spontaneous miscarriages in the presence of antiphospholipid antibodies (lupus anticoagulant, anticardiolipin) on testing; half have SLE.

CHAPTER 25 CORRELATION OF PHYSICAL SIGNS WITH RHEUMATOLOGICAL AND MUSCULOSKELETAL DISEASE   415

Examining for SLE

Systemic lupus erythematosus

FIGURE 25.9

1. **General inspection**
   Cushingoid appearance
   Weight
   Mental state
2. **Hands**
   Vasculitis
   Rash
   Arthropathy
3. **Arms**
   Livedo reticularis
   Purpura
   Proximal myopathy (active disease or steroids)
4. **Head**
   Alopecia, with or without scarring, lupus hairs
   Eyes—scleritis, cytoid lesions, etc.
   Mouth—ulcers, infection
   Rash—butterfly
   Cranial nerve lesions
   Cervical adenopathy
5. **Chest**
   Cardiovascular system—pericarditis
   Respiratory system—pleural effusion, pleurisy, pulmonary fibrosis, collapse or infection
6. **Abdomen**
   Hepatosplenomegaly
   Tenderness
7. **Hips**
   Aseptic necrosis
8. **Legs**
   Feet—red soles, small-joint synovitis
   Rash
   Ulcers over the malleoli (e.g. antiphospholipid syndrome)
   Proximal myopathy
   Neuropathy
   Mononeuritis multiplex
   Cerebellar ataxia
   Hemiplegia
9. **Other**
   Urine analysis (proteinuria)
   Blood pressure (hypertension)
   Temperature chart

TEXT BOX 25.2

may suggest psoriasis. A healed lesion may have marginal hyperpigmentation with central atrophy and depigmentation. The scalp, external ear and face are most commonly affected, but in some patients lesions may occur all over the arms and chest. Extensive annular or psoriaform lesions may indicate the presence of subacute cutaneous lupus.

After examining the face, feel for cervical lymphadenopathy, which is usually non-tender.

Chest

Signs of a pericardial rub (from pericarditis) may be found. In the respiratory examination a pleural rub (pleuritis) or signs suggesting the presence of a pleural effusion, pulmonary fibrosis, pulmonary collapse or pulmonary hypertension may be detected. Chest disease is probably most often secondary to an interstitial pneumonitis rather than to vasculitis of the lungs.

Abdomen

Splenomegaly, usually mild, can be detected in 10% of cases. Hepatomegaly (mild) may occur in uncomplicated cases. Chronic liver disease due to chronic hepatitis ('lupoid hepatitis') is a separate autoimmune disease rather than a variant of SLE.

Livedo reticularis

(Paller A, Mancini AJ. *Hurwitz clinical pediatric dermatology*, 4th edn. Philadelphia: Saunders, 2011.)

FIGURE 25.10

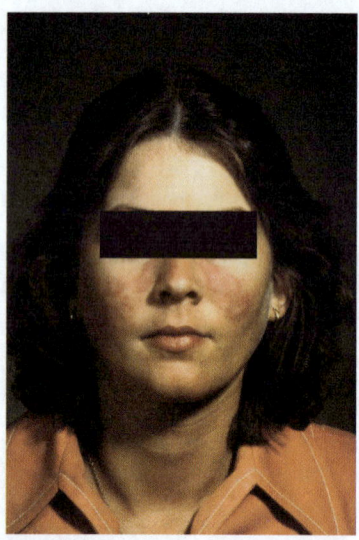

Butterfly rash of systemic lupus erythematosus

FIGURE 25.11

Hips

Examine the hip joint movements: in aseptic (avascular) necrosis there is pain on movement, with preservation of hip extension but loss of the other movements. This is due to ischaemia of the femoral head and may be related to steroid use or to the SLE itself.

Legs

Examine for proximal myopathy and peripheral neuropathy (mainly sensory).

Rarely there may be signs of hemiplegia, cerebellar ataxia or chorea.

Leg ulceration over the malleoli, due to vasculitis or the antiphospholipid syndrome,[1] is important. Very occasionally the toes may be gangrenous. There may be ankle oedema from the nephrotic syndrome or fluid retention from steroids. Livedo reticularis may be present on the legs.

Urine and blood pressure

Perform a urine analysis (for proteinuria and haematuria) and take the blood pressure (for hypertension). Renal disease is a common complication of SLE.

Temperature

Take the temperature, as fever is common in SLE, either from secondary infection or from the disease per se.

SYSTEMIC SCLEROSIS (SCLERODERMA AND CREST)

This is a disorder of connective tissue with variable cutaneous fibrosis and with abnormalities of the microvasculature of the fingers, gut, lungs, heart and kidneys. In diffuse systemic sclerosis there is more prominent skin sclerosis and these patients may have pulmonary fibrosis. In limited systemic sclerosis (**CREST** syndrome: Calcinosis, Raynaud's phenomenon, oEsophageal motility disturbance, Sclerodactyly and Telangiectasia), diffuse skin sclerosis and severe interstitial lung disease do not occur but patients are at risk of developing pulmonary hypertension.

General inspection

Look for cachexia due to dysphagia (from an oesophageal motility disturbance) or malabsorption (due to bacterial overgrowth; see Text box 25.3).

Skin changes in systemic sclerosis vary. There may be an early oedematous phase with non-tender pitting oedema of the hands, which appear tightly swollen. In patients with progressive disease the oedematous skin is replaced by indurated skin that appears thickened, hard and tight. This phase usually begins in the fingers (see List 25.1).

CHAPTER 25 CORRELATION OF PHYSICAL SIGNS WITH RHEUMATOLOGICAL AND MUSCULOSKELETAL DISEASE

Examining for systemic sclerosis (scleroderma)

Scleroderma

FIGURE 25.12

1. **General appearance** (Fig. 25.12)
   'Bird-like' facies
   Weight loss (malabsorption)
2. **Hands**
   CREST—calcinosis, atrophy distal tissue pulp (Raynaud's), sclerodactyly, telangiectasia, loss of finger pulp, necrosis
   Dilated capillary loops (nail folds)
   Tendon friction rubs
   Small-joint arthritis and tendon crepitus
   Fixed flexion deformity
   Hand function impaired
3. **Arms**
   Oedema (early), or skin thickening and tightening
   Pigmentation
   Vitiligo
   Hair loss
   Proximal myopathy
4. **Head**
   Alopecia
   Eyes—loss of eyebrows, anaemia, difficulty with closing
   Mouth—puckered ('purse string mouth'), reduced opening
   Pigmentation
   Telangiectasia
   Neck muscles—wasting and weakness
5. **Dysphagia**
6. **Chest**
   Tight skin ('Roman breastplate')
   Heart—signs of pulmonary hypertension, pericarditis, failure
   Lungs—fibrosis, reflux pneumonitis, chest infections
7. **Legs**
   Skin lesions
   Vasculitis
8. **Other**
   Blood pressure (hypertension with renal involvement)
   Urine analysis (proteinuria)
   Temperature chart (infection)
   Stool examination (steatorrhoea)

TEXT BOX 25.3

DIFFERENTIAL DIAGNOSIS OF THICKENED TETHERED SKIN

Systemic sclerosis (scleroderma), diffuse type; milder changes in limited cutaneous scleroderma

Mixed connective tissue disease (a distinct disorder with features of scleroderma, systemic lupus erythematosus, rheumatoid arthritis and myositis)

Eosinophilic fasciitis—widespread skin thickening due to inflammation of the fascia often following excessive muscle exercise; occurs in association with eosinophilia and hypergammaglobulinaemia

Localised morphea—heterogeneous group of disorders where there are small areas of sclerosis: most common type is morphea, which begins with large plaques of red or purple skin that are often painful and evolve into sclerotic areas that may regress spontaneously over years

Chemically induced: vinyl chloride, pentazocine, bleomycin

Pseudoscleroderma: porphyria cutanea tarda, acromegaly, carcinoid syndrome

Scleredema: thickened skin over the shoulders and upper back in diabetes mellitus

Graft versus host disease

Silicosis

Eosinophilic myalgia syndrome (L-tryptophan)

Toxic oil syndrome

LIST 25.1

Digital infarcts

FIGURE 25.13

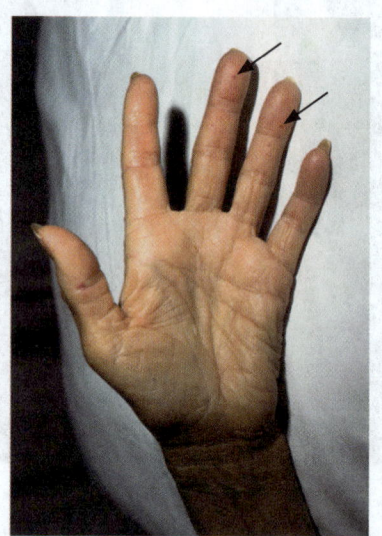

Telangiectasia of the hands in the CREST syndrome (arrows)

FIGURE 25.14

A summary of the physical signs that can be found in scleroderma is presented in Text box 25.3.

Hands

Examine the hands. Note particularly *calcinosis* (palpable nodules due to calcific deposits in the subcutaneous tissue of the fingers), *Raynaud's phenomenon* sometimes causing atrophy of the finger pulps (due to ischaemia; see Fig. 25.13), *sclerodactyly* (tightening of the skin of the fingers leading to tapering) and multiple large *telangiectasia* on the fingers (see Fig. 25.14).

Look for *contraction deformity of the fingers*, which is relatively common (see Fig. 25.15), and for synovitis, although this is uncommon. The nails can be affected by Raynaud's phenomenon. It can be useful to inspect the nail folds using a hand-held magnifying glass: in scleroderma you may see dilated capillary loops but this is not diagnostic. These are best viewed on the fourth digit. Tendon friction rubs may be present in patients with diffuse disease and suggest an adverse prognosis. Assessing hand function is important in this disease.

Arms

Determine the extent of skin tethering in the arms. If the skin thickening extends above the wrists to the

(a) and (b) Systemic sclerosis: signs in the hands. Sclerodactyly, tethered smooth skin, calcinosis and ulceration, atrophy of finger pulps due to Raynaud's phenomenon and fixed flexion deformities of the fingers

FIGURE 25.15

arms, legs or trunk, the diagnosis is *diffuse scleroderma* rather than *CREST*. If the skin thickening extends only to the elbows and face, this is called *limited scleroderma*. Assess for proximal myopathy due to myositis.

Face

The skin of the face is involved in progressive disease. There is loss of normal wrinkles and skinfolds as well as loss of the eyebrows. The face appears pinched and expressionless ('bird-like' facies). Inspect for malar telangiectasia and look for salt-and-pepper pigmentation. Ask the patient to close the eyes—skin tethering may make this incomplete. The eyes may be dry (Sjögren's syndrome), although this is uncommon, and the conjunctivae pale. There are a number of reasons for anaemia, including:

- the presence of chronic disease
- bleeding from oesophagitis
- watermelon stomach
- microangiopathic haemolytic anaemia.

Ask the patient to open the mouth fully. It may appear puckered and narrow. Inability to open the mouth so that there is more than 3 centimetres of clearance between the incisors indicates abnormal restriction.

Chest

Inspect the skin of the chest wall, which may have acquired a tight, thickened appearance, like ancient Roman breastplate armour.

Examine the lungs for pulmonary fibrosis, evidence of reflux pneumonitis or (rarely) a pleural effusion or alveolar cell carcinoma.

Examine the heart for pulmonary hypertension and cor pulmonale secondary to pulmonary fibrosis, or for pericarditis. Left ventricular failure may also occur owing to myocardial involvement.

Legs

Look for signs of vasculitis, ulceration and skin involvement. Peripheral neuropathy is rare.

Urinalysis and blood pressure

These are very important because renal involvement is common in scleroderma and is often associated with severe hypertension. Renal disease is one of the most common causes of death in scleroderma.

The stool

Look for evidence of steatorrhoea (due to malabsorption from bacterial overgrowth).

MIXED CONNECTIVE TISSUE DISEASE (MCTD)

Mixed connective tissue disease is an overlap syndrome with features of systemic sclerosis, SLE and sometimes polymyositis. It is a rare condition and affects women nine times as often as men. More than half of affected patients present with oedema and synovitis involving the hands. About a third of patients develop myositis and half have problems with oesophageal motility and develop interstitial lung disease (ILD). There may be a history of skin abnormalities including:

- photosensitivity
- malar rash
- sclerodactyly
- calcinosis
- telangiectasiae
- Gottren's papules.

Pleurisy and pericarditis are common. Sicca syndrome occurs in about half of patients. Kidney disease (membranous nephritis) occurs in 25%. Pulmonary hypertension occurs in 20% and these patients develop fatigue and increasing dyspnoea.

Examination

Examine as for systemic sclerosis and SLE. Look for proximal muscle weakness and tenderness (polymyositis). Signs of pulmonary hypertension indicate a worse prognosis.

NB. 30% of these patients have an underlying solid organ malignancy.

RHEUMATIC FEVER

Rheumatic fever is an inflammatory disease that is a delayed sequel to infection with group A beta-haemolytic *Streptococcus*; it is uncommon in Western nations today. It is diagnosed depending on the presence of major and minor criteria, plus evidence of recent streptococcal infection.

- Major criteria (manifestations)[3]
  - Carditis (causing tachycardia, murmurs, cardiac failure, pericarditis)
  - Polyarthritis, (polyarthralgia or aseptic monoarthritis in high-risk groups)
  - Chorea (p 600)
  - Erythema marginatum (see below)
  - Subcutaneous nodules (painless mobile swellings).
- Minor criteria (manifestations)
  - Fever
  - Polyarthralgia or aseptic monoarthritis
  - Acute phase proteins (ESR >30 mm/h or CRP >30 mg/L)
  - Prolonged PR interval on the ECG.

1. Definite initial episode=2 major **or** 1 major and 2 minor criteria **and** evidence of group A streptococcal infection (GAS).
2. Definite recurrent episode=2 major **or** 1 major and 1 minor **or** 3 minor criteria **and** evidence of GAS infection.
3. Probable first or recurrent episode=presentation that is 1 major or 1 minor criterion short or no streptococcal serology.

A high-risk population is one where rheumatic fever incidence is >30/100,000 5–14-year-old children.

Examining the patient with suspected rheumatic fever

First examine the large joints of the limbs for effusions and synovitis. Two or more joints must be involved (classically there is a transient migratory polyarthritis). Feel for subcutaneous nodules over bony prominences. Look for a rash. Erythema marginatum is a slightly raised pink or red rash that blanches with pressure. The red rings have a clear centre and round margins, and occur on the trunk and proximal limbs; the rash is not found on the face. Look for choreiform movements. These are sinuous dance-like movements. Their onset is usually delayed until about 3 months after the throat infection.

Now examine the cardiovascular system for any signs of pancarditis: (1) a pericardial rub due to pericarditis; (2) congestive cardiac failure due to myocarditis; (3) mitral or aortic regurgitation due to acute endocarditis.

Finally, take the temperature.

THE VASCULITIDES

This is a heterogeneous group of disorders characterised by inflammation and damage to blood vessels.[2] The

The vasculitides

Name	Vessels	Characteristics
Small-vessel vasculitis		
Wegener's* granulomatosis—now called granulomatosis with polyangiitis	Small-to-medium-sized capillaries, venules, arterioles, small arteries	Granulomatous inflammation affecting the respiratory tract, often with necrotising glomerulonephritis Saddle-nose deformity
Churg–Strauss syndrome (microscopic polyarteritis)	Small	Asthma, eosinophilia, skin nodules, mononeuritis multiplex, pulmonary infiltrates
Henoch–Schönlein purpura	Small	Children affected; purpura over buttocks, abdominal pain, arthritis of knee and ankle, nephritis (40%)
Microscopic polyangiitis	Small	Glomerulonephritis, alveolar haemorrhage, neuropathy, pleural effusions
Mixed essential cryoglobulinaemia	Small	Arthritis, palpable purpura of extremities, Raynaud's disease, neuropathy Hepatitis C common
Medium-sized vessel vasculitis		
Polyarteritis nodosa	Medium-sized to small	Myalgia, arthralgia, fever, palpable purpura, skin ulceration or infarction, weight loss, testicular tenderness, neuropathy (involvement of vasa nervorum), hypertension, renal infarction Hepatitis B associated
Kawasaki's disease	Medium-sized (coronary artery involvement)	Children affected; desquamating rash over extremities, strawberry tongue
Large-vessel vasculitis		
Giant cell arteritis (temporal arteritis; see Fig. 25.16)	Medium to large (temporal and ophthalmic arteries and their branches)	Localised headache, systemic symptoms, tenderness over the temporal artery, jaw pain, visual loss—posterior ciliary artery (age ≥50 years)
Takayasu's† disease	Large (aorta, brachial, carotid, ulnar and axillary arteries)	Systemic symptoms, claudication, loss of pulses (typically Asian race age ≤40 years)

*Frederich Wegener, a German pathologist, described this in 1936.
†Mikito Takayasu (1860–1938), a Japanese professor of ophthalmology.

TABLE 25.1

clinical features and major vessels involved are shown in Table 25.1.

SOFT-TISSUE RHEUMATISM

This includes a number of common, painful conditions that arise in soft tissue, often around a joint. The problem may be general (e.g. fibromyalgia) or restricted to a single anatomical region (e.g. tendon, tenosynovium, enthesis or bursa). There are a large number of these conditions; the more common ones are described here. There are a number of important associations:

- depression
- sleep disorder (obstructive sleep apnoea)
- irritable bowel syndrome.

It is important to exclude:

1. thyroid disease
2. diabetes mellitus
3. inflammatory arthritis
4. vitamin D deficiency.

Shoulder syndromes

Soft-tissue disorders of the shoulder are common and have certain particular clinical features.

Rotator cuff syndrome

Supraspinatus tendinitis is the most common form of rotator cuff syndrome. It is associated with degeneration and subsequent inflammation in the supraspinatus

Giant cell arteritis

(From Klippel JH, Dieppe PA, eds. *Rheumatology*, 2nd edn. Maryland Heights, MO: Mosby, 1997.)

FIGURE 25.16

tendon as it is compressed between the acromion and humeral head when the arm is raised. It mostly affects 40- to 50-year-olds. Symptoms may begin following unaccustomed physical activities such as gardening.

Examination

Examine the shoulder joint. Note pain on abduction of the arm (see Fig. 25.17), with a painful arc of movement between 60 and 120° of abduction. Involvement of other rotator cuff tendons causes similar painful movement. Biceps tendinitis is present in the majority of patients with a rotator cuff syndrome. Yergason's[g] sign for biceps tendinitis is helpful (LR+, 2.8).[4] The patient flexes the elbow to 90° and pronates the wrist. Hold the patient's wrists and try to prevent the patient's attempts to supinate the forearm. Inflammation of the head of the biceps causes pain in the shoulder as this muscle is the main supinator of the forearm.

Frozen shoulder

Capsulitis of the shoulder, or frozen shoulder, is associated with limitation of active and passive arm movements in all directions. It may follow immobilisation of the

Inflammation of the rotator cuff tendons may cause a 'painful arc' during abduction of the arm.

The initial movement (a) is painless but the next 90° of movement (b) causes pain. When the arm reaches full abduction (c) the pain eases as the pressure is taken off the rotator cuff apparatus

FIGURE 25.17

arm after a stroke. There is typically a sudden onset of shoulder pain, which is worse at night and radiates to the base of the neck and down the arm. Pain is made worse by shoulder movement and may be bilateral. Pain and stiffness usually subside over a period of months. Complete movement may not be regained.

Examination

Examine the shoulders. There is global restriction of both active and passive movement of the shoulder—that is, it is frozen.

---

[g] Robert Mosely Yergason (1885–1949), an American surgeon, described this sign in 1931.

Elbow epicondylitis (tennis and golfer's elbow)

Many contact and non-contact sports can cause physical injury, although serious injuries are rather uncommon with certain sports (e.g. synchronised swimming). There may be pain over the epicondyles of the elbow. The *lateral epicondyle* is the most often affected and is called 'tennis elbow'. Pain arises from the site of insertion of the extensor muscle tendons into the lateral epicondyle (enthesis). Involvement of the medial epicondyle at the site of insertion of the flexor tendons of the forearm causes medial epicondylitis—'golfer's elbow'. These conditions are also common in manual workers such as painters.

Examination

Examine for local tenderness over the lateral (see Fig. 25.18) or medial epicondyle (see Fig. 25.19). Ask the patient to extend the fingers against resistance (see Fig. 25.20). This will make the pain of lateral epicondylitis worse. Ask the patient to flex the fingers against resistance. This will exacerbate the pain of medial epicondylitis.

Tenosynovitis of the wrist

Inflammation of the synovial tubes in which tendons run can occur in patients with rheumatoid arthritis but also in otherwise healthy people. The cause is often unaccustomed repetitive movement. A common site for tenosynovitis is at the wrist, where it involves the long extensor and abductor tendons of the thumb (de Quervain's tenosynovitis; see Fig. 25.21).

Examination of the elbow—medial epicondylitis.

Local pressure over the medial epicondyle elicits pain. Symptoms are exacerbated by resisted flexion of the wrist and fingers

FIGURE 25.19

Examination of the elbow—lateral epicondylitis.

Looking for signs of lateral epicondylitis. Palpation over the forearm extensor muscle origin elicits pain. Straining the muscles by resisted extension of the wrist exacerbates the symptoms

FIGURE 25.18

Testing for lateral epicondylitis: 'Push your hand up against mine'

FIGURE 25.20

A patient with de Quervain's tenosynovitis.

There is characteristic swelling of the tendon sheath of the abductor pollicis brevis over the styloid process of the radius

FIGURE 25.21

Finkelstein's test

FIGURE 25.22

Examination

This reveals tenderness and swelling on the radial side of the wrist (radial styloid). There is pain on active or passive movement of the thumb. Confirm the diagnosis by performing Finkelstein's[h] test. Hold the patient's hand with the thumb tucked into the palm and then quickly turn the wrist into full ulnar deviation (see Fig. 25.22). An alternative approach that is reported to produce fewer false-positives involves gripping the patient's thumb rather than tucking the thumb into the palm.[5] Sharp pain will occur in the tendon sheath when the test is positive. Also examine the other common sites of tendon involvement: the flexor tendons of the fingers and the Achilles tendon.

---

[h] Harry Finkelstein (1865–1939), a surgeon at the Hospital for Joint Diseases, New York.

A red, swollen and painful prepatellar bursa.

(a) Anterior view; (b) lateral view

FIGURE 25.23

Bursitis

Bursae are found in areas exposed to mechanical strain or trauma, either at the site where muscle or tendon glides over bone or muscle, or superficially where bony prominences are exposed to mechanical stress. Bursitis usually occurs as a local soft-tissue inflammatory reaction to unusual mechanical pressure. It may be associated with rheumatoid arthritis, gout or sepsis. Common sites include the prepatellar area (housemaid's knee; see Fig. 25.23), over the olecranon (olecranon bursitis) and over the greater trochanter (trochanteric bursitis, often actually a tendinitis).

NERVE ENTRAPMENT SYNDROMES

Nerve entrapment syndromes are caused by compression of peripheral nerves at vulnerable sites and are associated

Carpal tunnel syndrome

Compression of the median nerve at the wrist is the most frequent form. This seems hardly surprising when one remembers that the carpal tunnel, sandwiched between the carpal bones and the carpal ligament, contains nine flexor tendons as well as the median nerve. These patients complain of numbness, pain and paraesthesiae in the median nerve distribution (the three radial fingers and the radial side of the ring finger). It can be a sign of early rheumatoid arthritis. Symptoms often wake patients from sleep and may radiate up the forearm (one-third of cases) and involve the fourth and fifth fingers and wrist but not the palm or dorsum of the hand—*classic* pattern. If the palms are involved the pattern is called *probable*. The largest group is idiopathic but overuse tenosynovitis of the flexor tendon sheaths at the wrist is also a cause. Fluid retention during pregnancy or from use of the oral contraceptive pill can also produce carpal tunnel symptoms. In addition, median nerve compression can occur in hypothyroidism, acromegaly and amyloidosis.

Examination

Symptoms can be reproduced by gentle percussion over the carpal tunnel (which begins at the distal wrist crease) while the wrist is held in extension (Tinel's sign—LR+, 1.8; LR−, 0.8). This sign is negative in up to 30% of patients with electrophysiologically proven median nerve compression. Prolonged (60 seconds) passive wrist flexion (Phalen's test) has a lower false-negative rate (LR+, 1.3; LR−, 0.7).[4] Ask the patient: 'What do you do with your hands when the feeling is there?' The *flick sign* is positive when the patient demonstrates a flicking movement with the wrist as if shaking a non-electronic thermometer (LR+ 29; LR− 0.1—but only in one study[6]). Look for wasting in the median nerve distribution and loss of motor (thenar muscle strength: weak thumb abduction) and sensory function (sensation over the thenar eminence, however, is usually preserved). These signs occur only in advanced cases.

Meralgia[i] paraesthetica

Compression of the lateral cutaneous nerve of the thigh causes paraesthesiae and sensory loss over the lateral side of the thigh. This entirely sensory nerve passes through the lateral part of the inguinal ligament only just medial to the anterior superior iliac spine. Here it is subject to compression in patients who are obese, wear tight or heavy belts or spend long periods sitting. Diabetes, pregnancy and trauma can also be causes of problems with the nerve.

Tarsal tunnel syndrome

This may be caused by compression of the posterior tibial nerve in its fibro-osseous canal formed by the flexor retinaculum and the tarsal bones. Symptoms include burning pain and paraesthesiae in the toe, sole and heel. Patients are often woken with pain at night and, as with the carpal tunnel syndrome, this may radiate upwards. Walking may improve the symptoms. Causes include diabetes, synovitis from rheumatoid arthritis, bony deformity and flexor tenosynovitis. Hypertrophy of the abductor hallucis muscle, which occurs in intemperate runners, is an occasional cause.

Examination

There is usually tenderness over the nerve posterior to the medial malleolus. There may be a positive Tinel's sign over the tarsal tunnel. Motor findings include weakness of toe flexion and of the intrinsic muscles of the foot.

Morton's 'neuroma'

This is caused by compression of one or more of the interdigital plantar nerves by the transverse metatarsal ligament. Patients complain of a burning pain or ache that extends distally from the affected web space to the toes (most often the third and fourth).

Metatarsalgia is a non-localised ache that spreads across the forefoot involving the area of some or all of the metatarsal heads. It can occur in normal feet after prolonged standing but also occurs in a number of other foot conditions (see List 25.2), and is often associated with poor-fitting shoes. *Morton's metatarsalgia* is interdigital nerve entrapment (usually between the third and fourth metatarsal bones). Patients describe burning pain between the metatarsal bones and may have numbness on the adjacent toes. They get relief by removing their shoes and massaging their foot.

---

[i] The Greek word *meros* means 'thigh' and *algia* means 'painful'.

> **CAUSES OF METATARSALGIA**
> - Tight or pointed shoes
> - Atrophy of metatarsal fat pad in elderly people
> - Plantar calluses
> - Metatarsophalangeal joint arthritis
> - Flat or cavus foot deformity
> - Overlapping toes
> - Interdigital entrapment
> - Hemiplegia
> - Peripheral vascular disease
>
> LIST 25.2

Examination

There is often tenderness between the involved metatarsal heads, and a painful nodule may be palpable.

Fibromyalgia syndrome

This syndrome is a common, frequently overlooked condition that mostly affects women in their 40s and 50s. It presents with a variable group of symptoms including widespread musculoskeletal aches and pains, and usually with symptoms of chronic fatigue. There are often cognitive symptoms—forgetting of words or difficulty in concentrating. The musculoskeletal pain is mostly axial (neck and back) and diffuse. It is made worse by stress or cold. Pain may be reported 'all over' unresponsive to anti-inflammatory drug treatment. The combination of pain and fatigue may cause the patient severe limitation. There is usually a poor sleep pattern. The patient wakes up feeling unrefreshed and more tired in the morning than later in the day. There is often intolerance to exercise. Days of exhaustion may follow any amount of exercise. Note that no abnormal pathology has been found in the joints, muscles or tendons of these patients.

Examination

Test for the characteristic multiple hyperalgesic tender points (see Fig. 25.24). These areas may be tender to finger pressure in normal people, but in affected patients there is marked tenderness and a definite withdrawal response. This response should be obtained in at least 11 of 18 sites in the upper and lower limbs and on both sides (i.e. it is widespread and symmetrical). Next examine for hyperalgesia at control sites such as the forehead or distal forearm, where it should be absent.

Frequent sites of localised tenderness in fibromyalgia.

18 tender point sites (test bilaterally) are:
1. Insertion of suboccipital muscle
2. Under lower sternocleidomastoid muscle
3. Insertion of supraspinatus muscle
4. Trapezius muscle (mid upper)
5. Near second costochondral junction
6. 2 centimetres distal to lateral epicondyle
7. At prominence of greater trochanter
8. Upper outer quadrant of buttock
9. At medial fat pad of knee

FIGURE 25.24

The diagnosis was based on the presence of multiple hyperalgesic tender sites (with negative control sites) but this is now thought to lead to overdiagnosis in women.[7] Current diagnostic criteria include:

- 3 months of self-reported pain at any of 19 different sites (widespread pain index [WPI]—1 point per site)
- fatigue
- waking unrefreshed
- cognitive symptoms—these three (fatigue, waking unrefreshed and cognitive symptoms) are scaled from 0 to 3 and the Symptoms Severity Scale (SSS) calculated
- a WPI >7 **and** SSS >5 or WPI 3–6 **and** SSS >9 is considered diagnostic of the condition.

Inflammatory and endocrine disease must be excluded.

T&O'C ESSENTIALS

1. The pattern of joint involvement can be a clue to the underlying rheumatological abnormality.
2. The diagnosis of carpal tunnel syndrome is suggested by a number of different tests, but asking the patient what he or she does when the symptoms are present often leads to a demonstration by the patient of the 'flick sign'.
3. The rotator cuff syndrome is a common presenting problem. Looking for the painful arc of movement can help make the diagnosis.
4. For patients with ankylosing spondylitis, serial measurements of movement of the spine and the occiput-to-wall distance help determine the progression of the disease.

OSCE REVISION TOPICS – RHEUMATOLOGICAL DISEASE

Use these topics, which commonly occur in the OSCE, to help with revision.

1. This woman has noticed problems with cold fingers associated with colour changes. Please examine her hands and anything else you think necessary. (pp 367, 416)
2. This woman has been diagnosed with systemic lupus erythematosus. Please examine her. (p 416)
3. This man has a very painful first metatarsophalangeal joint. Please examine him. (p 412)
4. This woman has had pain and stiffness in her shoulders. Please examine her. (pp 421, 426)

References

1. Grob JJ, Bonerandi JJ. Cutaneous manifestations associated with the presence of the lupus-anticoagulant. *J Am Acad Dermatol* 1986; 15:211–219. Antiphospholipid antibody syndrome can be associated with leg ulcers (that resemble pyoderma gangrenosum), livedo reticularis and fingertip ischaemia.
2. Stevens GL, Adelman HM, Wallach PM. Palpable purpura: an algorithmic approach. *Am Fam Phys* 1995; 52:1355–1362.
3. RHD Australia. Criteria. www.rhdaustralia.org.au.
4. McGee S. *Evidence-based clinical diagnosis*, 3rd edn. Philadelphia: Saunders, 2012.
5. Elliott BG. Finkelstein's test: a descriptive error that can produce a false-positive. *J Hand Surg Br* 1992; 17:481–482. Careful explanation of the performance of this test (which is often misunderstood) appears in this article. Movement with the thumb folded into the hand can produce a false-positive result.
6. Pryse-Phillips WE. Validation of a diagnostic sign in the diagnosis of carpal tunnel syndrome signs. *J Neurol Neurosurg Psychiatry* 1984; 47(8):870–872.
7. McBeth J, Mulvey MR. Fibromyalgia: mechanisms and potential impact of the ACR 2010 classification criteria. *Nat Rev Rheumatol* 2012; 8(2):108–116.

CHAPTER 26

A summary of the rheumatological examination and extending the rheumatological examination

Study sickness while you are well. THOMAS FULLER (1608–1661)

The rheumatological system: a suggested method using the GALS screening test

A modified **GALS** (gait, arms, legs and spine) assessment is a quick way to identify arthritis and mobility problems.[1,2]

Ask:

1. Have you been troubled by pain or stiffness in your back or muscles or joints? Where?
2. How are you affected by this? Can you walk up and down stairs? Can you get out of a chair easily? Can you dress and wash yourself?

Examine:

1. **Gait:** Ask the patient to walk to the end of the room, turn around and come back. Note the length of the stride, the smoothness of the walk and turning around, the stance, heel strike and arm swing. Is walking painful? Hemiplegic, Parkinsonian, foot drop and other neurological gaits should be obvious.
2. **Arms, legs and spine:**
   - *From behind:* look at the spine for scoliosis, muscle bulk of the shoulders, paraspinal muscles, gluteal muscles and calves; look at the iliac crests for loss of symmetry.
   - *From the side:* look for normal lordosis and thoracic kyphosis. Ask the patient to bend over and look for normal separation of lumbar spinous processes.
   - *From in front:* look for asymmetry or wasting of major muscle groups (shoulders, arms and quadriceps). Is there deformity of the knees, ankles or feet?

   When arthritis seems likely to be an important part of the case, take the time to test movement. Look for restricted, asymmetrical or painful movements.

3. **Spine:** Rotation: ask 'Turn your shoulders as far as you can to the right and now to the left.' Lateral flexion: ask 'Slide your hand down the side of your leg on the right side and now on the left.' Cervical spine—lateral flexion: ask 'Bend your right ear down towards your shoulder, now on the other side.' Flexion and extension: ask 'Look up and back as far as you can, now put your chin on your chest.'
4. **Shoulders (acromioclavicular, glenohumeral, sternoclavicular joints):** Ask 'Put your right hand on your back and reach up as far as you can as if to scratch your back. Now the left. Put your hands up behind your head and your elbows as far back as you can.'
5. **Elbows (extension):** Ask 'With your elbows straight, put your arms down beside you.'
6. **Hands and wrists:** Ask 'Straighten out your arms and hands in front of you.' Look for fixed flexion deformity of the fingers and swelling and deformity of the hands and wrists or wasting of the small muscles of the hands. Ask 'Turn your hands up the other way.' Look at the palms for swelling or muscle wasting. Is supination smooth and complete? Is there external rotation of the shoulder used to make up for limited supination? Ask 'Squeeze my fingers as hard as you can' (tests for grip strength). Ask 'Touch the tip of each finger with your thumb' (tests most finger joints).
7. **Legs and hips:** Ask the patient to lie down on the bed. Look at leg length and, if suspicious, measure true leg length from the anterior superior iliac spine to the medial malleolus and

TEXT BOX 26.1

> **The rheumatological system: a suggested method using the GALS screening test** *continued*
>
> apparent length from the umbilicus to the medial malleolus. Test knee flexion: ask 'Bend your knee and pull your foot up towards your bottom.' Meanwhile, put your hand on the patella and feel for crepitus. Test for osteoarthritis of the hip by internally rotating the hip. Flex the knee to 90° and move the foot laterally. Pain and limitation of movement occur early with osteoarthritis.
>
> 8. **Feet:** Look for arthritic changes, especially at the metatarsophalangeal joints, bunions, swelling, calluses, etc.
>
> The examination will have to be varied for very immobile patients, but with practice it can be performed rapidly. If a specific joint or group of joints is abnormal on screening, a more detailed targeted examination is indicated.

TEXT BOX 26.1

EXTENDING THE RHEUMATOLOGICAL SYSTEM EXAMINATION

Rheumatology investigations

Diagnosis in rheumatology relies on careful history taking and physical examination, and in many cases pattern recognition applied against accepted diagnostic criteria. Testing is undertaken to confirm the clinical diagnosis. Table 26.1 gives the current American College of Rheumatology (ACR) criteria for rheumatoid arthritis (RA)—a combination of clinical and laboratory findings.

Laboratory testing

Know your autoimmune antibodies. Testing includes the following:

- Antinuclear antibody (ANA) is positive in high titre in a number of autoimmune diseases including systemic lupus erythematosus (SLE) (95%), drug-induced lupus, mixed connective tissue disease, scleroderma and Sjögren's syndrome (and ANA is positive in at least 5% of healthy elderly patients). ANA is sensitive but not specific.
- If ANA is positive, testing for specific ANAs is helpful—for example, anti-double stranded DNA (specific for SLE), anti-U1-RNP (very sensitive for mixed connective tissue disease) and anticentromere antibody (CREST).
- Antineutrophil cytoplasmic antibodies (ANCA) can be perinuclear in pattern (p-ANCA; e.g. Churg–Strauss syndrome) or homogeneous in the neutrophil cytoplasm (c-ANCA; e.g. granulomatosis with polyangiitis [GPA]— Wegener's granulomatosis).
- Rheumatoid factor (RF, a polyclonal antibody of IgM and IgG classes) is present in only 70% of patients with rheumatoid arthritis and in 5% of unaffected people. Anti-cyclic citrullinated peptide (anti-CCP) is similar in sensitivity to RF for the diagnosis of RA but much more specific. It has largely replaced RF testing.
- Complement components (C4 and C3) are reduced in SLE.

ACR criteria for rheumatoid arthritis (RA)*	Score
A. Joints involved	
1 large joint (shoulder, elbow, hip, knee, ankle)	0
2–10 large joints	1
1–3 small joints (MCP, MTP, PIP, wrist)	2
4–10 small joints	3
>10 joints—at least one small	5
B. Serology	
RF negative, CCP antibodies negative	0
Low positive RF or CCP (1–3 times upper normal)	2
High positive RF or CCP	3
C. Acute-phase reactants	
ESR and CRP normal	1
Abnormal ESR or CRP	1
D. Duration	
<6 weeks	0
>6 weeks	1

CCP=cyclic citrullinated peptide; CRP=C-reactive protein; ESR=erythrocyte sedimentation rate; MCP=metacarpophalangeal; MTP=metatarsophalangeal; PIP=proximal interphalangeal; RF=rheumatoid factor.
*A score of 6 or more=definite rheumatoid arthritis.

(Neligan PC. *Plastivc surgery*, 3rd edn, 6 volume set, Elsevier, 2013.)

TABLE 26.1

- HLA-B27 is present in 90% of patients with ankylosing spondylitis and in up to 80% with reactive arthritis but is *not* used for diagnosis (up to 8% of the normal population are also HLA-B27 positive).

Joint aspiration is important to identify septic arthritis and sometimes gout and pseudogout.

Imaging

X-rays, computed tomography (CT) scans and magnetic resonance imaging (MRI) scans are now a standard part of the rheumatological investigation. Students need to be familiar with some of the more common changes in these tests and how they may be useful.

Plain X-rays may show the following in soft tissues and bones in different types of arthritis:

- soft-tissue swelling (e.g. pannus)
- deformity or enlargement of bone
- narrowing of the joint spaces due to loss of cartilage—focal in inflammatory arthritis and generalised in osteoarthritis (see Figs 26.1 and 26.2)
- cervical spine in RA (Fig. 26.3)
- joint erosion with areas of proliferation of bone (e.g. psoriatic; see Fig. 26.8 below) or without (e.g. rheumatoid arthritis; see Fig. 26.3)
- new bone formation (e.g. syndesmophytes (see Fig. 26.4), periosteal reaction, osteophytes)
- bone deformity (see Fig. 26.5)
- abnormal calcification of ligaments, cartilage, tendon or within joint spaces
- changes in bone density: osteosclerosis, increased density (e.g. at joint margins in osteoporosis), osteoporosis, decreased density (e.g. septic arthritis).

It is not usually necessary to X-ray all symptomatic joints; information about joint destruction and typical changes that help make the diagnosis can be obtained from selected X-rays. For example, a clinical presentation with a polyarthritis may warrant hand and foot X-rays, which, if they show erosion and a typical pattern (e.g. metatarsophalangeal [MTP] and metacarpophalangeal [MCP] involvement), can help make the diagnosis of rheumatoid arthritis (see Figs 26.6 and 26.7).

X-rays of the sacroiliac joints may reveal joint involvement in patients with some symptoms of

Osteoarthritis.

X-ray of the hands showing the typical findings of osteoarthritis with joint-space narrowing and proliferative changes in the distal joints. Also note erosive and destructive changes at multiple proximal interphalangeal (PIP) joints

(Courtesy Canberra Hospital X-ray library.)

FIGURE 26.1

Osteoarthritis.

Anteroposterior X-ray of the hip showing the features of osteoarthritis. The left side is more severely affected than the right; note sclerosis, osteophyte formation and asymmetrical joint-space narrowing

(Courtesy Canberra Hospital X-ray library.)

FIGURE 26.2

Rheumatoid arthritis.

Lateral X-ray of the cervical spine showing anterior subluxation of the anterior arch of the dens of the axis (C2, arrow)

(Courtesy Canberra Hospital X-ray library.)

FIGURE 26.3

ankylosing spondylitis before these joints are clinically abnormal.

CT scans and MRI scans: it must be kept in mind that CT scans expose patients to many times the radiation dose of plain X-rays, so they should be used only when they are likely to give information beyond what plain X-rays can show. MRI is often preferred when it is available.

CT scans and MRI scans give three-dimensional information about complicated joints and are especially useful for spinal problems. Examples of indications include:

- soft-tissue problems such as bursitis, tenosynovitis and rotator cuff tears
- suspected joint or soft-tissue infection
- intervertebral disc problems such as spinal cord compression or nerve root entrapment
- joint or associated soft-tissue or bony malignancy
- joint injury or damage such as knee problems in athletes or after trauma (see Figs 26.11, 26.12).

Ultrasound can be used to look for joint effusions, cysts and tendon thickening. However, it does not provide the spatial resolution of CT or MRI.

Nuclear scans using Tc-bisphosphonate can be useful for a number of specific problems, including detecting:

- metastases
- bone or joint infection
- stress fractures
- the extent of Paget's disease.

Ankylosing spondylitis.

Anteroposterior (a) and lateral (b) X-rays of the thoracic spine showing ankylosis of the sacroiliac joints, extensive syndesmophyte formation (short arrows) and squaring of the vertebral bodies (long arrows)
(Courtesy Canberra Hospital X-ray library.)

FIGURE 26.4

X-rays in specific rheumatological conditions

Ankylosing spondylitis
X-rays of the spine and sacroiliac joints (see Fig. 26.4) may show ankylosis (fusion) of the sacroiliac joints and 'squaring' of the vertebral bodies as a result of loss of their anterior corners and periostitis of their waists. 'Bridging syndesmophytes'[a] occur as a result of ossification of the fibres of the joint annulus. Severe disease causes the changes called *bamboo spine* visible on X-ray.

Reactive arthritis
The first attack of arthritis is associated with soft-tissue changes and subsequent attacks may lead to joint-space narrowing and proliferative erosions at the joint margins that show on X-ray. Changes in the sacroiliac joints and spine resemble those of ankylosing spondylitis except that the sacroiliac joint changes and spinal syndesmophytes tend to be asymmetrical. Calcaneal spurs—a result of plantar fasciitis—are characteristic.

Psoriatic arthritis
In mild cases X-rays are normal or show only joint-space narrowing and erosive changes. Unlike the X-rays of rheumatoid joints, the bone density is maintained and there may be sclerotic changes in the small bones (see Fig. 26.8). Ankylosis of peripheral joints and *arthritis mutilans* can occur in either condition. The involvement of the spine and sacroiliac joints is asymmetrical, as in reactive arthritis (see Fig. 26.9).

---
[a] A syndesmosis is a joint where the bones are joined by fibrous ligaments or sheets.

Haemophilia.

X-ray of the knee showing loss of joint space and some deformity of the adjacent bone. Although the tibia and femur are sclerotic adjacent to the destructive change, the bones are generally osteopenic with mild overgrowth of the epiphysis. Ask about the consequences of arthritis

(Courtesy Canberra Hospital X-ray library.)

FIGURE 26.5

Rheumatoid arthritis, early findings.

X-ray of the hands of a patient with early rheumatoid arthritis. Note erosions of the heads of the MCP joints and of the ulnar styloid, and reduced amounts of cartilage in the joint spaces

(Courtesy Canberra Hospital X-ray library.)

FIGURE 26.6

Rheumatoid arthritis, late findings.

X-ray of the hands of a patient with advanced rheumatoid arthritis. Note loss of joint space and destruction of the right carpal joints, subluxation of MCP and PIP joints, and Z deformity of the thumb. There are erosions of the PIP joints, a sign of active disease

(Courtesy Canberra Hospital X-ray library.)

FIGURE 26.7

Psoriatic arthritis.

X-ray of the wrist of a patient with psoriatic arthritis; note the 'pencil in cup' deformity (tapered proximal osseous surface and expanded base) of the distal bone of the fingers, early ankylosis [arrowhead] of the PIP joint of the right little finger and erosions with proliferative change of the little finger). Note also the lack of osteoporosis

(Courtesy Canberra Hospital X-ray library.)

FIGURE 26.8

Reactive arthritis.

X-ray of the pelvis of a patient showing loss of joint space in the sacroiliac joints (arrows)

FIGURE 26.9

Gout.

X-ray of the hands of a patient with severe gouty arthritis. Note multiple juxta-articular erosions with relative preservation of the joint space, and erosions with overhanging edges. There are large soft-tissue swellings over the distal interphalangeal joints of the index fingers

(Courtesy Canberra Hospital X-ray library.)

FIGURE 26.10

Gout
X-rays (see Fig. 26.10) show multiple juxta-articular erosions, which may obliterate the joint space.

Pseudogout
X-rays show joint-space narrowing, cyst formation under the cartilage and calcification of the joint cartilage (chondrocalcinosis). Chondrocalcinosis on X-ray is typical of pseudogout but is not always present.

Scans
Figs 26.11 and 26.12 show CT scans of changes in the knee.

CT scan showing a meniscal tear in the knee joint (arrow)

(From Resnick DR et al. *Internal derangement of joints*, 2nd edn. Philadelphia: Saunders, 2006.)

FIGURE 26.11

CHAPTER 26 A SUMMARY OF THE RHEUMATOLOGICAL EXAMINATION

CT scan showing a haemarthrosis of the knee (arrows)

(From Resnick DR et al. *Internal derangement of joints*, 2nd edn. Philadelphia: Saunders, 2006.)

FIGURE 26.12

> **T&O'C ESSENTIALS**
>
> 1. The GALS screening test is an excellent and quick way of assessing the effect of rheumatological disease on a patient's mobility.
> 2. Patterns of abnormality seen on plain X-rays of joints can be helpful in identifying the type of rheumatological disease.
> 3. CT and MRI scans can provide detailed structural information on joint abnormalities and are especially useful for the assessment of joint injuries.

References

1. Beattie KA, Bobba R, Bayoumi I et al. Validation of the GALS musculoskeletal screening exam for use in primary care: a pilot study. *BMC Musculoskelet Disord* 2008; 9:115. GALS is a useful tool in primary care.
2. Doherty M, Dacre J, Dieppe P, Snaith M. The 'GALS' locomotor screen. *Ann Rheum Dis* 1992; 51:1165–1169. Describes the GALS screen.

SECTION 8
The endocrine system

CHAPTER 27
The endocrine history

CHAPTER 28
The endocrine examination

CHAPTER 29
Correlation of physical signs and endocrine disease

CHAPTER 30
A summary of the endocrine examination and extending the endocrine examination

CHAPTER 27
The endocrine history

A physician is obligated to consider more than a diseased organ, more even than the whole man—he must view the man in his world. HARVEY CUSHING (1869–1939)

PRESENTING SYMPTOMS

Hormones control so many aspects of body function that the manifestations of endocrine disease are protean. Ask about:

- changes in body weight
- appetite
- bowel habit
- hair distribution
- pigmentation
- sweating
- height
- menstruation
- galactorrhoea (unexpected breast-milk production—in men and women)
- polydipsia
- polyuria
- lethargy
- headaches
- loss of libido and erectile dysfunction.

Back pain and loss of height caused by vertebral fractures may be symptoms and signs of osteoporosis, which has endocrine and non-endocrine causes. Many of these symptoms have other causes as well and must be carefully evaluated. On the other hand, the patient may know which endocrine organ or group of endocrine organs has been causing a problem. Histories of thyroid disease and diabetes mellitus are particularly common. A list of common symptoms associated with various endocrine diseases is presented in List 27.1. In this chapter some of the important symptoms associated with endocrine disease are discussed.

Changes in appetite and weight

An increased appetite associated with weight loss classically occurs in thyrotoxicosis (due to an increase in metabolic activity) and uncontrolled diabetes mellitus (due to loss of glucose in the urine). An increased appetite with weight gain may occur in Cushing's syndrome (effects of excessive glucocorticoids), hypoglycaemia and hypothalamic disease. A loss of appetite with weight loss can occur with adrenal insufficiency, but is also seen in anorexia nervosa and with gastrointestinal disease (particularly malignancy). A loss of appetite with weight gain can occur in hypothyroidism (reduced metabolic activity).

Changes in bowel habit

Diarrhoea and an increase in the frequency of bowel movements are associated with hyperthyroidism and adrenal insufficiency, whereas constipation may occur in hypothyroidism and hypercalcaemia. Autonomic dysfunction due to diabetes mellitus can result in diarrhoea or constipation.

Changes in sweating

Increased sweating is characteristic of hyperthyroidism, hypoglycaemia and acromegaly, but may also occur in anxiety states and at the menopause.

Changes in hair distribution

Hirsutism refers to an increased growth of body hair in women. The clinical evaluation and differential

> ### ENDOCRINE HISTORY
>
> **Major symptoms**
> Appetite and weight changes
> Disturbed defecation
> Sweating
> Change in hair distribution
> Lethargy
> Skin changes
> Pigmentation
> Stature
> Loss of libido, erectile dysfunction
> Menstruation
> Polyuria
> Lump in the neck (goitre)
>
> **Endocrine abnormalities and typical symptoms and signs**
>
> *Hypopituitarism:*
> - ACTH deficiency: chronic—as for Addison's disease but no excess pigmentation; acute—fatigue, hypotension, nausea or vomiting, weight loss
> - TSH deficiency: as for hypothyroidism
> - Gonadotrophin deficiency: women—infertility, osteoporosis, secondary amenorrhoea; men—testicular atrophy, infertility, decrease in body hair
> - Prolactin deficiency: failure of lactation for women
> - Growth hormone: loss of muscle mass, increased fat (especially central), increased cardiovascular risk, asthenia
>
> Vasopressin (anti-diuretic hormone [ADH]); polyuria, increased thirst, dilute urine, hypernatraemia, nocturia
>
> *Thyrotoxicosis:* preference for cooler weather, weight loss, increased appetite (hyperphagia), palpitations (especially at rest), increased sweating, nervousness, irritability, diarrhoea, amenorrhoea, muscle weakness, exertional dyspnoea, tremor
>
> *Hypothyroidism (myxoedema):* preference for warmer weather, lethargy, swelling of eyelids (oedema), hoarse voice, constipation, coarse skin, hypercarotenaemia, decreased relaxation phase of reflexes
>
> *Diabetes mellitus:* polyuria, polydipsia, thirst, blurred vision, weakness, infections, groin itch, rash (pruritus vulvae, balanitis), weight loss, tiredness, lethargy, disturbance of conscious state
>
> *Hypoglycaemia:* morning headaches, weight gain, seizures, sweating
>
> *Primary adrenal insufficiency:* pigmentation, tiredness, loss of weight, anorexia, nausea, diarrhoea, nocturia, postural hypotension, mental changes, seizures (hypotension, hypoglycaemia)
>
> *Acromegaly:* fatigue, weakness, increased sweating, heat intolerance, weight gain, enlarging hands and feet, enlarged and coarsened facial features, headaches, decreased vision, deepening of the voice, decreased libido, erectile dysfunction (impotence)
>
> *Cushing's syndrome:* truncal obesity, purple striae, moon-like facies, facial plethora, buffalo hump, myopathy, bruises, recurrent infections
>
> LIST 27.1

diagnosis are presented on page 475. The absence of facial hair in a man suggests hypogonadism, whereas temporal recession of the scalp hair in women occurs with androgen excess. The decrease in adrenal androgen production that occurs as a result of hypogonadism, hypopituitarism or adrenal insufficiency can cause loss of axillary and pubic hair in both sexes.

Lethargy

This common symptom can be due to a number of different diseases. Patients with hypothyroidism, Addison's disease or diabetes mellitus can present with this problem. Anaemia, connective tissue diseases, chronic infection (e.g. HIV, infective endocarditis), drugs (e.g. sedatives, diuretics causing electrolyte disturbances), chronic liver disease, chronic kidney disease and occult malignancy and depression may also result in lethargy.

Changes in the skin and nails

The skin becomes coarse, pale and dry in hypothyroidism, and dry and scaly in hypoparathyroidism. Flushing of the skin of the face and neck occurs in the carcinoid syndrome (due to the release of vasoactive peptides from the tumour). Soft-tissue overgrowth occurs in acromegaly and skin tags called molluscum fibrinosum may appear in the axillae. Acanthosis nigricans can also occur in acromegaly and in insulin-resistant states including Cushing's syndrome, polycystic ovarian syndrome and obesity. Xanthelasmata may be present in patients with diabetes mellitus, lipid disorders or hypothyroidism.

Onycholysis and rarely clubbing (called thyroid acropachy) and pretibial myxoedema may occur in Graves' disease. Cushing's syndrome is associated with spontaneous ecchymoses, thin skin and purple striae.

Changes in pigmentation

Increased pigmentation may be reported in primary adrenal insufficiency, Cushing's syndrome or acromegaly. Decreased pigmentation occurs in hypopituitarism. Localised depigmentation is characteristic of vitiligo (see Fig. 28.16), which may be associated with certain endocrine diseases such as Hashimoto's[a] disease and Addison's disease (autoimmune adrenal insufficiency) and other autoimmune conditions.

Changes in stature

Tallness may occur in children for constitutional reasons (tall parents) or, rarely, may reflect growth hormone excess (leading to gigantism), gonadotrophin deficiency, Klinefelter's[b] syndrome, Marfan's syndrome or generalised lipodystrophy. Short stature can also result from endocrine disease, as discussed on page 473. A loss of height of greater than 5 centimetres may indicate vertebral fractures and underlying osteoporosis.

Erectile dysfunction (impotence)

A persistent inability to attain or sustain penile erections may occasionally be due to primary hypogonadism or to secondary hypogonadism due to hyperprolactinaemia or hypopituitarism. More often, it is related to endothelial dysfunction (vascular disease) or emotional disorders (rule out depression). Autonomic neuropathy (e.g. in diabetes mellitus or alcoholism), spinal cord disease or testicular atrophy can also cause this problem.

Galactorrhoea

Hyperprolactinaemia (usually the result of a pituitary adenoma) can cause galactorrhoea in up to 80% of women and 30% of men. Galactorrhoea in men occurs from a normal-appearing male breast.

Menstruation

Failure to menstruate is termed *amenorrhoea*. *Primary amenorrhoea* is defined as a failure to start menstruating by 17 years of age. True primary amenorrhoea may result from ovarian failure (e.g. X chromosomal abnormalities such as Turner's syndrome), or from pituitary or hypothalamic disease (e.g. tumour, trauma or idiopathic disease). Excess androgen production or systemic disease (e.g. malabsorption, chronic kidney disease, obesity) can also result in primary amenorrhoea. Apparent primary amenorrhoea may also occur if menstrual flow cannot escape—for example, if there is an imperforate hymen.

Secondary amenorrhoea is defined as the cessation of menstruation for 6 months or more. Common causes include pregnancy, menopause, polycystic ovarian syndrome, hyperprolactinaemia, virilising syndromes or hypothalamic or pituitary disease. Use of the contraceptive pill, psychiatric disease and loss of weight of any cause, but especially as a result of anorexia nervosa, can also result in secondary amenorrhoea.

Polyuria

Polyuria is defined as a urine volume of more than 3 litres / day. Patients who report urinary frequency may find it difficult to tell whether large volumes of urine are being passed. Causes include diabetes mellitus (due to excessive filtration of glucose), diabetes insipidus (due to inadequate renal water conservation from a central deficiency of antidiuretic hormone, or a lack of renal responsiveness to this hormone), primary polydipsia—where a patient drinks excessive water (due to psychogenic or hypothalamic disease or drugs such as chlorpromazine or thioridazine or just simple eccentricity), hypercalcaemia and tubulointerstitial or cystic renal disease.

---

[a] Hakaru Hashimoto (1881–1934), a Japanese surgeon.
[b] Harry Fitch Klinefelter (1912–90), a Baltimore physician, described the condition when he was a medical student.

Criteria for diagnosis of the metabolic syndrome*	
Blood pressure	Systolic >130 mmHg Diastolic >85 mmHg or Current drug treatment for hypertension
Waist circumference	Men >102 cm Women >89 cm
Fasting triglycerides	>1.7 mmol/L or treated with drugs
HDL cholesterol	Men <1 mmol/L Women <1.3 mmol/L
Fasting glucose	>5.6 mmol/L or on drug treatment[†]

*3 out of 5 required for the diagnosis.
[†]World Health Organization (WHO)/International Diabetes Federation (IDF) criteria.

TABLE 27.1

RISK FACTORS FOR DIABETES (METABOLIC SYNDROME)

Metabolic syndrome is the term given to the coexistence of a group of risk factors for type 2 diabetes and cardiovascular disease. These include impaired glucose metabolism, obesity (central), hypertension and hyperlipidaemia (Table 27.1). Patients with metabolic syndrome have twice the risk of developing cardiovascular disease and five times the risk of developing type 2 diabetes.

PAST HISTORY AND TREATMENT

A previous history of any endocrine condition must be uncovered. This includes surgery on the neck. A partial thyroidectomy or radioiodine (^{131}I) treatment in the past can lead to eventual hypothyroidism. The same may apply to any radiation to the neck (e.g. for carcinoma). A woman may have been diagnosed with diabetes mellitus after the birth of a large baby. There may be a history of hypertension, which is occasionally due to an endocrine condition (e.g. phaeochromocytoma, Cushing's syndrome or Conn's syndrome). Previous thyroid surgery can be associated with hypoparathyroidism because of surgical damage to the parathyroid glands. Previous head injury may be a cause of pituitary or hypothalamic damage. Cranial irradiation for childhood leukaemia or brain tumours may eventually result in hypopituitarism.

Previous treatment of a patient's thyroid problems may have included the use of antithyroid drugs, thyroid hormone or radioactive iodine. Surgery on the adrenals or pituitary may have been performed and this may leave the patient with decreased adrenal or pituitary function.

Patients with diabetes mellitus have an important chronic condition. Treatment may be with diet, insulin, or drugs (e.g. metformin, sulphonylurea, glucagon-like insulinotropic peptide 1 [GLP-1] analogues). One must determine how well the patient understands the condition, and whether he or she understands the principles of the diabetic diet and adheres to it. Find out how the blood glucose levels are monitored and whether or not the patient adjusts the insulin dose. Most patients should be able to monitor their blood glucose levels at home using a glucose meter. There is now good evidence that tight control of blood glucose levels reduces the incidence of diabetic complications. Patients should have records of home blood glucose measurements, and may know the results of tests such as the haemoglobin A_{1c} (a surrogate marker of average blood glucose levels) and of tests of renal function and for protein in the urine.

The patient should be aware of the need for care of the feet and eyes to prevent complications. Most patients with diabetes have regular ophthalmological reviews, often using retinal photography. There may be a history of laser treatment or vascular endothelial growth factor (VEGF) inhibitor injections for proliferative diabetic retinopathy.

Patients with hypopituitarism or hypoadrenalism may be on glucocorticoid (steroid) replacement; the latter may also require mineralocorticoid replacement. Details of the patient's dosage schedule should be obtained.

Patients may know of a diagnosis of osteoporosis.[c] This may have been made following spontaneous fractures or as a result of screening tests for bone

---

[c] Although this is always called osteoporosis, it is often, at least partly, osteomalacia.

mineral density. Find out about treatment to prevent fractures.

The antiarrhythmic drug amiodarone contains iodine and quite commonly causes hypo- or hyperthyroidism. The risk is higher for patients with a history of thyroid disease.

SOCIAL HISTORY

Many of these conditions are chronic and their complications are serious. Ask how well the patient copes with various problems and the conditions at home and work, as this will have an important effect on the success of treatment.

FAMILY HISTORY

There may be a history in the family of thyroid disorders, autoimmune conditions or diabetes mellitus. Occasionally, a family history of a multiple endocrine neoplasia (MEN) syndrome may be obtained. These are rare autosomal-dominant conditions.

- MEN type I: manifests as primary hyperparathyroidism (>90%), pituitary tumours (20%) and gastrointestinal tumours (e.g. gastrinoma [70%]).
- MEN type II: should be considered if there is medullary thyroid cancer or phaeochromocytoma in the family.

T&O'C ESSENTIALS

1. The effects of endocrine disease are very varied. The history taken from a patient with suspected endocrine disease should cover the broad range of possible symptoms.
2. The history taken from the patient with diabetes mellitus must be complete as this disease can affect multiple systems. Include questions about the diagnosis, the symptoms of diabetes itself, current treatment and any of the numerous complications of the disease.
3. Questions to screen for certain common endocrine diseases (e.g. thyroid disease, diabetes mellitus, osteoporosis) should be a routine part of patient assessment.
4. Many endocrine diseases are chronic and may have a profound effect on a patient's life and work. This needs to be assessed.
5. Some symptoms traditionally associated with endocrine abnormalities (e.g. erectile dysfunction) are more often due to non-endocrinological disease.

OSCE REVISION TOPICS – THE ENDOCRINE HISTORY

Use these topics, which commonly occur in the OSCE, to help with revision.

1. Please take a history from this patient with a goitre. (pp 440, 448, 452)
2. Please take a history from this woman with recent weight gain. (p 440)
3. Please take a history from this man with loss of weight and polyuria. (pp 441, 464)
4. This woman has had galactorrhoea. Please take a history from her. (pp 441, 454)
5. This woman has developed weight gain and has difficulty getting up out of chairs. Please take an endocrine history from her. (pp 440, 459)

CHAPTER 28
The endocrine examination

The thyroid gland is that which when enlarged by disease gives rise to 'Derbyshire neck' or 'goitre'.
HUXLEY (1872)

A formal examination of the whole endocrine system is not routine. Usually, there will be some clue from the history and general inspection to indicate what specific endocrine disease should be pursued.

THE THYROID
The thyroid gland
Examination anatomy

Even when it is not enlarged, the thyroid[a] (see Fig. 28.1) is the largest endocrine gland (see Fig. 28.2). Enlargement is common, occurring in 10% of women and 2% of men and more commonly in iodine-deficient parts of the world. The normal gland lies anterior to the larynx and trachea and below the laryngeal prominence of the thyroid cartilage. It consists of a narrow isthmus in the middle line (anterior to the second to fourth tracheal rings and 1.5 centimetres in size) and two larger lateral lobes each about 4 centimetres long. Although the position of the larynx varies, the thyroid gland is almost always about 4 centimetres below the larynx.

Inspection

The normal thyroid may be just visible below the cricoid cartilage in a thin young person.[1,2] Usually only the isthmus is visible as a diffuse central swelling. Apparent enlargement (pseudogoitre) can occur as a result of the presence of a fat pad in the anterior and lateral part of the neck; this finding is more common in people who are overweight but can occur in those of normal weight. Enlargement of the gland, called a

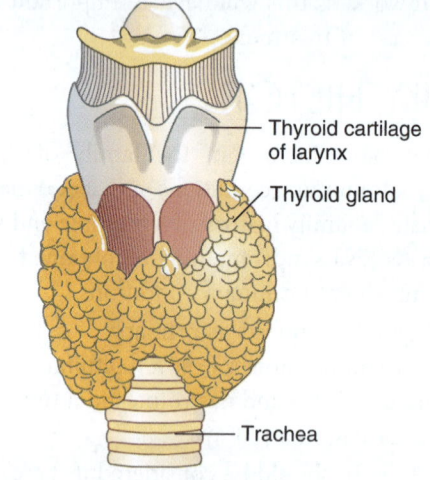

The anatomy of the thyroid

FIGURE 28.1

goitre,[b] should be apparent on inspection (see List 28.1, Good signs guide 28.1), especially if the patient extends the neck. Look at the front and sides of the neck and decide whether there is localised or general swelling of the gland. In healthy people the line between the cricoid cartilage and the suprasternal notch should be straight. An outward bulge suggests the presence of goitre (see Fig. 28.3). Remember that 80% of people with goitre are biochemically euthyroid, 10% are hypothyroid and 10% are hyperthyroid.

The temptation to begin touching a swelling as soon as it has been detected should be resisted until a glass of water has been procured. The patient takes sips from this repeatedly so that swallowing is possible without discomfort. Ask the patient to swallow, and watch the neck swelling carefully. Only a goitre or a thyroglossal

---

[a] The first person to distinguish an enlarged thyroid from cervical lymphadenopathy was the Roman medical writer Aulus Aurelius Cornelius Celsus (approx. 53 BC–AD 7). He is more famous for describing the four cardinal signs of inflammation: redness, swelling, heat and tenderness.

[b] From the Latin *guttur*, meaning 'throat'.

CHAPTER 28 THE ENDOCRINE EXAMINATION 445

> ### CAUSES OF NECK SWELLINGS
>
> **Midline**
>
> Goitre (moves up on swallowing)
>
> Thyroglossal cyst (moves on poking out the tongue with the jaw stationary)
>
> Submental lymph nodes
>
> **Lateral**
>
> Lymph nodes
>
> Salivary glands (e.g. stone, tumour)
> - Submandibular gland
> - Parotid gland (lower pole)
>
> Skin: sebaceous cyst or lipoma
>
> Lymphatics: cystic hygroma (translucent)
>
> Carotid artery: aneurysm or rarely tumour (pulsatile)
>
> Pharynx: pharyngeal pouch, or brachial arch remnant (brachial cyst)
>
> Parathyroid gland (very rare)
>
> LIST 28.1

GOOD SIGNS GUIDE 28.1
Accuracy in clinical assessment of grades of thyroid size (compared with ultrasound findings)

Size of gland	LR+	LR−
Normal ≤20 g	0.26	—
Up to twice normal (20–40 g)	2.6	—
More than twice normal (≥40 g)	13.0	—

(Jarløv AE, Hegedüs L, Gjørup T, Hansen JE. Accuracy of the clinical assessment of thyroid size. *Dan Med Bull* 1991; 38(1):87–89.)

The endocrine glands

FIGURE 28.2

cyst, because of attachment to the larynx, will rise during swallowing. The thyroid and trachea rise about 2 centimetres as the patient swallows; they pause for half a second and then descend. Some non-thyroid masses may rise slightly during swallowing but move up less than the trachea and fall again without pausing. A thyroid gland fixed by neoplastic infiltration may not rise on swallowing, but this is rare. Swallowing also allows the shape of the gland to be seen better.

Note whether an inferior border is visible as the gland rises. The thyroglossal cyst is a midline mass that can present at any age. It is an embryological

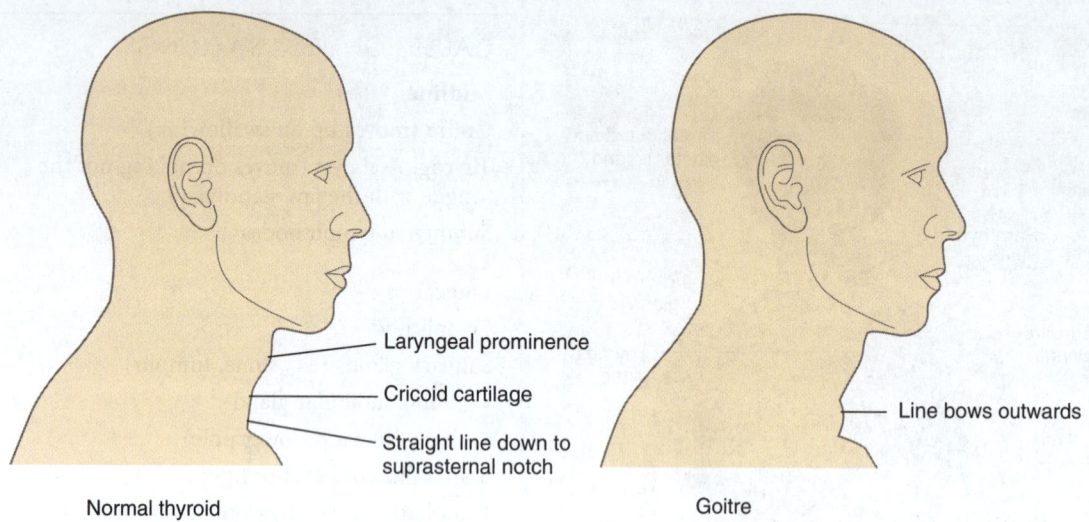

The thyroid and goitre
(Adapted from McGee S. *Evidence-based physical diagnosis*, 2nd edn, St Louis: Saunders, 2007.)

FIGURE 28.3

remnant of the thyroglossal duct. Characteristically it rises when the patient protrudes the tongue.

Inspect the skin of the neck carefully for scars. An old thyroidectomy scar forms a ring around the base of the neck in the position of a high necklace. More recent thyroid scars are much harder to detect because modern surgical techniques make them shorter and locate them in the crease of natural skinfold. Look for prominent veins. Dilated veins over the upper part of the chest wall, often accompanied by filling of the external jugular vein, suggest retrosternal extension of the goitre causing thoracic inlet obstruction. Rarely, redness of the skin over the gland occurs in cases of suppurative thyroiditis.

Palpation

Palpation is best begun from *behind* (see Fig. 28.4) but warn the patient first. Place both hands with the pulps of the fingers over the gland. The patient's neck should be slightly flexed so as to relax the sternocleidomastoid muscles. Feel systematically both lobes of the gland and its isthmus. Feel one side at a time; use one hand to retract the sternocleidomastoid muscle slightly to allow better access to the gland.

Consider the following:
- **Size:** only an approximate estimation is possible (see Fig. 28.5). Feel particularly carefully for a lower border, because its absence suggests retrosternal extension.
- **Shape:** note whether the gland is uniformly enlarged or irregular and whether the isthmus is affected. If a *nodule* that feels distinct from the remaining thyroid tissue is palpable, determine its location, size, consistency, tenderness and

Palpating the thyroid from behind while the patient swallows sips of water

FIGURE 28.4

Goitre.

(a) Large; (b) massive

FIGURE 28.5

> **DIFFERENTIAL DIAGNOSIS OF THYROID NODULES**
>
> 1. Carcinoma (5% of palpable nodules)—fixed to surrounding tissues, palpable lymph nodes, vocal cord paralysis, hard, especially if larger than 4 centimetres (most are, however, smaller than this)
> 2. Adenoma—mobile, no local associated features
> 3. Big nodule in a multinodular goitre—palpable multinodular goitre
>
> LIST 28.2

mobility. Also decide whether the whole gland feels nodular (multinodular goitre).

- **Consistency:** this may vary in different parts of the gland. Soft (but firmer than a fat pad) is normal; the gland is often firm in simple goitre and typically rubbery hard in Hashimoto's thyroiditis. A stony, hard node suggests carcinoma (see List 28.2), calcification in a cyst, fibrosis or Riedel's thyroiditis.
- **Tenderness:** this may be a feature of thyroiditis (subacute or rarely suppurative), or less often of a bleed into a cyst or carcinoma.
- **Mobility:** carcinoma may tether the gland.

- **A thrill:** this may be palpable over the gland, as occurs when the gland is unusually metabolically active (e.g. in thyrotoxicosis).

Repeat the assessment while the patient swallows.

Palpate the cervical lymph nodes. These may be involved in carcinoma of the thyroid.

Move to the *front*. Palpate again. Localised swellings may be more easily defined here. Note the position of the trachea, which may be displaced by a retrosternal gland.

Percussion

The upper part of the manubrium can be percussed from one side to the other. A change from resonant to dull indicates possible retrosternal goitre, but this is not a very reliable sign.

Auscultation

Listen over each lobe for a bruit (a swishing sound coinciding with systole). This is a sign of increased blood supply, which may occur in hyperthyroidism. The differential diagnosis also includes a carotid bruit (louder over the carotid itself) or a venous hum (obliterated by gentle pressure over the base of the neck). If there is a goitre, apply mild compression to the lateral lobes and listen again for stridor.

Pemberton's sign

Ask the patient to lift both arms as high as possible with the elbows close to the ears. Keep the arms raised for 1 minute or until signs of congestion appear. Wait, then search the face eagerly for signs of congestion (plethora) and cyanosis. Associated respiratory distress and inspiratory stridor may occur. Look at the neck

CAUSES OF GOITRE

Causes of a diffuse goitre (patient often euthyroid)
Idiopathic (majority)
Puberty or pregnancy
Thyroiditis
- Hashimoto's
- Subacute (gland usually tender)

Simple goitre (iodine deficiency)
Goitrogens—iodine excess, drugs (e.g. lithium)
Inborn errors of thyroid hormone synthesis (e.g. Pendred's* syndrome—an autosomal-recessive condition associated with nerve deafness)
Thyroid hormone resistance

Causes of a solitary thyroid nodule
Benign:
- Dominant nodule in a multinodular goitre
- Degeneration or haemorrhage into a colloid cyst or nodule
- Follicular adenoma
- Simple cyst (rare)

Malignant:
- Carcinoma—primary or secondary (rare)
- Lymphoma (rare)

*Vaughan Pendred (1869–1946), London physician.

LIST 28.3

QUESTIONS TO ASK THE PATIENT WITH SUSPECTED HYPERTHYROIDISM

! denotes symptoms for the possible diagnosis of an urgent or dangerous problem.

1. Have you any history of thyroid problems?
2. Have you a family history of thyrotoxicosis? (There is a familial incidence of Graves' disease and associated autoimmune conditions such as vitiligo, Addison's disease, pernicious anaemia, type 1 diabetes, myasthenia gravis and premature ovarian failure.)
3. Have you taken amiodarone or thyroxine?
4. Have you had recent exposure to iodine? (Iodinated X-ray contrast materials can precipitate thyrotoxicosis—usually in patients with an existing multinodular goitre.)
! 5. Have you had palpitations? (Thyrotoxicosis can present with atrial fibrillation, which may precipitate heart failure.)
6. Have you noticed insomnia, irritability or hyperactivity?
7. Have you had loss of weight, diarrhoea or increased stool frequency, increased sweating or heat intolerance?
8. Have you had muscle weakness? (Proximal muscle weakness is common and the patient may have noticed difficulty getting out of a chair.)
9. Have you had eye problems such as double vision, grittiness, redness or pain behind the eyes?

QUESTIONS BOX 28.1

veins for distension (venous congestion). Ask the patient to take a deep breath in through the mouth and listen for stridor. This is a test for thoracic inlet obstruction due to retrosternal goitre or any retrosternal mass.[3,c] (Lifting the arms up pulls the thoracic inlet upwards so that the goitre occupies more of this inflexible bony opening.) Examination of the thyroid should be part of every routine physical examination. Causes of goitre are outlined in List 28.3.

Hyperthyroidism (thyrotoxicosis)

Hyperthyroidism is a disease caused by excessive concentrations of thyroid hormones. The cause is usually overproduction by the gland but it may sometimes be due to accidental or deliberate use of thyroid hormone (thyroxine) tablets—*thyrotoxicosis factitia*. Thyroxine is sometimes taken by patients as a way of losing weight. The cause may be apparent in these cases if a careful history is taken (see Questions box 28.1). The antiarrhythmic drug *amiodarone*, which contains large

---
[c] The original description of Pemberton's sign required the arm to be raised for 1 minute. Many students perform this test inadequately as they do not wait long enough.

quantities of iodine, can cause thyrotoxicosis in up to 12% of patients in low-iodine-intake areas. Many of the clinical features of thyrotoxicosis are characterised by signs of sympathetic nervous system overactivity such as tremor, tachycardia and sweating. The explanation is not entirely clear. Catecholamine secretion is usually normal in hyperthyroidism; however, thyroid hormone potentiates the effects of catecholamines, possibly by increasing the number of adrenergic receptors in the tissues.

The most common cause of thyrotoxicosis in young people is Graves'[d] disease, an autoimmune disease where circulating immunoglobulins stimulate thyroid-stimulating hormone (TSH) receptors on the surface of the thyroid follicular cells (see List 28.5 below).

Examine a suspected case of thyrotoxicosis as follows.

Onycholysis (Plummer's nails)

FIGURE 28.6

General inspection

Look for signs of weight loss, anxiety and the frightened facies of thyrotoxicosis.

Hands

Ask the patient to put out his or her arms and look for a fine tremor (due to sympathetic overactivity). Laying a sheet of paper over the patient's fingers may more clearly demonstrate this tremor, to the amazement of less-experienced colleagues.

Look at the nails for *onycholysis* (Plummer's[e] nails; see Fig. 28.6). Onycholysis (where there is separation of the nail from its bed) is said to occur particularly on the ring finger, but can occur on all the fingernails and is apparently due to sympathetic overactivity. Inspect for thyroid acropathy (acropathy is another term for clubbing), seen rarely in Graves' disease but not with other causes of thyrotoxicosis.

Inspect for palmar erythema and feel the palms for warmth and sweatiness (sympathetic overactivity).

Take the pulse. Note the presence of sinus tachycardia (sympathetic overdrive) or atrial fibrillation (due to a shortened refractory period of atrial cells related to sympathetic drive and hormone-induced changes). The pulse may also have a collapsing character due to a high cardiac output.

Thyrotoxicosis: thyroid stare and exophthalmos

FIGURE 28.7

Arms

Ask the patient to raise the arms above the head. Inability to do this suggests proximal myopathy (muscle weakness). Tap the arm reflexes for abnormal briskness, especially in the relaxation phase.

Eyes

Examine the patient's eyes for exophthalmos, which is protrusion of the eyeball from the orbit (see Fig. 28.7 and List 28.4). This may be very obvious, but if not, look carefully at the sclerae, which in exophthalmos are not covered by the lower eyelid. Next look from behind over the patient's forehead for exophthalmos,

---

[d] Robert Graves (1796–1853), a Dublin physician.
[e] Henry Plummer (1874–1936), a physician at the Mayo Clinic in the United States.

> **CAUSES OF EXOPHTHALMOS**
>
> **Bilateral**
> Graves' disease
>
> **Unilateral**
> Tumours of the orbit (e.g. dermoid, optic nerve glioma, neurofibroma, granuloma)
> Cavernous sinus thrombosis
> Graves' disease
> Pseudotumours of the orbit
>
> LIST 28.4

where the eye will be visible anterior to the superior orbital margin. Now examine for the complications of proptosis, which include: (1) chemosis (oedema of the conjunctiva and injection of the sclera, particularly over the insertion of the lateral rectus), (2) conjunctivitis, (3) corneal ulceration (due to inability to close the eyelids), (4) optic atrophy (rare and possibly due to optic nerve stretching) and (5) ophthalmoplegia (the inferior rectus muscle power tends to be lost first, and later convergence is weakened).

There are TSH receptors on orbital muscles and biopsy of these patients shows lymphocyte infiltration. Exophthalmos occurs only in Graves' disease. It may precede the onset of thyrotoxicosis or may persist after the patient has become euthyroid. It is characterised by an inflammatory infiltrate of the orbital contents, but not of the globe itself. The orbital muscles are particularly affected, and an increase in their size accounts for most of the increased volume of the orbital contents and therefore for protrusion of the globe. It is due to an autoimmune abnormality. Treatment with radioactive iodine may worsen Graves' ophthalmopathy.

Next examine for the components of thyroid ophthalmopathy, which are related to sympathetic overactivity and are not specific for Graves' disease. Look for the thyroid stare (a frightened expression) and lid retraction (Dalrymple's[f] sign), where there is sclera visible above the iris. Test for lid lag (von Graefe's[g] sign) by asking the patient to follow your finger as it descends at a moderate rate from the upper to the lower part of the visual field. Descent of the upper lid lags behind descent of the eyeball.

If ptosis is present, one should rule out myasthenia gravis, which can be associated with autoimmune thyroid disease.

Neck

Examine for thyroid enlargement, which is usually detectable (in 60–90% of patients). In Graves' disease the gland is classically diffusely enlarged and is smooth and firm. An associated thrill is usually present, but this finding is not specific for thyrotoxicosis caused by Graves' disease. Absence of thyroid enlargement makes Graves' disease unlikely, but does not exclude it. Possible thyroid abnormalities in patients who are thyrotoxic but do not have Graves' disease include a toxic multinodular goitre, a solitary nodule (toxic adenoma) and painless, postpartum or subacute (de Quervain's[h]) thyroiditis. Patients with de Quervain's thyroiditis typically have a moderately enlarged firm and tender gland. Thyrotoxicosis may occur without any goitre, particularly in elderly patients. Alternatively, in hyperthyroidism due to a rare abnormality of trophoblastic tissue (a hydatidiform mole or choriocarcinoma of the testis or uterus), or excessive thyroid hormone replacement, the thyroid gland will not usually be palpable.

If a thyroidectomy scar is present, assess for hypoparathyroidism (Chvostek's[i] or Trousseau's[j] signs; p 471). These signs are most often present in the first few days after the operation.

Chest

Gynaecomastia (p 476) occurs occasionally. Examine the heart for systolic flow murmurs (due to increased cardiac output) and signs of congestive cardiac failure, which may be precipitated by thyrotoxicosis in older people.

Legs

Look first for pretibial myxoedema. This takes the form of bilateral firm, elevated dermal nodules and plaques,

---

[f] John Dalrymple (1803–52), a British ophthalmic surgeon.
[g] Friedrich von Graefe (1828–70), a professor of ophthalmology in Berlin, described this in 1864. He was one of the most famous ophthalmologists of the 19th century; Horner was one of his pupils. He died of tuberculosis at the age of 42.

[h] Fritz de Quervain (1868–1940), a professor of surgery in Berne, Switzerland.
[i] Franz Chvostek (1835–84), a Viennese physician.
[j] Armand Trousseau (1801–67), a Parisian physician.

which can be pink, brown or skin coloured. They are caused by mucopolysaccharide accumulation. Despite the name, this occurs only in Graves' disease and not in hypothyroidism. Test now for proximal myopathy and hyperreflexia in the legs, which is present in only about 25% of cases.

Hypothyroidism (myxoedema)

Hypothyroidism (deficiency of thyroid hormone) is due to primary disease of the thyroid or, less commonly, is secondary to pituitary or hypothalamic failure (see List 28.5). Myxoedema implies a more severe form of hypothyroidism. In myxoedema, for unknown reasons, hydrophilic mucopolysaccharides accumulate in the ground substance of tissues including the skin. This results in excessive interstitial fluid, which is relatively immobile, causing skin thickening and a doughy induration.

The symptoms of hypothyroidism are insidious but patients or their relatives may have noticed cold intolerance, muscle pains, oedema, constipation, a hoarse voice, dry skin, memory loss, depression or weight gain (see Questions box 28.2).

Examine the patient with suspected hypothyroidism as follows (see Good signs guide 28.2).

General inspection

Look for signs of obvious mental and physical sluggishness, or evidence of the very rare myxoedema madness. Hypothyroid speech is a feature in about

---

CAUSES OF THYROTOXICOSIS AND HYPOTHYROIDISM

Causes of thyrotoxicosis

PRIMARY

Graves' disease

Toxic multinodular goitre

Toxic uninodular goitre: usually a toxic adenoma

Hashimoto's thyroiditis (early in its course; later it produces hypothyroidism)

Subacute thyroiditis (transient)

Postpartum thyroiditis (non-tender)

Iodine-induced (Jod-Basedow* phenomenon—iodine given after a previously deficient diet)

SECONDARY

Pituitary (very rare): TSH hypersecretion

Hydatidiform moles or choriocarcinomas: hCG secretion (rare)

Struma ovarii (rare)

Drugs (e.g. excess thyroid hormone ingestion, amiodarone)

Causes of hypothyroidism

PRIMARY

Without a goitre (decreased or absent thyroid tissue):
- Idiopathic atrophy
- Treatment of thyrotoxicosis (e.g. ^{131}I, surgery)
- Agenesis or a lingual thyroid
- Unresponsiveness to TSH

With a goitre (decreased thyroid hormone synthesis):
- Chronic autoimmune diseases (e.g. Hashimoto's thyroiditis)
- Drugs (e.g. lithium, amiodarone)
- Inborn errors (enzyme deficiency)
- Endemic iodine deficiency or iodine-induced hypothyroidism

SECONDARY

Pituitary lesions (see List 28.7)

TERTIARY

Hypothalamic lesions

TRANSIENT

Thyroid hormone treatment withdrawn and not hypothyroid

Subacute thyroiditis

Postpartum thyroiditis

Post subtotal thyroidectomy

*Carl von Basedow (1799–1854), a German general practitioner, described this in 1840 (Jod=iodine in German).
hCG=human chorionic gonadotrophin; TSH=thyroid-stimulating hormone.

LIST 28.5

452 SECTION 8 THE ENDOCRINE SYSTEM

QUESTIONS TO ASK THE PATIENT WITH SUSPECTED HYPOTHYROIDISM

1. Have you found cold weather more difficult to cope with recently?
2. Have you had problems with constipation?
3. Have you gained weight?
4. Have you noticed that your skin has become dry?
5. Do you think your memory is not as good as it was? Have you felt depressed?
6. Do you think your voice has become hoarse? (Hypothyroid speech—characteristically slow and nasal—occurs in one-third of patients.)
7. Have you noticed swelling of your legs?

QUESTIONS BOX 28.2

GOOD SIGNS GUIDE 28.2
Hypothyroidism

Sign	LR+	LR−
SKIN		
Coarse	2.6	0.71
Cool and dry	5.1	0.69
Cold palms	1.6	0.82
Dry palms	1.5	0.80
Periorbital puffiness	3.2	0.61
Puffiness of wrists	3.1	0.80
Loss of eyebrow hair	1.95	0.83
SPEECH		
Hypothyroid speech	2.3	0.83
THYROID GLAND		
Goitre	2.6	0.68
PULSE		
<70 beats per minute	3.9	0.64

one-third of patients. This is characteristically slow, nasal and deep in pitch. Obesity is no more common than in euthyroid people.

Hands

Note peripheral cyanosis (due to reduced cardiac output) and swelling of the skin, which may appear cool and dry. The yellow discoloration of hypercarotenaemia (there is slowing down of hepatic metabolism of carotene) may be seen on the palms. Look for palmar crease pallor—anaemia may be due to: (1) chronic disease; (2) folate deficiency secondary to bacterial overgrowth, or vitamin B_{12} deficiency due to associated pernicious anaemia; or (3) iron deficiency due to menorrhagia.

Take the pulse, which may be of small volume and slow. Test for sensory loss, as the carpal tunnel is thickened in myxoedema.

Arms

Test for proximal myopathy (rare) and a 'hung-up' biceps or Achilles tendon reflex (see below).

Face

Inspect the patient's face (see Fig. 28.8). The skin, but not the sclerae, may appear yellow due to hypercarotenaemia.

Myxoedema

FIGURE 28.8

The skin may be generally thickened, and alopecia may be present, as may vitiligo (an associated autoimmune disease).

Inspect the eyes for periorbital oedema. Loss or thinning of the outer third of the eyebrows can occur in myxoedema but is also common in healthy people. Look for xanthelasmata (due to associated hypercholesterolaemia). Palpate for coolness and dryness of the skin and hair. There may be thinning of the scalp hair.

Look at the tongue for swelling. Ask the patient to speak, and listen for coarse, croaking, slow speech. Bilateral nerve deafness may occur with endemic or congenital hypothyroidism.

Thyroid gland

A primary decrease in thyroid hormone results in a compensatory oversecretion of TSH. A goitre will result if there is viable thyroid tissue.

Many cases of hypothyroidism are not associated with an enlarged gland as there is little thyroid tissue. The exceptions include severe iodine deficiency, enzyme deficiency (inborn errors of metabolism), late Hashimoto's disease and treated (with radioactive iodine) thyrotoxicosis (see List 28.5).

Chest

Examine the heart for a pericardial effusion and the lungs for pleural effusions.

Legs

There may be non-pitting oedema. Ask the patient to kneel on a chair with the ankles exposed. Tap the Achilles tendon with a reflex hammer. There is apparently normal (in fact, slightly slowed) contraction followed by delayed relaxation of the foot in hypothyroidism (the 'hung-up' reflex; see Fig. 28.11). Examine for signs of peripheral neuropathy and for other uncommon neurological abnormalities associated with hypothyroidism (see List 28.6).

THE PITUITARY
Examination anatomy

Although it is not placed where it can be examined directly, the neighbouring structures of this gland (see Fig. 28.9) can be affected by its enlargement (as a macroadenoma) and cause examination abnormalities. Microadenomas may cause signs as a result of their effect on hormonal activity. Posterior pituitary function is rarely affected, even with large macroadenomas.

> ### NEUROLOGICAL ASSOCIATIONS OF HYPOTHYROIDISM
>
> **Common**
> Entrapment: carpal tunnel, tarsal tunnel
> Delayed ankle jerks
> Muscle cramps
>
> **Uncommon**
> Peripheral neuropathy
> Proximal myopathy
> Hypokalaemic periodic paralysis
> Cerebellar syndrome
> Psychosis
> Coma
> Unmasking of myasthenia gravis
> Cerebrovascular disease
> High cerebrospinal fluid protein
> Nerve deafness
>
> LIST 28.6

- Superior to the gland lies the optic chiasm.
- Inferior to the gland lies the sphenoid bone and sphenoid (air) sinus.
- Laterally lie the cavernous (venous) sinuses, which contain the cranial nerves—III, IV, V and VI.

The gland has two parts: the anterior (adenohypophysis) and posterior (neurohypophysis). The anterior pituitary secretes six main hormones:

1. thyroid-stimulating hormone (TSH)
2. adrenocorticotrophic hormone (ACTH)
3. luteinising hormone (LH)
4. follicle-stimulating hormone (FSH)
5. growth hormone (GH)
6. prolactin.

The posterior pituitary secretes:

1. vasopressin (antidiuretic hormone [ADH])
2. oxytocin.

Pituitary tumours can present as a result of: (1) local effects such as headaches, or visual field loss and (2) changes in pituitary hormone secretion. (See

The cavernous sinus and its relationship with the cranial nerves and pituitary gland

FIGURE 28.9

Questions box 28.3.) These changes include: (1) excess growth hormone, causing acromegaly; (2) excess ACTH, causing Cushing's disease; (3) excess prolactin, causing galactorrhoea, impotence or secondary amenorrhoea; (4) excess TSH, causing hyperthyroidism; and (5) hormone deficiency (hypopituitarism, e.g. lost of gonadotropins causing sexual dysfunction).

Panhypopituitarism

Panhypopituitarism is a deficiency of most or all of the pituitary hormones and is usually due to a space-occupying lesion or destruction of the pituitary gland (see List 28.7). Hormone production is often lost in the following order:

1. GH (dwarfism in children, insulin sensitivity in adults)
2. prolactin (failure of lactation after delivery)
3. gonadotrophins (loss of secondary sexual characteristics, secondary amenorrhoea in women, loss of libido and infertility in men)
4. TSH (hypothyroidism)
5. ACTH (hypoadrenalism, with loss of secondary sexual hair due to decreased adrenal androgen production).

The posterior pituitary is usually spared in cases of pituitary adenoma. Loss of ADH results in profuse dilute urine output (diabetes insipidus).

However, isolated single hormonal deficiencies or multiple deficiencies may occur in any combination.

> **QUESTIONS TO ASK THE PATIENT WITH SUSPECTED PANHYPOPITUITARISM**
>
> 1. Have you had problems with lethargy, weakness and fatigue, or weight loss or poor appetite? (Adrenocorticoid deficiency)
> 2. Have you gained weight, found cold weather more intolerable or had constipation? (TSH deficiency)
> 3. (Men) Have you noticed reduced sexual interest (libido), reduced muscle strength, erectile dysfunction or had problems with infertility? (FSH deficiency)
> 4. (Women) Have you had cessation of periods or less bleeding during menstruation? (Oligomenorrhoea due to FSH deficiency)
> 5. Have you noticed reduced exercise ability and energy? (GH deficiency in adults)
> 6. Have you had headaches or visual disturbance? (Pituitary enlargement)
>
> QUESTIONS BOX 28.3

General inspection

The patient may be of short stature (failure of growth hormone secretion before growth is complete). Look for pallor of the skin (due to anaemia or occasionally

CAUSES OF HYPOPITUITARISM

Space-occupying lesion
- Pituitary tumour (non-secretory or secretory)
- Other tumours: craniopharyngioma, metastatic carcinoma
- Granulomata (e.g. sarcoid, tuberculosis)

Iatrogenic (e.g. surgery or irradiation)

Head injury

Sheehan's* syndrome (postpartum pituitary haemorrhage resulting in necrosis of the gland)

Empty sella syndrome (often an incidental MRI scan finding and not always associated with pituitary insufficiency)

Infarction or pituitary apoplexy

Idiopathic

Drug related (monoclonal antibodies to immune regulators)

*Harold Sheehan (1900–88), a professor of pathology in Liverpool, England, described the syndrome in 1937.
MRI=magnetic resonance imaging.

LIST 28.7

Secondary sexual development (Tanner stages 1–5)

These changes begin at puberty in response to pituitary gonadotrophins.

Males

Stage	
1	Preadolescent
2	Enlargement of testes and scrotum
3	Lengthening of penis
4	Increase in penis breadth, glans development and scrotal darkening
5	Adult: above, plus pubic hair spread to medial surface of the thighs

Females

Breasts		Pubic hair	
Stage		Stage	
1	Preadolescent	1	No pubic hair
2	Breast bud (elevation of breasts and papilla)	2	Sparse growth, mainly over the labia
3	Enlargement of breast and areola (no separation of contours)	3	Darker, coarser, more curled hairs but sparse over the junction of the pubes
4	Areola and papilla project above breast level (secondary mound)	4	Adult type but no hair spread to medial surface of thighs
5	Adult: areola is recessed and papilla projects	5	Adult: horizontal pattern and hair spread to medial thighs

TABLE 28.1

loss of α-melanocyte-stimulating hormone [MSH]) and fine-wrinkled skin and lack of body hair (due to gonadotrophin deficiency). There may be complete absence of the secondary sexual characteristics (see Table 28.1 and Figs 37.33 and 37.34 on p 679) if gonadotrophin failure occurred before puberty.

Face

Look at the face more closely. Multiple skin wrinkles around the eyes are characteristic of gonadotrophin deficiency. Inspect the forehead carefully for hypophysectomy scars—transfrontal scars will be apparent (see Fig. 28.10) but not transsphenoidal ones, as this operation is performed through the base of the nose, via an incision under the upper lip.

Examine the eyes (see Ch 32). The visual fields must be assessed for any defects, especially bitemporal hemianopia (an enlarging pituitary tumour may compress the optic chiasm), and the fundi examined for optic atrophy (optic nerve compression from a pituitary tumour). Assess the third, fourth, sixth and first divisions of the fifth cranial nerves, as these may be affected by extrapituitary tumour expansion into the cavernous sinus (see Fig. 28.9).

Feel the facial hair over the bearded area in men for normal beard growth (which is lost with gonadotrophin deficiency).

Chest

Go on to the chest. Look for skin pallor and for a decrease in nipple pigmentation. In men, decreased body hair (axillary and chest) may be present. In women, secondary breast atrophy may be found.

Genital region

Loss of pubic hair occurs in both sexes. In men, testicular atrophy may be present. Atrophied testes are characteristically small and firm. The normal-sized testis is about 15–25 mL in volume.

Acromegaly: common signs

FIGURE 28.10

Testing ankle jerks (second method—see also p 571).

This method best demonstrates the 'hung-up' reflexes of hypothyroidism. Look for rapid dorsiflexion followed by slow plantar flexion after the tendon is tapped

FIGURE 28.11

Ankle reflexes

Test for 'hung-up' jerks (see Fig. 28.11). These are an important sign of pituitary hypothyroidism. Occasionally, pituitary hypothyroid patients may be slightly overweight, but the classical myxoedematous appearance is usually absent.

Acromegaly

Acromegaly[k] is excessive secretion of growth hormone, typically due to an eosinophilic pituitary adenoma. Growth hormone stimulates the liver and other tissues to produce somatomedins, which in turn promote growth. Growth hormone is also a protein anabolic hormone exerting its effects at the ribosomal level, and it is diabetogenic as it exerts an anti-insulin effect in muscle and increases hepatic glucose release. The disease has a very gradual onset and patients may not have noticed symptoms. Most patients, however, have headache caused by stretching of the dura by the enlarging pituitary tumour.

Gigantism is the result of growth hormone hypersecretion occurring before puberty and fusion of the epiphyses. It results in massive skeletal as well as soft-tissue growth. Acromegaly occurs when the growth plates have fused, so that only soft-tissue and flat-bone enlargements are possible.

General inspection

The face and body habitus may be characteristic (see Figs 28.10 and 28.12).

Hands

Sit the patient on the side of the bed or in a chair and look at his or her hands. Notice a wide spade-like shape (due to soft-tissue and bony enlargement). Increased sweating and warmth of the palms may be noted. This is due to an increased metabolic rate. The skin may appear thickened. Changes of osteoarthritis in the hands are common and are due to skeletal overgrowth. Examine for median nerve entrapment, which can occur because of soft-tissue overgrowth in the carpal tunnel area.

---

[k] Acromegaly was first described by Pierre Marie in 1886 and was first called hyperpituitarism by Harvey Cushing in 1909. The acral parts are the hands and feet.

Acromegaly.

(a) This patient has outgrown three wedding rings; (b) skin tags; (c) macroglossia; (d) prognathism

FIGURE 28.12

Arms
Proximal myopathy may be present. Palpate behind the medial epicondyle (the 'funny bone') for ulnar nerve thickening.

Axillae
Carefully inspect the axillae for skin tags (called acrochordons, which are non-tender skin-coloured protrusions; see Fig. 28.12(b)). Summon up courage and feel for greasy skin. Look for acanthosis nigricans.

Face
Look for a large supraorbital ridge, which causes frontal bossing (this may also occur occasionally in Paget's disease, rickets, achondroplasia and hydrocephalus). The lips may be thickened.

Examine the eyes for visual field defects; classically there may be bitemporal hemianopia if the pituitary tumour is large. Look in the fundi for optic atrophy (due to nerve compression) and papilloedema (due to raised intracranial pressure with an extensive tumour). The presence of angioid streaks (red, brown or grey streaks that are three to five times the diameter of a retinal vein and appear to emanate from the optic disc) should also be sought: these are due to degeneration and fibrosis of Bruch's membrane. Also note hypertensive changes or diabetic changes in the fundus. Ocular palsies may occur with an extensive pituitary tumour.

Look in the mouth for an enlarged tongue that may not fit neatly between the teeth. The teeth themselves may be splayed and separated, with malocclusion as the jaw enlarges. The lower jaw may look square and firm (as it does on some American actors). When the jaw protrudes it is called prognathism.[1]

Neck
The thyroid may be diffusely enlarged or multinodular (all the internal organs may enlarge under the influence of growth hormone). Listen to the voice for hoarseness.

Chest
Look for coarse body hair and gynaecomastia. Examine the heart for signs of arrhythmias, cardiomegaly and congestive cardiac failure, which may be due to ischaemic heart disease, hypertension or cardiomyopathy (all more common in acromegaly).

Back
Inspect for kyphosis.

Abdomen
Examine for hepatic, splenic and renal enlargement, and look for testicular atrophy (the latter indicating gonadotrophin deficiency secondary to an enlarging pituitary tumour). Acromegaly may be associated with a mixed pituitary tumour, and resultant hyperprolactinaemia can also cause testicular atrophy.

Lower limbs
Look for signs of osteoarthritis in the hips especially, and knees (Ch 24), and for pseudogout. Foot drop may be present because of common peroneal nerve entrapment (p 576).

Signs of activity
Decide whether or not the disease is active. Signs of active disease include:
- large numbers of skin tags (however, these can occur commonly in healthy people in parts of the skin subject to friction, e.g. in the axillae, especially in people who are overweight)
- excessive sweating
- the presence of glycosuria
- increasing visual field loss
- enlarging goitre
- hypertension.

Note: Headache also suggests disease activity.

---

[1] From the Greek *pro* meaning 'forwards' and *gnathos* meaning 'jaw'.

Urinalysis and blood pressure
Test the urine for glucose, as excess growth hormone is diabetogenic in 25% of cases. Take the blood pressure to test for hypertension.

Other pituitary syndromes
Cushing's syndrome can occur as a result of excess pituitary ACTH secretion but has other causes as well. Hyperthyroidism can occur as a result of excess pituitary TSH production. Prolactinomas of the pituitary can cause galactorrhoea (production of milk) in both women and men.

THE ADRENALS
Cushing's syndrome
Cushing's syndrome is due to a chronic excess of glucocorticoids. Steroids have multiple effects on the body, due to stimulation of the DNA-dependent synthesis of select messenger ribonucleic acids (mRNAs). This leads to the formation of enzymes that alter cell function and result in increased protein catabolism and gluconeogenesis. Remember that Cushing's disease is specifically pituitary ACTH overproduction, whereas Cushing's syndrome is due to excessive steroid hormone production from any cause (see List 28.8, Good signs guide 28.3 and Questions box 28.4).

CAUSES OF CUSHING'S SYNDROME

Exogenous administration of excess steroids or ACTH (most common)

Adrenal hyperplasia
- Secondary to pituitary ACTH production (Cushing's disease)
    - Microadenoma
    - Macroadenoma
    - Pituitary–hypothalamic dysfunction
- Secondary to ACTH-producing tumours (e.g. small-cell lung carcinoma)

Adrenal neoplasia
- Adenoma
- Carcinoma (rare)

ACTH = adrenocorticotrophic hormone.

LIST 28.8

GOOD SIGNS GUIDE 28.3
Cushing's syndrome

Sign	LR+	LR−
VITAL SIGNS		
Hypertension	1.5	0.74
BODY HABITUS		
Moon face	1.7	0.05
Central obesity	3.7	0.17
General obesity	0.12	2.0
SKIN FINDINGS		
Thin skinfold	29.7	0.22
Plethora	2.7	0.25
Hirsutism	1.8	0.67
Ecchymoses	4.3	0.48
Red or purple striae	1.9	0.70
Acne	2.2	0.63
EXTREMITIES		
Proximal muscle weakness	3.95	0.45
Oedema	2.0	0.73

QUESTIONS TO ASK THE PATIENT WITH SUSPECTED CUSHING'S SYNDROME

! denotes symptoms for the possible diagnosis of an urgent or dangerous problem.

1. Have you gained a lot of weight recently? How much?
2. Do you bruise easily?
3. Has your skin become thin?
4. Have you had problems with acne?
! 5. Have you felt agitated and been unable to sleep?
6. Have you had problems with weakness of your muscles or difficulty getting up out of chairs? (Proximal myopathy)
7. Have you had problems maintaining erections (men) or had amenorrhoea (women)?
8. Have you been diagnosed with diabetes?

QUESTIONS BOX 28.4

Hands

Skinfold thickness is best assessed on the backs of the hands and may be reliable as a sign of Cushing's syndrome only in young women. The skinfold should be thicker than 1.8 millimetres.

Standing

Have the patient undress to the underpants and, if possible, stand up. Look from the front, back and sides. Note *moon-like facies* (see Fig. 28.13a) and *central obesity* (see Fig. 28.14). The limbs appear thin despite sometimes very gross truncal (mostly intra-abdominal rather than subcutaneous fat) obesity.[m] This is the characteristic fat distribution that occurs with steroid excess. *Bruising* may be present (due to loss of perivascular supporting tissue–protein catabolism). Look for excessive *pigmentation* on the extensor surfaces (because of MSH-like activity in the ACTH molecule). Ask the patient to squat at this point to test for *proximal myopathy*, due to mobilisation of muscle tissue or excessive urinary potassium loss. Look at the back for the *buffalo hump* (see Fig. 28.13b), which is due to fat deposition over the interscapular area. Palpate for bony *tenderness* of the vertebral bodies due to crush fractures from osteoporosis (due to inhibition by cortisol of osteoblastic maturation and function).

Sitting

Ask the patient to sit on the side of the bed, but remember that he or she may be suffering from steroid psychosis and refuses to do anything you ask.

Face and neck

Look for plethora (this occurs in the absence of polycythaemia, which, however, may also be present). The face may have a typical moon shape owing to fat deposition in the upper part. Inspect for acne and hirsutism (if adrenal androgen secretion is also increased). Telangiectasias may also be present. There may be periorbital oedema.

Examine the visual fields for signs of a pituitary tumour, and the fundi for optic atrophy, papilloedema and hypertensive or diabetic changes. Look for supraclavicular fat pads.

---

[m] The enthusiastic student can calculate the central obesity index. This is the sum of three truncal circumferences (neck, chest and waist) divided by six peripheral ones (arms, thighs and legs on both sides). A normal index is less than 1.

Cushing's syndrome.

(a) Moon face; (b) buffalo hump

(From Townsend C. *Sabiston's textbook of surgery*, 18th edn. Philadelphia: Saunders, 2007.)

FIGURE 28.13

Abdominal striae in a man with Cushing's syndrome

(From Townsend C. *Sabiston's textbook of surgery*, 18th edn. Philadelphia: Saunders, 2007.)

FIGURE 28.14

Abdomen

Ask the patient to lie in the bed on one pillow. Examine the abdomen for purple striae, which are due to weakening and disruption of collagen fibres in the dermis, leading to exposure of vascular subcutaneous tissues (see Fig. 28.14). In patients with Cushing's syndrome these are wider (1 centimetre) than those seen in people who have gained weight rapidly for other reasons. They may also be present near the axillae on the upper arms or on the inside of the thighs. Palpate for adrenal masses (rarely a large adrenal carcinoma will be palpable over the renal area). Palpate for hepatomegaly due to fat deposition or, rarely, to adrenal carcinoma deposits.

Legs

Palpate for oedema (due to salt and water retention). Look for bruising and poor wound healing.

Urinalysis and blood pressure

Test the urine for sugar (as steroids are diabetogenic; this is due to an increase in hepatic gluconeogenesis and an anti-insulin effect on peripheral tissues). Hypertension is common owing to salt and water retention (from the minerolacorticoid effect of cortisol) and possibly to increased angiotensin secretion or a direct effect on blood vessels.

Synthesis of signs

Certain signs are of some aetiological value in Cushing's syndrome:

- **Signs that suggest adrenal carcinoma may be the underlying cause:** (1) a palpable abdominal mass, (2) signs of virilisation in the female, (3) gynaecomastia in the male.
- **Signs that suggest ectopic ACTH production may be the cause:** (1) absence of the Cushingoid body habitus unless the responsible tumour has

CAUSES OF ADRENAL INSUFFICIENCY

Chronic
PRIMARY
Autoimmune adrenal disease
Infection (tuberculosis, HIV)
Granuloma
Following heparin therapy
Malignant infiltration
Haemochromatosis
Adrenoleucodystrophy

SECONDARY
Pituitary or hypothalamic disease

Acute
Septicaemia: meningococcal
Adrenalectomy
Any stress in a patient with chronic hypoadrenalism or abrupt cessation of prolonged high-dose steroid therapy

LIST 28.9

Palmar crease pigmentation in Addison's disease

FIGURE 28.15

Vitiligo involving the fingers

FIGURE 28.16

been slow growing and allowed time for Cushingoid features to develop, (2) more prominent oedema and hypertension, (3) marked muscle weakness. *Note:* When Cushing's is due to ectopic ACTH production from a small-cell carcinoma, the patient is much more likely to be male (LR+ 13) and the history to be of more rapid onset of the symptoms and signs (18 months: LR+ 15).[4]

- **Significance of hyperpigmentation:** this suggests an extra-adrenal tumour, or enlargement of an ACTH-secreting pituitary adenoma following adrenalectomy (Nelson's[n] syndrome).

Addison's disease

Addison's disease[o] is adrenocortical hypofunction with reduction in the secretion of glucocorticoids and mineralocorticoids. It is most often due to autoimmune disease of the adrenal glands. Other causes are outlined in List 28.9.

If this disease is suspected, look for cachexia. Then, with the patient undressed, look for pigmentation in the palmar creases (see Fig. 28.15), elbows, gums and buccal mucosa and genital area and in scars. This occurs because of compensatory MSH hypersecretion in primary hypoadrenalism (when there is adrenal disease), as ACTH has melanocyte-stimulating activity. Also inspect for vitiligo (localised hypomelanosis; see Fig. 28.16), an autoimmune disease that is commonly associated with autoimmune adrenal failure.

Take the blood pressure and test for postural hypotension. Remember that the rest of the autoimmune disease cluster may be associated with autoimmune adrenal failure (see Table 28.2).

---
[n] Warren Nelson (1906–64), an American endocrinologist.
[o] Thomas Addison (1793–1860) described the disease in 1849. Addison, Bright and Hodgkin made up the famous trio of physicians at Guy's Hospital, London.

A classification of conditions found in various combinations in autoimmune polyglandular syndromes

Type I (rare autosomal recessive)	Type II (more common, HLA DRB1, DQA1, DQB1)
1 Chronic mucocutaneous candidiasis	1 Insulin-requiring diabetes (type 1)
2 Hypoparathyroidism	2 Autoimmune thyroid disease
3 Addison's disease	3 Addison's disease
	4 Myasthenia gravis
	5 Pernicious anaemia
	6 Primary gonadal failure

TABLE 28.2

T&O'C ESSENTIALS

1. The endocrine examination is usually targeted at the likely endocrine disease suggested by the history.
2. The pituitary gland can cause endocrine disease anywhere in the body but headache and visual loss are important abnormalities caused by local effects in the brain.
3. Some endocrine conditions present as a 'spot' diagnosis (e.g. acromegaly, Cushing's syndrome, Addison's disease).
4. Always be on the lookout for subtle abnormalities of facial appearance or body habitus that may suggest endocrine disease: if you do not actively think about this in the first few seconds of general inspection, you will probably miss these abnormalities (and you should then kick yourself).

OSCE REVISION TOPICS – THE ENDOCRINE EXAMINATION

Use these topics, which commonly occur in the OSCE, to help with revision.

1. This man has been diagnosed with acromegaly. Please take a history from him. (p 456)
2. Please examine this man with acromegaly and try to decide whether there are signs of active disease. (p 456)
3. This woman has been diagnosed with Cushing's syndrome. Please examine her and outline the findings consistent with the condition. (p 459)
4. This man has a suspected pituitary abnormality. Please take a brief history from him and then perform a relevant examination. (p 453)

References

1. Alvi A, Johnson JT. The neck mass. A challenging differential diagnosis. *Postgrad Med* 1995; 97:87–90, 93–94. Reviews how the history and examination narrow the differential diagnosis.
2. Siminoski K. Does this patient have a goiter? *JAMA* 1995; 273:813–817. A guide to examining the thyroid.
3. Wallace C, Siminoski K. The Pemberton sign. *Ann Intern Med* 1996; 125:568–569. Describes the sign, due to a retrosternal goitre compressing cephalic venous inflow (and in some tracheal airflow).
4. McGee S. *Evidence-based physical diagnosis*, 3rd edn. Philadelphia: Saunders, 2012.

CHAPTER 29
Correlation of physical signs and endocrine disease

Remember, however, that every patient upon whom you wait will examine you critically and form an estimate of you by the way in which you conduct yourself at the bedside.

SIR WILLIAM OSLER (1849–1919)

DIABETES MELLITUS

Diabetes mellitus[a] is characterised by hyperglycaemia due to an absolute or a relative deficiency of insulin. The causes of diabetes are outlined in List 29.1. The disease can present with asymptomatic glycosuria detected on routine physical examination or with symptoms of diabetes (see List 27.1 on p 440), ranging from polyuria to coma as a result of diabetic ketoacidosis (see Questions box 29.1), or hyperosmolar hyperglycemia syndrome.

General inspection

Assess for evidence of dehydration because the osmotic diuresis caused by a glucose load in the urine can cause massive fluid loss. Note obesity (type 2 diabetics are usually obese) or signs of recent weight loss (this can be evidence of uncontrolled glycosuria).

Look for one of the abnormal endocrine facies (e.g. Cushing's syndrome or acromegaly) and for pigmentation (e.g. haemochromatosis—bronze diabetes) as these may cause secondary diabetes.

The patient may be comatose due to dehydration, acidosis or plasma hyperosmolality. Kussmaul's breathing ('air hunger') is present in diabetic ketoacidosis due to the acidosis (this occurs because fat metabolism is increased to compensate for the lack of availability of glucose; excess acetyl-coenzyme A is produced, which is converted in the liver to ketone bodies, and two of these are organic acids).

Lower limbs

Unlike most other systematic examinations, assessment of the patient with diabetes can profitably begin with the legs, as many of the major physical signs are to be found here. In particular, vascular and neurological abnormalities in the feet must not be missed.[1]

Inspection

Look at the skin. The skin of the feet and lower legs may be hairless and atrophied due to small-vessel vascular disease and resultant ischaemia (the mechanism is uncertain, but may be related to lipoprotein alterations in the vessel walls).

Note any leg *ulcers*, particularly on the toes or any area of the feet exposed to pressure (see Fig. 29.2). These ulcers are due to a combination of ischaemia and peripheral neuropathy (the cause of the neuropathy is unknown, but may be related to small-vessel ischaemia and glycosylation of neural proteins). Look at the ankles for signs of a Charcot's joint (grossly deformed disorganised joints, due to loss of proprioception or pain, or both; this leads to recurrent and unnoticed injury to the joint). Damage to the skin unprotected by pain sensation can also occur.

Look for superficial skin *infection*, such as boils, cellulitis and fungal infections. These are more common in patients with diabetes because of a combination of high tissue glucose levels and ischaemia, which provides a favourable environment for the growth of organisms.

Note any *pigmented scars* (late diabetic dermopathy). There may be small rounded plaques with raised borders lying in a linear fashion over the shins (diabetic dermopathy).

Necrobiosis lipoidica diabeticorum is a reasonably specific skin manifestation of diabetes mellitus, but is

---

[a] This disease was called diabetes by ancient Greek and Roman physicians because the word *diabetes* means a siphon, referring to the large urine volume. Rather courageously, they distinguished diabetes mellitus from diabetes insipidus by the sweet taste of the urine: *mellitus*, 'sweet, honeyed'; *insipidus*, 'tasteless'.

CAUSES OF DIABETES MELLITUS

Type 1
- Type 1A (autoimmune destruction of beta cells in the pancreas)
- Adult-onset type 1 (islet cell antibodies)

Type 2 (insulin deficiency and resistance)—by far the most common type of diabetes

Other types of diabetes
- Mutations leading to abnormalities of β-cell function
- Inherited defects of insulin action (e.g. lipoatrophic diabetes—characterised by generalised lipoatrophy, hepatomegaly, hirsutism, acanthosis nigricans, hyperpigmentation and hyperlipidaemia)
- Diseases of the exocrine pancreas (e.g. chronic pancreatitis, carcinoma, haemochromatosis)
- Endocrine abnormalities (e.g. acromegaly, Cushing's syndrome, phaeochromocytoma, glucagonoma, somatostatinoma)
- Drug-induced (e.g. steroids, the contraceptive pill, streptozotocin, diazoxide, phenytoin, thiazide diuretics)
- Infections (e.g. cytomegalovirus, coxsackie, congenital rubella)
- Rare forms of immune-mediated diabetes (e.g. anti-insulin receptor antibodies)
- Genetic abnormalities associated with diabetes (e.g. Down's syndrome, Klinefelter's syndrome, Turner's syndrome, cystic fibrosis)
- Stiff person syndrome (progressive muscle stiffness of axial muscles)

Gestational diabetes mellitus

LIST 29.1

QUESTIONS TO ASK THE DIABETIC PATIENT

! denotes symptoms for the possible diagnosis of an urgent or dangerous problem.

1. What was your age at the time diabetes was diagnosed?
2. Did you require insulin from the start?
3. What was the problem that led to the diagnosis? (Polyuria, thirst, weight loss, recurrent skin infections, screening assessment)
4. What previous and current drug treatment are you taking for diabetes?
5. What diet has been prescribed?
6. What blood glucose testing do you do? What are the usual results?
! 7. Have you had any problems with hypoglycaemia (low blood sugars)? Have you had episodes of sweating, confusion, malaise or unconsciousness?
8. Do you know what action should be taken if these acute symptoms (of hypo- or hyperglycaemia) occur?
9. Have you had ketoacidosis (very high blood glucose associated with acidosis) and needed admission to hospital? (Polyuria, dehydration, confusion, unconsciousness)
10. Have you had complications of diabetes—eyes, nerves, blood vessels, kidneys, erections (males)?
11. What regular testing has been performed for these problems?
12. How do you and your family cope with this chronic condition?
13. Have you been able to work?

QUESTIONS BOX 29.1

A summary of the examination of the patient with diabetes mellitus

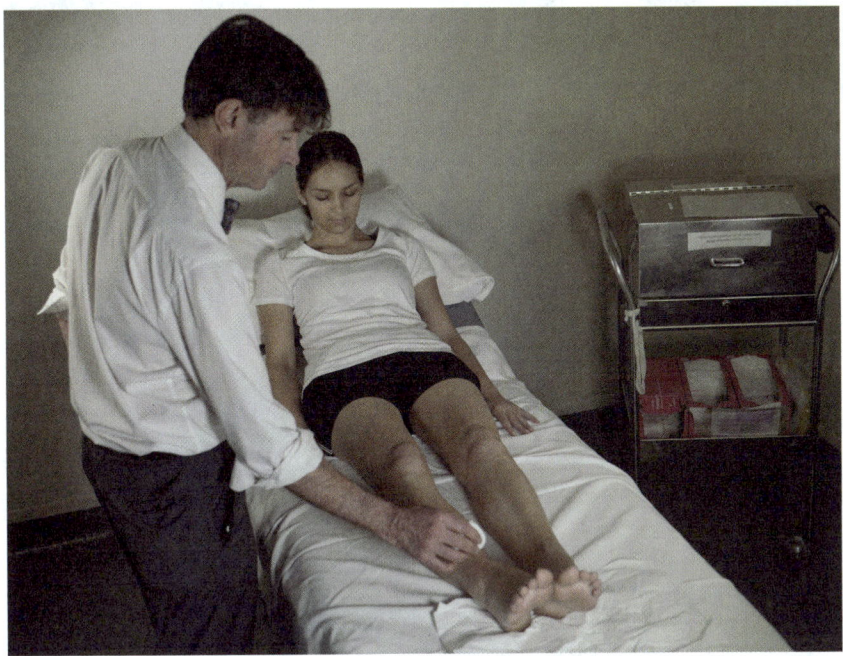

Diabetes mellitus

FIGURE 29.1

Lying

1. **General inspection**
   Weight—obesity
   Hydration
   Endocrine facies
   Pigmentation—haemochromatosis, etc.

2. **Legs**
   Inspect
   - Skin—necrobiosis, hair loss, infection, pigmented scars, atrophy, ulceration, injection sites
   - Muscle wasting

   Palpate
   - Temperature of feet (cold, blue due to 'small' or 'large' vessel disease, warm due to acute Charcot's joint)
   - Peripheral pulses

   Femoral (auscultate)
   Popliteal
   Posterior tibial
   Dorsalis pedis

3. **Arms**
   Inspect
   - Skin lesions (skin tags, acanthosis)

   Pulse

4. **Eyes**
   Fundi—cataracts, rubeosis, retinal disease
   III nerve palsy, other cranial nerves

5. **Mouth**
   Monilia
   Infection

6. **Neck**
   Carotid arteries—palpate, auscultate

7. **Chest**
   Signs of infection

8. **Abdomen**
   Liver—fat infiltration; rarely haemochromatosis
   Injection sites
   Neurological assessment
   - Femoral nerve mononeuritis
   - Peripheral neuropathy

9. **Other**
   Urine analysis—glycosuria, ketones, proteinuria
   Blood pressure—lying and standing
   Oedema
   Acetone on breath

TEXT BOX 29.1

Diabetic (neuropathic) ulcer

(From McDonald FS, ed. *Mayo Clinic images in internal medicine*, with permission. © Mayo Clinic Scientific Press and CRC Press. Reproduced by permission of Taylor and Francis Group, LLC, a division of Informa plc.)

FIGURE 29.2

Charcot's joint of left knee

FIGURE 29.4

Necrobiosis lipoidica diabeticorum

(From McDonald FS, ed. *Mayo Clinic images in internal medicine*, with permission. © Mayo Clinic Scientific Press and CRC Press. Reproduced by permission of Taylor and Francis Group, LLC, a division of Informa plc.)

FIGURE 29.3

rare (fewer than 1% of diabetics; see Fig. 29.3). It is most commonly found over the shins, where a central yellow scarred area is surrounded by a red margin when the condition is active. These plaques may ulcerate.

Look at the thighs for insulin injection sites. These may be associated with localised *fat atrophy* and *fat hypertrophy*, and may be related to impure insulin use, which causes a localised immune reaction (modern genetically engineered insulins have made these rare). Note any *quadriceps muscle wasting* due to femoral nerve mononeuropathy, which is called (inaccurately) diabetic amyotrophy.

Inspect the knees for Charcot's joints (see Fig. 29.4).

Palpation

Palpate any injection sites for fat atrophy or hypertrophy. Feel all the peripheral pulses and the temperature of the feet, and test the capillary return. Absent peripheral pulses, cold extremities and reduced capillary return are all evidence of peripheral vascular disease (Ch 6).

Neurological examination

Assess formally for peripheral neuropathy, including dorsal column loss (diabetic pseudotabes), and tap the reflexes. Test proximal muscle power (diabetic amyotrophy).

Monofilament testing for peripheral neuropathy in the feet
A nylon monofilament that buckles at a standard force (10 g) is useful to test sensation over the bottom of the feet. Ask the patient to close their eyes. Place the device perpendicular to the skin and apply pressure for 1 second (Fig. 29.5). Ask the patient to say 'Yes' if the pressure is felt. Test the arm so the patient understands, then test four sites: the 1st, 3rd and 5th

Monofilament testing for peripheral neuropathy in the feet

(Geralyn R. Spollett. Diabetic neuropathies: diagnosis and treatment. *Nursing Clinics of North America* 41:697–717, Fig. 1. Elsevier, December 2006. Copyright © 2006 Elsevier Inc. All rights reserved.)

FIGURE 29.5

metatarsal heads and the plantar surface of the distal hallux.

Upper limbs

Look at the nails for signs of *Candida* infection. Take the patient's blood pressure lying down and standing, as diabetic autonomic neuropathy can cause postural hypotension.

Face

Test visual acuity. This may be permanently impaired because of retinal disease or temporarily disturbed because of changes in the shape of the lens associated with hyperglycaemia and water retention. Look for Argyll Robertson pupils,[b] which are a rare complication of diabetes.

Using the ophthalmoscope, begin by examining for rubeosis (new blood vessel formation over the iris, which can cause glaucoma; see Fig. 29.6). Then note any cataracts, which are related to sorbitol deposition in the lens (when glucose is present in high concentrations

---

[b] Douglas Argyll Robertson (1837–1909), a Scottish ophthalmic surgeon and President of the Royal College of Surgeons, described these in 1869. The pupils are small, irregular and unequal, and react briskly to accommodation but not to light. Tertiary syphilis is another cause.

Rubeosis iridis.

Shows new vessels on the anterior surface of the iris. These are secondary to ischaemia (often due to diabetes)

(Courtesy of Dr Chris Kennedy and Professor Ian Constable, Lions Eye Institute, Perth.)

FIGURE 29.6

Diabetic retinopathy.

(a) Soft exudate (arrow) and small haemorrhages; (b) microaneurysms (dots), retinal haemorrhages (blots) and hard yellow exudates

(Courtesy of Dr Chris Kennedy and Professor Ian Constable, Lions Eye Institute, Perth.)

FIGURE 29.7

in the tissues it is converted to sorbitol by aldose reductase).

Now examine the retina, where many exciting changes may await the fundoscopist. There are two main types of retinal change in diabetes: non-proliferative and proliferative.

Non-proliferative changes (see Fig. 29.7) are directly related to ischaemia of blood vessels and include: (1) two types of haemorrhages—*dot haemorrhages*, which occur in the inner retinal layers, and *blot haemorrhages*, which are larger and occur more superficially in the nerve fibre layer; (2) *microaneurysms*, which are due to vessel wall damage; and (3) two types of exudates—*hard exudates*, which have straight edges, and *soft exudates* (cottonwool spots), which have a fluffy appearance.

Proliferative changes (see Fig. 29.8) are changes in blood vessels in response to ischaemia of the retina. They are characterised by new vessel formation, which can lead to vitreal haemorrhage, scar formation and eventually retinal detachment. The *detached retina* appears as an opalescent sheet that balloons forwards into the vitreous. The underlying choroid is visible through the detached retina as a bright red-coloured sheet. Look also for *laser scars* (small brown or yellow spots), which are secondary to photocoagulation of new vessels by laser therapy.

Assess the third, fourth and sixth cranial nerves. In particular, examine for diabetic third nerve palsy from ischaemia, which usually spares the pupil (as infarction of the third nerve affects the inner pupillary fibres more than the outer fibres; in this way it differs from compressive lesions, which have the opposite effect).

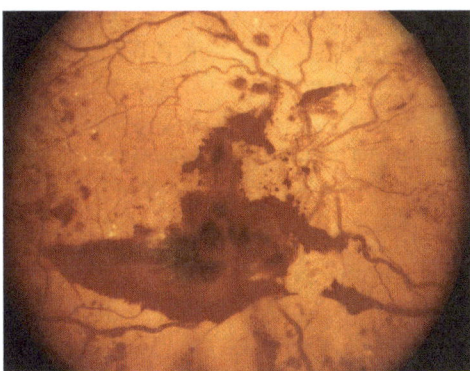

Proliferative diabetic retinopathy

(Courtesy of Dr Chris Kennedy and Professor Ian Constable, Lions Eye Institute, Perth.)

FIGURE 29.8

> ### TYPES OF HYPERPARATHYROIDISM
>
> **Primary**
> Adenoma (80%)
> Hyperplasia
> Carcinoma (rare)
>
> **Secondary**
> Hyperplasia following chronic renal failure
>
> **Tertiary (autonomous)**
> The appearance of autonomous hyperparathyroidism is a complication of secondary hyperparathyroidism
>
> LIST 29.2

Other cranial nerves may be affected sometimes because of cerebrovascular accidents (large-vessel atheroma). Rarely, *rhinocerebral mucormycosis* may develop in very poorly controlled diabetic patients, causing periorbital and perinasal swelling and cranial nerve palsies.

Look in the ears for evidence of infection. The rare *malignant otitis externa*, which is usually due to *Pseudomonas aeruginosa*, causes a mound of granulation tissue in the external canal, and facial nerve palsy in 50% of cases.

Look in the mouth for evidence of *Candida* infection or periodontal disease.

Neck and shoulders

Examine the carotid arteries for evidence of vascular disease. Rarely, there may be thickening of the skin of the upper back and shoulders (scleroedema diabeticorum—this diffuse cutaneous infiltration has a very different distribution from scleroderma, with which it is sometimes confused). Look for acanthosis nigricans and skin tags—which are associated with insulin resistance.

Abdomen

Palpate for hepatomegaly (fatty infiltration, or due to haemochromatosis). Look for signs of cirrhosis. Non-alcoholic steatohepatitis is an increasingly common cause of liver cirrhosis.

Urinalysis

Test for glucose and protein. Diabetic nephropathy (from glomerulonephritis, renal arterial disease or pyelonephritis) can cause proteinuria. The presence of nitrite and/or blood is of value as asymptomatic urinary tract infections can occur. In advanced disease there may be signs of chronic kidney disease.

CALCIUM METABOLISM

Primary hyperparathyroidism

This is due to excess parathyroid hormone (see List 29.2), which results in an increased serum calcium level, increased renal phosphate excretion and increased formation of 1,25-dihydroxycholecalciferol by activation of adenylcyclase in the bone and kidneys. Primary hyperparathyroidism causes problems with 'stones' (renal stones), 'bones' (osteopenia and pseudogout), 'abdominal groans' (constipation, peptic ulcer and pancreatitis) and 'psychological moans' (confusion) (see Questions box 29.2).

Other causes of hypercalcaemia are outlined in List 29.3.

General inspection

Note the mental state of the patient. Severe hypercalcaemia may cause cardiac arrhythmias, coma or convulsions. Assess hydration (polyuria from hypercalcaemia may cause dehydration).

> **QUESTIONS TO ASK THE PATIENT WITH SUSPECTED HYPERPARATHYROIDISM**
>
> ! denotes symptoms for the possible diagnosis of an urgent or dangerous problem.
>
> 1. Have you had kidney stones?
> 2. Have you had any fractures?
> 3. Have you been troubled by abdominal pain? Have you had constipation?
> 4. Have you been depressed or had hallucinations? (Psychiatric disorders)
> ! 5. Have you had episodes of confusion, irritability, extreme tiredness or even unconsciousness? (Neurological symptoms)
>
> QUESTIONS BOX 29.2

> **QUESTIONS TO ASK THE PATIENT WITH SUSPECTED HYPOCALCAEMIA**
>
> ! denotes symptoms for the possible diagnosis of an urgent or dangerous problem.
>
> 1. Have you recently had surgery to remove the parathyroid glands?
> 2. Have you had tingling around the mouth or in the fingers?
> 3. Have you had muscle cramps?
> ! 4. Have you had fits or seizures?
>
> QUESTIONS BOX 29.3

> **IMPORTANT CAUSES OF HYPERCALCAEMIA**
>
> Primary hyperparathyroidism
> Carcinoma (from bone metastases or humoral mediators)
> Thiazide diuretics
> Vitamin D excess
> Excessive production of vitamin D metabolites (e.g. sarcoidosis, granulomatous diseases, certain T-cell lymphomas)
> Thyrotoxicosis
> Associated with chronic kidney disease (e.g. severe secondary hyperparathyroidism)
> Multiple myeloma
> Familial hypocalciuric hypercalcaemia
> Prolonged immobilisation or space flight
>
> LIST 29.3

Face
Look in the patient's eyes for band keratopathy, which is rare.

Body and lower limbs
Palpate the patient's shoulders, sternum, ribs, spine and hips for bony tenderness, deformity or evidence of previous fractures. Test for proximal muscle weakness. Look for pseudogout. Take the blood pressure, as hypertension may occur.

Urinalysis
Test for blood in the urine (renal stones).

The MEN syndromes
The multiple endocrine neoplasias (MENs), types I and II, are autosomal dominant conditions. Hyperparathyroidism may be associated with both types. MEN type I (due to a mutation on chromosome 11) is associated with tumours of the parathyroid, pituitary and pancreatic islet cells. MEN type IIA (due to a mutation on chromosome 10 involving the *c-ret* proto-oncogene) is associated with medullary carcinoma of the thyroid, hyperparathyroidism and phaeochromocytoma. MEN type IIB is characterised by mucosal neuromas (often on the lips and tongue; see Fig. 29.9) and medullary carcinoma of the thyroid plus phaeochromocytoma.

Hypoparathyroidism
Hypoparathyroidism results in hypocalcaemia with neuromuscular consequences (tetany) (see Questions box 29.3). It is usually a postoperative complication after thyroidectomy, but can be idiopathic. Hypocalcaemia can also result from end-organ resistance to parathyroid hormone (pseudohypoparathyroidism; see List 29.4).

Multiple mucosal neuromas of the tongue

(From Melmed S. *Williams textbook of endocrinology*, 2nd edn. Saunders, 2011.)

FIGURE 29.9

CAUSES OF HYPOCALCAEMIA
Hypoparathyroidism: after thyroidectomy, idiopathic
Malabsorption
Deficiency of vitamin D
Chronic kidney disease
Acute pancreatitis
Pseudohypoparathyroidism
Magnesium deficiency
Hypocalcaemia of malignant disease

LIST 29.4

Look first for Trousseau's and Chvostek's signs. *Trousseau's sign* is elicited with a blood pressure cuff placed on the arm with the pressure raised above the patient's systolic pressure. Typical contraction of the hand occurs within 2 minutes when hypocalcaemia has caused neuromuscular irritability. The thumb becomes strongly adducted, and the fingers are extended, except at the metacarpophalangeal joints. The appearance is like that adopted by an obstetrician about to remove a placenta manually and is called the *main d'accoucheur*.

Chvostek's sign is performed by tapping gently over the facial (seventh) cranial nerve under the ear. The nerve is hyperexcitable in hypocalcaemia and a brisk muscular twitch occurs on the same side of the face.

Next test for hyperreflexia, which is again due to neuromuscular irritability.

Look at the nails for fragility and monilial infection. Note any dryness of the skin. Go to the face and look for deformity of the teeth. Examine the eyes for cataracts or papilloedema. These signs may all occur in idiopathic hypoparathyroidism, an autoimmune disease. Cataracts may also follow surgically induced hypoparathyroidism.

Pseudohypoparathyroidism

In pseudohypoparathyroidism the patients have tetany (due to hypocalcaemia) as well as typical skeletal abnormalities. These include short stature, a round face, a short neck, thin stocky build and very characteristically short fourth or fifth fingers or toes (due to metacarpal or metatarsal shortening; this can be unilateral or bilateral; see Fig. 29.10). Ask the patient to make a fist to demonstrate the characteristic clinical signs.

Pseudopseudohypoparathyroidism

This amusing name is given to a disease where there is no tetany (calcium concentration in the blood is normal), but the characteristic skeletal deformities are present.

OSTEOPOROSIS AND OSTEOMALACIA

These bone diseases have both endocrine and non-endocrine causes (see List 29.5). *Osteoporosis* is the result of insufficient bone production, which leads to a reduction in bone mass and an increased risk of fractures. Many cases are a result of the relative

Pseudohypoparathyroidism.

(a) Feet; (b) hands

(From McDonald FS, ed. *Mayo Clinic images in internal medicine*, with permission. © Mayo Clinic Scientific Press and CRC Press. Reproduced by permission of Taylor and Francis Group, LLC, a division of Informa plc.)

FIGURE 29.10

> **CAUSES OF AND RISK FACTORS FOR OSTEOPOROSIS AND OSTEOMALACIA**
>
> **Osteoporosis**
> GENERAL
> Females: menopause and being over 70 years of age
> Genetic factors
> Alcoholism
> Smoking
> Anorexia nervosa
>
> ENDOCRINE
> Hypogonadism
> Thyrotoxicosis
> Cushing's syndrome
> Hyperparathyroidism
>
> INFLAMMATORY DISEASE
> Rheumatoid arthritis
> Inflammatory bowel disease
>
> GASTROINTESTINAL DISEASE
> Malabsorption
> Chronic liver disease
>
> DRUGS
> Corticosteroids
> Anticonvulsants
> Heparin
>
> **Osteomalacia**
> Vitamin D deficiency, often due to lack of exposure to sunlight (e.g. nursing home patients, those who cover up from head to toe and dermatologists) or abnormalities of vitamin D metabolism
> Hypophosphataemia
> Inhibition of bone mineralisation caused by drugs
>
> LIST 29.5

hypogonadism that occurs with age, but often occur in combination with reduced vitamin D levels. Although the reduced bone mineral density that occurs in elderly people is called osteoporosis, it is usually at least partly the result of osteomalacia. In women, conditions that reduce oestrogen increase the risk: hypogonadism before menopause (e.g. due to anorexia nervosa), menopause, antioestrogenic drugs, smoking and being underweight.

Osteomalacia means defective bone mineralisation. It is usually due to low vitamin D levels, which lead to inadequate calcium absorption. This results in secondary hyperparathyroidism, which helps maintain serum calcium levels but at the expense of increased osteoclast activity and loss of calcium from the skeleton. When the condition occurs in childhood it causes rickets.

Many patients are asymptomatic but common symptoms (see Questions box 29.4) include unexpected fractures (especially of the vertebral bodies and associated with severe back pain, hip and wrist

QUESTIONS TO ASK THE PATIENT WITH KNOWN OR SUSPECTED OSTEOPOROSIS OR OSTEOMALACIA

1. Have you had an episode of severe back pain?
2. Is there a history of osteoporosis in your family?
3. Have you lost height?
4. Have you had any recent fractures (hips or wrist particularly)? Note if low-trauma.
5. Have you been a smoker? Do you drink alcohol?
6. Did you undergo menopause at an early age?
7. Have you had a DEXA scan?
8. Have you been treated with corticosteroids? (>7.5 mg prednisone for >3 months)
9. Are you normally physically active?
10. Have you had problems with arthritis (rheumatoid arthritis)? Diabetes? Coeliac disease?
11. Have you been prescribed treatment? What?

QUESTIONS BOX 29.4

The occiput-to-wall distance. The patient has severe ankylosing spondylitis

FIGURE 29.11

fractures); some people notice loss of height as a result of the development of thoracic kyphosis. The diagnosis may have been made from an X-ray taken for another reason or as a result of a screening bone mineral density (dual-energy X-ray absorptiometry [DEXA]) scan.

The examination

Measure the patient's height using a *stadiometer* (an upright bar with a sliding scale). Comparing this measured height with the patient's recollection of previous height measurements has been shown to be an accurate way of detecting a change in height. Thoracic kyphosis can be assessed, as is done for patients with ankylosing spondylitis, by measuring the occiput-to-wall distance (see Fig. 29.11). Inability of the patient when standing straight to touch the wall with the back of the head is considered abnormal (LR+, 3.8)[2] and serial measurements of the occiput-to-wall distance can be helpful in following the course of the disease.

Lumbar fractures can be assessed by measuring the *rib-to-pelvis* distance. Have the patient stand facing away from you with arms extended. Insert your fingers between the lower costal margin and the superior surface of the pelvis in the midaxillary line. Normally, more than two fingers can be inserted (LR+, 3.8).[3]

If the patient reports recent severe back pain, feel for tenderness over the spine. Remember, however, that fractures of the vertebral body may not cause localised tenderness—sometimes percussion over the area may elicit tenderness. Remember also that the differential diagnosis for these fractures includes malignancy (e.g. myeloma).

SYNDROMES ASSOCIATED WITH SHORT STATURE

These conditions begin in childhood but milder forms may not be diagnosed until adult life—for example, the woman with infertility found to have Turner's syndrome.

General inspection

First measure the height of the patient; in children this should be compared with percentile charts for age and sex. Look for the classical appearance of

Turner's syndrome

(From Wales JKH, Wit JM, Rogol AD. *Pediatric endocrinology and growth*, 2nd edn. Philadelphia: Saunders, 2003.)

FIGURE 29.12

Turner's syndrome (see Fig. 29.12), Down's syndrome, achondroplasia or rickets (see Fig. 29.13), which may explain the short stature. The height of parents and siblings should be checked as well.

Note any evidence of weight loss, including loose skinfolds, which may suggest a nutritional cause (starvation, malabsorption or protein loss). Look for signs of hypopituitarism or hypothyroidism, or steroid excess. Sexual precocity (early onset of secondary sexual characteristics) causes relative tallness at first but short stature later.

Chest

Examine for evidence of cyanotic congenital heart disease and pulmonary disease, such as cystic fibrosis.

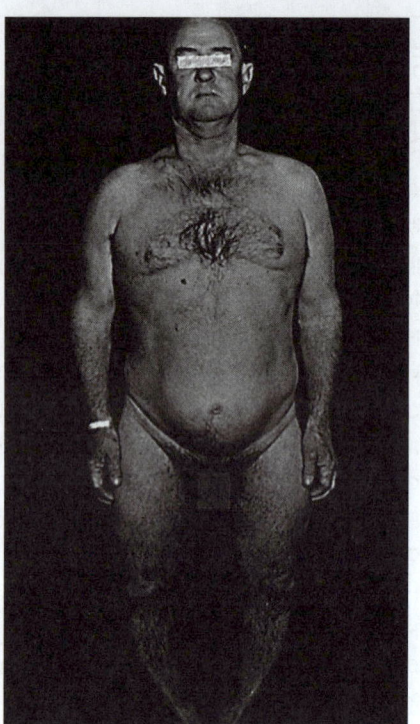

Rickets

FIGURE 29.13

Abdomen

Look for evidence of chronic liver or kidney disease (a cause of growth retardation when it occurs in children).

Turner's syndrome (45XO)

Sexual infantilism (failure of development of secondary sexual characteristics)—female genitalia (see Fig. 29.12) Look for:

- **upper limbs:** lymphoedema of the hands; short fourth metacarpal bones; hyperplastic nails; increased carrying angle; hypertension
- **facies:** micrognathia (small chin); epicanthic folds, ptosis; fish-like mouth; deformed or low-set ears; hearing loss
- **neck:** webbing of the neck; low hairline; redundant skinfolds on the back of the neck
- **chest:** widely spaced nipples (a shield-like chest); coarctation of the aorta
- **other:** pigmented naevi; keloid formation; lymphoedema of the legs.

Down's syndrome (Trisomy 21)
Look for:
- **facies:** oblique orbital fissures; conjunctivitis; Brushfield spots on the iris; small simple ears; flat nasal bridge; mouth hanging open; protruding tongue; narrow high-arched palate
- **hands:** short broad hands; incurving fifth finger; single palmar crease; hyperflexible joints
- **chest:** congenital heart disease; especially endocardial cushion defects
- **other:** straight pubic hair; gaps between the first and second toes; mental deficiency usually present.

Achondroplasia (dwarfism)
This is an autosomal dominant disease of cartilage caused by mutation of the fibroblast growth factor receptor gene. Short stature, short limbs, normal trunk, relatively large head, saddle-shaped nose, exaggerated lumbar lordosis and occasionally spinal cord compression are features. Look for:
- frontal bossing
- proximal myopathy of the arms and thighs
- bowing of the ulna, femur and tibia.

Rickets
This is defective mineralisation of the *growing* skeleton (see Fig. 29.13), due to lack of vitamin D (e.g. nutritional or chronic renal failure) or hypophosphataemia (e.g. renal tubular disorders). Look for:
- **upper limbs:** tetany; hypotonia, proximal myopathy; bowing of the radius and ulna
- **facies:** frontal bossing; parietal flattening
- **chest:** 'rickety rosary'—thickening of costochondral junctions; Harrison's groove—indentation of lower ribs at the diaphragmatic attachment
- **lower limbs:** bowing of femur and tibia; hypotonia, proximal myopathy; fractures.

HIRSUTISM
This is excessive hairiness in a woman beyond what is considered normal for her race (see List 29.6). It is usually caused by androgen (including testosterone)

> ### CAUSES OF HIRSUTISM
> Polycystic ovary syndrome (most common cause)
> Idiopathic
> Adrenal: androgen-secreting tumours (e.g. Cushing's syndrome, congenital adrenal hyperplasia, virilising tumour—more often a carcinoma than an adenoma)
> Ovarian: androgen-secreting tumour
> Drugs: phenytoin, diazoxide, streptomycin, minoxidil, anabolic steroids (e.g. testosterone)
> Other: acromegaly, porphyria cutanea tarda
>
> LIST 29.6

excess. In the examination of such a patient, it is important to decide whether virilisation is also present. Virilisation is the appearance of male secondary sexual characteristics (clitoromegaly, frontal hair recession, male body habitus and deepening of the voice) and indicates that excessive androgen is present.

General inspection
Ask the patient to undress to her underwear. Note the hair distribution over the face (see Fig. 29.14) and in the midline, front and back. In general, an obvious male balding pattern (a receding hairline), hair over the beard area or on the back and chest, and hair in the escutcheon (umbilicus to groin in the midline) is usually abnormal. Look for obvious acromegaly or Cushing's syndrome and for the skin changes of porphyria cutanea tarda.

Ask the patient to remove her underclothing and lie flat. Look for signs of virilism. These include breast atrophy and increased muscle bulk of the arms and legs, male pattern of pubic hair and enlargement of the clitoris. Look in the axillae; the patient with polycystic ovarian syndrome may have acanthosis nigricans (and associated insulin resistance).

Abdomen
Palpate for adrenal masses, polycystic ovaries or an ovarian tumour (these are rarely palpable).

Blood pressure
Hypertension occurs in the rare C11-hydroxylase deficiency, which is a virilising condition.

Hirsutism due to polycystic ovary syndrome

(From Black M. *Obstetric and gynecologic dermatology*, 3rd edn. Oxford: Mosby, 2008.)

FIGURE 29.14

Gynaecomastia.

This patient takes spironolactone for heart failure. Note the median sternotomy scar (black arrow) and defibrillator box (open arrow)

FIGURE 29.15

GYNAECOMASTIA

Gynaecomastia is 'true' enlargement of the male breasts (see Fig. 29.15).[4] Careful examination will detect up to 4 centimetres of palpable breast tissue in 30% of normal young men; this percentage increases with age. These men are unaware of any breast abnormality. Gynaecomastia occurs in up to 50% of adolescent boys, and also in elderly men in whom it is due to falling testosterone levels. Fat deposition ('false' enlargement) in obese men can be confused with gynaecomastia. In true gynaecomastia the normally flat male nipple protrudes. In false gynaecomastia the nipple remains soft and flat. The drug spironolactone is a common cause of painful gynaecomastia in men.

Examine the breasts (see Ch 41) for evidence of localised disease (e.g. malignancy, which is rare), tenderness, which indicates rapid growth, and any discharge from the nipple. Detection of breast tissue in men is best performed with the patient sitting up. Squeeze the breast behind the patient's nipple between the thumb and forefinger. Try to detect an edge between subcutaneous fat and true breast tissue. True breast tissue typically spreads from under the areolae and is mobile, rubbery and firm. Asymmetrical enlargement that is hard, fixed and associated with a bloody discharge from the nipple is suggestive of malignancy. The axillary lymph nodes must be examined for enlargement.

Examine the genitalia for sexual ambiguity and the testes for absence or a reduced size. Note any loss of secondary sexual characteristics.

Look especially for signs of *Klinefelter's syndrome* (see Fig. 29.16). These patients are tall, have decreased body hair and have characteristically small, firm testes.

Look also for signs of panhypopituitarism or chronic liver disease. Thyrotoxicosis can occasionally be a cause.

Finally, examine the visual fields and fundi for evidence of a pituitary tumour.

Causes of pathological gynaecomastia are summarised in List 29.7.

PAGET'S DISEASE

Paget's[c] disease (osteitis deformans) is characterised by excessive reabsorption of bone by osteoclasts and

---

[c] Sir James Paget (1814–99), a surgeon at St Bartholomew's Hospital, London, was also Queen Victoria's doctor.

CHAPTER 29 CORRELATION OF PHYSICAL SIGNS AND ENDOCRINE DISEASE   477

Klinefelter's syndrome: note the long limbs, narrow shoulders and chest, and small genitals

(From Grumbach MM, Hughes IA, Conte FA. Disorders of sex differentiation. In Larsen PR, Kronenberg HM, Melmed S, Polonsky KS, eds. *Williams textbook of endocrinology*, 10th edn. Philadelphia: Saunders, 2003.)

FIGURE 29.16

> ### CAUSES OF PATHOLOGICAL GYNAECOMASTIA
>
> **Increased oestrogen production**
> Leydig cell tumour (oestrogen)
> Adrenal carcinoma (oestrogen)
> Bronchial carcinoma (human chorionic gonadotrophin)
> Liver disease (increased conversion of oestrogen from androgens)
> Thyrotoxicosis (increased conversion of oestrogen from androgens)
> Starvation
>
> **Decreased androgen production (hypogonadal states)**
> Klinefelter's syndrome (see Fig. 29.16)
> Secondary testicular failure: orchitis, castration, trauma
>
> **Testicular feminisation syndrome**
>
> **Drugs**
> Oestrogen receptor binders: oestrogen, digoxin, marijuana
> Antiandrogens: spironolactone, cimetidine
> Anabolic steroid (exogenous testosterone) abuse
>
> LIST 29.7

compensatory disorganised deposition of new bone. It is possibly a disease of viral origin.

General inspection

Note short stature (due to bending of the long bones of the limbs) and any obvious deformity of the head and lower limbs.

Head and face

Inspect the scalp for enlargement in the frontal and parietal areas and measure the head circumference (>55 centimetres is usually abnormal). There may be prominent skull veins. Palpate for increased bony warmth and auscultate over the skull for systolic bruits. Both of these are due to increased vascularity of the skull vault. Oddly enough, bronchial breath sounds may be audible over the pagetic skull through the stethoscope. These are due to increased bone conduction of air. An area of very localised bony swelling and warmth may indicate development of a bony sarcoma (1% of cases of Paget's disease may develop this complication).

Examine the eyes. Assess visual acuity and visual fields, and look in the fundi for angioid streaks and optic atrophy. Retinitis pigmentosa occurs rather more rarely. Test for hearing loss (due to bony ossicle involvement or eighth nerve compression by bony enlargement).

Examine the remaining cranial nerves; all may be involved because of bony overgrowth of the foramina or be caused by basilar invagination (platybasia; where the posterior fossa becomes flat and the basal angle increased).

Neck

Patients with basilar invagination have a short neck and low hairline. The head is held in extension and neck movements are decreased. Assess the jugular venous pressure, as a high output cardiac failure may be present, particularly if there is coexistent ischaemic heart disease.

Heart

Examine for signs of cardiac failure.

Back

Inspect for kyphosis (due to vertebral involvement causing collapse of the vertebral bodies). Tap for localised tenderness, feel for warmth and auscultate for systolic bruits over the vertebral bodies.

Legs

Inspect for anterior bowing of the tibia and lateral bowing of the femur (see Fig. 29.17). Feel for bony warmth and tenderness. Note any changes of osteoarthritis in the hips and knees, which often coexist with Paget's disease. Note any localised warm swelling, which may indicate sarcoma.

Paget's disease, showing bowing of the tibia

FIGURE 29.17

Examine for evidence of paraplegia, which is uncommon but can occur because of cord compression by bone or vascular shunting in the spinal cord. Rarely, cerebellar signs may be present owing to platybasia.

Urinalysis

Check for blood in the urine (there is an increased incidence of renal stones in Paget's disease).

T&O'C ESSENTIALS

1. It is important to have a routine for examining a patient with diabetes mellitus. A quick screening examination will help detect any of the numerous complications of the disease.
2. Many endocrine abnormalities are suspected because of an abnormal facies or body habitus. This is likely to be missed unless you take a moment to step back and look at the patient as a whole.
3. Short stature is often genetic (it is the result of having short parents), but it is important to consider some of the endocrine and chromosomal causes if adolescents are unexpectedly shorter than their parents.
4. Endocrine diseases can affect any part of the body. A thorough general examination is necessary for these patients.

OSCE REVISION TOPICS (see the OSCE video Thyroid examination, no. 8 at Student CONSULT) – Endocrine system

Use these topics, which commonly occur in the OSCE, to help with revision.

1. This woman has type 2 diabetes. Please examine her. (p 465)
2. This woman is concerned that she has more body hair than is normal. Please examine her. (p 475)
3. This man has been diagnosed with Klinefelter's syndrome. Please examine him. (p 476)
4. This man has noticed an increase in the size of his hands. Please examine him. (p 456)
5. This woman has had type 1 diabetes for 30 years. Please examine her eyes, which have been dilated for you, and describe what you see. (pp 467, 776)

References

1. Edelson GW, Armstrong DG, Lavery LA, Ciacco G. The acutely infected diabetic foot is not adequately evaluated in an inpatient setting. *Arch Intern Med* 1996; 156:2372–2378. All patients evaluated had undergone a less than adequate foot examination. Of admitted patients, 31% did not have their pedal pulses documented and 60% were not evaluated for the presence or absence of protective sensation.
2. Siminoski K, Lee K, Warshawski R. Accuracy of physical examination for detection of thoracic vertebral fractures. *J Bone Miner Res* 2003; 18(suppl 2):S82.
3. Siminoski K, Warshawaski RS, Jen H, Lee KC. Accuracy of physical examination using the rib–pelvis distance for detection of lumbar vertebral fractures. *Am J Med* 2003; 115(3):233–236.
4. Braunstein GD. Gynecomastia. *N Engl J Med* 2007; 357:1229–1237. A good review.

CHAPTER 30

A summary of the endocrine examination and extending the endocrine examination

I learned a long time ago that minor surgery is when they do the operation on someone else, not you.
BILL WALTON

THE ENDOCRINE EXAMINATION: A SUGGESTED METHOD

Examining a patient with suspected endocrine disease is usually tailored to the clinical presentation. For example, for a patient with a possible goitre you need to define the mass properly to confirm that the thyroid is enlarged and identify its characteristics (including any retrosternal extension) and whether there are signs of thyrotoxicosis or alternatively hypothyroidism. Remember that thyrotoxicosis or hypothyroidism can be present in the *absence* of goitre (which you may suspect from your initial and important general inspection)! You may suspect Cushing's syndrome on first seeing the patient; your examination then needs to be tailored to look for the signs that will confirm your initial impression (or not). Remember that Cushing's syndrome and obesity can be difficult to differentiate even on initial biochemical testing. The astute clinician may also recognise one of the endocrine spot diagnoses (List 30.1) on first encountering the patient. On the other hand, diabetes mellitus may be diagnosed only after a routine blood glucose level has been measured, but if you know that the patient has diabetes you should routinely look for the complications of the disease as part of your clinical examination.

A summary of an approach to suspected endocrine disease is presented in Text box 30.1 as a guide, but the method must be tailored to the disease you suspect and you should not look for obviously irrelevant problems.

> **ENDOCRINE SPOT DIAGNOSES**
> 1. Acromegaly
> 2. Cushing's syndrome
> 3. Addison's disease
> 4. Thyrotoxicosis
> 5. Myxoedema
> 6. Panhypopituitarism
> 7. Virilisation
> 8. Paget's disease
>
> LIST 30.1

EXTENDING THE ENDOCRINE PHYSICAL EXAMINATION

Diagnostic testing

To interpret investigations for endocrine diseases you need to understand the physiology of hormonal regulation (the classic hormonal feedback cycles). Typically, biochemical testing is undertaken to identify the hormonal abnormality and then imaging may be performed to determine the anatomical lesion. Some introductory examples are given below.

Pituitary testing

Testing usually involves measuring the basal concentrations of the anterior pituitary hormones in the basal state (usually taken in the morning) and measuring the hormones produced by the target glands.

CHAPTER 30 A SUMMARY OF THE ENDOCRINE EXAMINATION AND EXTENDING THE ENDOCRINE EXAMINATION

The endocrine system: a suggested method of examination

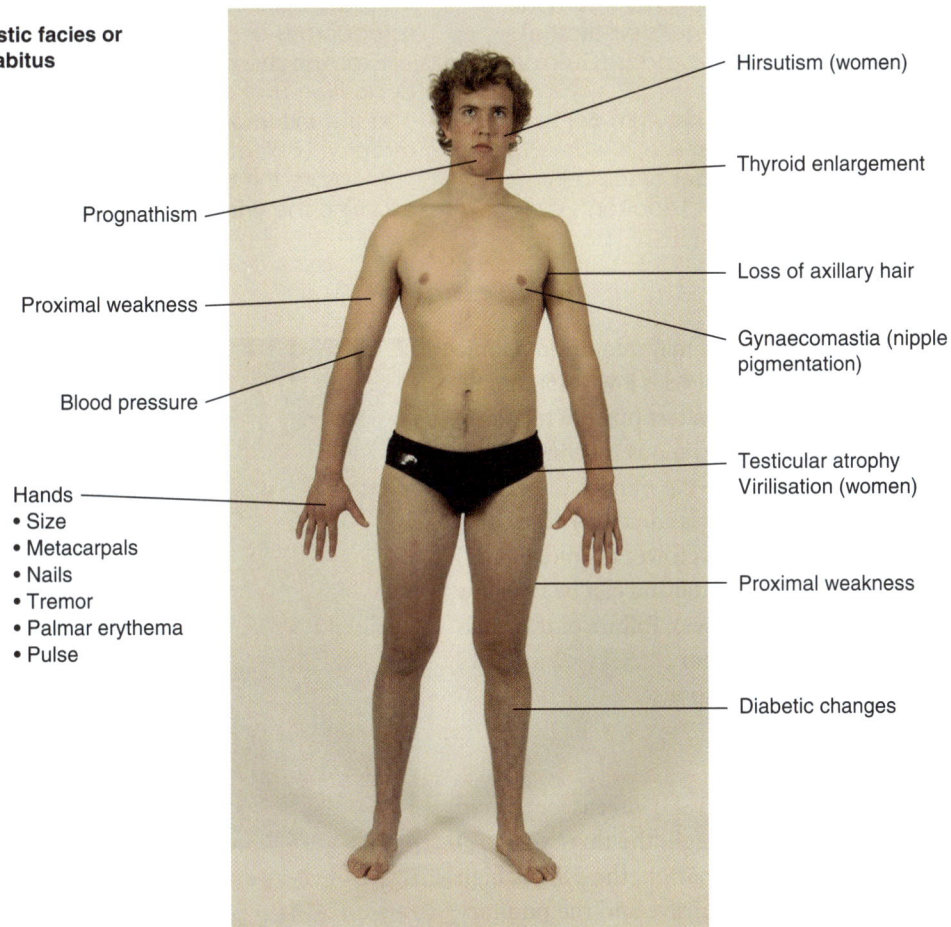

The endocrine examination

FIGURE 30.1

Inspect the patient for one of the diagnostic facies or body habitus. Look for thoracic kyphosis (vertebral fractures). If the diagnosis is obvious, proceed with the specific examination outlined previously. If not, examine as follows.

Pick up the patient's **hands**. Look at the overall size (acromegaly), length of the metacarpals (pseudohypoparathyroidism and pseudopseudo-hypoparathyroidism), for abnormalities of the nails (hyperthyroidism and hypothyroidism, and hypoparathyroidism), tremor, palmar erythema and sweating of the palms (hyperthyroidism).

Take the patient's pulse (thyroid disease) and blood pressure (hypertension in Cushing's syndrome, or postural hypotension in Addison's disease). Look for Trousseau's sign (tetany). Test for proximal muscle weakness (thyroid disease, Cushing's syndrome).

Go to the **axillae**. Look for loss of axillary hair (hypopituitarism) or acanthosis nigricans and skin tags (acromegaly).

Examine the **eyes** (hyperthyroidism) and the **fundi** (diabetes, acromegaly). Look at the **face** for hirsutism or fine-wrinkled hairless skin (panhypopituitarism). Note any skin greasiness, acne or plethora (Cushing's syndrome).

Look at the **mouth** for protrusion of the chin and enlargement of the tongue (acromegaly) or buccal pigmentation (Addison's disease).

TEXT BOX 30.1

Continued

The endocrine system: a suggested method of examination *continued*

Examine the **neck** for thyroid enlargement. Note any neck webbing (Turner's syndrome). Palpate for supraclavicular fat pads (Cushing's syndrome).

Inspect the **chest** wall for hirsutism or loss of body hair, reduction in breast size in women (panhypopituitarism) or gynaecomastia in men. Look for nipple pigmentation (Addison's disease).

Measure the occiput to wall distance if osteoporosis or osteomalacia is suspected.

Examine the **abdomen** for hirsutism, central fat deposition and purple striae (Cushing's syndrome) and the **external genitalia** for virilisation or atrophy. Look at the **legs** for diabetic changes.

Measure the body **weight** and **height**, and examine the **urine**.

TEXT BOX 30.1

The pituitary–adrenal axis may require dynamic testing. If the morning cortisol level is low (<150 nmol / L), a hypoglycaemia stimulation test (insulin tolerance test [ITT]) is performed. Intravenous insulin is given until the blood glucose level is <2.2 mmol / L. This will normally raise plasma cortisol (via adrenocorticotrophic hormone [ACTH] release) and growth hormone (GH) levels (which are usually pulsatile and can be very low in normal people between pulses). Failure of the levels to rise (peak cortisol <500 nmol / L, GH <9 mU / L) means a deficient pituitary response.

Thyroid function testing

Thyroid-stimulating hormone (TSH) screens for thyroid disease: if the TSH is low or high, the thyroxine (T_4) level is measured. In *hypothyroidism*, the TSH is high because the thyroid is unresponsive and the pituitary increases TSH production; the low T_4 level confirms the diagnosis. In *hyperthyroidism*, the TSH is low because the thyroid is producing thyroxine, which suppresses pituitary production of TSH; the high T_4 level confirms the diagnosis.

If a single nodule is detected on thyroid examination, it is important to check the TSH and order a thyroid nuclear scan. If the TSH is low, suggesting hyperthyroidism, thyroid scintigraphy can identify whether the nodule is hyperfunctioning (a 'hot' nodule; see Fig. 30.2) or not secreting (a 'cold' nodule)—the latter may be malignant and an ultrasound (see Fig. 30.3) is indicated.

From the ultrasound image one can tell whether the nodule is solid or not. If the nodule is solid and large (>1 centimetre) with worrying ultrasonographic features a fine-needle aspiration (FNA) under ultrasound guidance can help identify whether there is malignancy.

Nuclear scan of hot (secreting—unbroken arrow) and cold (non-secreting—broken arrow) thyroid nodules

(Herring W. *Learning radiology: recognising the basics*, 2nd edn. Philadelphia: Saunders, 2011.)

FIGURE 30.2

Blood glucose

A fasting blood glucose level (BGL) is usually ordered to make the diagnosis of diabetes mellitus. Do not forget the criteria for this diagnosis: a fasting (overnight) blood glucose level of 7.0 mmol / L or higher on at least two separate occasions, *or*, in the absence of fasting hyperglycaemia, a 2-hour postprandial glucose level of 11.1 mmol / L or higher. Fasting blood glucose levels between 6.1 and 7.0 mmol / L are considered to represent impaired fasting glucose levels. In a patient with symptoms of diabetes, a random BGL of ≥11.1 mmol / L or single fasting glucose reading above 7.0 mmol / L is diagnostic.

Ultrasound of a thyroid nodule.

A biopsy needle is visible

(Flint PW. *Cummings' otolaryngology: head & neck surgery*, 5th edn. Maryland Heights, MO: Mosby, 2010.)

FIGURE 30.3

A haemoglobin A_{1c} level can be used to identify the patient's average blood glucose level over the past 8–12 weeks. The test relies on the fact that glucose freely permeates red blood cells and attaches to haemoglobin (irreversibly); red cells live for 120 days. The management goal for most patients is to achieve normal or near-normal blood glucose levels as indicated by an A_{1c} of 52 mmol / L (<7%) in order to reduce the complications of diabetes. There is evidence that complications of diabetes may occur in some populations when the fasting glucose level is over 6.1 mmol / L. An A_{1c} level of ≥48 mmol / mol (≥6.5%) is consistent with a diagnosis of diabetes.

Cushing's syndrome

You may suspect this syndrome of cortisol excess clinically and this may be reinforced by routine blood tests (e.g. a low potassium with alkalosis, a high blood glucose level). You should then order special biochemical tests to screen for the diagnosis (midnight cortisol levels, 24-hour urine free cortisol or an overnight 1 mg dexamethasone suppression test where the morning cortisol level fails to suppress). To confirm the diagnosis, a higher-dose dexamethasone suppression test can be ordered and the ACTH level measured, followed, if indicated, by brain computed tomography (CT) or MRI scanning to identify whether there is a pituitary tumour (Cushing's disease; see Fig. 30.4). Adrenal disease (e.g. a cortisol-secreting adenoma; see Fig. 30.5) can also cause a Cushingoid appearance. Ectopic ACTH production (e.g. from a small-cell carcinoma of the lung), on the other hand, does not usually cause classical Cushingoid clinical features, but may cause pigmentation.

Addison's disease

You may suspect chronic adrenal insufficiency on routine blood tests (e.g. low sodium and high potassium on serum electrolytes). The diagnosis is biochemically confirmed by injecting synthetic ACTH and measuring the cortisol response (known as the synacthen test).

Bone disease

A number of bone diseases can occur because of underlying endocrine disease. Examples include fractures secondary to osteoporosis (reduced bone

MRI scans of brain pituitary adenoma (a) and empty sella (b)
(Melmed S. *Williams' textbook of endocrinology*, 12th edn. Philadelphia: Saunders, 2011.)

FIGURE 30.4

CT scan of an adrenal tumour with necrosis
(Adam A. *Grainger & Allison's diagnostic radiology*, 5th edn. Edinburgh: Churchill Livingstone, 2008.)

FIGURE 30.5

mineral density; see Fig. 30.6) and, more uncommonly, osteomalacia (vitamin D deficiency).

Bone densitometry using dual-energy X-ray absorptiometry (DEXA) assesses bone mineral density and is important to consider in patients who have had prolonged treatment with steroids or who have had fractures occur after minimal trauma. Review any available skeletal X-rays.

Measuring serum calcium, phosphate and alkaline phosphatase (an enzyme from bone as well as the liver) levels can help you to work out the likely bone disease. These tests are usually normal in osteoporosis. You can also measure the vitamin D level, which is usually low in osteomalacia.

If a high serum calcium level is found on routine testing or when evaluating for bone disease, a number of causes need to be considered, from parathyroid disease to excess vitamin D ingestion and malignancy. Make sure the raised calcium level is real—it may appear increased because of poor blood collection (haemoconcentration) or if the albumin is low. Primary hyperparathyroidism is an important cause of a raised calcium level (often due to a solitary parathyroid adenoma). If the parathyroid hormone (PTH) level is also raised, primary hyperparathyroidism is the most likely diagnosis. (In the setting of a truly raised serum calcium level, a PTH level in the high-normal range should alert you to this diagnosis, as PTH should be suppressed with a high calcium level.) If the PTH level is low, you need to search for other causes of the hypercalcaemia, especially malignancy.

CHAPTER 30 A SUMMARY OF THE ENDOCRINE EXAMINATION AND EXTENDING THE ENDOCRINE EXAMINATION

X-ray and CT scan of osteoporosis.

Note the reduced bone density

(Weissman BN. *Imaging of arthritis and metabolic bone disease,* 1st edn. Philadelphia: Mosby, 2009.)

FIGURE 30.6

T&O'C ESSENTIALS

1. The changes that occur with endocrine conditions such as hypothyroidism and acromegaly may be very gradual. They may seem obvious when a patient visits a new doctor.
2. Many symptoms of thyroid disease are not specific and a high index of suspicion is needed for the diagnosis to be considered.
3. Diabetes mellitus is the most common and important of the endocrine diseases.
4. Osteoporosis is very common in elderly people and an important cause of serious fractures. It should be routinely looked for.
5. Endocrine investigations are used to confirm an endocrine abnormality and imaging tests are often needed to identify the endocrine gland involved.

OSCE REVISION TOPICS – ENDOCRINE SYSTEM

Use these topics, which commonly occur in the OSCE, to help with revision.

1. This man has low blood pressure and pigmentation. Please examine him. What tests might you order? (p 483)
2. This man has diabetes. Discuss the investigations that might be useful in managing his condition. (p 482)
3. This woman is thought to have osteoporosis. How would you investigate her? (p 485)

SECTION 9

The nervous system

CHAPTER 31
The neurological history

CHAPTER 32
The neurological examination: the cranial nerves

CHAPTER 33
The neurological examination: speech and higher centres

CHAPTER 34
The neurological examination: the peripheral nervous system

CHAPTER 35
Correlation of physical signs and neurological syndromes and disease

CHAPTER 36
A summary of the neurological examination and extending the neurological examination

CHAPTER 31
The neurological history

Who could have foretold, from the structure of the brain, that wine could derange its functions?
HIPPOCRATES (460–375 BC)

STARTING OFF

As a preliminary to the neurological assessment, the clinician should obtain some biographical information from the patient, including age, place of birth, left- or right-handedness, occupation and level of education.

PRESENTING SYMPTOMS

The neurological history begins in detail with the presenting problem or problems (see List 31.1). The patient should be allowed to describe the symptoms in his or her own words to begin with, and then the clinician needs to ask questions to clarify information and obtain more detail. It is particularly important to ascertain the *temporal course of the illness*, as this may give important information about the underlying aetiology.

An acute onset of symptoms (seconds to minutes) is suggestive of a vascular or convulsive problem (e.g. the explosive severe headache of subarachnoid haemorrhage or the rapid onset of a seizure).

These episodes of sudden onset may feature a precipitating event (e.g. exercise) or warning (*aura*) may be present. The aura that precedes a seizure is in fact a partial (focal) seizure, and may be localising (e.g. auditory hallucinations, an unusual smell or taste, loss of speech or motor changes) or non-localising (e.g. a feeling of apprehension). The occurrence of an aura followed by sudden unconsciousness is very suggestive of the diagnosis of a complex partial seizure.

A *stroke*[a] usually causes symptoms that appear over seconds to minutes. However, symptoms may present when the patient wakes from sleep. The hallmark of stroke is *focal neurological dysfunction* arising from a localised insult to the brain, and reflects this area. Patients may be unable to move one side of the body (hemiplegia) or have difficulty with speech or swallowing. There may have been previous episodes. When there is resolution of the symptoms within

> **NEUROLOGICAL HISTORY**
>
> **Presenting symptoms***
> Headache, facial pain
> Neck or back pain
> Fits, faints or funny turns
> Dizziness or vertigo
> Disturbances of vision, hearing or smell
> Disturbances of gait
> Loss of or disturbed sensation, or weakness in limb(s)
> Disturbances of sphincter control (bladder, bowels)
> Involuntary movements or tremor
> Speech and swallowing disturbance
> Altered cognition
>
> **Risk factors for cerebrovascular disease**
> Hypertension
> Smoking
> Diabetes mellitus
> Hyperlipidaemia
> Atrial fibrillation, bacterial endocarditis, myocardial infarction (emboli)
> Haematological disease
> Family history of stroke
>
> *Note particularly the temporal course of the illness, whether symptoms suggest focal or diffuse disease and the likely level of involvement of the nervous system.
>
> LIST 31.1

---
[a] Less informatively called a cerebrovascular accident (CVA).

QUESTIONS TO ASK THE (NON-APHASIC) PATIENT WITH A POSSIBLE STROKE OR TRANSIENT ISCHAEMIC ATTACK

1. What have you noticed has been wrong?
2. How quickly did it come on? How long ago?
3. Has it improved or gone away now?
4. Have you ever had a stroke before? How did that affect you?
5. Have you had high blood pressure or cholesterol? (Risk factors)
6. Are you a diabetic? (Risk factor)
7. Do you smoke? (Risk factor)
8. Is there a history of strokes in your family?
9. Have you had palpitations or been told you have atrial fibrillation?
10. Have you been treated with blood-thinning drugs such as aspirin or warfarin?
11. Have you had fevers or a problem with a heart valve? (Endocarditis and embolic event)

QUESTIONS BOX 31.1

24 hours the episode is called a *transient ischaemic attack* (TIA),[b] though symptoms longer than an hour or two are typically associated with abnormality on imaging and are termed a stroke. The rapid onset of focal symptoms without seizure almost always has a vascular cause: infarction or haemorrhage. If the patient can answer questions it is important to ask about the onset of the symptoms and about risk factors for stroke (see Questions box 31.1).

The onset of weakness on one side of the body followed by resolution and a severe headache is characteristic of hemiplegic migraine, but in elderly patients especially there may be no headache. This makes the distinction from a transient ischaemic episode difficult.

A subacute onset occurs with infection (meningitis or encephalitis; hours to days) and inflammatory disorders (e.g. Guillain–Barré[c] syndrome—acute inflammatory polyradiculoneuropathy, myasthenia gravis, polymyositis; days to weeks).

A more insidious onset suggests that the underlying disorder may be related to either a tumour (weeks to months) or a degenerative process (months to years). Metabolic or toxic disorders may present with any of these time courses.

Based on the history (and physical examination), a judgement is made as to whether the disease process is *localised* or *diffuse*, and which *levels of the nervous system* are involved; the nervous system may be thought of as having four different levels:

1. the peripheral nervous system
2. the spinal cord
3. the posterior fossa (cerebellum and brainstem)
4. the cerebral hemisphere.

Consideration of the time course and the levels of involvement will usually lead to a logical differential diagnosis of the patient's symptoms. After detailed questions about the presenting problem, ask about previous neurological symptoms and about previous neurological diagnoses or investigations. The patient may know the results of CT or MRI brain scans performed in the past. A thorough neurological history will include routine questions about possible neurological symptoms (see Questions box 31.2). If the patient answers 'yes' to any of these, more-detailed questions about the nature of the problem and its time course are indicated.

Headache and facial pain

Headache is a very common symptom (see Questions box 31.3). It is important, as with any type of pain, to determine the character, severity, site, duration, frequency, radiation, aggravating and relieving factors and associated symptoms.[1,2] Unilateral headache that is preceded by flashing lights or zigzag lines and is associated with light hurting the eyes (photophobia) is likely to be a *migraine with an aura* ('classical migraine'); common migraine has no aura. Pain over

---

[b] If brain imaging shows an infarction or bleed the diagnosis is of a stroke rather than a TIA even if the symptoms are brief.

[c] Georges Guillain (1876–1961), Jean Alexandre Barré (1880–1967) and A Strohl described the syndrome in 1916; Strohl's name was dropped because of anti-German feeling during World War I.

QUESTIONS TO ASK THE PATIENT WITH A POSSIBLE NEUROLOGICAL PROBLEM

1. Can you tell me what has been happening to you?
2. Are you right- or left-handed?
3. Have you had problems with headaches?
4. Have you been dizzy or had problems with your balance?
5. Have you noticed trouble with your speech?
6. Have you had problems with your vision?
7. Have you had weakness in an arm or leg?
8. Have you ever had a seizure or a blackout?
9. Have you ever had a head injury?
10. Have you had any back problems?
11. Have you had any scans of your brain or spinal cord?
12. What medications have you been taking?
13. Have you had high blood pressure?
14. Is there a history of neurological or muscle problems in your family?
15. Do you drink alcohol?

QUESTIONS BOX 31.2

QUESTIONS TO ASK THE PATIENT WITH HEADACHE

1. What is it like (e.g. dull, sharp, throbbing or tight)?
2. Where do you feel it—at the front or back, on one side or in the face?
3. How severe is it and how long does it last?
! 4. Has it begun very suddenly and severely? (Subarachnoid haemorrhage)
5. Do you get any warning that it is about to start (e.g. flashing lights or zigzag lines in your vision)? (Migraine)
6. Is it associated with sensitivity to light (photophobia)? (Migraine)
7. Do you feel drowsy or nauseated? (Raised intracranial pressure)
! 8. Is the pain on one side over the temple and have you had double vision, pain in the jaw when chewing or any blurred vision? (Temporal arteritis)
9. Is the pain worse over your cheek bones? (Sinusitis)
10. Are the attacks likely to occur in clusters and associated with watering of one eye? (Cluster headache)
11. Is there a prolonged feeling of tightness over the head but no other symptoms? (Tension headache)
12. Did you drink large amounts of alcohol last night? (Hangover)

QUESTIONS BOX 31.3

one eye (or over the temple) lasting for minutes to hours, associated with lacrimation, rhinorrhoea and flushing of the forehead, and occurring in bouts that last several weeks a few times a year or less, is suggestive of *cluster headache*. These are described as the 'alarm clock' headache; it tends to wake patients from sleep at the same time each day during a cluster. They occur predominantly in males and patients often cannot stay still. Headache over the occiput and associated with neck stiffness may be from *cervical spondylosis*. *Coital headache* occurs during intercourse close to or during orgasm. This sudden severe headache affects middle-aged men. It is of sudden onset and lasts in its severe form for about 15 minutes and can persist as a milder discomfort for a few hours. There is no nausea or neck stiffness. It is benign, the cause is unknown and it needs to be distinguished from subarachnoid haemorrhage, which can also occur during sexual intercourse.

A generalised headache that is worse in the morning and is associated with drowsiness or vomiting may reflect *raised intracranial pressure*, whereas generalised headache associated with photophobia and fever as

GOOD SIGNS GUIDE 31.1
Temporal arteritis

Symptoms	LR+	LR−
Diplopia	3.5	0.96
Jaw claudication (pain in proximal jaw near the temporomandibular joint after brief chewing of tough food)	4.3	0.72
Scalp tenderness	1.7	0.73
Any headache	1.7	0.67
Visual disturbance (often sudden monocular blindness)	1.1	0.97

(Adapted from Simel DL, Rennie D. *The rational clinical examination: evidence-based diagnosis*. New York: McGraw-Hill, 2009, Table 49.7.)

Abnormal movements suggesting a seizure

Tonic	Stiffening of limbs or trunk with sustained muscle contraction
Clonic	Jerking movements, usually brief and waxing and waning in intensity
Tonic–clonic	Both types of movement usually beginning with tonic contractions
Atonic	Very sudden loss of tone throughout the body. The patient usually falls to the ground without warning and injury is common; these are characteristic of severe epilepsy syndromes and often accompanied by developmental delays
Myoclonic	Brief jerks of the limbs that often cause things to be dropped from the hands
Absence	There are no motor features. There is loss of awareness but not of motor tone

TABLE 31.1

well as with a stiff neck of more gradual onset may be due to *meningitis*. In patients over 50, a persistent unilateral headache over the temporal area associated with tenderness over the temporal artery and sometimes blurring of vision or diplopia suggests *temporal arteritis*.[3,4] This condition (see Good signs guide 31.1) is often associated with jaw claudication, or jaw pain during eating, which can lead to considerable loss of weight. Headache with pain or fullness behind the eyes or over the cheeks or forehead occurs in *acute sinusitis*. The dramatic and usually instantaneous onset of severe headache that is initially localised but becomes generalised and is associated with neck stiffness may be due to a *subarachnoid haemorrhage*. Morning headaches worse with coughing, especially in an obese patient, may be due to *idiopathic intracranial hypertension*; visual loss may occur.

Finally, the most frequent type of headache is episodic or chronic *tension-type headache*; this is commonly bilateral, occurs over the frontal, occipital or temporal areas and may be described as a sensation of tightness that lasts for hours and recurs often. It is not made worse by walking. There are usually no associated symptoms such as nausea, vomiting, weakness or paraesthesias (tingling in the limbs), and the headache does not usually wake the patient at night from sleep.

Remember the mnemonic **POUND** when trying to differentiate migraine headache from tension headache:

P ulsatile headache
4–72 h **O** urs duration
U nilateral, not bilateral
N ausea and/or vomiting
D isabling headache.

If there are 4–5 of these features, the LR+ for migraine is an impressive 24.[5]

Pain in the face can result from trigeminal neuralgia, temporomandibular arthritis, glaucoma, cluster headache, temporal arteritis, psychiatric disease, aneurysm of the internal carotid or posterior communicating artery, or the superior orbital fissure syndrome.

Faints and fits (see also p 66)

It is important to try to differentiate syncope (transient loss of consciousness) from *epilepsy* (see Questions box 31.4). However, primary syncopal events can cause a few clonic jerks in a significant number of cases[d] (see Table 31.1).

A detailed description of the episode can help identify the type of seizure. The prodrome is very

---

[d] The diagnosis of the cause of transient loss of consciousness can be difficult. Patients who have seen a cardiologist first are often told the cause is neurological, while those who have seen a neurologist first are often told that it is cardiac in origin.

QUESTIONS TO ASK THE PATIENT WITH SYNCOPE OR DIZZINESS

1. Did you lose consciousness completely? How long for?
2. Do you black out or feel dizzy when you stand up quickly? (Postural hypotension)
3. How often have episodes occurred?
4. Was the sensation more one of spinning? (Vertigo)
5. Did the episode occur during heavy exercise or when you got up to pass urine at night? (Exercise—suggests a left ventricular outflow tract obstruction such as aortic stenosis; pass urine at night—micturition syncope)
6. Have you injured yourself?
7. Do you get any warning? (A feeling of nausea and being in a stuffy room suggests a vasovagal episode; a strange smell or feeling of *déjà vu* suggests an aura and therefore a seizure)
8. Have you passed urine during the episode? (Seizure)
9. Have you bitten your tongue? (Seizure)
10. Has anyone seen an episode and noticed jerking movements (tonic–clonic movements)? (Makes a seizure more likely but can also occur with cardiac syncope)
11. Do you wake up feeling normal or drowsy? (Normal—cardiac syncope; drowsy—seizure)
12. What medications are you taking—any antihypertensive medications, cardiac antiarrhythmic drugs or antiepileptic drugs?

QUESTIONS BOX 31.4

QUESTIONS TO ASK THE PATIENT WITH DEFINITE OR SUSPECTED EPILEPSY

1. Has the diagnosis been confirmed? How? (e.g. typical features, investigations—EEG)
2. Has a cause been found? (e.g. developmental, abnormality on CT scan, trauma)
3. When was the last seizure? Was this during the day or during sleep?
4. How often have episodes occurred?
5. Have you ever injured yourself?
6. Did you lose consciousness?
7. Has drug treatment been started? Has it been successful? Have there been side effects of treatment?
8. Is it difficult for you to remember to take your tablets?
9. Do you drive? Have you been allowed to drive?
10. Has your work or education been affected?
11. Is there a family history of epilepsy?

QUESTIONS BOX 31.5

important; the sensation of a focal aura is often clearly different from that of presyncope. A witness may be able to describe the type of attack that occurred. A helpful friend or officious bystander may have recorded the episode on a mobile telephone. There are certain basic questions that should be asked of patients with confirmed or suspected epilepsy (Questions box 31.5).

There are two major classes of seizures:

1. focal (partial)
2. generalised.

Focal seizures are notable for symptoms localisable to a single part of the brain. They may be limited to a single part of the brain or body and not impair consciousness, in which case they are referred to as 'simple'. However, if seizure activity spreads through the brain, consciousness is often lost. These seizures are referred to as 'complex'. If the whole brain becomes involved with convulsive activity the seizure is called 'secondarily generalised'.

- The **aura**, mentioned above, is actually a simple focal seizure and it may resolve spontaneously or may spread and lead to loss of consciousness.

> **COMMON FORMS OF AURA**
>
> 1. A peculiar taste or smell
> 2. A feeling that something occurring has happened before; *'déjà vu'* or been heard before *'déjà entendu'*
> 3. A feeling that something happening has never happened before; *'jamais vu'*
> 4. The hearing of familiar music
> 5. A feeling of fear or anxiety welling up in the chest; this can make differentiating from a panic attack difficult
> 6. Visceral feelings such as nausea or abdominal pain
>
> LIST 31.2

- **Temporal lobe epilepsy** is the most common type of focal epilepsy. It may occur in the setting of temporal lobe sclerosis.
- **A focal dyscognitive seizure** may cause altered consciousness without collapse. Typically the patient begins to stare blankly and then to make automatic repetitive movements such as picking at the clothes or smacking the lips. It usually last only a few minutes and is followed by drowsiness or confusion. It may be preceded by an aura.
- **Focal motor seizures** arise in the primary motor cortex. Rhythmical jerking of the contralateral, face arm or leg occurs. The attacks may spread gradually from one place, e.g. the thumb. This has been called *Jacksonian*[e] epilepsy. If episodes are prolonged the patient may be left with paralysis of the affected limb for hours (Todd's[f] palsy).

Generalised tonic–clonic seizures (convulsions) cause abrupt loss of consciousness. They can begin with generalised EEG abnormalities at the onset, in which case they are called 'generalised', or after an aura[g] (see List 31.2), in which case they are called 'secondarily generalised'. Often the patient is incontinent of urine and faeces, and the tongue may be bitten, though these features are of limited diagnostic value in themselves.

Absence seizures are also generalised seizures, with synchronous, generalised electrical activity within the brain. They present in children and adolescents and may persist into adulthood. They are frequent (up to 200 times a day) brief episodes of loss of awareness often associated with staring. Major motor movements do not occur with this type of epilepsy. The presence of an aura or other focal symptoms (posturing, focal twitching, etc.) indicates that the seizures are *not* absences.

Other forms of generalised seizure include myoclonus (brief twitches or jerks, often present when tired and in the mornings) and atonic seizures.

Epilepsy in children (especially when characterised by atonic seizures) may be associated with developmental abnormalities and is often genetic. Epilepsy in adults previously considered idiopathic may also have a genetic basis, or may be the result of trauma, tumour or stroke.

> **T&O'C ESSENTIAL**
>
> *Remember: epilepsy is the condition of being affected by seizures; seizures are the epileptic events.*

Transient ischaemic attacks affecting the brainstem only rarely cause blackouts. They are generally associated with focal neurological symptoms or signs. Use of the term 'drop attacks' means the patient falls but there is no loss of consciousness. In either case the patient falls to the ground without premonition and the attacks are of brief duration. *Hypoglycaemia* can lead to episodes of loss of consciousness. Patients with hypoglycaemia may also report sweating, weakness and confusion before losing consciousness. They are usually diabetics who are taking insulin or an oral hypoglycaemic drug.

Sometimes bizarre, but often convincing, attacks of loss of consciousness occur in conversion disorder. These are referred to as psychogenic non-epileptic seizures (PNES). They do not respond to anticonvulsants, and a correct diagnosis is critical to prevent incorrect treatment (see List 31.3).

---

[e] John Hughlings Jackson (1835–1911) described this in 1863. He became the 'father of English neurology' after becoming interested in it after himself developing Bell's palsy. He did not like music, sport, eating or other people—a role model to avoid.

[f] Robert Todd (1809–60). He described this in 1856. He was a friend of Thomas Addison. He died with cirrhosis having advocated alcohol enthusiastically to his medical students as a panacea.

[g] Retrograde amnesia is common after a generalised seizure and the aura will not always be remembered.

FEATURES SUGGESTING PSYCHOGENIC NON-EPILEPTIC SEIZURE

1. Episodes are often prolonged, sometimes for over 30 minutes
2. Arching of the back (opisthotonus) is common
3. They often occur when there are witnesses (e.g. in the neurologist's waiting room)
4. Forced eye closure is common
5. Alternating planes of movement may occur (e.g. nodding and then shaking of the head)
6. Movements are not rhythmical
7. Incontinence and tongue biting are uncommon but may occur

LIST 31.3

The history and cause of vertigo

Symptoms	Likely diagnosis
Persistent vertigo without hearing loss	Vestibular neuronitis
Intermittent vertigo without hearing loss	Benign positioning vertigo
Persistent vertigo with hearing loss	Labyrinthitis
Intermittent vertigo and tinnitus with hearing loss	Ménière's disease

TABLE 31.2

Dizziness

It is important to determine what the patient means by the term *dizziness*.[h] In *vertigo*, there is a perceived sense of motion, of the surroundings or the person him- or herself.[6] When vertigo is severe it may not be possible for the patient to stand or walk, and associated symptoms of nausea, vomiting, pallor, sweating and headache may be present. The presence or absence of deafness and the time course of the vertigo can help with the diagnosis (see Table 31.2). Patients are not good at differentiating types of dizziness, so the associated features are important.

Vertigo can occur purely with movement, such as lying down, rolling over in bed and looking up or down. This paroxysmal positional vertigo can be due to underlying:

- benign paroxysmal positional vertigo (BPPV)—recurrent episodes of brief vertigo on moving the head in the direction of the involved canal; onset of dizziness on lying down or rolling over in bed is very suggestive
- migraine—vestibular migraine is a great mimic, and may be positional.

Causes of vertigo persisting longer than a few minutes and presenting with the head at rest include the 'peripheral vestibular lesions':

- vestibular neuronitis—non-positional vertigo due to inflammation of the acoustic nerve with normal hearing
- acute labyrinthitis—associated with hearing loss
- a stroke affecting the inner ear—sudden vertigo and hearing loss (occlusion of the labyrinthine artery)
- Ménière's[i] disease, which more often occurs in those over 50 years of age—the triad of episodic vertigo and tinnitus (ringing in the ears) and progressive deafness.

Central causes include:

- migraine—may last hours to days and can be nearly any pattern
- stroke—these patients usually have other symptoms such as diplopia, limb ataxia or sensory disturbance
- multiple sclerosis and cerebellar tumours.

Vestibular schwannoma only rarely causes vertigo because of its slow progression—patients more often present with progressive unilateral deafness with or without tinnitus.

Bilateral vestibular damage, such as that caused by aminoglycoside antibiotics, causes occilopsia rather than vertigo. This is due to loss of vestibular gaze stabilisation. The world seems to jump and slip, like bad handicam footage.

---

[h] The word comes from the Old English word *dysig*, meaning 'stupid'.

[i] Prosper Ménière (1799–1862), director of the Paris Institution for Deaf-Mutes, characterised this condition just before he died of postinfluenzal pneumonia. He was an expert on orchids and a friend of Victor Hugo and Honoré de Balzac. He added the grave accent on the second 'e' in his name; the acute accent on the first 'e' was added by his son.

Visual disturbances and deafness

Problems with vision can include double vision (diplopia), blurred vision (amblyopia), light intolerance (photophobia) and visual loss (p 509). The causes of deafness are summarised on page 531.

Disturbances of gait

Many neurological conditions can make walking difficult. These are described on page 577. Walking may also be abnormal when orthopaedic disease affects the lower limbs or spine. A bizarrely abnormal gait can sometimes be a sign of a conversion disorder (hysteria).

Disturbed sensation or weakness in the limbs

Pins and needles in the hands or feet may indicate nerve entrapment or a peripheral neuropathy (p 583) but can result from sensory pathway involvement at any level. The carpal tunnel syndrome is common: here there is median nerve entrapment, and patients experience pain and paraesthesias in the hand and wrist. Sometimes pain may extend to the arm and even to the shoulder, but paraesthesias are felt only in the fingers. These symptoms are usually worse at night and may be relieved by dangling the arm over the side of the bed or shaking the hand (the flick sign).

Nerve root, spinal cord and cerebral abnormalities can all cause disturbance of sensation and weakness.

Limb weakness can be caused by lesions at different levels in the motor system. There are a number of patterns of limb and muscle weakness:

- Upper motor neurone (UMN) weakness (p 580) is due to interruption of a neural pathway at a level above the anterior horn cell. The result is an increase in tone and peripheral reflexes. Interruption of this pathway has the greatest effect on the antigravity muscles and is called *pyramidal weakness*. There is little or no muscle wasting.
- Lower motor neurone (LMN) weakness (p 582) is due to a lesion that interrupts the reflex arc between the anterior horn cell and the muscle. There is a reduction in tone and reflexes, fasciculation (irregular contractions of small areas of muscle) may be seen and muscle wasting is prominent.
- Muscle disease causes weakness in a particular muscle or group of muscles. There is wasting and decreased tone, and the reflexes are reduced or absent.
- Disease at the neuromuscular junction (e.g. myasthenia gravis, p 593) causes generalised weakness, which worsens with repetition. The reflexes and tone are often normal.
- Non-organic weakness (e.g. due to hysteria) causes a non-anatomical pattern of weakness in association with normal tone and power and, unless there has been prolonged disuse, normal muscle bulk.

Tremor and involuntary movements

Tremor is a rhythmical movement (see Table 31.3). A slow tremor has, by definition, a rate between 3 Hz and 5 Hz. Rapid tremors are faster than 10 Hz.

Tremors can be described as resting, postural or action, and sometimes there are elements of each. *Resting* tremors are present mostly during relaxation of the muscles, and may not be noticed by the patient as much as by others. *Postural* tremors occur when the limbs are used, and may cause problems when the patient holds a cup or writes. *Action* ('*intention*') tremors occur with deliberate movement and become more pronounced towards the end of the action (they get worse towards the target).

Most tremors become worse with fatigue or anxiety. Shivering is a type of tremor brought on by cold. It is normal for there to be a fine tremor associated with holding a posture or performing a movement slowly. This is called a *physiological* tremor. It becomes more

Rates of tremors

Cause	Frequency (Hz)
Parkinson's disease	3–5
Essential/familial	4–7
Physiological	8–13

TABLE 31.3

obvious with fright and fatigue. It is often increased by the beta-agonist drugs used to treat asthma or by caffeine. Thyrotoxicosis is a cause of exaggeration of physiological tremor. These movements are very fine and may be difficult to see unless looked for specifically. *Benign essential (familial)* tremor is an inherited disorder (usually autosomal dominant) that causes postural tremor, but no other signs. The tremor is most easily seen when the patient's arms are stretched out; it can become worse during voluntary movements. It usually disappears when the muscles are at complete rest. It can involve the:

- head (34%)[j]
- arms (95%)
- voice (12%)
- lower limbs (30%).

Parkinson's[k] disease may present with a resting tremor (p 597). Intention (or target-seeking) tremor is due to cerebellar disease (p 595). *Chorea* involves involuntary jerky movements (p 600). Definitions of the terms used to describe movement disorders are shown in Table 31.4.

Speech and mental status

Speech may be disturbed by many different neurological diseases and is discussed on page 540. A number of different diseases can also result in delirium or dementia (see Ch 46).

PAST HEALTH

Enquire about a past history of meningitis or encephalitis, head or spinal injuries, a history of epilepsy or convulsions and any previous operations. Any past history of sexually transmitted infection (e.g. risk factors for HIV infection or syphilis) should be obtained. Ask about risk factors that may predispose to the development of cerebrovascular disease (see List 31.1). A previous diagnosis of peripheral vascular disease or of coronary artery disease indicates an increased risk of cerebrovascular disease. Chronic or paroxysmal atrial fibrillation is associated with a greatly increased risk of embolic stroke, especially for people over the age of 70.

Definitions of terms used to describe movement disorders

Akathesia	Motor restlessness; constant semipurposeful movements of the arms and legs
Asterixis	Sudden loss of muscle tone during sustained contraction of an outstretched limb
Athetosis	Writhing, slow sinuous movements, especially of the hands and wrists
Chorea	Jerky small rapid movements, often disguised by the patient with a purposeful final movement (e.g. the jerky upward arm movement is transformed into a voluntary movement to scratch the head)
Dyskinesia	Purposeless and continuous movements, often of the face and mouth; frequently a result of treatment with major tranquillisers for psychotic illness
Dystonia	Sustained contractions of groups of agonist and antagonist muscles, usually in flexion or extremes of extension; it results in bizarre postures
Hemiballismus	An exaggerated form of chorea involving one side of the body: there are wild flinging movements that can injure the patient (or bystanders)
Myoclonic jerk	A brief muscle contraction that causes a sudden purposeless jerking of a limb
Myokymia	A repeated contraction of a small muscle group; often involves the orbicularis oculi muscles
Tic	A repetitive irresistible movement that is purposeful or semipurposeful
Tremor	A rhythmical alternating movement

TABLE 31.4

MEDICATION HISTORY

Previous and current medications may be the cause of certain neurological or apparently neurological syndromes (see List 31.4).

Ask about treatment for neurological or psychiatric disorders with anticonvulsants, anti-Parkinsonian drugs, steroids, immunosuppressants, biological agents,

---

[j] Tremor involving the head is often called *titubation* from the Latin word *titubo—I stagger*. It can really be applied to tremor of any part of the body and the Latin word usually implies unsteadiness as a result of drunkenness—which is unfair as alcohol usually suppresses essential tremor.

[k] James Parkinson (1755–1824), an English general practitioner, published an essay on 'The shaking palsy' in 1817. He was nearly transported to Australia for reformist activities.

DRUGS AND NEUROLOGY

Antihypertensives
Therapeutic use: reduction of risk of stroke
Side effects: postural dizziness, syncope, depression (methyldopa)

Antiplatelet drugs and anticoagulants
Therapeutic use: reduction of risk of stroke
Side effect: cerebral haemorrhage

Statins
Therapeutic use: reduction in stroke risk
Side effect: myopathy

Major tranquillisers
Therapeutic use: treatment of psychoses
Side effects: ataxia, sedation, Parkinsonian tremor

Other neurological symptoms associated with drugs
Headache: nitrates, sildenafil
Deafness: aminoglycoside antibiotics, aspirin, frusemide
Peripheral neuropathy: amiodarone, isoniazid, metronidazole
Non-Parkinsonian tremor: lithium, sodium valproite, bronchodilators, amphetamines
Dysphagia: bisphosphonates
Confusion and loss of memory: major and minor tranquillisers, anticholinergic drugs (e.g. amitriptyline)
Seizures: pethidine

LIST 31.4

Examples of inherited neurological conditions

X-linked	Colour blindness, Duchenne's and Becker's muscular dystrophy, Leber's* optic atrophy
Autosomal dominant	Huntington's chorea, tuberous sclerosis, dystrophia myotonica
Autosomal recessive	Wilson's disease, Refsum's† disease, Freiderich's ataxia, Tay–Sachs'‡ disease
Increased incidence in families	Alzheimer's§ disease (autosomal dominant, increased risk with ApoE epsilon)

*Theodor Karl von Leber (1840–1917), a German ophthalmologist, professor of ophthalmology at Heidelberg. He began studying chemistry but was advised by Bunsen that there were too many chemists and so changed to studying medicine.
†Siguald Refsum (1907–91), a Norwegian neurologist. He described this in 1945, calling it heredotaxia hemerlopica polyneuritiformis. This may be an argument for the use of eponymous names.
‡Warren Tay (1843–1927), an English ophthalmologist, described the ophthalmological abnormalities of the condition. Bernard Sachs (1858–1944), an American neurologist and psychiatrist, described the neurological features in 1887. He studied in Germany and was a pupil of von Recklinghausen. The condition was originally called amaurotic family idiocy. This may be another reason to use eponymous names.
§Alois Alzheimer (1864–1915), a Bavarian neuropathologist, described the condition in 1906. His doctoral thesis was on the wax-producing glands of the ear.

TABLE 31.5

anticoagulants, antiplatelet agents and other drug treatment that may be associated with neurological problems; use of the contraceptive pill; and use of antihypertensive agents.

SOCIAL HISTORY

As smoking predisposes to cerebrovascular disease, the smoking history is relevant. It is useful to ask about occupation and exposure to toxins (e.g. heavy metals). Alcohol can also result in a number of neurological diseases (see List 1.3, p 18). Many neurological diseases affect people's ability to work and look after themselves.

In these cases, questions about financial security, living conditions and availability of help at home become very important.

FAMILY HISTORY

Any history of neurological or mental disease should be documented. A number of important neurological conditions are inherited (see Table 31.5).

T&O'C ESSENTIALS

1. Questions about the time course of a neurological illness can help with the diagnosis.
2. Neurological symptoms may occur before clinical signs.
3. In the absence of symptoms, abnormal examination findings are less likely to be significant.

4. The cause of dizziness may be obvious when a careful history has been taken.
5. Questioning of bystanders (e.g. for the presence of tonic–clonic movements) may be very helpful when an episode of unconsciousness is being assessed.
6. A video recording of a patient's seizure may be available for viewing.
7. The history will direct the relevant parts of the nervous system that need to be examined in detail.

OSCE REVISION TOPICS – THE NEUROLOGICAL HISTORY

Use these topics, which commonly occur in the OSCE, to help with revision.

1. This woman has been troubled by dizziness. Please take a history from her. (p 495)
2. This man has had recurrent syncopal episodes. Please take a history from him. (pp 66, 492)
3. This man has had a problem with headaches. Please take a history from him. (p 491)
4. This woman wakes at night with pain and tingling in her arm. Please take a history from her. (pp 380, 496)
5. This elderly woman has had problems with her speech. Please take a history from her. (p 540)
6. This man has had weakness in the legs. Please take a history from him. (p 496)
7. This man keeps dropping things. Please take a history from him. (p 496)

References

1. Sturm JW, Donnan GA. Diagnosis and investigation of headache. *Aust Fam Phys* 1998; 27:587–589. An accurate clinical history is the key to diagnosing the cause of headache.
2. Marks DR, Rapoport AM. Practical evaluation and diagnosis of headache. *Semin Neurol* 1997; 17:307–312. The history should include information about the onset, intensity, associated autonomic symptoms and trigger factors of headache. Special attention must be paid to the frequency of analgesic use, both prescription and over the counter, to identify analgesic rebound headache.
3. Hellmann D. Temporal arteritis: a cough, headache and tongue infarction. *JAMA* 2002; 287:2996–3000.
4. Smetana GW, Shmerling RH. Does this patient have temporal arteritis? *JAMA* 2002; 287:92–101.
5. Detsky ME, McDonald DR, Baerlocher MR. Does this patient with a headache have a migraine or need neuroimaging? *JAMA* 2006; 296:1274–1283.
6. Froehling DA, Silverstein MD, Mohr DN, Beatty CW. Does this dizzy patient have a serious form of vertigo? *JAMA* 1994; 271:385–388. Helps the clinician distinguish vertigo from other causes of dizziness.

CHAPTER 32

The neurological examination: general signs and the cranial nerves

When you have exhausted all possibilities, remember this: you haven't. THOMAS A. EDISON (1847–1931)

A PREAMBLE REGARDING THE NEUROLOGICAL EXAMINATION

The importance of clarity and simplicity when undertaking the neurological examination can't be overstated. Instructions to the patient should be short and simple, and physical demonstration of what you want the person to do is invaluable (except when testing speech and language). It is much easier to demonstrate a position you wish a person to hold, then to ask him or her to 'push up or down' than to give long strings of instructions. Patients will invariably get it wrong when given too many instructions to follow.

EXAMINATION ANATOMY

More than for any other system of the body, neurological diagnosis depends on localising the anatomical site of the lesion—in the brain, spinal cord or peripheral nerve. Fig. 32.1 shows the gross anatomy of the brain and the major functional areas.

The examination of the nervous system and the interpretation of findings require a lot of practice. In a *viva voce* examination, this system more than any other requires a polished technique. The signs need to be elicited carefully because the precise anatomical localisation of any lesions can often be determined this way. It is important, therefore, to remember some elementary neuroanatomy.

Examination can be long and difficult and it is said to take much of a day if absolutely everything that can be done (including psychometric assessment) is done. This is obviously impractical, but a screening examination that will uncover most signs takes only a relatively short time.

The functional areas of the brain

FIGURE 32.1

The following aspects of the examination should be attended to:

1. General, including examination for neck stiffness, assessment of the higher centres, speech and abnormal movements.
2. Cranial nerves I to XII.
3. Upper limbs. Motor system: inspection, tone, power, reflexes, coordination. Sensory system: pinprick sensation, proprioception, vibration sense, light touch.
4. Lower limbs: as for the upper limbs, but including assessment of walking (gait).
5. Skull and spine for local disease.
6. Carotid arteries for bruits.

GENERAL SIGNS

Consciousness

Note the level of consciousness. If the patient is unconscious,[a] look for responses to various stimuli (p 601).

Neck stiffness

Any patient with an acute neurological illness or who is febrile or has altered mental status must be assessed for signs of meningism.[1]

With the patient lying flat in bed, slip your hand under the occiput and gently flex the neck passively (i.e. without assistance from the patient). Bring the patient's chin up to approach the chest wall. The head, neck and shoulders will rise if there is true neck stiffness. Meningism may be caused by pyogenic or other infection of the meninges, or by blood in the subarachnoid space secondary to subarachnoid haemorrhage. There is resistance to neck flexion due to painful spasm of the extensor muscles of the neck. Other causes of resistance to neck flexion are characterised by an equal resistance to head rotation. They include:

1. cervical spondylosis
2. after cervical fusion
3. Parkinson's disease
4. raised intracranial pressure, especially if there is impending tonsillar herniation.

Brudzinski's[b] *sign* is spontaneous flexion of the hips during flexion of the neck by the examiner and indicates meningism.

Kernig's[c] *sign* should also be elicited if meningitis is suspected. Flex each hip in turn, then attempt to straighten the knee while keeping the hip flexed. This is greatly limited by spasm of the hamstrings (which in turn causes pain) when there is meningism due to an inflammatory exudate around the lumbar spinal roots.

Although the diagnostic value has been questioned (combined meningeal signs had a positive LR of 0.92 and a negative LR of 0.88),[1] these signs are useful clinically and they have good specificity. However, even the absence of all three items in the classical meningitis triad—**fever**, **headache** and **neck stiffness**—does not rule out meningitis (i.e. they are not very sensitive).[2]

Handedness

Shake the patient's hand and ask whether he or she is right- or left-handed. This is polite and allows you to assess the likely dominant hemisphere—94% of right-handed people and about 50% of left-handed people have a dominant left hemisphere. There is division of function between the two hemispheres, the most obvious distinction being that the dominant hemisphere controls language and mathematical functions.

Orientation

Test orientation in *person*, *place* and *time* by asking the patient his or her name, present location and the date (patients who have been in hospital for long periods often get the day wrong as one day seems very much like another in hospital). Disorientation is not a specific localising sign and may be acute and reversible (delirium) or chronic and irreversible (dementia). The Montreal Cognitive Assessment (MoCA) or mini-mental state examination (MMSE) are useful tools for documenting the progress of a confusional state or of dementia over time.

Next we focus on the head and neck—in particular, the cranial nerves. Subsequent chapters cover speech and the upper and lower limb neurological examinations.

THE CRANIAL NERVES

Examination anatomy

The cranial nerves[d] (see Fig. 32.2 and Table 32.1) arise as direct extensions of the brain (I and II) or from the brainstem (midbrain, pons and medulla)—see Figs 32.12, 32.21 and 32.38 respectively. They are numbered in the order that they arise, from rostral (top) to caudal (bottom). They are unable to be examined in strict order from CN I to XII as there are times that multiple

---

[a] If the patient in an OSCE exam is unconscious, it may be best to ask whether another patient can be provided.
[b] Josef Brudzinski (1874–1917), a Polish paediatrician, described this in 1909.
[c] Vladimir Kernig (1840–1917), a St Petersburg neurologist, described this in 1882.
[d] The anatomy and function of the cranial nerves was well established by the late 19th century. Galen identified at least seven of the cranial nerves in the 2nd century. These were probably the optic, the oculomotor, the sensory part of the trigeminal, the motor part of the trigeminal, the facial, the vestibular, the glossopharyngeal (including the vagus and accessory) and the hypoglossal nerves.

Cranial nerves

FIGURE 32.2

nerves contribute to a single element of neurological function, particularly with regard to the control of the eyes.

General inspection

If possible, position the patient so that he or she is sitting over the edge of the bed. Look at the patient's head, face and neck. Acromegaly (p 456), Paget's disease (p 476) or basilar invagination may be obvious. A careful *general inspection* may reveal signs that are easily missed when each cranial nerve is examined separately. This is particularly true of:
- ptosis (p 511)
- proptosis (p 774)
- pupillary inequality (p 511)
- skew deviation of the eyes
- facial asymmetry.

Inspect the whole scalp for craniotomy scars and the skin for neurofibromas (see Fig. 32.3). Look for

Subcutaneous neurofibromas in neurofibromatosis type I, associated with optic nerve and pontine gliomas (vestibular schwannomas, often called (incorrectly) acoustic neuromas occur in type II)

FIGURE 32.3

The cranial nerves

Cranial nerve	Name	Foramen	Fibres	Branches	Functions
I	Olfactory	Cribriform plate of the ethmoid bone	Sensory		Smell
II	Optic	Optic foramen	Sensory		Vision
III	Oculomotor	Superior orbital fissure	Motor		Extraocular muscles except superior oblique and lateral rectus; pupillary constriction
IV	Trochlear	Superior orbital fissure	Motor		Superior oblique
V	Trigeminal	V1 superior oblique fissure V2 foramen rotundum V3 foramen ovale	Motor and sensory	V1 ophthalmic V2 maxillary V3 mandibular	Sensation over the face; muscles of mastication
VI	Abducens	Superior orbital fissure	Motor		Lateral rectus muscle
VII	Facial	Internal acoustic meatus	Motor and sensory	Temporal Zygomatic Buccal Mandibular Cervical	Muscles of facial expression Stapedius muscle Taste sensation from anterior two-thirds of tongue
VIII	Vestibulocochlear	Internal acoustic meatus	Sensory		Balance and hearing
IX	Glossopharyngeal	Jugular foramen	Motor sensory and secretory		Sensation pharynx, ear, posterior third of tongue Secretory fibres to parotid Motor fibres to stylopharyngeus
X	Vagus	Jugular foramen	Motor and sensory		Sensation pharynx and larynx Muscles of pharynx, larynx and palate
XI	Accessory	Jugular foramen	Motor		Trapezius and sternocleidomastoid muscles
XII	Hypoglossal	Hypoglossal foramen	Motor		Muscles of the tongue

TABLE 32.1

skin lesions: for example, a capillary or cavernous haemangioma is seen on the face in the distribution of the trigeminal (V) nerve in the Sturge–Weber[e] syndrome. It is associated with an intracranial venous haemangioma of the leptomeninges and with seizures.

Herpes zoster (shingles) often appears in a nerve distribution as well as helping with the diagnosis of this painful rash. The characteristic distribution of the lesions demonstrates the anatomy of the nerve involved (see Figs 32.4 and 32.24).

---

[e] William Allen Sturge (1850–1919), a British physician, described this in 1879, and Frederick Parkes Weber (1863–1962), a London physician, described it in 1922.

Herpes zoster in the ophthalmic division of the facial nerve showing the nerve distribution

FIGURE 32.4

The cranial nerves are usually tested in approximately the order of their number.[3]

The first (olfactory) nerve
Examination anatomy
The first (olfactory) nerve[f] is a purely sensory nerve whose fibres arise in the mucous membrane of the nose and pass through the cribriform plate of the ethmoid bone to synapse in the olfactory bulb. From here the olfactory tract runs under the frontal lobe and terminates in the medial temporal lobe on the same side.

Examination of the nose and sense of smell
The first nerve is not tested routinely. If the patient complains of loss of smell (anosmia) or taste, or there are other signs suggesting a frontal or temporal lobe lesion, then it may be examined. Anosmic patients sometimes complain of loss of taste rather than loss of smell because the sense of smell plays a large part in the appreciation of taste.

Note the external appearance of the nose. Look for rash or deformity. Then examine the nasal vestibule by elevating the tip of the nose (in adults a speculum is usually needed to give an adequate view).

Test smell with a series of bottles containing essences of familiar smells, such as coffee, vanilla and peppermint (this is traditional, but not very reliable). Scratch and smell cards can be used somewhat more conveniently. Pungent substances such as ammonia should not be used, first because they upset the patient and second because noxious stimuli of this sort are detected by sensory fibres of the fifth (trigeminal) nerve. An easy way to test smell is to use the isopropyl alcohol wipes present in most hospital clinics. These have a distinctive and non-pungent smell.

Examination of the nasal passages must be performed if anosmia is present. Polyps and mucosal thickening may be seen and may explain the findings.

Causes of anosmia
Most cases of anosmia are bilateral. Causes include:
1. upper respiratory tract infection (most common)
2. smoking and increasing age
3. ethmoid tumours
4. basal skull fracture or frontal fracture, or after pituitary surgery
5. congenital—for example, Kallmann's syndrome (hypogonadotrophic hypogonadism)
6. meningioma of the olfactory groove
7. following meningitis.

The main unilateral causes are head trauma without a fracture, or an early meningioma of the olfactory groove.[g]

---

[f] Samuel von Sömmerring (1755–1830) is responsible for the modern classification of 12 cranial nerves. He separated the vestibulocochlear from the facial nerve, and the glossopharyngeal from the vagus and accessory nerve.

[g] Other abnormalities of smell are hyperosmia and parosmia. Hyperosmia is an increase in the sensitivity of the sense of smell. It is often a sign of psychosis or hysteria but may occur with migraine, during menstruation and in cases of encephalitis. Parosmia is a perversion of the sense of smell. It can occur following trauma to the head and in some psychoses. Olfactory hallucinations are more often than not a result of an organic lesion and suggest an irritating lesion in the olfactory cortex.

EXAMINING THE EYES

Dividing the ocular examination into individual cranial nerves is possible, but runs the risk of overlooking the multiple problems causing impairment of function that are not a result of cranial nerve abnormalities. For example, pathology can be:

- intraocular
- within muscles (such as in Graves' ophthalmopathy)
- at the neuromuscular junction (myasthenia gravis)
- in the sympathetic chain (Horner's syndrome)
- in the supranuclear brainstem (progressive supranuclear palsy)
- in a cerebral hemisphere (gaze palsy as a result of a frontal stroke).

For this reason, while using the cranial nerves as a framework, it is important to realise that the eyes are a 'window to the brain'. The cranial nerves involved in the ocular examination are:

II Optic nerve (and retina)—visual information to the brain

III Oculomotor nerve—most motor control, including pupillary constriction and eyelid control

IV Trochlear nerve—moves eye down and in, with intortion (twisting)

VI Abducens nerve—moves the eye out (abducts the eye as the name suggests)

VIII Vestibular component of the vestibulocochlear nerve—provides eye stabilisation within the head during movement and at rest

V_1 Ophthalmic division of the trigeminal nerve—sensation over the cornea and eyelid

VII Facial nerve—closes the eye.

The second (optic) nerve
Examination anatomy

The optic nerve is not really a nerve but an extension of fibres of the central nervous system that unites the retinas with the brain. It is purely sensory, contains about a million fibres and extends for about 5 centimetres (see Fig. 32.5), passing through the optic foramen close to the ophthalmic artery and joining the nerve from the other side at the base of the brain to form the optic chiasm. The spatial orientation of fibres from different parts of the fundus is preserved so that fibres from the lower part of the retina are found in the inferior part of the chiasm, and vice versa. Fibres from the temporal visual fields (i.e. projecting to the nasal halves of the retinas) cross in the chiasm, whereas those from the nasal visual fields (projecting to the lateral halves of the retinas) do not. Fibres for the light reflex from the optic chiasm finish in the superior colliculus, whence connections occur with both third nerve nuclei. The remainder of the fibres leaving the chiasm are concerned with vision and travel in the optic tract to the lateral geniculate body. From here the fibres form the optic radiation and pass through the posterior part of the internal capsule, finishing in the visual cortex of the occipital lobe. In their course they splay out so that fibres serving the lower quadrants course through the parietal lobe, and those for the upper quadrants traverse the temporal lobe. The result of the decussation of fibres in the optic chiasm is that fibres from the left visual field terminate in the right occipital lobe, and fibres from the right visual field terminate in the left occipital lobe.

History

The majority of visual symptoms involve reduction in visual acuity. These are discussed in detail with the physical examination findings. Some patients notice a more specific change, which will help direct the examination. Ask about the time course of the visual disturbance and whether it seems to involve the vision of one eye or one visual field. Sudden loss of vision in one eye (often described as an awareness of a curtain being drawn across the eye) may be due to an embolus to the retina. These are called *negative* visual symptoms. There is usually, but not always, spontaneous return of vision. This is termed *amaurosis fugax*. Migraine attacks may be preceded by subjective visual changes, including scintillating scotomas, photophobia, blurred vision or hemianopia. Visual hallucinations such as flashing lights and distortions of vision are called *positive* visual symptoms. They can also occur in migraine, retinal detachment or as the aura of an epileptic seizure.

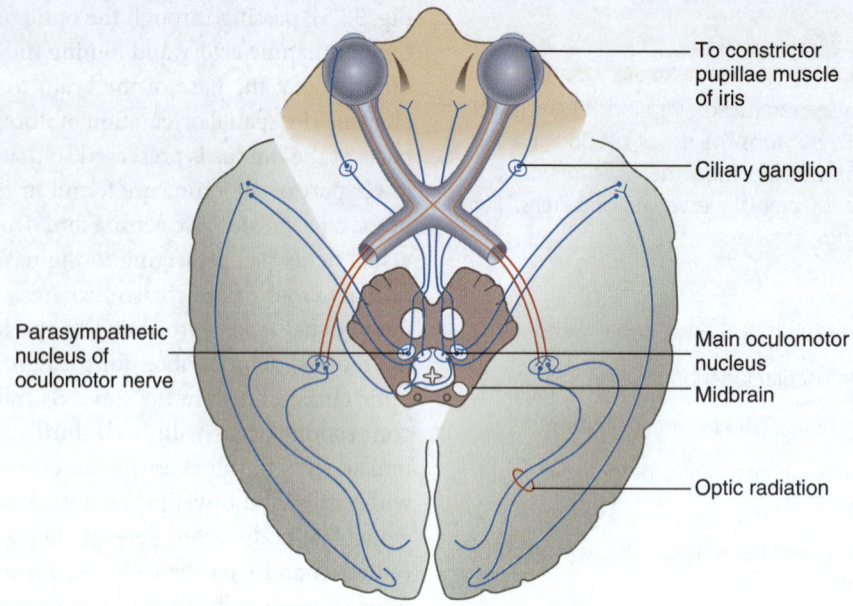

The optic pathways and visual reflexes
(Adapted from Snell RS, Westmoreland BF. *Clinical neuroanatomy for medical students*, 4th edition. Lippincott-Raven. 1997.)

FIGURE 32.5

More gradual loss of vision has many possible causes.

Examination
Assess visual acuity, visual fields and the fundi.

Visual acuity is tested with the patient wearing his or her spectacles, if used for reading or driving, as refractive errors are *not* considered to be cranial nerve abnormalities. Use a hand-held eye chart or a Snellen's chart[h] on the wall. Each eye is tested separately, while the other is covered by a small card.

Formal testing with a standard Snellen's chart requires the patient to be 6 metres from the chart. Unless a very large room is available, this is done using a mirror. Smaller charts are available, but care should be taken to keep them at the correct distance. Normal visual acuity is present when the line marked 6 can be read correctly with each eye (6/6 acuity. American readers may use the numbers 20/20 to denominate feet rather than metres). The examination will be quicker if the patient is asked to read the smallest line possible. If poor visual acuity improves when the patient is asked to read the chart through a pin-hole, refractive error is likely to be the cause. A patient who is unable to read even the largest letter of the chart should be asked to count fingers held up in front of each eye in turn, and if this is not possible, then perception of hand movement is tested. Failing this, test for light perception with a torch.

Any abnormality of the lens, cornea, fundus or optic nerve pathway can cause reduction in visual acuity:

- *Causes of bilateral blindness of rapid onset* include bilateral occipital lobe infarction, bilateral occipital lobe trauma, bilateral optic nerve damage (as with methyl alcohol poisoning) and somatisation or conversion reaction.[i]
- *Sudden blindness in one eye* can be due to retinal artery or vein occlusion, temporal arteritis (the artery may appear prominent and be tender to palpation; see Fig. 32.6), non-arteritic ischaemic optic neuropathy and optic neuritis. Patients

---

[h] Hermann Snellen (1834–1908), a Dutch ophthalmologist, invented this chart in 1862.

[i] No longer called hysterical, these types of illness behaviour are a response to psychological distress.

CHAPTER 32 THE NEUROLOGICAL EXAMINATION: GENERAL SIGNS AND THE CRANIAL NERVES   507

A visibly enlarged temporal artery in a patient with headache

(From Klippel JH, Dieppe PA, eds. *Rheumatology*, 2nd edn. Philadelphia: Mosby, 1997.)

FIGURE 32.6

Visual field testing: 'Tell me when you first see the red pin come into view'

FIGURE 32.7

often report single eye involvement even when the abnormality is homonymous (see below).

- *Bilateral blindness of gradual onset* may be caused by cataracts, acute glaucoma, macular degeneration, diabetic retinopathy (vitreous haemorrhages), bilateral optic nerve or chiasmal compression, and bilateral optic nerve damage—for example, tobacco *amblyopia* (blindness due to retinal disease).

Visual fields are examined by *confrontation* (see Fig. 32.7). Always remove a patient's spectacles first. Your head should be level with the patient's head. Use a red-tipped hat-pin. Test each eye separately. Hold the pin at arm's length with the coloured head upwards. It should be positioned halfway between you and the patient, and brought in from just outside your peripheral vision until the patient can see it. Make sure that the patient is staring directly at your eye and explain that he or she is looking for the first sight of the pin in the periphery of their vision. When the right eye is being tested the patient should look straight into your left eye. The patient's head should be at arm's length and the eye not being tested should be covered. The pin should be brought into the visual field from the four main directions (superotemporal, superonasal, inferotemporal, inferonasal), diagonally towards the centre of the field of vision.

Next the blind spot can be mapped out by asking about disappearance of the pin around the centre of the field of vision of each eye. Move the pin slowly across the field of vision. A large central scotoma will lead to its apparent temporary disappearance and then reappearance. Only a gross enlargement may be detectable.

The visual fields and optic pathways.

Numbers indicate sites of lesions producing field defects shown in Fig. 32.9

(Adapted from Snell RS, Westmoreland BF. *Clinical neuroanatomy for medical students*, 4th edition. Lippincott-Raven. 1997.)

FIGURE 32.8

1. **TUNNEL VISION**
   Concentric diminution, e.g. glaucoma, papilloedema, syphilis

2. **ENLARGED BLIND SPOT**
   Optic nerve head enlargement

3. **CENTRAL SCOTOMATA**
   Optic nerve head to chiasmal lesion, e.g. demyelination, toxic, vascular, nutritional

4. **UNILATERAL FIELD LOSS**
   Optic nerve lesion, e.g. vascular, tumour

5. **BITEMPORAL HEMIANOPIA**
   Optic chiasm lesion, e.g. pituitary tumour, sella meningioma

6. **HOMONYMOUS HEMIANOPIA**
   Optic tract to occipital cortex, e.g. vascular, tumour
   (NB: incomplete lesion results in macular (central) vision sparing)

7. **UPPER QUADRANT HOMONYMOUS HEMIANOPIA**
   Temporal lobe lesion, e.g. vascular, tumour

8. **LOWER QUADRANT HOMONYMOUS HEMIANOPIA**
   Parietal lobe lesion

Visual field defects with lesions at various levels along the optic pathway, at sites indicated in Fig. 32.8

(Adapted from Bickerstaff ER, Spillane JA. *Neurological examination in clinical practice*, 5th edn. Oxford: Blackwell, 1989.)

FIGURE 32.9

The red pin can also be used at this point to test for optic nerve pathology. Ask the patient to compare the colour of the pin when it is looked at with one eye covered at a time. The red colour will appear less intense or 'washed out' when the bad eye is used. Sometimes colour-test Ishihara[j] charts are also used.

If the patient has such poor acuity that a pin is difficult to see, map the fields with your fingers. You can also use your fingers to perform a quick screening test of the visual fields. Usually you hold up two fingers and bring them into the centre of vision in the four quadrants. Wiggle your fingers and ask the patient to say 'yes' when movement of the fingers is first seen. The following patterns of visual field loss may be detected (see Figs 32.8 and 32.9):

- *Concentric diminution of the field (tunnel vision)* may be caused by glaucoma, retinal abnormalities such as chorioretinitis or retinitis pigmentosa, or papilloedema as with migraine. Normally, even a reduced field of vision widens as objects are moved further away. Tubular diminution of the visual fields suggests a conversion reaction. There is always a small area close to the centre of the visual fields where there is no vision (the blind spot). This is the area where the optic disc is seen on fundoscopy and is the point where the optic nerve joins the

---
[j] Named after Shinobu Ishihara from Tokyo in 1917.

retina. The blind spot enlarges with papilloedema.

- *Central scotomata*, or *loss of central (macular) vision*, may be due to demyelination of the optic nerve (multiple sclerosis causes unilateral or asymmetrical bilateral scotomata); toxic causes, such as methyl alcohol (symmetrical bilateral scotomata); nutritional causes, such as tobacco or alcohol amblyopia (symmetrical central or centrocaecal scotomata); vascular lesions (unilateral); and gliomas of the optic nerve (unilateral).
- *Total unilateral visual loss* is due to a lesion of the optic nerve or to unilateral eye disease.
- *Bitemporal hemianopia* is due to a lesion that affects the centre of the optic chiasm, damaging fibres from the nasal halves of the retinas as they decussate. This will result in loss of both temporal halves of the visual fields. Causes include a pituitary tumour, a craniopharyngioma and a suprasellar meningioma.
- *Binasal hemianopia* is very rare and is due to bilateral lesions affecting the uncrossed optic fibres, such as atheroma of the internal carotid siphon.
- *Homonymous hemianopia* is due to a lesion that damages the optic tract or radiation, affecting the visual field on the right or left side. For example, left temporal and right nasal field loss will occur with a right-sided lesion. The exact nature of the defect depends on the site of interruption of the fibres. In the optic tract the defect is usually complete—there is no macular sparing. In the more posterior optic radiation the macular vision is usually spared if the cause is ischaemia, but not if a destructive process such as tumour or haemorrhage is responsible. The macular cortical area is thought to have some additional blood supply from the anterior and middle cerebral arteries.
- *Homonymous quadrantanopia* is loss of the upper or lower homonymous quadrants of the visual fields. This may be due to temporal lobe lesions (e.g. vascular lesions or tumours), which cause upper quadrantanopia, or parietal lobe lesions (e.g. vascular lesions or tumours), which cause lower quadrantanopia.

The presence of an abnormality has diagnostic value (LR+ 4.2–6.8),[4] but absence is largely unhelpful.

Fundoscopy begins not with examination of the fundus, but rather with visualisation of the cornea with the ophthalmoscope. Use your right eye to look in the patient's right eye, and vice versa. This prevents contact between the noses of the patient and the examiner in the midline. Keep your head vertical so that the patient can fix with the other eye.

Begin with the ophthalmoscope on the +20 lens setting, with the patient gazing into the distance. This prevents reflex pupil contraction, which occurs if the patient attempts to accommodate. Look first at the cornea and iris, and then at the lens. Large corneal ulcers may be visible, as may undulation of the rim of the iris, which is due to previous lens and lens capsule extraction and is called iridodonesis.[k]

By racking the ophthalmoscope down towards 0, the focus can be shifted towards the fundus. Opacities in the lens (cataracts) may prevent inspection of the fundus. When the retina is in focus, search first for the optic disc. This is done by following a large retinal vein back towards the disc. All these veins radiate from the optic disc.

The margins of the disc must be examined with care. The disc itself is usually a shallow cup with a clearly outlined rim. Loss of the normal depression of the optic disc will cause blurring at the margins and is called papilloedema (see Fig. 32.10(a)). It indicates raised intracranial pressure. If papilloedema is suspected, the retinal veins should be examined for spontaneous pulsations. When these are present raised intracranial pressure is excluded, but their absence does not prove the pressure is raised.[5] If the appearance of papilloedema is associated with demyelination in the anterior part of the optic nerve, it is called papillitis. These two can be distinguished because papillitis causes visual loss but papilloedema does not.

Next note the colour of the optic disc. Normally, it is a rich yellow colour in contrast to the rest of the fundus, which is a rich red colour. The fundus may be pigmented in some diseases and in patients with pigmented skin. When the optic disc has a pale insipid white colour, optic atrophy is usually present (see Fig. 32.10(b)).

---

[k] Modern cataract surgery leaves the lens capsule in place so that iridodonesis does not occur. A pity in some ways since it is a very nice word.

Fundoscopy in the neurological patient.

(a) Papilloedema; (b) optic atrophy; (c) grade 4 hypertensive retinopathy, with papilloedema, a 'macular star' of hard exudates collecting around the fovea, and retinal oedema

(Courtesy of Lions Eye Institute.)

FIGURE 32.10

Each of the four quadrants of the retina should be examined systematically for abnormalities. Look especially for diabetic and hypertensive changes (see Fig. 32.10(c)). Note haemorrhages or exudates, which may indicate infection such as cytomegalovirus (CMV), *Candida* or toxoplasmosis. Roth's spots are yellow-centred haemorrhages, which are a sign of endocarditis.

The third (oculomotor), fourth (trochlear) and sixth (abducens) nerves—the ocular nerves

Examination anatomy

The size of the pupils depends on a balance of parasympathetic and sympathetic innervation. The parasympathetic innervation to the eyes is supplied by the Edinger–Westphal[1] nucleus of the third nerve (stimulation of these fibres causes pupillary constriction: *miosis*). The sympathetic innervation to the eye (stimulation causes pupillary dilation: *mydriasis*) is as follows: fibres from the hypothalamus go to the ciliospinal centre in the spinal cord at C8, T1 and T2, where they synapse; from there second-order neurones exit via the anterior ramus in the thoracic trunk and synapse in the superior cervical ganglion in the neck; third-order neurones travel from here with the internal carotid artery to the eye. In addition, the pupillary reflexes (see Fig. 32.11) depend for their afferent limb on the optic nerve (see Fig. 32.5). Constriction of the pupil in response to light is relayed by the optic nerve and tract to the superior colliculus and then to the Edinger–Westphal nucleus of the third nerve in the midbrain (see Fig. 32.12). Efferent motor fibres from the oculomotor nucleus travel in the wall of the cavernous sinus, where they are in association with the fourth, the ophthalmic division of the fifth and the sixth cranial nerves (see Fig. 32.22 on p 522). These nerves leave the skull together through the superior orbital fissure. The iridoconstrictor fibres terminate in the ciliary ganglion, whence postganglionic fibres arise to innervate the iris. The rest of the third nerve supplies all the ocular muscles except the superior oblique (fourth nerve) and the lateral rectus (sixth

---

[1] Ludwig Edinger (1855–1918), a Frankfurt neurologist, and Carl Friedrich Otto Westphal (1833–90), a Berlin neurologist.

CHAPTER 32 THE NEUROLOGICAL EXAMINATION: GENERAL SIGNS AND THE CRANIAL NERVES   511

Cranial nerves II and III.

(a) The pupils: inspect for size and symmetry; (b) testing the pupillary reflex

FIGURE 32.11

nerve) muscles (see Fig. 32.13). The third nerve also supplies the levator palpebrae superioris, which elevates the eyelid.

Examination

Assess the pupils and movements of the eye.

The pupils

With the patient looking at an object at an intermediate distance, examine the pupils for size, shape, equality and regularity. Slight differences in pupil size (up to 20%) may be normal.[m]

Look for *ptosis* (drooping) of one or both eyelids. Remember that *ectropion* or drooping of the lower lid is a common degenerative problem in old age but can also be caused by a seventh nerve palsy or facial scarring. There is often eye irritation and watering associated with it because of defective tear drainage.

Test the *light reflex*. Using a pocket torch, shine the light from the side (so the patient does not focus on the light and accommodate) into one of the pupils to assess its reaction to light. Inspect both pupils and repeat this procedure on the other side. Normally, the pupil into which the light is shone constricts briskly—this is the *direct* response to light. Simultaneously, the other pupil constricts in the same way. This is called the *consensual* response to light.

Move the torch rapidly from pupil to pupil. If an eye has optic atrophy or reduced visual acuity from another

---

[m] Gross differences are abnormal and called anisocoria. A small amount of fluctuation in the size of the pupils is normal and called pupillary unrest. More-pronounced rhythmical contraction and dilation of the pupils is called hippus; this may follow recovery from a third nerve palsy or occur during sleepiness. This is not often of any significance and is not a localising sign except when it is present as a rare sign of severe aortic regurgitation.

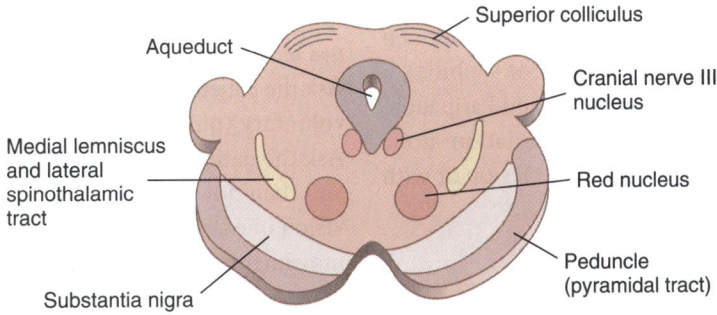

Anatomy of the midbrain

FIGURE 32.12

The eye muscles and nerve innervations

FIGURE 32.13

cause, the affected pupil will dilate paradoxically after a short time when the torch is moved from the normal eye to the abnormal eye. This is called a *relative afferent pupillary defect* (*RAPD* or the Marcus Gunn[n] pupillary sign). It occurs because an eye with even mildly reduced acuity has reduced afferent impulses so that the light reflex is decreased. When the light is shone from the normal eye to the abnormal one the pupil dilates, as reflex pupillary constriction in the abnormal eye is so reduced that relaxation after the consensual response dominates.

Now test *accommodation*. Ask the patient to look into the distance and then to focus his or her eyes on an object such as a finger or a white-tipped hat-pin brought to a point about 30 centimetres in front of the nose. There is normally constriction of both pupils—the accommodation response. It depends on a pathway from the visual association cortex descending to the third nerve nucleus. Causes of an absent light reflex with an intact accommodation reflex include a midbrain lesion (e.g. the Argyll Robertson pupil of syphilis), a ciliary ganglion lesion (e.g. Adie's[o] pupil) and Parinaud's[p] syndrome (p 520). Failure of accommodation alone may occur occasionally with a midbrain lesion or with cortical blindness.

Eye movements

There are four types of eye movements.

1. *Pursuit eye movements:* are used to follow a moving object. Watching a person walk by involves pursuit.
   - Controlled by the cerebellum and brainstem.
2. *Saccadic*[q]: are rapid movements from one point of fixation to another. Rapidly shifting gaze to someone calling out to you involves saccadic movements.
   - Controlled from the frontal lobe, brainstem and cerebellum.
3. *Convergence movements:* allow an object moving closer to the face to be followed. Needed to read a nearby book.
   - Controlled from the midbrain.
4. *Vestibulo-ocular reflex movements:* are used to compensate for movements of the head and enable fixation to be maintained, e.g. keeping your eyes on target while moving your head.
   - Controlled by vestibular organs and cerebellar and vestibular nuclei.

There are six eye muscles that move each eye, allowing horizontal, vertical and torsional movements. The evolutionary reason for this is that the muscles parallel the vestibular semicircular canals, with each muscle roughly in the plane of a vestibular canal. Fig. 32.13 illustrates the role for each muscle and its innervation. When any nerve fails (e.g. CN III) the eye movements of the affected eye are limited to those controlled by the unaffected nerves.

The full examination of eye movements includes assessment for:

- double vision (diplopia)
- nystagmus (see below).

Eye movements and diplopia

Ask the patient to look at the invaluable hat-pin.[r] Assess voluntary (pursuit) eye movements in both eyes first. Ask the patient to look laterally right and then left, up and then down (see Fig. 32.14). Ask if there is double vision in each direction, and look for failure of parallel movement. If diplopia is present, further testing is

---

[n] Robert Marcus Gunn (1850–1909), a London ophthalmologist, described the defect in 1883.
[o] William Adie (1886–1935), an Australian neurologist working in Britain, described this in 1931.
[p] Henri Parinaud (1844–1905), a French ophthalmologist, described this in 1889.

[q] From the French word meaning a jerking movement.
[r] The presence of these pins in the lapel of an expensive suit indicates the wearer is a neurologist.

Cranial nerves III, IV and VI: voluntary eye movements.

(a) 'Look to the left.' (b) 'Look to the right.' (c) 'Look up.' (d) 'Look down'

FIGURE 32.14

required (see section Advanced neurological eye examination).

Remember that the lateral rectus (sixth nerve) only moves the eyes horizontally outwards, whereas the medial rectus (third nerve) only moves the eyes horizontally inwards. The remainder of the muscle movements are a little more complicated. When the eye is abducted, the elevator is the superior rectus (third nerve), whereas the depressor is the inferior rectus (third nerve). When the eye is adducted, the elevator is the inferior oblique (third nerve), whereas the depressor is the superior oblique (fourth nerve; see Fig. 32.13). The practical upshot of all this is that the testing of pure movement (i.e. one muscle only) for elevation and depression is performed first with the eye adducted and then with it abducted. Therefore, ask the patient to follow the moving hat-pin, held 30–40 centimetres from the patient and moved in an H pattern, with both eyes and to say whether double images are seen in any direction.

The problem with testing in this way is that it is quite difficult for anyone to look up when the eyes are abducted or adducted and most people develop some diplopia when they try.[5] It is probably better to test vertical gaze with the patient staring straight ahead. The third nerve is still responsible for upward gaze. Horizontal movements will be abnormal for abduction on that side if there is a sixth nerve palsy and for adduction if there is a third nerve palsy. Moving the

---

[5] Humans began as hunters on the savanna; there were no predators threatening us from above, so our eye movements evolved to give us better horizontal movement than vertical movement. Elderly people have quite poor upward gaze.

> **TYPES OF NYSTAGMUS**
>
> 1. Physiological: (optokinetic nystagmus [OKN]) used to watch the scenery from a moving train
> 2. Retinal: (pendular) due to inability of the eyes to fixate (seen in established blindness)
> 3. Central: a result of abnormalities of cerebellar or vestibular connections
> 4. Peripheral: a result of lesions of the eighth nerve or the vestibular system of the ear
>
> LIST 32.1

pin in a cross pattern will enable this testing. Move the pin so that the patient looks down and to the right and then down and to the left. A fourth nerve palsy will lead to failure of movement and to diplopia on the side where the patient looks down and inwards.

Eye movements should be *conjugate* (parallel) to allow the eyes to fix on the same target for depth perception. Hold the hat-pin at arm's length from the patient to avoid superimposing convergence movements. Ask about double vision before testing, and if present, ensure it disappears with each eye covered. Diplopia that persists when one eye is covered (mononuclear diplopia) is uncommon.

Nystagmus

The eyes are normally maintained at rest in the midline by the balance of tone between opposing ocular muscles. Disturbance of this tone, which depends on impulses from the retina, the muscles of the eyes themselves and various vestibular and central connections, allows the eyes to drift in one direction. This drift is corrected by a quick movement (saccadic) back to the original position. When these movements occur repeatedly, **nystagmus** is said to be present (see List 32.1). The direction of the nystagmus is defined as that of the more apparent fast (correcting) movement, although it is the **slow drift that is abnormal**. Nystagmus from any cause tends to be accentuated by gaze in a direction away from the midline. In many instances nystagmus is not present when the eyes are at rest and is detected only when the eyes are deviated (gaze-evoked nystagmus). At the extremes of gaze, fine nystagmus is normal (physiological). Therefore, test for nystagmus by asking the patient to follow your pin out to 30° from the central gaze position.

Nystagmus may be jerky or pendular:

- **Jerky horizontal nystagmus** may be due to:
  - a vestibular lesion (drift is always to the side of the lesion, and intensity increases as the eye is moved away from this side—*Alexander's law*.[†] A torsional component may be present acutely.)
  - a cerebellar lesion (Can have a number of patterns. Typically drift is towards neutral due to failure of gaze holding. This results in *gaze-evoked nystagmus*, which changes direction; NB. Beats left looking left, right looking right. Cerebellar nystagmus often worsens with fixation [looking at a target].)
  - toxins (cerebellar toxicity), such as phenytoin and alcohol (may also cause vertical nystagmus)
  - internuclear ophthalmoplegia (see Fig. 32.15), which is present when there is nystagmus in the abducting eye and failure of adduction of the other (affected) side. This is due to a lesion of the medial longitudinal fasciculus. The most common cause in young adults with bilateral involvement is multiple sclerosis; in the elderly, vascular disease is an important cause.
- **Jerky vertical nystagmus** may be due to a cerebellar or brainstem lesion. Vertical nystagmus means nystagmus where the oscillations are in a vertical direction. Upbeat nystagmus suggests a lesion in the midbrain or floor of the fourth ventricle, whereas downbeat nystagmus suggests a foramen magnum lesion. Phenytoin or alcohol can also cause this abnormality. Downbeat nystagmus is often present when looking either left or right, though the nystagmus is vertical.
- **Pure torsional nystagmus** can be seen occasionally with the eye moving around the axis of the pupil in a clockwise or anticlockwise manner. When found in isolation this disconcerting finding always has a central cause.
- **Pendular nystagmus** is present when the nystagmus phases are equal in duration. Its cause

---

[†] Gustav Alexander (1873–1932), an Austrian otolaryngologist, described this in 1912.

Internuclear ophthalmoplegia.

(a) 'Look right' (normal). (b) 'Look left' (nystagmus left eye, failure of adduction right eye [affected side])

(From Compston A, McDonald I, Noseworthy J et al. *McAlpine's multiple sclerosis*, 4th edn. Edinburgh: Churchill Livingstone, 2006.)

FIGURE 32.15

may be retinal (decreased macular vision, e.g. albinism) or congenital. This condition is thought to occur as a result of poor vision or increased sensitivity to light. It develops in childhood and occurs as the patient performs searching movements in an attempt to fixate or improve the visual impulses.

A summary of how to approach the medical eye examination is provided in Chapter 42.

Advanced neurological eye examination
Test:
- pursuit (and if diplopia, the cross-cover test—see below)
- saccades
- convergence
- fatigability
- vestibular function.

If eye movements seem abnormal, further testing is indicated as set out below.

First, test **pursuit**, while asking about diplopia and watching for nystagmus. Move the target at only modest pace, and take your time. If you move too quickly, saccades (fast eye movements) will intrude. Move to about 30° of eye movement in a horizontal then a vertical direction. Watch for dysconjugate (the eyes do not move in parallel) eye movements and nystagmus. To test the individual elevator and depressor muscles, slowly draw an H or box shape, holding at each corner momentarily. Remember that muscles have a finite range, and that at extremes of gaze some nystagmus and separation of images are physiological.

If the patient has diplopia, there may be a clear loss of ocular motility on one or both sides. Diplopia is (in general) worst in the direction of muscle weakness. Common causes are listed below. However, the difference in movement between eyes that can cause diplopia may be only a degree or two. This may be difficult to detect without using the cross-cover test.

The cross-cover test

Diplopia that is not obvious so far may be revealed by the **cross-cover test** (Fig. 32.16).

1. Ask the patient to look at a target (e.g. your hat-pin), held at least 50 centimetres from the face. Initially this should be done in the neutral position (looking straight ahead).
2. Cover the patient's left eye with a card.
3. Uncover the left eye quickly and cover the right eye.
4. Look to see whether the left eye has had to change position (correct) to look at your target.
5. Repeat with the right eye.

If the eyes have made corrective saccades, they are misaligned. If the patient does not have diplopia this is called a *strabismus* (the patient may report a 'lazy eye'). Long-standing misalignment leads the brain to suppress one of the images it receives, so there is no diplopia. Correction in these patients occurs in the horizontal plane.[u]

---
[u] Vertical corrections suggest other pathology—ocular, neuromuscular or central.

An example of a cross-cover test used for a partial sixth nerve palsy on the right.

The patient had complained of double vision looking right, but the paretic eye was not easily appreciated. (a) When the left eye is covered, the right eye is able to fixate on the target. (b) However, when the cover is moved to cover the right eye, the left eye is excessively adducted and (c) a small corrective saccade (red arrow) is seen to refixate. (d) On switching the cover once again, the right eye is seen to make a larger corrective saccade (red arrow) from a relatively neutral position towards the target (a once again). This confirms that the paresis involves the right lateral rectus

FIGURE 32.16

If there is diplopia, the cross-cover test can help define the pathology. For example, if a patient has diplopia that is worst on left lateral gaze, perform cross-cover testing in this location. The paretic eye will correct to the target from a neutral position, whereas the normal eye will correct to the target from beyond the target. This immediately defines which eye is responsible.

Now test **saccades**, both horizontally and vertically. This is done by asking the patient to look between two targets (a finger and the hat-pin, or finger and thumb) held 6–10 centimetres apart. Look at the velocity of the saccades (your eyes should not be able to track the movement clearly), as well as the accuracy of saccades. Do they reach the target in a single fast movement? There may be multiple small saccades (*hypometric* saccades) or they may overshoot (*hypermetric* saccades).

These are features of cerebellar disease analogous to *past-pointing* with the hands.

There are conditions where horizontal and vertical saccades are affected differently from pursuit movements. A classic example is *progressive supranuclear palsy* (PSP), in which vertical saccades are often slowed before pursuit is lost.

Convergence is tested next. Ask the patient to look at the hat-pin placed about 50 centimetres away. Bring the pin slowly towards the patient and watch the eyes converge. Failure of this movement may occur with a third nerve lesion or eye muscle problems. Loss of convergence may occur with ageing, and as an early sign in PSP.

Test for fatigability. Myasthenia gravis is a great mimic of other eye movement disorders. Whenever the patient complains of diplopia, especially when nothing can be found objectively, it is worth testing for this. Fatigability refers to a progressive drop in muscle strength resulting from depletion of acetylcholine (the neurotransmitter) at the neuromuscular junction. With sustained muscle activation the weakness will become evident and diplopia may occur. Typically this increases as the patient attempts to hold the eye in the same position. Ptosis also often occurs. Test for this by holding a target up, 30–40° above the neutral position, and asking the patient to keep the gaze on the spot for 20–30 seconds. Ask whether there is double vision and watch for ptosis. If this occurs, rest the eyes and repeat to see whether recovery occurs, followed again by fatigue.

Sometimes there is ptosis or diplopia at rest, and this can be improved in the clinic by the *ice-pack* or *ice-on-eyes* test. Ask the patient to hold a glove containing ice with a little insulation (e.g. a thin cloth) over the eye, until it becomes uncomfortable. Resolution of diplopia or ptosis, followed by recurrence as the eye warms, is strongly suggestive of myasthenia gravis.

Vestibulo-ocular reflex (VOR)

The VOR is the fastest reflex in the body (8 milliseconds from signal to eye movement), and allows the eyes to stay on target when the head moves quickly. This powerful reflex can overcome voluntary deficits in pursuit and saccades so, for patients unable to cooperate for the testing of saccades, see whether they can fix on the spot and move the head in the opposite direction. This reflex can also drive eye movements in response to head movement in unconscious patients, though some medications can cause the VOR to disappear.

The **head impulse (thrust) test (HIT)**[v] (Fig. 32.17) allows assessment of vestibular integrity. Although it can be lost in brainstem lesions, it is typically present in a peripheral vestibular loss. The patient should watch a target, typically between the examiner's eyes, while the head is gently moved back and forward. Inability to fix at low velocities suggests bilateral vestibular *and* cerebellar failure. However, at high velocities, eye movements are driven by the VOR in isolation. Make fast, but small, turns of the head and watch the eyes. If there is loss of vestibular function the eyes will move with the head when turned towards the damaged side, and there will be a catch-up saccade back to the target.

---

[v] Described by G Michael Halmagyi and Ian Curthoys, of the neurology department, Royal Prince Alfred Hospital, Sydney.

Further vestibular assessment is discussed below as part of the eighth cranial nerve assessment.

Features of a third nerve lesion

These are complete ptosis (partial ptosis may occur with an incomplete lesion), divergent strabismus (eye 'down and out') and a dilated pupil that is unreactive both to direct light (the consensual reaction in the opposite normal eye is intact) and to accommodation (see Fig. 32.18). Always try to exclude a fourth (trochlear) nerve lesion when a third nerve lesion is present. One way to do this is by tilting the patient's head to the same side as the lesion. The affected eye will intort if the fourth nerve is intact. (Remember SIN—the *Superior* oblique *INtorts* the eye.)

Aetiology of a third nerve palsy

Third nerve lesions are most commonly related to trauma or are idiopathic. *Central causes* include vascular lesions in the brainstem, tumours and, rarely, demyelination. *Peripheral causes* include: (1) compressive lesions, such as an aneurysm (usually on the posterior communicating artery), tumour, basal meningitis, nasopharyngeal carcinoma or orbital lesions—for example, Tolosa–Hunt syndrome (superior orbital fissure syndrome—painful lesions of III, IV, VI and the first division of V), and (2) ischaemia or infarction, as in arteritis, diabetes mellitus and migraine.

Features of a fourth nerve lesion

Test this nerve by asking the patient to turn the eye in and then try to look down: a lesion results in paralysis of the superior oblique with weakness of downward (and outward) movement. The patient may walk around with his or her head tilted away from the lesion—that is, to the opposite shoulder (this allows the patient to maintain binocular vision).

An isolated fourth nerve palsy is rare and is usually idiopathic or related to trauma. It may occasionally occur with lesions of the cerebral peduncle.

Features of a sixth nerve lesion

These are failure of lateral movement, convergent strabismus and diplopia. These signs are maximal on looking to the affected side, and the images are horizontal and parallel to each other. The outermost

Head impulse (thrust) test.

(a and b) Normal head impulse test to the left; (c–e) abnormal to the right. Large green arrow denotes direction the head will be thrust. (a) Initial starting position places subject's head into cervical flexion; eyes are focused on the target. (b) Upon stopping the head thrust, the eyes are still on target and no corrective saccade is observed. In a and b, the subject's eyes stay fixed on the examiner's nose throughout the test. (c) Initial starting position places subject's head into cervical flexion; eyes are focused on the target. (d) As the head is thrust rapidly to the right, the eyes fall off the target and move with the head. (e) The subject must make a corrective saccade (small blue arrows) to bring the eyes back to the target of interest

(Adapted from Schubert MC et al. *Physical Therapy*, 2004; 84:151–158.)

FIGURE 32.17

image from the affected eye disappears on covering this eye (this image is usually also more blurred).

Aetiology of a sixth nerve palsy

Bilateral lesions may be due to trauma or to Wernicke's encephalopathy (a syndrome of ophthalmoplegia, confusion and ataxia, which is often associated with Korsakoff's psychosis due to thiamine deficiency). Mononeuritis multiplex and raised intracranial pressure are also causes of sixth nerve palsy.

Unilateral sixth nerve lesions are most commonly idiopathic or related to trauma. They may have a central (e.g. vascular lesion or tumour) or peripheral (e.g. raised intracranial pressure or diabetes mellitus) origin.

Abnormalities of conjugate gaze

Normal eye movements occur in an organised fashion so that the visual axes remain in the same plane throughout. There are centres for conjugate gaze in the frontal lobe for saccadic movements and in the

CHAPTER 32 THE NEUROLOGICAL EXAMINATION: GENERAL SIGNS AND THE CRANIAL NERVES 519

Third nerve palsy.

(a) Ahead, right eye down and out, ptosis. (b) Left failure of adduction (medial rectus). (c) Right abduction intact (lateral rectus [VI]). (d) Right up (failure of superior rectus [III]). (e) Left up (failure of interior oblique [III]). (f) Right down (failure of inferior rectus [III])

FIGURE 32.18

occipital lobe for pursuit movements. Conjugate movement to the right is controlled from the left side of the brain. From these centres fibres travel to the region of the sixth nerve nucleus, from which area the medial longitudinal fasciculus coordinates movement with the contralateral third nerve (medial rectus) nucleus (see Fig. 32.19). A brainstem lesion causes ipsilateral paralysis of horizontal conjugate gaze, and a frontal lobe lesion causes contralateral paralysis of horizontal conjugate gaze.

There are a number of possible causes for deviation of the eyes to one side. For example, *deviation of the eyes to the left* can result from:

1. a destructive lesion (usually vascular or neoplastic), which involves the pathways between the *left* frontal lobes and the oculomotor nuclei
2. a destructive lesion of the *right* side of the brainstem
3. an irritative lesion, such as an epileptic focus, of the *right* frontal lobe, which stimulates deviation of the eyes to the left.

Supranuclear palsy is loss of vertical or horizontal gaze, or both (see Fig. 32.20). The clinical features that distinguish this from third, fourth and sixth nerve palsies include:

1. Both eyes are affected.
2. Pupils may be fixed and are often unequal.
3. There is usually no diplopia.
4. The reflex eye movements—for example, on flexing and extending the neck—are usually intact.

In *progressive supranuclear palsy* (or Steele–Richardson–Olszewski syndrome[w]) there is loss of vertical and later of horizontal gaze, which is associated with extrapyramidal signs, neck rigidity and dementia. VOR eye movements on neck flexion and extension are preserved until late in the course of the disease.

Parinaud's syndrome is loss of vertical gaze often associated with nystagmus on attempted convergence (see below). There are pseudo-Argyll Robertson pupils. The causes of Parinaud's syndrome include a pinealoma, multiple sclerosis and vascular lesions.

Involuntary upward deviation of the eyes (*oculogyric crisis*) occurs with postencephalitic Parkinson's disease and may be seen in patients sensitive to phenothiazine derivatives or in patients on levodopa therapy.

One-and-a-half syndrome is rare but important to recognise. These patients have a horizontal gaze palsy when looking to one side (the 'one') plus impaired adduction on looking to the other side (the 'and-a-half'). Other features often include turning out (exotropia) of the eye opposite the side of the lesion (paralytic

(a) Horizontal and (b) vertical eye movements

(Adapted from Lance JW, McLeod JG. *A physiological approach to clinical neurology*, 3rd edn. London: Butterworth, 1981.)

FIGURE 32.19

[w] J Steele, J Richardson and J Olszewski, Canadian neurologists, described this in 1964.

Supranuclear palsy.

(a) Characteristic stare; (b) upward gaze (limited); (c) downward gaze (limited)
(From Liu GT, Volpe N, Galetta S. *Neuro-ophthalmology: diagnosis and management*. Philadelphia: Saunders, 2010.)

FIGURE 32.20

pontine exotropia). One-and-a-half syndrome can be caused by a stroke (infarct), plaque of multiple sclerosis or tumour in the dorsal pons.

Other causes of diplopia

- Infiltrative processes including Graves orbitopathy or malignancy may cause proptosis (bulging of the eye forward) and muscle weakness.
- Miller Fisher syndrome,[x] which is a variant of Guillain–Barré syndrome (p 583) may also mimic any single muscle palsy, though it is frequently more complex.

---

[x] Described in 1956 by C Miller Fisher, a Canadian neurologist. It presents with ataxia, ophthalmoplegia and areflexia.

- Mitochondrial pathologies may cause a generalised external ophthalmoplegia, usually with a ptosis.

The fifth (trigeminal) nerve
Examination anatomy

This nerve contains both sensory and motor fibres. Its motor nucleus and its sensory nucleus for touch lie in the pons (see Fig. 32.21), its proprioceptive nucleus lies in the midbrain, while its nucleus serving pain and temperature sensation descends through the medulla to reach the upper cervical cord. It is the largest of the cranial nerves.

The nerve itself leaves the pons from the cerebellopontine angle and runs over the temporal lobe

Anatomy of the pons

FIGURE 32.21

in the middle cranial fossa. At the petrous temporal bone the nerve forms the trigeminal (Gasserian[y]) ganglion and from here the three sensory divisions arise. The first (ophthalmic) division runs in the cavernous sinus with the third nerve and emerges from the superior orbital fissure to supply the skin of the forehead, the cornea and the conjunctiva. The second (maxillary) division emerges from the infraorbital foramen and supplies the skin in the middle of the face and the mucous membranes of the upper part of the mouth, the palate and the nasopharynx. The third and largest (mandibular) division runs with the motor part of the nerve, leaving the skull through the foramen ovale to supply the skin of the lower jaw and the mucous membranes of the lower part of the mouth (see Figs 32.22 and 32.23).

Pain and temperature fibres from the face run from the pons through the medulla as low as the upper cervical cord, terminating in the spinal tract nucleus as they descend. The second-order neurones arise in this nucleus and ascend again as the ventral trigeminothalamic tract. Touch and proprioceptive fibres terminate in the pontine or main sensory and mesencephalic nuclei, respectively, to form the dorsal and the ventral mesencephalic tracts. Because of this segregation in the brainstem, lesions of the medulla or upper spinal cord can cause a *dissociated sensory loss of the face*—loss of pain and temperature sensation, but retention of touch and proprioception.

The motor part of the nerve supplies the muscles of mastication.

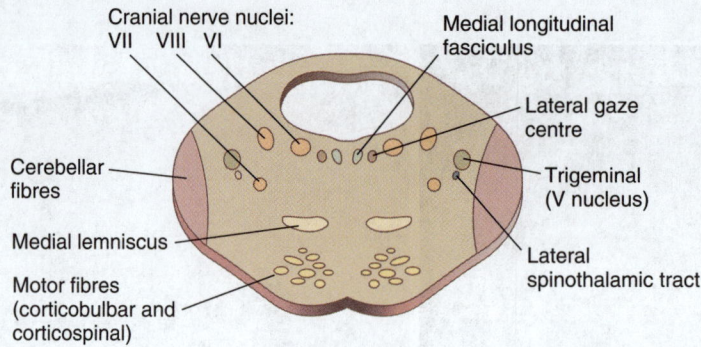

The trigeminal nerve (cranial nerve V)

FIGURE 32.22

History

Pain in the distribution of part of the trigeminal nerve is common. *Tic douloureux (trigeminal neuralgia)* is a sudden severe shooting pain in one of the divisions of the nerve. It is more common in elderly people. The occurrence in a young woman suggests multiple sclerosis. The pain is brief but very distressing. It may be precipitated by an activity such as eating or brushing the teeth. The pain is caused by a pontine lesion or by compression of the trigeminal nerve by a vascular abnormality. Pain due to sinusitis, dental abscess, malignant disease of the sinuses and herpes zoster may be felt in a trigeminal nerve distribution. Muscle

---

[y] Johann Laurenz Gasser (1723–65), a professor of anatomy in Vienna.

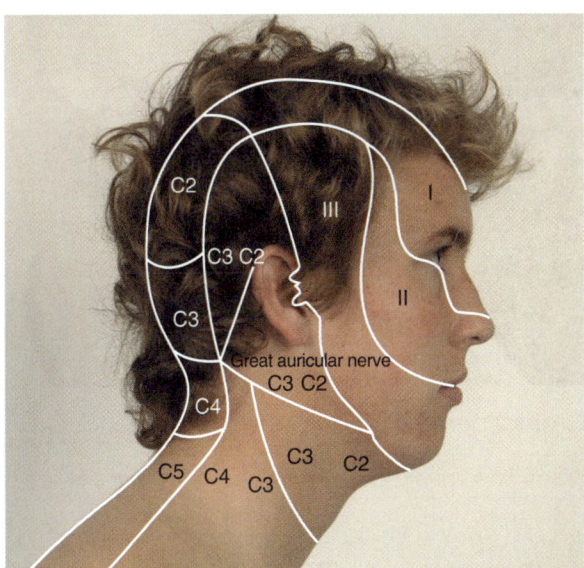

Dermatomes of the head and neck

FIGURE 32.23

(a) Facial sensation V, maxillary division: 'Does this feel sharp or blunt?'—test all three divisions on each side. (b) Herpes zoster in distribution of the maxillary nerve showing distribution of the nerve

FIGURE 32.24

weakness of the trigeminal nerve may lead the patient to complain of difficulty in eating or talking.

Examination

Test the *corneal reflex*. Lightly touch the cornea (*not* the conjunctiva) with a wisp of cottonwool brought to the eye from the side. Reflex blinking of *both* eyes is a normal response. Ask the patient whether he or she feels the touch of the cottonwool. The sensory component of the reflex is mediated by the ophthalmic division of the fifth nerve, whereas the reflex blink (motor) results from facial nerve innervation of the orbicularis oculi muscles. Absence of corneal sensation is associated with corneal ulceration.

Note: If blinking occurs only with the contralateral eye this indicates an ipsilateral seventh nerve palsy. The patient will then still feel the touch of the cottonwool on the cornea.

Test *facial sensation* in the three divisions of the nerve, comparing each side with the other (see Fig. 32.24(a)). Test with the sharp end of a new disposable neurological pin for pain sensation (never use an old pin and risk transmitting a blood-borne virus) or with something cool (the metal of a tuning fork or the end of your tendon hammer).[6] Temperature sensation is better tolerated than multiple pricks to the face. Apply the pin or metal lightly to the skin and ask the patient whether it feels sharp or dull or he or she can appreciate that the metal is cool. Some examiners ask patients to shut their eyes. Loss of sensation will result in the pinprick feeling dull or metal's feeling warmer (or occasionally 'very cold'). An area of dull sensation should be mapped by testing sensation progressively: testing should go *from the abnormal to the normal area*. Test also above the forehead progressively back over the top of the head. If the ophthalmic division is affected, sensation will return when the C2 dermatome is reached (see Fig. 32.23).

Cranial nerve V (motor): 'Clench your jaw'— feel the masseter muscles

FIGURE 32.25

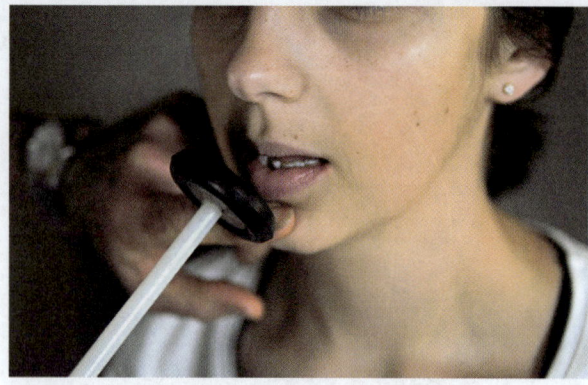

Cranial nerve V: the jaw jerk

FIGURE 32.26

It is important to exercise caution: too much pressure may leave a little trail of bloody spots, which is embarrassing.

Light touch can be tested with cottonwool, but typically yields little further information than temperature sensation.

Now examine the *motor division* of the nerve. Begin by inspecting for wasting of the temporal and masseter muscles. Ask the patient to clench the teeth, then palpate for contraction of the masseter above the mandible (see Fig. 32.25). The strength of these muscles can be tested by asking the patient to bite forcefully onto a wooden tongue depressor with the molar teeth. The depth of the teeth marks on each side gives an indication of the relative strength of the muscles. You can attempt to withdraw the tongue depressor as the patient bites it. A bite of normal strength will prevent this. Then get the patient to hold open the mouth (pterygoid muscles) while you attempt to force it shut. A unilateral lesion of the motor division causes the jaw to deviate towards the weak (affected) side.

Test the *jaw jerk* or *masseter reflex*. Ask the patient to let the mouth fall open slightly; place your finger on the tip of the jaw and tap it lightly with a tendon hammer (see Fig. 32.26). Normally, there is a slight closure of the mouth or no reaction at all. In an upper motor neurone lesion above the pons, the jaw jerk is greatly exaggerated. This is commonly seen in pseudobulbar palsy.[z]

Causes of a fifth nerve palsy

Central (pons, medulla and upper cervical cord) causes include a vascular lesion, tumour or syringobulbia. Peripheral (middle fossa) causes include an aneurysm, tumour (secondary or primary) or chronic meningitis. Trigeminal ganglion (petrous temporal bone) causes include a trigeminal neuroma, meningioma or fracture of the middle fossa. Cavernous sinus causes involve the ophthalmic division only and are usually associated with third, fourth and sixth nerve palsies. They include aneurysm, tumour or thrombosis.

Remember, if there is total loss of sensation in all three divisions of the nerve, this suggests that the level of the lesion is at the ganglion or the sensory root—for example, a schwannoma[aa] (see Fig. 32.27). If there is total sensory loss in one division only, this suggests a postganglionic lesion. The ophthalmic division is most commonly affected because it runs in the cavernous sinus and through the orbital fissure, where it is vulnerable to a number of different insults.

If there is dissociated sensory loss (loss of pain, but preservation of touch sensation), this suggests a

---

[z] Testing of the sneeze reflex is not routine. Here, stimulation or irritation of the nasal mucosa with a hair or small piece of string is followed by contraction of the muscles of the nasopharynx and thorax. The afferent limb of this arc is through the trigeminal nerve and the efferent limb through the facial, glossopharyngeal, vagus and trigeminal nerves, and the motor nerves of the cervical spine. The reflex centre is in the brainstem and upper spinal cord.

[aa] Although often called acoustic neuromas these are neither acoustic nor neuromas but rather vestibular schwannomas.

Cerebellopontine angle tumour.

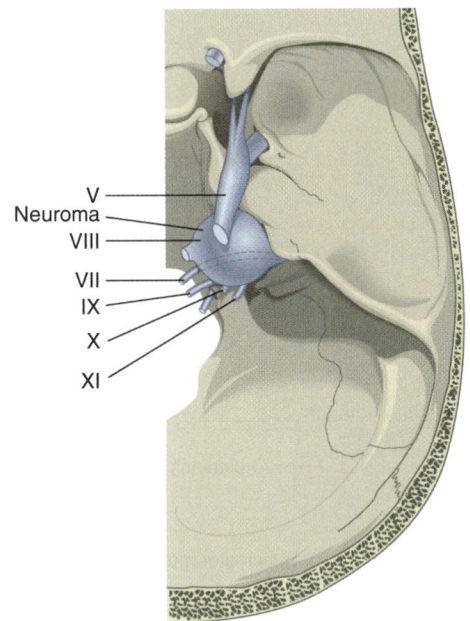

A schwannoma arising from the vestibulocochlear (VIII) nerve compresses adjacent structures, including the trigeminal (V) and facial (VII) nerves, the brainstem and the cerebellum (removed to permit the cranial nerves to be seen)

(Adapted from Simon RP, Aminoff MJ, Greenberg DA. *Clinical neurology*. Appleton & Lange, 1989. With permission of McGraw Hill, permission conveyed through Copyright Clearance Center, Inc.)

FIGURE 32.27

brainstem or upper cord lesion, such as syringobulbia, foramen magnum tumour or infarction in the territory of the posterior inferior cerebellar artery. If touch sensation is lost but pain sensation is preserved, this is usually due to an abnormality of the pontine nuclei, such as a vascular lesion or tumour. Motor loss can also be central or peripheral.

Irritative motor changes

Convulsive seizures that involve the precentral gyrus can include clenching of the jaw and biting of the tongue. Parkinson's disease and essential tremor can cause a rhythmic tremor of the lips or jaw. *Trismus* is a forceful clenching of the jaw that can occur in tetanus and encephalitis. The patient may be unable to open the mouth. Repetitive chewing and yawning movements can occur as an effect of antipsychotic drugs (*tardive orofacial dyskinesias*).

The seventh (facial) nerve
Examination anatomy

The seventh nerve nucleus lies in the pons next to the sixth cranial nerve nucleus (see Fig. 32.2). The nerve (see Fig. 32.28) leaves the pons with the eighth nerve through the cerebellopontine angle. After entering the facial canal it enlarges to become the geniculate ganglion. The branch that supplies the stapedius muscle is given off from within the facial canal. The chorda tympani (containing taste fibres from the anterior two-thirds of the tongue) joins the nerve in the facial canal. The seventh nerve leaves the skull via the stylomastoid foramen. It then passes through the middle of the parotid gland and supplies the muscles of facial expression. The frontalis muscle receives upper motor innervation bilaterally; the other muscles receive innervation from the contralateral cortex.

History

The patient may have noticed the onset of difficulty with speaking and keeping liquids in the mouth, or may have noticed facial asymmetry in the mirror. He or she may be aware of dryness of the eyes (decreased lacrimation) or the mouth (decreased salivary production). Paralysis of the stapedius muscle can cause *hyperacusis* or intolerance of loud or high-pitched sounds. Normal contraction of the stapedius muscle occurs in response to loud rebarbative noises such as popular music and dampens movement of the ossicles.

Examination

Inspect for *facial asymmetry*, as a seventh nerve palsy can cause unilateral drooping of the corner of the mouth, and smoothing of the wrinkled forehead and the nasolabial fold (see Fig. 32.29). However, symmetry may be maintained when facial nerve palsies are bilateral. Cosmetic botox use can cause confusing signs and it is worth asking about this if facial muscle power is abnormal.

Test the *muscle power*. Ask the patient to look up so as to wrinkle the forehead (see Fig. 32.30). Look for loss of wrinkling and feel the muscle strength by pushing down against the corrugation on each side. This movement is relatively preserved when there is

The facial nerve (cranial nerve VII).

Note: The branches of the facial nerve: 'Two zebras bit my car'—temporal, zygotic, buccal, mandibular, cervical

FIGURE 32.28

Left upper motor neurone facial weakness, showing drooping of the corner of the mouth, flattened nasolabial fold and sparing of the forehead; the lesion is in the right side of the brain

FIGURE 32.29

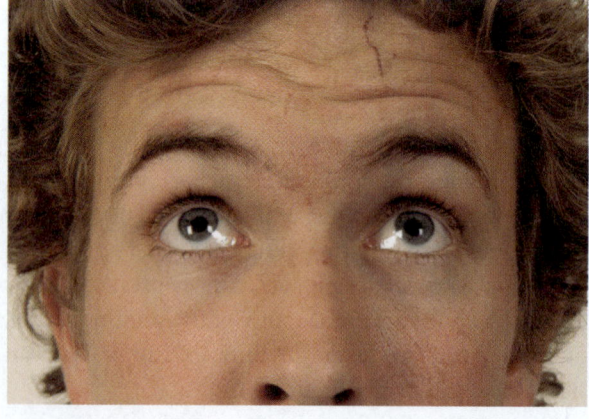

Cranial nerve VII: 'Look up to wrinkle your forehead' (normal)

FIGURE 32.30

Cranial nerve VII: 'Puff out your cheeks' (normal)

FIGURE 32.31

Cranial nerve VII: 'Shut your eyes tight and stop me opening them' (normal)

FIGURE 32.32

an upper motor neurone lesion (a lesion that occurs above the level of the brainstem nucleus) because of bilateral cortical representation of these muscles. The remaining muscles of facial expression are usually affected on the contralateral side of an upper motor neurone lesion, although occasionally the orbicularis oculi muscles are preserved. Ask the patient to puff out the cheeks (see Fig. 32.31). Look for asymmetry.

In a lower motor neurone lesion (at the level of the nucleus or nerve root), all muscles of facial expression are affected on the side of the lesion (though they need not be all *completely* paralysed).

Next, ask the patient to shut the eyes tightly (see Fig. 32.32). Compare how deeply the eyelashes are buried on the two sides and then try to force open each eye. Check whether Bell's[bb] phenomenon is evident. Bell's phenomenon is present in everyone, although not usually visible unless a person has a facial nerve palsy. In this case, when the patient attempts to shut the eye on the side of a lower motor neurone VII nerve palsy, there is upward movement of the eyeball and incomplete closure of the eyelid. Next ask the patient to grin (see Fig. 32.33) and compare the nasolabial grooves, which are smooth on the weak side.

Cranial nerve VII: 'Show me your teeth' (normal)

(Before asking this question, make sure the patient's teeth are not in a container beside the bed.)

FIGURE 32.33

[bb] Sir Charles Bell (1774–1842), a professor of anatomy at London's Royal College of Surgeons, later professor of surgery at Edinburgh, described facial nerve palsy in 1821.

If a lower motor neurone lesion is detected, check quickly for the ear and palatal vesicles of herpes zoster of the geniculate ganglion—the Ramsay Hunt[cc] syndrome.

A facial paralysis due to a cortical lesion may spare facial movements due to emotion such as crying or smiling, and indeed these movements may be exaggerated. The opposite abnormality (preservation of voluntary but loss of emotional movements) can also occur as a result of lesions in a number of areas, including the frontal lobes.

Examining for taste on the anterior two-thirds of the tongue is not usually required. If necessary, it can be tested by asking the patient to protrude the tongue to one side: sugar, vinegar, salt and quinine (sweet, sour, saline and bitter) are placed one at a time on each side of the tongue. The patient indicates the taste by pointing to a card with the various tastes listed on it. The mouth is rinsed with water between each sample.

Causes of a seventh (facial) nerve palsy

Vascular lesions or tumours are the common causes of **upper motor neurone lesions (supranuclear)**. Note that lesions of the frontal lobes may cause weakness of the emotional movements of the face alone; voluntary movements are preserved.

In **lower motor neurone lesions** *pontine* causes (often associated with CN V and VI lesions) include vascular lesions, tumours, syringobulbia and multiple sclerosis. *Posterior fossa* lesions include a schwannoma (VIII), a meningioma and chronic meningitis. At the level of the *petrous temporal bone* (Bell's palsy [an idiopathic acute paralysis of the nerve; see Fig. 32.34]), a fracture, the Ramsay Hunt syndrome or otitis media may occur, whereas the parotid gland may be affected by a tumour or sarcoidosis. Remember, Bell's palsy is the most common cause (up to 80%) of a facial nerve palsy.[dd]

Regrowth of the nerve fibres that occurs as the patient recovers from Bell's palsy can lead to aberrant connections. The most striking is the regrowth of fibres meant for the salivary gland to the lacrimal gland in up to 5% of patients. This leads to tear formation when a patient eats: crocodile tears.

Bilateral facial weakness may be due to the Guillain–Barré syndrome, sarcoidosis, bilateral parotid disease, Lyme disease or, rarely, mononeuritis multiplex. Myopathy, myasthenia gravis and botulism can also cause bilateral facial weakness, but in these cases it is not due to facial nerve involvement.

Unilateral loss of taste, without other abnormalities, can occur with middle-ear lesions involving the chorda tympani or lingual nerve, but these are very rare.

Irritative changes

Tonic and clonic movements of the facial muscles can occur in seizures. Various abnormal movements of the facial muscles can occur as a result of basal ganglia or extrapyramidal abnormalities. These include athetoid and dystonic movements. Irritative lesions in the brainstem can cause increased secretion of saliva (*sialorrhoea*). This can also occur in Parkinson's disease or accompany attacks of nausea.

Bell's palsy on the right side

(From McDonald FS, ed. *Mayo Clinic images in internal medicine*, with permission. © Mayo Clinic Scientific Press and CRC Press. Reproduced by permission of Taylor and Francis Group, LLC, a division of Informa plc.)

FIGURE 32.34

[cc] James Ramsay Hunt (1874–1937), an American neurologist.
[dd] A patient with an old Bell's palsy may exhibit *synkinesis*. When the patient blinks, the corner of the mouth twitches; when the lips are protruded, the affected eye closes.

Dix–Hallpike manoeuvre

(From Beran RG. *Neurology for general practitioners*. Sydney: Elsevier, 2012.)

FIGURE 32.35

The eighth (vestibulocochlear) nerve

Examination anatomy

The eighth (vestibulocochlear) nerve has two components: the **vestibular**, containing afferent fibres subserving balance and stabilisation of the eyes and the **cochlear**, with afferent fibres subserving hearing. Vestibular fibres begin in the utricle and semicircular canals, and join auditory fibres in the facial canal. They then enter the brainstem at the cerebellopontine angle. After entering the pons, vestibular fibres run widely throughout the brainstem and the cerebellum. Fibres for hearing originate in the organ of Corti[ee] and run to the cochlear nuclei in the pons. From here there is bilateral transmission to the medial geniculate[ff] bodies and thence to the superior gyrus of the temporal lobes.

History

Acute vertigo is a common presentation, and the history should be assessed as described in Chapter 31. If vertigo occurs only with movement, especially when lying on a bed, **benign paroxysmal positional (positioning) vertigo** (BPPV) is likely. Persistent dizziness with nystagmus while at rest is not a feature of BPPV.

Loss of hearing or tinnitus may have been noticed by the patient or complained of by his or her relatives or friends. Unilateral hearing loss is much more likely to be due to a nerve lesion and must be identified. Also find out whether this has been of gradual or sudden onset, whether there is a family history of deafness and whether the patient has had occupational or recreational exposure to loud noise (e.g. boilermaker, ageing rock musician) without hearing protection. There may be a history of trauma or recurrent ear infections.

Examination of vestibular function

If the patient complains of vertigo, an oculomotor examination should be undertaken as discussed for the cranial nerves III, IV and VI. If a patient has nystagmus, note that movement will always make them feel worse. A Dix–Hallpike test is likely to make them vomit, and is unlikely to be helpful.

However, in patients without nystagmus who complain of vertigo that is provoked by movement, especially when lying down or rolling over, the *Dix–Hallpike*[gg] *manoeuvre* should be performed (see Fig. 32.35 and the OCSE video at Student CONSULT). Have the patient sit up and explain what is about to occur. Help the patient to lie back so that the head lies at 45° to the side that is being tested, and hanging

---

[ee] Alfonso Corti (1822–88), an Italian anatomist, described this in 1851.
[ff] From the Latin *geniculus*—small knee, meaning bent at a sharp angle.

[gg] Charles Hallpike (1900–79) and MR Dix, English ear, nose and throat surgeons.

below the horizontal. This can often be achieved with a pillow behind the patient's back. Ask the patient to keep the eyes open. If the test is positive, after a short latent period, nystagmus occurs, in a waxing then waning pattern over seconds to a minute. This occurs in BPPV. It is due to abnormal *otoconia*[hh] within a semicircular canal and occurs, for example, following infection, trauma or vascular disease. The commoner type of BPPV results from otoconia in the posterior semicircular canal and is associated with *upbeating*—torsional nystagmus that beats towards the ground (*geotropic*). In the rarer horizontal canal BPPV, nystamus is horizontal and occurs on both sides with the Dix–Hallpike manoeuvre, but is worse on the affected side.

If there is no latent period, no waxing and waning or the nystagmus persists or is variable, this suggests that there may be a lesion of the brainstem (e.g. multiple sclerosis) or the cerebellum (e.g. metastatic carcinoma). More rarely there may be *cupulolithiasis*—otoconia stuck to the vestibular sensory organ.

Causes of vestibular abnormalities

Peripheral causes include:
- acute labyrinthitis, vestibular neuritis
- trauma.

In the brainstem:
- migraine
- vascular lesions
- tumours of the cerebellum or fourth ventricle
- demyelination.

Vertigo may be associated with temporal lobe dysfunction including:
- ischaemia
- complex partial seizures.

Examination of the ear and hearing

Look to see whether the patient is wearing a hearing aid; if so, remove it. Examine the pinna and look for scars behind the ears. Pull on the pinna gently (it is tender if the patient has external ear disease or temporomandibular joint disease). Feel for nodes (pre- and postauricular) that may indicate disease of the external auditory meatus.

Inspect the patient's external auditory meatus. The adult canal angulates, so in order to see the eardrum it is necessary to pull up and backwards on the auricle before inserting the otoscope. The normal eardrum (tympanic membrane) is pearly grey and concave. Look for wax or other obstructions, and inspect the eardrum for inflammation or perforation (see Ch 42).

Next, test hearing. A simple test involves covering the opposite auditory meatus with a finger, and moving it about as a distraction while whispering a number in the other ear. This should be standardised by the use of set numbers for different tones. For example, the number 68 is used to test high tone and 100 is used to test low tone. Whispering should be performed towards the end of expiration in an attempt to standardise the volume and at about 60 centimetres from the patient's ear. Your larynx should not vibrate if the whispering is soft enough. If partial deafness is suspected, know how to perform Rinné's and Weber's tests:

- **Rinné's**[ii] **test**—a 512 or 256 Hz vibrating tuning fork is placed on the mastoid process, behind the ear, and when the sound is no longer heard it is placed in line with the external meatus (see Fig. 32.36). Normally the note is audible at the external meatus. If the patient has nerve deafness, the note is audible at the external meatus, as air and bone conduction are reduced equally, so that air conduction is better (as is normal). This is termed Rinné-positive. If there is a conduction (middle-ear) deafness, no note is audible at the external meatus. This is termed Rinné negative.
- **Weber's**[jj] **test**—a vibrating 256 or 512 Hz tuning fork is positioned on the centre of the forehead (see Fig. 32.37). Normally the sound is heard in the centre of the forehead. Nerve deafness causes the sound to be heard better in the normal ear. A patient with conduction deafness finds the sound louder in the abnormal ear.

[hh] Calcium carbonate crystals, located on the saccule and utricle, which if loose may fall into the semicircular canals, causing BPPV.

[ii] Heinrich Adolf Rinné (1819–1968), a German ear specialist, described his test in 1855 using a 512 Hz fork.
[jj] Ernest Heinrich Weber (1795–1878), a German physiologist.

CHAPTER 32 THE NEUROLOGICAL EXAMINATION: GENERAL SIGNS AND THE CRANIAL NERVES   531

Cranial nerve VIII, Rinné's test: 'Where does it sound louder?'

FIGURE 32.36

Causes of deafness

Unilateral nerve deafness may be due to:
1. tumours, such as a schwannoma
2. trauma, such as fracture of the petrous temporal bone
3. vascular disease of the internal auditory artery (rare).

   Bilateral nerve deafness may be due to:
1. environmental exposure to noise
2. degeneration, such as presbyacusis
3. toxicity, such as aspirin, gentamicin or alcohol
4. infection, such as congenital rubella syndrome, acquired or congenital syphilis
5. Ménière's disease.

Brainstem disease is a rare cause of bilateral deafness. Conduction deafness may be due to:
1. wax
2. otitis media or effusion
3. otosclerosis
4. cholestatoma or other destructive lesion
5. Paget's disease of bone.

The ninth (glossopharyngeal) and tenth (vagus) nerves

Examination anatomy

These nerves have motor, sensory and autonomic functions. Nerve fibres from nuclei in the medulla (see Fig. 32.38) form multiple nerve rootlets as they exit the medulla. These join to form the ninth and tenth nerves, and also contribute to the eleventh nerve. The nerves emerge from the skull through the jugular foramen (see Fig. 32.39). The ninth nerve receives sensory fibres from the nasopharynx, the pharynx, the middle and inner ear and from the posterior third of the tongue (including taste fibres). It also carries secretory fibres to the parotid gland. The tenth nerve receives sensory fibres from the pharynx and the larynx, and innervates muscles of the pharynx, the larynx and the palate.

Cranial nerve VIII, Weber's test: 'Is the buzzing louder on one side?'

FIGURE 32.37

History

A lesion of the glossopharyngeal nerve may cause the patient no definite symptoms, but difficulty in swallowing dry foods may have been noticed.

Anatomy of the medulla.

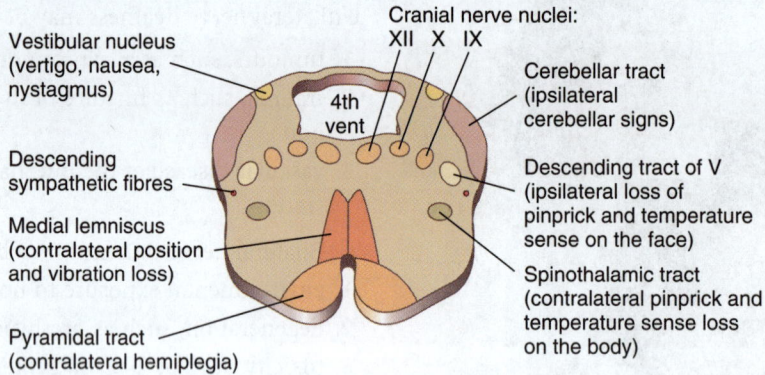

Shows correlation between lesions and clinical features

FIGURE 32.38

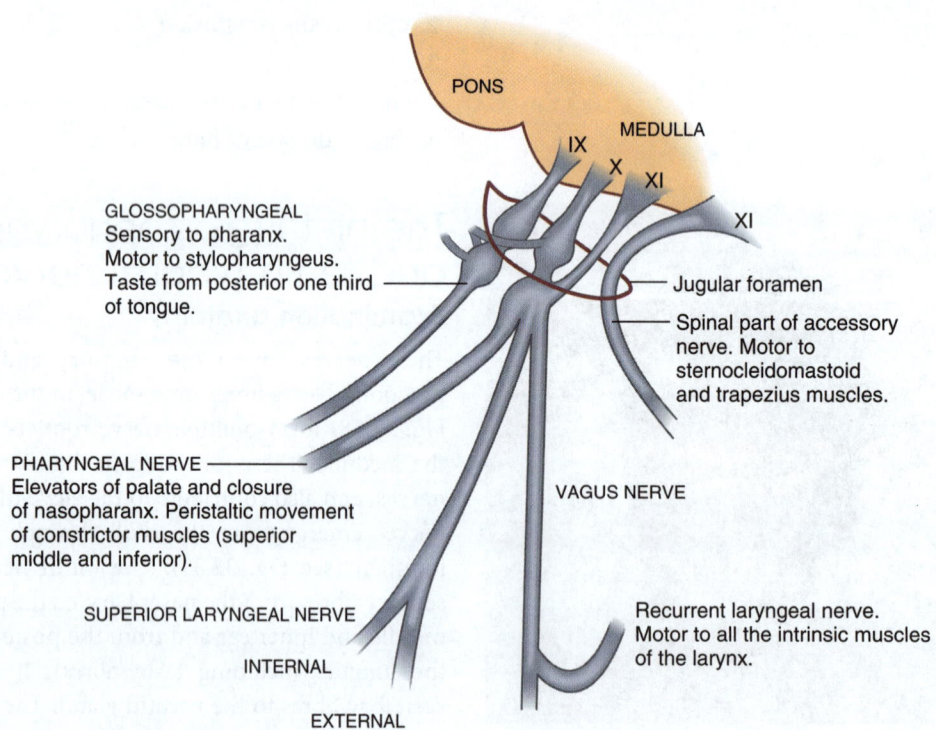

The lower cranial nerves—glossopharyngeal (IX), vagus (X) and accessory (XI)

(Adapted from Walton JN. *Brain's diseases of the nervous system*, 10th edn. Oxford: Oxford University Press, 1993.)

FIGURE 32.39

Cranial nerve X: 'Say "Ah"'—look for asymmetrical movement of the uvula

FIGURE 32.40

If contraction is absent and sensation is intact, this suggests a tenth nerve palsy. The most common cause of a reduced gag reflex is old age. Of more concern is the patient with an exaggerated but still normal reflex: this can lead to vomiting onto the examining clinician.

Ask the patient to speak in order to assess hoarseness (which may occur with a unilateral recurrent laryngeal nerve lesion), and then to cough. Listen for the characteristic bovine cough that occurs with recurrent laryngeal nerve lesions. It is not necessary routinely to test taste on the posterior third of the tongue (ninth nerve). A high-pitched 'eeee' sound is also a good test for vocal cord function.

Test the patient's ability to swallow a small amount of water and watch for regurgitation into the nose, or coughing. If bulbar function is obviously impaired, omit this step.

Causes of a ninth (glossopharyngeal) and tenth (vagus) nerve palsy

Central causes are vascular lesions (e.g. lateral medullary infarction, due to vertebral or posterior inferior cerebellar artery disease), tumours, syringobulbia and motor neurone disease. Peripheral (posterior fossa) lesions comprise aneurysms at the base of the skull, tumours, chronic meningitis or the Guillain–Barré syndrome.

The eleventh (accessory) nerve

Examination anatomy

The central portion of this nerve arises in the medulla close to the nuclei of the ninth, tenth and twelfth nerves and its spinal portion arises from the upper five cervical segments. It leaves the skull with the ninth and tenth nerves through the jugular foramen (see Fig. 32.39). Its central division provides motor fibres to the vagus and the spinal division innervates the trapezius and the sternocleidomastoid muscles. The motor fibres that supply the sternocleidomastoid muscle are thought to cross twice so that cortical control of the muscle is ipsilateral. This makes sense when one remembers that the muscle turns the head to the opposite side. This means that the hemisphere that receives information from and controls one side of the body also turns the head to face that side.

Glossopharyngeal neuralgia is a tic douloureux of the ninth nerve. The patient experiences sudden shooting pains that radiate from one side of the throat to the ear. There may be trigger areas in the throat and attacks can be brought on by chewing or swallowing.

Unilateral vagus nerve paralysis may cause difficulty in initiating the swallowing of solids and liquids, and hoarseness.

Examination

Ask the patient to open the mouth and inspect the palate with a torch. Note any displacement of the uvula. Then ask the patient to say 'Ah!' (see Fig. 32.40). Normally, the posterior edge of the soft palate—the *velum*[aa]—rises symmetrically. If the uvula is drawn to one side this indicates a unilateral tenth nerve palsy. Note that the uvula is drawn towards the normal side.[kk]

Testing for the *gag reflex* (CN IX is the sensory component and X the motor component) is traditional but not necessary.[7] A better alternative is to touch the back of the pharynx on each side (rather than the soft palate) with a spatula. The patient is asked whether the touch of the spatula (ninth) is felt each time. Normally, there is reflex contraction of the soft palate.

[kk] *Velum* means 'curtain' in Latin.

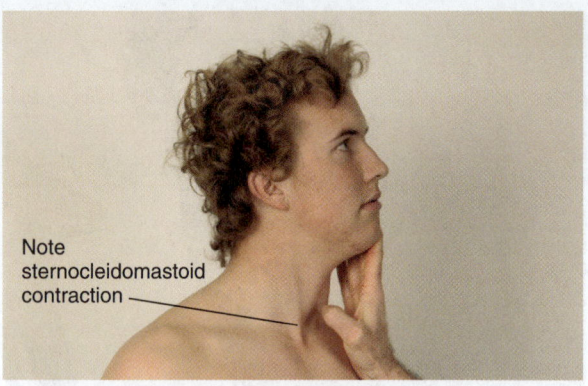

Cranial nerve XI: 'Turn your head against my hand'

FIGURE 32.42

(a) Cranial nerve XI: 'Shrug your shoulders—push up hard'. (b) Wasting of the left trapezius muscle

FIGURE 32.41

Examination

Ask the patient to shrug the shoulders (see Fig. 32.41). Feel the bulk of the trapezius muscles and attempt to push the shoulders down. Then instruct the patient to turn the head to the side against resistance (your hand; see Fig. 32.42). Remember that the right sternocleidomastoid turns the head to the left. Feel the muscle bulk of the sternocleidomastoids.

Weakness of these muscles is less common than cervical dystonia (*torticollis*), which is due to overactivity of multiple neck muscles. It is a complex movement disorder. The head appears turned to one side either permanently or in spasms. Ask the patient to turn the head to face forwards. This is usually possible at least briefly, but look to see whether he or she needs to use the hands to push the head straight.

Causes of eleventh nerve palsy

Unilateral causes are trauma involving the neck or the base of the skull, poliomyelitis, basilar invagination (platybasia), syringomyelia and tumours near the jugular foramen. Bilateral causes comprise motor neurone disease, poliomyelitis and the Guillain–Barré syndrome. *Note:* Bilateral sternocleidomastoid and trapezius weakness also occurs in muscular dystrophy (especially dystrophia myotonica).

The twelfth (hypoglossal) nerve

Examination anatomy

This nerve also arises from the medulla. It leaves the skull via the hypoglossal foramen. It is the motor nerve for the tongue.

History

The patient with bilateral hypoglossal nerve paresis may have noticed difficulty in swallowing and a sensation of choking if the tongue slips back into the throat. There are no sensory changes caused by hypoglossal nerve abnormalities, and unilateral disease rarely causes symptoms.

CHAPTER 32 **THE NEUROLOGICAL EXAMINATION: GENERAL SIGNS AND THE CRANIAL NERVES** 535

Fasciculations of the tongue in motor neurone disease

FIGURE 32.43

Cranial nerve XII: 'Stick out your tongue'

FIGURE 32.44

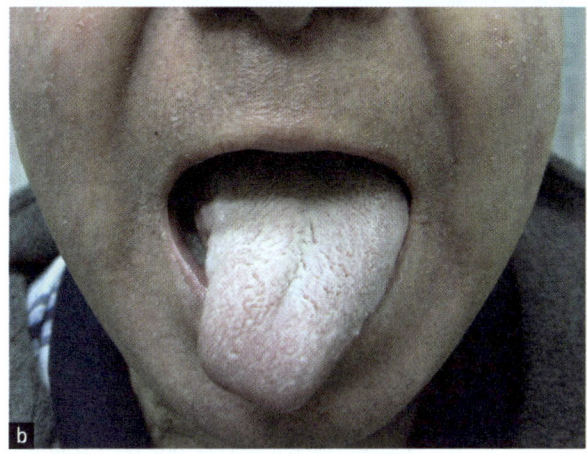

(a and b) Right hypoglossal (XII) nerve palsy—lower motor neurone lesion: 'Stick out your tongue'

FIGURE 32.45

Examination

Inspect the tongue at rest on the floor of the mouth. The normal tongue may move a little, especially when protruded, but is not wasted. Look for wasting and fasciculations (fine, irregular, non-rhythmical muscle fibre contractions). These signs indicate a lower motor neurone lesion. Fasciculations may be unilateral or bilateral (see Fig. 32.43).

Ask the patient to stick out the tongue (see Fig. 32.44), which may deviate towards the weaker (affected) side if there is a unilateral lower motor neurone lesion (see Fig. 32.45). The tongue, like the face and the palate, has a bilateral upper motor neurone innervation in most people, so a unilateral upper motor neurone lesion often causes no deviation.

A clinically obvious upper motor neurone lesion of the twelfth nerve is usually bilateral and results in a small immobile tongue. The combination of bilateral upper motor neurone lesions of the ninth, tenth and twelfth nerves is called pseudobulbar palsy.

A lower motor neurone lesion of the twelfth nerve causes fasciculation, wasting and weakness. If the lesion is bilateral, it causes dysarthria.

Movement disorders may affect the tongue. In Parkinson's disease there may be a coarse tremor of the tongue, made worse by speaking or protruding the tongue. Athetoid, choreiform and tardive dyskinesia can all involve the tongue. Patients with Huntington's chorea (disease) may have inability to keep the tongue protruded, termed *motor impersistence*.

Causes of twelfth nerve palsy

Bilateral upper motor neurone lesions may be due to vascular lesions, motor neurone disease or tumours, such as metastases to the base of the skull.

Unilateral lower motor neurone lesions with a *central* cause include vascular lesions, such as thrombosis of the vertebral artery, motor neurone disease and syringobulbia. *Peripheral* causes include: in the posterior fossa—aneurysms or tumours, chronic meningitis and trauma; in the upper neck—tumours or lymphadenopathy; and the Arnold–Chiari[ll] malformation. The Arnold–Chiari malformation is a congenital malformation of the base of the skull with herniation of a tongue of cerebellum and medulla into the spinal canal, causing lower cranial nerve palsies, cerebellar limb signs (due to tonsillar compression) and upper motor neurone signs in the legs.

Causes of bilateral lower motor neurone lesions include motor neurone disease, the Guillain–Barré syndrome, poliomyelitis and the Arnold–Chiari malformation.

Multiple cranial nerve lesions

The anatomical courses of the cranial nerves mean they can be affected in groups by single lesions that damage them when they run close to each other. Certain disease processes may also interfere with a number of the cranial nerves. There are a number of syndromes that result from abnormalities of groups of cranial nerves:

- Unilateral III, IV, V_1 and VI involvement suggests a lesion in the cavernous sinus.
- Unilateral V, VII and VIII involvement suggests a cerebellopontine angle lesion (usually a tumour).
- Unilateral IX, X and XI involvement suggests a jugular foramen lesion.
- Combined bilateral X, XI and XII involvement suggests bulbar palsy if lower motor neurone changes are present and pseudobulbar palsy if there are upper motor neurone signs. The clinical features of pseudobulbar and bulbar palsies are shown in Table 32.2, and the causes of multiple cranial nerve palsies are listed in List 32.2.
- Weakness of the eye and facial muscles that worsens with repeated contraction suggests myasthenia. Weakness of the eye muscles that does not conform to a cranial nerve distribution may be due to orbital myopathy. Here the pattern of weakness does not fit with any cranial nerve abnormality.

Head and neck

Inspect and palpate the skull for scars (previous surgery or trauma) and lumps, such as may be caused by a meningioma or a sarcoma. Auscultate the skull by placing the diaphragm of the stethoscope on the frontal bone, and then on the lateral occipital bones, and then

[ll] Julies Arnold (1835–1915) and Hans Chiari (1851–1916), German pathologists, described this in 1894.

Clinical features of pseudobulbar and bulbar palsies

Feature	Pseudobulbar (bilateral UMN lesions of IX, X and XII)	Bulbar (bilateral LMN lesions of IX, X and XII)
Gag reflex	Increased or normal	Absent
Tongue	Spastic	Wasted, fasciculations
Jaw jerk	Increased	Absent or normal
Speech	Spastic dysarthria	Nasal
Other causes	Bilateral limb UMN (long tract) signs	Signs of the underlying cause (e.g. limb fasciculations)
	Labile emotions	Normal emotions
	Bilateral cerebrovascular disease (e.g. both internal capsules)	Motor neurone disease
	Multiple sclerosis	Guillain–Barré syndrome
	Motor neurone disease	Poliomyelitis
		Brainstem infarction

LMN = lower motor neurone; UMN = upper motor neurone.

TABLE 32.2

CAUSES OF MULTIPLE CRANIAL NERVE PALSIES

Nasopharyngeal carcinoma

Chronic meningitis (e.g. carcinoma, haematological malignancy, tuberculosis, sarcoidosis)

Guillain–Barré syndrome (spares sensory nerves)

Brainstem lesions—these are usually due to vascular disease causing crossed sensory or motor paralysis (i.e. cranial nerve signs on one side and contralateral long tract signs); patients with a brainstem tumour (e.g. in the cerebellopontine angle) may also have similar signs

Arnold–Chiari malformation

Trauma

Paget's disease

Mononeuritis multiplex (rarely) (e.g. diabetes mellitus)

LIST 32.2

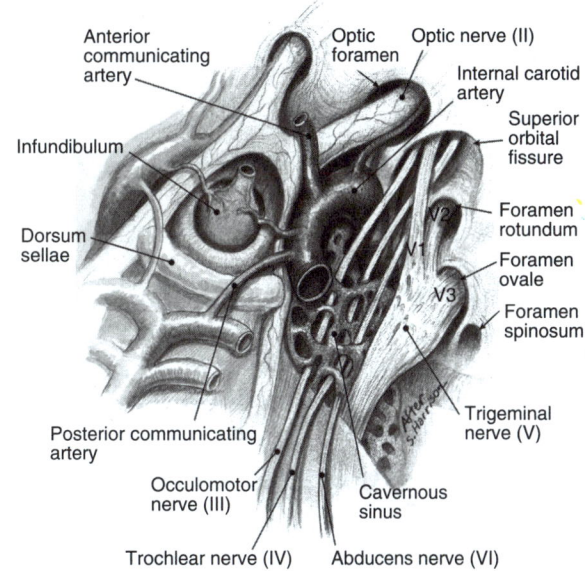

Anatomy of the carotid artery
(Ducic Y. Operative techniques in otolaryngology. *Head and Neck Surgery* 2010; 21(1):9–18.)

FIGURE 32.46

place the bell over each eye (with the opposite eye open). Ask the patient to hold his or her breath each time. Bruits heard over the skull may be due to an arteriovenous malformation, advanced Paget's disease or a vascular meningioma, or they may be conducted from the carotids.

Carotid bruits
Examination anatomy

The left common carotid artery arises directly from the aorta and the right arises from the brachiocephalic artery, which is the first branch of the aortic arch. The common carotids run up from the level of the sternoclavicular joint and back through the neck to divide at the level of the upper border of the thyroid cartilage into the external and internal carotids. The external carotids continue to the parotid glands where they terminate and branch into the superficial temporal and mandibular arteries. The internal carotid climbs to the base of the skull and enters it via the carotid canal in the temporal bone (see Fig. 32.46).

It is traditional to listen for carotid bruits with the bell of the stethoscope placed somewhere between the angle of the jaw and the upper end of the thyroid cartilage, but no method has been shown to be better than any other.

Carotid bruits are common, being found in 20% of children and 1% of adults. They are more common in patients with increased cardiac output (anaemia, thyrotoxicosis and haemodialysis fistula). They must be distinguished from the conducted murmur of aortic stenosis (louder over the praecordium) and from venous hums (diastolic component and abolished by gentle pressure on the neck above the stethoscope).

The significance of a bruit is its association with carotid artery stenosis and stroke. The LR+ for significant carotid stenosis (70–99% stenosis by Doppler ultrasound) is about 4.[8] In symptomatic patients (ipsilateral previous transient ischaemic attack or stroke) a bruit predicts significant stenosis with a very similar LR+. The absence of a bruit does not rule out a significant lesion.

There is general agreement that the presence of a bruit indicates an increased risk of atherosclerotic disease and in younger patients (<75), at least, an increase in risk of stroke to an annual incidence of 1–3%.[9] However, as the correct treatment of these patients has not been established, various groups have recommended that asymptomatic patients should *not* be examined for the presence of a carotid bruit lest its discovery cause unnecessary alarm and tests.[10]

T&O'C ESSENTIALS

1. The detailed neurological examination can proceed only when level of consciousness, orientation and left- or right-handedness have been established.
2. Remember throughout the neurological examination that symmetry is your friend: always compare both sides of the body.
3. The cranial nerve examination is complicated and constant practice is essential if the examination is to at least appear proficient.
4. Experience with many different cranial nerve abnormalities is the only way these lesions can be correctly diagnosed in OSCEs. It is very difficult, for example, to diagnose a third nerve palsy if you see it for the first time in an examination.
5. If an abnormality of eye movements does not fit with a cranial nerve or multiple cranial nerve pathology, consider an ocular myopathy or myasthenia gravis.
6. The presence of fasciculation of the tongue is very specific for a lower motor neurone twelfth nerve palsy, often due to motor neurone disease. It is easily missed unless time is taken to look for it.
7. Remember that carotid bruits are common and their detection has a poor sensitivity for clinically relevant carotid stenosis in asymptomatic people.

OSCE EXAMPLE – INTRODUCTION (STEM)*

'This patient is a volunteer actor, but let us assume that he has had a stroke that has affected his vision. Please examine his second, third, fourth and sixth cranial nerves.'

	N = not attempted	1 = attempted	2 = performed satisfactorily
Greets patient, introduces self, explains what he or she will be doing (briefly).			
Washes hands or uses an alcohol-based hand rub.			
Asks whether patient is comfortable sitting over edge of bed or in chair. Takes time to stand back and look at patient and then at eyes. Meanwhile, asks patient whether he or she wears spectacles or contact lenses.			
Tests visual acuity using Snellen chart (with patient's spectacles on).			
Tests visual fields by confrontation including checking for visual inattention.			
Looks at pupils for size and inequality.			
Tests light reflexes direct and consensual with torch.			

OSCE EXAMPLE – **INTRODUCTION (STEM)*** *continued*			
	N=not attempted	1= attempted	2= performed satisfactorily
Tests for relative afferent pupil defect (Marcus Gunn phenomenon)			
Tests convergence.			
Asks about diplopia and knows to test each eye separately if answer is 'yes'.			
Assesses eye movements and looks for nystagmus.			
Cross-cover test if diplopia.			
Looks at eyelids for ptosis, inequality, and lid retraction.			
Asks to perform ophthalmoscopy (may be given result: normal).			
Informs patient at each stage about what is to happen.			
Is polite and pleasant to patient throughout, despite nervousness.			
Washes hands.			
Examiners' comments In a case like this there are unlikely to be any abnormal findings. The examiners are therefore especially interested in the student's technique and understanding of the reasons the examination is conducted in the way that it is. It is not necessary to perform the examination in exactly this order but no major step should be left out. The stem in this case contains important information. The patient is an actor, so abnormal findings are unlikely. The examiners have asked for the examination of specific cranial nerves, so it is important not to waste time on examining other nerves. Note the emphasis in the examining sheet on hand-washing and a considerate approach to the patient.			

*This is usually written on the marking sheet and is standardised for each case to avoid misleading any student.

References

1. Thomas KE, Hasbun R, Jekel J et al. The diagnostic accuracy of Kernig's sign, Brudzinski's sign, and nuchal rigidity in adults with suspected meningitis. *Clin Infect Dis* 2002; 35:46–52.
2. Van de Beek D, De Gans J, Spanjaard L et al. Clinical features and prognostic factors in adults with bacterial meningitis. *N Engl J Med* 2004; 351(18):1849–1859.
3. Steinberg D. Scientific neurology and the history of the clinical examination of the cranial nerves. *Semin Neurol* 2002; 22:349–356. An interesting historical review that explains the background to the modern understanding of cranial nerve function and structure.
4. McGee S. *Evidence-based physical diagnosis*, 3rd edn. St Louis: Saunders, 2012.
5. Levin DE. The clinical significance of spontaneous pulsations of the retinal vein. *Arch Neurol* 1978; 35:37–40. Elevated intracranial pressure is excluded if pulsations are observed in the retinal veins. However, the absence of pulsations in the retinal veins does not necessarily mean that intracranial pressure is elevated.
6. Nelson KR. Use new pins for each neurologic examination [Letter]. *New Engl J Med* 1986; 314:581. A cautionary tale.
7. Ruffin R, Rachootin P. Gag reflex in disease [Letter]. *Chest* 1987; 92:1130. This suggests that many normal people may have an absent gag reflex.
8. De Virgilio C, Toosie K, Arnell T et al. Asymptomatic carotid artery stenosis screening in patients with lower extremity atherosclerosis: a prospective study. *Ann Vasc Surg* 1997; 11(4):374–377.
9. US Preventive Services Task Force. *Screening for asymptomatic carotid artery stenosis. Guide to clinical preventive services*, 2nd edn. Baltimore: Lippincott Williams & Wilkins, 1996, 53–61.
10. Pickett CA, Jackson JL, Hemann BA, Atwood JE. Carotid bruits and cerebrovascular disease risk: a meta-analysis. *Stroke* 2010; 41(10):2295–2302. The presence of a carotid bruit does signify an increased stroke risk but does not identify critical carotid stenosis. Absence of a carotid bruit on auscultation cannot exclude carotid stenosis.

CHAPTER 33

The neurological examination: speech and higher centres

Thus the thoughtes and counsailes of the minde and spirit are discovered and manifested by speech.
JOHN MILTON (1608–74)

By the time the general and neurological history has been taken, the presence of any disorder of speech is likely to be apparent.

SPEECH

It is important to distinguish between *dysphasia* (dominant higher centre disorder in the use of symbols for communication—language), *dysarthria* (difficulty with articulation) and *dysphonia* (altered quality of the voice with reduction in volume as a result of vocal cord disease). If the nature of the abnormality is not obvious, before going on to the compartmentalised tests below, first ask the patient to talk freely—*propositional* or *free* speech. In a normal clinical encounter this will have already come from history taking. However, at times when the clinical interaction is difficult it is worth moving to an early examination of language before proceeding. In *viva voce* examinations or OSCEs, a structured approach is essential to ensure you can identify the problem correctly.

Dysphasia

Dysphasia is often described as expressive or receptive, though it can also be characterised as fluent or non-fluent.[a] Although the cardinal types of dysphasia are listed below, often features are mixed, which is why a structured approach to examining speech is important (List 33.1). *Non-fluent aphasia* is slow, effortful and often has significant patient frustration (imagine trying to communicate with only a rudimentary knowledge of English). Words are often nouns or verbs, though

> **CLASSIFICATION OF DYPHASIAS**
> 1. Expressive dysphasia = Broca's dysphasia = motor dysphasia = typically non-fluent
> 2. Receptive dysphasia = Wernicke's dysphasia = sensory dysphasia = typically fluent
> 3. Nominal dysphasia = dysnomic dysphasia
>
> LIST 33.1

there may be paraphasic errors. In contrast, *fluent aphasia* is often flowing with frequent errors and content is often poor. Patients with fluent aphasia are often mistakenly thought to be simply confused, once again demonstrating the importance of structured language assessment.[1]

1. **Receptive (posterior) dysphasia.** This is where the patient cannot understand the spoken word (*auditory dysphasia*) or the written word (*alexia*). This condition is suggested when the patient is unable to understand any commands or questions, or to recognise written words in the absence of deafness or blindness. Speech is fluent but disorganised. It occurs with a lesion (infarction, haemorrhage or space-occupying tumour) in the dominant hemisphere in the posterior part of the first temporal gyrus (Wernicke's[b] area).

2. **Expressive (anterior) dysphasia.** This is present when the patient understands, but cannot answer

---
[a] The terms dysphasia and aphasia are sometimes used synonymously but aphasia really means a complete absence of speech.

[b] Karl Wernicke (1848–1904), a professor of neurology at Breslau, described receptive aphasia in 1874. He was killed while riding his bicycle.

appropriately. Speech is non-fluent. This occurs with a lesion in the posterior part of the dominant third frontal gyrus (Broca's[c] area). Certain types of speech may be retained by these patients. These include *automatic speech*: the patient may be able to recite word series such as the days of the week or letters of the alphabet. Sometimes *emotional speech* may be preserved so that when frustrated or upset the patient may be able to swear fluently. In the same way the patient may be able to sing familiar songs while being unable to speak the words. It is important to remember that unless the lesion responsible for these defects is very large there may be no reduction in the patient's higher intellectual functions, memory or judgement. Some patients may incorrectly be considered as psychotic because of their disorganised speech.

3. **Nominal dysphasia.** All types of dysphasia may cause difficulty in naming objects. There is also a specific type of nominal dysphasia, whereby objects cannot be named (e.g. the nib of a pen) but other aspects of speech are normal. The patient may use long sentences to overcome failure to find the correct word (circumlocution). It occurs with a lesion of the dominant posterior temporoparietal area. Other causes include encephalopathy or the intracranial pressure effects of a distinct space-occupying lesion; it may also occur in the recovery phase from any dysphasia. Its localising value is therefore doubtful.

4. **Conductive dysphasia.** This is present when the patient repeats statements and names objects poorly, but can follow commands. It is thought to be caused by a lesion of the arcuate fasciculus and/or other fibres linking Wernicke's and Broca's areas.

> **EXAMINATION OF A PATIENT WITH DYSPHASIA**
>
> **Fluent speech (usually receptive, conductive or nominal aphasia)**
>
> 1. *Name objects.* Patients with nominal, conductive or receptive aphasia will name objects poorly.
> 2. *Repetition.* Conductive and receptive aphasic patients cannot repeat 'no ifs, ands or buts'.
> 3. *Comprehension.* Only receptive aphasic patients cannot follow commands (verbal or written): 'Touch your nose, then your chin and then your ear'.
> 4. *Reading.* Conductive and receptive aphasic patients may have difficulty (dyslexia).
> 5. *Writing.* Conductive aphasic patients have impaired writing (dysgraphia) whereas receptive aphasic patients have abnormal content of writing. Patients with dominant frontal lobe lesions may also have dysgraphia.
>
> **Non-fluent speech (usually expressive aphasia)**
>
> 1. *Naming of objects.* This is poor but may be better than spontaneous speech.
> 2. *Repetition.* This may be possible with great effort. Phrase repetition (e.g. 'No ifs, ands or buts') is poor.
> 3. *Comprehension.* Often mildly impaired despite popular belief, but written and verbal commands are followed.
> 4. *Reading.* Patients may have dyslexia.
> 5. *Writing.* Dysgraphia may be present.
> 6. *Look for hemiparesis.* The arm is more affected than the leg.
> 7. As patients are usually aware of their deficit they are often frustrated and depressed.
>
> LIST 33.2

Examination of speech (List 33.2)

First assess *comprehension*. If the patient cannot understand you, then further examination is near impossible! Ensure that you (or relatives) do not give the patient cues with body language. Start with a simple command—'Close your eyes'. Give another simple command—'Show me your tongue'. Then increase the difficulty, for example 'Touch your right ear with your left hand' (also tests for left–right agnosia), 'Touch your nose, then your chin, then your forehead' and 'Point to the ceiling *after* you point to the floor' (stress *after*).

Next test *repetition*. Start simple and increase complexity as in every step. 'Blue sky' and 'green grass' are useful starting points. 'Hippopotamus' is an early screen for dysarthria. Next give a longer phrase such

---
[c] Pierre Broca (1824–80), a professor of surgery at Paris, described this area in 1861. He described muscular dystrophy before Duchenne.

Assessing free speech: instruct the patient to 'describe what you see'

FIGURE 33.1

as 'We went to the circus and had a good time'. 'No ifs, ands, or buts' is very difficult for many patients and may indicate other cognitive issues aside from language.

Next comes *naming*. A hand has many layers of complexity from 'hand' to 'thumb' to 'ring finger' (ask which one—which also helps with finger agnosia) to 'knuckles'. Similarly a 'shirt' also has a 'collar', 'sleeve' and 'cuff' in order of difficulty.

Finally, *free speech* can be tested (if this has not already been done—see above). This can be remarkably difficult in an exam situation. Asking the patient to describe you is fraught with danger. The exam room is often small, featureless and drab. Asking about hobbies may reveal very brief answers such as 'I like footy'. Instead, it is often good to have a detailed image to show the patient, and ask him or her to describe it (see Fig. 33.1). This allows assessment of fluency of speech, as well as giving initial insight into visual function. Alternatively, the patient can be asked about a day-to-day task such as 'Explain the steps in getting dressed'. This helps assess planning.

Interpretation of the findings

If the patient's speech is fluent, but conveys information with paraphasic errors, such as 'treen' for 'train' (i.e. using a word of similar sound or spelling to the one intended),[d] the main possibilities are nominal, receptive and conductive dysphasia. Test for these by asking the patient to name an object, repeat a statement after you and then follow commands. If these are abnormal, ask the patient to read and write, but remember that some patients may be illiterate.

If the speech is slow, hesitant and non-fluent, expressive dysphasia is more likely and exactly the same procedure is followed. It is important to note that many dysphasias will have mixed elements. Large lesions in the dominant hemisphere may cause global dysphasia.

Dysprosody is the loss of the normal ups and downs in speech, without a change in the content from a non-dominant hemisphere lesion. This is not dysphasia, but may be noticed while examining speech carefully.

Dysarthria

Here there is no disorder of the content of speech but a difficulty with articulation. It can occur because of abnormalities at a number of levels. Upper motor neurone lesions of the cranial nerves, extrapyramidal

---

[d] Sometimes a word of similar meaning is used (e.g. 'go' for 'start');; this is called *semantic paraphrasia*.

conditions (e.g. Parkinson's disease) and cerebellar lesions cause disturbances to the rhythm of speech.

Ask the patient to say a word like 'hippopotamus', or a phrase such as 'British Constitution' or 'Peter Piper picked a peck of pickled peppers'.

Pseudobulbar palsy is an upper motor neurone weakness that causes a spastic dysarthria (it sounds as if the patient is trying to squeeze out words from tight lips), paralysis of the facial muscles and difficulty in chewing and swallowing. The cause is infarction in both internal capsules. This causes interruption of the descending pyramidal tracts to the brainstem motor nuclei. The jaw jerk is usually increased. These patients tend to be very emotional and laugh and cry inappropriately. Their facial expressions become very animated at these times in contrast to their inability to control their facial expressions voluntarily.[e] This phenomenon occurs because the nuclei that control motor responses to emotion do not reside in the motor cortex.

Patients who have bilateral lesions of the ninth and tenth cranial nerves are at risk of aspirating fluids or solids into their lungs if they try to eat or drink. Certain bedside tests can be performed to see whether it is safe for them to eat or drink. These traditionally include testing the level of consciousness, the gag reflex, pharyngeal sensation and swallowing water. The water-swallowing test involves asking the patient to sip 5–10 mL of water repeatedly. Coughing or choking makes the test positive.

Bulbar palsies cause a nasal speech, whereas *facial muscle weakness* causes slurred speech. *Extrapyramidal disease* can be responsible for monotonous speech, as it causes bradykinesia and muscular rigidity. Other causes of dysarthria include alcohol intoxication and *cerebellar disease*. These result in loss of coordination and slow, slurred and often explosive speech, or speech broken up into syllables, called *scanning speech*.

Mouth ulceration or disease may occasionally mimic dysarthria. Each of these causes must be considered and examined for as appropriate.

Dysphonia

This is alteration of the sound of the voice, such as huskiness of the voice with decreased volume. It may be due to laryngeal disease (e.g. following a viral infection or a tumour of the vocal cord) or to recurrent laryngeal nerve palsy.

THE CEREBRAL HEMISPHERES

Parietal, temporal and frontal lobe functions are tested if the patient is disoriented or has dysphasia, or if cognitive decline (dementia) is suspected. If the patient has a receptive aphasia, however, these tests cannot be performed. Their examination is otherwise not routine (see List 33.3).

Parietal lobe function

The parietal lobe is concerned with the reception and analysis of sensory information.

Dominant lobe signs

A lesion of the dominant parietal lobe in the angular gyrus causes a distinct clinical syndrome called Gerstmann's[f] syndrome. Test for this in the following manner.

1. Ask the patient to perform simple arithmetical calculations—for example, serial 7s (take 7 from 100, then 7 from the answer, and so on). The inability to do this with at least partial accuracy is called *acalculia*.
2. Ask the patient to write—inability is called *agraphia*.
3. Test for left–right disorientation by asking the patient to show you his or her right and then left hand. If this is correctly performed, ask the patient to touch his or her left ear with the right hand and vice versa. Inability to do this is called *left–right disorientation*.
4. Ask the patient to name his or her fingers—inability to do this is called *finger agnosia*. This inability may extend to identification of the examiner's fingers. The agnosias are receptive defects involving the inability to understand the meaning of stimulations of different types.

A mnemonic for these four dominant parietal lobe signs is **AALF**:

---

[e] This syndrome should probably be called 'pseudo-pontine-bulbar palsy' as the motor nuclei of the fifth and seventh nerves are in the pons, not the medulla (bulbs).

[f] Josef Gerstmann (1887–1969), an Austrian-born neuropsychiatrist who worked in the United States.

SYMPTOMS AND SIGNS IN HIGHER CENTRE DYSFUNCTION

Parietal lobe

Dysphasia (dominant)

Acalculia,* agraphia,* left–right disorientation,* finger agnosia*

Sensory and visual inattention,† construction and dressing apraxia,† spatial neglect and inattention,† lower quadrantic hemianopia,‡ astereognosis‡

Seizures

Temporal lobe

Memory loss

Upper quadrantic hemianopia

Dysphasia (receptive if dominant lobe)

Seizures

Frontal lobe

Personality change

Primitive reflexes (e.g. grasp, pout)

Anosmia

Optic nerve compression (optic atrophy)

Gait apraxia

Leg weakness (parasagittal)

Loss of micturition control

Dysphasia (expressive), dysgraphia

Seizures

Occipital lobe

Homonymous hemianopia

Alexia (inability to read; word blindness)

Seizures (flashing light aura)

*Gerstmann's syndrome: dominant hemisphere parietal lobe only.
†Non-dominant parietal lobe signs.
‡Non-localising parietal lobe signs.

LIST 33.3

A calculia
A graphia
L eft–right disorientation
F inger agnosia.

Remember that Gerstmann's syndrome can be diagnosed only if the higher centres are intact. A demented patient would not be able to perform many of these tests.

Agraphaesthesia: 'What number have I drawn?' Patient's reply: 'One'.

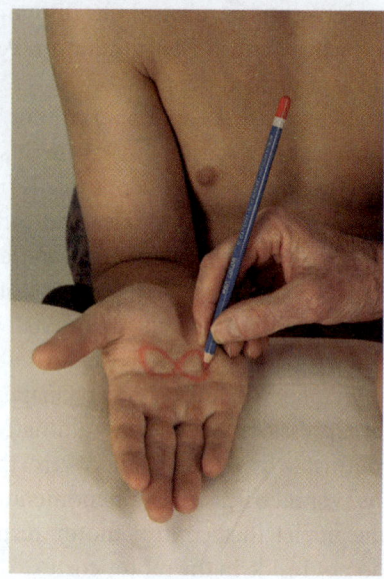

Avoid the use of an indelible pencil

FIGURE 33.2

Non-dominant and non-localising parietal lobe signs (cortical sensation)

Cortical sensations are those that require processing at a higher level than simple sensation. They rely on an intact simple sensation, especially touch and pinprick.

- *Graphaesthesia* is the ability to recognise numbers or letters drawn on the skin. Use a pointed object or pencil to draw numbers on the skin (see Fig. 33.2).
- Look for *sensory* and *visual inattention/extinction*. When one arm or leg is tested at a time, sensation is normal, but when both sides are tested simultaneously the sensation is appreciated only on the normal side. Touch the patient (with their eyes shut, not yours) first on one hand and then on the other, and then on both together. Ask on which side the touch is felt. The normal response is 'both' when stimulation is applied to each side. It is important that the hands be touched simultaneously. Similarly visual fields are normal, but with bilateral visual stimulation only one side

is perceived. A right-sided parietal lesion will lead to inattention on the left side and vice versa. This is often tested as routine during visual field (cranial nerves) and peripheral sensory testing.
- Formal *visual field testing* is also important, as parietal, temporal and occipital lesions can give distinctive defects.
- Examine now for *astereognosis* (*tactile agnosia*), which is the inability, with eyes closed, to recognise an object placed in the hand when the ordinary sensory modalities are intact. A parietal lobe lesion results in astereognosis on the opposite side.
- *Agraphaesthesia* may also be present; this is the inability to appreciate a number drawn on the hand on the opposite side to a parietal lesion (see Fig. 33.2).
- *Two-point discrimination* testing involves the ability to distinguish a single point from two points close together (see Fig. 33.3). The minimal separation that can be distinguished is about 3 centimetres on the hand or foot and 0.6 centimetres on the fingertips. A compass can be used for this test. Ask the patient to shut the eyes and then say whether one or two points can be felt. Bring the compass points closer together and test intermittently with just one point.

- Examine for *dressing* and *constructional apraxia*. Dressing apraxia is tested by taking the patient's pyjama top or cardigan, turning it inside out and asking him or her to put it back on. Patients with a non-dominant parietal lobe lesion may find this impossible to do. Constructional apraxia is tested by asking the patient to copy an object that you have drawn (e.g. a tree or a house—see Fig. 33.4(a) and (b)).
- Next test *spatial neglect* by asking the patient to fill in the numbers on an empty clock face (see Fig. 33.4(c)). Patients with a right parietal lesion may fill in numbers only on the left side (the other side of the clock face is ignored). Spatial neglect also occurs with dominant parietal lobe lesions, but is less common.

Temporal lobe function

This lobe is concerned with short-term and long-term memory. Test short-term memory by the name, address, flower test—ask the patient to remember a name, address and the names of three flowers, and repeat them immediately. Then ask the patient 5 minutes later to repeat the names again. Test long-term memory by asking, for example, what year World War II ended. Memory may be impaired in dementia from any cause.

An alert patient with a severe memory disturbance may make up stories to fill any gaps in his or her memory. This is called *confabulation* and is typical of the syndrome of *Korsakoff's*[g] *psychosis* (amnesic dementia). Confabulation can be tested by asking the patient whether he or she has met you before. However, be prepared for the very long, detailed and completely false story that may follow.

Korsakoff's psychosis occurs most commonly in alcoholics owing to thiamine deficiency (where there is loss of nerve cells in the thalamic nuclei and mammillary bodies), and rarely with thalamic stroke, head injury, tumour, anoxic encephalopathy or encephalitis. It is characterised by retrograde amnesia (memory loss for events before the onset of the illness) and an inability to memorise new information, in a patient who is alert, responsive and capable of problem solving.

Two-point discrimination: 'Can you feel one point or two?'

FIGURE 33.3

---

[9] Sergei Sergeyevich Korsakoff (1853–1900), a Russian psychiatrist and great humanitarian, described the syndrome in 1887.

Lower figures show (a and b) constructional apraxia and (c) spatial neglect

FIGURE 33.4

Frontal lobe function

Frontal lobe damage as a result of tumours or surgery (or both), or diffuse disease such as dementia or HIV infection, may cause changes in emotion, memory, judgement, carelessness about personal habits and *disinhibition*. There may be persistent or alternating irritability and euphoria.[h] These features may be clear when the history is taken but may need to be reinforced by interviewing relatives or friends. Changes of this sort in a previously reserved personality may be obvious and very distressing to relatives.

First assess the *primitive reflexes*. There is controversy concerning their significance; they are not normally present in adults but may reappear in normal old age.[2] The presence of an isolated primitive reflex may not be abnormal, but multiple primitive reflexes are usually associated with diffuse cerebral disease involving the frontal lobes and frontal association areas more than other parts of the brain. Dementia, encephalopathy and neoplasms are all possible causes.

1. *Grasp reflex:* run your fingers across the palm of the patient's hand, which will grasp your fingers involuntarily on the side contralateral to the lesion.
2. *Palmomental reflex:* ipsilateral contraction of the ipsilateral mentalis muscle occurs when you stroke the thenar eminence firmly with a key or thumbnail. Contraction of the mentalis causes protrusion and lifting of the lower lip. This is best considered as the beginning of a wince in response to pain. The response can also be elicited by painful stimulus to other parts of the body. The response is bilateral in about 50% of cases. A unilateral lesion does not necessarily correspond to the side of the lesion in the brain.
3. *Pout and snout reflexes:* stroking or tapping with the tendon hammer over or above the upper lip induces pouting movements of the lips. This can occur with many intracranial lesions. The sucking reflex is an extension of this. The stimulation may produce sucking, chewing and swallowing movements. It is not a localising sign.

Next ask the patient to *interpret a proverb*, such as 'A rolling stone gathers no moss'. Patients with frontal lobe disease give concrete explanations of proverbs. Test for loss of smell (*anosmia*) and for *gait apraxia*, where there is marked unsteadiness in walking, which

---

[h] Euphoria may cause a lack of seriousness, and the repetition of bad jokes and puns (*witzelsucht*).

can be bizarre—the feet typically behave as if glued to the floor, causing a strange shuffling gait. Look in the *fundi*; you may rarely see optic atrophy on the side of a frontal lobe space-occupying lesion caused by compression of the optic nerve, and papilloedema on the opposite side due to secondarily raised intracranial pressure (Foster Kennedy[i] syndrome).

T&O'C ESSENTIALS

1. Methodical assessment of speech can help localise the anatomical site of the abnormality.
2. Know how to assess dominant parietal lobe function (test for acalculia, agraphia, left–right disorientation and finger agnosia).
3. The presence of a number of primitive reflexes suggests frontal lobe dysfunction.

OSCE REVISION TOPICS – SPEECH AND HIGHER CENTRES

Use these topics, which commonly occur in the OSCE, to help with revision.

1. Please examine the speech of this patient who has had difficulty with words recently. (p 541)
2. Please assess this patient for frontal lobe abnormalities. (p 546)
3. Please show on this volunteer patient how you would assess the parietal lobes. (p 543)

References

1. Damasio AR. Aphasia. *N Engl J Med* 1992; 326:531–539. A very detailed review.
2. Forgotten symptoms and primitive signs (editorial). *Lancet* 1987; 1:841–842. This puts many of the frontal lobe signs into perspective and suggests they are sometimes of only historical interest.

---

[i] Robert Foster Kennedy (1884–1952), a New York neurologist.

CHAPTER 34

The neurological examination: the peripheral nervous system

System; any complexure or combination of many things acting together. SAMUEL JOHNSON, A Dictionary of the English Language (1775)

LIMBS AND TRUNK

History

The patient may present with symptoms that are purely or predominantly sensory or motor (see Questions box 34.1), or related to disorders of movement such as tremor. Sensory symptoms include pain, numbness and paraesthesias (tingling or pins and needles). It is important to find out whether there is involvement of more than one modality, something the patient may not have noticed. The distribution, time of onset and duration may give clues to the aetiology of the symptoms or at least as to where the sensory examination should be concentrated.

QUESTIONS TO ASK THE PATIENT WITH MUSCLE WEAKNESS

1. Have you felt weakness on both sides of the body? (Suggests spinal cord disease, myopathy or myasthenia gravis)
2. Is the weakness just on one side of the body or face? (Transient ischaemic attack or stroke)
3. Has the weakness affected just an arm or a leg or part of a limb? (Peripheral neuropathy or radiculopathy, stroke or multiple sclerosis)
4. Have you had trouble getting up from a chair, brushing your hair or lifting your head? (Proximal muscle weakness—myasthenia gravis, diabetic amyotrophy [involves lower limbs], polymyositis)
5. Have you had trouble swallowing or difficulty in speaking? (Myasthenia gravis, polymyositis)
6. Have you noticed double vision? (Myasthenia gravis, cranial nerve mononeuritis multiplex)
7. Are you taking any medications? (Steroid-induced proximal myopathy)
8. Have you had problems with your neck or back, or with severe arthritis? (Radiculopathy)
9. Have you had a cancer diagnosed at any stage? (Paraneoplastic, Eaton–Lambert syndrome)
10. Is there any problem like this in your family? (Familial myopathy, Charcot–Marie–Tooth disease)
11. Have you had HIV infection? (Various neurological lesions and drug reactions)
12. Have you ever had multiple sclerosis diagnosed?
13. Are you a diabetic? (Mononeuritis multiplex, amyotrophy)

QUESTIONS BOX 34.1

A family history of a similar problem may help provide the diagnosis in conditions such as muscular dystrophy. A previous injury may be responsible, for example, for a peripheral nerve problem but not remembered until asked about specifically.

Ask the patient about medications that can be a cause of neuropathy such as chemotherapeutic agents, metronidazole and amiodarone. Steroids can cause proximal muscle weakness. Alcohol excess is associated with neuropathy and occasionally strict vegans can become vitamin B_{12} deficient. Travel to countries where Lyme disease or leprosy are endemic may be relevant.

Examination anatomy

Muscle weakness has five major causes:

1. Pyramidal or upper motor neurone weakness, which is caused by a lesion in the brain proximal to the 'pyramids' in the brainstem. This is where the nerve fibres decussate or cross to the other side before travelling down the spinal cord (see Fig. 34.1).
2. Lower motor neurone weakness, which is caused by a nerve lesion within the spinal cord or peripheral nerve.

Motor neurone lesions

(Adapted from Lance JG, McLeod JW. *A physiological approach to clinical neurology*, 3rd edn. London: Butterworth, 1981.)

FIGURE 34.1

3. Abnormalities of the neuromuscular junction (myasthenia gravis).
4. Muscle disease.
5. Functional weakness (conversion reaction).

General examination approach

It is most important to have a set order of examination of the limbs for neurological signs so that nothing important is omitted. The following scheme is a standard approach.

1. Motor system
   General inspection
   - Posture
   - Muscle bulk
   - Abnormal movements
   - Fasciculations

   Tone
   Power
   Reflexes
   Coordination
2. Sensory system
   Pain and temperature
   Vibration and proprioception
   ±Light touch

Testing for arm drift: 'Shut your eyes and hold your arms out straight. Now turn your palms upwards'

FIGURE 34.2

General inspection

Remember to look for *asymmetry*.

1. Stand back and look at the patient for an *abnormal posture*—for example, one due to hemiplegia caused by a stroke. In this case, the upper limb is flexed and there is adduction and pronation of the arm, while the lower limb is extended.
2. Look for *muscle wasting*, which indicates a denervated muscle, a primary muscle disease or disuse atrophy. Compare one side with the other for wasting and try to work out which muscle groups are involved (proximal, distal or generalised, symmetrical or asymmetrical).
3. Inspect for *abnormal movements*, such as tremor of the wrist or arm.
4. Inspect the *skin*—for example, for evidence of neurofibromatosis, cutaneous angiomata in a segmental distribution (associated with syringomyelia) or herpes zoster. Look for scars from old injuries or surgical treatment. Note the presence of a urinary catheter.

Upper limbs

Motor system[a]

General

Shake hands with the patient and introduce yourself. A patient who cannot relax his or her hand grip has myotonia (an inability to relax the muscles after voluntary contraction). The most common cause of this is the muscle disease dystrophia myotonica (p 591). Once your hand has been extracted from the patient's, and after pausing briefly for the vitally important general inspection, ask the patient to undress so that the arms and shoulder girdles are completely exposed.

Sit the patient over the edge of the bed if this is possible. Next ask the patient to hold out both hands, palms upwards, with the arms extended and the eyes closed (see Fig. 34.2). Watch the arms for evidence of drifting (movement of one or both arms from the initial

---
[a] Aretaeus of Cappadocia reasoned, in AD 150, that the nerves cross (decussate) between the brain and the periphery and that injury to the right side of the head causes abnormalities of the left side of the body.

> **CAUSES (DIFFERENTIAL DIAGNOSIS) OF FASCICULATIONS**
>
> Motor neurone disease
> Motor root compression
> Peripheral neuropathy (e.g. diabetic)
> Primary myopathy
> Thyrotoxicosis
>
> *Note:* Myokymia resembles coarse fasciculation of the same muscle group and is particularly common in the orbicularis oculi muscles, where it is usually benign. Focal myokymia, however, often represents brainstem disease (e.g. multiple sclerosis or glioma).
> Fibrillation is seen only on the electromyogram.
>
> LIST 34.1

neutral position). There are only three causes of arm drift:

1. *Upper motor neurone (pyramidal) weakness:* the drift of the affected limb(s) here is due to muscle weakness and tends to be in a downward direction. The drifting typically starts distally with the fingers and spreads proximally. There may be slow pronation of the wrist and flexion of the fingers and elbow.
2. *Cerebellar disease:* the drift here is usually upwards. It also includes slow pronation of the wrist and elbow.
3. *Loss of proprioception:* the drift here (pseudoathetosis) is really a searching movement and usually affects only the fingers. It is due to loss of joint position sense and can be in any direction.

Fasciculations

Ask the patient to relax the arms and rest them on his or her lap. Inspect the large muscle groups for *fasciculations* (see List 34.1). These are irregular contractions of small areas of muscle that have no rhythmical pattern. Fasciculation may be coarse or fine and is present at rest, but not during voluntary movement.[b] If present with weakness and wasting, fasciculation indicates

---

[b] If no fasciculation is seen, tapping over the bulk of the brachioradialis and biceps muscles with the finger or with a tendon hammer and watching again has been recommended, but this is controversial. Most neurologists do not do this. The reason is that fasciculations are spontaneous. Any muscle movement from a local stimulus is not spontaneous. Even if they occur, they may have nothing to do with fasciculations.

degeneration of the lower motor neurone. It is usually benign if not associated with other signs of a motor lesion.

Tone

Tone is tested at both the wrists and the elbows. Rotation of the wrists with supination and pronation of the elbow joints (supporting the patient's elbow with one hand and holding the hand with the other) is performed passively (the examiner does the work), and the patient should be told to relax to allow you to move the joints freely.

When you raise and then drop the patient's arm, it will fall suddenly if tone is reduced. With experience it is possible to decide whether tone is normal or increased (hypertonic, as in an upper motor neurone or extrapyramidal lesion). Hypotonia is a difficult clinical sign to elicit and probably not helpful in the assessment of a lower motor neurone lesion. Most elderly people find it difficult not to try to help you and to relax their muscles completely. This leads to an increase in tone in all directions of movement, which increases with the speed of movement and with encouragement to relax. This is called *gegenhalte*[c] or *paratonia*. When it is severe it may be a result of frontal lobe or diffuse cerebrovascular disease. If the joints are moved unpredictably and at different rates or if the patient is distracted (e.g. by being asked to count backwards from 100) it may be reduced. Young people who are able to relax their muscle completely have little or no tone and hypotonia cannot be diagnosed in these people.

The cogwheel rigidity of Parkinson's disease is another abnormality of tone in the upper limbs. It is best assessed by having the patient move the other arm up and down as you move the hand and forearm, testing tone at the wrist and elbow. It is the result of rigidity and superimposed tremor.

Myotonia as described above is also an abnormality of tone that is worse after active movement. In these patients, tone is usually normal at rest but after sudden movements there may be a great increase in tone and the patient is unable to relax the muscle. Tapping over the body of a myotonic muscle causes a dimple of contraction, which only slowly disappears (*percussion myotonia*). This is best tested by tapping the thenar

---

[c] From the German meaning 'counterpressure' or 'standing your ground'.

eminence or by asking the patient to make a tight fist and then open the hand quickly. The opening of the fist is very slow when the muscles are myotonic.

Power

Muscle strength is assessed by gauging your ability to overcome the patient's full voluntary muscle resistance. Test this joint by joint, one side at a time, holding either side of the joint to isolate the movement in question. To decide whether the power is normal, the patient's age, sex and build should be taken into account. Power is graded based on the maximum observed (no matter how briefly), according to the following modified British Medical Research Council scheme (although this lacks sensitivity at the higher grades because work against gravity may make up only a small component of a muscle's function [e.g. the finger flexors]):

- 0   Complete paralysis (no movement).
- 1   Flicker of contraction possible.
- 2   Movement is possible when gravity is excluded.
- 3   Movement is possible against gravity but not if any further resistance is added.
- 4− Slight movement against resistance.
- 4   Moderate movement against resistance.
- 4+ Submaximal movement against resistance.
- 5   Normal power.[d]

If power is reduced, decide whether this is symmetrical or asymmetrical, whether it involves only particular muscle groups or whether it is proximal, distal or general. Sometimes painful joint or muscle disease may interfere with the assessment (see Ch 23). Asymmetrical muscle weakness is most often the result of a peripheral nerve, brachial plexus or root lesion or an upper motor neurone lesion. As each movement is tested, the important muscles involved should be observed or palpated.

Shoulder

- *Abduction*—mostly deltoid and supraspinatus—(C5, C6): the patient should abduct the arm with the elbow flexed and resist your attempt to push it down (see Fig. 34.3a).
- *Adduction*—mostly pectoralis major and latissimus dorsi—(C6–C8): the patient should

Testing power—shoulder (test each arm separately)

FIGURE 34.3

adduct the arm with the elbow flexed and not allow you to push it to the side (see Fig. 34.3b).

Elbow

- *Flexion*—biceps and brachialis—(C5, C6): the patient should bend the elbow and pull so as not to let you straighten it out (see Fig. 34.4).
- *Extension*—triceps brachii—(C7, C8): the patient should partly bend the elbow and push so as not to let you bend it further (see Fig. 34.5).

Wrist

- *Flexion*—flexor carpi ulnaris and radialis—(C6, C7): the patient should bend the wrist and not allow you to straighten it. Hold the arm just above the wrist.

---

[d] You should not be able to overcome a normal adult patient's power, at least in the legs.

CHAPTER 34 THE NEUROLOGICAL EXAMINATION: THE PERIPHERAL NERVOUS SYSTEM   553

Testing power—elbow flexion: 'Stop me straightening your elbow' (test each arm separately)

FIGURE 34.4

Testing power—wrist extension: 'Stop me bending your wrist'

FIGURE 34.6

Testing power—elbow extension: 'Stop me bending your elbow' (test each arm separately)

FIGURE 34.5

- *Extension*—extensor carpi group—(C7, C8): the patient should extend the wrist and not allow you to bend it (see Fig. 34.6).

Fingers

- *Extension*—extensor digitorum communis, extensor indicis and extensor digiti minimi—(C7, C8): the patient should straighten the fingers and not allow you to push them down (push with the side of your hand across the patient's metacarpophalangeal [MCP] joints).
- *Flexion*—flexor digitorum profundus and sublimis—(C7, C8): the patient squeezes two of your fingers (see Fig. 34.7).
- *Abduction*—dorsal interossei—(C8, T1): the patient should spread out the fingers and not allow you to push them together (see Fig. 34.8).
- *Adduction*—volar interossei—(C8, T1): the patient holds the fingers together and tries to prevent you from separating them further. Alternatively the patient holds a piece of paper between the fingers, and you try to pull it out.

Reflexes

The sudden stretching of a muscle usually evokes brisk contraction of that muscle or muscle group. This reflex is usually mediated via a neural pathway synapsing in the spinal cord. It is subject to regulation via pathways from the brain. As the reflex is a response to stretching of a muscle, it is correctly called a muscle stretch reflex rather than a tendon reflex. The tendon merely transmits stretch to the muscle.

Tendon hammers are available in a number of designs. Sir William Gowers[e] used the ulnar side of

Testing power—finger flexion: 'Squeeze my fingers hard' (don't offer more than two fingers)

FIGURE 34.7

Testing power—finger abduction: 'Stop me pushing your fingers together'

FIGURE 34.8

his hand or part of his stethoscope. In Australia and the United Kingdom, the Queen Square hammer[f] is in common use (see Fig. 34.9). The Taylor hammer is popular in the United States; it is shaped like a tomahawk and has a broad rubber edge for most tendons and a more pointed side for the cutaneous reflexes.

Reflexes are graded from absent to greatly increased (see Table 34.1). Remember that patients who are very anxious or are thyrotoxic may have a general increase in the briskness of their reflexes.

Make sure the patient is resting comfortably with the elbows flexed and the hands lying pronated on the lap and not overlapping one another. To test the **biceps jerk** (C5, C6), place one forefinger on the biceps tendon and tap this with the tendon hammer (see Fig. 34.10). The hammer should be held near its end and the head allowed to fall with gravity onto the positioned forefinger. You will soon learn not to hit too hard. Normally, if the

A Queen Square patellar hammer—'triceps jerk'

FIGURE 34.9

Classification of muscle stretch reflexes	
0	Absent
+	Present but reduced
++	Normal
+++	Increased, possibly normal
++++	Greatly increased, often associated with clonus

TABLE 34.1

---

[e] Sir William Gowers (1845–1915), a professor of clinical medicine at University College Hospital, London, and neurologist to the National Hospital for Nervous Diseases, Queen Square, London. He was also an artist who illustrated his own books and had paintings exhibited at the Royal Academy.

[f] The Queen Square hammer was invented by Miss Wintle, staff nurse at Queen Square. She made hammers from brass wheels covered by a ring pessary and mounted on a bamboo handle; she sold these to medical students and resident medical officers.

The triceps jerk examination

FIGURE 34.11

The biceps jerk examination

FIGURE 34.10

reflex arc is intact, there is a brisk contraction of the biceps muscle with flexion of the forearm at the elbow, followed by prompt relaxation. Practice will help you decide whether the response is within the normal range. When a reflex is greatly exaggerated, it can be elicited away from the usual zone.

If a reflex appears to be absent, always test following a *reinforcement manoeuvre*. For example, ask the patient to clench the teeth tightly just before you let the hammer fall. Various mechanisms have been identified to explain reinforcement, but it works partly as a distraction, especially if the reflex is absent, because an anxious patient has contracted opposing muscle groups. Merely talking to the patient may provide enough distraction for the reflex to be elicited. Sometimes normal reflexes can be elicited only after reinforcement, but they should still be symmetrical.

An increased jerk occurs with an upper motor neurone lesion. A decreased or absent reflex occurs with a breach in any part of the reflex motor arc—the muscle itself (e.g. myopathy), the motor nerve (e.g. neuropathy), the anterior spinal cord root (e.g. spondylosis), the anterior horn cell (e.g. poliomyelitis) or the sensory arc (sensory root or sensory nerve).

To test the **triceps jerk** (C7, C8), support the elbow with one hand and tap over the triceps tendon (see Fig. 34.11). Normally, triceps contraction results in forearm extension.

To test the **brachioradialis (supinator) jerk** (C5, C6), strike the lower end of the radius just above the wrist (see Fig. 34.12). To avoid hurting the patient by striking the radial nerve directly, place your own first two fingers over this spot and then strike your fingers, as with the biceps jerk. Normally, contraction of the brachioradialis causes flexion of the elbow.

If elbow extension and finger flexion are the only response when the patient's wrist is tapped, the response is said to be inverted, known as the *inverted brachioradialis (supinator) jerk*. The triceps contraction causes elbow extension instead of the usual elbow flexion. This is associated with an absent biceps jerk and an exaggerated triceps jerk. It indicates a spinal cord lesion at the C5 or C6 level due, for example, to compression (e.g. disc prolapse), trauma or syringomyelia. It occurs

The supinator jerk strike zone

FIGURE 34.12

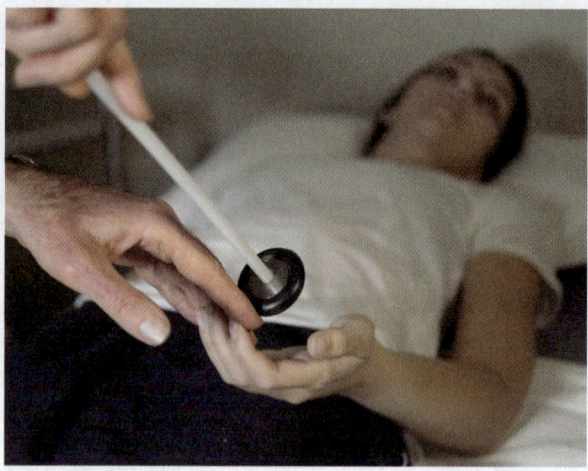

The finger jerk examination

FIGURE 34.13

because a lower motor neurone lesion at C5 or C6 is combined with an upper motor neurone lesion affecting the reflexes below this level.

To test **finger jerks** (C8), the patient rests the hand palm upwards, with the fingers slightly flexed. Place your hand over the patient's and strike the hammer over your fingers (see Fig. 34.13). Normally, slight flexion of all the patient's fingers occurs.

Coordination

The cerebellum has multiple connections (afferent and efferent) to sensory pathways, brainstem nuclei, the thalamus and the cerebral cortex. Via these connections the cerebellum plays an integral role in coordinating voluntary movement. A standard series of simple tests is used to test coordination. Always demonstrate these movements for the patient's benefit.

Finger–nose test

Ask the patient to touch his or her nose with the index finger and then turn the finger around and touch your outstretched forefinger at nearly full extension of the shoulder and elbow (see Fig. 34.14). The test should be done at first slowly and then briskly, and repeated a number of times with the patient's eyes open and later closed. Slight resistance to the patient's movements by you pushing on his or her forearm during the test may unmask less-severe abnormalities.

Look for the following abnormalities: (1) intention (not *intentional*) tremor, which is tremor increasing as the target is approached (there is no tremor at

Finger–nose test: 'Touch your nose with your forefinger and then reach out and touch my finger'

FIGURE 34.14

rest), and (2) past-pointing, where the patient's finger overshoots the target towards the side of cerebellar abnormality. These abnormalities occur with cerebellar disease.

Rapidly alternating movements

Ask the patient to pronate and supinate his or her hand on the dorsum of the other hand as rapidly as possible

Testing for dysdiadochokinesis in the upper limbs: 'Turn your hand over, backwards and forwards on the other one, as quickly and smoothly as you can'

FIGURE 34.15

Pain and temperature pathways

(Adapted from Snell RS, Westmoreland BF. *Clinical neuroanatomy for medical students*, 4th edition. Lippincott-Raven. 1997.)

FIGURE 34.16

(see Fig. 34.15). This movement is slow and clumsy in cerebellar disease and is called dysdiadochokinesis.[g]

Rapidly alternating movements may also be affected in extrapyramidal disorders (e.g. Parkinson's disease) and in pyramidal disorders (e.g. internal capsule infarction).

Rebound

Ask the patient to lift the arms rapidly from the sides and then stop. Hypotonia due to cerebellar disease causes delay in stopping the arms. This method of demonstrating rebound is preferable to the more often used one where the patient flexes the arm at the elbow against the examiner's resistance. When the examiner suddenly lets go, violent flexion of the arm may occur and, unless prevented, the patient can strike himself or herself in the face. Therefore, only medical students trained in self-defence should use this method.[h]

Muscle weakness may also cause clumsiness, but motor testing should have revealed any impairment of this sort.

The sensory system

When examining the sensory system, less is more. The more time spent, the more that subjective and irrelevant subtle differences will be noticed, and the more confused you will become. Start distally and work proximally. It is seldom of value to map sensation over every square centimetre of skin.[1]

Spinothalamic pathway (pain and temperature)

Pain and temperature fibres enter the spinal cord and cross, a few segments higher, to the opposite spinothalamic tract (see Fig. 34.16). This tract ascends to the brainstem.

Pain (pinprick) testing

Using a new pin,[2] demonstrate to the patient that this induces a relatively sharp sensation by touching lightly a normal area, such as the anterior chest wall. Then ask the patient to say whether the pinprick feels sharp or dull. Begin distally and work proximally. Test in each dermatome—the area of skin supplied by a vertebral spinal segment (see Fig. 34.17). Also compare

---

[g] Actually, dysdiadochokinesis is the inability to perform alternating movements of both wrists with the arms and forefingers extended. *Diadochi* is a Greek word meaning 'succession'. The problem here is with successive movements. The Diadochi were the successors of Alexander the Great. They divided his empire.

[h] Nick Talley has a black belt in Tae Kwon Do and Tang Soo Do.

Testing for pinprick (pain) sensation with a disposable neurology pin: 'Does this feel sharp or blunt?'

FIGURE 34.17

Vibration and joint position sense pathways

(Adapted from Snell RS, Westmoreland BF. *Clinical neuroanatomy for medical students*, 4th edition. Lippincott-Raven. 1997.)

FIGURE 34.18

right with left in the same dermatome. Map out the extent of any area of dullness. Always do this by going from the area of dullness to the area of normal sensation (hence distal to proximal in most neuropathies).

Temperature testing

Cold sensation can be tested with a metal object, such as a tuning fork or metal end of the tendon hammer. Absence of ability to feel heat is almost always associated with inability to feel cold. Start distally and rapidly move proximally asking whether the temperature changes. Temperature sensation testing is often better tolerated by patients than pain sensation testing and neurologists consider it more helpful—though they may go on to do this to confirm temperature findings.

Posterior columns (vibration and proprioception[i])

These fibres enter and ascend ipsilaterally in the posterior columns of the spinal cord to the nucleus gracilis and nucleus cuneatus in the medulla, where they decussate (see Fig. 34.18).

Vibration testing

Use a 128 Hz (not a 256 Hz) tuning fork. Ask the patient to close the eyes, and place the vibrating tuning fork on one of the distal interphalangeal joints. Patients who have no experience with testing may let out a surprised exclamation. This confirms normal vibration sensation in that hand. The patient may describe a feeling of vibration, buzzing or may even gesture with their hands. Deaden the tuning fork with your hand; the patient should be able to say exactly when this occurs. Compare one side with the other. If vibration sense is reduced or absent, test over the ulnar head at the wrist, then the elbows (over the olecranon) and then the shoulders to determine the level of abnormality. Although the tuning fork is traditionally placed only over bony prominences, vibration sense is just as good over soft tissues.

Proprioception testing

Use the distal interphalangeal joint of the patient's little finger. When the patient has his or her eyes open, grasp the distal phalanx from the sides (not the top and bottom) and move it up and down to demonstrate these positions. Start with big movements so the patient gets the idea, and progress to smaller movements. Then ask the patient to close the eyes while these manoeuvres are repeated randomly. Normally, movement through even a few degrees is detectable, and should be reported

---

[i] In 1826 Sir Charles Bell recognised that there was a 'sixth sense', which was later called proprioception. Vibration sense had been recognised in the 16th century and tests for it were developed in the 19th century by Rinné and others. Rydel and Seiffer found that vibration sense and proprioception were carried in the posterior columns of the spinal cord.

correctly. If there is an abnormality, proceed to test the wrists and elbows similarly. As a rule, sense of position is lost before sense of movement, and the little finger is affected before the thumb.

Light-touch testing

Some fibres travel in the posterior columns (i.e. ipsilaterally) and the rest cross the middle line to travel in the anterior spinothalamic tract (i.e. contralaterally). For this reason, light touch is of the least discriminating value. It is often omitted, except for bilateral touching with the fingers to assess for inattention or neglect (Ch 33). Irritation of light-touch receptors is probably responsible for paraesthesias—for example, following ischaemia of a limb.

Test light touch by touching the skin with a wisp of cottonwool. Ask the patient to shut the eyes and say 'yes' when the touch is felt. Do not stroke the skin because this moves hair fibres. Test each dermatome,[j] comparing left and right sides.

Interpretation of sensory abnormalities

Try to fit the distribution of any sensory loss into a dermatome (due to a spinal cord or nerve root lesion), a single peripheral nerve territory, a peripheral neuropathy pattern (glove distribution, p 583) or a hemisensory loss (due to spinal cord or upper brainstem or thalamic lesion).

Sensory dermatomes of the upper limb (see Fig. 34.19) can be recognised by memorising the following rough guide:

- C5 supplies the shoulder tip and outer part of the upper arm.
- C6 supplies the lateral aspect of the forearm and thumb.
- C7 supplies the middle finger.
- C8 supplies the little finger.
- T1 supplies the medial aspect of the upper arm and the elbow.

Examination of the peripheral nerves of the upper limb

A lesion of a peripheral nerve causes a characteristic motor and sensory loss.[3] Peripheral nerve lesions may have local causes, such as trauma or compression, or may be part of a mononeuritis multiplex, where more than one nerve is affected by systemic disease.

The radial nerve (C5–C8)

This is the *motor nerve* supplying the triceps and brachioradialis and the extensor muscles of the hand. The characteristic deformity that results from radial nerve injury is *wrist drop* (see Fig. 34.20). To demonstrate this, if it is not already obvious, get the patient to flex the elbow, pronate the forearm and extend the wrist and fingers. If a lesion occurs above the upper third of the upper arm, the triceps muscle is also affected. Therefore, test elbow extension, which will be absent if the lesion is high.

Test *sensation* using a pin over the area of the anatomical snuff box. Sensation here is lost with a radial nerve lesion before the bifurcation into posterior interosseous and superficial radial nerves at the elbow (see Fig. 34.21).

The median nerve (C6–T1)

This nerve contains the *motor* supply to all the muscles on the front of the forearm except the flexor carpi ulnaris and the ulnar half of the flexor digitorum profundus. It also supplies the following short muscles of the hand—LOAF:

L ateral two lumbricals
O pponens pollicis
A bductor pollicis brevis
F lexor pollicis brevis (in many people).

Lesion at the wrist (carpal tunnel)[4,5]

Use the pen-touching test to assess for weakness of the abductor pollicis brevis. Ask the patient to lay the hand flat, palm upwards on the table, and attempt to abduct the thumb vertically to touch your pen held above it (see Fig. 34.22). This may be impossible if there is a median nerve palsy at the wrist or above. Remember, however, that most patients with the carpal tunnel syndrome have normal power and may indeed have symptoms but no signs at all. Feel at the wrist for a thickened median nerve (e.g. sarcoid, leprosy).

Lesion in the cubital fossa

Ochsner's clasping test[k] (for loss of flexor digitorum sublimis): ask the patient to clasp the hands firmly together (see Fig. 34.23(a))—the index finger on the

---

[j] The human dermatomes (which he called pain spots) were first mapped by Sir Henry Head (1861–1940). He was most famous for his experimental cutting of his own radial nerve. This enabled him to chart the order of return of the sensory modalities.

[k] Albert Ochsner (1858–1925), an American surgeon of Swiss extraction, who claimed descent from Andreas Vesalius, the great anatomist.

SECTION 9 THE NERVOUS SYSTEM

Dermatomes of the upper limb and trunk.

(a) The dermatomes explained. (b) The distribution of the dermatomes makes more sense if we are thought of as quadrupedal. (c) Herpes zoster of the C8 dermatome showing its distribution

((c) Courtesy of Dr A Watson, Infectious Diseases Department, The Canberra Hospital.)

FIGURE 34.19

CHAPTER 34 THE NEUROLOGICAL EXAMINATION: THE PERIPHERAL NERVOUS SYSTEM   561

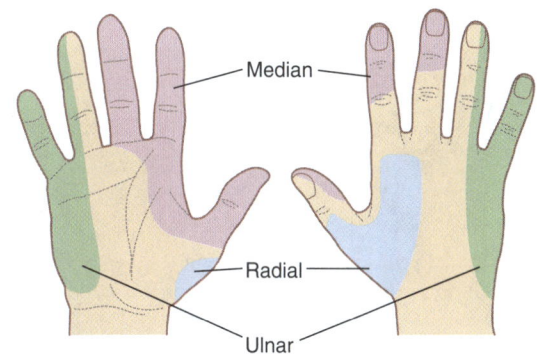

Average loss of pain sensation (pinprick) with lesions of the major nerves of the upper limbs

FIGURE 34.21

(a) Typical appearance of a left radial nerve palsy with wrist drop. (b) Even with the wrist supported, the patient is still unable to actively extend their fingers and thumb at the MCP joints

(From Jones Neil F and Machado Gustavo R. Functional hand reconstruction tendon transfers for radial, median, and ulnar nerve injuries: current surgical techniques. *Clin Plastic Surg* 2011; 38 (4):621–642. Copyright ©Elsevier.)

FIGURE 34.20

Pen-touching test for loss of abductor pollicis brevis: 'Lift your thumb straight up to touch my pen'

FIGURE 34.22

affected side fails to flex with a lesion in the cubital fossa or higher (see Fig. 34.23(b)).

For the *sensory* component of the median nerve, test pinprick sensation over the hand. The constant area of loss includes the palmar aspect of the thumb, the index finger, the middle finger and the lateral half of the ring finger (see Fig. 34.21). The palm is spared in median nerve lesions in the carpal tunnel.

The ulnar nerve (C8–T1)

This nerve contains the *motor* supply to all the small muscles of the hand (except the LOAF muscles), the flexor carpi ulnaris and the ulnar half of the flexor digitorum profundus. Look for wasting of the small muscles of the hand and for partial clawing of the little and ring fingers (a claw-like hand). Clawing is hyperextension at the metacarpophalangeal joints and flexion of the interphalangeal joints. Note that clawing is more pronounced with an ulnar nerve lesion at the wrist, as a lesion at or above the elbow also causes loss

Ochsner's clasping test.

(a) Normal; (b) abnormal due to loss of function of the flexor digitorum (simulated demonstration)

FIGURE 34.23

Motor neurone disease.

Shows wasting of the small muscles of the hand

FIGURE 34.24

> **CAUSES (DIFFERENTIAL DIAGNOSIS) OF A TRUE CLAW HAND (ALL FINGERS CLAWED)**
>
> Ulnar and median nerve lesion (ulnar nerve palsy alone causes a claw-like hand)
> Brachial plexus lesion (C8–T1)
> Other neurological disease (e.g. syringomyelia, polio)
> Ischaemic contracture (late and severe)
> Rheumatoid arthritis (advanced, untreated disease)
>
> LIST 34.2

of the flexor digitorum profundus, and therefore less flexion of the interphalangeal joints. This is the 'ulnar nerve paradox', in that a more distal lesion causes greater deformity. Also, feel at the elbow for a thickened ulna nerve.

Froment's[1] sign

Ask the patient to grasp a piece of paper between the thumb and lateral aspect of the forefinger with each hand. The affected thumb will flex because of loss of the adductor of the thumb.

---
[1] Jules Froment (1878–1946), a professor of medicine in Lyons, France, described the sign in 1915.

Causes of a true claw hand are shown in List 34.2, while causes of wasting of the small muscles of the hand are shown in List 34.3; see also Fig. 34.24.

For the *sensory* component of the ulnar nerve, test for pinprick loss over the palmar and dorsal aspects of the little finger and the medial half of the ring finger (see Fig. 34.21).

The brachial plexus

Brachial plexus lesions vary from mild to complete; motor and/or sensory fibres may be involved. Nerve roots form trunks, which divide into cords and then form peripheral nerves (see Tables 34.2 and 34.3). The anatomy is shown in Fig. 34.25.

CAUSES (DIFFERENTIAL DIAGNOSIS) OF WASTING OF THE SMALL MUSCLES OF THE HAND

Spinal cord lesions

Syringomyelia

Cervical spondylosis with compression of the C8 segment

Tumour

Trauma

Anterior horn cell disease

Motor neurone disease, poliomyelitis

Spinal muscular atrophies (e.g. Kugelberg–Welander* disease)

Root lesion

C8 compression

Lower trunk brachial plexus lesion

Thoracic outlet syndromes

Trauma, radiation, infiltration, inflammation

Peripheral nerve lesions

Median and ulnar nerve lesions

Peripheral motor neuropathy

Myopathy

Dystrophia myotonica—forearms are more affected than the hands

Distal myopathy

Trophic disorders

Arthropathies (disuse)

Ischaemia, including vasculitis

Shoulder hand syndrome

Note: Distinguishing an ulnar nerve lesion from a C8 root / lower trunk brachial plexus lesion depends on remembering that sensory loss with a C8 lesion extends proximal to the wrist, and the thenar muscles are involved with a C8 root or lower trunk brachial plexus lesion. Distinguishing a C8 root from a lower trunk brachial plexus lesion is difficult clinically, but the presence of a Horner's syndrome or an axillary mass suggests the brachial plexus is affected.

*Eric Klas Kugelberg (1913–83), a professor of clinical neurophysiology at the Karolinska Institute in Stockholm, and Lisa Welander (1909–2001) described this in 1956. Lisa Welander was Sweden's first female professor of neurology.

LIST 34.3

Nerve roots and brachial plexus trunks

Nerve roots	Trunks	Muscles supplied
C5 and 6	Upper	Shoulder (especially biceps and deltoid)
C7	Middle	Triceps and some forearm muscles
C8 and T1	Lower	Hand and some forearm muscles

TABLE 34.2

Brachial plexus cords, nerves and their supplied muscles

Cords	Nerves formed	Muscles supplied
Lateral	Musculocutaneous, median	Biceps, pronator teres, flexor carpi radialis
Medial	Median and ulnar	Hand muscles
Posterior	Axillary and radial	Deltoid, triceps and forearm extensors

TABLE 34.3

Patients with brachial plexus lesions may complain of pain or weakness in the shoulders or arms. Pain is often prominent, especially when there has been nerve root avulsion. A neurological cause is more likely if there is dull pain that is difficult to localise, if the pain is not related to limb movement and is worse at night and if there is no associated tenderness. The patient may be unable to get comfortable. An orthopaedic or traumatic cause is more likely if the pain is much worse with movement, or there are signs of inflammation, joint deformity or local tenderness. Most plexus lesions are supraclavicular (i.e. proximal), especially when they occur after trauma. When infraclavicular (i.e. distal) lesions occur, they are usually less severe.

Examine the arms and shoulder girdle (see List 34.4). Remember that the dorsal scapular nerve (which supplies the rhomboid muscles) comes from the C5 nerve root proximal to the upper trunk, and so rhomboid function is usually spared in upper trunk lesions. Typical lesions of the brachial plexus are described in List 34.5. The cervical rib syndrome may cause a lower brachial plexus lesion (see List 34.6). Table 34.4 suggests a scheme for distinguishing between plexus and nerve root lesions.

The brachial plexus
(Adapted from Chusid JG. *Correlative neuroanatomy and functional neurology*, 19th edn. Los Altos: Lange Medical, 1985.)

FIGURE 34.25

SHOULDER GIRDLE EXAMINATION

Method

Abnormalities are likely to be due to a muscular dystrophy, single nerve or a root lesion. Inspect each muscle, palpate its bulk and test function as follows:

1. Trapezius (XI, C3, C4): ask the patient to elevate the shoulders against resistance and look for winging of the upper scapula.
2. Serratus anterior (C5–C7): ask the patient to push the hands against the wall and look for winging of the lower scapula.
3. Rhomboids (C4, C5): ask the patient to pull both shoulder blades together with the hands on the hips.
4. Supraspinatus (C5, C6): ask the patient to abduct the arms from the sides against resistance.
5. Infraspinatus (C5, C6): ask the patient to rotate the upper arms externally against resistance with the elbows flexed at the sides.
6. Teres major (C5–C7): ask the patient to rotate the upper arms internally against resistance.
7. Latissimus dorsi (C7, C8): ask the patient to pull the elbows into the sides against resistance.
8. Pectoralis major, clavicular head (C5–C8): ask the patient to lift the upper arms above the horizontal and push them forwards against resistance.
9. Pectoralis major, sternocostal part (C6–T1) and pectoralis minor (C7): ask the patient to adduct the upper arms against resistance.
10. Deltoid (C5, C6) (and axillary nerve): ask the patient to abduct the arms against resistance.

LIST 34.4

BRACHIAL PLEXUS LESIONS

Complete lesion (rare)
1. Lower motor neurone signs affect the whole arm
2. Sensory loss (whole limb)
3. Horner's syndrome (an important clue)

Note: This is often painful.

Upper lesion (Erb Duchenne*) (C5, C6)
1. Loss of shoulder movement and elbow flexion—the hand is held in the waiter's tip position
2. Sensory loss over the lateral aspect of the arm and the forearm

Lower lesion (Klumpke†) (C8, T1)
1. True claw hand with paralysis of all the intrinsic muscles
2. Sensory loss along the ulnar side of the hand and the forearm
3. Horner's syndrome

*Wilhelm Heinrich Erb (1840–1921), Germany's greatest neurologist.
†Auguste Déjérine-Klumpke (1859–1927), a French neurologist, described this lesion as a student. She was an American, but was educated in Switzerland. As a final-year student she married the great French neurologist Jules Déjérine.

LIST 34.5

Distinguishing between brachial plexus lesions and nerve root compression

	Plexus	Root
Previous trauma	Some types	Occasionally
Insidious onset	Some types	Usually
Neck pain	No	Yes
Unilateral interscapular pain	No	Yes
Weakness	Often severe	Mild–moderate
Pattern of weakness	Usually shoulder and biceps or hand	Most commonly triceps (C7 lesions, the most commonly affected root)

TABLE 34.4

CERVICAL RIB SYNDROME

Clinical features
1. Weakness and wasting of the small muscles of the hand (claw hand)
2. C8 and T1 sensory loss
3. Unequal radial pulses and blood pressure
4. Subclavian bruits on arm manoeuvring (may be present in healthy people)
5. Palpable cervical rib in the neck (uncommon)

LIST 34.6

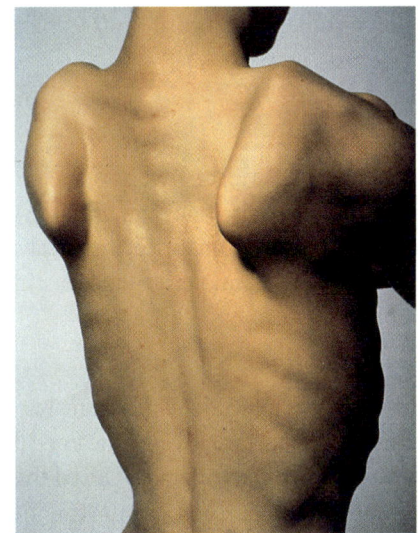

Winging of the scapulae, often a result of muscular dystrophy

(From Mir MA. *Atlas of clinical diagnosis*, 2nd edn. Edinburgh: Saunders, 2003.)

FIGURE 34.26

Ask the patient to stand facing away from you with the arms and hands stretched out to touch and push against the wall. Winging of the scapulae is seen typically in fascioscapular–humeral dystrophy (see Fig. 34.26).

Causes of brachial plexus lesions include:
- inflammation and infection, autoimmune disorders (more often upper plexus)
- radiotherapy (more often upper plexus)
- cancer (more often lower plexus)—cancer causes a brachial plexus lesion by local invasion; the

lower trunk is usually affected first. These plexus lesions are usually painful and progress rapidly. Weakness and sensory loss are both present
- trauma: direct (motor vehicle crash, surgery including sternotomy, lacerations and gunshots), traction (birth injuries, motor vehicle crashes, sporting injuries such as rugby tackles—more often upper plexus), chronic compression (thoracic outlet, 'backpack palsy', fractures with bone displacement).

Lower limbs

Begin by testing *gait*, if this is possible (see p 577).

Inspect the legs with the patient lying in bed with the legs and thighs entirely exposed (place a towel over the groin). Note whether there is a urinary catheter present, which may indicate that there is spinal cord compression or other spinal cord disease, particularly multiple sclerosis.

The motor system

Fasciculations and muscle wasting

Inspect for fasciculations. Look for muscle wasting. Feel the muscle bulk of the quadriceps and calves. Then run a hand along each shin, feeling for wasting of the anterior tibial muscles.

Tone

Test tone at the knees and ankles. Place one hand under a chosen knee and then abruptly pull the knee upwards, causing flexion. When the patient is relaxed this should occur without resistance. Then, supporting the thigh, flex and extend the knee at increasing velocity, feeling for resistance to muscle stretch (tone). Tone in the legs may also be tested by sitting the patient with legs hanging freely over the edge of the bed. Raise one of the patient's legs to the horizontal and then suddenly let go. The leg will oscillate up to half a dozen times in a healthy person who is completely relaxed. If hypotonia is present, as occurs in cerebellar disease, the oscillations will be wider and more prolonged. If increased tone or spasticity is present, the movements will be irregular and jerky.

Next test for *clonus* of the ankle and knee. This is a sustained rhythmical contraction of the muscles when put under sudden stretch. It is due to hypertonia from an upper motor neurone lesion. It represents an increase in reflex excitability (from increased alpha motor neurone activity).

Sharply dorsiflex the foot with the knee bent and the thigh externally rotated. When ankle clonus is present, recurrent ankle plantar flexion movement occurs. This may persist for as long as you sustain dorsiflexion of the ankle. Test for patellar clonus by resting a hand on the lower part of the quadriceps with the knee extended and moving the patella down sharply. Sustained rhythmical contraction of the quadriceps occurs as long as the downward stretch is maintained.

Power

Test power next.

Hip

- *Flexion*—psoas and iliacus muscles—(L2, L3): ask the patient to lift up the straight leg and not let you push it down (having placed your hand above the knee; see Fig. 34.27).
- *Extension*—gluteus maximus—(L5, S1, S2): ask the patient to keep the leg down and not let you pull it up from underneath the calf or ankle (see Fig. 34.28).
- *Abduction*—gluteus medius and minimus, sartorius and tensor fasciae latae—(L4, L5, S1): ask the patient to abduct the leg and not let you push it in (see Fig. 34.29).

Testing power—hip flexion: 'Lift your leg up and don't let me push it down'

FIGURE 34.27

Testing power—hip extension: 'Push your heel down and don't let me pull it up'

FIGURE 34.28

Testing power—hip adduction: 'Don't let me push your hip out'; pull hard

FIGURE 34.30

Testing power—hip abduction: 'Don't let me push your hip in'

FIGURE 34.29

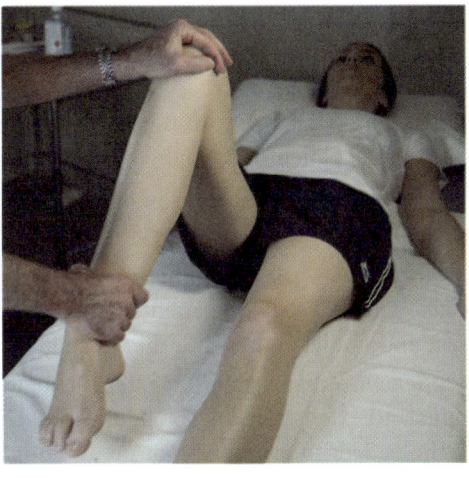

Testing power—knee flexion: 'Bend your knee and don't let me straighten it'; pull hard

FIGURE 34.31

- *Adduction*—adductors longus, brevis and magnus—(L2, L3, L4): ask the patient to keep the leg adducted and not let you push it out (see Fig. 34.30).

Knee

- *Flexion*—hamstrings (biceps femoris, semimembranosus, semitendinosus)—(L5, S1): ask the patient to bend the knee and not let you straighten it (see Fig. 34.31). If there is doubt about the real strength of knee flexion, it should be tested with the patient in the prone position. Here possible help from hip flexion is prevented and the muscles can be palpated during contraction.
- *Extension*—quadriceps femoris (this muscle is three times as strong as its antagonists, the

Testing power—knee extension: 'Straighten your knee and don't let me bend it'; push hard

FIGURE 34.32

Testing power—ankle, plantar flexion: 'Don't let me push your foot up'

FIGURE 34.33

hamstrings)—(L3, L4): with the knee slightly bent, ask the patient to straighten the knee and not let you bend it (see Fig. 34.32).

Ankle
- *Plantar flexion*—gastrocnemius, plantaris, soleus—(S1, S2): ask the patient to push the foot down and not let you push it up (see Fig. 34.33).
- *Dorsiflexion*—tibialis anterior, extensor digitorum longus and extensor hallucis longus—(L4, L5): ask the patient to bring the foot up and not let you push it down (see Fig. 34.34). The power of the ankle joint can also be tested by having the patient stand up on the toes (plantar flexion) or on the heels (dorsiflexion); these movements may also be limited if coordination is impaired.

Tarsal joint
- *Eversion*—peroneus longus and brevis, and extensor digitorum longus—(L5, S1): evert the foot for the patient and ask him or her to hold it there (see Fig. 34.35).
- *Inversion*—tibialis posterior, gastrocnemius and hallucis longus—(L5, S1): invert the foot for the patient and ask him or her to hold it there (see Fig. 34.36).

Testing power—ankle, dorsiflexion: 'Don't let me push your foot down'

FIGURE 34.34

Non-organic or functional unilateral limb weakness may be detected by Hoover's test. Normally, when a patient attempts to resist movement, the contralateral limb works to support the effort. For example, when a patient attempts to extend the leg against resistance, the other leg pushes down into the bed. If this movement is absent, Hoover's[m] sign is positive.

---

[m] Charles Hoover also described an important sign of chronic obstructive pulmonary disease.

Quick test of lower limb power

The clinician in a hurry can test lower limb power quickly by asking the patient to:

1. stand up on his or her toes (S1) (see Fig. 34.37(a))
2. stand up on the heels (L4, L5) (see Fig. 34.37(b))
3. squat and stand again (L3, L4) (see Fig. 34.37(c)).

This tests ankle, knee and hip power. Inability to perform any of the tests suggests a need to test more formally.

Testing power—ankle (tarsal joint) eversion: 'Stop me turning your foot inwards'

FIGURE 34.35

Testing power—ankle (tarsal joint) inversion: 'Stop me turning your foot outwards'

FIGURE 34.36

Quick test of lower limb power.

(a) 'Stand up on your toes.' (b) 'Now lift up on your heels.' (c) 'Now squat and stand up again.'

FIGURE 34.37

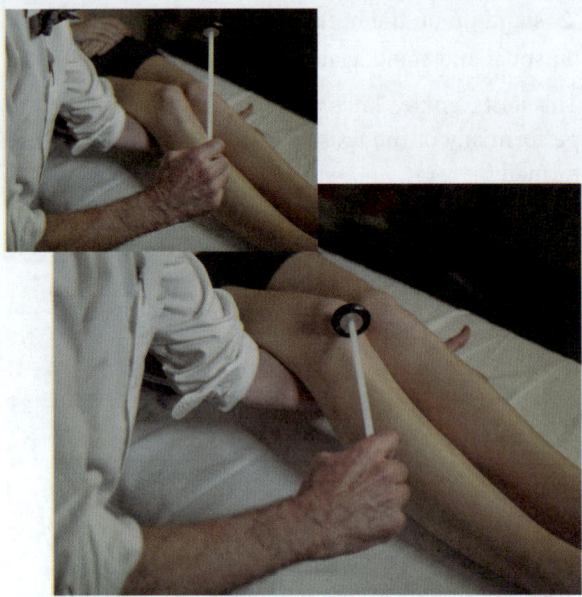

The knee jerk examination

FIGURE 34.38

The knee jerk with reinforcement: 'Grip your fingers and pull your hands apart'

FIGURE 34.39

Reflexes

Test the following reflexes.

Knee jerk (L3, L4)

Slide one arm under the patient's knees so that they are slightly bent and supported. The tendon hammer is allowed to fall onto the infrapatellar tendon (see Fig. 34.38). Normally, contraction of the quadriceps causes extension of the knee. Compare the two sides. If the knee jerk appears to be absent on one or both sides, it should be tested again following a reinforcement manoeuvre. Ask the patient to interlock the fingers and then pull apart hard at the moment before the hammer strikes the tendon (Jendrassik's manoeuvre;[n] see Fig. 34.39). This manoeuvre has been shown to restore an apparently absent ankle jerk in 70% of elderly people. A reinforcement manoeuvre such as this, or teeth-clenching or grasping an object, should be used if there is difficulty eliciting any of the muscle stretch reflexes.

Ankle jerk (S1, S2)

Have the foot in the mid-position at the ankle with the knee bent, the thigh externally rotated on the bed and the foot held in dorsiflexion by you. Allow the hammer to fall on the Achilles tendon (see Fig. 34.40). The normal response is plantar flexion of the foot with contraction of the gastrocnemius muscle. Again, test with reinforcement if appropriate. This reflex can also be tested with the patient kneeling or by tapping the sole of the foot.[6]

Plantar reflex (L5, S1, S2)

After telling the patient what is going to happen, use a blunt object (such as the key to an expensive car) to stroke up the lateral aspect of the sole and curve inwards before it reaches the toes, moving towards the middle metatarsophalangeal (MTP) joint (see Fig. 34.41). The patient's foot should be in the same position as for testing the ankle jerk. The normal response is flexion of the big toe at the MTP joint in patients over 1 year of age. The extensor (Babinski[o])[7] response is abnormal and is characterised by extension of the big toe at the MTP joint (the upgoing toe) and fanning of the other toes. This indicates an upper motor neurone (pyramidal)

---

[n] Ernst Jendrassik (1858–1921), a Budapest physician.

[o] Josef Babinski (1857–1932), a Parisian neurologist of Polish extraction, described this sign in 1896. Somatisation disorders vary in their nature according to fashion. In the 19th century, hysterical paralysis was common. Babinski, while strolling through his ward, casually stroked the soles of the feet of two patients in adjoining beds (this would probably lead to his being struck off the medical register today). He noticed that the big toe of the woman thought to have hysterical paralysis moved down and that of the woman whose paralysis was thought genuine and due to a stroke moved up. The sign was probably first described by Ernst Remak in 1893. Babinski was a famous gourmet and assistant to Charcot.

CHAPTER 34 THE NEUROLOGICAL EXAMINATION: THE PERIPHERAL NERVOUS SYSTEM 571

The ankle jerk (first method, see also p 456): the examiner dorsiflexes the foot slightly to stretch the tendon

FIGURE 34.40

The heel–shin test: 'Run your heel down your shin smoothly and quickly'

FIGURE 34.42

lesion, although the test's reliability can be relatively poor. Bilateral upgoing toes may also be found after a generalised seizure, or in a patient in a coma.

Coordination

Test for cerebellar disease with three manoeuvres.

Heel–shin test

Ask the patient to run the heel of one foot up and down the opposite shin at a moderate pace and as accurately as possible (see Fig. 34.42). In cerebellar disease the heel wobbles all over the place, with oscillations from side to side and overshooting. Closing the eyes makes little difference to this in cerebellar disease, but if there is posterior column loss the movements are made worse when the eyes are shut—that is, there is 'sensory ataxia'.

Toe–finger test

Unfortunately, a toe–nose test is not a practical way of assessing the lower limbs, so a toe–finger test is used. Ask the patient to lift the foot (with the knee bent) and touch your finger with the big toe. Look for intention tremor.

Foot-tapping test

Rapidly alternating movements are tested by getting the patient to tap the sole of the foot quickly on your hand or to tap the heel on the opposite shin. Look for loss of rhythmicity.

The plantar reflex examination

FIGURE 34.41

Testing pinprick (pain) sensation in the lower limbs (do not draw blood with the pin)

FIGURE 34.43

The sensory system

As for the upper limb, test for pain or cold sensation or both, first in each dermatome, starting distally and comparing the right with the left side (see Fig. 34.43). Map out any abnormality and decide on the pattern of loss.

Then test vibration sense over the great toe or malleoli or both and, if it is absent there, on the knees and if necessary on the anterior superior iliac spines (see Fig. 34.44). Next test proprioception, using the big toes (see Fig. 34.45) and, if necessary, the knees and hips.

Finally, test light touch bilaterally for neglect. Light touch can also be tested using a twirl of cottonwool or a microfibre tester (see Fig. 34.46). This sensation is especially protective against the development of ulcers in the feet.

Dermatomes

Memorise the following rough guide (see Fig. 34.47):
- L2 supplies the upper anterior thigh.
- L3 supplies the area around the front of the knee.
- L4 supplies the medial aspect of the leg.
- L5 supplies the lateral aspect of the leg and the medial side of the dorsum of the foot.
- S1 supplies the heel and most of the sole.
- S2 supplies the posterior aspect of the thigh.
- S3, S4 and S5 supply concentric rings around the anus.

Sensory levels

If there is peripheral sensory loss in the leg, attempt to map out the upper level with a pin, moving up at 5-centimetre intervals initially, from the leg to the abdomen, until the patient reports it to be sharp. This may involve testing over the abdominal or even the chest dermatomes. Establishing a sensory level on the trunk indicates the spinal cord level that is affected. Remember, a level of hyperaesthesia (increased sensitivity) often occurs above the sensory level and it is the upper level of this that should be determined, as it usually indicates the highest affected spinal segment. Also remember that the level of a vertebral body only corresponds to the spinal cord level in the upper cervical cord because the spinal cord is shorter than the spinal canal. The C8 spinal segment lies opposite the C7 vertebra. In the upper thoracic cord there is a difference of about two segments and in the midthoracic cord it is three segments. All the lumbosacral segments are opposite the T11 to L1 vertebrae.

The superficial or cutaneous reflexes

These reflexes occur in response to light touch or scratching of the skin or mucous membranes. The stimulus is more superficial than the tendon (muscle stretch) reflexes. As a rule these reflexes occur more slowly after the stimulus, are less constantly present and fatigue more easily.

Examples include the palmar or grasp reflex, the abdominal reflexes, the cremasteric reflex and the plantar responses.

The abdominal reflexes (epigastric T6–T9, midabdominal T9–T11, lower abdominal T11–L1) (See the OSCE video Abdominal reflexes at Student CONSULT)

Test these by lightly stroking the abdominal wall diagonally towards the umbilicus in each of the four quadrants of the abdomen (see Fig. 34.48). Reflex contractions of the abdominal wall are *absent* in upper motor neurone lesions above the segmental level and also in patients who have had surgical

Testing vibration sense in the lower limbs.

(a) Strike a 128 Hz tuning fork confidently on your thenar eminence. (b) Demonstrate the vibration of the tuning fork on the patient's sternum: 'Can you feel this vibration?' (c) Place the tuning fork on the great toe: 'Can you feel the vibration there? Tell me when it stops.' (d) If vibration sense is absent on the great toe, try testing on the patella. (e) If vibration sense is absent at the knee, try testing on the anterior superior iliac spine

FIGURE 34.44

SECTION 9 THE NERVOUS SYSTEM

Position sense: 'Shut your eyes and tell me whether I have moved your toe up or down'

FIGURE 34.45

Testing touch sensation with a monofilament. Cotton wool can be used as an alternative but do not stroke the skin

FIGURE 34.46

operations interrupting the nerves. They disappear in coma and deep sleep, and during anaesthesia. They are usually difficult to elicit in obese patients and can also be absent in some healthy people (20%). Their absence in the presence of increased tendon reflexes is suggestive of corticospinal tract abnormality.

The cremasteric reflexes (L1–L2)

Stroke the inner part of the thigh in a downward direction; normally contraction of the cremasteric muscle pulls up the scrotum and testis on the side stroked. It may be absent in elderly men and in those with a hydrocele or varicocele, or after an episode of orchitis. This is seldom tested, unless there are specific concerns about this region (e.g. from the history or because of a known L1, L2 lesion).

Saddle sensation and anal reflex

Test now for saddle sensation if a cauda equina lesion is suspected (e.g. because of urinary or faecal incontinence). The only sensory loss may be on the buttocks or around the anus (S3–S5). In this case also test the anal reflex (S2–S4): normal contraction of the external sphincter in response to pinprick of the perianal skin is abolished in patients with a lesion of the sacral segments of the cauda equina. If, however, the lowest sacral segments are spared but the higher ones are involved, this suggests that there is an intrinsic cord lesion.

Spine

Examine the spine with the patient standing. Look and feel for:

- scars
- scoliosis
- a midline pit or patch of hair (spina bifida)
- tenderness (malignancy or infection).

Ask the patient to lie down and perform the straight-leg-raising test (tests for disc herniation, which causes pain in the sciatic nerve distribution—p 575).

CHAPTER 34 THE NEUROLOGICAL EXAMINATION: THE PERIPHERAL NERVOUS SYSTEM

Dermatomes of the lower limbs

FIGURE 34.47

Abdominal reflex: stroke towards the umbilicus from each quadrant and watch for abdominal muscle contraction

FIGURE 34.48

Examination of the peripheral nerves of the lower limb

Lateral cutaneous nerve of the thigh

Test for sensory loss (see Fig. 34.49). A lesion of this nerve usually occurs because of entrapment between the inguinal ligament and the anterior superior iliac spine. It is more common in people who are overweight and in those who spend much of their time sitting (e.g. truck drivers, public servants). It causes a sensory loss over the lateral aspect of the thigh with no motor loss detectable. If painful, it is called *meralgia paraesthetica*.

Femoral nerve (L2, L3, L4)

Test for weakness of knee extension (quadriceps paralysis). Hip flexion weakness is only slight, and adductor strength is preserved. The knee jerk is absent. The sensory loss involves the inner aspect of the thigh and leg (see Fig. 34.50).

Sciatic nerve (L4, L5, S1, S2)

This nerve supplies all the muscles below the knee and the hamstrings. Test for loss of power below the knee resulting in a foot drop (plantar-flexed foot) and for weakness of knee flexion. Test the reflexes: with a sciatic nerve lesion the knee jerk is intact but the ankle jerk and plantar response are absent. Test sensation on the posterior thigh, the lateral and posterior calf,

576 SECTION 9 THE NERVOUS SYSTEM

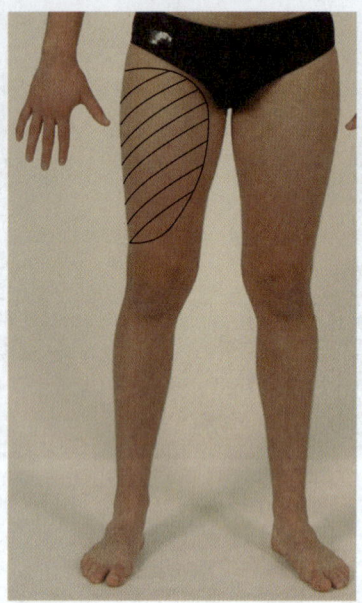

Distribution of the lateral cutaneous nerve of the thigh

FIGURE 34.49

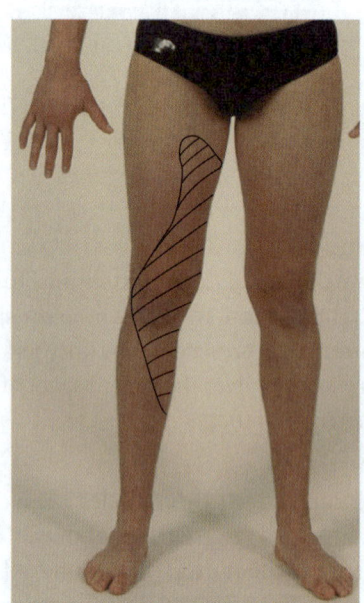

Sensory distribution of the femoral nerve

FIGURE 34.50

Sensory distribution of the sciatic nerve

FIGURE 34.51

and the foot (lost with a proximal nerve lesion; see Fig. 34.51).

Common peroneal nerve (L4, L5, S1)

This is a major terminal branch of the sciatic nerve. It supplies the anterior and lateral compartment muscles of the leg (see Fig. 34.52). On inspection one may notice a foot drop (see List 34.7 and Fig. 34.53). Test for weakness of dorsiflexion and eversion. Test the reflexes, which will all be intact. Test for sensory loss. There may be only minimal sensory loss over the lateral aspect of the dorsum of the foot. Note that these findings can be confused with an L5 root lesion,

CHAPTER 34 THE NEUROLOGICAL EXAMINATION: THE PERIPHERAL NERVOUS SYSTEM   577

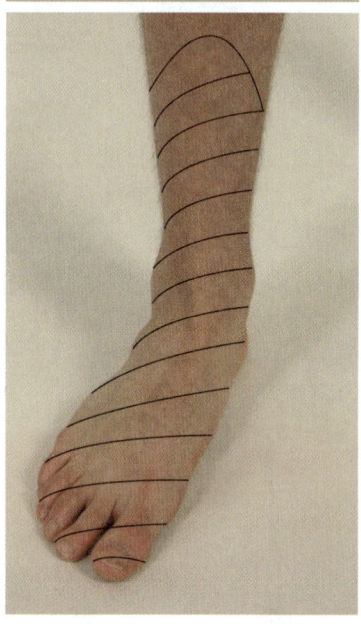

Sensory distribution of the common peroneal nerve (compression at the fibular neck)

FIGURE 34.52

> **CAUSES (DIFFERENTIAL DIAGNOSIS) OF FOOT DROP**
>
> Common peroneal nerve palsy
> Sciatic nerve palsy
> Lumbosacral plexus lesion
> L4, L5 root lesion
> Peripheral motor neuropathy
> Distal myopathy
> Motor neurone disease
> Stroke—anterior cerebral artery or lacunar syndrome ('ataxic hemiparesis')
>
> LIST 34.7

but the latter includes weakness of knee flexion and loss of foot inversion as well as sensory loss in the L5 distribution.

Gait

Make sure the patient's legs are clearly visible. Ask the patient to walk normally for a few metres and turn around quickly and walk back and then walk heel to toe to exclude a midline cerebellar lesion (see Fig. 34.54). Ask the patient to walk on the toes (an S1 lesion will make this difficult or impossible) and then on the heels (an L4 or L5 lesion causing foot drop will make this difficult or impossible).

Test for proximal myopathy by asking the patient to squat and then stand up, or to sit in a low chair and then stand.

To test *station* (Romberg[p] test), ask the patient to stand erect with the feet together and the eyes open (see Fig. 34.55(a)) and then, once the patient is stable, to close the eyes (see Fig. 34.55(b)). Compare the steadiness shown with the eyes open, then closed for up to 1 minute. Even in the absence of neurological disease a person may be slightly unsteady with the eyes closed, but the sign is positive if marked unsteadiness occurs to the point where the patient looks likely to fall. Normal people can maintain this position easily for 60 seconds. The Romberg test is positive when unsteadiness increases with eye closure. This is usually seen with the loss of proprioceptive sensation; unsteadiness is worse when visual information about position is removed.

Marked unsteadiness with the eyes open is seen with severe proprioceptive loss, cerebellar or vestibular dysfunction.

Gait disorders are summarised in List 34.8.

---

[p] Moritz Heinrich von Romberg (1795–1873), a Berlin professor, wrote the first modern neurology textbook. His original description of the sign was of patients with tabes dorsalis (dorsal column disease caused by syphilis).

(a) Foot drop: the patient lifts the affected leg high in the air to prevent the foot scraping on the ground. (b) Shoe supports to prevent foot drop

FIGURE 34.53

Cerebellar testing—heel–toe walking

FIGURE 34.54

Romberg test.

(a) 'Stand with your feet together.' (b) 'Now shut your eyes. I won't let you fall.'

FIGURE 34.55

GAIT DISORDERS

Hemiplegia: the foot is plantar flexed and the leg is swung in a lateral arc

Spastic paraparesis: scissors gait

Parkinson's disease:
- Hesitation in starting
- Shuffling
- Freezing
- Festination
- Propulsion
- Retropulsion

Cerebellar: a drunken gait that is wide-based or reeling on a narrow base; the patient staggers towards the affected side if there is a unilateral cerebellar hemisphere lesion

Posterior column lesion: clumsy slapping down of the feet on a broad base

Foot drop: high-stepping gait

Proximal myopathy: waddling gait

Prefrontal lobe (apraxic): feet appear glued to the floor when erect, but move more easily when the patient is supine

Conversion disorder (hysteria): characterised by a bizarre, inconsistent gait

LIST 34.8

T&O'C ESSENTIALS

1. *Compare both sides and observe any lack of symmetry in the limb examination.*
2. *Reflexes are best thought of as being present, increased or absent; more specific grades are not really useful.*
3. *There are large normal variations in tone.*
4. *There are even more variations in pinprick sensation and sometimes one can say only that the findings on examination are not useful.*

OSCE REVISION TOPICS – THE PERIPHERAL NERVOUS SYSTEM

Use these topics, which commonly occur in the OSCE, to help with revision.

1. This man has noticed a problem with balance. Please examine his lower limbs from a cerebellar aspect. (pp 571, 577)
2. This man has difficulty lifting his right foot when he walks. Please examine him. (pp 566, 577)
3. Please assess the reflexes in this man's lower limbs. (p 570)
4. Please test the power in this woman's arms. (p 552)
5. This woman has been noticed to have wasting of the small muscles of her left hand. Please examine her. (pp 550, 559)

References

1. Freeman C, Okun MS. Origins of the sensory examination in neurology. *Semin Neurol* 2002; 22:399–407.
2. Nelson KR. Use new pins for each neurologic examination [Letter]. *New Engl J Med* 1986; 314:581. A cautionary tale.
3. Medical Research Council. *Aids to the investigation of peripheral nerve injury*. London: Her Majesty's Stationery Office, 1972. Presents, in a clear and straightforward manner, bedside methods for testing the innervation of all important muscles. An invaluable guide.
4. Katz JN, Larson MG, Sabra A et al. The carpal tunnel syndrome: diagnostic utility of the history and physical examination findings. *Ann Intern Med* 1990; 112:321–327. Unfortunately, individual symptoms and signs have limited diagnostic usefulness. Tinel's sign appears to be of little value.
5. D'Arcy DA, McGee S. The rational clinical examination. Does this patient have carpal tunnel syndrome? *JAMA* 2000; 283:3110–3117. Weak thumb abduction and self-reported sensory symptoms (drawn on a diagram) are useful to predict abnormal median nerve conduction testing.
6. Schwartz RS, Morris JG, Crimmins D et al. A comparison of two methods of eliciting the ankle jerk. *Aust NZ J Med* 1990; 20:116–119. The ankle jerk can be tested by tapping the sole of the foot.
7. Lance JW. The Babinski sign. *J Neurol Neurosurg Psychiatry* 2002; 73(4):360–362. A clear explanation of the history and clinical relevance of this most important of neurological signs.

CHAPTER 35
Correlation of physical signs and neurological syndromes and disease

Knowledge is a process of piling up facts; wisdom lies in their simplification.
MARTIN H FISCHER (1879–1962)

UPPER MOTOR NEURONE LESIONS

In neurology a clinical diagnosis is made by defining the deficit that is present, deciding on its anatomical level and then considering the likely causes. It is important to be able to distinguish *upper motor neurone* signs from *lower motor neurone* signs (see Fig. 34.1 on p 549 and List 35.3 on p 583). The former occur when a lesion has interrupted a neural pathway at a level above the anterior horn cell—for example, motor pathways in the cerebral cortex, internal capsule, cerebral peduncles, brainstem or spinal cord. When this occurs there is greater weakness of abductors and extensors in the upper limb, and of flexors and abductors in the lower limb, as the normal function of this pathway is to mediate voluntary contraction of the antigravity muscles. All muscles, however, are usually weaker than normal. Muscle wasting is slight or absent, probably because there is no loss of trophic factors normally released from the lower motor neurone. The disuse that results from severe weakness may, however, cause some atrophy.

Upper motor neurone signs occur when the lesion is in the brain or spinal cord above the level of the lower motor neurone (see List 35.1).

Spasticity occurs because of destruction of the corticoreticulospinal tract, resulting in stretch reflex hyperactivity.

Monoplegia is paralysis affecting only one limb, when there is a motor cortex or partial internal capsule lesion. *Hemiplegia* affects one side of the body owing to a lesion affecting projection of pathways from the contralateral motor cortex.

Paraplegia affects both legs, whereas *quadriplegia* affects all four limbs and is the result of spinal cord trauma or, less often, a brainstem lesion (e.g. basilar artery thrombosis).

Causes of hemiplegia (upper motor neurone lesion)
Vascular disease (stroke or TIA)

Thrombosis, embolism or haemorrhage occur in specific vascular territories (see Fig. 35.1).[1,2] The deficit usually progresses over a period of minutes, but continuing deterioration may occur over hours or days as a result of oedema or haemorrhage around or into the infarct. A transient ischaemic attack (TIA) is an episode of *focal neurological disturbance attributable to a transient vascular occlusion*, without evidence of stroke on imaging. Typically this lasts no more than an hour or two, and the historical benchmark of 24 hours was probably inappropriately long. If any neurological symptoms persist, the episode is *not* a TIA. Lesions in the territory of the *internal carotid artery* result in hemiplegia on the opposite side of the body if a large

---

LEVEL OF UPPER MOTOR NEURONE LESION

1. Leg affected: L1 or above
2. Arm affected: C3 or above
3. Face affected: pons or above
4. Diplopia: midbrain or above

LIST 35.1

Anatomy of the circle of Willis, showing the functional importance of the arterial blood supply

(Adapted from Weiner HL, Levitt LP. *Neurology for the house officer*, 6th edn. Baltimore: Williams & Wilkins, 2000.)

FIGURE 35.1

area of the internal capsule or hemisphere is involved. Homonymous hemianopia, hemianaesthesia and dysphasia may occur (see Table 35.1). Stenosis of the internal carotid artery in the neck may be associated with a bruit.[3]

Haemorrhagic strokes often involve the internal capsule and putamen (causing a contralateral hemiparesis and often sensory loss) or the thalamus (causing a contralateral hemianaesthesia).[2]

Lesions in the territory of the *vertebrobasilar artery* may produce cranial nerve palsies, cerebellar signs, Horner's syndrome and sensory loss, as well as upper motor neurone signs (often bilateral because of the close proximity of structures in the brainstem). For example, a lesion in the midbrain may be associated with a third nerve paralysis and upper motor neurone signs on the opposite side. Hemianaesthesia and homonymous hemianopia may occur if the posterior

Intracerebral thrombosis or embolism: clinical features

Middle cerebral artery	Posterior cerebral artery	Anterior cerebral artery	Vertebral/basilar (brainstem)
Main branch	**Main branch***		
Infarction middle third of hemisphere: UMN face, UMN arm>leg; homonymous hemianopia; dysphasia or non-dominant hemisphere signs (depends on side); cortical sensory loss	Infarction of thalamus and occipital cortex: hemianaesthesia (loss of all modalities); homonymous hemianopia (complete); colour blindness	UMN leg>arm; cortical sensory loss leg only; (if corpus callosum affected) urinary incontinence	'Crossed' motor/sensory (e.g. left face, right arm); bilateral extremity motor/sensory; Horner's syndrome; cerebellar signs; lower cranial nerve signs
Perforating artery			
Internal capsule infarction: UMN face, UMN arm>leg			

UMN = upper motor neurone lesion.
*Effects are variable because of anastomoses with distal middle cerebral artery branches and supply from posterior communicating artery, but one would examine particularly for occipital and temporal lobe dysfunction.

TABLE 35.1

cerebral arteries are affected. An important syndrome to recognise is the *lateral medullary syndrome* (see List 35.2). This syndrome demonstrates the importance of examining pain and temperature rather than light touch. Atheroma in the ascending aorta is increasingly recognised as a source of cerebral emboli.

Cerebral abscesses and mycotic aneurysms may also cause hemiplegia.

Compressive and infiltrative lesions

Tumours tend to occur in the lobes of the brain, and focal signs will depend on the tumour site. Signs localised to the parietal, temporal, occipital or frontal lobe suggest this disease process. There may, however, be false localising signs in the presence of raised intracranial pressure—for example, a unilateral or bilateral sixth nerve palsy (because of the nerve's long intracranial path). Papilloedema is usually associated if there is raised intracranial pressure.

Demyelinating disease

Multiple sclerosis (MS) results in lesions in different areas, usually with a relapsing and remitting course.

Infection

Human immunodeficiency virus (HIV) infection is an important cause of neurological problems, including upper motor neurone syndromes.

LATERAL MEDULLARY SYNDROME (WALLENBERG'S* SYNDROME)

Occlusion of the vertebral or posterior inferior cerebellar or lateral medullary arteries causes ipsilateral and 'crossed' neurological signs:

- Cerebellar signs (ipsilateral)
- Horner's syndrome (ipsilateral)
- Lower cranial nerves (IX, X)—palate and vocal cord weakness (ipsilateral)
- Facial sensory loss of pain (ipsilateral)
- Arm and leg sensory loss of pain (contralateral)
- No upper motor neurone weakness

*Adolf Wallenberg (1862–1942), a professor of medicine in Danzig.

LIST 35.2

LOWER MOTOR NEURONE LESIONS

Lower motor neurone lesions interrupt the spinal reflex arc and therefore cause muscle wasting, reduced or absent reflexes and sometimes fasciculations. This results from a lesion of the spinal motor neurones, motor root or peripheral nerve (see List 35.3).

UPPER AND LOWER MOTOR NEURONE LESIONS

Signs of upper motor neurone (pyramidal) lesions

- Weakness is present in all muscle groups, but in the lower limb it may be more marked in the flexor and abductor muscles. In the upper limb, weakness may be most marked in the abductors and extensors. There is very little muscle wasting.
- Spasticity: increased tone is present (may be clasp-knife) and often associated with clonus.
- The reflexes are increased except for the superficial reflexes (e.g. abdominal), which are absent.
- There is an extensor (Babinski) plantar response (upgoing toe).

Signs of lower motor neurone lesions

- Weakness may be more obvious distally than proximally, and the flexor and extensor muscles are equally involved. Wasting is a prominent feature.
- Tone is reduced.
- The reflexes are reduced and the plantar response is normal or absent.
- Fasciculations may be present.

LIST 35.3

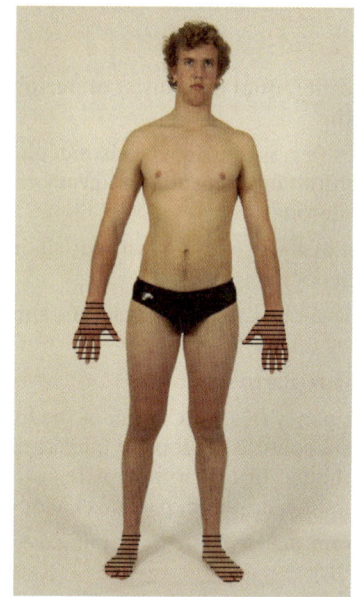

Peripheral neuropathy: glove and stocking sensory loss

FIGURE 35.2

MOTOR NEURONE DISEASE

This disease of unknown aetiology results in pathological changes in the anterior horn cells, the motor nuclei of the medulla and the descending tracts. It therefore causes a combination of upper motor neurone and lower motor neurone signs, although one type may predominate.

Importantly, fasciculations are almost always present. The muscle stretch reflexes are usually present (often increased) until late in the course of the disease, and there are rarely any objective sensory changes (15–20% of patients report sensory symptoms).

PERIPHERAL NEUROPATHY

Distal parts of the nerves are usually involved first because of their distance from the cell bodies, causing a distal loss of sensation or motor function, or both, in the limbs. A typical sensory change is a symmetrical 'glove and stocking' loss (though the hands should not be involved until the neuropathy reaches the level of the knees) of pain and temperature, proprioception and vibration modalities (see Fig. 35.2). This is unlike the pattern found with individual nerve or nerve root disease, which should be suspected if sensory loss is asymmetrical or confined to one limb. Peripheral muscle weakness may be present owing to motor nerve involvement. Occasionally, motor neuropathy may occur without sensory change. In the latter case, reflexes are reduced but may not be absent in the distal parts of the limbs (see List 35.4).

GUILLAIN–BARRÉ SYNDROME (ACUTE INFLAMMATORY POLYRADICULONEU-ROPATHY)

This disease, with an immune basis, may begin 7–10 days after an infective illness, commonly *Campylobacter*

PERIPHERAL NEUROPATHY

Causes (differential diagnosis) of peripheral neuropathy

1. Drugs (e.g. isoniazid, vincristine, phenytoin, nitrofurantoin, cisplatinum, heavy metals, amiodarone)
2. Alcohol abuse (with or without vitamin B_1 deficiency)
3. Metabolic (e.g. diabetes mellitus, chronic kidney disease)
4. Guillain–Barré syndrome
5. Malignancy (e.g. carcinoma of the lung [paraneoplastic neuropathy], leukaemia, lymphoma) or chemotherapy (e.g. vincristine, cisplatin, paclitaxel, etoposide)
6. Vitamin deficiency (e.g. B_{12}) or excess (e.g. B_6)
7. Connective tissue disease or vasculitis (e.g. PAN, SLE)
8. Hereditary (e.g. hereditary motor and sensory neuropathy)
9. Other (e.g. amyloidosis, HIV infection)
10. Idiopathic

Causes of a predominant motor neuropathy

1. Guillain–Barré syndrome, chronic inflammatory polyradiculoneuropathy
2. Hereditary motor and sensory neuropathy
3. Diabetes mellitus
4. Other (e.g. acute intermittent porphyria, lead poisoning, diphtheria, multifocal motor neuropathy with conduction block)

Causes of a painful peripheral neuropathy

1. Diabetes mellitus
2. Alcohol
3. Vitamin B_1 or B_{12} deficiency
4. Carcinoma
5. Porphyria
6. Arsenic or thallium poisoning

HIV = human immunodeficiency virus; PAN = polyarteritis nodosa; SLE = systemic lupus erythematosus.

LIST 35.4

jejuni gastroenteritis. It results in flaccid proximal and distal muscle paralysis, which typically ascends from the lower to the upper limbs. The reflexes are reduced or absent. Back pain is common owing to radiculitis (inflammation of the nerve roots). The cranial nerves can be affected; occasionally disease is confined to these. Sensory loss is common, though it is frequently patchy on testing. Unlike in transverse myelitis, the sphincters are little affected. Weakness of the respiratory muscles can be fatal but the disease is usually self-limiting. HIV infection can cause a similar syndrome. It is important that the patient's respiratory function be assessed regularly by measuring the forced expiratory volume in the first second (FEV_1) and the forced vital capacity (FVC). A decline in these can lead to respiratory failure and death.

MULTIPLE SCLEROSIS

This disease with unknown cause is characterised by scattered areas of inflammation in the central nervous system (CNS). A careful history is necessary as the diagnosis of MS depends on the occurrence of at least two neurological episodes separated in time and place within the CNS; see List 35.5.

The signs can be very variable. Look particularly for signs of spastic paraparesis and posterior column sensory loss as well as cerebellar signs. Examine the cranial nerves. Look carefully for loss of visual acuity, optic atrophy, papillitis and scotomata (usually central). *Internuclear ophthalmoplegia* is an important sign and is almost diagnostic in a young adult. It is weakness of adduction in one eye as a result of damage to the ipsilateral medial longitudinal fasciculus; there may be nystagmus in the abducting eye. Bilateral internuclear ophthalmoplegia is almost always caused by MS.

Other cranial nerves may rarely be affected (III, IV, V, VI, VII, pseudobulbar palsy) by lesions within the brainstem. Charcot's triad for MS consists of nystagmus, cerebellar (intention) tremor and scanning speech, but occurs in only 10% of patients.

Ask about Lhermitte's[a] sign (an electric shock-like sensation in the limbs or trunk following neck flexion).

---

[a] Jacques Jean Lhermitte (1877–1939), a French neurologist and neuropsychiatrist.

> **CLINICAL MANIFESTATIONS SUGGESTIVE OF MULTIPLE SCLEROSIS**
>
> Internuclear ophthalmoplegia (see Fig. 32.15 on p 515) (affected eye—weak adduction; other eye—horizontal nystagmus on abduction)
>
> Optic neuritis (central visual loss, eye pain, pale optic disc)
>
> Relative afferent pupillary defect (Marcus Gunn pupil)
>
> Upper motor neurone weakness
>
> Cerebellar signs
>
> Posterior columns sensory loss
>
> Faecal/urinary incontinence
>
> LIST 35.5

> **MONONEURITIS MULTIPLEX**
>
> **Definition**
> Mononeuritis multiplex refers to the separate involvement of more than one peripheral (or less often cranial) nerve by a single disease.
>
> **Acute causes (usually vascular)**
> Polyarteritis nodosa
> Diabetes mellitus
> Connective tissue disease (e.g. rheumatoid arthritis, systemic lupus erythematosus)
>
> **Chronic causes**
> Multiple compressive neuropathies
> Sarcoidosis
> Acromegaly
> HIV infection
> Leprosy
> Lyme disease
> Others (e.g. carcinoma—rare)
>
> HIV = human immunodeficiency virus.
>
> LIST 35.6

This can also be caused by other disorders of the cervical spine, such as subacute combined degeneration of the cord, cervical spondylosis, cervical cord tumour, foramen magnum tumours, from nitrous oxide abuse and from mantle irradiation. Uhthoff's[b] phenomenon is a worsening of symptoms in the setting of hotter temperatures or exercise. This commonly occurs in MS but also in peripheral disorders like myasthenia gravis.

THICKENED PERIPHERAL NERVES

If there is evidence of a peripheral nerve lesion, peripheral neuropathy or a mononeuritis multiplex (see List 35.6), palpate for thickened nerves. The median nerve at the wrist, the ulnar nerve at the elbow, the greater auricular nerve in the neck and the common peroneal nerve at the head of the fibula are the most easily accessible. If nerves are thickened, consider the following diagnoses:

- acromegaly
- amyloidosis
- chronic inflammatory demyelinating polyradiculoneuropathy
- leprosy

- hereditary motor and sensory neuropathy (autosomal dominant; see List 35.10 on p 592)
- other (e.g. sarcoidosis, diabetes mellitus, neurofibromatosis).

SPINAL CORD COMPRESSION

It is important to remember that a spinal cord lesion causes lower motor neurone signs at the level of the lesion and upper motor neurone signs below that level (see List 35.7). Do not forget the spinal cord's anatomy and vascular supply (see Fig. 35.3). Examine any suspected case as follows.

After carefully examining the lower limbs (see above) determine the level of any sensory impairment (see Table 35.2). Then examine the back for signs of a local lesion. Look for deformity, scars and neurofibromas. Palpate for vertebral tenderness and auscultate down the spine for bruits. Next examine the upper limbs and cranial nerves to determine the upper level, if this is not already obvious.

---
[b] Wilhelm Uhthoff (1853–1927) was a German ophthalmologist who described this phenomenon in 1890.

IMPORTANT MOTOR AND REFLEX CHANGES OF SPINAL CORD COMPRESSION

(See Figs 35.5 to 35.7 for sensory changes.)

Upper cervical
- Upper motor neurone signs in the upper and lower limbs

C5
- Lower motor neurone weakness and wasting of rhomboids, deltoids, biceps and brachioradialis
- Upper motor neurone signs affecting the rest of the upper and all the lower limbs; the biceps jerk is lost and the brachioradialis jerk is inverted

C8
- Lower motor neurone weakness and wasting of the intrinsic muscles of the hand
- Upper motor neurone signs in the lower limbs

Midthoracic
- Intercostal paralysis
- Upper motor neurone signs in the lower limbs
- Loss of upper abdominal reflexes at T7 and T8

T10–T11
- Loss of the lower abdominal reflexes and upward displacement of the umbilicus
- Upper motor neurone signs in the lower limbs

L1
- Cremasteric reflex is lost (normal abdominal reflexes)
- Upper motor neurone signs in the lower limbs

L4
- Lower motor neurone weakness and wasting of the quadriceps
- Knee jerks lost
- Ankle jerks may be hyperreflexic with extensor plantar response (upgoing toes), but more often the whole conus is involved, causing a lower motor neurone lesion

L5–S1
- Lower motor neurone weakness of knee flexion and hip extension (S1) and abduction (L5), plus calf and foot muscles
- Knee jerks present
- No ankle jerks or plantar responses
- Anal reflex present

S3–S4
- No anal reflex
- Saddle sensory loss
- Normal lower limbs

Causes of spinal cord compression

1. Vertebral
   - Spondylosis
   - Trauma
   - Prolapse of a disc
   - Tumour
   - Infection
2. Outside the dura
   - Lymphoma, metastases
   - Infection (e.g. abscess)
3. Within the dura but extramedullary
   - Tumour (e.g. meningioma, neurofibroma)
4. Intramedullary*
   - Tumour (e.g. glioma, ependymoma)
   - Syringomyelia
   - Haematomyelia

*Lower motor neurone signs may extend for several segments, and spastic paralysis occurs late, unlike the situation with extramedullary lesions.

LIST 35.7

Anatomy and vascular supply of the spinal cord.

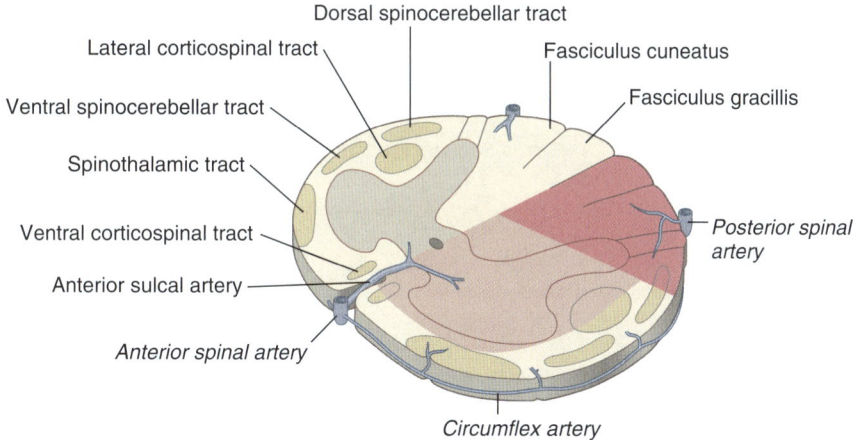

Note: Anterior spinal artery occlusion spares posterior column function

FIGURE 35.3

Important patterns of abnormal sensation

Sign	Location of lesion
Total unilateral loss of all forms of sensation	Thalamus or upper brainstem (extensive lesion)
Pain and temperature loss on one side of the face and opposite side of the body	Medulla involving descending nucleus of the spinal tract of the fifth nerve and ascending spinothalamic tract (lateral medullary lesion; see Fig. 35.9)
Bilateral loss of all forms of sensation below a definite level	Spinal cord lesion (if only pain and temperature affected: anterior cord lesion)
Unilateral loss of pain and temperature below a definite level	Partial unilateral spinal cord lesion on opposite side (Brown-Séquard syndrome; see Fig. 35.8)
Loss of pain and temperature over several segments but normal sensation above and below	Intrinsic spinal cord lesion near its centre anteriorly (involves the crossing fibres)—e.g. syringomyelia, intrinsic cord tumour (*note:* more posterior lesions cause proprioceptive loss)
Loss of sensation over many segments with sacral sparing	Intrinsic cord compression more likely
Saddle sensory loss (lowest sacral segments)	Cauda equina lesion (touch preserved in conus medullaris lesions)
Loss of position and vibration sense only	Posterior column lesion
Glove and stocking loss (hands and feet)	Peripheral neuropathy
Loss of all forms of sensation over a well-defined body part only	Posterior root lesion (purely sensory) or peripheral nerve (often motor abnormality associated)

TABLE 35.2

Spinal cord syndromes

(Adapted from Brazis PW. *Localisation in clinical neurology*, Philadelphia: Lippincott, Williams & Wilkins, 2001.)

FIGURE 35.4

IMPORTANT SPINAL CORD SYNDROMES

(See Figs 35.4–35.8.)

Brown-Séquard syndrome[c]

Clinical features are shown in Fig. 35.8. These signs result from hemisection of the cord.

- **Motor changes:** (1) upper motor neurone signs below the hemisection on the same side as the lesion; (2) lower motor neurone signs at the level of the hemisection on the same side.
- **Sensory changes:** (1) pain and temperature loss on the opposite side to the lesion—note that the upper level of sensory loss is usually a few segments below the level of the lesion; (2) vibration and proprioception loss occur on the same side; (3) detection of light touch is often normal.
- **Causes:** (1) multiple sclerosis, (2) angioma, (3) trauma, (4) myelitis, and (5) postradiation myelopathy.

Subacute combined degeneration of the cord (vitamin B$_{12}$ deficiency)

Clinical features are: (1) posterior column loss symmetrically (vibration and joint position sense), causing an ataxic gait, and (2) upper motor neurone signs in the lower limbs symmetrically with absent ankle reflexes; knee reflexes may be absent or, more often, exaggerated. There may also be (3) peripheral

---

[c] Charles Edouard Brown-Séquard (1817–94) succeeded Claude Bernard at the College de France. He was the son of an American sea captain (pirate) and a French woman. He was born in Mauritius at a time when it was under British rule. With this background he roved around the world, working in Paris, Mauritius, London and New York. His syndrome usually arose from failed murder attempts. Traditionally Mauritian cane cutters, when trying to murder someone, used a very long thin knife that was slipped between the ribs from behind, to cut the aorta or penetrate the heart. Only such a knife could have caused a cord hemitransection.

Sensory loss with transverse section of the spinal cord

FIGURE 35.5

Pattern of sensory loss with intrinsic spinal cord disease.

For example, central tumour or less commonly with extrinsic compression of the spinal cord—sacrum is spared

FIGURE 35.6

sensory neuropathy (less common and mild), (4) optic atrophy, and (5) dementia.

Dissociated sensory loss

This usually indicates spinal cord disease but may occur with a peripheral neuropathy.
- **Causes of spinothalamic loss only:** (1) syringomyelia, (2) Brown-Séquard syndrome (contralateral leg), (3) anterior spinal artery thrombosis, (4) lateral medullary syndrome (contralateral to the other signs; see Fig. 35.9), and (5) small-fibre peripheral neuropathy (e.g. diabetes mellitus, amyloid).
- **Causes of dorsal column loss only:** (1) subacute combined degeneration, (2) Brown-Séquard syndrome (ipsilateral leg), (3) spinocerebellar degeneration (e.g. Friedreich's[d] ataxia), (4) multiple sclerosis, (5) tabes dorsalis, (6) peripheral neuropathy (e.g. diabetes mellitus, hypothyroidism), and (7) sensory neuronopathy (a dorsal root ganglionopathy that may be caused by carcinoma, diabetes mellitus or Sjögren's syndrome).

Syringomyelia (a central cavity in the spinal cord)

- **Clinical triad:** (1) loss of pain and temperature over the neck, shoulders and arms (a 'cape' distribution), (2) amyotrophy (atrophy and areflexia) of the arms, and (3) upper motor neurone signs in the lower limbs.

There may also be thoracic scoliosis due to asymmetrical weakness of the paravertebral muscles.

---

[d] Nicholaus Friedreich (1825–82), a German physician, described this in 1863. He was professor of pathology at Heidelberg. Pes cavus is also called Friedreich's foot.

Conus medullaris or cauda equina lesion—saddle anaesthesia

FIGURE 35.7

Brown-Séquard syndrome.

Loss of pain and temperature on the opposite side to the lesion, with loss of vibration and proprioception on the same side as the lesion

FIGURE 35.8

An extensor plantar response plus absent knee and ankle jerks

- **Causes:** (1) subacute combined degeneration of the cord (B_{12} deficiency), (2) conus medullaris lesion, (3) combination of an upper motor neurone lesion with cauda equina compression or peripheral neuropathy, such as a stroke in a diabetic, (4) syphilis (taboparesis), (5) Friedreich's ataxia, (6) motor neurone disease, and (7) human T-cell lymphotrophic virus I (HTLV-I) infection.

A summary of the features that differentiate intramedullary from extramedullary cord lesions is presented in Table 35.3.

MYOPATHY

Muscle weakness can be due to individual peripheral nerve lesions, mononeuritis multiplex, peripheral neuropathy or spinal cord disease. Each of these has

Differentiating intramedullary from extramedullary cord lesions

Intramedullary	Extramedullary
Root pains rare	Root pains common
Late onset of corticospinal signs	Early onset of corticospinal signs
Lower motor neurone signs extend for several segments	Lower motor neurone signs localised
Dissociated sensory loss (pain and temperature) may be present	Brown-Séquard syndrome if lateral cord compression
Normal or minimally altered cerebrospinal fluid findings May have sacral sparing	Early, marked cerebrospinal fluid abnormalities

TABLE 35.3

CHAPTER 35 CORRELATION OF PHYSICAL SIGNS AND NEUROLOGICAL SYNDROMES AND DISEASE

Pattern of sensory loss in the lateral medullary syndrome

FIGURE 35.9

> **CAUSES (DIFFERENTIAL DIAGNOSIS) OF PROXIMAL WEAKNESS AND MYOPATHY**
>
> **Causes of proximal weakness**
>
> Myopathy
>
> Neuromuscular junction disease (e.g. myasthenia gravis)
>
> Neurogenic (e.g. motor neurone disease, polyradiculopathy, Kugelberg–Welander disease [proximal muscle wasting and fasciculation due to anterior horn cell disease—autosomal recessive])
>
> **Causes of myopathy**
>
> Hereditary muscular dystrophy (see List 35.9)
>
> Congenital myopathies (rare)
>
> Acquired myopathy (mnemonic, PACE, PODS):
>
> P olymyositis or dermatomyositis (see Fig. 35.11)
>
> A lcohol, AIDS (HIV infection)
>
> C arcinoma
>
> E ndocrine (e.g. hyperthyroidism, hypothyroidism, Cushing's syndrome, acromegaly, hypopituitarism)
>
> P eriodic paralysis (hyperkalaemic, hypokalaemic or normokalaemic)
>
> O steomalacia
>
> D rugs (e.g. statins, chloroquine, steroids)
>
> S arcoidosis
>
> *Note:* Causes of proximal myopathy with a peripheral neuropathy include:
> - paraneoplastic syndrome
> - alcohol
> - hypothyroidism
> - connective tissue diseases.
>
> AIDS = acquired immunodeficiency syndrome; HIV = human immunodeficiency virus.
>
> LIST 35.8

a characteristic pattern. Primary disease of muscle (myopathy) causes weakness *without* sensory loss. The motor weakness is similar to that of the lower motor neurone type. There are two major patterns: proximal myopathy and distal myopathy.

Proximal myopathy is the more common form. On examination there is proximal muscle wasting and weakness (see Lists 35.8 and 35.9 and Figs 35.10 and 35.11). Reflexes involving these muscles may be reduced. This can be caused by genetic (e.g. muscular dystrophy) or acquired disease. *Distal myopathy* also occurs and is always genetic, although peripheral neuropathy is a much more common cause of distal muscle weakness. If the distal limbs are affected, consider hereditary motor and sensory neuropathy (see List 35.10). Motor neurone disease also causes weakness without any sensory loss.

DYSTROPHIA MYOTONICA

If this disease (which is inherited as an autosomal dominant condition) is suspected because of an inability on the part of the patient to let go when shaking hands (myotonia), or because general inspection reveals the characteristic appearance (see Fig. 35.12), examine as follows.

Observe the face for frontal baldness (the patient may be wearing a wig), the expressionless triangular facies, atrophy of the temporalis muscle and partial ptosis. Thick spectacles, a traditional sign of this disease, are not often seen now because of lens replacement

> **MUSCULAR DYSTROPHIES**
>
> 1. Duchenne's* (pseudohypertrophic)
>   - Affects only males (X-linked recessive)
>   - Calves and deltoids: hypertrophied early, weak later
>   - Proximal weakness: early
>   - Dilated cardiomyopathy
> 2. Becker[†]
>   - Affects only males (X-linked recessive)
>   - Similar clinical features to Duchenne's except for less heart disease, a later onset and less-rapid progression
> 3. Limb girdle
>   - Males or females (autosomal recessive), onset in the third decade
>   - Shoulder or pelvic girdle affected
>   - Face and heart usually spared
> 4. Facioscapulohumeral
>   - Males or females (autosomal dominant)
>   - Facial and pectoral weakness with hypertrophy of deltoids
> 5. Dystrophia myotonica (autosomal dominant)
>
> *Guillaume Duchenne (1806–75), a brilliant eccentric who founded French neurology. He died of a stroke.
> [†]Peter Becker (1908–2000), a German professor of genetics.
>
> LIST 35.9

> **FEATURES OF HEREDITARY MOTOR AND SENSORY NEUROPATHY (CHARCOT–MARIE–TOOTH* DISEASE)**
>
> 1. Pes cavus (short-arched feet)
> 2. Distal muscle atrophy due to peripheral nerve degeneration; this does not usually extend above the elbows or above the middle third of the thighs; peroneal muscle atrophy gives the legs the shape of an inverted champagne bottle
> 3. Absent reflexes
> 4. Slight or no sensory loss in the limbs
> 5. Thickened nerves
> 6. Optic atrophy, Argyll Robertson pupils (rare)
>
> *Jean Martin Charcot (1825–93), a Parisian physician and neurologist; Pierre Marie (1853–1940), a Parisian neurologist and Charcot's greatest pupil; Howard Henry Tooth (1856–1926), a London physician, who described the condition independently in 1886. Type I is usually autosomal dominant.
>
> LIST 35.10

surgery. The eyes should still be examined, as these patients can develop characteristic iridescent cataracts and subcapsular fine deposits.

Look at the neck for atrophy of the sternocleidomastoid muscles and then test neck flexion (neck flexion is weak, whereas extension is normal).

Go to the upper limbs. Shake hands and test for percussion myotonia. Tapping over the thenar eminence causes contraction and then slow relaxation of the abductor pollicis brevis. Examine the arms for signs of wasting and weakness distally (the forearms are usually affected first) and proximally. There are no sensory changes.

Go to the chest and look for gynaecomastia (uncommon). Examine the cardiovascular system for cardiomyopathy. Next palpate the testes for atrophy. Examine the lower limbs. The tibial nerves are affected first. Always ask to test the urine for sugar (diabetes mellitus is associated with this disease).

Fascioscapular muscular dystrophy

(From Mir MA. *Atlas of clinical diagnosis*, 2nd edn. Edinburgh: Saunders, 2003.)

FIGURE 35.10

Dermatomyositis.

(a) Gottren's sign in dermatomyositis—heliotrope (lilac-coloured) flat-topped papules, which occur over the knuckles, but may also be seen over the elbows or knees and may ulcerate. (b) Dermatomyositis may also cause a heliotrope rash on the face (especially on the eyelids, upper cheeks and forehead), periorbital oedema, erythema, maculopapular eruptions and scaling dermatitis. Dermatomyositis and the closely related condition polymyositis are idiopathic myopathies. Up to 10% of adult patients with dermatomyositis may have an underlying malignancy. (c) Heliotrope in flower

((a) and (b) From McDonald FS, ed. *Mayo Clinic images in internal medicine*, with permission. © Mayo Clinic Scientific Press and CRC Press. Reproduced by permission of Taylor and Francis Group, LLC, a division of Informa plc.)

FIGURE 35.11

Note: Muscle myotonia can also occur in the hereditary diseases myotonia congenita (autosomal dominant or recessive) and hereditary paramyotonia (autosomal dominant cold-induced myotonia).

MYASTHENIA GRAVIS

Myasthenia gravis is an autoimmune disease of the neuromuscular junction. There are circulating antibodies against acetylcholine receptors. It differs from the proximal myopathies in that muscle power decreases with use. There is little muscle wasting and no sensory change.

About 65% of patients present with ocular symptoms including diplopia and drooping eyelids. Patients (or their students, if the patient is a university lecturer) may report that their speech becomes unintelligible during prolonged speaking.

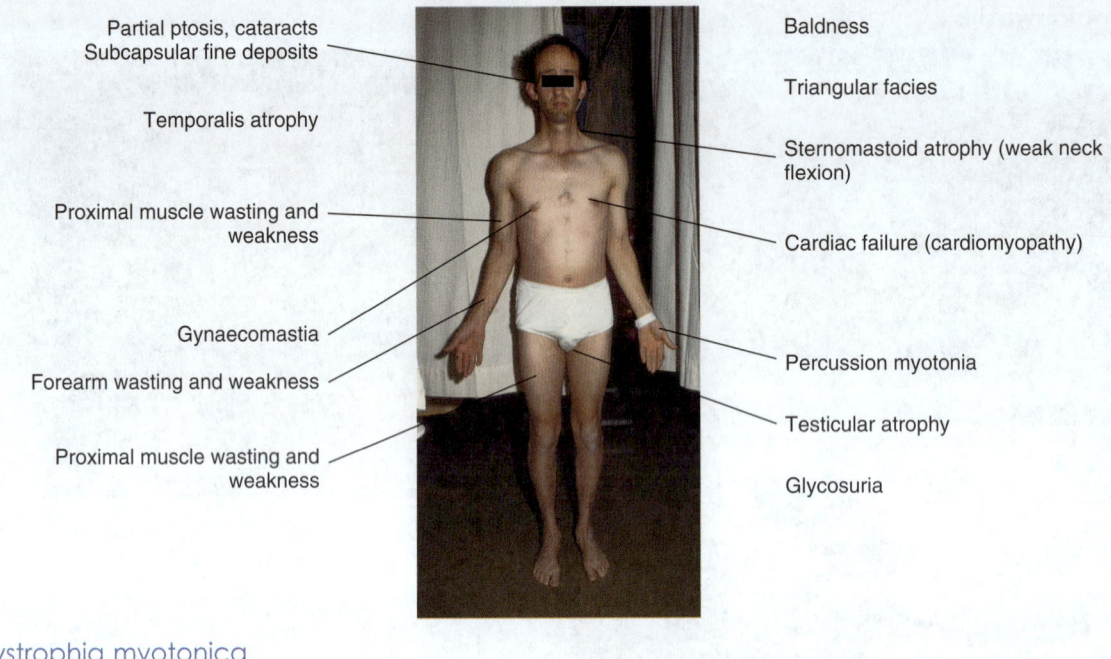

Dystrophia myotonica

FIGURE 35.12

It is necessary to test for muscle fatigue. Test the oculomotor muscles by asking the patient to sustain an upward gaze by looking up at the ceiling for 1 minute, and watch for progressive ptosis (see Fig. 35.13). Test for the peek sign for orbicularis oculi weakness. Ask the patient to close the eyes; if positive, within 30 seconds the lid margin will begin to separate, showing the sclera. This test strongly increases the likelihood of myasthenia (LR+, 30.0; LR−, 0.88).[4] Weakness of facial muscles is also common but less often reported by the patient. The *transverse smile* sign may present. Weakness of the levator muscles of the mouth makes an attempt at prolonged smiling look more like a grimace. To elicit this sign, tell the patient a series of mildly amusing anecdotes and watch the face carefully.

Then test the proximal limb girdle muscles—ask the patient to hold the arms above the head. You can repeatedly press the abducted arms down until they weaken. Power will decrease with repeated muscle contraction. Consider an ice-pack test (p 517).

Look for a thymectomy scar (over the sternum)—thymectomy is often undertaken as treatment for generalised myasthenia.

Bilateral ptosis after upward gaze in myasthenia gravis

FIGURE 35.13

CHAPTER 35 **CORRELATION OF PHYSICAL SIGNS AND NEUROLOGICAL SYNDROMES AND DISEASE** 595

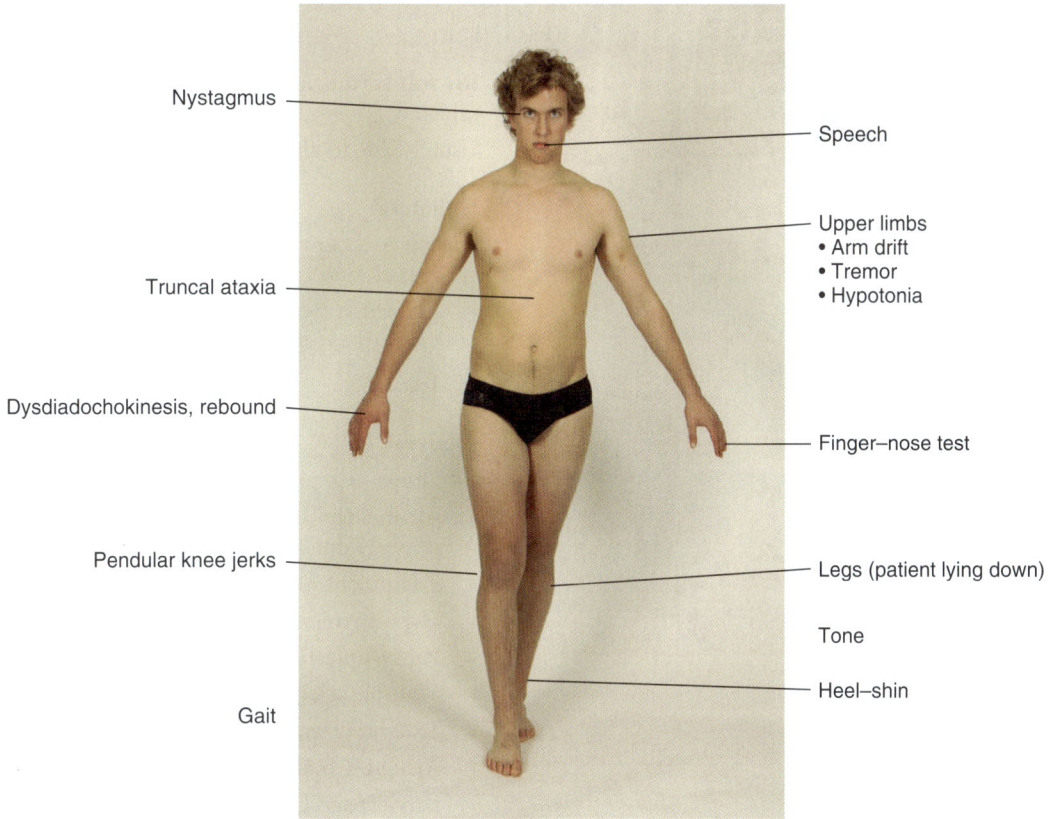

The cerebellar examination

FIGURE 35.14

THE CEREBELLUM

If the patient complains of clumsiness or problems with coordination of movement, a cerebellar examination is indicated (see Fig. 35.14). Signs of cerebellar disease occur on the same side as the lesion in the brain. This is because most cerebellar fibres cross twice in the brainstem, both on entry to and on exit from the cerebellum. Proceed as follows with the examination.

Look first for nystagmus—usually jerky horizontal nystagmus with increased amplitude on looking towards the side of the lesion. The direction of fast movement is the side of the lesion. There may also be upbeat nystagmus. Assess for hypometric or hypermetric saccades, and difficulty with smooth pursuit. Assess speech next. Ask the patient to say 'Hippopotamus' or 'West Register Street' (see Fig. 35.15). Cerebellar speech is jerky, explosive and loud, with an irregular separation of syllables.

Go to the upper limbs. Ask the patient to extend the arms and look for upward arm drift due to hypotonia of the agonist muscles. Test the tone. Hypotonia[e] is due to loss of a facilitatory influence on the spinal motor neurones.

Next perform the finger–nose test. The patient touches the nose, then rotates the finger and touches your finger (see Fig. 34.14 on p 556). Note any intention tremor (tremor that increases as the target is approached—this is due to loss of cerebellar connections in the brainstem)

---

[e] The concepts of hypotonia, rebound and pendular jerks in cerebellar disease stem from Gordon Holmes' 1917 description of signs in acute unilateral cerebellar disease. They may well not exist in other cerebellar problems. Students will, however, still be expected to know how to test for these signs.

West Register Street, Edinburgh

FIGURE 35.15

CAUSES OF CEREBELLAR DISEASE

Rostral vermis lesion (only lower limbs affected)

Usually due to alcohol

Unilateral
- Space-occupying lesion (tumour, abscess, granuloma)
- Ischaemia (vertebrobasilar disease)
- Multiple sclerosis
- Trauma

Bilateral
- Drugs (e.g. phenytoin)
- Alcohol (both acutely and chronically, possibly due to thiamine deficiency)
- Friedreich's ataxia / spinocerebellar ataxias
- Hypothyroidism
- Paraneoplastic syndrome
- Multiple sclerosis
- Trauma ('punch drunk')
- Arnold–Chiari malformation
- Large space-occupying lesion, cerebrovascular disease

Midline
- Paraneoplastic syndrome
- Midline tumour

LIST 35.11

and past-pointing (the patient overshoots the target). Test rapidly alternating movements: the patient taps alternately the palm and back of one hand on the other hand or thigh; inability to perform this movement smoothly is called *dysdiadochokinesis* (see Fig. 34.15 on p 557). Now test rebound: ask the patient to lift the arms quickly from the sides, then stop (incoordination of antagonist and agonist action causes the patient to be unable to stop the arms). Before testing, always demonstrate these movements for the patient's benefit.

Go on to examine the legs. Again, test the tone here. Then perform the heel–shin test looking for accuracy of fine movement when the patient slides the heel down the shin slowly on each side for several cycles (see Fig. 34.42 on p 571). Then ask the patient to lift the big toe up to touch your finger, and look for intention tremor and past-pointing. Ask the patient then to tap each heel on the other shin.

Test for truncal ataxia by asking the patient to fold the arms and sit up. While the patient is sitting, ask him or her to put the legs over the side of the bed and test for pendular knee jerks (the lower leg continues to swing a number of times before coming to rest—this is evidence of hypotonia).

Test gait (the patient will stagger towards the affected side if there is a unilateral cerebellar hemisphere lesion). If there is an obvious unilateral cerebellar problem, examine the cranial nerves for evidence of a cerebellopontine angle tumour (fifth, seventh and eighth nerves affected) or the lateral medullary syndrome, and auscultate over the cerebellum.

Always look in the fundi for papilloedema. Next examine for peripheral signs of malignant disease and for vascular disease (carotid or vertebral bruits). Examine the base of the skull for scars from previous neurosurgery.

If there is evidence of a midline lesion, such as truncal ataxia, abnormal heel–toe walking or abnormal speech, consider either a midline tumour or a paraneoplastic syndrome (see List 35.11). If there is

> ### CLINICAL FEATURES OF FRIEDREICH'S ATAXIA (AUTOSOMAL RECESSIVE)
>
> This is usually a young person with:
> 1. Cerebellar signs (bilateral) including nystagmus
> 2. Pes cavus;* cocking of the toes; kyphoscoliosis
> 3. Upper motor neurone signs in the limbs (although reflexes are absent)
> 4. Peripheral neuropathy
> 5. Posterior column loss in the limbs
> 6. Cardiomyopathy (ECG abnormalities occur in more than 50% of cases)
> 7. Diabetes mellitus (common)
> 8. Optic atrophy (uncommon)
> 9. Normal mentation
>
> *Other causes of pes cavus include hereditary motor and sensory neuropathy, spinocerebellar degeneration or neuropathies in childhood.
>
> LIST 35.12

> ### CAUSES OF SPASTIC AND ATAXIC PARAPARESIS (UPPER MOTOR NEURONE AND CEREBELLAR SIGNS COMBINED)
>
> **In adolescence**
> Spinocerebellar ataxia (e.g. Marie's spastic ataxia)
>
> **In young adults**
> Multiple sclerosis
> Spinocerebellar ataxia
> Syphilitic meningomyelitis
> Arnold–Chiari malformation or other lesion at the craniospinal junction
>
> **In later life**
> Multiple sclerosis
> Syringomyelia
> Infarction (in upper pons or internal capsule on one side—'ataxic hemiparesis')
> Lesion at the craniospinal junction (e.g. meningioma)
>
> *Note:* Unrelated diseases that are relatively common (e.g. cervical spondylosis and cerebellar degeneration from alcohol) may cause a similar clinical picture.
>
> LIST 35.13

bilateral disease, look for signs of multiple sclerosis, Friedreich's ataxia (pes cavus is the most helpful initial clue; see List 35.12) and hypothyroidism (rare). Alcoholic cerebellar degeneration (which affects the anterior lobe of the cerebellar vermis) classically spares the arms. If there are, in addition, upper motor neurone signs, consider the causes in List 35.13.

Remember that there are important reciprocal connections between the cerebellum and the parietal and frontal lobes. These explain the problems that cerebellar abnormalities can cause with functions other than coordination. Loss of verbal fluency, grammatical problems with speech and difficulty with memory and planning can all sometimes be features of cerebellar disease.

PARKINSON'S DISEASE

This is a common extrapyramidal disease of middle to old age (1% of people older than 65) where there is degeneration of the substantia nigra and its pathways. It is typically asymmetrical at first. This results in dopamine deficiency and a relative excess of cholinergic transmission in the caudate nucleus and putamen, which causes excessive supraspinal excitatory drive. There may be a history of insidious and asymmetrical onset. Non-specific symptoms (sleep abnormalities, constipation, depression and dementia) may precede or accompany the classic tremor.

Examine as follows.[5]

Inspection

Note the lack of facial expression, which leads to a mask-like facies. The posture is characteristically flexed and there are few spontaneous movements.

Gait and movements

Ask the patient to rise from a chair, walk, turn quickly, stop and start.

The characteristic gait is described as *shuffling*—there are small steps, and the patient hardly raises the feet from the ground. There is often difficulty in initiating walking, but once it begins the patient hurries (festination) and has difficulty stopping. The Parkinsonian patient seems always to be trying to catch up with the centre of gravity. There is a lack of the normal arm swing. Walking heel to toe will be difficult (see Fig. 34.54 on p 578).

Testing for *propulsion* or *retropulsion* (propulsion involves pushing the patient from behind and retropulsion pushing from in front) is of uncertain value and must be done with some caution because the patient may be unable to stop and may fall over. You can stand behind the patient and pull him or her backwards, but should stand braced to catch the patient.

Bradykinesia (a decrease in the speed and amplitude of complex movements) may be the result of a lesion in the nigrostriatal pathway (a dopaminergic pathway), which affects connections between the caudate nucleus, the putamen and the motor cortex, causing abnormal movement programming and abnormal recruitment of single motor units. Two simple tests (see Fig. 35.16) for this are *finger tapping* and *twiddling*. Ask the patient to tap the fingers in turn onto a surface repeatedly, quickly and with both hands at once. Twiddling is rotating the hands around each other in front of the body. These movements are slow and clumsy in Parkinsonian patients but obviously depend on motor and cerebellar function as well. Difficulty in getting out of a chair can be another sign of bradykinesia and patients also often have difficulty turning over in bed.

Kinesia paradoxica is the striking ability of a patient to perform rapid movements (especially if startled) but not slow ones; for example, the patient may be able to run down the stairs in response to a fire alarm but be unable to stop at the bottom—this is *not* a recommended test.

Tremor

Have the patient return to bed. Look for a *resting* tremor, which is often asymmetrical. The characteristic movement is described as pill rolling. Movement of the fingers at the metacarpophalangeal joints is combined with the movements of the thumb. Various attending movements may also occur at the wrist. On finger–nose testing the resting tremor decreases, but a faster-action tremor may supervene.

Tremor can be facilitated by getting the patient to perform 'serial 7s'—take 7 from 100, then 7 from the answer and so forth (mental stimulation)—or to move the contralateral limb (e.g. by rapidly opposing the contralateral thumb and fingers). Other types of tremor are summarised in List 35.14.

Tone

Test the tone at both wrists. The characteristic increase in tone is called cogwheel or plastic (lead pipe) rigidity. Tone is increased with an interrupted nature, the muscles giving way with a series of jerks. If hypertonia is not obvious, obtain reinforcement by asking the patient to turn the head from side to side or to wave the contralateral arm. Cogwheel rigidity occurs because the exaggerated stretch reflex is interrupted by tremor.

Remember, the signs should be asymmetrical early in the course of Parkinson's disease.

Face

There may be *titubation* (tremor) of the head, absence of blinking, dribbling of saliva and lack of facial expression. Test the *glabellar tap* (reflex): keeping your

Detecting bradykinesia.

(a) Tapping the fingers; (b) twiddling

FIGURE 35.16

CHAPTER 35 CORRELATION OF PHYSICAL SIGNS AND NEUROLOGICAL SYNDROMES AND DISEASE

> ### A CLASSIFICATION OF NON-PHYSIOLOGICAL TREMOR*
>
> 1. Resting tremor
> 2. Parkinson's disease
> 3. Dystonic tremor
> 4. Postural/action tremor: present throughout movement; the following most often cause a static or postural tremor of the outstretched arms:
>   - Idiopathic (most common)
>   - Anxiety
>   - Drugs
>   - Familial
>   - Thyrotoxicosis
> 5. Essential/familial
> 6. Intention tremor (cerebellar disease): increases towards the target
> 7. Midbrain ('red nucleus') tremor: abduction–adduction movements of upper limbs with flexion–extension of wrists (usually associated with intention tremor)
>
> *Tremor is a rhythmic oscillation of a part of the body around a fixed point.
> *Note:* Flapping (asterixis) is not strictly a tremor but rather a sudden brief loss of tone in hepatic failure, cardiac failure, respiratory failure or renal failure (metabolic encephalopathies).
>
> LIST 35.14

(a) and (b) The glabellar tap (Wilson's sign)

FIGURE 35.17

finger out of the patient's line of vision, tap the middle of the patient's forehead (glabella) with your middle finger (see Fig. 35.17). This sign is positive when the patient continues to blink as long as you tap. Normal people blink only a couple of times and then stop. The glabellar reflex is a primitive reflex that is also frequently present in frontal lobe disease.

Assess *speech*, which is typically monotonous, soft and faint, lacking intonation. Sometimes palilalia is present; this is repetition of the end of a word (the opposite of stuttering).

Now test ocular movements, particularly for *weakness of vertical gaze*. Early loss of vertical saccades and convergence should raise the possibility of progressive supranuclear palsy. This group of patients may look Parkinsonian superficially, but have marked rigidity, early dementia and frequent falls. These people develop loss of downward gaze first, then loss of upward gaze and finally loss of horizontal gaze. Their prognosis is significantly worse.

Feel the brow for greasiness (seborrhoea) or sweating, which is due to associated autonomic dysfunction. Orthostatic hypotension may also be present for the same reason.

The palmomental reflex is commonly present in these patients and tends to be more prominent in those with severe akinesia. Dementia is present in 30% of patients.

Writing

Ask the patient to write his or her name and address. *Micrographia* (small writing) is characteristic. The patient may also be unable to do this because of the development of dementia, a late manifestation. Test the higher centres if appropriate.

Good signs guide 35.1 lists the likelihood ratios of the major signs.

Causes of Parkinson's syndrome

These are shown in List 35.15.

> **GOOD SIGNS GUIDE 35.1**
> **Parkinson's disease**
>
> | Sign | LR+ | LR− |
> |---|---|---|
> | Rigidity, tremor and bradykinesia all present | 2.2 | 0.5 |
> | Tremor alone | 1.5 | 0.47 |
> | Rigidity | 2.8 | 0.38 |
> | Glabellar tap | 4.5 | 0.13 |
> | Voice softer | 3.7 | 0.25 |
> | Difficulty with heel to toe | 2.9 | 0.32 |
>
> (Adapted from Simel DL, Rennie D. *The rational clinical examination: evidence-based diagnosis*. New York: McGraw-Hill, 2009, Table 38.3.)

> **CAUSES OF PARKINSON'S SYNDROME**
>
> **Idiopathic:** Parkinson's disease
> **Drugs** (e.g. phenothiazines, methyldopa)
> **Postencephalitis** (now very rare)
> **Other:** toxins (carbon monoxide, manganese), Wilson's disease, progressive supranuclear palsy, Steele–Richardson syndrome, Shy–Drager syndrome, syphilis, tumour (e.g. giant frontal meningioma)
> **Atherosclerosis** is a controversial cause
>
> LIST 35.15

OTHER EXTRAPYRAMIDAL MOVEMENT DISORDERS (DYSKINESIA)

Chorea

Here there is a lesion of the corpus striatum, which causes non-repetitive, abrupt, involuntary flowing dance-like movements.[f] These may be unilateral or generalised. Often the patient attempts to disguise this by completing the involuntary movements with a voluntary one. In this disease, dopaminergic pathways dominate over cholinergic transmissions.

Chorea can usefully be distinguished from hemiballismus, athetosis and pseudoathetosis. *Hemiballismus* is due to a subthalamic lesion on the side opposite the movement disorder. It causes unilateral wild, throwing movements of the proximal joints. There may be skin excoriation due to limb trauma. These movements may persist during sleep. *Athetosis* or *dystonia* is due to a lesion of the outer segment of the putamen and causes slow sinuous writhing distal movements that are present at rest. *Pseudoathetosis* is a description given to athetoid movements in the fingers in patients with severe proprioceptive loss (these are especially prominent when the eyes are shut).

If the patient has chorea or if chorea is suspected, proceed as follows. First shake hands. There may be tremor and dystonia superimposed on lack of sustained handgrip ('milkmaid's grip'). Ask the patient to hold out the hands, then look for a choreic (dystonic) posture. This typically involves finger and thumb hyperextension and wrist flexion.

Go to the face and look at the eyes for exophthalmos (thyrotoxicosis), Kayser–Fleischer rings (Wilson's disease) and conjunctival injection (polycythaemia). Ask the patient to poke out the tongue and note frequent retraction of the tongue (serpentine movements). Look for skin rashes (e.g. systemic lupus erythematosus, vasculitis). If the patient is a young girl, examine the heart for signs of rheumatic fever (Sydenham's[g] chorea).

Test the reflexes. The abdominal reflexes are usually brisk, but tendon reflexes are reduced and may be pendular (because of hypotonia).

Assess the higher centres for dementia (Huntington's[h] chorea).

Causes of chorea are shown in List 35.16.

Dystonia

The patient manifests an involuntary abnormal posture with excessive co-contraction of antagonist muscles. Dystonia may be focal (e.g. spasmodic torticollis), segmental or generalised. Other forms of movement disorder may be present (e.g. myoclonic dystonia). The acute onset of dystonia is seen most commonly as a side

---

[f] Sydenham's chorea is also called *St Vitus' dance*. St Vitus, a martyr, died in about 303. He is the patron saint of epileptics and of patients with Sydenham's chorea.

[g] Thomas Sydenham (1624–89) was a captain in Cromwell's army and became the most famous English physician of his time, providing clinical descriptions of gout (from which he suffered), fevers, hysteria and venereal disease. He was called the Father of English Clinical Medicine.

[h] George Huntington (1850–1916), an American general practitioner. He described this disease in his only clinical paper in 1872, when he was 22.

> **CAUSES OF CHOREA**
>
> Drugs (e.g. excess levodopa, phenothiazines, the contraceptive pill, phenytoin)
>
> Huntington's disease (autosomal dominant)
>
> Sydenham's chorea (rheumatic fever) and other postinfectious states (both rare)
>
> Senility
>
> Wilson's disease
>
> Kernicterus (rare)
>
> Vasculitis or connective tissue disease (e.g. systemic lupus erythematosus—very rare)
>
> Thyrotoxicosis (very rare)
>
> Polycythaemia or other hyperviscosity syndromes (very rare)
>
> Viral encephalitis (very rare)
>
> LIST 35.16

effect of various drugs (e.g. levodopa, phenothiazines, metoclopramide).

Tics and de la Tourette's syndrome

Tics are brief, rapid movements that interrupt normal movements. Patients can suppress them to some extent, but often at the expense of later outbursts. They may begin as an automatic or voluntary reaction to a local stimulus or external anxiety and then become compulsive. For example, an episode of conjunctivitis might lead to a blinking tic that continues after the stimulus has gone. The facial muscles, eyes and mouth are often affected and spasmodic rotation of the head is a common form. Respiratory tics include sneezing, coughing and hiccup. Simple tics usually begin in childhood and resolve or diminish in adult life.

Complicated motor tics that begin in childhood, last for more than a year and involve vocal tics suggest de la Tourette's syndrome.[i] Vocal tics include repetition of other people's speech (*echolalia*) and, rarely, the explosive use of obscenities (*coprolalia*). The patient feels an increasing urge to carry out the movement or vocal tic and increasing discomfort until he or she gives in to it.[j] Common associations include:

- obsessive compulsive disorder
- attention deficit disorder
- mood disorders.

THE UNCONSCIOUS PATIENT

The rapid and efficient examination of the unconscious patient is important. The word **COMA** provides a mnemonic for four major groups of causes of unconsciousness:

C O_2 narcosis (respiratory failure: uncommon)

O verdose (e.g. tranquillisers, alcohol, salicylates, carbon monoxide, antidepressants)

M etabolic (e.g. hypoglycaemia, diabetic ketoacidosis, end stage renal disease, hypothyroidism, hepatic coma, hypercalcaemia, adrenal failure)

A poplexy (e.g. head injury, stroke [infarction or haemorrhage], subdural or extradural haematoma, meningitis, encephalitis, epilepsy).

Coma occurs when the reticular formation is damaged by a lesion or metabolic abnormality, or when the cortex is diffusely damaged.

General inspection

Remember **ABC**:

A irway

B reathing

C irculation.

Airway and breathing

Look to see whether the patient is breathing, as indicated by chest wall movement. If not, urgent attention is required, including clearing the airway and providing ventilation.

Note particularly the pattern of breathing (see Table 9.4 on p 170). Important signs to look for are Cheyne–Stokes respiration (the rate and depth of respiration waxes and wanes often to the point of ceasing altogether for periods, which may indicate diencephalic injury, but is not specific), irregular ataxic breathing (Biot's breathing, from an advanced brainstem lesion) and deep

---

[i] Georges Albert Edouard Brutus Gilles de la Tourette, a French neurologist 1857–1904, described this condition in 1884 and called it *maladie des tics*. It was renamed 'maladie Gilles de la Tourette' by Charcot. De la Tourette was shot in the head by a former patient in 1893.

[j] Dr Samuel Johnson is a famous de la Tourette patient (at least in retrospect).

rapid respiration (e.g. Kussmaul breathing, secondary to a metabolic acidosis, as in diabetes mellitus).

Circulation

Look for signs of shock, dehydration and cyanosis. A typical cherry-red colour occurs rarely in cases of carbon monoxide poisoning. Take the pulse rate and blood pressure.

Posture

Look for signs of trauma. Note any neck hyperextension (from meningism in children or cerebellar tonsillar herniation).

Look for:

1. A *decerebrate* or extensor posture, which may be held spontaneously or occur in response to stimuli, and which suggests severe midbrain disease. The arms are held extended and internally rotated and the legs are extended.
2. A *decorticate* or flexor posture, which suggests a lesion above the brainstem. It can be unilateral or bilateral. There is flexion and internal rotation of the arms and extension of the legs.

Involuntary movements

Recurrent or continuous convulsions, which may be focal or generalised, suggest status epilepticus. Myoclonic jerks can occur after hypoxic injury and as a result of metabolic encephalopathy. Remember that complex partial seizure status epilepticus can cause a reduced level of consciousness without convulsive movements.

Level of consciousness

Tickle the patient's nose with cottonwool and watch for facial movements. This is less likely to harm the patient than the traditional method of firmly pressing the knuckles over the patient's sternum to cause pain.

Determine the level of consciousness. *Coma* is unconsciousness with a reduced response to external stimuli. Coma in which the patient responds semipurposefully is considered light. In deep coma there is no response to any stimuli and no reflexes are present (it is usually due to a brainstem or pontine lesion, although drug overdose, such as with barbiturates, can be responsible). *Stupor* is unconsciousness, but the patient can be aroused. Purposeful movements occur in response to painful stimuli. *Drowsiness* resembles normal sleepiness. The patient can be fairly easily roused to normal wakefulness, but when left alone falls asleep again.

It is most useful to score the depth of coma, as changes in the level of consciousness can then be judged more objectively. The Glasgow Coma Scale (see Table 35.4) is used to assess the depth of coma more accurately; record the subscores and total scores.

Glasgow coma scale

Add up the score for 1, 2 and 3. Score of 4 or less = very poor prognosis; score >11 = good prognosis for recovery.

1.	Eyes	Open	Spontaneously	4
			To loud verbal command	3
			To pain	2
		No response		1
2.	Best motor response	To verbal command	Obeys	6
		To painful stimuli	Localises pain	5
			Flexion—withdrawal	4
			Abnormal flexion posturing	3
			Extension posturing	2
			No response	1
3.	Best verbal response		Oriented	5
			Confused, disoriented	4
			Inappropriate words	3
			Incomprehensible sounds	2
			None	1

TABLE 35.4

Horner's syndrome.

Note ipsilateral right-sided ptosis and pupillary miosis (constriction)

(From Yanoff M, Duker J. *Ophthalmology*, 3rd edn. Maryland Heights, MO: Mosby, 2008.)

FIGURE 35.18

Neck

If there is no evidence of neck trauma, assess for neck stiffness and Kernig's sign (for meningitis or subarachnoid haemorrhage).

Head and face

Inspect and palpate for head injuries, including Battle's[k] sign (bruising behind the ear indicating a fracture of the base of the skull). Look for facial asymmetry (i.e. facial weakness). The paralysed side of the face will be sucked in and out with respiration. A painful stimulus (e.g. pressing the supraorbital notch) may produce grimacing and make facial asymmetry more obvious. Note jaundice (e.g. hepatic coma) or manifestations of myxoedema.

Eyes

Inspect the pupils. Very small pupils (but reactive to light) occur in pontine lesions and with narcotic overdoses. One small pupil occurs in Horner's syndrome (e.g. as part of the lateral medullary syndrome or in hypothalamus injury; see Fig. 35.18). Two midpoint non-reactive pupils suggest midbrain disease, anoxia or drugs (anticholinergics). One dilated pupil suggests a subdural haematoma, raised intracranial pressure (unilateral tentorial herniation) or a subarachnoid haemorrhage from a posterior communicating artery aneurysm. Widely dilated pupils may occur when increased intracranial pressure and coning cause secondary brainstem haemorrhage, or with anticholinergic drugs.

Conjunctival haemorrhage suggests skull fracture. Look in the fundi for papilloedema, diabetic or hypertensive retinopathy, or subhyaloid haemorrhage. The locked-in syndrome is rare; in a lower brainstem lesion patients are awake but can control only their eye movements (see p 876).

Look at the position of the eyes. Particular cranial nerve palsies may cause deviation of an eye in various directions. The sixth nerve is particularly vulnerable to damage because of its long intracranial course. Deviation of both eyes to one side in the unconscious patient may be due to a destructive lesion in a cerebral hemisphere, which causes fixed deviation towards the side of the lesion. An irritative (epileptic) focus causes the direction of gaze to be away from the lesion. Upward or downward eye deviation suggests a brainstem problem. Trapping of the globe or extraocular muscles by fracture may also lead to an abnormal eye position or to an abnormal eye movement.

Assess the *vestibulo-ocular reflex* by lifting the patient's eyelids and rolling the head from side to side. When vestibular reflexes are intact (i.e. an intact brainstem), the eyes maintain their fixation as if looking at an object in the distance, but change their position relative to the head. This has been referred to as the 'doll's eye phenomenon'. Brainstem lesions or drugs affecting the brainstem cause the eyes to move with the head, so that fixation is not maintained.

Ears and nostrils

Look for any bleeding or drainage of cerebrospinal fluid (the latter indicating a skull fracture). A watery discharge can be simply tested for glucose. The presence of glucose confirms that it is cerebrospinal fluid.

Tongue and mouth

Trauma may indicate a previous seizure, and corrosion around the mouth may indicate ingestion of a corrosive poison. Gum hyperplasia suggests that the patient may be taking phenytoin for epilepsy. Smell the breath for evidence of alcohol poisoning, diabetic ketosis, hepatic coma or uraemia. Remember that alcohol ingestion

---

[k] William Battle (1855–1936), a surgeon at St Thomas's Hospital, London.

may be associated with head injury. Test the gag reflex; its absence may indicate brainstem disease or deep coma, but is not a specific sign. Bite marks on the tongue suggest that an epileptic seizure may have been the cause of unconsciousness.

Upper and lower limbs

Look for injection marks (drug addiction, diabetes mellitus). Test tone in the normal way and by picking up the arm and letting it fall. Compare each side, assessing for evidence of hemiplegia. In coma and acute cerebral hemiplegia, the muscle stretch reflexes may be normal or reduced at first on the paralysed side. Later the muscle stretch reflexes become increased and the cutaneous reflexes are absent.

Test for pain sensation by placing a pen over a distal finger or toe just below the nail bed. Press firmly and note whether there is arm or leg withdrawal. Test all limbs. There will be no response to pain if sensation is absent or if the coma is deep. If sensation is intact but the limb is paralysed, there may be grimacing with movement of the other limbs.

The presence of grimacing or purposeful movements is important. Segmental reflexes alone can cause the limb to move in response to pain.

Body

Look for signs of trauma. Examine the heart, lungs and abdomen.

Urine

Note whether there is incontinence. Test the urine for glucose and ketones (diabetic ketoacidosis), protein (chronic kidney disease) and blood (trauma).

Blood glucose

Always prick the patient's finger, place a drop of blood on an impregnated test strip and test for hypoglycaemia or hyperglycaemia. If this cannot be done immediately, give the patient a bolus of intravenous glucose anyway (which will not usually harm the patient in diabetic ketoacidosis, but will save the life of a patient with hypoglycaemia). If there is any suspicion of Wernicke's encephalopathy, thiamine must be given as well.

Temperature

Hypothermia (e.g. exposure or hypothyroidism) or fever (e.g. meningitis) must be looked for.

Stomach contents

While protecting the airway, examine stomach contents by inserting a nasogastric tube and consider washing out the stomach if a drug overdose is suspected, or if no other diagnosis is obvious. (Gastric lavage is recommended for only a minority of ingestions.)

> **T&O'C ESSENTIALS**
>
> 1. The diagnosis of Parkinson's disease is a clinical one.
> 2. If told to examine a patient who has difficulty in walking, ask him or her to walk, rather than beginning with a neurological examination of the lower limbs.
> 3. Try to decide from the physical signs whether a problem of weakness is due to muscle disease, peripheral nerve abnormalities or a cerebral problem.
> 4. The distribution of sensory loss should help to distinguish a peripheral neuropathy from a nerve root or peripheral nerve problem.

OSCE REVISION TOPICS – NEUROLOGICAL SYNDROMES AND DISORDERS

Use these topics, which commonly occur in the OSCE, to help with revision.

1. This man has noticed a problem with slurred speech. Please examine him. (p 595)
2. This woman has had difficulty in walking. Please examine her. (p 577)
3. This woman has noticed numbness in her feet. Please examine her. (p 583)
4. This woman reports difficulty getting out of chairs. Please examine her. (p 590)
5. Explain and demonstrate on this mannequin how you would assess an unconscious patient. (p 601)

References

1. Goldstein LB, Matchar DB. The Rational Clinical Examination. Clinical assessment of stroke. *JAMA* 1994; 271:1114–1120. Discusses the limitations of physical examination in identifying the lesion.

2. Runchey S, McGee S. Does this patient have a hemorrhagic stroke? Clinical findings distinguishing hemorrhagic stroke from ischemic stroke. *JAMA* 2010; 303(22):2280–2286. Nothing works well enough to avoid neuroimaging, but a history of headache, seizures and vomiting and finding neck stiffness and hypertension increase the probability of a subarachnoid haemorrhage. Finding a carotid bruit decreases the likelihood.

3. Sauve JS, Laupacis A, Ostbyte T et al. The Rational Clinical Examination. Does this patient have a clinically important carotid bruit? *JAMA* 1993; 270:2843–2846. Describes how to interpret the findings of a carotid bruit. Distinguishing high-grade from moderate symptomatic carotid stenosis based on the bruit itself is difficult and the absence of a bruit does not mean the absence of a significant carotid stenosis.

4. Scherer K, Bedlack RS, Simel DL. Does this patient have myasthenia gravis? *JAMA* 2005; 293:1906–1914. Speech failure when speaking over a prolonged period and the peek test increases the likelihood of myasthenia; their absence is unhelpful.

5. Rao G, Fisch L, Srinivason S et al. Does this patient have Parkinson disease? *JAMA* 2003; 289:347–353. Rigidity, the glabella tap and walking (heel–toe) seem to be useful signs of Parkinsonism.

CHAPTER 36

A summary of the neurological examination and extending the neurological examination

A conclusion is the place where you got tired of thinking. MARTIN H FISCHER (1879–1962)

Examining the nervous system: a suggested method

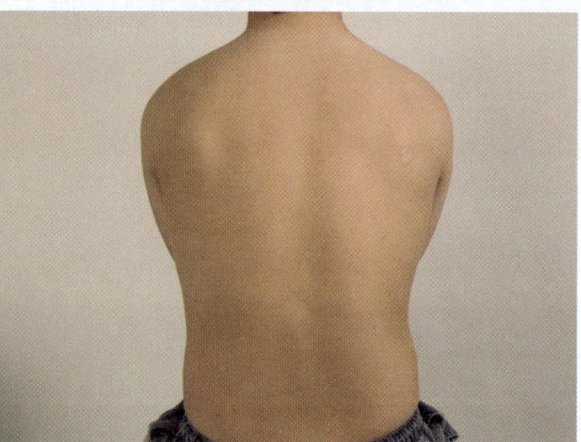

The nervous system examination

FIGURE 36.1

1. **HIGHER CENTRES EXAMINATION**
   Lying or sitting
   a. General inspection
      Obvious cranial nerve or limb lesions
      Ask patient about right- or left-handedness, level of education
      Shake hands
   b. Orientation
      Time
      Place
      Person
   c. Speech (simple to complex)
      Comprehension
      Repetition
      Name objects (nominal dysphasia)
      Describe a picture

   d. Parietal lobes
      Dominant (Gerstmann's syndrome)
      ○ Acalculia (mental arithmetic)
      ○ Agraphia (write)
      ○ Left–right disorientation
      ○ Finger agnosia (name fingers)
      Non-dominant
      ○ Dressing apraxia
      Both
      ○ Sensory inattention
      ○ Visual inattention
      ○ Cortical sensory loss (loss of graphaesthesia, two-point discrimination, joint position sense and stereognosis)
      ○ Constructional apraxia

TEXT BOX 36.1

Examining the nervous system: a suggested method *continued*

    e. Memory (temporal lobe)
       Short term (e.g. 3–5 words)
       Long term
    f. Frontal lobe
       Reflexes—grasp—pout—palmar—mental
       Proverb interpretation
       Smell
       Fundi
       Gait
    g. Other
       Visual fields
       Bruits
       Blood pressure, etc.

2. **NECK STIFFNESS AND KERNIG'S SIGN**

3. **CRANIAL NERVES**
   - II   Visual acuity and fields; fundoscopy
   - III, IV, VI Pupils and eye movements
   - V   Corneal reflexes, jaw jerk
   - VII   Facial muscles
   - VIII   Hearing
   - IX, X   Palate and gag
   - XI   Trapezius and sternocleidomastoids
   - XII   Tongue

4. **UPPER LIMBS EXAMINATION**
   a. General inspection (patient sitting to begin with)
      Scars
      Skin (e.g. neurofibromata, café-au-lait)
      Abnormal movements
   b. Shake hands
   c. Motor system
      Inspect arms, shoulder girdle—extend both arms
        ○ Wasting
        ○ Fasciculation
        ○ Tremor
        ○ Drift
      Palpate
        ○ Muscle bulk
        ○ Muscle tenderness
      Tone
        ○ Wrist
        ○ Elbow
      Power
        ○ Shoulder
        ○ Elbow
        ○ Wrist
        ○ Fingers
        ○ Ulnar, median nerve function
      Reflexes
        ○ Biceps
        ○ Triceps
        ○ Supinator
        ○ Finger
      Coordination
        ○ Finger–nose test—intention tremor, past-pointing
        ○ Dysdiadochokinesis
        ○ Rebound
   d. Sensory system
      Pain (pinprick)
      Cold (tuning fork/tendon hammer end)
      Vibration (128 Hz tuning fork)
      Proprioception—distal interphalangeal joint (each hand)
      ± Light touch (cottonwool)
   e. Other
      Thickened nerves (wrist, elbow)
      Axillae
      Neck
      Lower limbs
      Cranial nerves
      Urine analysis, etc.

5. **LOWER LIMBS EXAMINATION**
   Patient lying
   a. General inspection
      Scars, skin
      Urinary catheter
   b. Gait
   c. Motor system
      Inspect
        ○ Wasting
        ○ Fasciculation
        ○ Tremor
      Palpate
        ○ Muscle bulk
        ○ Muscle tenderness
      Tone
        ○ Knee—and test for clonus
        ○ Ankle—and test for clonus
      Power
        ○ Hip
        ○ Knee
        ○ Ankle
        ○ Foot
      Reflexes
        ○ Knee
        ○ Ankle
        ○ Plantar
      Coordination
        ○ Heel–shin test
        ○ Toe–finger test
        ○ Foot-tapping test

TEXT BOX 36.1

Continued

| Examining the nervous system: a suggested method *continued* |

d. Sensory system
   Pain
   Cold (tuning fork/tendon hammer)
   Vibration
   Proprioception
   ± Light touch
e. Saddle region sensation

f. Anal reflex
g. Back
   Deformity
   Scars
   Tenderness
   Bruits

TEXT BOX 36.1

EXTENDING THE NEUROLOGICAL EXAMINATION

Handedness, orientation and speech

Ask the patient whether he or she is right- or left-handed. As a screening assessment, ask for the patient's name, present location and the date. Next ask the patient to name an object you are pointing at and then have him or her point to a named object in the room, to test for dysphasia. Ask the patient to say 'British Constitution' to test for dysarthria.

Neck stiffness and Kernig's sign

Ask the patient to lie flat and attempt gently to flex the patient's head by placing a hand under the occiput. Flex the patient's hip with the knee bent and then attempt to straighten the leg.

Cranial nerves

The patient should sit over the edge of the bed if possible. Begin by general inspection of the head and neck looking for craniotomy scars, neurofibromas, facial asymmetry, ptosis, proptosis, skew deviation of the eyes or inequality of the pupils.

The second nerve

Test visual acuity with the patient wearing his or her spectacles. Each eye is tested separately, while the other is covered with a small card.

Visual field charts.

Both eyes superimposed. The blind spot is indicated in a darker colour

(From Stamper RL. *Visual field interpretation. Becker-Shaffer's diagnosis and therapy of the glaucomas*, 8th edn. St Louis, MO: Mosby, 2009.)

FIGURE 36.2

Examine the visual fields by confrontation using a hat-pin or fingers. Your head should be level with the patient's head. Each eye is tested separately. If visual acuity is very poor, the visual fields (Fig. 36.2) are mapped using the fingers.

Look into the fundi.

The third, fourth and sixth nerves

Look at the pupils, noting the shape, relative sizes and any associated ptosis. Use a pocket torch and shine the light from the side to gauge the reaction of the pupils to light. Assess quickly both the direct and the consensual responses. Look for an afferent pupillary defect by moving the torch in an arc from pupil to pupil. Test accommodation by asking the patient to look into the distance and then at the hat-pin or your finger held about 30 centimetres from the patient's nose.

Assess eye movements with both eyes first, getting the patient to follow the pin in each direction. Test saccadic movements horizontally and vertically. Look for failure of movement and for nystagmus. Ask about diplopia in each direction. Do a head impulse test (see Fig. 32.17, p 518) horizontally if there is nystagmus suggestive of a peripheral lesion.

The fifth nerve

Test the corneal reflexes gently and ask the patient if he or she can feel the touch of a piece of cottonwool on the cornea. The sensory component of this reflex is nerve V and the motor component is VII.

Test facial sensation in the three divisions: ophthalmic, maxillary and mandibular. Test pain sensation with the pin first and map any area of sensory loss from dull to sharp. Test light touch as well so that sensory dissociation can be detected if present.

Examine the motor division of the fifth nerve by asking the patient to clench the teeth while you feel the masseter muscles. Then get the patient to open the mouth while you attempt to force it closed; this is not possible if the pterygoid muscles are working. A unilateral lesion causes the jaw to deviate towards the weak (affected) side.

Test the jaw jerk. This is increased in cases of pseudobulbar palsy.

The seventh nerve

Test the muscles of facial expression. Ask the patient to look up and wrinkle the forehead. Look for loss of wrinkling and feel the muscle strength by pushing down on each side. This is preserved in upper motor neurone lesions because of bilateral cortical representation of these muscles.

Next ask the patient to shut the eyes tightly and compare the two sides. Tell the patient to grin and compare the nasolabial grooves.

The eighth nerve

Ask the patient to repeat a number you have softly whispered 60 centimetres away from each ear. Examine the external auditory canals and the eardrums if this is indicated. Do a Dix–Hallpike test if the history suggests benign paroxysmal positional vertigo (BPPV).

The ninth and tenth nerves

Look at the palate and note any uvular displacement. Ask the patient to say 'Ah' and look for symmetrical movement of the soft palate. A unilateral lesion causes the uvula to be drawn towards the unaffected (normal) side. Test gently for sensation on the palate (the ninth nerve). Ask the patient to speak to assess hoarseness, and to cough. A bovine cough suggests bilateral recurrent laryngeal nerve lesions.

The twelfth nerve

While examining the mouth, inspect the tongue for wasting and fasciculation. Next ask the patient to protrude the tongue. With a unilateral lesion the tongue deviates towards the weaker (affected) side.

The eleventh nerve

Look for torticollis and test the sternocleidomastoid and trapezius muscles. Ask the patient to shrug the shoulders and feel the trapezius as you push the shoulders down. Then ask the patient to turn his or her head against resistance and also feel the bulk of the sternocleidomastoid. Then examine the skull and auscultate for carotid bruits.

Upper limbs

Shake the patient's hand firmly. Ask him or her to sit over the side of the bed facing you, if possible.

Examine the *motor system* systematically every time. Inspect first for wasting (both proximally and distally) and fasciculations. Do not forget to include the shoulder girdle in your inspection.

Ask the patient to hold both hands out (palms up) with the arms extended and close the eyes. Look for drifting of one or both arms (upper motor neurone weakness, cerebellar lesion or posterior column loss). Also note any tremor or pseudoathetosis due to proprioceptive loss.

Feel the muscle bulk next, both proximally and distally, and note any muscle tenderness.

Test tone at the wrists and elbows by passively moving the joints at varying velocities.

Assess power at the shoulders, elbows, wrists and fingers.

If indicated, test for an ulnar nerve lesion (Froment's sign) and a median nerve lesion (pen-touching test).

Examine the reflexes: biceps (C5, C6), triceps (C7, C8) and brachioradialis (C5, C6).

Assess coordination with finger–nose testing and look for dysdiadochokinesis and rebound.

Motor weakness can be due to an upper motor neurone lesion, a lower motor neurone lesion or a myopathy. If there is evidence of a lower motor neurone lesion, consider anterior horn cell, nerve root or brachial plexus lesions, peripheral nerve lesions or a motor peripheral neuropathy.

Examine the *sensory system* after motor testing, because this can be time consuming.

First test the spinothalamic pathway (pain and temperature). Confirm any abnormality with pinprick. Demonstrate to the patient the sharpness of a pin on the anterior chest wall or forehead. Then ask him or her to close the eyes and tell you whether the sensation is sharp or dull. Start proximally and test each dermatome working distally to proximally. Map the abnormal area. As you are assessing, try to fit any sensory loss into dermatomal (cord or nerve root lesion), peripheral nerve, peripheral neuropathy (glove) or hemisensory (cortical or cord) distribution. Test cold sensation and quickly work distally to proximally covering all dermatomes.[a]

Next test the posterior column pathway (vibration and proprioception). Use a 128 Hz tuning fork to assess vibration sense. Place the vibrating fork on a distal interphalangeal joint when the patient has the eyes closed and ask what can be felt. To confirm, ask the patient to tell you when the vibration ceases and then, after a short wait, stop the vibrations. If the patient has deficient sensation, test at the wrist, then at the elbow and then at the shoulder.

Examine proprioception with the distal interphalangeal joint of the little finger. When the patient has the eyes open, grasp the distal phalanx from the sides and move it up and down to demonstrate; then ask the patient to close the eyes and repeat the manoeuvre. Normally, movement through even a few degrees is detectable, and the patient can tell whether it is up or down. If there is an abnormality, test larger movements and then proceed to test the wrist and elbows similarly if necessary.

Test sensation bilaterally simultaneously with touch from your fingers, assessing for extinction or neglect. Light touch can be done with cottonwool, but is seldom of value when other modalities have been tested.

Feel for thickened nerves—the ulnar at the elbow, the median at the wrist and the radial at the wrist—and feel the axillae if there is evidence of a proximal lesion. Note any scars, and finally examine the neck if relevant.

Lower limbs

Test the stance and gait first if possible. Then put the patient in bed with the legs entirely exposed. Place a towel over the groin—note whether a urinary catheter is present.

Look for muscle wasting and fasciculations. Note any tremor. Feel the muscle bulk of the quadriceps and run your hand up each shin, feeling for wasting of the anterior tibial muscles.

Test tone at the knees and ankles. Test clonus at this time. Push the lower end of the quadriceps sharply down towards the knee. Sustained rhythmical contractions indicate an upper motor neurone lesion. Also test the ankle by sharply dorsiflexing the foot with the knee bent and the thigh externally rotated.

Assess power next at the hips, knees and ankles.

Elicit the reflexes: knee (L3, L4), ankle (S1, S2) and plantar responses (L5, S1, S2).

Test coordination with the heel–shin test, toe–finger test and tapping of the feet.

Examine the sensory system as for the upper limbs: pinprick and cold, then vibration and proprioception, and then light touch if required. If there is a peripheral sensory loss, attempt to establish a sensory level by moving the pin or cold tuning fork up the leg and onto the abdomen and, if necessary, onto the chest. Examine sensation in the saddle region and test the anal reflex (S2, S3, S4).

Go to the back. Look for deformity, scars and neurofibromas. Palpate for tenderness over the vertebral bodies and auscultate for bruits. Perform the straight leg-raising test.

---

[a] Remember that many neurologists recommend starting with temperature testing. Students can do either first but must appear proficient at both.

DIAGNOSTIC TESTING

Neurological diagnosis depends on the history and examination. Imaging can confirm the location of the lesion and the likely pathology. Special testing is guided by the clinical setting.

Lumbar puncture

If acute meningitis is suspected, or less often if a CT of the brain is negative but you clinically suspect a subarachnoid haemorrhage, a *lumbar puncture* (LP) is indicated. An LP may also help in the diagnosis of certain neurological diseases, such as carcinomatous meningitis, tuberculous meningitis, central nervous system syphilis or vasculitis, idiopathic intracranial hypertension (pseudotumour cerebri) or normal-pressure hydrocephalus. An LP may also be helpful in diagnosing multiple sclerosis, Guillain–Barré syndrome or a paraneoplastic syndrome.

If there is papilloedema on fundoscopy or focal neurological signs (e.g. one side is weak), or the patient is immunocompromised, a computed tomography (CT) or magnetic resonance imaging (MRI) scan of the brain should be undertaken beforehand so as to exclude raised intracranial pressure (because of the risk of cerebral herniation after an LP in this setting).

The cerebrospinal fluid (CSF) is sent for Gram staining and culture as well as cell count and differential, protein and glucose testing. Additional molecular tests for *Neisseria meningitidis*, *Streptococcus pnueumoniae*, *Haemophilus influenzae* type B, *Listeria monocytogenes*, *Mycobacterium tuberculosis*, herpes simplex and varicella can be performed when indicated. Cryptococcal antigen, syphilis serology and fungal serology can be tested if necessary.

Neurological imaging

CT and MRI scans have revolutionised neurological investigations. These techniques are generally non-invasive, although CT scans expose patients to moderately large doses of radiation and both types of scans are often used with contrast agents, which can affect some patients. MRI scans cannot be performed on patients with magnetic metal implants (e.g. most pacemakers).

Interpretation of the scans often requires the assessment of multiple planes and slices or of three-dimensional reconstructions.

Some common examples of important diagnostic scans are shown in Figs 36.3–36.10.

Embolic stroke.

CT scan shows an ischaemic stroke on the right (left side of the image—white arrow) and a haemorrhage on the left (right side of the image—black arrow)

(From Crawford M, DiMarco J, Paulus W. *Cardiology*, 3rd edn. St Louis, MO: Mosby, 2009.)

FIGURE 36.3

Haemorrhagic stroke.

These CT scans without contrast injection ((a) and (b)) show low-density changes confined to the deep subcortical regions in a patient with acute left-sided weakness. The image in (c) taken 2 days later shows extensive haemorrhage within the area of infarction, which has ruptured into the ventricular system

(From Haaga J. *CT and MRI of the whole body*, 5th edn. St Louis, MO: Mosby, 2008.)

FIGURE 36.4

Multiple sclerosis.

The lesions of multiple sclerosis on MRI tend to involve the periventricular area, the corpus callosum and the optic nerves (solid white arrows). (a) The lesions produce discrete, globular foci of high-signal intensity (white) on T2-weighted MRI scans. (b) Ovoid lesions with their long axis perpendicular to the ventricular surface are called Dawson's fingers (solid white arrows)

(From Herring W. *Learning radiology: recognising the basics*, 2nd edn. Philadelphia: Saunders, 2011.)

FIGURE 36.5

Cerebellar tumour.

This is the typical appearance of a brain tumour on MRI, in this case a cerebellar medulloblastoma. (a) The tumour has a low signal on spin-echo T1-weighted images. (b) After injection of gadolinium (a contrast agent) the tumour enhances avidly, indicating a breakdown of the blood–brain barrier

(From Adam A. *Grainger & Allison's diagnostic radiology*, 5th edn. Edinburgh: Churchill Livingstone, 2008.)

FIGURE 36.6

Brain abscess.

This gadolinium-enhanced MRI scan shows a multiloculated ring-enhancing lesion caused by *Nocardia* infection

(From Goldman L. *Goldman's Cecil medicine*, 24th edn. Philadelphia: Saunders, 2011.)

FIGURE 36.7

Cerebral atrophy.

In this CT scan, note the expanded sulci (arrow), the shrunken gyri and the retraction of the cerebral cortex from the inner table of the skull. The ventricles have expanded

(From Kaufman D. *Clinical neurology for psychiatrists*, 6th edn. Philadelphia: Saunders, 2006.)

FIGURE 36.8

Cerebral aneurysm.

MRI scan showing a partly thrombosed giant aneurysm

(From Layon AJ. *Textbook of neurointensive care*, 1st edn. Philadelphia: Saunders, 2003.)

FIGURE 36.9

Spinal cord tumour.

An MRI scan showing an intradural and partly extradural right L3 schwannoma. (a) Axial and (b) coronal T1-weighted images with gadolinium contrast. Note the large lobular tumour extending into the spinal canal and compressing the spinal cord (arrows)

(From Adam A. *Grainger & Allison's diagnostic radiology*, 5th edn. Edinburgh: Churchill Livingstone, 2008.)

FIGURE 36.10

T&O'C ESSENTIALS

1. The neurological examination can be long and complicated. It should usually be directed at the area suggested by the history, but a screening general examination should also be carried out.
2. Considerable practice is necessary if the neurological examination is to be performed accurately (especially when you are also being examined).
3. Symmetry is the student's friend. Always compare one side with the other when testing strength, reflexes and so on. Asymmetry helps you to localise the site of a lesion.
4. The routine of the various parts of the examination should become familiar to you so that you can put the signs together as they are found, rather than worrying about what to do next at each stage.
5. Expert neurologists strive to (and can) accurately localise the site of a lesion likely to have caused a particular combination of signs.
6. Neurological localisation is most often firmly established by CT and MRI scanning. MRI is more accurate for brainstem lesions, which CT can miss. Using these cross-sectional imaging techniques it is often possible to determine the cause of the lesion (e.g. infection, tumour), as well as its position in the central nervous system.

clinical examination

A guide to specialty examinations

8th edition

VOLUME TWO

clinical examination

A guide to specialty examinations

8th edition

VOLUME TWO

NICHOLAS J TALLEY

MBBS (Hons)(NSW), MD (NSW), PhD (Syd), MMedSci (Clin Epi)(Newc.),
FRACP, FAFPHM, FAHMS, FRCP (Lond. & Edin.), FACP, FACG, AGAF, FAMS, FRCPI (Hon)
Laureate Professor and Pro Vice-Chancellor, Global Research, University of Newcastle, NSW, Australia
Senior Staff Specialist, John Hunter Hospital, Newcastle, NSW, Australia
Professor of Medicine, Professor of Epidemiology, Joint Supplemental Consultant Gastroenterology
and Health Sciences Research, Mayo Clinic, Rochester, MN, United States; Professor of Medicine,
University of North Carolina, United States; Foreign Guest Professor, Karolinska Institute, Sweden; Past
President, Royal Australasian College of Physicians

SIMON O'CONNOR

FRACP, DDU, FCSANZ
Cardiologist, The Canberra Hospital, Canberra, ACT, Australia
Clinical Senior Lecturer, Australian National University Medical School, Canberra, ACT, Australia

ELSEVIER

ELSEVIER

Elsevier Australia. ACN 001 002 357
(a division of Reed International Books Australia Pty Ltd)
Tower 1, 475 Victoria Avenue, Chatswood, NSW 2067

This edition ©2018 Elsevier Australia. 1st edition ©1988, 2nd edition ©1992, 3rd edition ©1996, 4th edition ©2001, 5th edition ©2006, 6th edition ©2010, 7th edition ©2014 Elsevier Australia

All rights reserved. No part of this publication may be reproduced or transmitted in any form or by any means, electronic or mechanical, including photocopying, recording, or any information storage and retrieval system, without permission in writing from the publisher. Details on how to seek permission, further information about the Publisher's permissions policies and our arrangements with organizations such as the Copyright Clearance Center and the Copyright Licensing Agency, can be found at our website: www.elsevier.com/permissions.

This book and the individual contributions contained in it are protected under copyright by the Publisher (other than as may be noted herein).

ISBN: 978-0-7295-4289-0

Notice

Practitioners and researchers must always rely on their own experience and knowledge in evaluating and using any information, methods, compounds or experiments described herein. Because of rapid advances in the medical sciences, in particular, independent verification of diagnoses and drug dosages should be made. To the fullest extent of the law, no responsibility is assumed by Elsevier, authors, editors or contributors for any injury and/or damage to persons or property as a matter of products liability, negligence or otherwise, or from any use or operation of any methods, products, instructions, or ideas contained in the material herein.

Although all advertising material is expected to conform to ethical (medical) standards, inclusion in this publication does not constitute a guarantee or endorsement of the quality or the value of such product or the claims made of it by its manufacturer.

National Library of Australia Cataloging-in-Publication Data

 A catalogue record for this book is available from the National Library of Australia

Senior Content Strategist: Larissa Norrie
Content Development Specialist: Lauren Santos
Project Manager: Devendran Kannan
Edited by Chris Wyard
Proofread by Annabel Adair
Design by Natalie Bowra
Index by Innodata Indexing
Typeset by Toppan BestSet Premedia Ltd.
Printed in China

Foreword by Sarah Dalton

The more things change, the more they stay the same. We live in a world where healthcare stands to be significantly disrupted by artificial intelligence, machine learning and big data but at the same time as doctors we have a fundamental responsibility to connect with our patients, to hear their stories and to diagnose and treat their conditions with wisdom and compassion. So, no matter how precise medicine can become, the foundations of taking a history and performing a comprehensive physical examination have never been more important.

Clinical Examination by Talley and O'Connor has been widely recognised as providing the cornerstone to learning physical diagnoses over many decades. It is with some pride that I have kept my original first edition that accompanied me throughout medical school all those years ago. The words of wisdom then are just as true today—that 'treatment of the patient begins the moment one reaches the bedside'. But even more true, at this time heralded by over-diagnosis and over-investigation in healthcare, is the need to use the simplest, most effective and arguably most reliable of all investigative approaches—a good history and physical examination.

In this most recent iteration, the authors have expanded their repertoire and turned their tried and tested formula to all medical specialties, ranging from paediatric medicine to specific approaches to ears, eyes, nose and throat assessments. The companion series offers the same structured approach to diagnoses, highlighting important differences and bringing a wealth of information destined to prepare any candidate admirably for a short or long case in these areas. The text outlines tips and tricks designed to demystify the sometimes challenging task of assessing neonates and children, discussing a range of approaches from maternal health assessment to talking to adolescents and their families.

Most doctors care for young people at some point in their career, and young people with medical conditions most definitely grow up. Thankfully our patients are living longer and living better, but caring for chronic and complex conditions means we all need some understanding of specialty issues. Many doctors do not feel particularly well prepared for this challenge, making this text relevant to all clinicians. Whilst there is much we do not know about the future of medicine, one thing we know for certain is that healthy young people create healthy futures. From little things, big things grow.

Dr Sarah Dalton
BMed MAppMgt(Hlth) FRACP
Paediatric Emergency Physician,
The Children's Hospital at Westmead
President, Division of Paediatrics and Child Health,
The Royal Australasian College of Physicians

Foreword by David Ellwood

The clinical practice of Obstetrics & Gynaecology (O&G) presents medical students with challenges and opportunities. It is, by its very nature, a very practical discipline of medicine and for this reason many students will enjoy their clinical attachments immensely. O&G has enormous breadth and depth and to understand many common presentations requires a detailed knowledge of pelvic anatomy, reproductive physiology, microbiology and psychology, as well as many other branches of clinical medicine. But the standard approaches to the patient of history and examination bring with them some unique difficulties in terms of clinical skills development. Virtually all examinations are intimate, and history taking must embrace the fact that there are significant psychosocial aspects of both gynaecological and obstetric problems.

This second volume of the well-known Talley & O'Connor's *Clinical Examination* (8th Edition) contains separate chapters on gynaecological and obstetric history and examination. They can both be read separately as stand-alone aids for students, but will also complement each other when read together as there are many areas of overlap. Both are clear, concise, and contain many practical tips which will be valuable for both the junior medical student encountering these clinical experiences for the first time, as well as the more senior student revising for final examinations. The frameworks for history taking and examination, and the many clear illustrations, go a long way to demystifying the subject matter.

It is especially important for the medical student to understand some of the complexities of O&G practice. The clinical etiquette around intimate gynaecological and obstetric examination is extremely important, including the use of chaperones. Understanding the interface between a woman's gynaecological and sexual health wellbeing, and how this is impacted by psychological factors, is also vital. In modern O&G, much of the information that used to be derived from clinical examination is now obtained by the liberal use of ultrasound, but there are many times when both are essential and an appreciation of how this works in practice is essential. These chapters manage to provide clear and practical advice across all of these areas.

Finally, the diligent student of medicine will know that volumes such as this, important though they are, are only companions to learning, and it is the patient from whom most can be learned. Armed with this practical guide, students should be very well-equipped to take advantage of all of their clinical learning opportunities, which will ultimately be for the good of the women who they encounter in the future as patients.

David Ellwood
Professor of Obstetrics and Gynaecology

Contents

Foreword by Sarah Dalton — v
Foreword by David Ellwood — vi
Preface — xx
Acknowledgements — xxi
Clinical methods: an historical perspective — xxiii
The Hippocratic oath — xxv

VOLUME ONE

SECTION 1
THE GENERAL PRINCIPLES OF HISTORY TAKING AND PHYSICAL EXAMINATION — 1

CHAPTER 1
The general principles of history taking — 3

T&O'C essentials — 3
Bedside manner and establishing rapport — 3
Obtaining the history — 5
Introductory questions — 6
T&O'C essentials — 6
Presenting (principal) symptom — 7
History of the presenting illness — 7
  Current symptoms — 7
  Associated symptoms — 8
  The effect of the illness — 12
Drug and treatment history — 12
Past history — 14
  Additional history for the female patient — 15
Social history — 15
T&O'C essentials — 15
  Upbringing and education level — 15
  Marital status, social support and living conditions — 15
  Diet and exercise — 16
  Occupation and hobbies — 16
  Overseas travel — 16
  Smoking — 16
  Alcohol use — 17
  Analgesics and street drugs — 18
  Mood — 19
  Sexual history — 19
Family history — 19
Systems review — 19
Skills in history taking — 20
T&O'C essentials — 20
References — 21

CHAPTER 2
Advanced history taking — 22

Taking a good history — 22
The differential diagnosis — 22
Fundamental considerations when taking the history — 22
Personal history taking — 23
  Common general symptoms — 24
  Sexual history — 27
  Reproductive history — 27
Cross-cultural history taking — 28
The 'uncooperative' or 'difficult' patient — 28
Self-harming and Münchhausen's syndrome — 29
History taking for the maintenance of good health — 29
The elderly patient — 31
  Activities of daily living — 31
  Polypharmacy — 32
  Adherence — 32
  Mental state — 32
  Specific problems in the elderly — 33
  Advance care planning (advance health directives) — 33
Patient confidentiality — 33
Evidence-based history taking and differential diagnosis — 33
The clinical assessment — 34
Concluding the consultation — 34
T&O'C essentials — 35
References — 35

CHAPTER 3
The general principles of physical examination — 37

- Clinical examination — 38
- How to start — 38
  - Hand washing — 38
- First impressions — 39
  - Vital signs — 40
  - Facies — 40
  - Jaundice — 40
  - Cyanosis — 41
  - Pallor — 44
  - Hair — 45
- Weight, body habitus and posture — 45
- Hydration — 46
- The hands and nails — 48
- Temperature — 49
- Smell — 50
- Preparing the patient for examination — 51
- Advanced concepts: evidence-based clinical examination — 51
  - Inter-observer agreement (reliability) and the κ-statistic — 53
- T&O'C essentials — 54
- Introduction to the OSCE — 55
- References — 56

SECTION 2
THE CARDIOVASCULAR SYSTEM — 57

CHAPTER 4
The cardiovascular history — 59

- Presenting symptoms — 59
  - Chest pain — 59
  - Dyspnoea — 63
  - Ankle swelling — 64
  - Palpitations — 64
  - Syncope, presyncope and dizziness — 66
  - Fatigue — 67
  - Intermittent claudication and peripheral vascular disease — 67
- Risk factors for coronary artery disease — 68
- Drug and treatment history — 70
- Past history — 70
- Social history — 71
- Family history — 71
- T&O'C essentials — 71
- OSCE example – CVS history — 72
- OSCE revision topics – CVS history — 72
- References — 72

CHAPTER 5
The cardiac examination — 74

- Examination anatomy — 74
- Positioning the patient — 75
- General appearance — 76
- Hands — 79
- Arterial pulse — 81
  - Rate of pulse — 83
  - Rhythm — 83
  - Radiofemoral and radial–radial delay — 83
  - Character and volume — 84
  - Condition of the vessel wall — 84
- Blood pressure — 84
  - Measuring the blood pressure with the sphygmomanometer — 86
  - Variations in blood pressure — 88
  - High blood pressure — 88
  - Postural blood pressure — 88
- Face — 89
- Neck — 89
  - Carotid arteries — 89
  - Jugular venous pressure — 90
- Praecordium — 92
  - Inspection — 92
  - Palpation — 93
  - Percussion — 95
  - Auscultation — 95
  - Abnormalities of the heart sounds — 97
  - Murmurs of the heart — 100
  - Auscultation of the neck — 105
- The back — 106
- The abdomen and legs — 106
- T&O'C essentials — 107
- OSCE example – CVS examination — 107
- OSCE revision topics – CVS examination — 108
- References — 108

CHAPTER 6
The limb examination and peripheral vascular disease — 109

- Examination anatomy — 109
  - Arms — 109
  - Legs — 109
  - Lower limbs — 109
- Peripheral vascular disease — 113
- Acute arterial occlusion — 114
- Deep venous thrombosis — 115
- Varicose veins — 115
- Chronic venous disease — 116
- T&O'C essentials — 117
- OSCE example – peripheral vascular disease — 117

OSCE revision topics	118
References	118

CHAPTER 7
Correlation of physical signs disease and cardiovascular disease — 119

Cardiac failure	119
Left ventricular failure (LVF)	119
Right ventricular failure (RVF)	120
Chest pain	121
Myocardial infarction or acute coronary syndrome	121
Pulmonary embolism	122
Acute aortic dissection	122
Pericardial disease	122
Acute pericarditis	122
Chronic constrictive pericarditis	123
Acute cardiac tamponade	123
Infective endocarditis	123
Systemic hypertension	124
Causes of systemic hypertension	125
Complications of hypertension	125
Malignant (accelerated) hypertension	125
Pulmonary hypertension	125
Causes of pulmonary hypertension	126
Innocent murmurs	126
Valve diseases of the left heart	126
Mitral stenosis	126
Mitral regurgitation (chronic)	128
Acute mitral regurgitation	129
Mitral valve prolapse (MVP, systolic-click murmur syndrome)	130
Aortic stenosis (AS)	130
Aortic regurgitation	131
Valve diseases of the right heart	135
Tricuspid stenosis	135
Tricuspid regurgitation (TR)	136
Pulmonary stenosis (in adults)	137
Pulmonary regurgitation	137
Prosthetic heart valves	137
Cardiomyopathy	137
Hypertrophic cardiomyopathy	137
Dilated cardiomyopathy	139
Restrictive cardiomyopathy	139
Acyanotic congenital heart disease	139
Ventricular septal defect	139
Atrial septal defect	139
Patent ductus arteriosus	141
Coarctation of the aorta	141
Ebstein's anomaly	141
Cyanotic congenital heart disease	142
Eisenmenger's syndrome (pulmonary hypertension and a right-to-left shunt)	142
Fallot's syndrome	142
'Grown-up' congenital heart disease	143
Fallot's syndrome	143
Transposition of the great arteries	143
T&O'C essentials	143
OSCE example – cardiovascular examination	144
OSCE revision topics – cardiovascular examination	144
References	144

CHAPTER 8
A summary of the cardiovascular examination and extending the cardiovascular examination — 145

Extending the cardiovascular physical examination	147
The chest X-ray: a systematic approach	147
The echocardiogram	151
T&O'C essentials	159
OSCE revision topics	159

SECTION 3
THE RESPIRATORY SYSTEM — 161

CHAPTER 9
The respiratory history — 163

Presenting symptoms	163
Cough and sputum	163
Haemoptysis	165
Breathlessness (dyspnoea)	165
Wheeze	168
Chest pain	168
Other presenting symptoms	168
Current treatment	169
Past history	171
Occupational history	171
Social history	172
Family history	173
T&O'C essentials	173
OSCE revision topics – the respiratory history	173
References	173

CHAPTER 10
The respiratory examination — 174

Examination anatomy	174
Positioning the patient	174
General appearance	174
Dyspnoea	174
Characteristic signs of COPD	175

CONTENTS

Cyanosis	177
Character of the cough	177
Sputum	177
Stridor	177
Hoarseness	177
Hands	177
Clubbing	178
Staining	178
Wasting and weakness	178
Pulse rate	178
Flapping tremor (asterixis)	178
Face	178
Trachea	179
Chest	180
Inspection	180
Palpation	182
Percussion	184
Auscultation	184
The heart	188
The abdomen	188
Other	188
Pemberton's sign	188
Legs	188
Respiratory rate on exercise	188
Temperature	188
T&O'C essentials	188
OSCE revision topics – the respiratory examination	189
References	189

CHAPTER 11
Correlation of physical signs and respiratory disease — 190

Respiratory distress: respiratory failure	190
Consolidation (lobar pneumonia)	190
Symptoms	191
Signs	191
Causes of community-acquired pneumonia	192
Atelectasis (collapse)	192
Signs	192
Causes	192
Pleural effusion	192
Signs	192
Causes	192
Yellow nail syndrome	193
Pneumothorax	193
Signs	193
Causes	193
Tension pneumothorax	194
Signs	194
Causes	194
Bronchiectasis	194
Signs	194
Causes	194
Bronchial asthma	194
Signs	194
Chronic obstructive pulmonary disease (COPD)	195
Signs	195
Causes of generalised emphysema	196
Chronic bronchitis	196
Signs	196
Causes	196
Interstitial lung disease (ILD)	196
Signs	197
Causes	197
Tuberculosis (TB)	197
Primary tuberculosis	197
Postprimary tuberculosis	197
Miliary tuberculosis	197
Mediastinal compression	197
Signs	198
Carcinoma of the lung	198
Respiratory and chest signs	198
Apical (Pancoast's) tumour	198
Distant metastases	198
Non-metastatic extrapulmonary manifestations	198
Sarcoidosis	199
Pulmonary signs	199
Extrapulmonary signs	199
Pulmonary embolism (PE)	199
Signs	200
T&O'C essentials	200
OSCE revision topics – respiratory disease	200
References	200

CHAPTER 12
A summary of the respiratory examination and extending the respiratory examination — 201

Extending the respiratory physical examination	203
Bedside assessment of lung function	203
The chest X-ray and computed tomography (CT) scan in respiratory medicine	206
Chest X-ray checklist	206
T&O'C essentials	213
OSCE revision topics – respiratory investigations	213
References	213

SECTION 4
THE GASTROINTESTINAL SYSTEM 215

CHAPTER 13
The gastrointestinal history 217

- Presenting symptoms 217
  - Abdominal pain 217
  - Patterns of pain 218
  - Appetite and weight change 218
  - Early satiation and postprandial fullness 218
  - Nausea and vomiting 218
  - Heartburn and acid regurgitation (gastro-oesophageal reflux disease—GORD) 219
  - Dysphagia 220
  - Diarrhoea 222
  - Constipation 223
  - Mucus 224
  - Bleeding 224
  - Jaundice 225
  - Pruritus 225
  - Abdominal bloating and swelling 225
  - Lethargy 226
- Treatment 226
- Past history 227
- Social history 227
- Family history 227
- T&O'C essentials 227
- OSCE revision topics – the gastrointestinal history 228
- References 228

CHAPTER 14
The gastrointestinal examination 229

- Examination anatomy 229
- Positioning the patient 230
- General appearance 230
  - Jaundice 230
  - Weight and wasting 231
  - Skin 231
  - Mental state 234
- Hands 235
  - Nails 235
  - Palms 235
  - Hepatic flap (asterixis) 236
- Arms 237
- Face 238
  - Eyes 238
  - Salivary glands 239
  - Mouth 240
- Neck and chest 243
- Abdomen 244
  - Inspection 244
  - Palpation 248
  - Percussion 257
  - Ascites 258
  - Auscultation 260
- Hernias 261
  - Examination anatomy 261
  - Hernias in the groin 262
  - Epigastric hernia 264
  - Incisional hernias 264
- Rectal examination 264
  - The pelvic floor—special tests for pelvic floor dysfunction 267
  - Ending the rectal exam 267
  - Testing of the stools for blood 267
- Other 268
- Examination of the gastrointestinal contents 268
  - Faeces 268
  - Vomitus 269
- Urinalysis 269
- T&O'C essentials 271
- OSCE revision topics – the gastrointestinal examination 271
- References 271

CHAPTER 15
Correlation of physical signs and gastrointestinal disease 272

- Examination of the acute abdomen 272
- T&O'C essential 273
  - Acute abdomen after blunt trauma 274
- Liver disease 274
  - Signs 275
- Portal hypertension 275
  - Signs 275
  - Causes 275
- Hepatic encephalopathy 275
  - Grading 275
  - Causes 275
- Dysphagia 276
  - Signs 276
- Gastrointestinal bleeding 276
  - Assessing degree of blood loss 276
  - Determining the possible bleeding site 277
- Inflammatory bowel disease 277
  - Ulcerative colitis 277
  - Crohn's disease 279

xii CONTENTS

Malabsorption and nutritional status	279
Signs	*280*
Causes	*280*
Classification of malabsorption	*280*
T&O'C essentials	**281**
References	**281**

CHAPTER 16
A summary of the gastrointestinal examination and extending the gastrointestinal examination — 282

Extending the gastrointestinal examination	284
Endoscopy	*284*
Biochemistry	*285*
Imaging the gastrointestinal system	285
Abdominal X-rays	*285*
Abdominal ultrasound	*287*
CT of the abdomen	*289*
T&O'C essentials	**294**
Revision OSCEs	**294**

SECTION 5
THE GENITOURINARY SYSTEM — 295

CHAPTER 17
The genitourinary history — 297

Presenting symptoms	297
Change in appearance of the urine	*298*
Urinary tract infection	*298*
Urinary obstruction	*300*
Urinary incontinence	*300*
Chronic kidney disease	*300*
Menstrual and sexual history	303
Treatment	304
Past history	304
Social history	304
Family history	304
T&O'C essentials	**304**
OSCE revision topics – genitourinary history	**305**
References	**305**

CHAPTER 18
The genitourinary examination — 306

Examination anatomy	306
The examination	306
General appearance	306
Hands	306
Arms	307
Face	309
Neck	310
Chest	310
The abdominal examination	310
Inspection	*310*
Palpation	*310*
Ballotting	*311*
Percussion	*311*
Auscultation	*312*
Rectal and pelvic examination	*312*
The back	312
Legs	312
Blood pressure	313
Fundi	313
Male genitalia	313
Differential diagnosis of a scrotal mass	*314*
T&O'C essentials	**315**
OSCE revision topics – genitourinary examination	**316**
References	**316**

CHAPTER 19
A summary of the examination of chronic kidney disease and extending the genitourinary examination — 317

Extending the genitourinary examination	319
Investigations	*319*
T&O'C essentials	**326**
OSCE revision topics	**326**
Reference	**326**

SECTION 6
THE HAEMATOLOGICAL SYSTEM — 327

CHAPTER 20
The haematological history — 329

Haematological disorders	329
Presenting symptoms	329
Red cell abnormalities	*329*
Clotting and bleeding	*330*
Recurrent infection	*333*
Treatment history to ask about	333
Past history	333
Social history	334
Family history	334
T&O'C essentials	**334**
OSCE revision topics	**334**

CHAPTER 21
The haematological examination — 335

Examination anatomy	335
General appearance	335
Hands	335

Forearms	339
Epitrochlear nodes	339
Axillary nodes	339
Face	340
Cervical and supraclavicular nodes	341
Bone tenderness	342
The abdominal examination	343
Inguinal nodes	345
Legs	345
Fundi	346
T&O'C essentials	347
References	347

CHAPTER 22
A summary of the haematological examination and extending the haematological examination — 348

Extending the haematological physical examination	350
Haematology tests	350
Examination of the peripheral blood film	350
Anaemia	350
Pancytopenia	354
Acute leukaemia	354
Chronic leukaemia	355
Myeloproliferative disease	355
Lymphoma	357
Multiple myeloma	358
Haematological imaging	358
T&O'C essentials	360
OSCE revision topics – the haematological system	360

SECTION 7
THE RHEUMATOLOGICAL SYSTEM — 361

CHAPTER 23
The rheumatological history — 363

Presenting symptoms	363
Peripheral joints	363
T&O'C essential	365
Back pain	365
Limb pain	366
Raynaud's phenomenon	367
Dry eyes and mouth	367
Red eyes	368
Systemic symptoms	368
Treatment history	368
Past history	368
Social history	369
Family history	369
T&O'C essentials	369
OSCE revision topics – the rheumatological history	369
References	369

CHAPTER 24
The rheumatological examination — 370

Examination anatomy	370
General inspection	370
Principles of joint examination	372
Look	372
Feel	373
Move	373
Measure	374
Assessment of individual joints	374
Hands and wrists	374
T&O'C essentials	375
Elbows	383
Shoulders	384
Temporomandibular joints	388
Neck	388
Thoracolumbar spine and sacroiliac joints	392
Hips	395
Knees	399
Ankles and feet	403
T&O'C essentials	407
OSCE revision topics – the rheumatological examination	407
References	407

CHAPTER 25
Correlation of physical signs with rheumatological and musculoskeletal disease — 408

Rheumatoid arthritis	408
General inspection	408
Hands	408
Wrists	408
Elbows	408
Shoulders and axillae	408
Eyes	408
Parotids	409
Mouth	409
Temporomandibular joints	410
Neck	410
Chest	410
Heart	410
Abdomen	410
Lower limbs	410
Ankles and feet	410

Seronegative spondyloarthritides	410
Ankylosing spondylitis	*411*
Reactive arthritis	*411*
Psoriatic arthritis	*412*
Enteropathic arthritis	*412*
Gouty arthritis	412
Calcium pyrophosphate arthritis (pseudogout)	413
Calcium hydroxyapatite arthritis	413
Osteoarthritis	413
Systemic lupus erythematosus	414
General inspection	*414*
Hands	*414*
Forearms	*414*
Head and neck	*414*
Chest	*415*
Abdomen	*415*
Hips	*416*
Legs	*416*
Urine and blood pressure	*416*
Temperature	*416*
Systemic sclerosis (scleroderma and CREST)	416
General inspection	*416*
Hands	*418*
Arms	*418*
Face	*419*
Chest	*419*
Legs	*419*
Urinalysis and blood pressure	*419*
The stool	*419*
Mixed connective tissue disease (MCTD)	420
Examination	*420*
Rheumatic fever	420
Examining the patient with suspected rheumatic fever	*420*
The vasculitides	420
Soft-tissue rheumatism	421
Shoulder syndromes	*421*
Elbow epicondylitis (tennis and golfer's elbow)	*423*
Tenosynovitis of the wrist	*423*
Bursitis	*424*
Nerve entrapment syndromes	424
Carpal tunnel syndrome	*425*
Meralgia paraesthetica	*425*
Tarsal tunnel syndrome	*425*
Morton's 'neuroma'	*425*
Fibromyalgia syndrome	*426*
T&O'C essentials	**427**
OSCE revision topics – rheumatological disease	427
References	427

CHAPTER 26
A summary of the rheumatological examination and extending the rheumatological examination — 428

Extending the rheumatological system examination	429
Rheumatology investigations	*429*
Imaging	*430*
T&O'C essentials	435
References	435

SECTION 8
THE ENDOCRINE SYSTEM — 437

CHAPTER 27
The endocrine history — 439

Presenting symptoms	439
Changes in appetite and weight	*439*
Changes in bowel habit	*439*
Changes in sweating	*439*
Changes in hair distribution	*439*
Lethargy	*440*
Changes in the skin and nails	*440*
Changes in pigmentation	*441*
Changes in stature	*441*
Erectile dysfunction (impotence)	*441*
Galactorrhoea	*441*
Menstruation	*441*
Polyuria	*441*
Risk factors for diabetes (metabolic syndrome)	442
Past history and treatment	442
Social history	443
Family history	443
T&O'C essentials	443
OSCE revision topics – the endocrine history	443

CHAPTER 28
The endocrine examination — 444

The thyroid	444
The thyroid gland	*444*
Hyperthyroidism (thyrotoxicosis)	*448*
Hypothyroidism (myxoedema)	*451*
The pituitary	453
Examination anatomy	*453*
Panhypopituitarism	*454*

Acromegaly	*456*
Other pituitary syndromes	*458*
The adrenals	458
Cushing's syndrome	*458*
Addison's disease	*461*
T&O'C essentials	462
OSCE revision topics – the endocrine examination	462
References	462

CHAPTER 29
Correlation of physical signs and endocrine disease — 463

Diabetes mellitus	463
Calcium metabolism	469
Primary hyperparathyroidism	*469*
The MEN syndromes	*470*
Hypoparathyroidism	*470*
Osteoporosis and osteomalacia	471
Syndromes associated with short stature	473
Turner's syndrome (45XO)	*474*
Down's syndrome (Trisomy 21)	*475*
Achondroplasia (dwarfism)	*475*
Rickets	*475*
Hirsutism	475
Gynaecomastia	476
Paget's disease	476
T&O'C essentials	478
OSCE revision topics – endocrine system	479
References	479

CHAPTER 30
A summary of the endocrine examination and extending the endocrine examination — 480

The endocrine examination: a suggested method	480
Extending the endocrine physical examination	480
Diagnostic testing	*480*
T&O'C essentials	486
OSCE revision topics – endocrine system	486

SECTION 9
THE NERVOUS SYSTEM — 487

CHAPTER 31
The neurological history — 489

Starting off	489
Presenting symptoms	489
Headache and facial pain	*490*
Faints and fits	*492*
T&O'C essential	*494*
Dizziness	*495*
Visual disturbances and deafness	*496*
Disturbances of gait	*496*
Disturbed sensation or weakness in the limbs	*496*
Tremor and involuntary movements	*496*
Speech and mental status	*497*
Past health	497
Medication history	497
Social history	498
Family history	498
T&O'C essentials	498
OSCE revision topics – the neurological history	499
References	499

CHAPTER 32
The neurological examination: general signs and the cranial nerves — 500

A preamble regarding the neurological examination	500
Examination anatomy	500
General signs	501
Consciousness	*501*
Neck stiffness	*501*
Handedness	*501*
Orientation	*501*
The cranial nerves	501
The first (olfactory) nerve	*504*
The second (optic) nerve	*505*
The third (oculomotor), fourth (trochlear) and sixth (abducens) nerves—the ocular nerves	*510*
The fifth (trigeminal) nerve	*521*
The seventh (facial) nerve	*525*
The eighth (vestibulocochlear) nerve	*529*
The ninth (glossopharyngeal) and tenth (vagus) nerves	*531*
The eleventh (accessory) nerve	*533*
The twelfth (hypoglossal) nerve	*534*
Multiple cranial nerve lesions	*536*
Carotid bruits	*537*
T&O'C essentials	538
OSCE example – introduction (STEM)	538
References	539

CHAPTER 33
The neurological examination: speech and higher centres — 540

Speech	540
Dysphasia	*540*

Dysarthria	*542*
Dysphonia	*543*
The cerebral hemispheres	543
Parietal lobe function	*543*
Temporal lobe function	*545*
Frontal lobe function	*546*
T&O'C essentials	**547**
OSCE revision topics – speech and higher centres	**547**
References	**547**

CHAPTER 34
The neurological examination: the peripheral nervous system — 548

Limbs and trunk	548
History	*548*
Examination anatomy	*549*
General examination approach	*550*
General inspection	*550*
Upper limbs	*550*
Lower limbs	*566*
Gait	*577*
T&O'C essentials	**579**
OSCE revision topics – the peripheral nervous system	**579**
References	**579**

CHAPTER 35
Correlation of physical signs and neurological syndromes and disease — 580

Upper motor neurone lesions	580
Causes of hemiplegia (upper motor neurone lesion)	*580*
Lower motor neurone lesions	582
Motor neurone disease	583
Peripheral neuropathy	583
Guillain–Barré syndrome (acute inflammatory polyradiculoneuropathy)	583
Multiple sclerosis	584
Thickened peripheral nerves	585
Spinal cord compression	585
Important spinal cord syndromes	588
Brown-Séquard syndrome	*588*
Subacute combined degeneration of the cord (vitamin B_{12} deficiency)	*588*
Dissociated sensory loss	*589*
Syringomyelia (a central cavity in the spinal cord)	*589*
An extensor plantar response plus absent knee and ankle jerks	*590*
Myopathy	590
Dystrophia myotonica	591
Myasthenia gravis	593
The cerebellum	595
Parkinson's disease	597
Inspection	*597*
Gait and movements	*597*
Tremor	*598*
Tone	*598*
Face	*598*
Writing	*599*
Causes of Parkinson's syndrome	*599*
Other extrapyramidal movement disorders (dyskinesia)	600
Chorea	*600*
Dystonia	*600*
Tics and de la Tourette's syndrome	*601*
The unconscious patient	601
General inspection	*601*
Level of consciousness	*602*
Neck	*603*
Head and face	*603*
Upper and lower limbs	*604*
Body	*604*
Urine	*604*
Blood glucose	*604*
Temperature	*604*
Stomach contents	*604*
T&O'C essentials	**604**
OSCE revision topics – neurological syndromes and disorders	**604**
References	**605**

CHAPTER 36
A summary of the neurological examination and extending the neurological examination — 606

Extending the neurological examination	608
Handedness, orientation and speech	*608*
Neck stiffness and Kernig's sign	*608*
Cranial nerves	*608*
Upper limbs	*609*
Lower limbs	*610*
Diagnostic testing	611
Lumbar puncture	*611*
Neurological imaging	*611*
T&O'C essentials	**615**

VOLUME TWO

SECTION 10
PAEDIATRIC AND NEONATAL HISTORY AND EXAMINATION — 617

CHAPTER 37
The paediatric history and examination — 619

- Principles of paediatric history taking and examination — 619
- Paediatric history taking — 619
  - History-taking sequence — 620
- General physical examination — 622
  - Preparing for the examination — 622
  - Examination — 622
- T&O'C essentials — 682
- OSCE revision topics – the paediatric history and examination — 682
- References — 683

CHAPTER 38
The neonatal history and examination — 684

- The history — 684
  - Maternal health — 684
  - Other family history — 685
  - History of the pregnancy, labour and delivery — 685
- The physical examination — 687
  - Preparing for the physical examination — 688
  - Measurements — 689
  - Head-to-toe assessment — 696
  - Gestational age — 723
- T&O'C essentials — 723
- OSCE revision topics – the neonatal history and examination — 724
- References — 724

SECTION 11
WOMEN'S HEALTH HISTORY AND EXAMINATION — 727

CHAPTER 39
The obstetric history and examination — 729

- The obstetric history — 729
- Early pregnancy symptoms — 729
  - Amenorrhoea — 729
  - Breast changes — 730
  - Nausea and vomiting — 730
- Minor symptoms in pregnancy — 730
  - Hyperemesis gravidarum — 730
  - Heartburn and acid regurgitation — 730
  - Constipation — 730
  - Back pain — 731
  - Pubic symphysis pain — 731
  - Vaginal discharge — 731
  - Pruritus — 731
  - Neuropathies — 731
  - Tiredness — 731
  - Breathlessness — 731
  - Palpitations — 731
- Major symptoms in pregnancy — 731
  - Change in fetal movements — 731
  - Vaginal bleeding — 732
  - Rupture of membranes — 732
  - Abdominal pain — 732
  - Headache — 732
  - Oedema — 732
- History — 732
  - Current pregnancy history — 734
  - Past obstetric history — 734
  - Past gynaecological history — 734
  - Past medical history — 734
  - Treatment history — 734
  - Social history — 735
  - Family history — 736
- Examination anatomy — 736
- Examination — 736
  - Positioning the patient — 736
  - General appearance — 736
  - Observations — 737
  - The abdomen: mother and fetal findings — 737
  - The genitals — 738
  - The lower limbs — 740
  - Urinalysis — 741
  - Obstetric ultrasound: a systematic approach — 741
- T&O'C essentials — 742
- OSCE revision topics – the obstetric history and examination — 742
- References — 742

CHAPTER 40
The gynaecological history and examination — 743

- History — 743
  - Presenting symptoms — 743
  - Menstrual history — 744
  - Sexual history — 750
  - Previous gynaecological history — 750
  - Previous medical history — 750
  - Family and social history — 750
- Examination — 752
  - Examination of the breasts — 752
  - Examination of the abdomen — 752

xviii CONTENTS

    Pelvic examination   752
    Rectal examination   762
OSCE revision topics – the gynaecological history and examination   762
T&O'C essentials   762
References   762

CHAPTER 41
The breasts: history and examination   763

    Examination anatomy   763
    History   763
    Examination   764
        Inspection   764
        Palpation   765
    Evaluation of a breast lump   766
T&O'C essentials   766
OSCE revision topics – the breasts   767
References   767

SECTION 12
SPECIALTY SYSTEM HISTORY AND EXAMINATION   769

CHAPTER 42
The eyes, ears, nose and throat   771

    Eyes   771
        Examination anatomy   771
        History   772
        Examination method   772
T&O'C essentials   775
T&O'C essentials   776
        Diplopia   778
        Horner's syndrome   778
        Iritis   780
        Glaucoma   780
        Shingles   781
        Eyelid   781
    Ears   782
        Examination anatomy   782
        History   783
        Examination method   785
T&O'C essentials   788
    Nose and sinuses   788
        Examination anatomy   788
        History   789
        Examination method   790
        Sinusitis   790
    Mouth and throat   791
        Examination anatomy   791
        History   792
        Examination method   792
        Pharyngitis   794
        Supraglottitis (epiglottitis)   795
    Common investigations   795
T&O'C essentials   796
OSCE examples   797
OSCE revision topics – eyes, ears, nose and throat   798
References   798

CHAPTER 43
The skin and lumps   799

    Examination anatomy   799
    Dermatological history   800
    General principles of physical examination of the skin   801
    How to approach the clinical diagnosis of a lump   804
    Correlation of physical signs and skin disease   806
        Pruritus   806
        Erythrosquamous eruptions   807
        Blistering eruptions   809
        Erythroderma   813
        Livedo reticularis   814
        Pustular and crusted lesions   814
        Dermal plaques   815
        Erythema nodosum   816
        Erythema multiforme (EM)   816
        Cellulitis and erysipelas   817
        Folliculitis, furuncles and carbuncles   818
        Other infections   818
        Hyperpigmentation, hypopigmentation and depigmentation   819
        Flushing and sweating   819
        Skin tumours   821
    The nails   823
T&O'C essentials   824
OSCE example – skin   825
References   825

CHAPTER 44
The older person assessment   826

    History taking in older persons: special considerations   826
    Physical examination in older persons: special considerations   830
        Dementia screening   833
OSCE revision topics – assessment of the geriatric patient   833
References   833

CHAPTER 45
Approaching infectious diseases — 834

- Pyrexia of unknown origin — 834
  - *History* — 835
  - *Examination* — 835
  - *Clinical scenarios for unexplained fever* — 836
- HIV infection and AIDS — 836
  - *History* — 837
  - *Examination* — 838
- T&O'C essentials — 840
- OSCE revision topics – infectious diseases — 841
- References — 841

SECTION 13
MENTAL HEALTH HISTORY AND EXAMINATION — 843

CHAPTER 46
The psychiatric history and mental state examination — 845

- The history — 845
- Obtaining the history — 846
  - *Introductory questions* — 846
  - *History of the presenting illness* — 846
  - *Past history and treatment history* — 851
  - *Family history* — 853
  - *Social and personal history* — 853
  - *Premorbid personality* — 854
- The mental state examination — 854
- The diagnosis — 854
- Examples of important psychiatric illnesses — 859
  - *Disorders that lead to physical illness* — 859
  - *Schizophrenia* — 860
  - *Depression* — 861
  - *Anxiety disorders* — 862
  - *Post-traumatic stress disorder (PTSD)* — 862
  - *Obsessive–compulsive disorder (OCD)* — 863
- T&O'C essentials — 863
- OSCE revision topics – the psychiatric history and the mental state examination — 863
- References — 863

SECTION 14
ACUTE CARE AND END OF LIFE — 865

CHAPTER 47
The acutely ill patient — 867

- Initial assessment — 867
- Level of consciousness — 867
- Delirium — 867
- Further examination — 868

- OSCE example – emergency care — 872
- References — 872

CHAPTER 48
The pre-anaesthetic medical evaluation (PAME) — 873

- The history — 873
  - *Cardiovascular history* — 873
  - *The respiratory history* — 874
  - *Other* — 874
- The examination — 874

CHAPTER 49
Assessment of death — 875

- Assessment — 875
  - *Do-not-resuscitate (DNR) orders* — 875
  - *Do not misdiagnose death* — 875
  - *Examining a suspected death* — 875
- Informing relatives — 876
- Completing the death certificate — 876
- Postmortem — 877
- Organ donation — 877

SECTION 15
ADULT HISTORY TAKING AND EXAMINATION IN THE WARDS AND CLINICS — 879

CHAPTER 50
Writing and presenting the adult history and physical examination — 881

- History — 881
- Physical examination (PE) — 882
- Provisional diagnosis — 882
- Problem list and plans — 882
- Continuation notes — 882
- Presentation — 882
- Reference — 885

CHAPTER 51
A suggested method for a rapid screening adult physical examination — 886

- Hands and arms — 886
- Face — 886
- Front of the neck — 886
- Chest — 886
- Back of the chest and neck — 886
- Abdomen — 887
- Legs — 887
- Neurological examination — 887
- Completing the examination — 888

Index — I-1

Preface

Acquire the art of detachment, the virtue of method, and the quality of thoroughness, but above all the grace of humility.

Ask not what disease the person has, but rather what person the disease has.

Sir William Osler

Welcome to the new edition of *Clinical Examination*, which has been carefully revised and updated. Clinical skills are the foundation of clinical medicine, most importantly history taking and physical examination. In most cases, a good history and physical examination will lead you to make the correct diagnosis, and this is critical—your diagnosis will more often than not seal the fate of your patient and, assuming you are correct, take them down the optimal management path.

In order to make a correct diagnosis you need to assemble all the facts at hand. Blindly ordering tests in the absence of the clinical history and relevant examination often leads to serious errors. It is distressingly common for tests to be ordered and referrals made without an adequate history or even a cursory examination of the patient. The wrong diagnosis can cause harm and distress that lasts a lifetime.

Clinical Examination is designed to take students on an exciting journey from acquiring core skills to an advanced level, applying a strong evidence-based focus. We have taken a systematic approach because recognition of all the facts aids accurate diagnosis. The patient presenting with, for example, heart disease may have not only objective changes of disease when listening to the heart but also relevant findings in the hands, arms, face, abdomen and legs that can guide identification of the underlying disease process and prognosis. Diagnosticians are great medical detectives who apply rigorous methodology to uncover the truth, solve a puzzle and commence the healing process.

Our book is not a traditional undergraduate textbook and we are proud of its distinctive features. Learning must be fun! Unlike most other similar textbooks, ours is deliberately laced with humour and historical anecdotes that generations of students have told us enhance the learning experience. Another distinguishing feature is that every chapter in this book has undergone peer review, just as you would expect would occur for any published journal article. We have believed from the beginning that peer review is integral to ensuring the highest possible standards and maximising the value of a core textbook. In this edition based on the peer review process we have made revisions, excluded irrelevant material and added updates where appropriate. Videos demonstrating techniques enhance the learning experience, and the e-book format supports learning from a tablet or computer anywhere and anytime. We are also proud of this book being current and as evidence based as is possible, with updated chapter references and annotations so readers can dive deeper into any of the literature that interests them. We want students at all levels to know there are many limitations and gaps (all crying out for more research), and to remain curious and excited about medicine as they learn.

Clinical skills can be mastered only by practice and you should aim to see as many cases as you can while studying from this or any book. You will learn from your patients your entire career if only you take the time to listen and observe.

Great clinicians are made not born, and everyone practising medicine needs to master clinical skills. Thank you to all those who have provided us with expert input as we have made our revisions. We also thank all of our colleagues and patients who educate us daily, and the legion of students who have written to us, including those who have pointed out omissions or mistakes (real or perceived).

Nicholas J Talley
Simon O'Connor
Newcastle and Canberra
July 2017

Acknowledgements

This book provides an evidence-based account of clinical skills. We are very grateful for the reviews, comments and suggestions from the many outstanding colleagues over the years who have helped us to develop and refine this book. All chapters have again been peer reviewed, a hallmark of our books, and we have taken great care to revise the material based on the detailed reviews obtained. We take responsibility for any errors or omissions.

We would like to especially acknowledge **Professor Ian Symonds**, Dean of Medicine, University of Adelaide, and **Professor Kichu Nair**, Professor of Medicine and Associate Dean Continuing Medical Professional Development, University of Newcastle, for producing the videos for the OSCEs.

Dr Tom Wellings, Staff Specialist in Neurology, John Hunter Hospital, provided expert input into the neurology chapters for this edition. **Dr Philip McManis** provided invaluable input into neurology for earlier editions.

Dr A Manoharan and **Dr J Isbister** provided the original blood film photographs and the accompanying text. **Associate Professor L Schreiber** provided the original section on soft-tissue rheumatology. We have revised and updated all of these sections again.

We thank **Professor Alex Ford** (Leeds Teaching Hospitals Trust, UK) and his team for their systematic review of the evidence supporting (or refuting) key clinical signs that has been retained.

Professor Brian Kelly, Dean of Medicine at the University of Newcastle, provided valuable comments on the psychiatry chapter.

Thank you to **Dr Malcolm Thomson** who provided a number of the X-rays and scans for this title. Others have been provided by the Medical Imaging Department at the Canberra Hospital X-ray Library. We would like to thank **Associate Professor Lindsay Rowe**, Staff Specialist Radiologist at the John Hunter Hospital, for preparing the text and images within the gastrointestinal system section retained from the last edition.

Associate Professor S Posen, **Associate Professor IPC Murray**, **Dr G Bauer**, **Dr E Wilmshurst**, **Dr J Stiel** and **Dr J Webb** helped us obtain many of the original photographs in earlier editions. We would like to acknowledge and thank **Glenn McCulloch** for the photographs he supplied for this title. A set of photographs come from the Mayo Clinic library and from FS McDonald (editor), *Mayo Clinic images in internal medicine: self-assessment for board exam review* (Mayo Clinic Scientific Press, Rochester MN & CRC Press, Boca Raton FL, 2004). We would like to thank the following from Mayo Clinic College of Medicine for their kind assistance in selecting additional photographic material: **Dr Ashok M Patel**, **Dr Ayalew Tefferi**, **Dr Mark R Pittelkow** and **Dr Eric L Matteson**. We would also like to acknowledge **Coleman Productions** who provided new photographs.

Dr Michael Potter and **Dr Stephen Brienesse** provided assistance with the clinical examination photographs.

Elsevier Australia and the authors also extend their appreciation to the following reviewers for their comments and insights on the entire manuscript:

REVIEWERS

Jessica Bale, BMedRadSc, MBBS, Conjoint Lecturer (Dermatology), University of Newcastle, NSW, Australia

Andrew Boyle, MBBS, PhD, FRACP, Professor of Cardiovascular Medicine, University of Newcastle and John Hunter Hospital, Newcastle, NSW, Australia

Judi Errey, BSc, MBBS, MRACGP, Senior Lecturer and Clinical Coordinator, University of Tasmania, TAS, Australia

Tom Goodsall, BSc, MBBS (Hons), Advanced Trainee Gastroenterology and General Medicine, John Hunter Hospital, NSW, Australia

Hadia Haikal-Mukhtar, MBBS (Melb), BSc Hons (Melb), LLB Hons (Melb), FRACGP, Dip Ger Med (Melb), Grad Cert Health Prof Ed (Monash), Head of Auburn Clinical School, School of Medicine, Sydney, University of Notre Dame Australia, NSW, Australia

Adam Harris, MBChB, MMed, Conjoint lecturer at the University of Newcastle, NSW, Australia

Rohan Jayasinghe, MBBS (Sydney; 1st Class Honours), FRACP, FCSANZ, PhD (UNSW), MSpM(UNSW), MBA(Newcastle), Medical Director, Cardiology Department, Gold Coast University Hospital, QLD, Australia; Professor of Cardiology, Griffith University, QLD, Australia; Clinical Professor of Medicine, Macquarie University, Sydney, NSW, Australia

Kelvin Kong, BSc MBBS (UNSW), FRACS (OHNS), VMO John Hunter Hospital, NSW, Australia

Kypros Kyprianou, MBBS, FRACP, Grad Dip Med Ed., Consultant Paediatrician, Monash Children's Hospital and Senior Lecturer, University of Melbourne, VIC, Australia

Judy Luu, MBBS, FRACP, MIPH, Staff Specialist, John Hunter Hospital, NSW; Conjoint Lecturer, University of Newcastle, NSW, Australia

Joy Lyneham, PhD, Associate Professor, Faculty of Health and Medicine, University of Newcastle, NSW, Australia

Genevieve McKew, MBBS, FRACP, FRCPA, Staff Specialist, Concord Repatriation General Hospital and Clinical Lecturer, Concord Clinical School University of Sydney, NSW, Australia

Balakrishnan R Nair (Kichu), AM MBBS, MD (Newcastle) FRACP, FRCPE, FRCPG, FRCPI, FANZSGM, GradDip Epid, Professor of Medicine and Deputy Dean (Clinical Affairs), School of Medicine and Public Health, Newcastle, Australia; Director, Centre for Medical Professional Development HNE Local Health District, Adjunct Professor University of New England, Armidale, Australia

Christine O'Neill, MBBS(Hons), FRACS, MS, VMO General Surgeon, John Hunter Hospital, Newcastle, NSW, Australia

Steven Oakley, MBBS, FRACP, PhD, Staff Specialist Rheumatologist, John Hunter Hospital, Newcastle, Australia; Conjoint Associate Professor, School of Medicine and Public Health, University of Newcastle, Australia

Robert Pickles, BMed (Hons), FRACP, Senior Staff Specialist Infectious Diseases and General Medicine, John Hunter Hospital, NSW, Australia; Conjoint Associate Professor, School of Medicine and Public Health, University of Newcastle, NSW, Australia

Philip Rowlings, MBBS, FRACP, FRCPA, MS, Director of Haematology, Calvary Mater Newcastle and John Hunter Hospital, NSW, Australia; Senior Staff Specialist Pathology North-Hunter, Professor of Medicine, University of Newcastle, Australia

Josephine Thomas, BMBS, FRACP, Senior Lecturer, University of Adelaide, SA, Australia

Alicia Thornton, BSc, MBBS (Hons), Conjoint Lecturer (Dermatology), University of Newcastle, NSW, Australia

Scott Twaddell, BMed, FRACP, FCCP, Senior Staff Specialist, Department of Respiratory and Sleep Medicine, John Hunter Hospital, NSW, Australia

Martin Veysey, MBBS, MD, MRCP(UK), FRACP, MClinEd, Professor of Gastroenterology, Hull York Medical School, UK

Tom Wellings, BSc(Med), MBBS, FRACP, Staff Specialist Neurologist, John Hunter Hospital, NSW, Australia

CONTRIBUTORS

Joerg Mattes, MBBS, MD, PhD, FRACP, Senior Staff Specialist, John Hunter Children's Hospital and Professor of Paediatrics, University of Newcastle, NSW, Australia

Bryony Ross, B.Biomed.Sc, MBBS, FRACP, FRCPA, Staff Specialist, Calvary Mater Newcastle, John Hunter Children's Hospital and Pathology North, NSW Australia; Conjoint Lecturer, School of Medicine and Public Health, University of Newcastle, NSW, Australia

Ian Symonds, MD, MMedSci, FRCOG, FRANZCOG, Dean of Medicine, University of Adelaide, SA, Australia

Clinical methods: an historical perspective

The best physician is the one who is able to differentiate the possible and the impossible.

Herophilus of Alexandria (335–280BC)

Since classical Greek times interrogation of the patient has been considered most important because disease was, and still is, viewed in terms of the discomfort it causes. However, the current emphasis on the use of history taking and physical examination for diagnosis developed only in the 19th century. Although the terms 'symptoms and signs' have been part of the medical vocabulary since the revival of classical medicine, until relatively recently they were used synonymously. During the 19th century, the distinction between *symptoms* (subjective complaints, which the clinician learns from the patient's account of his or her feelings) and *signs* (objective morbid changes detectable by the clinician) evolved. Until the 19th century, diagnosis was empirical and based on the classical Greek belief that all disease had a single cause: an imbalance of the four humours (yellow bile, black bile, blood and phlegm). Indeed the Royal College of Physicians, founded in London in 1518, believed that clinical experience without classical learning was useless, and physicians who were College members were fined if they ascribed to any other view. At the time of Hippocrates (460?–375BC), observation (inspection) and feeling (palpation) had a place in the examination of patients. The ancient Greeks, for example, noticed that patients with jaundice often had an enlarged liver that was firm and irregular. Shaking a patient and listening for a fluid splash was also recognised by the Greeks. Herophilus of Alexandria (335–280BC) described a method of taking the pulse in the 4th century BC. However, it was Galen of Pergamum (AD130–200) who established the pulse as one of the major physical signs, and it continued to have this important role up to the 18th century, with minute variations being recorded. These variations were erroneously considered to indicate changes in the body's harmony. William Harvey's (1578–1657) studies of the human circulation, published in 1628, had little effect on the general understanding of the value of the pulse as a sign. Sanctorius (1561–1636) was the first to time the pulse using a clock, while John Floyer (1649–1734) invented the pulse watch in 1707 and made regular observations of the pulse rate. Abnormalities in heart rate were described in diabetes mellitus in 1776 and in thyrotoxicosis in 1786. Fever was studied by Hippocrates and was originally regarded as an entity rather than a sign of disease. The thermoscope was devised by Sanctorius in 1625. In association with Gabriel Fahrenheit (1686–1736), Hermann Boerhaave (1668–1738) introduced the thermometer as a research instrument and this was produced commercially in the middle of the 18th century. In the 13th century Johannes Actuarius (d. 1283) used a graduated glass to examine the urine. In Harvey's time a specimen of urine was sometimes looked at (inspected) and even tasted, and was considered to reveal secrets about the body. Harvey recorded that sugar diabetes (mellitus) and dropsy (oedema) could be diagnosed in this way. The detection of protein in the urine, which Frederik Dekkers (1644–1720) first described in 1673, was ignored until Richard Bright (1789–1858) demonstrated its importance in renal disease. Although Celsus described and valued measurements such as weighing and measuring a patient in the 1st century AD, these methods became widely used only in the 20th century. A renaissance in clinical methods began with the concept of Battista Morgagni (1682–1771) that disease was not generalised but rather arose in organs, a conclusion published in 1761. Leopold Auenbrugger invented chest tapping (percussion) to detect disease in the same year. Van Swieten, his teacher, in fact used percussion to detect ascites. The technique was forgotten for nearly half a century until Jean Corvisart (1755–1821) translated Auenbrugger's work in 1808.

The next big step occurred with René Laënnec (1781–1826), a student of Corvisart. He invented the stethoscope in 1816 (at first merely a roll of stiff paper) as an aid to diagnosing heart and lung disease by listening (auscultation). This revolutionised chest examination, partly because it made the chest accessible in patients too modest to allow a direct application of the examiner's ear to the chest wall, as well as allowing accurate clinicopathological correlations. William Stokes (1804–78) published the first treatise in English on the use of the stethoscope in 1825. Josef Skoda's (1805–81) investigations of the value of these clinical methods led to their widespread and enthusiastic adoption after he published his results in 1839. These advances helped lead to a change in the practice of medicine. Bedside teaching was first introduced in the Renaissance by Montanus (1498–1552) in Padua in 1543. In the 17th century, physicians based their opinion on a history provided by an apothecary (assistant) and rarely saw the patients themselves. Thomas Sydenham (1624–89) began to practise more modern bedside medicine, basing his treatment on experience and not theory, but it was not until a century later that the scientific method brought a systematic approach to clinical diagnosis.

This change began in the hospitals of Paris after the French Revolution, with recognition of the work of Morgagni, Corvisart, Laënnec and others. Influenced by the philosophy of the Enlightenment, which suggested that a rational approach to all problems was possible, the Paris Clinical School combined physical examination with autopsy as the basis of clinical medicine. The methods of this school were first applied abroad in Dublin, where Robert Graves (1796–1853) and William Stokes worked. Later, at Guy's Hospital in London, the famous trio of Richard Bright, Thomas Addison (1793–1860) and Thomas Hodgkin (1798–1866) made their important contributions. In 1869 Samuel Wilks (1824–1911) wrote on the nail changes in disease and the signs he described remain important. Carl Wunderlich's (1815–77) work changed the concept of temperature from a disease in itself to a symptom of disease. Spectacular advances in physiology, pathology, pharmacology and the discovery of microbiology in the latter half of the 19th century led to the development of the new 'clinical and laboratory medicine', which is the rapidly advancing medicine of the present day. The modern systematic approach to diagnosis, with which this book deals, is still, however, based on taking the history and examining the patient by looking (inspecting), feeling (palpating), tapping (percussing) and listening (auscultating).

Suggested reading

Reiser SJ. The clinical record in medicine. Part I: Learning from cases. *Ann Intern Med* 1991; 114:902–907.

Bordage G. Where are the history and the physical? *Can Med Assoc J* 1995; 152:1595–1598.

McDonald C. Medical heuristics: the silent adjudicators of clinical practice. *Ann Intern Med* 1996; 124:56–62.

The Hippocratic oath

I swear by Apollo the physician, and Aesculapius, and Hygieia, and Panacea, and all the gods and goddesses that, according to my ability and judgment, I will keep this Oath and this stipulation: To reckon him who taught me this Art equally dear to me as my parents, to share my substance with him and relieve his necessities if required; to look upon his offspring in the same footing as my own brother, and to teach them this Art, if they shall wish to learn it, without fee or stipulation, and that by precept, lecture, and every other mode of instruction, I will impart a knowledge of the Art to my own sons and those of my teachers, and to disciples bound by a stipulation and oath according to the law of medicine, but to none others. I will follow that system of regimen which, according to my ability and judgment, I consider for the benefit of my patients, and abstain from whatever is deleterious and mischievous. I will give no deadly medicine to any if asked, nor suggest any such counsel; and in like manner I will not give a woman a pessary to produce abortion. With purity and with holiness I will pass my life and practise my Art. I will not cut persons laboring under the stone, but will leave this to be done by men who are practitioners of this work. Into whatever houses I enter I will go into them for the benefit of the sick and will abstain from every voluntary act of mischief and corruption; and further from the seduction of females or males, of freemen and slaves. Whatever, in connection with my professional practice, or not in connection with it, I may see or hear in the lives of men which ought not to be spoken of abroad I will not divulge, as reckoning that all such should be kept secret. While I continue to keep this Oath unviolated may it be granted to me to enjoy life and the practice of the Art, respected by all men, in all times! But should I trespass and violate this Oath, may the reverse be my lot!

Hippocrates, born on the Island of Cos (c.460–357 BC) is agreed by everyone to be the father of medicine. He is said to have lived to the age of 109. Many of the statements in this ancient oath remain relevant today, while others, such as euthanasia and abortion, remain controversial. The seduction of slaves, however, is less of a problem.

SECTION 10
Paediatric and neonatal history and examination

CHAPTER 37
The paediatric history and examination
Joerg Mattes and Bryony Ross

CHAPTER 38
The neonatal history and examination
Joerg Mattes and Bryony Ross

CHAPTER 37
The paediatric history and examination
Joerg Mattes and Bryony Ross

Medicine cannot exist without observation of the patient. HIPPOCRATES (460?–357BC)

PRINCIPLES OF PAEDIATRIC HISTORY TAKING AND EXAMINATION

Children are not simply little adults: the history taking and physical examination of these little people needs to be tailored to their specific needs. Like the neonatal examination (and often more so) physical examination in childhood is opportunistic: trying slavishly to follow a set sequence will almost always end in frustration and tears for the clinician, the parents and, most importantly, the child. Much of the paediatric examination is, however, identical or very similar to that of the adult. To avoid unnecessary repetition, this chapter focuses mainly on where the paediatric examination differs from that of the adult examination.

In contrast to the neonatal examination, there is no consensus regarding the timing and regularity of the paediatric examination. Many clinicians use the immunisation schedule as a convenient routine for the evaluation of children in their care. The American Academy of Paediatrics suggests that every school-aged child should have a complete physical examination and health evaluation every 1–2 years.[1]

The principal aims of well-child examination in school-aged children (kindergarten to early adolescence) are:[2]
- promoting health
- detecting disease
- counselling to prevent injury and future health problems.

It is generally accepted that children should have a physical examination every time they present to a clinician. These examinations should not be restricted to the part of the body considered to be the basis of the presenting complaint, although they should be concentrated on that area or body system, as in adults. The purpose and scope of the examination need to be explained to the parents and child (particularly to adolescents) and should take into account their level of understanding. If any part of the examination will be physically or psychologically uncomfortable, the parents and child should be informed in advance.[3]

PAEDIATRIC HISTORY TAKING

The paediatric history is somewhat unique in medicine in that in most cases it is given by someone other than the patient—this is usually one or both parents. Children and teenagers, however, have much to say—their input in the history is extremely useful. It is important to involve children in this process, but their level of maturity must be taken into account. If the child is old enough to have some understanding of what is going on, it is best to direct simple questions to the child but in many cases to expect that the parent will answer or even repeat the question to the child, almost as an interpreter. In many cases it may be preferable to interview adolescents without their parents at some point. Reassuring the adolescent at the start of the consultation that matters discussed will be kept confidential is a must.[4] Equally important, however, is also explaining to the adolescent when this confidentiality *may* be broken. (See 'Screening of development and social interactions' below and Table 37.1.)

HEADSSS assessment	
Home	Who, where, recent moves, relationships, violence
Education and employment	Where, attendance, year, performance, relationships, supports, recent moves, bullying, disciplinary actions, future plans, work details
Eating	Weight (heaviest, lightest, recent changes), dieting, exercise, menstrual history, restricted eating, binging, purging
Activities	Outside of school: sport, organised groups, clubs, parties, TV/computer use
Alcohol and drugs	Cigarettes, alcohol and illicit drug use by friends, family and patient, patterns and frequency of use, regrets from using substances, how use is financed, problems it has caused
Sexuality	Close relationships, sexual experiences, number of partners (total and in the last 3 months), gender of sexual partners (don't assume sexual preferences), uncomfortable situations/sexual abuse, risk of pregnancy and previous pregnancies (relevant to males as well as females), contraception, condoms, sexually transmissible infections (STIs)
Suicide, depression and self-harm	Presence and frequency of feeling down or sad as well as current feelings (e.g. 'How do you feel in yourself at the moment on a scale of 1 to 10?'), actions when down, supports, self-harm (thoughts and actions), suicide (thoughts, attempts, plans and means), hopes for future
Safety from injury and violence	Serious injuries, use of safety gear for sports and driving, riding with an intoxicated driver, exposure to violence at school and in neighbourhood, online (cyber) safety; for high-risk youths: carrying or use of weapons, other criminal behaviour, incarceration of family or friends

(Royal Children's Hospital, Melbourne, Australia, *Clinical Practice Guideline on Engaging with and assessing the adolescent patient*, [Internet, cited 15th March 2017], Available from: www.rch.org.au/clinicalguide/guideline_index/Engaging_with_and_assessing_the_adolescent_patient/#headds.)

TABLE 37.1

History-taking sequence

1. Review the history of the presenting chief complaints under the following headings using the mnemonic **SIC**:
   S ymptoms [severity, frequency, triggers, treatments]
   I nvestigations
   C omplications.
2. Then address any other concerns raised by the patient or the parents.
3. Perform a systems review, which is useful to cover any information that may have been omitted. It is often easiest for this to be remembered as a 'top-to-toe' checklist of questions to ask the carer (and the child as appropriate, according to the developmental stage) or young person (see Text box 37.1).
4. Next collect the antenatal and birth history (see Ch 38).
5. Ask about medications (including dose, frequency and adherence), relevant environmental exposures (e.g. tobacco smoke).
6. Ask whether immunisations are up to date (see www.immunise.health.gov.au for the current Australian vaccination schedule).
7. Find out whether there are any known drug allergies. Ask about other allergies and/or intolerances. Ask specifically about food allergies, asthma, eczema and hay fever.
   Ask whether there is a family history of inherited diseases. Are the child's parents related (consanguinity)?
8. Have there been unexplained premature deaths in the family?
9. Explore the psychosocial history by asking questions using the mnemonic **BEST CARE**:
   BEhavioural history: this should cover any unusual behaviours (such as frequent temper tantrums), sleep disturbances or phobias, and toileting problems (such as encopresis[a] and bed wetting).
   Screening of development and social interactions: a quick developmental surveillance in the school-aged child should

---
[a] Faecal incontinence of psychological cause.

The top-to-toe checklist

System	Sample questions
Head	Does your child have headaches? Has your child ever hurt his or her head?
Eyes	Does your child have blurred vision or double vision?
Ears	Have your child's ears been sore? Has your child ever had an ear infection or muck coming out of the ears?
Nose	Does your child have problems with a bleeding nose? Does anything other than snot ever come out of your child's nose? (Discharge) Does your child snore loudly?
Mouth and throat	Has your child ever had trouble swallowing food or drinks? Does your child brush their teeth after eating?
Neck	Have you ever noticed any lumps in your child's neck? If so, were they sore? Stable in size on growing? (Lymphadenopathy) Does your child have trouble keeping their neck straight? (Torticollis)
Chest	Does your child get more short of breath than his or her friends when playing sport? Does your child get wheezy? Does your child have problems with a cough? Does your child cough anything up?
Abdomen	Does your child often vomit or get pains in the tummy? Has your child had problems with runny poo when going to the toilet? Does your child sometimes find it difficult to do a poo?
Genitourinary	Does your child have pain when passing urine? Has there ever been blood in your child's urine? *For girls:* Have you ever noticed any discharge from your vagina? At what age did your periods begin? Tell me about your periods: are they painful? Do they occur regularly? Is there much blood? Are you sexually active?
Endocrine	Has your child been drinking more water lately? Does your child need to urinate at night? Has your child had more or less energy lately?
Neurological	Has your child had problems with dizziness? Tell me what it feels like. Has your child ever had a fit? Have you noticed weakness in your child's arms or legs?
Skin	Has your child had any rashes on the skin? Are they itchy? Does your child get many bruises?

TEXT BOX 37.1

cover school performance, vision, hearing, speech, gross- and fine-motor function, and social interaction. A more structured screening can be of particular importance in adolescents (HEADSSS assessment). Ideally, this should be performed without the parents present and, again, concepts around confidentiality should be explained and respected (see Table 37.1).

Typical day: asking the parents to describe a typical day can give an idea of their living conditions and social history. Also check the child's habits regarding physical activity, food and diet, sleep, dental care practices and safety (e.g. use of bike helmets, seatbelts).

Coping with hospitalisation and / or disease: explore how well the parents understand the current situation and their expectations for the future.

Access to healthcare: find out whether the family lives in a remote area, or has transport available.

Relationships: discuss how members of the family get on with each other, extended family support and any alternative care arrangements. Is the child in foster care? Who are the primary carers? Does the child spend time between family members?

Effect of illness on the child and family: find out how limitations in physical, cognitive, emotional, and social functioning and the dependence on services impact on the child, siblings and parents. This is particularly important in children and teenagers with chronic medical and/or neurodevelopmental conditions (e.g. cerebral palsy, autism, Down's syndrome).

10. Conclude the history by ensuring that you and the family have a shared understanding of what the main issues are. Ask the family whether there are any other concerns or issues that haven't been covered so far.

GENERAL PHYSICAL EXAMINATION

(For a general summary see Text box 37.2.)

Preparing for the examination

Before you start the physical examination, roll up your sleeves to above the elbow. Hand hygiene is crucial for the prevention of cross-infection and nosocomial[b] infections. Clean your hands and forearms with ethanol-based hand disinfectant or soap and water before and after contact with children, before and after any procedure or exposure to bodily fluids and after touching the child's surroundings. It is generally advised that you do not sit on the patient's bed when you see the child as a hospital inpatient. However, a child-friendly approach may sometimes necessitate that this rule be broken. Ideally, one should wear examination gloves and other personal protective equipment when indicated so as to avoid cross-infection. Clean your examination tools (e.g. stethoscope) thoroughly with appropriate antimicrobial agents before and after use as recommended by the manufacturer.

Moving a settled, happy child from the parent's lap to start an examination may cause significant distress. This can make an already potentially challenging examination all the more difficult! Feel free to begin the examination where the child is most comfortable. **Engaging the child with play, and establishing rapport, is a key first step.** In an ideal situation, the child should be examined undressed to his or her underwear, but this may not always be possible for small children and may cause significant distress to the adolescent patient. It is preferable for the parents to undress the young child when this is necessary.

Always consider examining adolescents fully clothed, and ask them to undress only if necessary for particular parts of the examination (e.g. the skin). Sometimes getting the older child to change in private into a hospital-type gown may help. Parents should be present for the examination of a child. Always offer to have a chaperone present for physical examination of an adolescent if the child does not want the parents present or they are absent.[3]

Examination
Observation

Much information can be gathered by observing the young child, either sitting in the parent's lap or playing on the floor. Assess the child's state of wellbeing (does the child look sick or well, under- or overnourished? How active is he or she?). Note any asymmetry of movement or abnormal posturing, and evaluate the child's skin colour and breathing pattern. Observe the way the child interacts with the parents and with other people.

Take time to allow the child to become acquainted and comfortable with you. As mentioned, much of the examination can be performed with the child in the parent's lap—usually the place where the child is likely to feel the most safe. Be prepared to play with, be silly with and interact with the child in a friendly, calm and quiet manner wherever possible. Some age-appropriate toys (well cleaned between patients) can be very helpful; when all else fails, using a bubble wand to blow a few well-timed bubbles should soothe and win over even the most upset child. Never forget to warm your hands before touching a child.

Whereas the young child may be most comfortable on the parent's lap, slightly older children usually sit

---

[b] This means an infection acquired when a person is under medical care—usually in hospital.

The paediatric history and examination: a suggested method

1. **Preparation**
   a. Wash your hands.
   b. Wear personal protective equipment (PPE) if indicated.
2. **Measurements**
   a. Document the child's weight, height and head circumference and plot on the appropriate growth chart.
   b. Calculate body mass index (BMI) in the older child.
   c. Look for disproportional growth.
   d. Measure vital parameters (blood pressure, pulse and respiratory rate, temperature).
3. **General inspection**
   Observe the child, either sitting in the parent's lap or playing to assess the child's state of wellbeing, asymmetry of movement, abnormal posturing and spontaneous movements.
4. **Upper and lower limbs**
   a. Examine limbs individually and then compare for size disparity and deformities, swelling, tenderness, tone, strength, flexibility and range of movement.
   b. Inspect nails and palms.
5. **Back**
   Inspect spine for neural tube defects, scoliosis and lumbar hyperlordosis.
6. **Skin**
   Look out for petechiae, bruising, rash, lesions and masses.
7. **Head**
   a. Inspect hair.
   b. Palpate for craniosynostosis, bony and soft-tissue masses.
8. **Neck**
   a. Feel for nodes and masses.
   b. Palpate the thyroid gland.
   c. Check range of active movement.
9. **Face and dysmorphology**
   a. Note face shape and symmetry.
   b. Carefully inspect eyes, nose, mandible, mouth and lips for dysmorphic features.
   c. Look out for cleft lip and palate and check size of tongue.
   d. Note abnormal ear size and shape or unusual folding.
10. **Neurological system**
    a. Examine cranial nerves.
    b. Perform 180° examination in infants and small children.
    c. Examine gait.
    d. Determine tone, power, reflexes, coordination and sensation at all four extremities.
11. **Developmental assessment**
    Assess vision, hearing, fine-motor and gross-motor skills, social interaction and language.
12. **Lymphatic system**
    Assess for lymphadenopathy, large spleen and tonsils.
13. **Respiratory and cardiac systems**
    a. Inspect chest for deformity and scars and signs of respiratory distress.
    b. Auscultate for stridor, wheeze and crackles.
    c. Percuss for dullness or hyperresonance.
    d. Check capillary refill.
    e. Palpate pulses of all four limbs and localise the apex heartbeat.
    f. Auscultate the heart sounds.
14. **Abdominal system**
    a. Inspect for distension, epigastric peristalsis, masses and scars.
    b. Auscultate for bowel sounds and bruits.
    c. Palpate for masses, tenderness and organomegaly.
    d. Percuss for ascites and to measure organ size.
15. **Genitourinary system**
    a. Inspect skin for lesions and location of the urethral meatus.
    b. Palpate the scrotum for both testes, hernias and abnormal masses.
    c. Visualise the labia, clitoris, urethral meatus and vaginal introitus.
    d. Inspect the anus.
    e. Tanner staging.
16. **Ear, nose and throat (last, but not least)**
    a. Inspect ears for size, shape and position, and malformations.
    b. Perform otoscopy.
    c. Examine the mouth for stomatitis, ulcers, pallor and cyanosis.
    d. Visualise the oropharynx and palatine tonsils.

TEXT BOX 37.2

happily on an examination table or bed with the examiner to one side and the parents to the other side. Approach the child in a friendly, gentle, patient way. Asking the child to show you his or her hands and praising the child for doing so often builds some trust, which allows you to start with some non-frightening palpation (e.g. brachial pulses) and gentle manoeuvres (e.g. turning the hands and inspecting the palms) before proceeding to the head-to-toe examination. Lastly, if in the hospital setting, much can be gained by a quick glance and visual exploration of the room, especially for children and teenagers with chronic medical conditions or prolonged hospital stays.

Measurements

In addition to documenting the child's **weight**, **height** and **head circumference** at the well-child examinations, it is prudent to check and document these measurements every time the child presents for review. These measurements are crucially important for the detection of serious pathologies and the monitoring of growth and development. Plot the results on the appropriate growth charts: it is generally standard practice to use gender-specific, height-for-age, weight-for-age and head-circumference charts (see Fig. 37.1). There are special growth charts for children with certain syndromic diagnoses (e.g. Down's syndrome).

For children who do not walk, recumbent length is measured rather than height. A sitting height can also be useful in some situations (see below). It is best to use a stable, accurate, fixed measuring device wherever possible.

For an accurate weight to be determined, children should be undressed (underwear for older children; nappy for infants). The nappy weight needs to be considered when calculating the accurate weight. Also do not forget to remove the child's shoes and socks.

A method for measuring an accurate head circumference is outlined in Chapter 38. It may be important to measure the head circumference of both parents if benign familial macrocephaly is suspected. Head shape and craniosynostosis are explained later in this chapter.

Body mass index (BMI; see Ch 3) and waist circumference are used less in children than in adults, but can be useful tools, particularly in adolescents. BMI and growth velocity centile charts are available from the World Health Organization and should be used wherever possible. Recent studies suggest that **waist circumference** may be more useful than BMI for the assessment of Indigenous children.[5]

Other anthropometric measurements that may be useful, particularly in children who are at risk of growth failure (e.g. children with feeding difficulties, chronic illness or social difficulties), include mid-upper arm circumference and skinfold measurements, although these are rarely performed in routine practice.

Mid-upper arm circumference: first remove any clothing that may be covering the child's arm. Estimate the midpoint of the arm and use a tape measure to determine the circumference. This is usually easier with the arm lying flat against the patient's side and with the tape neither too tight nor too loose. A measurement of less than 11 centimetres in a child over 6 months old usually indicates malnutrition.[6]

Skinfold measurements: these are usually taken from the triceps and subscapular region. Using a skinfold calliper, measure the thickness of a fold of skin and underlying subcutaneous tissue (*not* muscle; see Fig. 37.2). Skinfold measurements can be compared with population averages.

Measuring the triceps skinfold

(From Wilson SF, Giddens JF. *Health assessment for nursing practice*, 4th edn. St Louis, MO: Mosby, 2009.)

FIGURE 37.2

Text continued on p 633

CHAPTER 37 THE PAEDIATRIC HISTORY AND EXAMINATION 625

FIGURE 37.1

FIGURE 37.1, cont'd

CHAPTER 37 THE PAEDIATRIC HISTORY AND EXAMINATION 627

FIGURE 37.1, cont'd

FIGURE 37.1, cont'd

CHAPTER 37 THE PAEDIATRIC HISTORY AND EXAMINATION 629

FIGURE 37.1, cont'd

630 SECTION 10 PAEDIATRIC AND NEONATAL HISTORY AND EXAMINATION

Weight-for-age GIRLS
Birth to 5 years (percentiles)

WHO Child Growth Standards

FIGURE 37.1, cont'd

CHAPTER 37 THE PAEDIATRIC HISTORY AND EXAMINATION 631

FIGURE 37.1, cont'd

632 SECTION 10 PAEDIATRIC AND NEONATAL HISTORY AND EXAMINATION

FIGURE 37.1, cont'd

Tall and short stature

Once a child's height (or length) is accurately measured and plotted, three further considerations need to take place: (1) is the child tall or short (above or below the upper/lower centiles for age and sex), (2) what is the trend or trajectory over time, and (3) what are the biological parents' heights?

The mid-parental height can be determined to give an idea of the child's growth potential:

For males:
$$\frac{(\text{mother's height in cm} + \text{father's height in cm}) + 13\,\text{cm}}{2}$$

For females:
$$\frac{(\text{mother's height in cm} + \text{father's height in cm}) - 13\,\text{cm}}{2}$$

The child would be expected to grow to within 2 standard deviations, or approximately 9 centimetres, of the number obtained from this equation.

When performing routine measurements in children, look for disproportionate growth and be aware of the extra measurements that can be taken (e.g. **upper and lower segment lengths**) if this is suspected. This is particularly important if there are concerns that the child may have short stature (e.g. caused by a 'chondroplasic' disorder). For example, a child with 'achrondroplasia' may have a normal sitting height, but have a marked reduction in standing height. Generally, at birth the normal upper-to-lower segment ratio is 1.7:1 and by the age of 10 the segments should be equal (and remain so into adulthood).[7]

Measurement of upper and lower segment lengths: the lower segment is measured from the symphysis pubis to the floor in the standing child; to calculate the upper segment, subtract the lower segment length from the total height.

In most children with short stature the cause is hereditary short stature, so parental height should always be taken into account. As with other growth parameters, if a child's height was previously within a healthy range and is now crossing height centiles *downwards* this is usually more cause for concern than a child who has followed the same, albeit lower, centile.

A wide range of diagnoses are associated with short stature, including nutritional deficiencies (see below), chromosomal abnormalities (such as trisomy 21 or Turner's syndrome), skeletal dysplasias (such as achondroplasia), metabolic disorders (e.g. Hunter's or Hurler's syndrome), endocrinopathies (such as hypothyroidism, Cushing's syndrome or primary pituitary disease) and iatrogenic causes (such as craniospinal irradiation in childhood for malignancy).

Pathological tall stature is less common, but causes include Klinefelter's syndrome, Marfan's syndrome, gigantism, thyrotoxicosis and Beckwith–Wiedemann syndrome.

Vital signs

These (blood pressure, pulse and respiratory rates, temperature) should be measured at each presentation, particularly if the child is unwell.

Blood pressure

The American Academy of Pediatrics recommends routine blood pressure measurements for children from the age of 3 years.[8] The blood pressure cuff should be appropriate for the child's size (the width of the cuff bladder should equal 40% of the mid-upper arm circumference; see Fig. 37.3(a) and (b)).[9] It is best measured after the child has been sitting quietly for 5 minutes, although this is seldom possible in practice. An automatic sphygmomanometer is often used for screening, but auscultation is more precise. Listen with the diaphragm of the stethoscope over the brachial artery pulse, proximal and medial to the cubital fossa (see Fig. 37.3(c)). Systolic pressure is indicated by the appearance of the first Korotkoff sound and diastolic by the fifth Korotkoff sound (the cessation of all sound) (pp 82, 669).

Hypertension is not common in children and is usually indicative of an underlying disease, such as renal disease or cardiovascular disease. However, primary hypertension is increasingly seen in morbidly obese children and adolescents.[10] One should compare a patient's systolic and diastolic measurements with

634 SECTION 10 PAEDIATRIC AND NEONATAL HISTORY AND EXAMINATION

(a, b) Determining the proper cuff size.
(c) Measuring the blood pressure

(From Hockenberry MJ, Wilson D. *Wong's essentials of pediatric nursing*, 8th edn. St Louis, MO: Mosby, 2009.)

FIGURE 37.3

Blood pressure values requiring further evaluation, according to age and sex

	Male Systolic (mmHg)	Male Diastolic (mmHg)	Female Systolic (mmHg)	Female Diastolic (mmHg)
3	100	59	100	61
4	102	62	101	64
5	104	65	103	66
6	105	68	104	68
7	106	70	106	69
8	107	71	108	71
9	109	72	110	72
10	111	73	112	73
11	113	74	114	74
12	115	74	116	75
13	117	75	117	76
14	120	75	119	77
15	120	76	120	78
16	120	78	120	78
17	120	80	120	78
18	120	80	120	80

(Kaelber DC, Pickett F. Simple table to identify children and adolescents needing further evaluation of blood pressure. *Pediatrics* 2009; 123:e972e4. With permission of the American Academy of Pediatrics.)

TABLE 37.2

population data tables—that are age, sex and sometimes height matched—in order to diagnose hypertension accurately.[11]

Hypotension is also uncommon in children, but it warrants rapid evaluation to exclude hypovolaemia or sepsis, which can lead to shock (circulatory failure; see Table 37.2). Remember, hypotension is a *late sign* in critically ill children with other signs often present prior to hypotension (e.g. tachycardia, pallor, mottled skin).

Pulse and respiratory rates
In childhood, a **wide pulse pressure** may be seen in patients with patent ductus arteriosus, aortic regurgitation and hyperthyroidism. The most common causes of a **narrow pulse pressure** are subaortic and aortic valve stenosis. Again, it is better to count the pulse than to use an automated system, and the pulse is usually easily palpated in most children, so there are

no excuses. Many clinicians find the brachial or femoral pulses easier to feel in infants and small children, although the radial or carotid pulse can also be used. It is particularly hard to feel a carotid pulse in infants and small children as they have a proportionally large head and a small, short neck.

The **heart rate** changes with age. Figure 37.4 shows the range of resting heart rates for children of different ages.

Accurate **respiratory rate** determination can also be tricky in children and ideally should be taken when the child is awake but at rest (see Fig. 37.5). By far the most common cause of an elevated respiratory rate in children is respiratory disease, but severe infection and cardiac and metabolic disorders should be considered. Toxins and raised intracranial pressure can depress the respiratory rate.

Pulse oximetry is becoming more and more common in the routine assessment of children (and almost universal as part of the neonatal examination—see Ch 38) and this allows for a simple, non-invasive and reasonably accurate estimation of arterial oxygen saturation.[11] Normal oxygen saturation (S_aO_2) values in paediatrics have not been established and are known to vary with altitude, but it is generally accepted that in healthy children (at sea level) the normal range for S_aO_2 is 97–100%.[12]

Temperature

There is considerable debate about the best method for checking the temperature in infants and children. It is important to remember that there can be a significant difference in each recording with different thermometers.[13] It used to be common practice to measure children's temperatures in the rectum, but this experience can be frightening for small children and may be psychologically harmful for older children.[14] Taking the temperature in the axilla is a reasonable alternative but **tympanic thermometry** is now commonly used. It is easy and quick to take the temperature from the ear and the reading is closely correlated with core body temperature (see Table 37.3 for normal values). Mercury thermometers should be avoided, and an oral temperature should be considered only in children who are capable of understanding the procedure (from about 6 years of age).

Specific physical examinations

Upper and lower limbs (legs and arms)

When examining the upper and lower limbs, remember to examine the limbs individually and then to compare

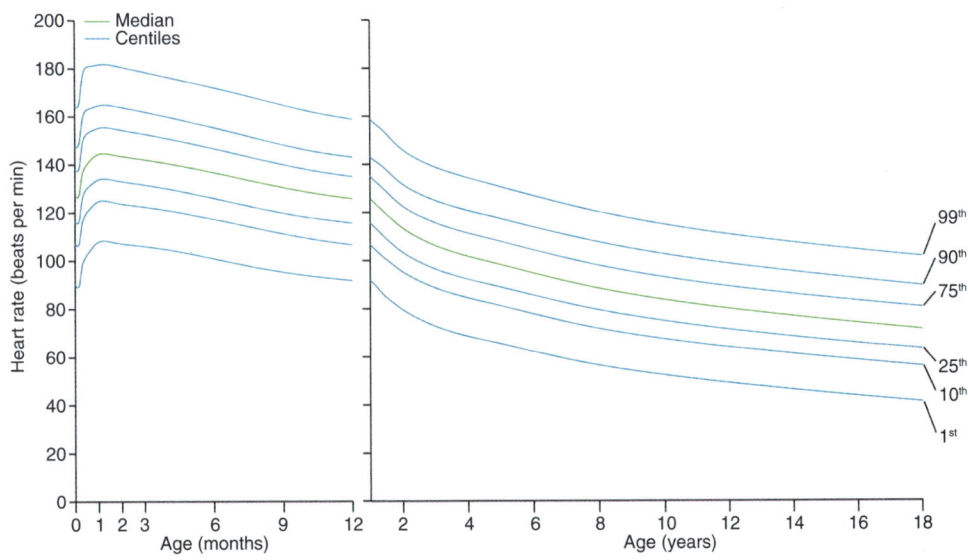

Heart rate and age

(From Fleming S, Thompson M, Stevens R et al. Normal ranges of heart rate and respiratory rate in children from birth to 18 years of age: a systematic review of observational studies. *Lancet* 2011; 377(9770):1011–1018, with permission.)

FIGURE 37.4

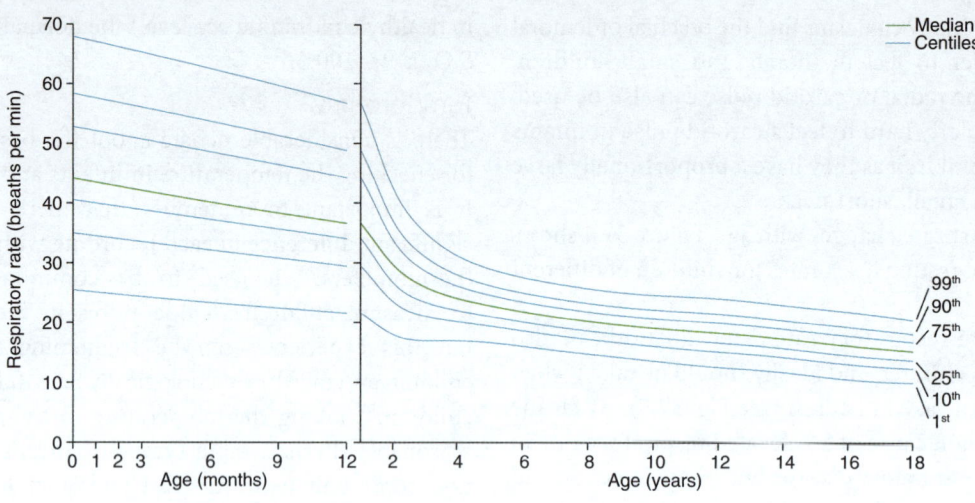

Respiratory rate and age

(From Fleming S, Thompson M, Stevens R et al. Normal ranges of heart rate and respiratory rate in children from birth to 18 years of age: a systematic review of observational studies. *Lancet* 2011; 377(9770):1011–1018, with permission.)

FIGURE 37.5

Normal temperatures at different sites

Body site	Type of thermometer	Normal range, mean (°C)	Elevated body temperature or fever (°C)
Axilla	Hg in glass, electronic	34.7–37.3, 36.4	37.4
Sublingual	Hg in glass, electronic	35.5–37.5, 36.6	37.6
Rectal	Hg in glass, electronic	36.6–37.9, 37.0	38.0
Ear	Infrared emission	35.7–37.5, 36.6	37.6

(Chamberlain JM, Terndrup TE. New light on ear thermometer readings. *Contemp Pediatr* 1994; 11(3):66–76.)

TABLE 37.3

both limbs, particularly when checking for size disparity (e.g. hemihyperplasia). Ask the child whether he or she is sore anywhere before beginning the examination.

Look

On the dorsal surface of the hands, examine the skin, joints and nails before turning the hands over to examine the palms, taking particular care to check the palmar creases. Examine the nails for any abnormalities (e.g. pitted nails in psoriasis, fungal infection) and the interdigital webbing for any lesions (e.g. scabies).

Feel

Note any areas of increased heat (particularly over joints), tenderness (e.g. dermatomyositis) or swelling. A hot, swollen joint with limited and/or painful movement could signify septic arthritis, juvenile arthritis or rheumatic fever (the latter especially in the Indigenous child population).

Move and measure

Gently move the wrist and finger joints through their respective ranges of motion, looking for flexibility, asymmetry and any unusual positions. Thus if there appears to be restriction of movement in any joint, make a note of the degree of movement possible.

If there is a suggestion of hypermobility, consider calculating the Beighton score in children over the age of 6 years:

1. One point if while standing forwards bending the patient can place his or her palms on the ground with legs straight
2. One point for each elbow that bends backwards
3. One point for each knee that bends backwards
4. One point for each thumb that touches the forearm when bent backwards
5. One point for each little finger that bends backwards beyond 90° (see Fig. 37.6).

This score can be used to formulate whether the child has **benign joint hypermobility syndrome (BJHS)** using the Brighton criteria (http://hypermobility.org/help-advice/hypermobility-syndromes/the-brighton-score/) or needs further investigation for other conditions associated with joint hypermobility (e.g. Marfan's syndrome, Ehlers–Danlos syndrome).

Examine the feet in a similar manner.

Look
Examine the proximal upper and lower limbs for asymmetry and deformity.

Feel
Note muscle bulk (atrophy, hypertrophy), swelling, heat and tenderness.

Move and measure
Measure tone, strength, flexibility and range of movement.

Look for any bony or joint deformities, masses or dysmorphic features. Deformities of the feet and knee are quite common. See Chapter 38 to review common deformities of the foot. The main deformities seen at the knee are genu varum (bow legs) (see Fig. 37.7) and genu valgum (knock-knees), both of which *may be normal at certain ages* (i.e. physiologically normal or normal, non-pathological, anatomical variation) and usually correct spontaneously (see Fig. 37.7(c)). Unilateral deformity, however, is less likely to be physiological and requires investigation.

Genu varum (bow legs; see Fig. 37.7)
Genu varum is common in normal children under the age of 2 years.

Ask the child to stand with the feet together and measure the **intercondylar** distance.

Pathological causes include rickets, skeletal dysplasias or Blout's disease (unilateral closure of the proximal medial tibial growth plate).

Genu valgum (knock-knees; see Fig. 37.8)
Genu valgum is common in normal young children (usually between the ages of 3 and 7 years).

Ask the child to stand and compare the limb lengths, then measure the **intermalleolar** distance.

If this condition is persistent beyond the age of 7 or increasing deformity is seen before this age, underlying causes should be sought (again, rickets and skeletal dysplasia are the usual cause).

Adolescent genu valgum is an idiopathic disorder seen after the age of 8 years.

Calculating the Beighton score

((c) Hypermobility Syndromes Association, http://hypermobility.org/help-advice/hypermobility-syndromes/beighton-score.)

FIGURE 37.6

638 SECTION 10 PAEDIATRIC AND NEONATAL HISTORY AND EXAMINATION

(a, b) Genu varum; (c) shows the same toddler in (b), with the deformity corrected

((a) and (b) from Scoles P. *Pediatric orthopedics in clinical practice*. Chicago: Year Book Medical Publishers, 1982, p 84; (c) from Macnicol MF. *Orthopaedics and Trauma* 2010; 24(5):369–380.)

FIGURE 37.7

Genu valgum

(From Macnicol MF. *Orthopaed Trauma* 2010; 24(5):369–380.)

FIGURE 37.8

CHAPTER 37 THE PAEDIATRIC HISTORY AND EXAMINATION 639

In-toeing

(From Harris E. The intoeing child: etiology, prognosis, and current treatment options. *Clin Podiatr Med Surg* 2013; 30(4):531–565.)

FIGURE 37.9

Leg length discrepancy

(From Herring JA. *Tachdjian's pediatric orthopaedics*. Philadelphia: Saunders, 2008, Ch 24, pp 1191–1271.)

FIGURE 37.10

Look for **toeing in** (**metatarsus varus**; see Fig. 37.9), which is physiological in the young child (aged 2 to 5 years), but may require correction in the older child, and **toeing out** (**metatarsus valgus**), which may require surgical correction as it *does not* self-correct with time.[15]

If there is limitation of **movement**, consider whether this is due to pain, weakness, contractures or spasticity.

It is also useful to **measure** for **limb length** discrepancies, although a small discrepancy (up to 2 centimetres) is common once patients have reached adulthood. There are two measurements traditionally used for this purpose:

1. *The true leg length*: measure from the anterior superior iliac spine to the medial malleolus.
2. *The apparent leg length*: measure from the pubic symphysis to the medial malleolus.

Clinically, it is more reliable to assess the posterior iliac crest level while the child stands with the knees and hips extended and to use blocks placed under the foot until the pelvis is level (then measure the height of the block; see Fig. 37.10).

Limb length discrepancies (true leg length discrepancy >2 cm) can be seen in hemihypertrophy syndromes such as Beckwith–Wiedemann syndrome.

Back

When examining the back, ensure that the entire length of the spine is uncovered. Examine the child standing, with the feet together and the arms at the sides. **Look** for obvious **neural tube defects** (meningocele and meningomyelocele; see Fig. 38.7) and any asymmetry, skin lesions or masses. Check whether the shoulders, scapulae and pelvic rims are symmetrical. Have the child bend over to touch the toes to assess the level of the pelvis. Palpate along the vertebral column, which should form a straight line from the base of the neck to the gluteal cleft, looking for tenderness or any defects in the bony spine (**spina bifida occulta**).

Lumbar hyperlordosis is sometimes seen in children between the ages of 8 and 10 years. It is usually

Thoracic kyphosis. Note the sharp break in the contour of a child with kyphosis

(From Behrman RE. *Nelson textbook of pediatrics*, 14th edn. Philadelphia: Saunders, 1992.)

FIGURE 37.11

Right thoracic idiopathic scoliosis

(From Graham JM. *Smith's recognizable patterns of human deformation*. Philadelphia: Elsevier, 2007, Ch 20, pp 107–110.)

FIGURE 37.12

physiological and resolves spontaneously.[16] Structural hyperkyphosis (Scheuermann's disease) is the most common kyphotic deformity in adolescence (see Fig. 37.11). In these patients, the kyphosis will be fixed and can be seen on hyperextension as well as with forward flexion.[17]

Scoliosis (lateral curvature of the spine; see Fig. 37.12) is by far the most common spinal abnormality seen in children and adolescents. Always consider a functional scoliosis caused by leg length discrepancy—this will correct as the child bends forwards. Early-onset scoliosis occurs before the age of 5 years and is more likely to progress as the child ages and to lead to cardiovascular problems.[16] This form of scoliosis is also more likely to be associated with an underlying pathology. Thus, associated anomalies should be sought (e.g. intraspinal, cardiovascular, urogenital). Late-onset (older than 5 years of age) scoliosis is much more common and much more likely to be idiopathic. Finish the back examination by inspecting the buttocks. Flattened buttocks and shortening of the gluteal cleft may be seen in sacral agenesis. Check for sacral dimples, hair tufts and skin lesions (these are other potential signs of spina bifida occulta—see Ch 38).

An excellent resource of information for the musculoskletal examination of children is pGALS—paediatric Gait Arms Legs and Spine, by Foster and Jandial.[18]

Skin

Look at the skin for:
- colour (pallor, plethora, jaundice, carotinaemia)
- any lesions (location, colour, raised or flat, diffuse or localised)
- haemorrhages (ecchymoses, petechiae, purpura)
- peripheral stigmata of systemic disease (e.g. spider naevi in liver disease, telangiectasia in ataxia-telangiectasia).

Skin lesions can be referred to as either primary (first change to occur in the skin because of disease; see Table 37.4) or secondary (caused by external factors that may evolve from primary lesions; see Table 37.5).

Primary skin lesions	
Macules	Small, flat areas of change in skin colour <1 cm (e.g. freckles)
Patches	Larger, flat areas of colour change (e.g. port-wine stain)
Papules	Elevated lesions <1 cm (e.g. molluscum contagiosum)
Plaques	Raised lesions >1 cm; the surface area is greater than the elevation (e.g. psoriasis)
Nodules	Circumscribed, elevated lesions displaying both depth and elevation; larger than pustules (e.g. capillary haemangioma)
Vesicles	Small, raised cavities containing fluid (<1 cm) (e.g. chicken pox)
Bullae	Larger (>1 cm) fluid-filled lesions (e.g. bullous impetigo)
Pustules	Similar to vesicles, but filled with pus (e.g. pustular psoriasis)
Wheal	Raised lesions that are transient and caused by dilation of local blood vessels (e.g. urticaria)
Comedones	Plugs of clumped keratin and sebum in a hair follicle (e.g. acne)
Burrows	Linear tunnels made by mites in the epidermis (e.g. scabies)
Telangiectasia	Dilated (permanently) superficial blood vessels in the skin

(Modified from Goldbloom RB. *Pediatric clinical skills*. Philadelphia: Saunders, 2010.)

TABLE 37.4

Secondary skin lesions	
Scaling	Accumulation of desquamating skin cells (e.g. ichthyosis)
Crusts	Accumulations of dried exudates or transudate (e.g. infected eczema)
Excoriations	Linear breaks in the skin (e.g. scratches seen in scabies)
Fissures	Linear cracks in the skin (e.g. cracked heels)
Erosions	Circumscribed loss of the superficial layer
Ulcer	Circumscribed loss of tissue that extends into the dermis to subcutaneous tissue or even deeper
Atrophy	Thinning of the skin layers (e.g. postradiation skin changes)
Scars	Fibrous tissue repairs of skin that has been damaged below the level of the epidermis

(Modified from Goldbloom RB. *Pediatric clinical skills*. Philadelphia: Saunders, 2010.)

TABLE 37.5

Many benign skin lesions are commonly seen in childhood (e.g. warts, epidermal cysts, pyogenic granulomata) and require no specific treatment. Bruising in babies is an unexpected finding and requires further investigation (e.g. coagulopathy, non-accidental injury). Although below-knee bruising in cruising[c] children is more common, this should prompt concerns if the bruises are located in *atypical* areas such as the buttocks, hands and trunk and a plausible mechanism is not identified. (See later in the chapter regarding examination for suspected child abuse.)

Palpate the skin to feel for areas of rough, dry skin. Eczema typically presents on the face in an infant, the extensor surfaces in a young child and the flexor surfaces in an older child. Examine the groin, particularly if the child is still in nappies (nappy rash or napkin dermatitis).

Look for vascular lesions (ask the parents about 'birthmarks'), which, although relatively common, may be of clinical significance. Infantile **haemangiomas** are benign vascular tumours (see Fig. 37.13) that have a period of growth (proliferation) but eventually (over 90%) self-resolve (involute) spontaneously by the time the child is 9 years old. Thus, they do not require treatment unless they are extensive, increase in size or are in a problematic area (e.g. perioral, periorbital, anogenital, laryngeal).[19] These lesions need to be differentiated from vascular malformations, which neither *proliferate* nor *involute* (see Table 37.6).

The presence of cervicofacial or more than five cutaneous haemangiomas may indicate the presence of airway or visceral haemangiomas. The infantile vascular lesions associated with **Sturge–Weber syndrome** and **Klippel–Trenaunay syndrome** are detailed in Chapter 38, but remember that these vascular lesions grow in proportion to the child and often require treatment.

Malignant skin lesions (squamous cell carcinomas, basal cell carcinomas, melanomas) are very uncommon

---
[c] Cruising is where an infant, prior to walking independently, uses furniture or other sturdy objects to hold onto and walk, often sideways.

Haemangioma of the cheek.

(a) Initial presentation at 2 weeks; (b, c) in proliferative phase at 2 months; (d, e) in involuting phase at 18 months; (f, g) in involuted phase at 6 years. Steroid treatment was used in infancy and surgery has been avoided

(From Leon-Villapalos J. Understanding vascular anomalies: a common language for doctors. *Surgery* 2012; 30(8):427–434, with permission.)

FIGURE 37.13

in children, but should be considered in adolescence. Also note any hypopigmented lesions (see Fig. 37.14), which can be benign (previous scarring, vitiligo) or may indicate an underlying disorder such as **tuberous sclerosis (TS)**. Note the number of lesions in particular, because most children with one to three hypopigmented macules will *not* be at risk of TS.[19] Facial angiofibromas (see Fig. 37.15) are classic skin lesions seen in patients with TS, but these are not usually seen prior to puberty. Check also for forehead plaques, shagreen patches (see Fig. 37.16), ungual fibromas and gingival fibromas in these children.

Café-au-lait spots (see Fig. 37.17) are very common in the general population (found in up to 15%), but

CHAPTER 37 THE PAEDIATRIC HISTORY AND EXAMINATION   643

Haemangiomas and vascular malformations

Childhood haemangiomas	Vascular malformations
Development in first to fourth week of life, growth in the first 12 months	Established at birth, often later manifestation
Obligate regression phase	No tendency to regression, increasing ectasia more common while lacking true progression
Usually not completely compressible	Often compressible, differences in circumference and length, temperature differences
Histology: proliferation of endothelial cells, increase in number of mast cells	Histology: ectatic vessels, occluded vessels, variable vessel wall thickness or disturbed vessel wall architecture
High blood flow	Usually low blood flow, high in arteriovenous fistulae
Muscle and skeletal involvement rare	Muscle and skeletal involvement frequent

(Hohenleutner U, Landthaler M, Hamm H, Sebastian G. Hemangiomas of infancy and childhood. *J Dtsch Dermatol Ges* 2007; 5(4):334–338. ©John Wiley & Sons.)

TABLE 37.6

Hypopigmented lesion in tuberous sclerosis (TS)

(From Winn R. *Youmans neurological surgery*, 6th edn. Philadelphia: Saunders, 2011.)

FIGURE 37.14

Clinical image of the lesions before the start of treatment. Multiple facial angiofibromas predominantly affecting the cheeks, with a prominent erythematous base

(From Valerón-Almazán P. Topical rapamycin solution to treat multiple facial angiofibromas in a patient with tuberous sclerosis. *Dermatology* (Actas Dermo-Sifiliográficas, English edn) 2010; 103(2):165–167. Copyright ©2010 Elsevier España, S.L. and AEDV.)

FIGURE 37.15

(a) Ashleaf macules are often present at birth or noted early in infancy. (b) Confetti hypopigmentation typically becomes more common over time. (c) Shagreen patch: large shagreen patches may be congenital, whereas smaller ones typically develop over time. (d) Gingival fibromas are a less common feature, but occasionally develop in young children

(From Morrell DS, Burkhart CN, Siegel D. In Eichenfield L, Eichenfield L, Frieden I, eds. *Neonatal dermatology*, 2nd edn. Philadelphia: Saunders, 2008, Ch 26, pp 477–501.)

FIGURE 37.16

six or more spots rarely occur in a patient without **neurofibromatosis type 1** (NF1; see Fig. 37.18); and conversely, patients with NF1 rarely have fewer than six café-au-lait spots.[20] Always remember to check for axillary freckling in patients with suspected NF1 (see Fig. 37.19), as this is usually present after 5 years of age.

Head

Examine the **hair**. Look for areas of alopecia. It is common for babies to have a 'bald spot' from lying in one position. Look for the oily, flaky scalp of 'cradle cap' (seborrhoeic dermatitis). Other causes of dry, flaky scalp include atopic dermatitis or tinea capitis. Some rare genetic disorders have clues in the hair: 'kinky hair' (twisted, fragile hair) can be seen in Menkes disease, or discoloration (e.g. a single white forelock) can be found in in Waardenburg's syndrome.

Measure the **head circumference**. If this is not within the normal range, also measure the head circumference of the parents and any siblings. Use a non-stretching tape to measure around the head at the widest point.

A small head (**microcephaly**) generally means a small brain. Causes can be familial or genetic. Secondary causes include congenital infection, hypoxic–ischaemic encephalopathy and fetal alcohol syndrome. Many

CHAPTER 37 THE PAEDIATRIC HISTORY AND EXAMINATION   645

Café-au-lait macules on the thigh of a child

(From Boyd KP, Korf BR, Bruce R et al. Neurofibromatosis type 1. *J Am Acad Dermatol* 2009; 61(1):1–14.)

FIGURE 37.17

Cutaneous neurofibromas

(From Boyd KP, Korf BR, Bruce R et al. Neurofibromatosis type 1. *J Am Acad Dermatol* 2009; 61(1):1–14.)

FIGURE 37.18

Bilateral axillary freckling

(From Boyd KP, Korf BR, Bruce R et al. Neurofibromatosis type 1. *J Am Acad Dermatol* 2009; 61(1):1–14.)

FIGURE 37.19

paediatric syndromes such as Down's syndrome, Rett's syndrome and Edwards' syndrome are also associated with microcephaly.

A large head (**macrocephaly**) does not always mean a large brain. It may be the result of an enlarged brain (megalencephaly), but can also be due to fluid accumulation within the skull (hydrocephalus), porencephaly[d] or enlargement of the skull itself due to rickets, thalassaemia or osteogenesis imperfecta. Macrocephaly may be familial, secondary to metabolic disorders like Tay–Sachs disease, mucopolysaccharidoses (e.g. Hunter's or Hurler's syndrome), or syndromic (e.g. as a result of Soto's syndrome or neurofibromatosis).

If hydrocephalus is suspected in an infant or a small child, check for a bulging fontanel while the child is seated, prominent scalp veins and 'sun-setting' eyes (this failure of upward gaze means the child will have proportionally more conjunctiva visible *above* the iris than below). Smaller children are much more tolerant of increased intracranial pressure (and therefore may present late with massive hydrocephalus) than older children, who have fused cranial sutures.

Head shape should also be assessed (see Fig. 37.20). The most commonly seen head shape abnormality is positional plagiocephaly (an asymmetrical, flattened deformity of the skull secondary to positioning). Occipital plagiocephaly has been increasingly seen as parents have been encouraged to place their infants on their backs to sleep to decrease the risk of sudden infant death syndrome (SIDS).

Craniosynostosis (the premature fusion of the cranial sutures) is much less common and may occur as an isolated event or as part of a recognised

---

[d] A developmental abnormality whereby one of the lateral ventricles communicates with the surface of the brain.

Diagnostic features of craniosynostosis.

(a) Schematic diagram showing positions of the major cranial sutures. (b) CT scan (vertex view of skull) showing major sutures; anterior is at top. (c, d) Sagittal synostosis: note the long, narrow head. (e, f) Metopic synostosis: note hypotelorism and the triangular profile of the forehead. (g, h) Bicoronal synostosis: broad, flattened head. (i, j) Right unicoronal synostosis: note the flattened brow and anterior position of the ear on the affected side, deviation of the nasal tip and prominent brow on the unaffected side. Congenital anomalies of the feet or hands characteristic of (k) Pfeiffer's syndrome, (l) Apert's syndrome and (m) craniofrontonasal syndrome. (n) Crouzonoid facial appearance. (o) Severe hypertelorism, grooved nasal tip and left unicoronal synostosis in craniofrontonasal syndrome. (p) Ptosis and left unicoronal synostosis in Saethre–Chotzen syndrome. (q) Positional plagiocephaly: prominence on the right anteriorly and the left posteriorly, with right ear anterior and parallelogram shape to the skull. (r) CT reconstruction showing left unicoronal synostosis. (s) CT reconstruction showing clover-leaf skull. (t) CT venogram showing abnormal venous drainage in multisuture syndromic craniosynostosis

(Reprinted by permission from Macmillan Publishers Ltd. Johnson David & Wilkie Andrew. (c) 2011. Craniosynostosis. Eur J Hum Genet. Apr; 19(4): 369–376.)

FIGURE 37.20

syndrome (e.g. Crouzon's or Apert's syndrome).[21] The most common single suture synostosis involves the sagittal suture, but may also be seen at the coronal, metopic and lambdoid sutures. As these abnormalities may be associated with complications that affect the sensory, respiratory and neurological systems, it is important that they are recognised early and referred for treatment.[22]

Palpate over the skull for bony lumps (e.g. exostoses) and soft-tissue lumps (e.g. haemangiomas or cysts). Palpate the fontanels if still open (see Ch 38).

Examine the neck. As well as palpating for lymph nodes (see later in this chapter), look for cervical masses such as cystic hygromas, thyroglossal cysts or epidermoid cysts, which present with painless, soft or semifirm swellings. **Thyroglossal cysts** are most commonly localised in the midline at or below the level of the hyoid bone and move upwards when the tongue is protruded.[23] Epidermoid cysts are found on the floor of the mouth and superior to the hyoid bone.

Look for a **webbed neck**, which suggests Turner's syndrome (see Fig. 37.21) or Noonan's syndrome; if found, look for decreased lateral rotation, which is seen in both syndromes. A **short neck** may be seen in several syndromes (e.g. Hurler's syndrome and Klippel–Feil syndrome) as well as in congenital hypothyroidism.

Finally, palpate for the **thyroid gland**. This lies on either side of the trachea, below the thyroid cartilage, and is best felt by standing behind the patient and placing your hands gently on either side of the patient's neck. Ask the patient to swallow and the thyroid will move upwards. This is really only possible in the older cooperative child, however; it can be very difficult to examine the neck of an infant owing to the relative size of the head compared with the neck. Also, not surprisingly, small children usually will not tolerate an examiner standing behind them putting their hands around their neck! Try to examine the thyroid with the patient sitting and facing you if that approach is more likely to be successful.

Ear, nose and throat

It is particularly important to be proficient in the ear, nose and throat (ENT) examination as infections in these organs are some of the most common presentations for children. **This is a key skill in the paediatric examination.**

Look at the size, shape and position of the ears. Check for malformations and any preauricular tags or pits, which can be associated with hearing loss but are usually benign. **Palpate** over the tragus and pinna, which may be tender if the child has otitis externa, and over the mastoid behind the ear if mastoiditis is suspected. Mastoiditis, if present, may also push the pinna of the ear forwards, giving the child a lop-sided appearance. Infection and inflammation of the skin of the ears and the ear canal (e.g. eczema, bacterial or fungal otitis externa) are quite common. Children are also predisposed to middle ear infections. A hyperaemic (red), inflamed, bulging tympanic membrane, with loss of the light reflex (see Ch 32, Fig. 42.16), may signify **acute otitis media (AOM)** (also called otitis media with effusion—OME; see Ch 42). While genetic, infectious, immunological and environmental factors all play a role in this predisposition, the shape of the eustachian tube itself, which is shorter and less angled in children (see Fig. 37.22), means that it is easier for organisms to migrate from the nasopharynx to the middle ear and more difficult for the middle ear to drain.[22]

Although **otoscopy** should not hurt unless it is done incorrectly, it can be quite upsetting for younger children and is best performed while they are seated on their parent's lap—**and at the end of the examination.** If necessary, have the parent lock the child's lower limbs securely between their thighs (or even wrap a leg across the child's legs) and use his or her arms to embrace the child warmly, holding them tight against their chest,

Webbed neck in Turner's syndrome

(From Bouloux PM. Self-assessment picture tests. *Medicine*, vol 1. St Louis, MO: Mosby, 1996; Goljan EF. *Rapid review laboratory testing in clinical medicine*. St Louis, MO: Mosby, 2008.)

FIGURE 37.21

Comparison of the eustachian tubes in children and adults

(From Hockenberry MJ, Wilson D. *Wong's nursing care of infants and children*, 9th edn. St Louis, MO: Mosby, 2011.)

FIGURE 37.22

whilst simultaneously holding down the child's arms and head.

Ensure that you hold the otoscope with part of your hand touching the child's head so that it can move with any movements of their head to prevent injuring the tympanic membrane (see Fig. 37.23). Tips for otoscopes come in various sizes; use one that fits comfortably in the ear canal but also allows visualisation of the drum. Generally, to visualise the ear canal and eardrum adequately, gently pull the pinna downwards if the child is under the age of 2 years, and upwards and backwards if older than 2 years.[7] Take note of the ear canal as the otoscope enters the ear. Look for swelling and erythema. Bear in mind that earwax can build up in the canal and make visualisation of the tympanic membrane difficult or even impossible.

Finally, examine the eardrum itself (see Figs 37.24 and 37.25). Normally, this is a pale-pink colour, although previous infections and perforations can cause scarring. If the eustachian tube is blocked, the drum may be under negative pressure and may be retracted away from you. Retraction is also seen in chronic otitis media with effusion. If there is pus behind the drum, as in acute otitis media, it can take on a red or yellow colour and may be bulging.

Examine the shape and position of the **nose**, and look for signs of inflammation and rhinorrhoea. Palpate over the bony and cartilaginous surfaces of the nose feeling for lumps, pain and swelling. Look inside the nose. If there is pain, look for lesions or ulcers. Look for blood and the site of haemorrhage (often a large vessel is seen in 'Little's area' in children with recurrent

Positioning of examiner's hands for otoscopic examination. Note that the little finger of the hand holding the otoscope is braced against the child's head. (The examiner is left-handed.) The first two fingers of the other hand retract the pinna, while the remaining fingers are wrapped around the bulb of the insufflator, prepared to squeeze the bulb if the examination warrants

(From Swartz MH. *Textbook of physical diagnosis: history and examination*, 6th edn. Philadelphia: Saunders, 2009.)

FIGURE 37.23

epistaxis—see Ch 42). An inflamed mucosa suggests allergy, while the presence of polyps suggests cystic fibrosis. Look for a foreign body (e.g. beads, food—or pretty much anything!). In a general paediatrics setting, an otoscope can be used for this, and if a more detailed examination is required then referral to an ENT surgeon is necessary for nasal endoscopy.

Examination of the **mouth** and **throat** is fundamental in paediatrics and is one of the most common examinations in everyday practice. Again, the best place for this examination is with the child sitting in the parent's lap. It is usually best to position the child facing forwards with one of the parent's arms across the child's arms and the other hand on the child's forehead, preventing the child's head from moving. Initially, look at the lips and mouth. Check for lesions such as ulcers or angular stomatitis. Look for pallor or cyanosis and

Tympanic membrane landmarks

(From Seidel HM, Ball JW, Dains JE et al. *Mosby's guide to physical examination*, 7th edn. St Louis, MO: Mosby, 2011.)

FIGURE 37.24

Acute otitis media.

(a) This is the textbook picture: an erythematous, opaque, bulging tympanic membrane. The light reflex is reduced, and the landmarks are partially obscured. Mobility is markedly reduced. (b) In this acutely febrile child who complained of otalgia, the presence of both air and fluid formed bubbles separated by greyish-yellow menisci. Even though the drum was not injected, this finding, combined with fever and otalgia, is consistent with acute infection. (c) In this child the tympanic membrane was injected at the periphery, and a yellow purulent effusion caused the inferior portion to bulge outwards. Mobility was markedly reduced

((a) From Hawke M, Yellon RF. *Zitelli and Davis' atlas of pediatric physical diagnosis*, 6th edn. Philadelphia: Saunders, 2012.)

FIGURE 37.25

for any anatomical defects such as a cleft lip. Ask the child to show you the teeth. Note the position and signs of dental decay, which remains the most common chronic disease in children. In a cooperative (or older) child, examine the sublingual space (under the tongue), looking particularly for where the lingual frenulum attaches to the tongue. If possible, examine the buccal mucosa and look for the opening of the salivary ducts.

To visualise the **oropharynx**, a tongue depressor is often needed to move the tongue down and out of the way, and parental cooperation can be critical at this stage. Check the hard and soft palates, looking in

Pharyngotonsillitis.

This common syndrome has several causative pathogens and a wide spectrum of severity. (a) The diffuse tonsillar and pharyngeal erythema seen here is a non-specific finding that can be produced by a variety of pathogens. (b) This intense erythema, seen in association with acute tonsillar enlargement and palatal petechiae, is highly suggestive of group A *Streptococcus* β-haemolytic infection, although other pathogens can produce these findings. (c) This picture of exudative tonsillitis is most commonly seen with either group A streptococcal or Epstein–Barr virus infection

(From Yellon RF, McBride TP, Davis HW. Otolaryngology. In: Zitelli BJ, Davis HW (eds). *Atlas of pediatric physical diagnosis*, 4th edn. St Louis, MO: Mosby, 2002, p 852.)

FIGURE 37.26

particular for defects, including midline cleft palate defects. Inspect the uvula: a bifid uvula may be a sign of a submucous cleft along with a thin translucent bluish or white strip of lining (mucosa). If seen, palpate the hard palate looking for a defect or notch at the base of the uvula.

The palatine tonsils are commonly enlarged in children and are generally easily visualised after about 9 months of age. Look for erythema and exudate if infection is suspected (see Fig. 37.26). Unilateral tonsillar enlargement may indicate a tonsillar abscess or, much less commonly, lymphoma. Also look at the pharynx itself for erythema and exudate.

Face and dysmorphology

The goal is to determine whether the size, shape and position of a physical feature is a normal variant versus a minor or major anomaly, which can be quite challenging on occasions. **An empathic approach is clearly needed**, as the parents are often the first to realise their child 'looks different'. The list below is not exhaustive but outlines some common facial dysmorphisms that suggest particular diagnoses. Importantly the *entire clinical picture* needs to be taken into account as single, isolated facial anomalies may be more likely to be normal anatomical variation *without* a syndromic diagnosis.

Careful examination of the **face** (in association with other features) may reveal the presence of a syndromic or genetic abnormality (see Tables 37.7 and 37.8).[24] Note the general shape of the face (e.g. broad or round). Look for asymmetry (e.g. CHARGE syndrome, Goldenhar's syndrome), coarse features (e.g. metabolic disorders such as mucopolysaccharidoses), midface hypoplasia (e.g. fetal alcohol syndrome) and expression (e.g. the expressionless facies of congenital myotonic dystrophy).

Look at the shape of the **forehead**: is it prominent, broad, short or bossed? Is the hairline high or low? Look at the prominence of the supraorbital ridges and the eyebrows and note the bushy and singular eyebrows (synophrys) of Cornelia de Lange's syndrome.

Examine the **eyes**. Look for coloboma (defects in which tissue is missing from various parts of the structure of the eye). These may be seen in the eyelids, iris, lens and macula and even in the optic nerve (e.g. CHARGE syndrome). Look at the colour of the sclerae, which are bluish in osteogenesis imperfecta, and the

Select syndromes with dysmorphic features	
Condition	**Selected distinctive features**
1p36 deletion syndrome	Deep-set eyes, straight eyebrows, flat midface
17q21.31 microdeletion syndrome	Long face, narrow palpebral fissures, bulbous nasal tip, large low-set ears
22q deletion syndrome	Short palpebral fissures, broad midnose, long tapered fingers
9q22.3 microdeletion syndrome	Large size, macrocephaly, small mouth, thin upper lip
9q34 microdeletion syndrome	Long eyebrows with synophrys, upturned nose, short philtrum, low-set ears
Angelman's syndrome	Large mouth, prominent jaw
ATRX	Hypertelorism, short philtrum, macrostomia, everted lower lip
Cardiofaciocutaneous syndrome	Sparse coarse hair, high forehead, relative macrocephaly, hyperkeratotic macules
CHARGE syndrome	Dysplastic ears, which are often asymmetrical; unilateral facial palsy
Coffin–Lowry syndrome	Full lips, with the upper lip being rounded with minimal vermilion peaks; 'puffy' tapered fingers
Cornelia de Lange's syndrome	Synophrys with arched eyebrows, ill-defined alae, thin lips with downturned mouth
Costello syndrome	'Coarse' appearance, sparse curly hair, deep palmar creases
Fetal alcohol syndrome	Short palpebral fissures, flat philtrum, relatively thin upper lip
Kabuki syndrome	Long palpebral fissures, prominent ears, fetal finger pads
Mowat–Wilson syndrome	Deeply set eyes, round nasal tip, uplifted earlobes
Noonan's syndrome	Hypertelorism, deeply grooved philtrum
Prader–Willi syndrome	Narrow forehead, 'upslanting' palpebral fissures, small hands and feet
Smith–Magenis syndrome	Short philtrum with upturned upper lip, flat midface
Soto's syndrome	Macrocephaly, high forehead, 'downslanting' palpebral fissures
Williams syndrome	Periorbital puffiness, anteverted nares, full lips

ATRX = alpha-thalassemia syndrome, X-linked.

(Toriello HV. Role of the dysmorphologic evaluation in the child with developmental delay. *Pediatr Clin North Am* 2008; 55(5):1085–1098.)

TABLE 37.7

iris, which appears bicoloured (heterochromic) in Waardenburg's syndrome. Look for hypertelorism (widely spaced eyes)[e,f] (e.g. Apert's syndrome) and, if suspected, measure the inner and outer canthal distances. Hypotelorism (closely spaced eyes) is a strong indicator for abnormal brain development.[24] Examine the eyelids looking for ptosis (e.g. Noonan's syndrome), and check for ectropion (whereby the eyelids appear everted, as in Kabuki syndrome) or entropion (whereby the eyelids are turned inwards, as in DiGeorge's syndrome). Look for the presence of epicanthal folds and note whether the palpebral fissures slant upwards as in Down's syndrome or downwards as in Treacher Collins syndrome.

Look at the shape and size of the **nose**, particularly for a flat nasal bridge, which is common in many syndromes. The philtrum may be long, as in Cornelia de Lange's syndrome, or smooth, as in fetal alcohol syndrome. Assess the mandible for micrognathia (small jaw) and prognathia (forward position of mandible relative to maxilla). Micrognathia, glossoptosis (tongue further back in mouth), and cleft palate occur in Pierre Robin sequence. Note the size of the mouth, which may be enlarged in Angelman's syndrome, and the size of the lips, which may be thin, as in the thin upper lip of fetal alcohol syndrome. Look for a cleft of the lip or palate and check for the high-arched palate of Marfan's

---

[e] This is one of numerous parts of the paediatric examination that it is recommended should be left until the end.
[f] This means an abnormally large separation of parts of the body. It is most often used to mean abnormal separation of the eye sockets caused by enlargement of the sphenoid bone.

Select metabolic conditions with dysmorphic features

Condition	Dysmorphic features
Arginino succinic aciduria	Alopecia, brittle hair
Congenital disorders of glycosylation	Lipodystrophy, high nasal bridge, prominent jaw, inverted nipples
D-2-hydroxy glutaric aciduria	Macrocephaly, epicanthal folds, coarse facial features, single transverse palmar crease
Glutaric aciduria type I	Prenatal- or postnatal-onset macrocephaly, facial grimacing
Glutaric aciduria type II	High forehead, depressed nasal bridge, short nose, single transverse palmar crease
GM$_1$ gangliosidosis	Coarse facial features, expressionless face, hirsutism on forehead, long philtrum
Homocystinuria	Tall and thin, depigmented hair
I-cell disease	Similar to mucopolysaccharidosis but earlier onset
Kearns–Sayre syndrome	Progressive ptosis, short stature
Menkes syndrome	Depigmented, kinky or brittle hair; abnormal eyebrow hair
Methylmalonic acidaemia	High forehead, broad nasal bridge, epicanthal folds, long smooth philtrum, triangular mouth
Mucolipidosis III	Hirsutism, synophrys, coarse facial features
Mucopolysaccharidosis	Macrocephaly, coarse facial features, frontal bossing, prominent eyes, depressed nasal bridge, thick lips
Multiple carboxylase deficiency	Alopecia, sparse eyebrows and eyelashes
Multiple sulfatase deficiency	Postnatal microcephaly, coarse facial features, prominent eyes
Propionic acidaemia	Frontal bossing, depressed nasal bridge, epicanthal folds, open mouth with downturned corners
Pyruvate dehydrogenase deficiency	Frontal bossing, short nose, long philtrum, thin upper lip
Smith–Lemli–Opitz syndrome	High forehead, ptosis, epicanthal folds, short nose, micrognathia, syndactyly of toes 2–3
Zellweger's syndrome	High forehead, large fontanels, abnormal ears, broad nasal bridge, hypoplastic supraorbital ridges

(Toriello HV. Role of the dysmorphologic evaluation in the child with developmental delay. *Pediatr Clin North America* 2008; 55(5):1085–1098.)

TABLE 37.8

syndrome. Look for macroglossia suggestive of Down's syndrome or Beckwith–Wiedemann syndrome.

The **ears** may be large, as in fragile X syndrome, or small, as in Down's syndrome. Check whether the ears are abnormal in shape or position. Inspect the pinna for unusual folding and the earlobes for size and creases (e.g. Beckwith–Wiedemann syndrome) and for preauricular pits and tags (may be normal anatomical variation; may or may not be associated with hearing issues).

An excellent online source of information on diagnosis, genetic testing, management and genetic counselling of patients and families can be found at GeneReviews™ (www.ncbi.nlm.nih.gov/books/NBK1116), a peer-reviewed and regularly updated site. Another useful site is Genetics Home Reference (http://ghr.nlm.nih.gov).

Neurological examination

Much of the neurological examination in older children is essentially identical to that in an adult. Examining the upper and lower limbs for tone, power, deep tendon reflexes, coordination and sensation and examining the gait are unchanged, as are the cerebellar examination, much of the cranial nerve (CN) examination and the ophthalmological examination (see Chs 32–34 for a detailed explanation of these examinations). In infants and younger children, keen observation and interactive play can reveal much with respect to their developing neurological system.

Cranial nerves

CN I (olfactory nerve)
In infants: not generally able to be tested.

In older children: ask the child to close the eyes and identify a common scent (e.g. vanilla).

CN II (optic nerve)
Always remember to examine each eye individually.

In infants:

Perform fundoscopy.

Perform the swinging torch test (this tests CN II [afferent] and CN III [efferent]).

- Use a torch to shine a light onto the pupil, then move the light to the other pupil and look closely for a change in pupillary diameter.
- A defect in CN II (afferent pupillary defect) will result in less constriction of both pupils when light is shone into the affected eye; subsequently shining the light into the normal eye will result in the pupils constricting even further.

Visual fields: cannot be tested reliably.

Visual acuity: cannot be tested reliably.

In older children:

Perform fundoscopy.

Perform the swinging torch test (as above).

Visual fields:

- Have an assistant (often the parent) distract the child while you bring a toy (traditionally red in colour) from behind them into the visual field.
- The child should notice the toy and respond as soon as the toy is perpendicular to the outer canthus of the eye.
- For an older child, ask him or her to cover up one eye with the hand and focus on your nose and tell you how many fingers he or she can see being held up into each of the four visual quadrants (identical to the examination in an adult).

Visual acuity:

- For smaller children, offer small interesting objects for them to pick up (raisins or hundreds-and-thousands are particularly well received) but ensure they do not put them into their mouth and choke on it—as a bonus, this also tests fine-motor function.
- For older children, use an age-appropriate vision chart (see Fig. 37.27).

CN III, IV and VI (oculomotor, trochlear and abducens)
These three cranial nerves are examined together as they all innervate muscles of the face: the superior oblique by CN IV, the lateral rectus by CN VI and the medial rectus, superior rectus, inferior rectus and inferior oblique by CN III.

For infants:

Look for ptosis (CN III) and, if seen, look for a constricted pupil on the affected side (e.g. Horner's syndrome).

Looking at the infant front-on, move your head from left to right and watch him or her fix and follow your face. Alternatively, use a picture of a face for the infant's eyes to follow, held about arm's length from the infant.

For older children:

Use a finger puppet or toy for the child to focus on and move this through the lateral, medial, upper and lower visual fields. Observe the eye movements.

In school-aged children, it is often useful to use a torch, so that you can observe the light reflection centred on both pupils.

If there is any diplopia, ask where the two images are most widely separated.

The false image (the outer image) can be determined by having the child close each eye. This can also help determine which muscle is paretic.

CN V (trigeminal)
For infants:

Observe the infant feeding and palpate over the masseter muscles as he or she sucks.

For older children:

Observe and palpate the masseter muscles while the child clenches the teeth together.

Test sensation in the ophthalmic, maxillary and mandibular divisions of the trigeminal nerve as you would in an adult.

The jaw jerk *can* be elicited by placing your thumb over the child's chin while the mouth is slightly open. Tap on your thumb with a

654 SECTION 10 PAEDIATRIC AND NEONATAL HISTORY AND EXAMINATION

Age-appropriate visual acuity charts

(Snellen visual acuity chart, *Clinical Neurology: A Primer*, Figure 4.2, 2010, Elsevier Australia; Picture visual acuity chart, *Ophthalmic Assistant*, The Ninth Edition, Fig. 8.4, 2013, Elsevier Inc; Visual acuity charts designed for use with children, *Clinical Procedures in Primary Eye Care*, Fourth Edition, Figure. 3.2, 2014, Elsevier Limited.)

FIGURE 37.27

tendon hammer and the mouth should close. An upper motor neurone lesion is suggested by a brisk mouth closure. It is really only in older children that this reflex can be elicited, as most children will not let you come anywhere near their faces with the hammer.

CN VII (facial)
For infants:
  Observing the child's face during the examination is usually sufficient.
  Look for drooling out of the weak side of the mouth. Subtle changes are more pronounced when the infant is crying or laughing.

For older children:
  Ask the child to smile, raise the eyebrows, close the eyes and show the teeth.
  Ask the child to blow on a toy or finger puppet.

The corneal reflex (CN V afferent and CN VII efferent) is rarely tested in children, but if there is serious concern, it is best to perform this by gently blowing on the eye. Use your hand to protect the other eye during the procedure.

CN VIII (cochlear and vestibular)
For infants: generally, if there is serious concern, formal audiometry should be arranged.

For older children: test as you would for an adult, including Weber's and Rinne's tests if appropriate (see Ch 32).

CN IX and X (glossopharyngeal and vagus)
For infants:

Observe the palate if (when) the child cries at any stage during the examination.

Listen for b, d and k sounds when the child is speaking, as children with defective palate movement often have difficulty producing these sounds.

For older children:

In practice, this is usually limited to asking the child to open up and say 'Ah' and observing palate movements.

Again, listen for b, d and k sounds when the child is speaking.

It is not recommended to test routinely for the gag reflex in children unless there is a history suggestive of swallowing difficulties or palate dysfunction. Be aware that children with a sensitive gag reflex may well vomit during this procedure.

CN XI (spinal accessory)
For infants:

Lay the infant supine on an examination table, with your arm underneath the shoulders providing support. Push gently on the head laterally and the infant should resist this movement.

Palpate the sternocleidomastoid muscles bilaterally.

For older children: as in the adult, have the child push against your hand with his or her mandible, and while you palpate the contralateral sternocleidomastoid muscle.

CN XII (hypoglossal)
For infants: examination in this age group is fairly limited—assess for tongue fasciculation and movement of the tongue if possible during the examination.

For older children: ask the child to poke the tongue out at you and to imitate you as you move your tongue from side to side (most children love this).

Motor and cerebellar examination

The majority of the motor and cerebellar examination in smaller children is best performed using a combination of observation and play. Have the child reach overhead to grasp a toy and then manipulate small objects (blocks, balls, etc.). This gives you an indication of proximal and distal strength in the upper limbs. If things are going particularly well, you can perform the **wheelbarrow test**: have the child begin on his or her hands and knees, then lift and hold the child's legs under your arms while the child 'walks' forwards on the hands. For older children, test power in the upper and lower limbs as you would in an adult.

Watch the child walk and climb stairs, or jump and hop; for the smaller child, note the infant's ability to bear weight while standing supported. These all give a good indication of strength in the lower limbs. In fact, the **gait examination** is probably the quickest and easiest test of gross-motor function in children. Where appropriate, perform a gait examination for older children as you would in the adult.

Ask the child to lie on the floor (supine) and to stand up as quickly as possible: a child with proximal weakness may roll onto the abdomen and 'climb up' his or her legs using the strength in the upper limbs (Gower's sign; see Fig. 37.28). This is usually seen in Duchenne's muscular dystrophy, but also may be seen in children with other myopathies and dystrophies (e.g. spinal muscular atrophy, Becker's muscular dystrophy or steroid myopathy).

Examining **tone** in children is of particular significance. The clinical presentation prompting examination includes the 'floppy' infant, the child with abnormal gait or the child with delayed motor milestones. In these children, inherited neuromuscular disorders must always be considered, although numerous other conditions (e.g. infectious, autoimmune, vascular) can have a similar presentation. Features from the history and examination can guide diagnosis; for example, normal-looking muscle bulk (or even pseudohypertrophy, particularly of the calves) coupled with decreased muscle tone and strength may indicate Duchenne's or Becker's muscular dystrophy.

If weakness is found during the physical examination, an attempt should be made to differentiate between an upper motor neurone (UMN) lesion, which usually presents with hypertonia, hyperreflexia, clonus, spasticity and a positive Babinski's sign (after the age of 1 year), and a lower motor neurone (LMN) lesion, where the child has hypotonia and hyporeflexia.[20] For infants, this differentiation is described as 'floppy

Gower's sign

(Menezes MP, North KN. Inherited neuromuscular disorders: pathway to diagnosis. *Journal of Paediatrics and Child Health* 2012; 48(6):458–465 © John Wiley & Sons.)

FIGURE 37.28

weak' (an infant with a disorder of the LMN, e.g. spinal muscular atrophy) or 'floppy strong' (an infant with central weakness and hence UMN signs, e.g. cerebral palsy).[20] **Cerebral palsy** is an umbrella term for a group of non-progressive clinical conditions, ranging in severity, whose key characteristic is that of **motor abnormalities** of tone, movement and posture. It occurs due to an abnormality or 'insult' in the developing brain.

Start by assessing tone in the arms and legs by moving the joints passively at the wrists, elbows, knees and ankles. As well as assessing for hypotonia, note any rigidity or spasticity. A few simple manoeuvres are particularly useful in demonstrating tone and strength in infants and small children, particularly when looking for reduced tone.[25] This is called the **180° examination** (see Fig. 37.29).

Measurers of hypotonia.

(a) 'Pull to sit', (b) scarf sign, (c) shoulder suspension and (d) ventral suspension
(From Bodensteiner JB. The evaluation of the hypotonic infant. *Semin Pediatr Neurol* 2008; 15(1):10–20.)

FIGURE 37.29

1. *The 180° examination:* Begin with the infant or small child lying supine on a firm surface.

    Note the resting posture and positioning and look for movement of the arms and legs (voluntary and involuntary), symmetry of movements and general level of alertness.

2. *'Scarf sign':* take the child's hand and pull it (gently) across his or her chest so that the elbow is underneath the chin.

    This tests appendicular tone in the shoulders, but remember that this is also reflective of the child's level of alertness (a child in a deep sleep may appear to have lower tone).

    In the hypotonic child the elbow can be easily pulled beyond the middle line with minimal resistance.

3. *'Pull to sit':* grasp the child's hands and pull the child gently into a sitting position.

    This tests axial tone of the neck and back and appendicular tone of the shoulder and arms.

    Normal newborns will have a head lag, but this should not be present after 2–3 months of age (always remember to use the corrected age for premature infants, who may have lower tone than term infants).

4. *'Shoulder suspension':* lift the child up by holding him or her under the arms.

    This gives an indication of head control, appendicular tone and strength. It is also useful for looking for scissoring of the lower limbs, which is seen in cerebral palsy.

    The hypotonic child tends to slip through your hands (take particular care when performing this procedure).

    While performing this manoeuvre, it is also useful to 'stand' the child up on the flat surface. This helps to demonstrate hypotonia and weakness, but also inappropriate early weight-bearing, as seen in children with UMN lesions (as in cerebral palsy).

5. *'Ventral suspension':* lift the child up and hold him or her with a hand under the chest and abdomen.

    Again, this gives an idea of head control and appendicular tone and strength.

    With severe hypotonia, the child adopts a floppy 'C' shape. Conversely, there may be increased extensor tone in children with UMN lesions (as in cerebral palsy).

6. Lay the child prone on a firm surface.

    Position in the classic 'tummy time' pose, with the child's hands placed palms down on the bed on either side of the shoulders, with elbows flexed.

    Once again, this gives an idea of head control, appendicular tone and strength.

Coordination can be tested in older children in a similar way to testing in adults, often by asking the child to touch your finger and then his or her nose. Remember to hold your finger at arm's length away from the child, so that any tremor can be seen.

Test for sensation in the upper and lower limbs in the older child as it is performed in adults; infants or young children are generally unable to understand and follow commands (or have a long enough attention span) for this to be feasible.

Testing deep tendon reflexes in infants and children is also essentially identical to that in adults. In the smaller child, many paediatricians place their finger over the tendon and tap on that with the tendon hammer, rather than risk hurting the child.

There are some excellent videos detailing the paediatric neurological exam at http://library.med.utah.edu/pedineurologicexam/html/introduction.html.

Developmental assessment

The developmental assessment is what truly differentiates the paediatric examination from examination of the adult. The developmental kit, with all its amusing toys and paraphernalia, clearly separates paediatric doctors from their adult colleagues with their boring briefcases.

Developmental assessment is increasingly important in paediatrics as it has evolved from acute care, particularly the treatment of infectious diseases, to 'a near revolution of successful preventive care measures that have improved the health and prognosis of children and created the expectation of longer, safer lives'.[26] Added to this are the increasing numbers of surviving extremely premature infants, for whom disability, ranging in severity, is not uncommon. The care of children with developmental disabilities remains a major challenge, requiring regular follow-up and early intervention to maximise outcomes.[27]

Although it is not expected that every doctor who examines children should be able to complete a full developmental assessment, it is imperative that doctors who regularly examine children are familiar with the common developmental milestones and can quickly and accurately assess for delay.

Remember that development progresses in an orderly fashion from cephalic to caudal: head control precedes trunk control, which in turn progresses to standing and eventually to locomotion. Many assessment tools are used to monitor development. Most extremely premature infants are now monitored at regular intervals using the Bayley Scales of Infant Development or the Griffiths Scale. These and many other assessment tools take into account four key fields: **gross motor**, **fine motor** (including vision), **speech** (including hearing), and **social and interpersonal** development. Delays in any of these areas should be cause for concern and require follow-up and possibly referral to appropriate services. Generally, however, manipulative or fine-motor development is more important than gross-motor development. A child's level of alertness and interest in his or her surroundings is most important in the assessment of **cognition**.[28]

Much of the developmental assessment can be completed by **observation**: watch how the child plays with toys; watch their interaction with other children, family and clinicians. In this way it can be easier to gauge children's social development by the way they interact with their parents, with you and with their surroundings. **Listen** for any vocalisations or words that children make throughout the examination, whether they can follow any commands given and make note of any of their interactions with you (smiling, waving, pushing you away, etc.).

Developmental examination
Begin the formal part of the developmental assessment by testing vision and hearing, as the assessment will need to be modified extensively if these senses are impaired. Before starting, some developmental milestones may be elicited on history: can the infant roll, sit, crawl, pull to stand, cruise or walk independently? Can the infant suck his or her fist, reach for objects, swap objects from hand to hand, feed self, stack blocks, wave? Can the infant understand simple words like 'yes', 'no', 'milk', 'mummy'? How many words do infants have; can they put two or three words together; can they be understood by strangers? Do they make good eye contact, share things they are enjoying, socialise with other children? Do they know colours, animals, parts of the face? Do they point to things they want, things they are interested in, things they want to share with you? The answers to these questions can then guide the developmental examination.

Vision is relatively easy to assess: hold out a toy for a small child to fix on and follow. If the child's response appears normal, place much smaller items in the palm of your hand for the child to see, reach for and grasp (the classic is to use hundreds-and-thousands). For older children, ask him or her to read aloud from a book. Very young infants often prefer a face—yours or the parents'—rather than a toy.

Assessing **hearing** in an infant or a small child is a little more tricky and requires a cooperative child, preferably held in the parent's lap, and an assistant with a toy that makes a noise (like a bell or a squeaky toy). Have the assistant stand behind the child out of the child's line of sight. Distract the child using a toy that does not make any noise and, once you are sure you have the child's attention, hide this toy behind your back. The assistant should then make a sound with the noisy toy next to the child's ear. Note whether the child's expression changes or the child turns towards the sound. Check each ear in turn. In an older child, you should have an idea of the child's level of hearing from speaking and interacting with him or her throughout the examination.

Fine-motor skill is usually assessed next. If the child was able to grasp the hundreds-and-thousands in the visual test, this indicates that the child has a **pincer grip**. Watching the child play will also give you an idea of fine-motor skills: shaking a rattle, stacking blocks, threading beads on a string, rolling a ball and miming eating using a knife and fork are all good tests of fine-motor skills.

Moving on to **gross-motor skills**, consider checking the primitive reflexes in an infant (see Ch 38) and complete the *180° examination* described earlier. In an older child, the **standard gait examination** can be used to assess gross-motor skills.

Finally, summarise your findings and determine whether there is isolated delay or global delay. Remember to always ask the parents whether there are any particular areas of development that they are concerned about.

Table 37.9 is a general guideline for development over the first 5 years of life. It is included to give you a rough idea of the childhood development milestones expected at different ages. There is large variability in the range of normal for childhood development and these guidelines are not meant to be followed strictly. If there are any concerns about a child's development, formal testing using a verified scale (e.g. the Denver Developmental Screening Test or Bayley's scales) should be used.

Lymphatic and immune system

History: frequent coughs and colds (even up to 10 a year) in an otherwise normally developing, normally growing child may not necessarily signify an immune disorder but rather recurrent exposures to common childhood viruses that children often grow out of. Recurrent invasive bacterial infections, frequent hospitalisations, significant lethargy, night sweats, weight loss, bone or joint pain and rashes (e.g. petechiae) may herald more sinister diseases of the immune and haematopoietic systems.

Parents are often concerned about **adenoidal and tonsillar hypertrophy**. This is usually assumed to be the cause of a great variety of persistent ENT or respiratory problems but, except for obstructive sleep apnoea,[g] a causal relationship between these immune organs and illness is poorly established. Thus, always explore the sleeping history, particularly whether symptoms of obstructive sleep apnoea such as loud snoring and abnormal breathing or breathing efforts during sleep have been observed by the parents. This problem is sometimes associated with daytime somnolence and behavioural problems.

Examination: lymphadenopathy (small, <1 cm, non-tender, freely mobile lymph nodes) is *extremely* common in younger children, particularly in the head and neck region (see List 37.1).[29]

The location of the lymphadenopathy will often give a clue to its aetiology. Cervical lymph node enlargement is more commonly caused by infection, whereas supraclavicular lymphadenopathy, particularly when large and unilateral, is more likely to be malignant. If lymphadenopathy is localised, ensure that the region drained by the nodes is examined for evidence of infection or inflammation. Note the size, shape and

---

[g] Repeated cessation of breathing due to upper airway obstruction, particularly in rapid eye movement (REM) sleep.

> **CAUSES OF LYMPHADENOPATHY IN CHILDREN**
>
> - Viral, bacterial, protozoal or fungal infection
> - Autoimmune disorders (systemic lupus erythematosus, sarcoidosis, Kawasaki's disease)
> - Primary malignancy (lymphoma)
> - Secondary malignant infiltration (much less common in children)
>
> (Motyckova G, Steensma DP. Why does my patient have lymphadenopathy or splenomegaly? *Hematolol/Oncol Clin North Am* 2012; 26(2):395–408.)
>
> **LIST 37.1**

A guide to developmental assessment

Age	Gross motor	Vision/fine motor	Hearing/speech	Personal/social
6 weeks	Symmetrical limb movements Ventral: head in line with body briefly Supine: fencing posture Automatic stepping and walking	Fixes and follows to 90° Turns to light Grasp reflex	Cries/coos Startles to noise	Smiles
3 months	Moves limbs vigorously No head lag Back: lumbar curvature only Prone: lifts upper chest up	Fixes and follows to 180° Plays with own hands Holds rattle placed in hand	Quietens to mother's voice Turns to sound	Laughs and squeals

TABLE 37.9

A guide to developmental assessment *continued*

Age	Gross motor	Vision/fine motor	Hearing/speech	Personal/social
6 months	Sits without support Lifts chest up on extended arms Grasps feet Rolls from front to back Downward parachute reflex	Palmar grasp Transfers objects Shakes rattle Mouths objects	Turns to quiet sound Says vowels and syllables	Laughs and screams Not shy
9 months	Tripod sits: rights self if pushed and can reach for toy steadily Rolls back to front Pulls to standing Stands holding on Forward parachute reflex (7 months)	Reaches for small objects Rolls balls Points with index finger Early pincer grip Looks for fallen objects Releases toys	Distraction hearing test Says 'mama', 'dada' non-specifically	Chews biscuit Stranger anxiety Plays 'peek-a-boo' Understands 'no' and 'bye-bye'
12 months	Cruises around furniture Walks if held, may take a few steps unsupported	Neat pincer grip Casting objects Bangs cubes together	Knows own name Understands simple commands Says a few words	Finger-feeds Waves 'bye' Finds hidden object
15 months	Broad-based gait Kneels Pushes wheeled toy	Sees small objects Builds tower of 2 bricks To and fro scribble	Speaks 2–6 words Communicates wishes and obeys commands	Uses cup and spoon
18 months	Steady purposeful walk Runs, squats Walks carrying toy Pushes/pulls Creeps downstairs	Circular scribble Points to pictures in book Turns pages of book Hand preference	Speaks 6–20 words	Points to named body parts Feeds independently Domestic mimicry Symbolic play alone Takes off socks and shoes
2 years	Kicks ball Walks up and down stairs holding on	Builds tower of 6 bricks Copies vertical line	Uses 2–3 word sentences Uses pivotal grammar Uses question words	Feeds with fork and spoon Begins toilet training Has temper tantrums
3 years	Walks up stairs one foot per step, down with two Walks on tip-toes Throws ball Pedals tricycle	Builds tower of 9 bricks Builds train and bridge with bricks if shown Copies circle	Gives first and last name Knows sex Recognises colours Pure tone audiometry	Washes hands and brushes teeth Eats with fork and spoon (+/− knife) Make-believe play Likes hearing and telling stories
4 years	Walks up and down stairs one foot per step Hops	Builds steps of bricks Copies cross Draws man	Counts to 10 or more	Able to undress
5 years	Skips Catches ball Runs on toes	Copies triangle	Asks 'how' and 'when' questions Uses grammatical speech	Uses knife and fork Able to put on clothes and to do up large buttons

(Stephenson T, Wallace H, Thomson A. *Clinical paediatrics for postgraduate examinations*. Edinburgh: Churchill Livingstone, 2003.)

TABLE 37.9

Lymph node groups of the head and neck
(Modified from www.netterimages.com. In Som PM, Curtin HD. *Head and neck imaging*, 5th edn. St Louis, MO: Mosby, 2011, with permission.)

FIGURE 37.30

---

consistence of any enlarged node and whether it is tender or warm to touch. It is particularly important to determine whether the node is freely movable or fixed to underlying structures. Fixed nodes or groups of nodes matted together are particularly suspect and *less likely* to be benign.

You need to have a system for reviewing the different lymph node groups to ensure that none are forgotten. It is usually easiest to have the child in the parent's lap facing you.

Start at the head (see Fig. 37.30) and examine bilaterally for the pre- and postauricular nodes, followed by the occipital and posterior cervical nodes at the back of the neck. Feel under the angle of the jaw for the superior cervical, submaxillary and submental nodes. Feel along the sternocleidomastoids bilaterally, followed by the supraclavicular nodes.

The axilla (see Fig. 37.31) is palpated next: feel high up into the apex and along the lateral, medial and pectoral surfaces. This usually elicits gales of laughter in most children and can be quite difficult if the child is ticklish. Feel for the epitrochlear nodes, although these are not commonly palpable in children. Ensure that the child's arm is bent at 90° and palpate around the head of the medial epicondyle of the humerus (see Fig. 37.31).

Palpate along the inguinal crease for any nodes and into the femoral triangle. It is not uncommon to be able to palpate small (<1 cm) nodes in the inguinal region, but it is less common to feel nodes in the femoral triangle.[7] Lastly, feel behind the knees for the popliteal nodes.

The spleen and the tonsils are also part of the lymphatic system and should be examined: these are

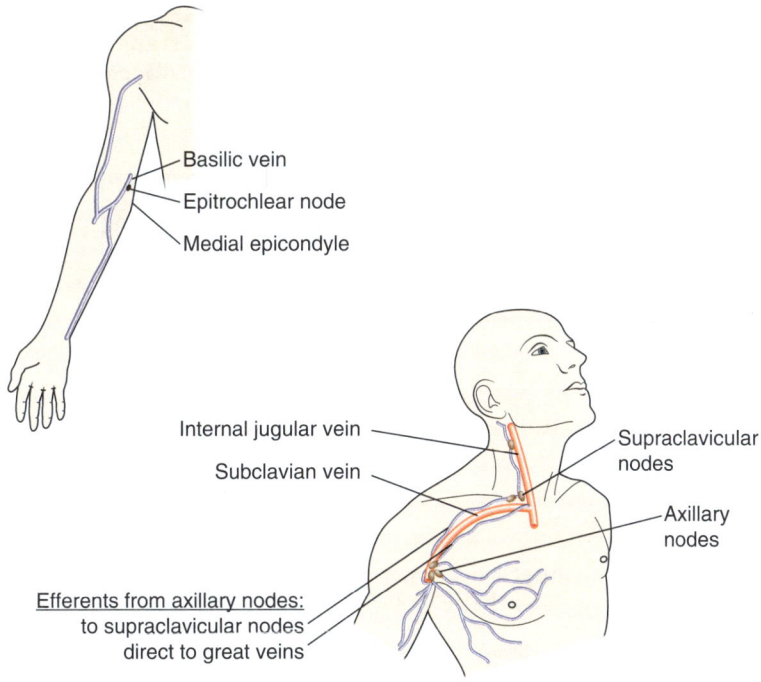

Examining the epitrochlear and the axillary nodes

(From McGee S. *Evidence-based physical diagnosis*. 3rd edn. Philadelphia: Saunders, 2012, pp 215–226.)

FIGURE 37.31

covered in the abdominal examination and the ENT examination, respectively.

Respiratory and cardiovascular system

Common symptoms

Ask the parents or an older child what the main problem has been.

Establish with each symptom whether it is acute (less than 3 weeks' duration), chronic (more than 3 months' duration) or recurrent (with variable symptom-free episodes).

Respiratory noises (wheeze, stridor and/or grunting) are symptoms that are suggestive of some degree of respiratory disease or cardiovascular failure (see Table 37.10). The parents may have noticed laboured breathing, difficult feeding, weight loss, diaphoresis or rapid breathing.

Noisy breathing is extremely common but distinguishing the different noises from each other can be difficult when gathering the history from the parents.[30] Ascertain from the parents whether the noises occur episodically or continuously and are present acutely or chronically. Some parents can specify whether the respiratory noise is more pronounced during inspiration or expiration.

Cough is also very common (see Questions box 37.1) and in an otherwise healthy child may not warrant specific investigation unless prolonged (>3 weeks).[31]

History

A detailed history will help narrow the large list of differential diagnoses.

An episodic dry cough with wheeze and shortness of breath triggered by viruses, cold air exposure (winter,

---

QUESTIONS TO ASK ABOUT A CHILD'S COUGH

1. Is the cough dry or wet?
2. Does it occur at night or during exercise?
3. Does anything seem to bring it on?

QUESTIONS BOX 37.1

Site of origin and differential diagnoses of common respiratory breathing noises

Respiratory breathing noise	Site of origin	Differential diagnoses — Acute	Differential diagnoses — Chronic
Expiratory wheeze or stridor	Intrathoracic	Virus-induced wheezy illness Bronchiolitis (infants) Viral pneumonitis Foreign body in lower airways Asthma attack	Asthma Tracheomalacia Bronchomalacia Chronic lung disease of prematurity (infants) Cystic fibrosis
Inspiratory or biphasic stridor	Extrathoracic or extra- and intrathoracic	Laryngotracheitis (infectious, pseudomembranous, spasmodic croup) Epiglottitis Foreign body in trachea/oesophagus	Laryngomalacia Tracheomalacia Vascular rings and slings Haemangioma Vocal cord paralysis Subglottic stenosis Laryngeal web Laryngeal warts Gastro-oesophageal reflux Rare congenital lesions of the larynx and trachea
Rattle (often confused with wheeze)	Intra- or extrathoracic or both	Upper and/or lower respiratory tract infection	Protracted bronchitis Aspiration Suppurative lung disease (cystic fibrosis, primary ciliary dyskinesia, immune deficiencies, bronchiectasis of unknown aetiology) Anatomical airway malformations
Snore (stertor)	Oronasopharynx	Tonsillitis Pharyngitis	Adenoidal/tonsillar hypertrophy
Snuffle/snort	Nasopharynx	Infectious rhinitis/head cold (coryza)	Allergic rhinitis
Grunt	Alveoli/lung parenchyma	Respiratory distress syndrome/hyaline membrane disease Pneumonia	Chronic lung disease Interstitial lung disease

(Modified from Mellis C. Respiratory noises: how useful are they clinically? *Pediatr Clin North Am* 2009; 56(1):1–17, ix.)

TABLE 37.10

night-time), exercise, allergen exposure (house dust mites, pollen, animals) and/or weather change suggests asthma.

Pertussis should be considered when there is a more persistent spasmodic (paroxysmal: occurring in bouts), choking, repetitive cough with a whooping inspiratory sound, even if the child is vaccinated. Unvaccinated small babies with whooping cough often present with cyanotic coughing spells, which may terminate with life-threatening apnoeic episodes (cessation of respiration longer than 20 seconds).

A dry, honking and loud cough in the absence of any other symptoms that occurred after a non-specific chest infection and is not heard at night likely constitutes a psychogenic (habitual) cough.

Persistent cough (and wheeze) after a choking episode that has occurred after a child has had access to small objects (e.g. peanuts) suggests foreign body aspiration.

Many children have recurrent cough as the chief symptom of frequent episodes of respiratory infections. It is not uncommon for healthy preschoolers to have eight to ten mild respiratory infections ('common colds') per year.

However, a history of two or more bouts of lobar pneumonia in a short interval, confirmed by chest

X-ray, suggests the possibility of aspiration, abnormal immune function or suppurative lung disease. Ask about associated problems, such as:

- poor weight gain, steatorrhoea (cystic fibrosis)
- severe infections of other tissues such as meningitis, skin, intra-abdominal abscesses or osteomyelitis (immunoglobulin deficiency)
- detection of unusual pathogens such as *Pneumocystis jiroveci (previously carinii)*, *Serratia marcescens*, *Candida* (e.g. cellular immune deficiency) and *Aspergillus*.

Ask about **rapid breathing** (tachypnoea) or **difficult breathing** (dyspnoea). These are important features of respiratory distress, which is a common indicator of a respiratory, cardiac or circulatory problem in children. In young infants particularly there may also be neurological and metabolic causes (see Ch 38). Respiratory distress may rapidly worsen and result in life-threatening respiratory failure (type 1: hypoxia with normocapnia; type 2: hypoxia and hypercapnia) or cardiocirculatory failure (inadequate tissue perfusion; see Table 37.11).

Ask the parents of small infants about feeding duration (normally less than 20 minutes), frequency (6–8 times per day in fully breastfed or bottle-fed babies) and fluid intake (normally 100–150 mL/kg per 24 hours of oral feeds in infants of less than 10 kg).

Parents may have noticed **squatting** (rare nowadays) in children with cyanotic heart defects because this position improves systemic oxygen saturation by reducing the right-to-left shunt. Ask about cyanosis, although this can be difficult for parents to recognise. Hypercyanotic (blue) spells are easily recognised medical emergencies and always require specialist involvement in the long-term management.

If **chest pain** has been the problem, careful questioning can help in the assessment (see Questions box 37.2).

Breathlessness during exercise raises the possibility of heart disease. If the onset is recent, a cardiomyopathy or episode of myocarditis is a possibility. Gradually worsening symptoms may indicate congenital heart disease. Shortness of breath directly after physical activity in association with respiratory noises (cough, wheeze) is a typical symptom of exercise-induced asthma.

> ### QUESTIONS TO ASK THE CHILD WITH CHEST PAIN
>
> 1. What is the pain like? Is it sharp and worse when you take big breaths? (Pleuritic or sometimes muscular pain) Is it stabbing? (Musculoskeletal) Is it dull and heavy? (Myocardial ischaemia—very rare in children)
> 2. Where do you feel the pain? (Left- or right-sided pain is unlikely to be cardiac)
> 3. Does the pain go to anywhere else? (To the back with aortic dissection or musculoskeletal pain)
> 4. How bad is it? Does it keep you awake at night?
> 5. Does it come on with exercise?
> 6. Are you sore to touch anywhere on the chest?
>
> QUESTIONS BOX 37.2

Fainting (syncope) and **dizziness** are not uncommon symptoms in older children (see Questions box 37.3).

Palpitations may have been noticed by the child, or the parents may have found an abnormal heart rate (see Questions box 37.4).

Most importantly, beware of the **three Cs** of serious infection and illness:

- Concerns from the parents that the current illness is different from previous illnesses (if mum says he is sick, he is sick)
- Changes in behaviour by the child (e.g. crying, drowsiness, moaning or inconsolability)
- your Clinical instinct that something is wrong.

Examination

The respiratory and cardiovascular examination is of particular significance in paediatrics because it can detect clinical features that identify a seriously ill child (see Table 37.11). Note that some important warning signs are already found in the history and on careful inspection. **Palpation** (starting with the hands and proceeding in an opportunistic fashion) and **auscultation** are usually done next. Sometimes, in a quiet, sleeping

QUESTIONS TO ASK A CHILD WHO HAS BEEN DIZZY OR SYNCOPAL

1. Did you black out altogether? (Syncope) Did you get any warning? What did you feel before you blacked out? Did you notice an odd sensation or a funny smell? (Aura) Did you hurt yourself?
2. Did anyone see it happen? Did you notice any funny shaking movements? (Seizure)
3. Did you bite your tongue or pass urine while you were blacked out? (Seizure)
4. Did you feel strange or sleepy when you woke up? (Postictal symptoms)
5. Did it come on after you stood up suddenly? (Postural hypotension)
6. Did you feel sick in the stomach or sweaty before it happened? (Vasovagal episode)
7. Had you just seen something upsetting, like an accident? (Vasovagal)
8. Had you been coughing badly just before it happened? (Tussive syncope)
9. Are you a diabetic? (Hypoglycaemia)
10. Was there a feeling of spinning or turning? (Vertigo)

QUESTIONS BOX 37.3

QUESTIONS TO ASK THE CHILD ABOUT PALPITATIONS

1. Do you think you can feel your heart beating abnormally?
2. Is it beating fast? A bit faster than normal, or faster than it has ever gone before? (Supraventricular tachycardia)
3. Does it seem to be steady or is it missing and jumping? (Ectopic beats or, if fast, atrial fibrillation)
4. Have you or your parents ever counted how fast it is?
5. Does it start very suddenly? (Supraventricular tachycardia, which often begins in teenagers)
6. Do you feel dizzy or faint when it happens?
7. Have you had any other problems with your heart? (Congenital heart disease is associated with atrial and ventricular arrhythmias)
8. Is there a history of sudden death in your family? (Inherited *channelopathies*, e.g. long QT interval syndrome)

QUESTIONS BOX 37.4

---

infant, *auscultation* may be done first. **Percussion** and particularly inspection of the oral cavity may upset a young child, so these are best left until last.

Look at the child carefully to pick up unusual posturing or body habitus (see List 37.2).

Inspect the chest for:
- signs of respiratory distress such as chest in-drawings (intercostal or subcostal recessions), tracheal tug and nasal flaring
- abnormally shaped chest (e.g. bell-shaped, unilateral or bilateral lung hypoplasia; see Ch 38)
- symmetrical expansion and any deformities such as a pectus excavatum or pectus carinatum (see Ch 10)

BODY HABITUS ABNORMALITIES TO NOTE ON GENERAL INSPECTION

- Marfanoid (risk of aortic dilation, dissection)
- Cushingoid (hypertension)
- Dysmorphic features (webbed neck, short stature and commonly cardiac malformations in Turner's syndrome)
- Developmental delay (supravalvular aortic stenosis with Williams–Beuren syndrome)

LIST 37.2

Respiratory distress and associated signs and symptoms

Impaired function	Possible signs/symptoms	Aetiology

Cardiac/circulatory	Tachypnoea, sweating, fatigue, impaired tolerance to physical activity, poor feeding, failure to thrive, cyanosis, pallor, weak pulses, prolonged capillary refill, low/high blood pressure, tachycardia/bradycardia, murmur, subcostal recessions	Congenital heart disease:
		   left-to-right shunt causing fluid overload (e.g. ventricular septal defect, persistent ductus arteriosus)
		   right-to-left shunt causing cyanosis (e.g. tetralogy of Fallot, transposition of the great arteries)
		   stenoses causing obstruction (e.g. coarctation of the aorta, aortic stenosis, pulmonary stenosis)
		Acquired heart disease, e.g.:
		   Kawasaki's disease (myocardial infarction)
		   rheumatic fever (mitral stenosis)
		   drug-induced cardiomyopathy
		   cardiac tamponade
		   pericarditis
		   myocarditis
		Cardiac arrhythmias, e.g.:
		   pre-excitation syndromes (Wolff–Parkinson–White syndrome)
		   supraventricular tachycardia
		   AV block
		Circulatory, e.g.:
		   hypertension
		   dehydration
		   blood loss
		   anaphylaxis
		   septicaemia
		   neurogenic

Respiratory	Respiratory noises, reduced or prolonged or added breath sounds, tachypnoea/dyspnoea, tachycardia, subcostal recessions, failure to thrive, tracheal tug, nasal flaring	Obstructive lung disease (airway resistance increased [reduced airway patency]):
		   upper airway (e.g. croup, epiglottitis, choanal atresia, piriform aperture stenosis, adenoidal hypertrophy)
		   lower airways (e.g. bronchiolitis, wheezy illness, asthma, cystic fibrosis)
		Restrictive lung disease (lung compliance reduced [stiff lungs]):
		   respiratory distress syndrome
		   pneumonia
		   hypersensitivity/viral pneumonitis
		   interstitial lung disease/lung fibrosis
		   scoliosis/kyphosis
		   neuromuscular disease
		   pulmonary oedema (mixed cardiac and respiratory)
		Other:
		   pneumothorax
		   trauma (flail chest)

TABLE 37.11

- signs of hyperinflation (e.g. barrel chest with increased anterior–posterior chest diameter)
- a horizontal groove along the lower border of the thorax corresponding to the insertion of the diaphragm (Harrison's sulcus), which signifies increased contractile activity of the diaphragm (e.g. in chronic asthma) or rachitic rosary as a result of vitamin D deficiency
- left-sided chest prominence, which can be due to cardiac enlargement.

Look out for any thoracic scars (including on the back) that may indicate previous surgery. A midline sternotomy scar suggests complex surgery for congenital heart disease in the past, whereas a left-sided thoracotomy scar may indicate persistent ductus arteriosus, aortic coarctation repair, or—similar to a right-sided thoracotomy—pulmonary artery banding (palliative reduction of excessive pulmonary blood flow), Blalock–Taussig[h] shunt (palliative systemic-to-pulmonary shunt to increase impaired pulmonary blood flow) or non-cardiac surgery (e.g. removal of congenital pulmonary airway malformation).

Assess for the presence of acrocyanosis (nailbeds) or central cyanosis (mouth and tongue at the end of the examination in young children; see also Ch 38). Cyanosis may be present only in the lower extremities in patients with aortic coarctation or a persistent ductus arteriosus complicated by pulmonary hypertension and reversal of the shunt.

Arrange for the measurement of oxygen saturation employing pulse oximetry if available or you are in doubt, and expose to 100% oxygen (hyperoxygenation test; see Ch 38). Check for dental caries and pallor while inspecting the oral cavity. Pallor can also be detected by inspecting the conjunctivae and palmar creases. Common causes of pallor include:

- low haemoglobin levels (with increased pulse rate)
- poor cardiac output (weak pulse, prolonged capillary refill and sometimes bradycardia).

There may be koilonychia if the cause is iron deficiency, hypertension if the cause is renal disease, or a recent history of erythema infectiosum ('fifth disease') with bone marrow suppression.

Clubbing is present when there is an increase in the angle between the nail and the skin overlying the distal phalanx (>160°).[7] This is caused by proliferation of subungual tissue at the root of the nail and can easily be detected when it exceeds 180° by holding both thumbs back to back with the fingertips and interphalangeal joints aligned. With clubbing, the elongated, diamond-shaped opening that is normally apparent is lost (Schamroth's sign, p 80). Applying pressure onto the root of a clubbed nail produces movement towards the bone ('floating nail').

Look out for rarities such as splinter haemorrhages and Osler's nodes (infective endocarditis), tuberous and tendon xanthomata (familial hypercholesterolaemia), absent thumbs (Holt–Oram syndrome) or absent radii. Bending of the fifth finger (clinodactyly) occurs in many genetic conditions (Russell–Silver syndrome, Down's syndrome, pseudohypoparathyroidism) but is also seen in the general population.

Heart and circulation

Feel the brachial pulses in the antecubital fossa of both upper limbs using your first and second index fingers. Determine:

- rate (see Table 37.12)
- rhythm (regularly irregular: coupled extrasystoles; irregularly irregular: ectopic beats [more common], atrial fibrillation [less common])
- volume (full: persistent ductus arteriosus, aortic regurgitation; shallow: left ventricular outflow tract obstruction, cardiac/circulatory failure)
- presence of pulsus paradoxus, which is an exaggeration of the physiological decrease in

Proposed normal values for heart rate per minute

Age range (years)	Pediatric advanced life support, American Heart Association	Advanced paediatric life support, Advanced Life Support Group
0–1	100–190*	110–160
1–2	100–190	100–150
2–5	60–140	95–140
5–10	60–140	80–120
10–12	60–100	80–120
12–18	60–100	60–100

*PALS provides separate ranges for infants up to 3 months, and for those between 3 months and 2 years of age.

(American Heart Association; Ralston M, Hazinski FM, Zaritsky AL, Schexnayder FM. *PALS provider manual*. Dallas: American Heart Association, 2006; Advanced Life Support Group (Manchester England). *Pre-hospital paediatric life support: a practical approach to the out-of-hospital emergency care of children*. Oxford: BMJ Books/Blackwell, 2005.)

TABLE 37.12

---

[h] In 1938 Helen Taussig, a paediatric cardiologist, approached Alfred Blalock, the Chief of Surgery at Johns Hopkins, to create a ductus-like anastomosis between the left subclavian and pulmonary artery. Coincidentally, a young surgical technician named Vivien Thomas in Dr Blalock's laboratory had already performed this work successfully in dogs. He stood behind Blalock during the first surgery performed in a 15-month-old girl with tetralogy of Fallot in 1944 to provide procedural advice. The technical oversight of Vivien Thomas contributed to one of the most dramatic progresses in 20th century paediatric cardiology.

systolic blood pressure during inspiration (greater than 10 mmHg). On palpation, the pulses are fainter during inspiration and this can be found with severe airways obstruction (e.g. in asthma or croup) or reduced left ventricular filling (e.g. cardiac tamponade or pericarditis). It must be quantified with a stethoscope and blood pressure cuff.

The femoral pulses must be checked at some stage but in chubby babies this requires patience. Thus, feel the groins only towards the end of the examination. Absence of the femoral pulses or a radiofemoral delay raises suspicion of the presence of aortic coarctation.

Test the capillary refill time by pressing your index finger onto the child's chest for 5 seconds. This inhibits skin perfusion and leaves a pale area, which should regain its colour (refill) within 2–3 seconds. A prolonged capillary refill indicates poor peripheral perfusion, which is most commonly caused by:

- septicaemia
- dehydration, or
- heart failure.

Assess the location and quality of the impulse of the apex beat, which should be located in the fourth intercostal space approximately on the left midclavicular line. Feel for a vibration under your right hand held onto the left lower sternal border (ventricular septal defect, VSD) and left upper sternal edge (pulmonary valve stenosis). A parasternal impulse may be felt when there is right ventricular hypertrophy (e.g. tetralogy of Fallot). In infants you can feel for impulse and thrill by pressing the first and second digits of your right hand onto the left lower sternal border (next to the xiphoid process) and the second intercostal space (above the pulmonary valve area). Next, place your index finger into the suprasternal notch to search for a thrill caused by aortic stenosis.

Proceed to auscultation of heart sounds using the diaphragm of a good-quality paediatric stethoscope and then make your way backwards with the bell to search for murmurs of low frequency. At least four praecordial areas should be auscultated:

- apical or mitral area (fourth intercostal space between the midclavicular and anterior axillary lines)
- tricuspid area (left lower sternal border [LLSB] in the fourth intercostal space)
- pulmonary area (left upper sternal border [LUSB] in the second intercostal space)
- aortic area (right upper sternal border [RUSB] in the second intercostal space).

If a murmur is present, then assess as follows using the mnemonic **CARDIO**:

C haracter of the sound or murmur

A rea where the sound is the loudest

R adiation of the sound into other areas

D egree or **I**ntensity of the loudness of the sound or murmur

O ccurrence of the sound or murmur in the cardiac cycle.

Character of the sound or murmur
Normal
The first heart sound (S_1) marks the closure of the mitral and tricuspid valves and is louder than the second heart sound (S_2). S_1 is not split except above the tricuspid area where it may be closely split. S_2 is produced by closure of the aortic (A_2) and pulmonary (P_2) valves. S_2 is split in inspiration but there is no split or only a close split in expiration above the pulmonary area.

Innocent systolic (between S_1 and S_2) vibratory ejection murmurs are common (Still's murmur) and have a musical character (like twanging a piece of tense string). There are also systolic flow ejection murmurs, which are not musical (medium-pitched) but they are never harsh or coarse. They may be innocent if S_2 is normal. They are also heard with atrial septal defect (ASD) (p 77), but then there is also a fixed splitting of S_2.

Abnormal
1. *Heart sounds.* If the intensity of S_1 varies from beat-to-beat variation, there may be complete atrioventricular heart block present. This causes dissociation between closure of the valve leaflets and ventricle contractions. This sign can be useful in distinguishing complete heart block from sinus bradycardia.

   An absent or faint S_1 is found when the PR interval is prolonged. A fixed split of S_2 is found with ASD and pulmonary valve stenosis. However, ASD is associated with a systolic flow murmur (medium-pitched), while pulmonary valve stenosis leads to a systolic obstructive murmur (low-pitched, harsh, coarse).

A third heart sound (S_3) can be found in normal children with hyperdynamic circulation, but a fourth heart sound (S_4) is always abnormal.

2. *Murmurs.* A systolic regurgitant murmur is non-musical and has a high-pitched sound character like breath sounds or blowing. A systolic ejection murmur due to valvular stenosis is also non-musical but low-pitched, meaning it sounds harsh or coarse, and is usually quite loud and easily heard. Almost any diastolic murmur or continuous murmur is pathological except for a venous hum. A venous hum arises from the neck and disappears when the patient is supine or when gentle pressure is applied to the base of the neck.

3. *Clicks and rubs.* Clicks at the beginning of systole directly after S_1 are generated by the opening of the heart valves and are heard in aortic or pulmonary stenosis. A midsystolic click is pathognomonic for mitral valve prolapse.

A pericardial friction rub is a scratchy sound heard at the left sternal border and usually has one systolic and two diastolic components. It can occur with pericarditis or after cardiac surgery. A mediastinal crunch (Hamman's sign: a crackly, crunchy, bubbly sound) can be heard with mediastinal emphysema[i] after chest injury or thoracic surgery.

Area where the sound is the loudest

The suggested sequence of auscultation is the mitral, tricuspid, pulmonary and aortic areas with the diaphragm of the stethoscope first to detect high- and medium-pitched murmurs and then in the reverse direction with the bell for low-pitched murmurs.

Radiation of the sound into other areas

A thrill in the suprasternal notch may be palpable in aortic stenosis. The harsh systolic obstructive murmur found with pulmonary valve stenosis radiates into the back, whereas the high-pitched blowing systolic regurgitant murmur with mitral valve regurgitation may be auscultated in the axilla.

Degree or intensity of the loudness of the sound or murmur

This can be measured by grading the loudness from 1 to 6 for systolic and 1 to 4 for diastolic murmurs. For instance, a grade 1 murmur is extremely faint, whereas a grade 3 murmur is loud. With a grade 4 murmur a thrill is also palpable and with a grade 6 murmur you would not need a stethoscope to hear it. Importantly, innocent murmurs are not loud and never have a thrill (see below).

Timing of the occurrence of the sound or murmur in the cardiac cycle

A systolic regurgitant murmur (usually high-pitched, blowing) commences immediately *with* S_1 and concludes only with S_2 (pan- or holosystolic); for example, it is observed in mitral or tricuspid valve regurgitation. In contrast, systolic obstructive ejection murmurs (low-pitched, harsh) commence *after* S_1 (small pause between S_1 and murmur). They have a crescendo–decrescendo occurrence, meaning that their intensity increases and then decreases before S_2. Ejection murmurs can occur in early, mid or late systole and are heard with, for instance, aortic and pulmonary valve stenosis. Diastolic regurgitant murmurs commence *with* S_2 and are high-pitched with aortic regurgitation (high pressure gradient) and low-pitched with pulmonary regurgitation (low pressure gradient) but they are not pandiastolic. In contrast, diastolic obstructive murmurs commence *after* S_2 and have a crescendo–decrescendo occurrence. In mitral valve stenosis, they occur in late diastole and have a low-pitched rumbling character. There are also occasionally short mid-diastolic flow murmurs (medium-pitched) in severe VSD, ASD, tricuspid or mitral valve regurgitation due to markedly increased flow volume.

Many healthy children have a heart murmur and several types of **innocent murmurs** are reported (see Table 37.13). Innocent murmurs are not harsh and occur in systole but are not pansystolic. They are not loud and they may further diminish in intensity in different positions. Usually they are localised with no radiation except for the pulmonary branch murmur of infancy. Patients with murmurs with these characteristics can usually be reassured, especially if there are no cardiac symptoms. In neonates, however, the absence of a murmur never excludes structural heart disease.

Pathological murmurs may be due to congenital or acquired heart defects (<1% in the general population). If they are not recognised and treated they can lead to progressive limitation and premature death. Consider the following features suggestive of pathological murmurs:

---

[i] Air in the mediastinum.

Characteristics of innocent murmurs in childhood

Origin (term)	Character	Area	Radiation	Degree/intensity	Occurrence
Left ventricular outflow tract (Still's murmur)	Non-harsh	LLSB	No	Less than grade 3	Early systole, diminishes with inspiration, sitting, standing
Right ventricular outflow tract (pulmonary flow murmur)	Non-harsh	LUSB	No	Less than grade 3	Early systole, diminishes with inspiration, sitting, standing
Pulmonary branch murmur of infancy	Non-harsh	LUSB RUSB	Axillae and back	Less than grade 3	Early systole
Supraclavicular arterial/carotid bruit	Non-harsh	Neck	No	Less than grade 3	Early systole, diminishes with neck extension
Superior vena cava (cervical venous hum)	Machinery-like	Right infraclavicular	No	Often grade 3	Continuous, disappears with supine position or light pressure on jugular vein

TABLE 37.13

- harsh character
- loud (grade 3 or more)
- pansystolic, diastolic or continuous (if not disappearing in supine position)
- associated with ejection clicks
- associated with abnormal S_2 sound
- associated with other abnormal cardiac findings.

Table 37.14 summarises potential auscultation notes for some more common structural heart defects in childhood (see also Ch 38 for ventricular and atrial septal defect and persistent ductus arteriosus, which are equally relevant to older children).

Mitral valve prolapse is common (2–3% in children) and may be associated with connective tissue disorders (Marfan's syndrome, Ehlers–Danlos syndrome, Stickler's syndrome) or other structural abnormalities. On auscultation the characteristic feature is of one or more midsystolic clicks best heard at the cardiac apex. These become louder when the child stands up and may be followed by a murmur of mitral regurgitation.

During auscultation decide again whether the cardiac rhythm is regular or irregular. Count the heart rate over 15 seconds and check the normal range (see Table 37.12).

Measure the blood pressure (also lower extremities if there is no femoral pulse or radiofemoral delay) and liver size (see below) and assess for periorbital, sacral and pretibial oedema to complete the cardiovascular examination.

Lungs

Respiratory rate

Count the respiratory rate over one full minute by assessing both chest movements and breath sounds. Although percentile charts are published (see Fig. 37.1), it is more common in clinical practice to employ the proposed ranges of normal that are best suited to a specific region and are endorsed by local policy (see Table 37.15).

Rapid breathing (tachypnoea) and reduced breathing (hypopnoea, apnoea) are signs of respiratory failure. They are red flags indicating severe illness. List 37.3 outlines important differential diagnoses of rapid breathing often associated with **type 1 respiratory failure** where there is a ventilation/perfusion mismatch and a fall in oxygenation. List 37.4 outlines important differential diagnoses of reduced breathing often associated with **type 2 respiratory failure** where there is inadequate ventilation and a fall in oxygenation is associated with a rise in carbon dioxide levels.

Auscultation findings in common structural heart diseases

Cause	CARDIO	
Pulmonary valve stenosis (0.8:1000 [50% with other lesions])	C A R D I O	Ejection click, murmur low pitch, harsh Left upper sternal border Back Variable Crescendo–decrescendo (ejection) midsystolic murmur (the later the peak intensity, the greater the obstruction), S_2 widely split proportionate to severity of obstruction (P_2 delayed)
Aortic valve stenosis (1:2500–1:25,000)	C A R D I O	Ejection click, murmur low pitch, harsh Right upper sternal border Into the neck, thrill suprasternal notch Variable, usually grade 4 or more Crescendo–decrescendo (ejection) midsystolic murmur, S_2 narrowly split proportionate to severity of obstruction (A_2 delayed) Early diastolic regurgitation murmur common
Mitral valve stenosis (rare)	C A R D I O	Low-pitched, rumbling Apex in left lateral decubitus position None Grade 1 to 2 Diastolic murmur
Mitral valve regurgitation	C A R D I O	High-pitched, blowing Apex Axilla Less than grade 3 Pansystolic murmur, soft/absent S_1, loud S_2 (with pulmonary hypertension), diastolic flow murmur (in severe cases) due to increased flow volume

(Keane JF, Lock JE, Fyler DC, Nadas AS. *Nadas' pediatric cardiology*. Philadelphia: Saunders, 2006.)

TABLE 37.14

IMPORTANT DIFFERENTIAL DIAGNOSES OF RAPID BREATHING OFTEN ASSOCIATED WITH TYPE 1 RESPIRATORY FAILURE

- Structural (pleural/lung/abdomen) abnormalities (pneumothorax, pleural effusion, ascites, interstitial lung disease, diaphragmatic hernia/paresis)
- Infection and inflammation (pneumonia, pneumonitis, bronchitis, tracheitis, bronchiolitis, asthma)
- Cardiocirculatory failure (congenital heart disease, arrhythmias, pneumomediastinum, pericardial effusion, septicaemia, metabolic disease, severe anaemia)

LIST 37.3

IMPORTANT DIFFERENTIAL DIAGNOSES OF REDUCED BREATHING OFTEN ASSOCIATED WITH TYPE 2 RESPIRATORY FAILURE

- Obstruction of upper/lower airways (infection [croup, epiglottitis], inflammation [asthma], congenital/anatomical)
- Central hypoventilation (CNS infections, respiratory infections in young infants, extreme obesity, apnoea of prematurity [diagnosis of exclusion], head trauma, brainstem compression, metabolic disturbances)
- Neuromuscular impairment (congenital/genetic diseases, drugs/intoxication, metabolic disturbances)

LIST 37.4

Proposed normal values for respiratory rate per minute

Age range (years)	Pediatric advanced life support, American Heart Association	Advanced paediatric life support, Advanced Life Support Group
0–2	30–60	30–40
2–3	24–40	25–35
3–5	24–40	25–30
5–12	20–24	20–25
12–18	12–20	15–20

(American Heart Association; Ralston M, Hazinski FM, Zaritsky AL, Schexnayder FM. *PALS provider manual.* Dallas: American Heart Association, 2006. Advanced Life Support Group (Manchester England). *Pre-hospital paediatric life support: a practical approach to the out-of-hospital emergency care of children.* Oxford: BMJ Books / Blackwell, 2005.)

TABLE 37.15

Trachea and chest wall
Verify the position of the trachea in the midline with your index finger by gently palpating the trachea in the suprasternal (jugular) notch while placing your first finger and third finger onto the clavicles on either side of the clavicular notch of the manubrium sterni. Shifting of the trachea signifies an increase in the intrathoracic pressure, which may be the result of:

- air (a tension pneumothorax, congenital lobar emphysema, congenital pulmonary airway malformation)
- fluid (a volume increase due to effusion, haemorrhage in the contralateral hemithorax)
- collapse (a volume decrease [atelectasis] on the same side [the ipsilateral hemithorax]).

Check the chest wall for subcutaneous air (pneumomediastinum +/− pneumothorax), which results in crackling under the skin with palpation.

Auscultation
Next auscultate the lung sounds in a pragmatic fashion:

1. anterior: compare right versus left upper sternal border (upper lobes), lower sternal border (middle lobe right, lingular segment left) and lateral lower chest (lower lobes)
2. posterior: compare right versus left in the upper (upper lobes), median and lower chest (between spine and scapula)
3. laterally (all lower lobes).

Lung sounds are bronchovesicular in young infants. They are of medium pitch and volume and equal in expiration and inspiration. In older children they are vesicular. Vesicular breath sounds are low-pitched and soft and louder and longer in inspiration. Listen for reduced breath sounds (for causes see Ch 38). Bronchial breath sounds are high-pitched, loud and more prominent in expiration. They can normally be heard over the trachea but not over healthy lung areas. They may be heard over consolidated lungs.

Prolonged expiration is a sign of lower airway obstruction and is characteristic of asthma. **Prolonged inspiration** is characteristic of viral croup (infectious laryngotracheitis). These children also have stridor due to upper airway obstruction and collapse (for other causes of stridor, see Ch 38).

If **stridor** is audible during inspiration and expiration, it is an ominous sign indicating severe obstruction or obstruction at multiple sites with the potential to progress rapidly to complete airway obstruction and death.

Grunting is produced at the start of expiration when air is forced against a closed glottis to prevent small-airway collapse. It is heard in association with respiratory distress. **Wheeze** is more high-pitched and musical sounding and may be monophonic or polyphonic. Wheeze is usually heard during expiration and is associated with lower airway obstruction (e.g. asthma in older children). If an infant presents with wheeze, coryza, signs of respiratory distress and inspiratory fine crackles it is suggestive of a virus-induced infection of the terminal airways (**bronchiolitis**), which causes small-airway obstruction, lung hyperinflation and collapsed lung areas. These are often mistaken for consolidation.

The diagnosis of asthma is difficult to make in young children, even if they present with apparently typical features (episodic wheeze, cough and shortness of breath). First, young children are more prone to wheeze when they have a respiratory virus infection (e.g. bronchiolitis in the first 2 years of life). Half of them will outgrow this predisposition by the age of 3 years. Second, children born with hypoplastic lungs and airways as a result of maternal smoking during pregnancy or of prematurity are prone to these symptoms but improve as their lungs grow. Third, there are many other causes of wheeze in early life, including structural airway anomalies such as broncho- and tracheomalacia, and cystic fibrosis. Thus, it is sensible to consider a wide range of differential diagnoses if severe and frequent wheezy illnesses occur, unless a compelling case for asthma can be made based on clinical presentation and response to specific treatment.[1]

Crackles are non-musical interrupted lung sounds of short duration that may occur at any time during inspiration or expiration. Crackles may be high-pitched (fine) or of variable pitch (coarse). They are produced by abrupt opening of closed airways during inspiration.[32] This means that crackles heard during early inspiration originate from the abrupt opening of larger airways, whereas those generated during late inspiration come from the terminal bronchioli or alveoli and are a sign of bronchiolitis, pneumonitis or pneumonia.[33] Place your stethoscope on the child's neck to distinguish coarse lung crackles from conducted upper airway sounds due to upper airway secretions if they are heard in both lungs.

Percussion, chest expansion and vocal fremitus

Percussion can be very helpful in localised processes of the lung to describe the extent of dullness. Dullness to percussion can be the result of consolidation, collapse (atelectasis) or fluid in the pleural space. An increased percussion note (hyperresonance) suggests unilateral hyperinflation due to a unilateral pneumothorax; when associated with wheeze it may be the result of a foreign body in the main bronchus.

Chest expansion is not routinely measured but may be assessed by percussion (p 95).

Vocal fremitus can be tested in older children.

The respiratory examination is completed with an assessment of the ear, nose and throat (see above).

Gastrointestinal system: abdomen

Examination of the abdomen is central to assessment of the gastrointestinal system. Remember, however, that examination of other systems can provide very important (and sometimes the only) clues to pathologies that are primarily localised in the abdomen. Assessment of nutrition is part of the abdominal and gastrointestinal examination. This includes a medical history (see Table 37.16) and a physical examination focused on detecting significant loss of subcutaneous fat (face, arms, chest, buttocks), muscle wasting (temples, shoulders, thighs, knees, calves) and peripheral oedema (pretibial, sacral).

Nutrition-focused medical history

Domain	Indicators of potential impairment in nutritional status
Growth	Below third percentile Crossing percentiles downwards in serial measurements (may be normal in first 2 years of life and puberty if shifting towards fiftieth percentile) Reduced weight-to-length percentile ratio Unintentional weight loss (5–10% moderate; >10% severe) Rapid weight loss
Dietary intake	Appetite ('fussy' eater) Frequency (decreases with age) and amount (increases with age) of food Feeding problems (uncoordinated swallow) Restrictions (parent-perceived food intolerance versus specialist-diagnosed allergy)
Functional impairment	Activity Power/strength
Metabolic stress	Infection (gastroenteritis, sepsis, pneumonia) Inflammation (pancreatitis) Endocrine disorders (hyperthyroidism, diabetes) Trauma Surgery (bowel resection)
Abdominal symptoms	Frequent vomiting Gastro-oesophageal reflux Constipation Pain Nausea Diarrhoea

TABLE 37.16

Positioning the patient

Ask the child to lie flat in the supine position with the arms placed alongside their body and the feet together. The abdomen and inguinal region should be fully exposed; use a sheet to cover the external genitalia in older children. The external genitalia should be inspected routinely in young children so that important abnormalities such as testicular torsion, undescended testes and penile malformations are not missed. A toddler may be unwilling to lie flat and may become upset if you (or the parent) try to insist. Young children may, however, sit quietly in the parent's lap and let the parent proceed with undressing them. Remember that rather than the crying agile toddler, it is the unusually quiet child with paucity of movements and suspected illness who is of greatest concern and who requires most urgent assessment.

Inspection

Begin with inspection. Imagine a vertical line and a perpendicular horizontal line running through the umbilicus to 'divide' the abdomen into four quadrants (right upper, right lower, left upper, left lower) and describe the location of any abnormality. The abdomen often appears as if it is generally distended in toddlers owing to their physiological lumbar lordosis. Abdominal distension may be observed with the following:

- ascites (liver disease, cardiac failure, malnutrition, protein-losing enteropathy)
- malabsorption (coeliac disease, food allergy, lactase or sucrase–isomaltase deficiency and intolerance, glucose–galactose malabsorption)
- maldigestion (pancreatic insufficiency in cystic fibrosis and Shwachman–Diamond syndrome, impaired bile flow in chronic liver disease)
- solid organomegaly (hepatic or haematological or infectious splenic disorders)
- urogenital malformations (obstructive uropathy due to urethral valves)
- tumours (haemangioma, nephroblastoma, neuroblastoma)
- cysts (polycystic kidney disease), abscess (paratyphoid in appendicitis)
- mechanical (bowel obstruction due to impacted meconium or stool, intussusception, malrotation with volvulus, intestinal atresias, inflammatory or postsurgical adhesions) or paralytic ileus (infections [gastroenteritis, appendicitis], postsurgery, ischaemia, electrolyte imbalances [low potassium])
- umbilical hernia and diastasis recti (separation of the left and right rectus abdominis muscles).

Epigastric peristalsis may be visible owing to hypertrophic pyloric stenosis, which typically manifests after the neonatal period with projectile vomiting and life-threatening dehydration. A paucity of abdominal wall movements during respiration may be due to significant abdominal pain. A depressed abdomen with bowel sounds in the chest indicates a congenital or acquired (trauma) diaphragmatic defect. Assess for the asymmetry caused by an abdominal mass and the bulging flanks that result from ascites. If inguinal swelling is observed, it is commonly—but not always—caused by a hernia (see Ch 38). Carefully attempt to reduce the hernia at the end of the examination. A hernia is an indication for prompt surgical review (and if not reducible this is urgent). Note any abdominal scars indicating past surgical operations that may be relevant to the current major problem. Carefully inspect the skin for jaundice, discoloration, rashes, petechiae, bruising and spider naevi (see also Ch 38).

Auscultation

Auscultation of the abdomen is usually performed to assess bowel sounds and to listen for vascular bruits. It is generally felt that auscultation should take place before palpation, as this may alter bowel sounds. There is a lack of evidence that palpation alters bowel sounds but conventions in medicine are hard to alter. Auscultation requires patience, cooperation from the child (and the parent) and, in the case of bruits, a quiet room.

Begin by listening in the right upper quadrant over the liver for bruits or rubs. Bruits can occasionally be heard in children with hepatic haemangiomas. Bowel sounds from the overlying segments of bowel will often be heard in all quadrants. Next, move to the left upper quadrant to similarly listen over the spleen for bruits or rubs. Auscultate the left and right lower quadrants for inguinal bruits, before moving to the periumbilical region, where aortic and renal bruits are most commonly heard.[7] If a renal bruit is suspected, listen within 2 centimetres of the midline, halfway between the umbilicus and the xiphoid process. Remember that a renal bruit may be associated with hypertension as a result of renal artery stenosis so measure the blood pressure. Bruits are caused by turbulent flow through major blood vessels. Aortic bruits are usually heard only in systole, whereas **venous hums** are continuous.

To conclude that no bowel sounds can be heard, you need to have listened for several minutes and in several different areas of the abdomen. **Bowel sounds** that can be heard without a stethoscope are referred to as borborygmi. The complete absence of bowel sounds in the setting of abdominal pathology is an ominous sign that usually implies a paralytic ileus.[34] Increased or 'active' bowel sounds may be heard in patients with gastroenteritis, and when obstruction is present they often have a high-pitched or 'tinkling' quality.

Although auscultation is a commonly practised part of the paediatric abdominal examination, there is very little evidence of its value in the literature. Thankfully, what evidence can be found shows that bowel sounds have high specificity but low sensitivity in diagnosing abdominal obstruction.[35] This means that if abnormal sounds are heard, obstruction is likely, *but* the presence of normal bowel sounds will not accurately exclude bowel obstruction.

Palpation

Occasionally it is helpful to flex the knees or put a cushion under the neck in older children. This may help relax the abdominal muscles. First palpate all abdominal quadrants superficially and away from any tenderness. Remember to look at the child's face—not your hands—for any sign that the examination is painful. There is little you can do about a child's giggling during palpation except to try to divert his or her attention to something else. Giggling at least suggests that the examination is not painful. Next palpate more deeply with slow rather than poking movements. If you can feel a mass, assess it for tenderness and size and try to define its borders. This can also be done by percussion. Feel the surface and decide whether it is flat or nodular and whether the texture is soft or firm. If not completed previously, listen for bruits. A firm mass deep in the right lower abdominal quadrant (iliac fossa) is often due to faecal loading. This will disappear after bowel movements.

To palpate the **liver**, begin in the right iliac fossa using one hand in toddlers and infants and, if preferred, both hands in older children. Advance towards the right hypochondrium, which is the area below the right costal margin, and then across to the epigastrium to feel the liver edge, which is usually palpable just below the costal margin in older children or 1–2 centimetres below in younger children. The liver edge can be confirmed and the liver span can be determined with percussion using a tape measure. This may help you to decide whether the liver is enlarged (hepatomegaly) or pushed downwards (liver ptosis) by lung hyperinflation or a pleural effusion.

To palpate the **spleen**, begin in the *left* iliac fossa and advance towards the left costal margin. This is different from the adult examination. Remember that an enlarged spleen in older children (as in adults) can extend into the right iliac fossa. An enlarged spleen may be painful upon palpation so be very gentle. The tip of the spleen can often be felt in normal young children just below the left costal margin, particularly during inspiration, and in the right lateral decubitus position. If splenomegaly is suspected, it is important to ensure that you cannot palpate over the mass in the cranial direction, that you can feel a notch along the medial border and that the percussion note is dull.

Next palpate for **kidney enlargement** or cysts. Causes include hydronephrosis due to obstructive uropathy, polycystic kidneys and tumours such as nephroblastoma and neuroblastoma. Palpation is performed with two hands, one positioned beneath the flank and the other anteriorly in line with the first hand. The kidney may be felt during inspiration and can be trapped (ballotted) by pushing up with the hand under the flank and catching the kidney as it rises with the other hand.

Percussion

In children, abdominal percussion is used mostly to assess organ size and to check for ascites, but it is also useful in detecting mass lesions and areas of tenderness. Generally, fluid such as ascites or urine in the bladder or mass lesions will elicit a dull sound, whereas an air-filled structure like gas within the bowel will elicit a resonant note on percussion. Techniques are not different from those used in adults (see Ch 14), but be gentle, sensible and opportunistic in your approach.

Genitourinary system and Tanner staging

Genitourinary examination is not routinely performed in children, and in many instances, including suspected child sexual abuse, should be carried out only by a clinician who is well trained in this area. For small children, the parent should always be present; if an older child or adolescent is uncomfortable having the parent act as a chaperone, another appropriate chaperone should be provided. The examination for ambiguous genitalia is covered briefly in Chapter 38.

Genital examination in males

Check that the scrotum contains both testes, which should also be of similar size. Orchidometer beads can be used to estimate testicular size. Examine the skin for any unusual lesions and visualise the urethral meatus. Examine the glans for hypospadias

Hypospadias with the abnormal displaced urethral opening located in (a) the glans, (b, c) distal end of the penile shaft, (d) midshaft, (e) scrotum and (f) perineum

(From Baskin LS. Hypospadias and urethral development. *J Urol* 2000; 163:951–956.)

FIGURE 37.32

(see Fig. 37.32): in this condition, the urethral meatus may be displaced ventrally, anywhere within the glans, the shaft of the penis, the scrotum or even the perineum.

Palpate the scrotum for hernias, abnormal masses such as a varicocele or testicular enlargement (e.g. as a result of acute lymphoblastic leukaemia), and ensure that there is no pain or swelling of the testes that would suggest torsion. If a hydrocele is suspected, transilluminate the scrotum (see Fig. 18.11 on p 315). Check bilaterally for **inguinal hernia**. **Penile length** should be assessed as part of Tanner staging (see below). Care should be taken to ensure that the examination is not painful.

Genital examination in females

Proper visualisation of the female genitalia is usually easiest with the patient lying supine with the legs abducted at the hips. Again, care should be taken to ensure that this examination is not painful. If necessary, the labia can be separated to review the clitoris, the urethral meatus and the vaginal introitus. If clitoral enlargement is present, consider androgen stimulation as a result of congenital adrenal hyperplasia or disorders of sex development. Examine for labial adhesions and soft-tissue masses such as urethral prolapse, prolapsed ectopic ureterocele or paraurethral cysts. Check to ensure that the patient does not have an imperforate hymen or the associated hydrocolpos.

Internal examination (using a speculum) is almost never indicated in young girls and specialist advice should be sought before attempting this, even in the postpubertal female.

Anal and rectal examination

Anal and rectal examination is fairly similar for all age groups. Check for an anteriorly placed anus, skin tags, haemorrhoids (uncommon in children) and anal fissures, which can be caused by constipation or inflammatory bowel disease. Although inspection can be very important and informative, rectal examination is almost never indicated in children.

Tanner staging in puberty

Genital examination in children and adolescents may be performed as part of a pubertal assessment. In the 1960s Tanner and colleagues developed a staging system that is still used today (with minor modifications) to assess progression through puberty in both sexes (see Tables 37.17 and 37.18). Generally, enlargement of the testes is the first physical evidence of puberty in males (~98%) and the appearance of palpable breast tissue under the areola is the first physical evidence of puberty in females (~80%; see Fig. 37.33). In the remainder of adolescents, pubic hair is the first physical evidence (see Fig. 37.34).[7] For a quick screening it is often sufficient to show the child Tanner staging illustrations and ask where they see their current stage best represented.

Physical examination for suspected child abuse (see Text box 37.3)

Unfortunately, child abuse is one of the leading causes of injury-related mortality in infants and children,[36] and those of us who regularly examine children need to be able to recognise potentially abused children (see Table 37.19 and List 37.5) and treat them at first presentation to prevent significant morbidity and mortality.

Physical abuse should always be a differential for injuries in children. Suspicion may be raised during history taking, particularly if the caregiver has no explanation for the child's injuries, the explanation changes over time or there is a delay in seeking care.

Classification of sexual maturity in girls

SMR stage	Pubic hair	Breasts
1	Preadolescent	Preadolescent
2	Sparse, lightly pigmented, straight, medial border of labia	Breast and papilla elevated as small mound; diameter of areola increased
3	Darker, beginning to curl, increased amount	Breast and areola enlarged, no contour separation
4	Coarse, curly, abundant, but less than in adult	Areola and papilla form secondary mound
5	Adult feminine triangle, spread to medial surface of thighs	Mature, nipple projects, areola part of general breast contour

SMR = sexual maturity rating.

(Republished with permission of John Wiley & Sons Inc, from Tanner JM. *Growth at adolescence*, 2nd edn. Oxford, Blackwell Scientific/Wiley, 1962, permission conveyed through Copyright Clearance Center, Inc.)

TABLE 37.17

Classification of sexual maturity in boys

SMR stage	Pubic hair	Penis	Testes
1	None	Preadolescent	Preadolescent
2	Scanty, long, slightly pigmented	Minimal change/enlargement	Enlarged scrotum, pink, texture altered
3	Darker, starting to curl, small amount	Lengthens	Larger
4	Resembles adult type, but less quantity; coarse, curly	Larger; glans and breadth increase in size	Larger, scrotum dark
5	Adult distribution, spread to medial surface of thighs	Adult size	Adult size

SMR = sexual maturity rating.

(Republished with permission of John Wiley & Sons Inc, from Tanner JM. *Growth at adolescence*, 2nd edn. Oxford, Blackwell Scientific/Wiley, 1962, permission conveyed through Copyright Clearance Center, Inc.)

TABLE 37.18

CHAPTER 37 THE PAEDIATRIC HISTORY AND EXAMINATION 679

Sexual maturity ratings (1–5) of breast changes in adolescent girls

(From Behrman RE, Kliegman RM, St Geme JW et al. *Nelson textbook of pediatrics*, 17th edn. Philadelphia: Saunders, 2004.)

FIGURE 37.33

Sexual maturity ratings (2–5) of pubic hair changes in adolescent (a) boys and (b) girls

(From Behrman RE, Kliegman RM, St Geme JW et al. *Nelson textbook of pediatrics*, 17th edn. Philadelphia: Saunders, 2004.)

FIGURE 37.34

Assessing for suspected child abuse: a suggested method

1. Observe hygiene status, nutritional status, affect and behaviour.
2. Look carefully for bruising, lacerations, abrasions, scars, soft-tissue swelling and musculoskeletal deformities.
3. Palpate fontanels.
4. Inspect the oral cavity for dental caries, palatal petechiae and injuries to the lip and lingual frenula.
5. Inspect the eyes for subconjunctival haemorrhage and consider fundoscopy.
6. Palpate for bony pain or callus formation.
7. Perform the abdominal examination for tenderness or guarding.
8. Perform the genitourinary examination if required.
9. Complete the neurological examination.
10. Assess development.
11. Perform otoscopy.
12. Document meticulously.

TEXT BOX 37.3

> ### CLUES IN THE EVALUATION OF NON-ACCIDENTAL TRAUMA IN CHILDREN
>
> Suspect non-accidental trauma if the answer is 'yes' to any of the following questions
>
> - Is there an unusual distribution or location of lesions?
> - Is there a pattern of bruises or marks?
> - Can a bleeding disorder or collagen disease be ruled out as a cause of the lesions?
> - If there is a bite or handprint bruise, is it adult size?
> - If there is a burn, are the margins clearly demarcated with uniform depth of burn?
> - If there is a burn, is there a stocking and glove distribution?
> - Are there lesions of various healing stages or ages?
> - Is the reported mechanism of injury inconsistent with the extent of trauma?
>
> (McDonald KC. Child abuse: approach and management. *Am Fam Physician* 2007; 75(2):221–228.)
>
> LIST 37.5

Risk factors for child maltreatment

Caregiver factors	Criminal history, inappropriate expectations of the child, mental health history, misconceptions about child care, misperceptions about child development, substance abuse
Child factors	Behaviour problems, medical fragility, non-biological relationship to carer, prematurity, special needs
Family and environmental factors	High local unemployment rates, intimate partner violence in the home, poverty, social isolation or lack of support

(Reprinted with permission from Child Abuse: Approach and Management, January 15, 2007, Vol 75, No 2, American Family Physician Copyright © 2007 *American Academy of Family Physicians*. All Rights Reserved.)

TABLE 37.19

Always remember that when children disclose about abuse they are almost never lying. As clinicians, it is our duty to protect children from potential harm and act accordingly.

As part of routine paediatric practice, children are sometimes referred for examination by an order of a child welfare agency. These children require complete examination, rather than focusing on the area in question (e.g. bruising). Bear in mind that in preverbal children a physical examination is insufficient, and imaging (e.g. skeletal survey) and other investigations (e.g. blood tests) are usually required.

The rationale for physical examination is three-fold:
1. to assess the extent of the injury and to formulate a management plan
2. to provide a sense of safety for the child
3. to provide documentation that may be used as evidence.

Start (as always) by documenting the child's growth parameters, and ensure that appropriate documentation is completed (including clinical photography if indicated). Use a bodygram (see Fig. 37.35) if photography is not being performed to document any visible findings. Note the child's appearance, hygiene, nutritional status, affect (e.g. frightened, friendly) and behaviour throughout the examination. Also make note of the parent's behaviour during the examination, if present.

Examine the child for:
- bruising
- lacerations
- abrasions
- scars
- soft-tissue swellings
- musculoskeletal deformities.

Document the size and location of any abnormality seen. It is mandatory to check for lesions that may be present under the child's clothes and do not forget to move the hair to visualise the scalp. Remember that it can be quite difficult to differentiate bruising from other, innocent, skin discolorations (e.g. café-au-lait spots, pigmented birthmarks); when in doubt, reschedule a repeat examination for several days later. Palpate along the limbs for any tenderness or swelling. Look for redundant skinfolds secondary to weight loss, poor muscle bulk and other signs of malnutrition and neglect such as severe nappy rash.

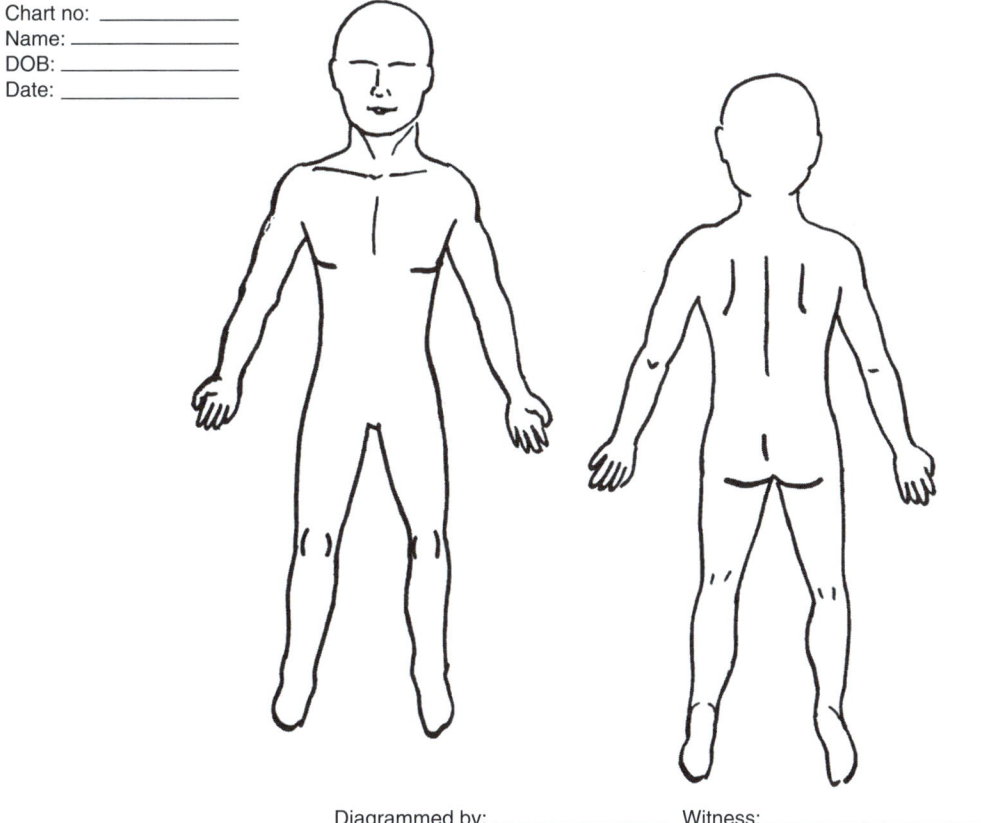

Bodygram

(From Legano L, McHugh MT, Palusci VJ. Child abuse and neglect. *Curr Probl Pediatr Adolesc Health Care* 2009; 39(2):e26–e31.)

FIGURE 37.35

Palpate the fontanel in infants, as an intracranial haemorrhage or cerebral oedema may present with a bulging or tense fontanel. Examine the oral cavity for dental caries, palatal petechiae and injuries to the lip and lingual frenulum. Examine the eyes for subconjunctival haemorrhage. Examine the retina by fundoscopy and consider whether dilated indirect fundoscopy (usually performed by an ophthalmologist) is required. Perform otoscopy looking for haemotympanum or a perforated eardrum and check over the mastoids for bruising.

Palpate over the chest (particularly looking for callus formation and crepitus due to rib fractures) and perform an abdominal examination noting any tenderness or guarding. Genitourinary examination should be performed, but kept minimally invasive. External examination is sufficient in girls; and the penis and scrotum should be carefully visualised in boys to check for injuries or bruising.

Perform a neurological examination, but be aware that further imaging is required in very young children if intracranial haemorrhage is to be ruled out. Perform a developmental examination in any child suspected of being neglected.

Meticulously document all your findings and arrange any medical treatments that may be required. Be aware that this documentation may be required as evidence in child protection and even criminal investigations.

T&O'C ESSENTIALS

1. Children are not simply little adults: history taking and physical examination need to be tailored to their specific needs.
2. Much information can be gathered by observing the child.
3. Be gentle and opportunistic but as thorough as possible in conducting the examination.
4. Do not make up clinical signs or disregard them if they are detected with appropriate certainty.
5. Perform less-pleasant assessments (e.g. ear, nose, throat) at the end of the examination.
6. Height, weight and head circumference should always be assessed and recorded.
7. Differentiate between physiological conditions often seen in childhood (e.g. lumbar hyperlordosis) and pathological conditions (e.g. scoliosis).
8. Careful inspection of the face, eyes, ears and oral cavity may reveal the presence of a syndromic or genetic abnormality.
9. The majority of the neurological examination in smaller children is best performed using a combination of observation and play.
10. The respiratory and cardiovascular examinations are of particular significance in paediatrics because they can identify a seriously ill child.
11. The genitourinary examination is not routinely performed in children.
12. Physical abuse should always be a differential for injuries in children.

OSCE REVISION TOPICS – THE PAEDIATRIC HISTORY AND EXAMINATION

Use these topics, which commonly occur in the OSCE, to help with revision.

1. This child's parent is concerned that he is much shorter than his brother was at the same age. Please examine him. (p 624)
2. This child has an unusual-shaped head. Please examine her. (p 644)
3. Please perform a developmental assessment on this child and give an estimate of the child's developmental age. (p 659)
4. The community nurse is concerned that this child is 'floppy'. Please perform a 180° examination. (p 658)
5. Please examine this child's cranial nerves. (p 653)
6. A general practitioner has noticed that this child has clubbing. Please examine her. (p 668)
7. Please examine this child who has been noted to have a murmur. (p 669)
8. This child's teacher has noticed some unusual bruising. Please examine the child. (pp 641, 678)
9. This child's parent has noticed that his abdomen is more distended than usual. Please examine the child. (p 674)
10. Please examine this child's ears as his parents have noticed some purulent discharge. (p 647)

References

1. Cook DE, Andringa CL, Hess KL. et al. School health examinations. *Pediatrics* 1981; 67(4):576–577.
2. Riley M, Locke AB, Skye EP. Health maintenance in school-aged children: Part I. History, physical examination, screening, and immunizations. *Am Fam Physician* 2011; 83(6):683–688.
3. Committee on Practice and Ambulatory Medicine. The use of chaperones during the physical examination of the pediatric patient. *Pediatrics* 1996; 98(6):1202.
4. Britto MT, Tivorsak TL, Slap GB. Adolescents' needs for health care privacy. *Pediatrics* 2010; 126(6):e1469–e1476.
5. Watts K, Bell LM, Byrne SM et al. Waist circumference predicts cardiovascular risk in young Australian children. *J Paediatr Child Health* 2008; 44(12):709–715.
6. Owen GM. Measurement, recording, and assessment of skinfold thickness in childhood and adolescence: report of a small meeting. *Am J Clin Nutr* 1982; 35(3):629–638.
7. Walker HK, Hall WD, Hurst JW. *Clinical methods: the history, physical, and laboratory examinations*. Oxford: Butterworth–Heinemann, 1990.
8. US Dept of Health and Human Sciences. The fourth report on the diagnosis, evaluation, and treatment of high blood pressure in children and adolescents. *Pediatrics* 2004; 114(2 suppl 4th report):555–576.
9. National High Blood Pressure Education Program Working Group on Hypertension Control in Children and Adolescents. Update on the 1987 task force report on high blood pressure in children and adolescents: a working group report from the national high blood pressure education program. *Pediatrics* 1996; 98(4):649–658.
10. Kavey RE, Daniels SR, Flynn JT. Management of high blood pressure in children and adolescents. *Cardiol Clin* 2010; 28(4):597–607.
11. Kaelber DC, Pickett F. Simple table to identify children and adolescents needing further evaluation of blood pressure. *Pediatrics* 2009; 123(6) e972–e974.
12. Fouzas S, Priftis KN, Anthracopoulos MB. Pulse oximetry in pediatric practice. *Pediatrics* 2011; 128(4):740–752.
13. Devrim I, Kara A, Ceyhan M et al. Measurement accuracy of fever by tympanic and axillary thermometry. *Pediatr Emerg Care* 2007; 23(1):16–19.
14. El-Radhi AS, Barry W. Thermometry in paediatric practice. *Arch Dis Child* 2006; 91(4):351–356.
15. Fabry G. Clinical practice. Static, axial, and rotational deformities of the lower extremities in children. *Eur J Pediatr* 2010; 169(5):529–534.
16. Fabry G. Clinical practice: the spine from birth to adolescence. *Eur J Pediatr* 2009; 168(12):1415–1420.
17. Houghton KM. Review for the generalist: evaluation of low back pain in children and adolescents. *Pediatr Rheumatol* 2010; 8(28):1546–1696.
18. Foster HE, Jandial S. pGALS – paediatric Gait Arms Legs and Spine: a simple examination of the musculoskeletal system. *Pediatr Rheumatol* 2013; 11:44. A good resource for paediatric musculoskeletal exam.
19. Hohenleutner U, Landthaler M, Hamm H, Sebastian G. Hemangiomas of infancy and childhood. *J Dtsch Dermatol Ges* 2007; 5(4):334–338.
20. Menezes MP, North KN. Inherited neuromuscular disorders: pathway to diagnosis. *J Paediatr Child Health* 2012; 48(6):458–465.
21. Forrest CR, Hopper RA. Craniofacial syndromes and surgery. *Plast Reconstr Surg* 2013; 131(1):86e–109e.
22. Rothman R, Owens T, Simel DL. Does this child have acute otitis media? *JAMA* 2003; 290(12):1633–1640.
23. Park YW. Evaluation of neck masses in children. *Am Fam Physician* 1995; 51(8):1904–1912.
24. Toriello HV. Role of the dysmorphologic evaluation in the child with developmental delay. *Pediatr Clin North Am* 2008; 55(5):1085–1098, xi.
25. Bodensteiner JB. The evaluation of the hypotonic infant. *Semin Pediatr Neurol* 2008; 15(1):10–20.
26. Miller JW. Screening children for developmental behavioral problems: principles for the practitioner. *Prim Care* 2007; 34(2):177–201; abstract v.
27. Wood NS, Marlow N, Costeloe K et al. Neurologic and developmental disability after extremely preterm birth. EPICure Study Group. *N Engl J Med* 2000; 343(6):378–384.
28. Stephenson T, Wallace H, Thomson A. *Clinical paediatrics for postgraduate examinations*. Edinburgh: Churchill Livingstone, 2003.
29. Motyckova G, Steensma DP. Why does my patient have lymphadenopathy or splenomegaly? *Hematol Oncol Clin North Am* 2012; 26(2):395–408.
30. Mellis C. Respiratory noises: how useful are they clinically? *Pediatr Clin North Am* 2009; 56(1):1–17, ix.
31. Shields MD, Bush A, Everard ML et al. BTS guidelines: Recommendations for the assessment and management of cough in children. *Thorax* 2008; 63:iii1–iii15.
32. Forgacs P. Crackles and wheezes. *Lancet* 1967; 2(7508):203–205.
33. Nath AR, Capel LH. Inspiratory crackles and mechanical events of breathing. *Thorax* 1974; 29(6):695–698.
34. Goldbloom RB. *Pediatric clinical skills*. Philadelphia: Saunders, 2010.
35. Böhner H, Yang Q, Franke C et al. Simple data from history and physical examination help to exclude bowel obstruction and to avoid radiographic studies in patients with acute abdominal pain. *Eur J Surg* 1998; 164(10):777–784.
36. McDonald KC. Child abuse: approach and management. *Am Fam Physician* 2007; 75(2):221–228.

CHAPTER 38

The neonatal history and examination

Joerg Mattes and Bryony Ross

The important thing is to make the lesson of each case tell on your education. The value of experience is not in seeing much, but in seeing wisely. SIR WILLIAM OSLER (1849–1919)

Neonates are very different from adult and even paediatric patients. They are very fragile, cannot cooperate in their examination and cannot give you a history.[a] The usual systematic approach to the history taking and examination is often not possible and an *opportunistic* method must be adopted. This means that history taking may have to wait until the parents, hospital staff or relatives are available and the examination must be fitted around the infant's feeding schedule, need for sleep and mood.

THE HISTORY

In many cases, history taking begins with a review of the maternal and infant medical records (if available) and the gathering of information from clinical staff, and then progresses to an interview with the parents. As with history taking for the adult, your approach needs to be methodical. There may not be a presenting complaint, but asking about problems that may have occurred during the pregnancy or delivery is an important aspect of the history taking.

Remember that this is usually a happy but anxious time for new parents. They must be approached with understanding and patience. Allow enough time for the interview and respect their privacy and sensitivities of various sorts. Parents' worries must always be taken seriously and dealt with respectfully, even when they seem insignificant from a medical point of view.[b]

First, introduce yourself to the parents and congratulate them on the birth of their child. Explain the reasons for the neonatal assessment and tell them how it will be carried out. Ask for their consent wherever possible.

Maternal health

Assemble a comprehensive history by asking about the mother's current and past medical and surgical history. This should identify any chronic illnesses that could affect the baby's health (see Table 38.1). If the mother has an acute or a chronic illness, ask questions around the mnemonic **SIC**:

Symptoms (severity, frequency, triggers, treatments)

Investigations

Complications.

A maternal illness may affect the mother's ability to look after her baby and directly affect the baby's health.

Next, ascertain the mother's health, lifestyle and psychosocial background using the mnemonic **HeLP**:

Health status

Lifestyle

Psychosocial background.

Of particular relevance is substance use (see Table 38.2). Also assess nutrition and immunisation status and possible mental health problems. Ask tactfully what the parents know about neonatal health and safety by keeping in mind the mnemonic **CARE**:

Coping with parenthood (e.g. understanding the baby's nutritional needs and sudden infant death syndrome [SIDS] risk factors)

---

[a] Paediatrics has been compared, rather unkindly, to veterinary medicine by adult physicians.
[b] Experienced parents' opinions should always be taken seriously.

Mother's medical and surgical history

Mother	Effect on baby
Endocrine system, e.g: Diabetes[2] Hypo/hyperthyroidism[3]	Macrosomia (birth weight >4000 g), birth trauma, jaundice, seizures (hypoglycaemia, hypocalcaemia), plethora (polycythaemia), birth trauma, major congenital anomalies, cardiomyopathy Premature birth, SGA, thyroid enlargement
Immune system, e.g: Lupus erythematosus[4] Asthma[5]	Stillbirth, neonatal deaths, premature birth, SGA, thrombotic events Premature birth, low birth weight
Inborn errors of metabolism, e.g: Hyperphenylalaninaemia[6]	Microcephaly,* murmurs/cyanosis (congenital heart disease)
Cardiovascular/renal system, e.g: Hypertension	Pulmonary complications, sepsis, prematurity
Medications, e.g: Valproate[7] SSRIs[8]	Neural tube defects, hypospadias,** cardiac defects and oral clefts Respiratory, motor, central nervous system and gastrointestinal symptoms (SSRI neonatal behaviour syndrome)

*Small head size.
**An abnormality of the urethra such that it opens on the ventral surface of the penis or on the perineum or into the vagina.
SGA = small for gestational age; SSRIs = selective serotonin reuptake inhibitors.

TABLE 38.1

Access to healthcare practitioners and social support
Relationships and conflicts
Effects of illness on the child's health.

Other family history

Ask briefly about serious or possibly inherited illnesses in other family members, particularly siblings.

QUESTIONS TO ASK THE MOTHER ABOUT HER PREGNANCY AND DELIVERY

1. What type of antenatal screening did you have? (Ultrasound, amniocentesis)
2. Did you have problems with high blood pressure during your pregnancy? Was pre-eclampsia diagnosed?
3. Did you have any blood group incompatibility problems?
4. Did you have any bladder or kidney infections?
5. Was your baby delivered at full term?
6. How was your baby's health during delivery?
7. Was there any mention of meconium staining during delivery? (A sign of fetal distress)
8. Did you have a vaginal delivery or a caesarean section?

QUESTIONS BOX 38.1

History of the pregnancy, labour and delivery

This should include questions about:

- antenatal screening (e.g. serology, ultrasound, amniocentesis), pregnancy
- birth-related complications and operations (e.g. pre-eclampsia [hypertension and proteinuria], rhesus/ABO incompatibility [blood group])
- infections (urinary tract infections, group B *Streptococcus* colonisation)
- fetal wellbeing (blood-flow patterns, biophysical profiles such as cardiotocography)
- vaginal bleeding, amniotic fluid (amount and aspect) and type of delivery (vaginal or caesarian section)—see Questions boxes 38.1 and 38.2.

Enquire about the baby's health status at birth (5-minute Apgar score [see Table 38.3], any resuscitation required, medical support, treatments, birth weight, length, head circumference), immunisation status

Mother's health, life and psychosocial background (HeLP)	
Mother	**Effect on baby**
Infections[9–13], e.g.:	
HIV	Increased risk of sepsis and infections if HIV positive
Toxoplasmosis	Hepatosplenomegaly, lymphadenopathy, chorioretinitis, seizures, hydrocephalus, SGA
Syphilis	Stillbirth, hepatomegaly, lymphadenopathy, maculopapular/vesicular rash, rhinitis
Rubella	Sensorineural hearing loss, ocular abnormalities (glaucoma, retinopathy, cataract), congenital heart disease, central nervous system (hyperoxygenation S) abnormalities, SGA
Cytomegalovirus	Hepatosplenomegaly, petechiae, microcephaly, chorioretinitis, sensorineural hearing loss, SGA
Parvovirus B19 (fifth disease)	Non-immune fetal hydrops,* myocarditis, hepatitis
Varicella-zoster	Skin scarring, eye defects, limb hypoplasia, premature birth, SGA
Listeriosis	Pneumonia, sepsis or meningitis
Herpes simplex	Local skin, eye and mouth infections with vesicular lesions, CNS infections
Obesity (BMI >30 kg/m^2)	Macrosomia/LGA, premature birth, neural tube defects, congenital heart disease, omphalocele**
Antenatal drug use[14] Nicotine	SIDS, SGA, asthma, ADHD
Marijuana	Decreased self-quieting ability, fine tremors, increased hand-to-mouth activity, sleep pattern changes
Methadone	Strabism,*** NAS: respiratory distress increased tone, tremors, seizures poor feeding, vomiting, regurgitation, diarrhoea sweating
Heroin	NAS, increased perinatal mortality, SGA, ADHD
Cocaine	Genitourinary malformations, CNS symptoms, SGA
Amphetamines	Congenital CNS, cardiovascular, limb defects, oral clefts, neurobehavioural effects
Hallucinogens	Congenital cardiovascular and kidney defects
Alcohol	Fetal alcohol spectrum disorder with developmental delay, ADHD, characteristic facial appearance, SGA (small eyes, flattened nasal bridge, maxillary hypoplasia, shortened palpebral fissures, short upturned nose, smooth philtrum, small upper lip)

*Increased amniotic fluid, a sign of fetal heart failure.
**A hernia into the umbilical cord and then umbilicus.
***Squint.
ADHD = attention deficit hyperactivity disorder; BMI = body mass index; HIV = human immunodeficiency virus; LGA = large for gestational age; NAS = neonatal abstinence syndrome; SGA = small for gestational age; SIDS = sudden infant death syndrome.

TABLE 38.2

and prophylaxis (hepatitis B, vitamin K) and current nutrition (breastfed/bottle-fed, frequency, amounts, weight gain).

Any bilious vomiting warrants immediate further investigation. Meconium should be passed within the first 48 hours. This pasty green substance consists of desquamated epithelial cells, mucus, bile, lanugo (fine hair that covers the fetus and is swallowed as it falls off before birth) and vernix caseosa (a white cheesy material that coats the fetal skin), which collects in the fetal bowel and is passed after birth. When meconium is passed in utero it is usually a sign of fetal distress or hypoxia.

Predictors of severe illness in the medical history of the newborn include a history of difficult feeding, reduced feeding ability, weak sucking, lethargy,

> **QUESTIONS TO ASK THE MOTHER ABOUT THE BABY'S HEALTH AT BIRTH AND EARLY LIFE**
>
> ❗ denotes a potentially serious symptom
>
> 1. Do you know your baby's Apgar score?
> 2. What was your baby's birth weight?
> 3. Has your baby been given vitamin K or any vaccinations yet?
> 4. Are you breastfeeding? How are you managing?
> ❗ 5. Is your baby able to suck strongly?
> ❗ 6. Has your baby had any convulsions?
> ❗ 7. Does your baby seem breathless when feeding?
> ❗ 8. Has your baby had any bilious vomiting? (Bowel obstruction)
>
> QUESTIONS BOX 38.2

Normal umbilical cord vessel configuration with two arteries on the right and one vein on the left

(From Harding S. *Rennie & Roberton's textbook of neonatology*. Philadelphia: Elsevier, 2012.)

FIGURE 38.1

convulsions, fast or difficult breathing and abnormal behaviour.[16–18]

Obtain results of the placental examination (size, membranes, vessels, infarcts, clots) and umbilical cord, which usually has two arteries and one vein (see Fig. 38.1). If the cord has only one of each (1% of all deliveries), there is a 60% increased risk of associated anomalies in major organ systems (most commonly the kidneys).[19] Most of this information can be gathered by reviewing the mother and baby's medical records or by consultation with clinical staff.

THE PHYSICAL EXAMINATION

It is generally accepted that all neonates should have an immediate health check after birth, followed by a more detailed physical examination in the first 3 days of life.[20] Repeat physical examination is recommended at 6–8 weeks of age. The principal aims of the neonatal examination are to:

1. detect congenital anomalies and illnesses, insufficient perinatal adaptation to extrauterine life and adverse effects resulting from birth
2. discuss the results and limitations of the assessment with the parents in a tactful and sympathetic manner
3. arrange for appropriate follow-up examinations and management.

One- and five-minute Apgar values*	
Appearance	0 = blue or pale 1 = blue extremities only 2 = pink (no cyanosis)
Pulse	0 = absent 1 = less than 100 beats per minute 2 = more than 100 beats per minute
Grimace	0 = no response when stimulated 1 = grimace when stimulated 2 = cry/pull away when stimulated
Activity	0 = no muscle tone 1 = flexor tone 2 = flexor tone resisting extension
Respiration	0 = absent 1 = irregular/gasping 2 = regular/crying

*Rapid assessment of the newborn immediately after birth (1 minute and 5 minutes after birth and each 5 minutes thereafter in a severely depressed neonate) was devised by Dr Virginia Apgar (1909–74), leading to a drastic reduction in infant mortality.[15]

(Apgar V. A proposal for a new method of evaluation of the newborn infant. *Curr Res Anesth Analg* 1953; 32(4):260–267; republished *Anesth Analg* 2015; 120(5):1056–1059.)

TABLE 38.3

Examination of the neonate: a suggested method

1. **Preparation**
   Wash your hands and put on gloves if indicated.
   Undress the baby to the nappy but make sure that he or she is kept warm.
   Never leave the baby unattended on the examination table.
   Explain to parents what you are doing.

2. **Measurements**
   Weigh the baby without the nappy or weigh the nappy separately and subtract.
   Measure the baby's length (called height in adults).
   Measure the baby's head circumference.
   Plot these on the appropriate growth charts.
   Take the baby's temperature.

3. **Inspection**
   Posture and spontaneous movements
   Muscle fasciculations
   Dysmorphic features: face, hands and feet
   Asymmetry: muscles, limbs, leg creases
   Jaundice
   Cyanosis
   Skin
     Naevi
     Erythema or vesicles (suggesting infection)
     Skin tumours
   Head and spine
     Shape
     Sutures
     Fontanels
     Signs of spina bifida
   Eyes
     Size
     Sclerae
     Pupils
     Movements
     Dysmorphic features
   Ears
     Abnormal position
     Skin tags
     Auditory canal
   Nose
     Asymmetry
     Nasal flaring or respiratory distress
     Nasal cavity
   Mouth
     Jaw size
     Tongue size
     Cleft palate or lip
   Neck
     Torticollis
     Abnormal skinfolds
   Chest
     Deformity
     Stridor, wheezing or grunting
     Apex beat and heart sounds
     Lung sounds
   Abdomen and genitals
     Inspection, distension, umbilicus
     Palpation
     Auscultation
     Hernias
     Testes and scrotum
     Penis
     Female genitalia
     Anus
   Limbs
     Symmetry
     Deformity
     The hips
   Central nervous system
     Posture
     Tone
     Developmental reflexes

TEXT BOX 38.1

A method for the examination of the neonate is given in Text box 38.1.

Preparing for the physical examination

A structured yet flexible head-to-toe approach is essential for the identification of serious pathologies and for differentiating them from benign variations or from what is expected during the physiological transition from intra- to extrauterine life. The newborn should not be examined immediately after a large feed, as this may cause vomiting, or when hungry as the baby is likely to cry. Exposure to bright light and cold environments may cause discomfort to the neonate.

Before you start the examination, remove your jewellery and/or watch and roll up your sleeves to above the elbow. Hand hygiene is crucial for the prevention of cross-infection and nosocomial infection in newborn infants.[21] Clean your hands and forearms with soap and water or an ethanol-based hand disinfectant before and after contact with the baby, before and after any

(a) The five moments for hand hygiene, and (b) use of personal protective equipment as indicated are extremely effective measures to prevent cross-infection

((a) Based on 'My 5 moments for hand hygiene', www.who.int/gpsc/5may/background/5moments/en/index.html, ©World Health Organization, 2009.)

FIGURE 38.2

procedure or exposure to bodily fluids, and after touching the baby's surroundings (see Fig. 38.2(a)). Wear examination gloves and other personal protective equipment when indicated to avoid cross-infection (see Fig. 38.2(b)). Clean your examination tools (e.g. stethoscope) thoroughly with the appropriate antimicrobial agents before and after use.

Usually, newborns cannot turn but they may be able to move rather dangerously sidewards on the examination table. This should be explained to the parents. It is imperative to create barriers on both sides of the baby (e.g. the wall and yourself) or to secure the baby gently with your hand during the examination. Never step away without asking someone else to watch the infant. Alternatively, carry the baby with you.

Measurements

Measurements of weight, length and occipitofrontal head circumference are important for the detection of serious pathologies and for monitoring growth and development. To obtain the bare weight, fully undress the neonate (including the nappy) and use an electronic baby scale. Never leave the baby unattended on the scales as they may fall off and injure themselves. If the room is too cold, use a heating lamp. Alternatively, you can measure the baby covered with a preweighed towel.

Use a newborn stadiometer (also called a head-board) to measure length. To obtain exact measurements a helper is required. Hold both the neonate's feet on the footpiece with one hand, fully extend the neonate's legs gently and slide the headpiece horizontally to rest (gently) on top of the neonate's head.

To measure head circumference use a non-stretching tape measure around the neonate's head at the widest point. This is usually achieved by placing the end of the tape measure on the middle of the forehead just above the palpebral fissures, then wrapping it around the temporal bones beneath the auricular helices and the most posterior portion of the occipital bone. Occipitofrontal circumference measurements should be taken until there is a variation of less than 0.5 centimetres between two repeated measurements.

Plot the results on growth charts that are most suitable for your location. The WHO *Child growth standards* (2006) charts (see Fig. 38.3) are based on data from term, breastfed and healthy infants born to non-smoking mothers in six countries (United States, Norway, India, Ghana, Brazil and Oman) and may be appropriate for term babies (see www.who.int/childgrowth/en/). The Fenton growth charts may be suitable for premature neonates (see www.biomedcentral.com/1471-2431/3/13/figure/F2). Note that other growth charts are available for premature babies (e.g. Babson and Benda,[22] Lubchenco et al[23] and Dancis et al[24]) and for infants with specific genetic conditions (e.g. for trisomy 21[25]).

Text continued on p 696

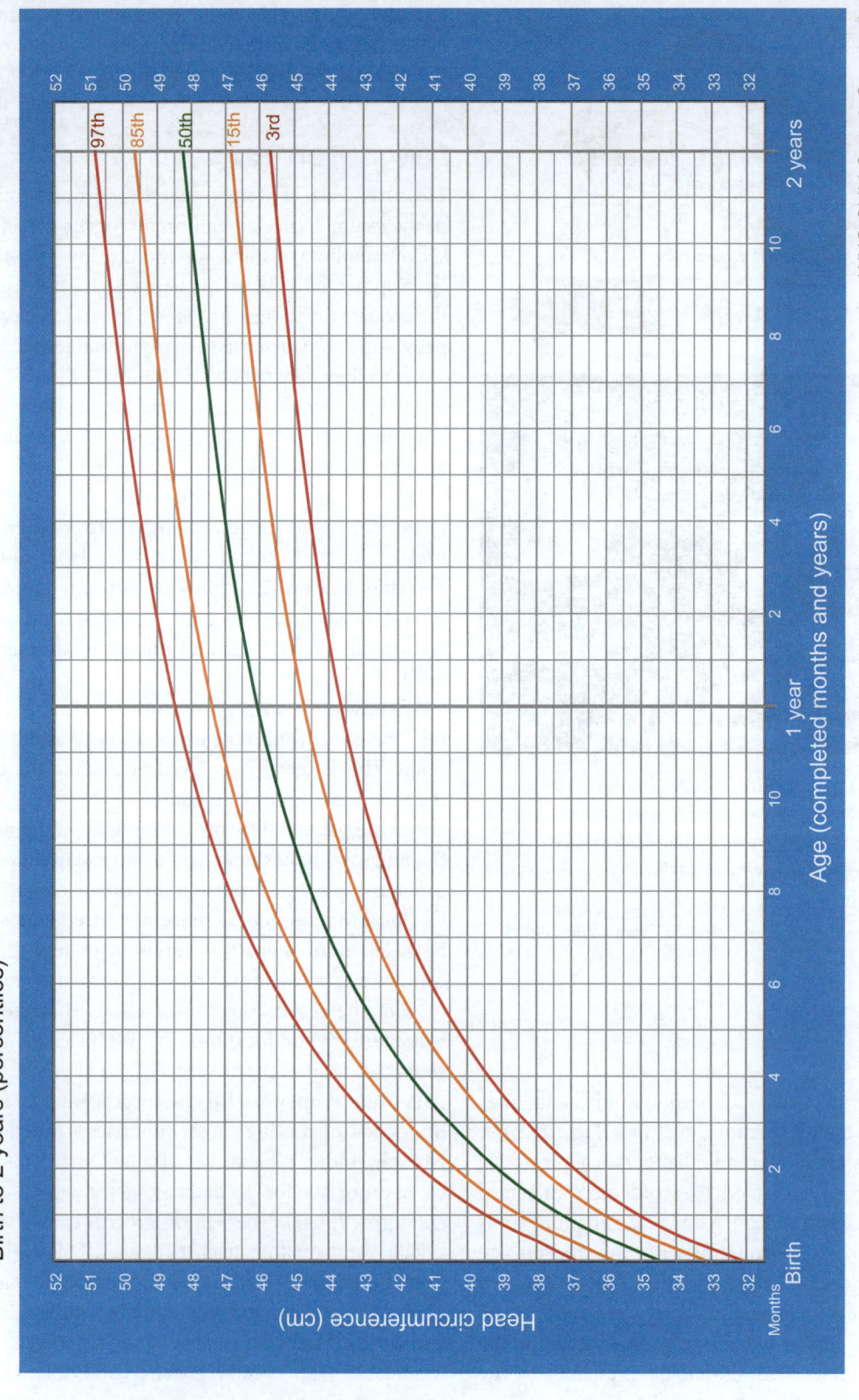

Growth charts for term infants
(Reprinted from World Health Organisation Child Growth Standard Charts, http://www.who.int/childgrowth/standards/en/.)

FIGURE 38.3

CHAPTER 38 THE NEONATAL HISTORY AND EXAMINATION 691

FIGURE 38.3, cont'd

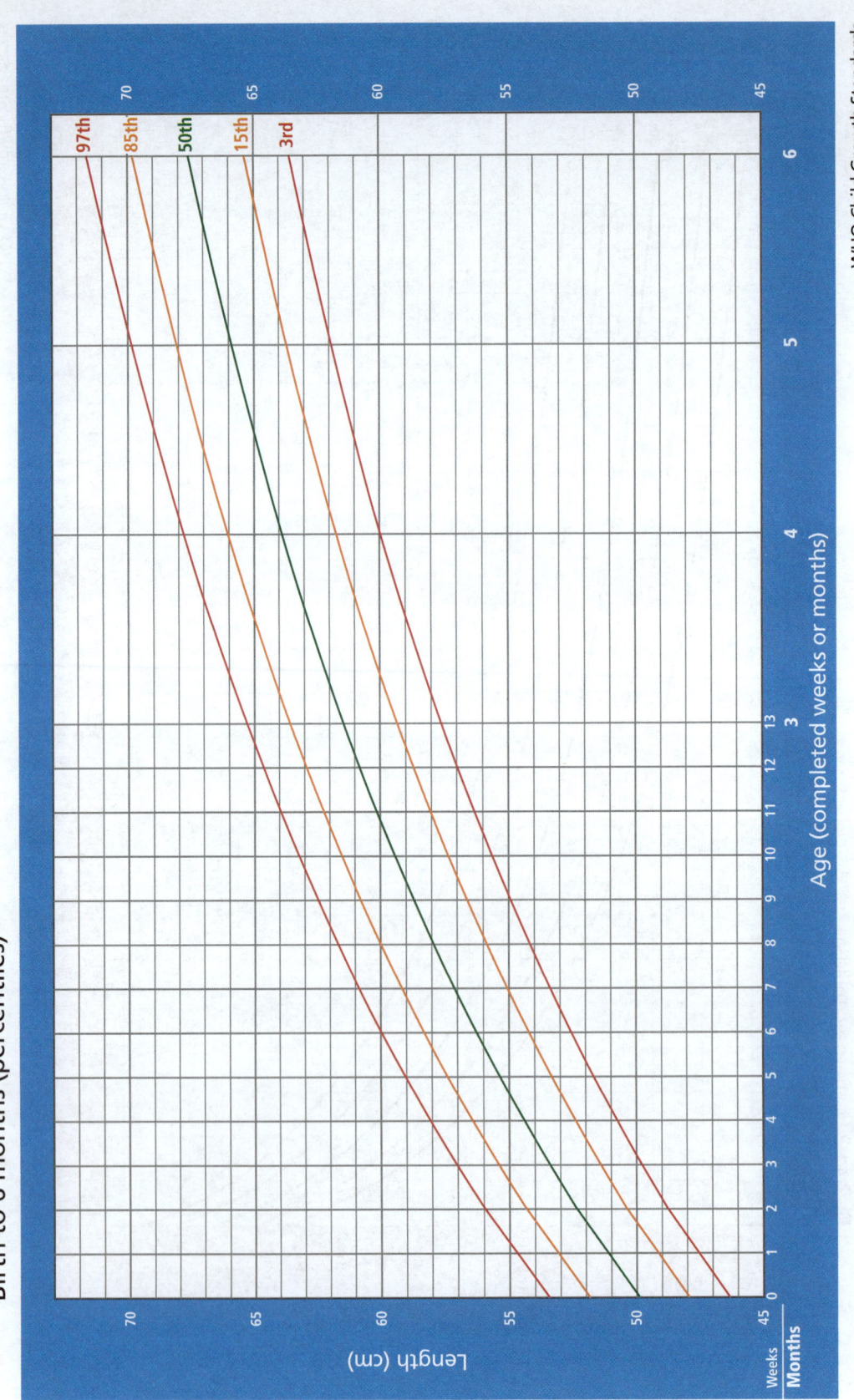

FIGURE 38.3, cont'd

CHAPTER 38 THE NEONATAL HISTORY AND EXAMINATION 693

FIGURE 38.3, cont'd

694 SECTION 10 PAEDIATRIC AND NEONATAL HISTORY AND EXAMINATION

FIGURE 38.3, cont'd

CHAPTER 38 THE NEONATAL HISTORY AND EXAMINATION 695

FIGURE 38.3, cont'd

Small for gestational age (**SGA**) is most commonly defined as a birth weight below the tenth percentile, whereas large for gestational age (**LGA**) is defined as a birth weight above the ninetieth percentile corrected for gestational age. A baby can be constitutionally small (e.g. small parents) or pathologically small (fetal, maternal, placental factors). If pathological SGA is potentially present, determine whether the newborn has symmetrical intrauterine growth restriction (weight, length and head circumference <tenth percentile). This indicates slow growth development throughout pregnancy present from a very early stage. Common causes are:

- intrauterine infections
- maternal drug abuse
- anaemia
- chromosomal abnormalities in the fetus.

Thus, symmetrical SGA is often associated with other clinical signs and serious long-term sequelae (see Tables 38.1 and 38.2). In contrast, asymmetrical intrauterine growth restriction leads to a disproportionate reduction in weight only (<tenth percentile) and indicates impaired growth development in the third trimester. Common causes are:

- pre-eclampsia
- placental insufficiency
- multiple gestation
- maternal age >35 years.

As the subcutaneous fat layer is underdeveloped, these neonates are at increased risk of hypoglycaemia, hypocalcaemia, polycythaemia, fetal distress and hypoxia.

A common cause of LGA is gestational diabetes, which has the potential to lead to serious complications if not recognised and managed appropriately (see Table 38.1).

Head-to-toe assessment
Posture and spontaneous movements

Observe the baby's posture and any spontaneous movements. Newborns perform flexion in the upper and lower limbs and symmetrical alternating movements involving all extremities. Deviation from this pattern may indicate birth injuries, deformities, or neurological or genetic abnormalities. A lack of spontaneous movements, which occur only on stimulation, is associated with a marked risk of severe illness.[18]

Generalised paucity of movements

If the baby is in a frog-leg position and there is a paucity of limb movements, this suggests reduced muscle tone and power (floppy infant). A history of polyhydramnios[c] and poor fetal movements may indicate congenital hypotonia and a problem with motor neurones that travel from the anterior horn of the spinal cord to the muscles (lower motor neurone lesions such as spinal muscular atrophy), motor end plate (e.g. congenital myasthenia gravis, botulism), or muscles (congenital myopathy, muscular dystrophy, infections).

Look for muscle fasciculations, especially of the tongue, and remember to test for a lack of tendon reflexes (biceps, triceps, brachioradialis, knee and ankle) that is suspicious for a lower motor neurone lesion. In the first 6 months of life upper motor neurone abnormalities are often associated with reduced muscle tone rather than spasticity (see List 38.1). The presence of increased muscle tone ('stiff limbs') indicates the possibility of severe illness in the newborn.[18] In older babies, an upper motor neurone lesion should be suspected if there is scissoring of the lower limbs and flexion of the thumbs.

Localised paucity of movements

Asymmetry in power and tone may indicate a focal upper or lower (e.g. brachial plexus palsies) motor

---

CAUSES OF UPPER MOTOR NEURONE WEAKNESS IN INFANTS

Generalised
- Hypoxic encephalopathy due to birth asphyxia
- Metabolic disturbances, infections
- Chromosomal abnormalities

Asymmetrical
- Cerebrovascular accident or haemorrhage
- Intracranial
- Spinal malformation

LIST 38.1

---

[c] Increased amniotic fluid volume.

Neonatal brachial plexus palsies

Brachial plexus palsy	Brachial trunk/spinal root	Clinical signs
Duchenne–Erb	Upper/C5–C6	'Waiter's tip' posture with arm adducted and internally rotated, elbow extended, forearm pronated, wrist and fingers flexed
Middle trunk	Middle/C7	Elbow flexed
Klumpke	Lower/C8–T1	'Claw hand' posture with arm supinated, elbow flexed, wrist extended, hyperextension of the metacarpophalangeal joints, flexion of the interphalangeal joints
Complete	Upper+middle+lower/C5–T1	'Flail limb' (all above) plus possibly Horner's syndrome

(Adapted from Alfonso I, Alfonso DT, Papazian O. Focal upper extremity neuropathy in neonates. *Semin Pediatr Neurol* [Review] 2000; 7(1):4–14; Klumpke A. Klumpke's paralysis. 1885. *Clin Orthop Rel Res* [Biography Classical Article Historical Article Portraits] 1999; (368):3–4.)

TABLE 38.4

(a) Duchenne–Erb: this infant demonstrates the characteristic posture of the limply adducted and internally rotated arm. (b, c) Infant with Klumpke palsy involving the lower segments of C7 and T1. Note the different posture of the arm compared with the Erb palsy, and the claw-hand deformity

((a) From Brozanski BS. *Zitelli and Davis' atlas of pediatric physical diagnosis*. Philadelphia: Saunders, 2012, with permission; (b, c) courtesy of Dr Michael Painter, Children's Hospital of Pittsburgh.)

FIGURE 38.4

neurone lesion (see Table 38.4 and Fig. 38.4). Brachial plexus lesions occur most commonly during birth (e.g. as a result of shoulder dystocia,[d] which increases the risk 100-fold). Note the size of the hand and arm, the muscle bulk and the presence of joint contractures because injuries can affect normal growth and development of the affected arm.

Respiratory distress could indicate phrenic nerve palsy. Horner's syndrome (miosis, ptosis, anhidrosis) suggests injury to the T1 spinal root proximal to the point where the sympathetic nerve fibres have separated from the somatic motor nerve fibres. Beware of other abnormalities such as clavicular and humeral fractures, torticollis,[e] cephalohaematoma (see Fig. 38.5) and facial nerve palsy (see Fig. 38.6).

---

[d] A difficult birth because the width of the shoulders causes obstruction.

[e] Twisting of the head to one side, often as a result of spasm of one sternocleidomastoid muscle.

Cephalohaematoma is a subperiosteal haemorrhage and thus limited by the suture lines due to a ruptured vessel within the space between the periosteum and the skull. When finger pressure is applied a bulge forms that disappears once the pressure is released

(From Galbraith SS. In Eichenfield L, Eichenfield L, Frieden I, eds. *Neonatal dermatology*, 2nd edn. Philadelphia: Saunders, 2008.)

FIGURE 38.5

Facial nerve palsy right side

(From Cameron C. *J Cystic Fibrosis* 2006; 6(3):241–243. Figure 1 Photograph of patient on initial admission demonstrating right-sided facial paralysis. ©2006 European Cystic Fibrosis Society.)

FIGURE 38.6

Spine and skull

Inspect the spine carefully for soft-tissue masses and any failure of bony fusion in the posterior midline of the vertebral column (dysraphism), a result of abnormal fusion of the embryonic sacral neural tube. These abnormalities of spinal fusion—lumbosacral meningoceles, myeloceles, myelocystoceles and meningomyeloceles[f] (called spina bifida cystica)—are usually diagnosed before birth by routine fetal ultrasound (see Fig. 38.7). These babies are at risk of infection and should be examined only by clinicians wearing sterile gloves. The associated neurological deficit depends on the localisation of the spinal dysraphic[g] lesion (see Table 38.5).

Hydrocephalus is an increase in the volume of cerebrospinal fluid, usually due to obstruction of drainage pathways; it is a common complication of meningomyelocele (see List 38.2).

The presence of inspiratory stridor, abnormal cry and difficulty with swallowing suggests lower cranial

Localisation of meningomyelocele and neurological deficits

Level of dysraphic spinal lesion	Neurological deficit
Above L3	Combination of upper and lower motor neurone lesions with flaccid (less commonly spastic) paraplegia, areflexia (less commonly hyperreflexia), sensory deficits according to dermatomes affected, bladder and rectal incontinence
L4 and below	Preservation of hip flexors, adductors, extensors
S1 and below	Preservation of feet dorsiflexors, hip extensors, knee flexors
S3 and below	Normal motor function in hip and knee, variable ankle plantar flexor strength, variable bladder and rectal incontinence, saddle anaesthesia

TABLE 38.5

---

[f] The longer the name, the more layers of tissue are present in the defect.
[g] This means defective formation of a seam or ridge between two symmetrical halves of the body.

Various forms of spina bifida.

(a) Meningocele contains meninges and spinal fluid. There are usually no neurological defects or hydrocephalus. (b) Myelomenigocele also contains spinal cord. (c) Myelocystocele is caused by an attachment of the posterior spinal cord to the ectoderm and shows abnormal fluid collection within the cord (hydromelia/syringomelia). (d) Myelocele is a cyst anterior to the spinal cord

(From Benda CE. *Developmental disorders of mentation and cerebral palsies*. New York: Grune & Stratton, 1952.)

FIGURE 38.7

> ### SIGNS OF HYDROCEPHALUS
> - Increased head circumference
> - A large bulging fontanel and wide skull sutures
> - Dilated scalp veins
> - Loss of upward conjugate gaze with visible sclera between the upper eyelid and iris (setting-sun sign)
> - A hyperresonant percussion note of the skullcap (be gentle)
>
> LIST 38.2

Low sacral dimple

(From Herring JA. *Tachdjian's pediatric orthopaedics: from the Texas Scottish Rite Hospital for Children*. Philadelphia: Saunders, 2008.)

FIGURE 38.8

nerve palsies (bulbar palsy); and apnoeic episodes indicate impaired brainstem function, which is the leading cause of death in these infants.

Spinal and lower extremity deformities and joint contractures are common in patients with spina bifida. If a midline dermal dimple or sinus is present (see Fig. 38.8), measure the depth of the dimple and the distance from the anal verge. An occult spina bifida should be excluded by ultrasound[26] or magnetic resonance imaging (MRI) if the dimple is deeper than 0.5 centimetres, its location is greater than 2.5 centimetres from the anus or a naevus, haemangioma, lipoma or hairy patch is present.[27]

Abnormal limb movements

Jerky limb movements

Sudden brief jerks of the extremities (myoclonus) may be **benign** if they occur only during sleep (non-rapid eye movement [NREM] sleep), are sensitive to stimulation and stop abruptly when the neonate wakes, resolve in the first months of life and are not explained by other disorders. It is important to distinguish benign neonatal sleep myoclonus from other types of jerks that may indicate serious pathologies. Horizontal deviation of the eyes and blinking of the eyelid may indicate seizure activity. In these babies, jerks or abnormal tone of the extremities and orobuccal movements such as grimacing, tongue smacking and extranutritional sucking may be observed (mnemonic: EEG—Eyes, Extremities, Grimacing). Dysregulation of the autonomic nervous system with apnoeic spells and increased heart rate in isolation or combination with loss of muscle tone (limbs becoming limp) may be the only sign of neonatal seizures.[16]

Jittery limb movements

Jitters are common in the first days of life and refer to rhythmic tremors of equal amplitude as a presentation of excited neuromuscular activity (jitteriness/tremulousness). They are sensitive to stimulation and can easily be interrupted by gentle flexion or holding of the involved extremities. If persistent or exaggerated they can indicate hypoglycaemia, hypocalcaemia, abstinence syndrome, sepsis and birth asphyxia.

The skin

Inspect the skin from head to toe. The normal colour of fair-skinned newborns is pink. A bluish appearance of the hands and feet (acrocyanosis) is common in the first days of life. A number of skin changes without pathological relevance are often present. These include:

- erythema toxicum (see Fig. 38.9(a))
- sebaceous hyperplasia (see Fig. 38.9(b))
- miliae—tiny epidermal cysts, probably the result of blocked pilosebaceous opening (see Fig. 38.9(c and d))
- salmon patches/angel's kiss (naevus simplex; see Fig. 38.9(e))
- hyperpigmentations ('Mongolian spots'; see Fig. 38.9(f)).

However, generalised rashes and blister can be caused by life-threatening disease in neonates.

However, a generalised erythematous rash and fluid-filled small blisters (vesicles) or large blisters (bullae) with exfoliation of the skin on gentle rubbing (Nikolskys sign—due to toxic epidermal necrolysis) is suggestive of '*Staphylococcus aureus*' infection (called Ritters disease of the newborn or *Staphylococcus* scalded skin syndrome). Less generalised blisters (bullous impetigo) or erythematous papules (non-bullous impetigo) are more commonly seen and caused by *Staphylococcus* and *Streptococcus* spp. The occurrence of vesicles with surrounding erythema in the face or scalp that develop into pustules filled with purulent or cloudy material in a baby who had a vaginal delivery is indicative of neonatal herpes.

Large pigmented naevi are caused by a benign proliferation of melanocytes but they need to be monitored for changes in size and shape that might indicate the development of malignancy.[28] Port-wine stains (naevus flammeus) are dark-red or purple skin patches with well-defined borders and can be associated with other abnormalities (e.g. Sturge–Weber syndrome).

Haemangiomas of infancy are benign and present as a superficial nascent (new) lesion consisting of small dilated blood vessels (capillary telangiectasias) surrounded by a pale halo (see Fig. 38.10(a)), a pale or erythematous macule or a bruise or scratch.[29] Superficial haemangiomas that have progressed from a nascent into a proliferative stage show a strawberry-like appearance with a raised, bright-red and lobulated dermis and may feel warm. A colour change from bright red to grey may indicate shrinkage (involution), which usually starts centrally.[29] A deep haemangioma originating from the subcutis appears as a soft mass with a dusky or bluish colour (see Fig. 38.10(b)) but it can be difficult to distinguish clinically from other vascular malformations. Be aware that the presence of haemangiomas on the face or neck is associated with haemangiomas of the airway and that more than five cutaneous haemangiomas anywhere else is associated with visceral haemangiomas.

Visible jaundice develops with a total serum bilirubin of greater than 6 mg/dL or 102.6 mmol/L (1 mg/dL=17.1 mmol/L). However, it is difficult to estimate the severity of hyperbilirubinaemia by the visual assessment of jaundice.[30] Physiological jaundice is not usually evident in the first 24 hours of life (e.g. less than 6 mg/dL) but peaks at day 3 to day 5 after birth, does not exceed 15 mg/dL and resolves within a week's time in term newborns and within 2 weeks in premature babies. However, some neonates develop excessive hyperbilirubinaemia, which requires careful monitoring and potentially treatment (see List 38.3).

If significant jaundice is present, look for signs of or associated factors that can lead to excessive red blood cell breakdown (haemolysis) such as:

- excessive bruising and cephalohaematoma (e.g. birth trauma)
- splenomegaly (e.g. associated with spherocytosis)
- pallor

(a) Erythema toxicum; (b) sebaceous hyperplasia; (c, d) miliae; (e) naevus simplex and (f) hyperpigmentations

((a, b and d) from Kliegman RM, Jenson HB, Behrman RE, Stanton BF. *Nelson's textbook of pediatrics*, 18th edn. Philadelphia: Saunders Elsevier, 2007; (c) from Seidel HM, Ball JW, Danis JE, Benedict GW. *Mosby's guide to physical examination*, 6th edn. St Louis, MO: Mosby Elsevier, 2006; (e) from Habif T. *Clinical dermatology*, 4th edn. St Louis, MO: Mosby, 2004; (f) from Lemmi FO, Lemmi CAE. *Physical assessment findings CD-ROM*, Philadelphia: Saunders, 2000.)

FIGURE 38.9

- generalised oedema and signs of heart failure (e.g. severe anaemia as a result of rhesus/ABO incompatibility)
- macrosomia and plethora (e.g. polycythaemia)
- African American or Asian descent (e.g. glucose-6-phosphate dehydrogenase deficiency).

Also assess for signs of impaired bilirubin elimination, such as:

- functional or mechanical bowel obstruction (e.g. increased enterohepatic bilirubin circulation)
- hepatomegaly (e.g. hepatitis, infection)

(a) Superficial nascent and (b) deep proliferating haemangioma

(From Drolet BA. Infantile hemangiomas: an emerging health issue linked to an increased rate of low birth weight infants. *J Pediatr* 2008; 153(5):712–715.e1.)

FIGURE 38.10

SIGNS OF EXCESSIVE HYPERBILIRUBINAEMIA*

- Poor feeding
- Lethargy
- Opisthotonus (spasm of the back muscles leads to dramatic arching of the back and extension of the head)
- Irritability
- High-pitched crying
- Apnoea
- Seizures (acute bilirubin encephalopathy)
- Sensorineural hearing loss
- Motor delay
- Extrapyramidal signs
- Gaze palsy
- Dental dysplasia

*Bilirubin deposition in the basal ganglia and its associated neurological signs are called kernicterus.

LIST 38.3

(a) Petechiae and (b) mottling

((a) From Weston WL. *Color textbook of pediatric dermatology*, 4th edn. St Louis, MO: Mosby, 2007; (b) from Murphy CC. Late-onset pediatric glaucoma associated with cutis marmorata telangiectatica congenita managed with Molteno implant surgery: case report and review of the literature. *J AAPOS* 2007; 11(5):519–521, with permission.)

FIGURE 38.11

- pale chalky stools and dark urine staining the nappy (e.g. cholestasis, biliary atresia).

Search for petechiae, which do not empty and disappear when pressed (see Fig. 38.11(a)); if generalised, they may indicate neonatal thrombocytopenia.

Poor perfusion of the peripheries (hypothermia, sepsis, heart failure, hypovolaemia) is suggested by uneven discoloured skin patches (mottling; see Fig. 38.11(b)).

More than six café-au-lait spots, each with a size greater than 5 millimetres, is a diagnostic feature of neurofibromatosis type 1 (see Ch 37).

Temperature

A baby who is cold to touch may be very ill. Measure the body temperature in the axilla and if it is abnormal (less than 35.5°C [hypothermia] or more than 37.5°C [hyperthermia]) it is best remeasured in the rectum. Hypothermia and increased body temperature are strong predictors of severe illness in newborn infants.[16,18]

Head

Shape

The head of the newborn is moulded by the baby's intrauterine position and passage through the birth canal. A baby lying in the breech position has its head positioned against the fundus of the uterus, which results in a flatter-appearing top (vertex) and elongation of the occipitofrontal diameter. A baby born head first (cephalic delivery) usually has a shorter biparietal diameter and a more prominent-appearing top. Reassure parents that prominent moulding usually disappears in a couple of days even if bony ridges are palpable owing to a slight overlap of skull bones.

Inspect the head for

- any signs of swelling and bruising (haematoma)
- lacerations and abrasions (birth injuries)
- asymmetry and protuberances (craniosynostosis, see below)
- abnormal hair growth and pigmentation (see Table 38.6)[31]
- scalp defects (e.g. aplasia cutis)
- caput succedaneum, an area of subcutaneous serosanguineous effusion that is pitting and crosses the cranial sutures, which must be distinguished from
- cephalohaematoma (see Fig. 38.5), a haemorrhage between the periosteum and the skull (which is non-pitting and is limited by the suture lines).

Caput succedaneum resolves within 2 weeks whereas swelling caused by frank haemorrhage may persist for months or even longer if calcification occurs.

Sutures

Feel along the four suture lines for palpable ridges, which may indicate premature fusion of the skull bones (*craniosynostosis*). The metopic suture is the line where the frontal skull bones meet; it extends from the anterior fontanel down the middle of the forehead towards the nose. *Metopic synostosis* results in the development of a triangular-shaped forehead when viewed from above (*trigonocephaly*). The coronal suture marks the point where the frontal and parietal skull bones on each side meet; it extends from ear to ear. Bilateral synostosis leads to a short anterior–posterior and increased transverse head diameter (*brachycephaly*), whereas unilateral synostosis will result in anterior *plagiocephaly*. The sagittal suture line is formed by the two parietal bones; it extends from the anterior to the posterior fontanel. Premature fusion results in a long, narrow head shape and is the most common synostosis (*scaphocephaly*). The lambdoidal suture is the space between the two parietal bones and the single occipital bone and if fused it leads to a trapezoid-shaped head with flattening of the occipital region on one side (posterior *plagiocephaly*). Note, however, that the most common—and self-resolving—presentation, that of posterior plagiocephaly, is caused by positional moulding due to the fetus' position in utero, which may be exacerbated by the infant's preference for placing the head on the same side during sleep. *Oxycephaly* (turricephaly) is the premature fusion of all cranial sutures. Craniosynostoses may be seen in association with Apert's, Crouzon's, Saethre–Chotzen, Pfeiffer's or Carpenter's syndrome.

Fontanels

Next, palpate the anterior and posterior fontanels for fullness and size. The anterior fontanel is a diamond-shaped opening of the skull at the point where the frontal and parietal skull bones meet at the junction between the metopic, sagittal and coronal suture lines. The mean area of the anterior fontanel is 220 mm^2 (2.5th to 97.5th centile: 164 to 276 mm^2) in term newborns[32] and is expected to be closed at 18 months of age. The size can be determined by introducing the index finger into each of the four bony corners of the fontanel, marking them with a small circular ink dot immediately distal to the finger, transferring the four dots onto paper by firmly pressing it onto the skin and calculating the area (see Fig. 38.12). The posterior fontanel is triangle shaped, situated at the junction of the sagittal and lambdoidal suture lines and is closed by 3 months of age. **Large or bulging fontanels** may indicate raised intracranial pressure (see List 38.4) whereas an increase in size without fullness is observed in neonates with bony and endocrine abnormalities (see List 38.5).[33] Premature closure of the fontanels may be associated with craniosynostoses (see above). Auscultate for bruits, which can be heard with intracranial aneurysmal malformations (e.g. of the vein of Galen, the great cerebral vein).[34]

Face

Eyes (see Text box 38.2)

Examination of the eyes has the potential to disturb the infant and may best be done last. However, remember that this examination will become virtually impossible if you have made the baby cry.

Conditions that threaten normal sight may require urgent intervention.

Inspect the upper face and orbits for possible dysmorphic features (e.g. short palpebral fissures,

Scalp hair characteristics in neonates and potential clinical significance

Hair abnormality	Potentially associated conditions
Hypopigmentation	
White forelock	Waardenburg's syndrome (abnormal iris pigmentation, cochlear deafness) Piebaldism
Silvery metallic sheen	Chediak–Higashi syndrome (immune deficiency, metabolic disease, partial or complete albinism) Prader–Willi syndrome (deletion 15q11-q13) Piebaldism Ectrodactyly–ectodermal dysplasia–cleft (EEC) syndrome Cross (oculocerebral hypopigmentation) syndrome Nutritional deficiency, inborn error of metabolism (phenylketonuria)
Light coloured	Oculocutaneous albinism
Generalised	Chediak–Higashi syndrome
Hypotrichosis / alopecia*	
Localised	Birth trauma, infection, extravasation of intravenous medication Aplasia cutis congenita Naevus
Generalised	Ectodermal dysplasia Ichthyosis Nutritional deficiencies (zinc, vitamins B_6 and B_{12}, biotinidase) Inborn errors of metabolism (homocystinuria, congenital hypothyroidism)
Hypertrichosis**	
Localised	Naevus, encephalocele, meningocele
Generalised	Cornelia de Lange's syndrome Coffin–Siris syndrome Hurler's syndrome (mucopolysaccharidosis type I) Edwards' syndrome (trisomy 18) Fetal hydantoin and alcohol syndrome Congenital hypertrichosis lanuginosa
Abnormal hairline	
Low frontal hairline	Costello's syndrome Cornelia de Lange's syndrome Coffin–Siris syndrome Fanconi's syndrome Fetal hydantoin syndrome Noonan's syndrome
Low posterior hairline	Turner's syndrome Kabuki syndrome Cornelia de Lange's syndrome Fetal hydantoin syndrome

*Too little hair.
**Too much hair.

(Furdon SA, Clark DA. Scalp hair characteristics in the newborn infant. *Adv Neonatal Care* [Review] 2003; 3(6):286–296.)

TABLE 38.6

---

epicanthic folds, flat nasal bridge). Look for ptosis (often due to a third cranial nerve palsy), inability to close the eye (the result of a seventh cranial nerve palsy due to birth trauma) or displacement due to a haemangioma or birth trauma. The size of the eyes may be unequal or enlarged (e.g. *buphthalmos*[h] due to increased intraocular pressure—glaucoma),

---

[h] From the Greek words meaning the eye of an ox. Increased intraocular pressure changes the shape of the cornea, enlarging its diameter.

Calculation of anterior fontanel area

(Davies DP, Ansari BM, Cooke TJ. Anterior fontanelle size in the neonate. *Archives of Disease in Childhood* 1975; 50(1):81–3 with permission from BMJ Publishing Group Ltd.)

FIGURE 38.12

A summary of the neonatal eye examination

Dysmorphic features—epicanthic fold, short palpebral fissures,* flat nasal bridge

Movements—conjugate gaze abnormality; strabismus—consider cranial nerve injury

Ptosis—consider third nerve palsy

Inability to close eye completely—consider seventh nerve palsy

Enlargement of an eye (*buphthalmos*)—glaucoma

Scleral colour—jaundice, osteogenesis imperfecta

Conjunctivae—injected (conjunctivitis, glaucoma, haemorrhage)

Watery eyes—blocked lacrimal duct, conjunctivitis

Irises—hypopigmented (albinism)

Corneas—cloudy (ulcers, oedema, trauma)

Pupils—asymmetrical (amblyopia-blindness, third nerve palsy), irregular (coloboma), opaque (cataract, retinal abnormality)

Abnormal gaze—cranial nerve abnormality

*Palpebra is the Latin word for eyelid.

TEXT BOX 38.2

CAUSES OF LARGE BULGING FONTANELS

- Hydrocephalus
- Haemorrhage
- Meningitis
- Tumour

LIST 38.4

CAUSES OF LARGE NON-BULGING FONTANELS

- Small for gestational age
- Osteogenesis imperfecta
- Achondroplasia
- Russell–Silver syndrome[34]
- Hypothyroidism
- Hypophosphataemia

LIST 38.5

---

the sclerae may be blue (premature birth or *osteogenesis imperfecta*) or yellow (jaundice), the conjunctivae injected (glaucoma or subconjunctival haemorrhage; see Fig. 38.13[35]), the irises hypopigmented (oculocutaneous albinism), the cornea cloudy (e.g. metabolic causes, ulcers, transient oedema, trauma tears, dermoids; see Fig. 38.14(a)), the pupils asymmetrical (e.g. amblyopia, ocular motor nerve palsy), not round (e.g. coloboma[i]) or opaque (leucocoria due to cataract, retinoblastoma; see Fig. 38.14(b)). Watery eyes may result from nasolacrimal duct stenosis (see Fig. 38.15(a)), which can be associated with cyst formation (dacrocystocele) if the inferior or superior ducts are obstructed. Purulent discharge, however, suggests bacterial infection unless proven otherwise by negative cultures (e.g. *Chlamydia trachomatis* or *Neisseria gonorrhoeae* conjunctivitis).

Observe the baby's vertical and horizontal gaze by moving your face within the baby's visual field. Avoid talking or making noises at the same time. It is common for neonates to lose track intermittently and require readjustment. Look for dysconjugate eye movements

---

[i] A congenital defect in the iris, retina, choroid and/or optic nerve.

CHAPTER 38 THE NEONATAL HISTORY AND EXAMINATION   707

Subconjunctival haemorrhage and petechiae at the forehead commonly as a result from changes in cephalic venous pressure[35]

(From Goldbloom RB. *Pediatric clinical skills*, 4th edn. Philadelphia: Saunders, 2011, pp 38–55.)

FIGURE 38.13

(a) Haziness of the cornea in front of the pupils and involving the iris, versus (b) an opacity behind the pupils

((a) From Krachmer JH, Mannis MJ, Holland EJ. *Cornea*, 3rd edn. Philadelphia: Elsevier Saunders, 2011.)

FIGURE 38.14

(*squint* or *strabismus*[j]) and determine whether these are transiently noticeable (e.g. when falling asleep or waking up) or fixed (e.g. as a result of cranial nerve damage due to birth trauma). A convergent squint can be the result of lateral rectus muscle weakness due to a sixth cranial nerve palsy.

Use an ophthalmoscope to assess papillary and red reflexes. Darken the room and face the neonate away from any light sources such as windows. Select a small viewing aperture at the front of the ophthalmoscope and dial up the '0' lens with your index finger on the side of the ophthalmoscope (no lens correction). Hold the ophthalmoscope with your right hand vertically in front of your right eye and direct the light beam laterally towards the baby's right and left eye from a distance of approximately 15 centimetres. Pupils should be **e**qual **a**nd **r**eactive to **l**ight (**PEARL**). The red reflex is a light reflection from the retina and a lack of the reflex is suggestive of lens opacities (e.g. cataract), retinal abnormalities such as haemorrhage or detachment, or retinoblastoma. On closer inspection, the retina should appear yellow-white, grey or red depending on pigmentation.

Ears

Look for periauricular pits and skin tags, which are common findings. The presence of these increases the risk of hearing impairment five-fold. Hearing loss can be detected by hearing screening (e.g. transient-evoked otoacoustic emissions or auditory brainstem response audiometry).[36]

Note the position of the ear. Approximately 30% of the auricle (pinna) should be positioned above an

---

[j] These words mean the same thing. When one eye looks at an object the other may look too far inwards (convergent strabismus), too far outwards (divergent strabismus) or too far up or down (vertical strabismus).

Acute dacryocystitis in a 4-week-old child with redness and swelling of left upper and lower lids and a prominent nasolacrimal sac

(From Krachmer JH, Mannis MJ, Holland EJ. *Cornea*, 3rd edn. Philadelphia: Elsevier Saunders, 2011.)

FIGURE 38.15

Low-set and hypoplastic right ear

(From Corrin B. *Pathology of the lungs*. Philadelphia: Elsevier Saunders, 2011 (courtesy of the late Dr AH Cameron, Birmingham, UK).)

FIGURE 38.16

imaginary line drawn from the inner and outer canthus[k] to the occipital bone. The ear is clearly low set (see Fig. 38.16) if the upper margin of the ear helix is below the eye level and this may be associated with chromosomal anomalies.

Inspection of the tympanic membranes with an otoscope is not performed routinely because the ear canals may be obscured by vernix[l] or blood. Applying a positive pressure using a pneumatic otoscope prevents the collapse of the cartilaginous auricular meatus for better visualisation of the tympanic membrane, which is greyer, thicker and more vascular in newborns than in older children.[37] Middle ear effusions are commonly seen but resolve in the first 3 days of life in most neonates.[38]

Nose

Inspect the external nose for any deformity and asymmetry of the nasal bridge and nares, which can affect nasal airway patency. Nasal flaring may indicate respiratory distress. Infants are preferential nose breathers and bilateral nasal airway patency should therefore be verified, particularly in those babies with signs of respiratory distress or apnoeic spells. The presence of cyanosis exacerbated by feeding and relieved by crying suggests nasal obstruction, which may be due to:

- choanal[m] atresia—posterior nasal obstruction
- piriform aperture[n] stenosis—anterior obstruction
- dacryocystoceles[o] with intranasal extension.

Inspect both nasal passages by inserting the tip of the otoscope a few millimetres into the anterior nasal apertures to assess for nasal septum deviation and uncommon masses (e.g. encephalocele, dermoid cysts, haemangiomas).

Several functional tests have been described. For example, look for movement of thin cotton fibres, or for condensation on metal or a mirror held beneath each nostril. Alternatively, close the baby's mouth and one nasal aperture with your left thumb and index finger and auscultate for airflow sounds with a stethoscope held beneath the other nostril (and vice versa).[39] If in any doubt, check patency by gently trying to pass a nasogastric feeding tube (e.g. 6 French, 2

---

[k] The angle formed by the junction of the eyelids, also called the palpebral angle.
[l] This greasy deposit covers a baby's skin at birth. It consists of skin scales and fine hairs. The full name is vernix caseosa and comes from the Latin words for varnish and cheese.
[m] Choana means funnel and these are the funnel-shaped openings between the nose and the nasopharynx.
[n] Piriform means pear shaped; this is the bony opening of the nose.
[o] This is a protrusion of the lacrimal sac.

millimetres) through each nasal aperture into the hypopharynx. However, partial obstruction (e.g. piriform aperture stenosis) cannot be excluded with these manoeuvres. Non-structural abnormalities such as mucosal oedema may also cause nasal obstruction. Clear nasal discharge is commonly caused by a virus-induced upper respiratory tract infection (and very rarely by a cranial cerebrospinal fluid leak), whereas purulent discharge may indicate a bacterial aetiology.

Mouth

Inspect the mandibles from the front and sides to identify lower facial asymmetry and abnormal jaw size. A Pierre Robin[p] sequence is suggested by a proportionally small mandible (*micrognathia*), which includes posterior displacement of the tongue into the pharynx (*glossoptosis*) and airway obstruction. It may be associated with a cleft palate.[40]

If you have made the baby cry, look for the symmetrical opening of the mouth and for apparently unrestricted side and forward mobility. This excludes temporomandibular joint fixation (ankylosis).[41]

Note the presence of lip cyanosis and a cleft lip or any other dysmorphic features (e.g. small upper lip and smooth philtrum in fetal alcohol spectrum disorder).

Inspect the oral cavity for cleft palate and a bifid uvula, which may occasionally indicate a submucous cleft. Cleft lip and palate interfere with swallowing and feeding, whereas the clinical relevance of a submucous cleft may surface only later in life with symptoms of velopharyngeal[q] insufficiency (nasal regurgitation, recurrent ear infections, hypernasality of speech). Exclusion of a cleft palate requires palpation of the hard and soft palate with the index finger and while wearing an examination glove. Prevent full closure of the mouth during the examination of the palate as strong sucking by the neonate otherwise precludes assessment of the soft palate.

Small white cysts at the junction between the soft and hard palates or the gum (Epstein's pearls; see Fig. 38.17(a)) are common and harmless if they do not interfere with function (e.g. feeding). Natal (present at birth) or neonatal (erupting in the first month of life) teeth, mostly lower central incisors, are often loose and show enamel hypoplasia, making extraction the treatment of choice.[42] Assess the size of the tongue (e.g. *aglossia* or *microglossia*, which is associated with micrognathia; and *macroglossia*, which is associated with Beckwith–Wiedemann, Down's syndrome or hypothyroidism). Look at its position (e.g. for glossoptosis) and mobility (e.g. tongue tie [lingual frenulum[r]]; see Fig. 38.17(b)).[43] The need for treatment of ankyloglossia can be assessed using standardised score sheets. Look beneath the tongue for sublingual (central) cyanosis.

Neck

Examine the neck for symmetry and abnormal skinfolds. **Loose nuchal[s] skin** can be seen in several conditions (e.g. intrauterine lymphoedema, Down's syndrome, Noonan's syndrome and Turner's syndrome; see Fig. 38.18).

Look at the sternocleidomastoid muscles for unilateral shortening or swelling to rule out congenital torticollis. In this condition the head tilts towards the affected side while the chin points to the opposite side. Turn the baby's head gently from side to side as far as the neck will allow. The full range of movement is restricted when torticollis is present.

Look for cervical masses (e.g. cystic hygromas,[t] thyroglossal cysts, epidermoid cysts), which present with painless, soft or semifirm swellings. In newborn infants, cystic hygromas are most commonly found in the posterior cervical space on one side and vary in size. Large ones may cause compromise to the airway and extend into the mediastinum or face.[44] Thyroglossal cysts are most commonly localised in the midline at or below the level of the hyoid bone and move upwards with tongue protrusion.[45] Epidermoid cysts are found at the floor of the mouth and superior to the hyoid bone. Isolated palpable cervical lymph nodes (up to 12 millimetres in diameter) are common in healthy newborns but warrant documentation and follow-up.[46]

A short and asymmetrical neck may indicate maldeveloped cervical vertebrae (Klippel–Feil syndrome).

---

[p] This sequence includes micrognathia, cleft palate, glossoptosis and sometimes glaucoma and retinal detachment.

[q] A velum is a sail or curtain in Latin and refers here to the posterior part of the soft palate.

[r] The Latin word for a bridle.

[s] The *nucha* is the nape of the neck.

[t] This is a cystic cavity arising from distended lymphatics.

Oral examination in the neonate.

(a) Epstein's pearls of the hard palate. (b) An infant with ankyloglossia (tongue-tie). Note the short frenulum, which extends to the tip of the tongue. Ankyloglossia interferes with protrusion of the tongue and may make breastfeeding difficult

((a) From Metry DW. *Neonatal dermatology*. Philadelphia: Saunders, 2008, with permission. (b) Courtesy of Dr Evelyn Jain, Lakeview Breastfeeding Clinic, Calgary, Alberta, Canada; from: Moore KL. *The developing human*. Philadelphia: Saunders, 2013.)

FIGURE 38.17

Clinical photographs show several physical manifestations associated with Turner's syndrome. (a) In this newborn a webbed neck with low hairline, shield chest with widespread nipples, abnormal ears, and micrognathia are seen. (b) The low-set posterior hairline can be better appreciated in this older child who also has protruding ears. The newborn shown in (a) also had prominent lymphoedema of the hands and feet

(From Zitelli BJ, McIntire SC, Nowalk AJ. *Atlas of pediatric physical diagnosis*, 6th edn. Philadelphia: Saunders, 2012 (Figure 1.25 a and b).)

FIGURE 38.18

Chest and cardiovascular system

Approximately half of the evidence-based clinical signs best identifying severe illness in newborn infants can be detected during a chest examination.[16] Note that the sequence of 'look, listen and feel' will change in an opportunistic fashion during the examination. If you have made the baby cry, auscultation may be impossible.

Inspect the chest for symmetrical expansion and any deformities. These may be acquired (fracture or pneumothorax) or congenital (pectus or dystrophy). A depressed sternum (pectus excavatum—funnel chest; see Fig. 38.19) is the most commonly observed congenital deformity.[47] A protuberance of the sternum (pectus carinatum—pigeon chest) may be symmetrical or affect only one side of the chest wall, which results in asymmetry with sternal rotation and depression of the contralateral site of the chest wall. A narrow chest due to the intrauterine failure of chest wall growth (e.g. Jeune's syndrome [asphyxiating thoracic dystrophy], Poland's syndrome [hypoplasia of the chest wall variably involving soft tissues, muscles and ribs], Ellis–van Creveld syndrome [chondroectodermal dysplasia]) may be associated with bilateral lung hypoplasia. Unilateral lung hypoplasia is commonly observed with a left-sided diaphragmatic hernia.

Count the respiratory rate over one full minute (normal is 40–60 breaths per minute) by assessing both chest movements and breath sounds. Fast breathing (tachypnoea) predicts severe illness moderately well.[16]

Assess for intermittent upper airway obstruction (e.g. Pierre Robin sequence, choanal atresia, tracheo- or laryngomalacia). These babies cannot move air sufficiently despite normal or increased respiratory efforts. Asymmetry in chest movements suggests that phrenic nerve palsy has caused unilateral paralysis of the diaphragm. If you have made the baby cry, use the opportunity to note the presence of abnormal crying (e.g. weak or hoarse). Paradoxical inward movements of the chest and outward movements of the abdomen during inspiration are normal in newborns, particularly in sleep when chest compliance increases.

Episodes of periodic breathing (normal breathing for as long as 20 seconds followed by an apnoeic period of less than 10 seconds) that occur at least three times in succession[48] are normal in newborn infants. However, **apnoeas** defined as cessations of airflow for longer than 20 seconds (or associated with oxygen desaturation or bradycardia)[49] in a term neonate are commonly a manifestation of serious potentially life-threatening illnesses requiring urgent evaluation and intervention.[50]

Look carefully for other signs of respiratory distress such as nasal flaring, intercostal and subcostal chest recessions, tracheal tug and grunting. Central cyanosis occurs when the amount of deoxygenated haemoglobin is greater than 3 g/dL or so.[51] The aetiology may be a right-to-left shunt due to pulmonary or intracardiac conditions.

Central cyanosis is associated with low partial arterial oxygen pressure (P_aO_2) and a variable degree of reduction in the percentage of haemoglobin saturated with oxygen (S_aO_2), which depends on the total haemoglobin concentration.[51] For example, a severely anaemic neonate with a total haemoglobin of 8 g/dL will appear cyanosed only if the S_aO_2 is less than 63%, whereas a polycythaemic infant with a total haemoglobin of 25 g/dL will appear cyanosed with a S_aO_2 of 88%.[51] It is important to remember that peripheral cyanosis (acrocyanosis) in the first days of life is common and usually without any pathological relevance.

Chest

Test the capillary refill time by pressing your index finger onto the neonate's chest for 2 seconds. This inhibits skin perfusion and leaves a pale area, which should regain its colour (refill) within 2 seconds. A prolonged capillary refill indicates poor peripheral

Pectus excavatum

(From Hebra A. *Semin Thorac Cardiovasc Surg* 2009; 21(1):76–84.)

FIGURE 38.19

> **CAUSES OF INCREASED CAPILLARY REFILL TIME**
>
> - Low body temperature
> - Cardiac failure (consider congenital heart disease)
> - Infection (pneumonia, meningitis, urinary tract infection, omphalitis)
> - Anaemia (haemolysis or bleeding)
> - Dehydration (feeding difficulties or vomiting)
>
> LIST 38.6

Situs explained

Situs	Commonly associated abnormalities
Levocardia + situs inversus abdominalis	Complex congenital heart disease
Dextrocardia + situs inversus abdominalis	Primary ciliary dyskinesis
Dextrocardia + abdominal situs solitus	Atrial or ventricular septal defects

TABLE 38.7

perfusion (see List 38.6). Feel the brachial and femoral pulses on all four extremities. These will be diminished if the baby has heart failure and bounding if he or she has a patent ductus arteriosus. Coarctation of the aorta (without cardiac failure) results in weak or absent femoral pulses only.

Heart

Assess the location, size and quality of the impulse of the heart apex beat, which should be located in the fourth intercostal space approximately on the left midclavicular line in the case of the normal arrangement of the heart (left-sided, levocardia).[52] An increased size may indicate ventricular dilation, and a forceful beat ventricular hypertrophy.

Note that when the heart is on the correct side (levocardia) but the abdominal organs are inverted (situs inversus abdominalis; see Table 38.7) there is commonly congenital heart disease.[53,54] In contrast, a cardiac apex located on the right side (dextrocardia) in association with situs inversus abdominalis (situs inversus totalis) usually occurs without structural heart defects but can be associated with primary ciliary dyskinesia leading to bronchiectasis and chronic sinusitis in later life (Kartagener's syndrome).[55] Dextrocardia in combination with normal arrangement of the abdominal organs (abdominal situs solitus[u]) is commonly associated with left-to-right shunts at the atrial or ventricular level.[53] Dextroposition of the heart is acquired (e.g. left diaphragmatic hernia, pneumothorax, congenital lung emphysema, congenital cystic adenomatoid malformation), in which case breath sounds on the left side are often reduced or absent.

Approximately 1% of newborns have a murmur and about half of them have structural heart defects even if they are asymptomatic.[56] A murmur may not be heard at birth and may develop after a couple of days. Conversely, it may disappear in the first hours of life (e.g. a patent ductus arteriosus) or in the first months of life (e.g. a muscular ventricular septum defect) even though the structural abnormality remains. Start by feeling for a vibration under your hand (a palpable thrill is consistent with a murmur of grade 4 or more) held onto the left upper sternal edge (pulmonary stenosis) and left lower sternal border (ventricular septal defect). A left parasternal impulse or lift may be felt with right ventricular hypertrophy (e.g. tetralogy of Fallot).

While auscultating decide whether the cardiac rhythm is regular or irregular. Count the heart rate over 15 seconds. Normal is between 120 and 160 beats per minute in an active neonate.

Proceed to auscultation of heart sounds using the diaphragm at first and then the bell of the stethoscope. At least four praecordial areas should be auscultated: the apical or mitral area (fourth intercostal space between the midclavicular and anterior axillary lines), the tricuspid area (left lower sternal border in the fourth intercostal space), the pulmonary area (left upper sternal border; second intercostal space) and the aortic area (right upper sternal border; second intercostal space).

Listen for any murmurs and if present aim at assessing the mnemonic **CARDIO**:

Character of the sound

Area of the sound where they are best heard

Radiation of the sound into other areas

---

[u] Solitus means accustomed or usual in Latin.

Degree or **I**ntensity of the loudness of the sound
Occurrence of the sound in the cardiac cycle.

Table 38.8 summarises potential auscultation notes for some common congenital structural heart defects.[57] Clearly, assessment of heart murmurs in infants for the purpose of identifying the underpinning structural abnormality is challenging (e.g. due to the faster heart and respiratory rate and lack of cooperation as compared with older children). Thus, the absence of a murmur in a neonate does not necessarily exclude serious cardiac disease. The sensitivity of the examination for the detection of congenital heart disease can be markedly increased when combined with measurement of peripheral cutaneous oxygen saturation (S_pO_2) employing pulse oximetry.[58]

If central cyanosis is present (see Table 38.9) or there is any doubt about its presence, perform a preductal (right arm) and postductal (either foot) S_pO_2 measurement employing pulse oximetry. These should both be 95% or above[59] but may be lower (91–96%) at altitudes greater than 2000 metres.[60]

Auscultation findings in common congenital heart diseases[58]

Cause	CARDIO	
Ventricular septal defect (3:1000 persistent [mostly membranous defect]; 50:1000 spontaneously closing [mostly muscular defect])	C	High frequency if very restrictive/small Low frequency (harsh) if moderately restrictive/large
	A	Left lower sternal border
	R	Back
	D	Systole at least grade 2 (faint but immediately audible) or greater (3 moderately loud, 4 loud with thrill, 5 audible with rim of stethoscope, 6 audible with stethoscope raised off the chest)
	I	Diastole grade 1 to 2 (out of 4)
	O	Early systolic if restrictive (small) Pansystolic murmur (moderately large) Mid-diastolic flow mitral murmur/rumble if very large
Isolated patent ductus arteriosus (1:2000 to 1:5000)	C	Machinery
	A	Left upper sternal border
	R	Suprasternal notch, left infraclavicular region +/– thrill
	D	Variable (systole grade 1 to 6)
	I	
	O	Pansystolic tricuspid valve regurgitation murmur Diastolic decrescendo pulmonic regurgitation murmur +/– systolic aortic ejection murmur; S_2 may not be audible ('buried' in the murmur)
Atrium septum defect (1:1000)	C	Harsh
	A	Systolic murmur: left upper sternal border +/– palpable click Diastolic murmur: left lower sternal border
	R	Back
	D	Systole grade 2, diastole grade 1 to 2
	I	
	O	Crescendo–decrescendo pulmonic ejection murmur Early-diastolic tricuspid flow murmur if large Loud, wide split and fixed S_2
Tetralogy of Fallot (3:10,000)	C	Harsh
	A	Left upper sternal border
	R	Lung fields, back
	D	Variable
	I	
	O	Crescendo–decrescendo pulmonic ejection murmur, single S_2

(Based on Keane JF, Lock JE, Fyler DC, Nadas AS. *Nadas' pediatric cardiology*. 2nd edn. Philadelphia: Saunders, 2006.)

TABLE 38.8

Causes of right-to-left shunt leading to central cyanosis in the first weeks of life

Intrapulmonary (2 Ps)	Persistent pulmonary hypertension of the neonate
	Pulmonary arteriovenous malformations
Intracardiac (5 Ts and others)	Transposition of the great arteries
	Tetralogy of Fallot
	Total anomalous pulmonary venous return
	Truncus arteriosus
	Tricuspid atresia
	Ebstein's anomaly (abnormal tricuspid valve)
	Pulmonary atresia
	Hypoplastic left heart
	Atrioventricular canal defect

TABLE 38.9

Reduced postductal S_pO_2 indicates right-to-left shunting through a patent ductus arteriosus, which may be caused by duct-dependent congenital heart disease. This means the patent ductus is required to maintain circulation. Causes include tricuspid atresia and transposition of the great arteries. It can also be caused by duct-independent congenital heart disease such as a tetralogy of Fallot.

A hyperoxygenation test may be useful to distinguish between structural heart defects and pulmonary diseases if echocardiography is not immediately available. To perform this test, the infant is exposed via a facemask to 100% oxygen over 10 minutes followed by an assessment of the partial pressure of oxygen in arterial blood (P_aO_2) pre- and postductally (e.g. right radial and umbilical artery, respectively). Failure of significant improvement in P_aO_2 on exposure to oxygen suggests congenital heart disease, although pulmonary diseases with a large right-to-left shunt may also fail to respond to hyperoxygenation.

Blood pressure is not routinely measured in healthy neonates, but non-invasive oscillometric measurements should be performed in ill infants. However, the accuracy of this method fails in very premature hypotensive and critically ill babies and invasive measurement via an arterial catheter may thus be required.[61]

Lungs

Continue the chest examination with auscultation of the lung sounds, which are bronchovesicular (medium pitch and volume, equally in expiration and inspiration) unlike the vesicular (low pitch and soft, dominant in inspiration) sounds heard in adults.[37] Listen for reduced breath sounds, which may be due to:

- collapse (atelectasis)
- fluid collection (effusion)
- intra-alveolar fluid collection (consolidation)
- diaphragmatic hernia
- pneumothorax in pleural space
- emphysema
- obstruction.

Listen also for bronchial breath sounds, which are high-pitched, loud and dominant in expiration. They are normally present when auscultation is performed over the trachea but when heard elsewhere indicate consolidation or interstitial lung disease.

Prolonged breath sounds are a sign of airway obstruction. Added breath sounds include **stridor**, which is a harsh continuous sound often audible without the stethoscope. Stridor may be heard during inspiration if an obstruction is localised outside of the chest wall. Causes include:

- laryngomalacia[v]
- infection
- gastro-oesophageal reflux
- subglottic stenosis due to a web, cyst or haemangioma
- vocal cord paralysis
- enlarged thyroid.

Stridor that occurs during expiration may be due to intrathoracic obstruction. Causes include:

- tracheomalacia
- bronchomalacia

due, for instance, to a vascular ring.

Stridor that occurs in both expiration and inspiration may be a result of severe obstruction or obstruction at multiple sites.

Grunting is produced at the start of expiration when air is forced against a closed glottis. This is in an attempt

---
[v] Softening and destruction of the cartilage of the trachea.

Conditions manifesting with respiratory distress in neonates[37]		
Respiratory	Parenchymal	Respiratory distress syndrome, transient tachypnoea, pneumonia, aspiration syndrome, persistent or primary pulmonary hypertension, pulmonary oedema/haemorrhage, lung hypoplasia, lobar emphysema, interstitial lung disease
	Extraparenchymal	Nasal, laryngeal, tracheal or bronchial obstruction, pneumothorax, haemothorax, chylothorax, pleural effusion
Cardiovascular	Structural	Congenital heart disease, cardiomyopathy, large aneurysm, haemangioma, vascular malformation
	Non-structural	Septicaemia, hypovolaemia, arrhythmia, anaemia, polycythaemia, methaemoglobinaemia
Neurological	Central/cranial	Asphyxia, pain, seizure, hydrocephalus, infection (meningitis, encephalitis), haemorrhage, aneurysmal malformation, cerebrovascular accident (stroke), drugs, maternal sedation
	Peripheral	Diaphragmatic and vocal cord paralysis, neonatal myasthenia gravis, spinal muscular atrophy, drugs
Abdominal		Diaphragmatic hernia, necrotising enterocolitis, large tumours, pneumoperitoneum
Metabolic		Hypo/hyperthermia, hypoglycaemia, metabolic alkaloses (e.g. hyperammonaemia), organic aciduria, hypocalcaemia

(Based on Fletcher MA. *Physical diagnosis in neonatology*. Philadelphia: Lippincott-Raven, 1998.)

TABLE 38.10

to prevent small airway collapse during expiration by generating a positive airway pressure and is not pathognomonic for a specific condition. It may indicate (like tachypnoea, apnoeas and cyanosis) respiratory distress, which has an extremely wide range of differential diagnoses in neonates (see Table 38.10).

Wheeze is more high-pitched and musical sounding and is usually heard during expiration only. However, wheeze may also occur during inspiration (it is then called biphasic) if airway obstruction is very severe.

Crackles are non-musical interrupted lung sounds of short duration that may occur at any time during inspiration or expiration. Crackles may be high-pitched (fine) or of variable pitch (coarse). They are sometimes unwisely referred to as râles or crepitations. Inspiratory crackles are produced by the abrupt opening of closed airways.[62] Thus crackles during early inspiration may be assumed to originate from the abrupt opening of larger airways, while those generated during late inspiration may stem from terminal bronchioli or alveoli (e.g. as a result of bronchiolitis or pneumonia).[63]

Percussion is not part of the routine examination in neonates but may potentially be helpful in a few circumstances (e.g. unilateral pneumothorax versus effusion).

Gastrointestinal and urogenital systems

Remove the nappy (if not done beforehand) and inspect it for the presence of meconium (first stool), which should be passed in the first 48 hours in healthy term newborns.[64]

Inspect the abdomen for vertical bulging (diastasis recti;[w] see Fig. 38.20) or general distension, which may indicate bowel obstruction. Functional causes of bowel obstruction include:

- Hirschsprung's disease
- hypoganglionosis
- neuronal intestinal dysplasia type B
- megacystis–microcolon–intestinal hypoperistalsis syndrome.

Mechanical causes include:
- duodenal atresia
- anal atresia
- meconium plug syndrome
- meconium ileus as a result of cystic fibrosis.[65]

---
[w] A weakness of the rectus sheath.

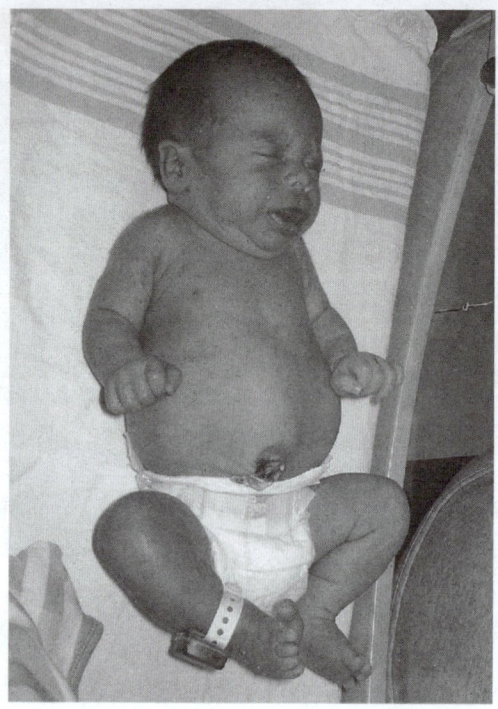

A premature newborn with Beckwith–Wiedemann syndrome, macroglossia, and rectus diastasis

(From Gleason CA, Devaskar S. *Avery's diseases of the newborn*, 9th edn. Philadelphia: Elsevier, 2012.)

FIGURE 38.20

(a) Omphalitis and (b) umbilical hernia

(From (a) Püttgen KB, *Pediatric dermatology*: Expert Consult—Online and Print, Elsevier, 2013; Chapter 2, 14–67. (b) Seidel HM, Ball JW, Dains JE et al. *Mosby's guide to physical examination*, 7th edn. St Louis, MO: Mosby, 2011, pp 482–534.)

FIGURE 38.21

You may be fortunate enough to see the baby vomiting. If not, ask to see any vomitus, which should have been kept by the helpful staff or parents. Bilious vomiting, in particular, raises the suspicion of the presence of gastrointestinal obstruction. However, bile is not seen if an obstruction is proximal to the ampulla of Vater[x] (causes include oesophageal atresia and proximal duodenal atresia). Early vomiting associated with respiratory distress is highly suggestive of oesophageal atresia, which is commonly associated with a tracheo-oesophageal fistula (TOF). This results in aspiration of gastric contents into the lungs.

Identify the umbilical vein (one) and the umbilical arteries (two) and look for signs of infection (omphalitis; see Fig. 38.21(a)) or an umbilical hernia (see Fig. 38.21(b)). Inspect the inguinal areas for swelling, which may indicate an inguinal hernia or the presence of an inguinal ovary or testis. Look for a concave or scaphoid contour of the abdomen, which is seen when its contents have moved into the chest as a result of a diaphragmatic hernia.

Look carefully for the presence and position of the anus, as the presence of faeces does not exclude anal atresia.

Palpate the abdomen gently for masses, which may be a result of organomegaly or tumours. Palpate the liver, which can be felt up to 2 centimetres below

---

[x] The joint opening of the pancreatic and common bile duct into the distal part of the duodenum.

the rib cage on the right side, while the tip of the spleen may be felt below the left rib cage in healthy newborns with situs solitus abdominalis. Feel for abdominal masses and the bladder. The upper edge of a full bladder can be verified with percussion and should be below the umbilicus; otherwise, further investigations for causes leading to urinary retention (e.g. urethral valves, drugs, dysraphic spinal lesion) and appropriate intervention are urgently warranted. Inspect the back for spinal dysraphism (spina bifida).

Percuss the abdomen. Masses and fluid have a dull percussion note, whereas an obstructed abdomen will generally be resonant.

Next listen for bowel sounds. They should be easily heard. They may be increased if there is mechanical bowel obstruction or heard clearly in the chest if the baby has a diaphragmatic hernia. Auscultate for renal bruits.

Inguinal region and genitals

If an inguinal hernia has been seen on inspection an attempt should be made to see whether it is reducible, using gentle pressure in the direction of the inguinal canal. However, if the hernia is non-reducible or appears to be painful, incarceration of herniated bowel, ovary or testis should be considered (a surgical emergency). Advise parents to be very vigilant for reducibility and pain if a hernia is detected.

If the scrotum is empty and an inguinal or suprascrotal testis (size 1.0–1.5 centimetres) can be palpated, try carefully to manipulate the testis into the scrotum. A retractable testis that remains in the scrotum for some time is a normal finding. A testis that immediately returns into the original position is an undescended testis, which requires further management to prevent infertility and increased risk for malignancy. If a testis is impalpable that may be because it is located in the abdomen (undescended), too small to be found by you (atrophic) or absent (e.g. in combination with ambiguous genitalia, see below).

Scrotum and penis

Examine the scrotum. Discoloration of the scrotum may occur as a result of ischaemia due to testicular torsion, which is another surgical emergency. A large painless fluctuant scrotum can be assessed with a torch (see Fig. 18.11 on p 315) to demonstrate translucency of light due to fluid accumulation (hydrocele). This occurs in 2%–5% of baby boys. It often resolves spontaneously in the first year of life but may require correction if persistent.

Examine the penis. A length of less than 2.5 centimetres is abnormal. Do not withdraw the foreskin (prepuce) for routine inspection of the urethral meatus because adherence to the glans penis is normal in infants. However, an abnormal opening of the prepuce on the ventral side of the penis is often associated with malposition of the urethral meatus (hypospadias). The urethral meatus should also be inspected if there is bending of the penis (chordee) or the neonate does not pass urine. A urethral meatus that opens at the dorsum of the penis in association with a marked chordee is a severe but rare penile abnormality that requires urgent assessment of associated renal tract abnormalities (by ultrasound).

Female genitalia

Inspect the female genitalia for the presence of normal labia majora, which should not be fused but cover the labia minora in term newborns. The clitoris is found at the upper border of the labia minora and the urethra is visible below, with the hymen below that. Inspect for any skin tags or mucoid cysts. Effects of maternal hormones regularly cause mucoid vaginal discharge, occasionally mixed with blood, which is normal in the first days of life.

Ambiguous genitalia

Ambiguous genitalia are a medical emergency and can be a cause of great psychosocial distress to the family. Congenital adrenal hyperplasia (CAH) secondary to 21-hydroxylase deficiency (less commonly 11-hydroxylase, 3β-hydroxysteroid dehydrogenase) causes overvirilisation (labial fusion, clitoral enlargement, joint vagina and urethra [urogenital sinus]) leading to masculinised external genitalia in female (karyotype 46, XX) neonates. Babies with 21-hydroxylase deficiency are at risk of life-threatening salt wasting.

Neonates with syndromes such as Smith–Lemli–Opitz (microcephaly, syndactyly, cleft palate, hypospadias, growth retardation) and **VACTERL** (vertebral abnormalities, anal atresia, cardiac abnormalities, TOF, oesophageal atresia, renal abnormalities, limb defects) may show variable degrees of genital ambiguity.

Developmental dysplasia of the hip in an older infant with rigid spine myopathy. Aberrantly increased muscular forces resulted in postnatal hip dislocation, evident as (a) tight hips with limited abduction, (b) upper leg length discrepancy with uneven knee height and (c) asymmetric thigh creases

(From Graham JM. *Smith's recognizable patterns of human deformation*. Philadelphia: Elsevier, 2007, pp 69–76.)

FIGURE 38.22

Musculoskeletal system

Limbs

Examine the upper and lower limbs for symmetry, in particular symmetry of the leg creases (asymmetry is a sign of congenital hip dysplasia; see Fig. 38.22), muscle bulk, range of motion and strength. Look for spontaneous symmetrical movements and consider nerve damage or long-bone fractures sustained during the birth process (clavicle and humeral fractures are the most common). Compared with term infants, premature infants are at higher risk of birth-associated fractures, particularly multiple fractures.[66]

Upper limbs

Examine the hands and forearms for dysmorphic features. Causes of anomalies can be genetic (e.g. Diamond–Blackfan anaemia), environmental (amniotic bands, congenital infection) or unknown. Around half of all cases with multiple anomalies will be due to a known syndrome and more than a hundred recognised syndromes are described with hand anomalies (see Table 38.11, Fig. 38.23).[67,68] The term *malformation* is preferred if the cause of the anomaly is unknown.

When examining the hands, remember to examine each hand separately and then both hands together to compare them, particularly when checking for size disparity (e.g. hemihyperplasia). On the dorsal surface, examine the skin, joints and nails before turning the hands over to examine the palms, taking particular care to check the palmar creases. Gently move the wrist and finger joints through their respective ranges of motion, looking for flexibility, asymmetry and any unusual positions.

Lower limbs

As with the hands, systematically examine the skin, joints and nails of the feet before moving on to the soles of each foot. Examine for symmetry and any unusual positioning or skinfolds, and gently move each joint through its respective ranges of motion. Common newborn foot abnormalities include:

- metatarsus adductus
- clubfoot deformity
- calcaneovalgus (flexible flatfoot)
- congenital vertical talus (rigid flatfoot)
- multiple digital deformities (polydactyly, syndactyly)
- overlapping toes
- amniotic bands.[69]

It is particularly important in children with congenital foot deformities that careful and repeated hip examinations are performed, as developmental dysplasia

Proposed classification of upper limb malformations[67] and frequencies[68]	
Type	**Malformations**
Type I: Failure of formation: Transverse arrest Longitudinal arrest	Amputations at any level from shoulder to phalanx (7%) Preaxial: varying degrees of hypoplasia of the thumb (4%) or radius (1%) Central: divided into typical and atypical types of cleft hand Postaxial: varying degrees of ulnar hypoplasia to hypothenar hypoplasia Intercalated longitudinal arrest: various types of phocomelia* (<1%)
Type II: Failure of differentiation: Soft tissue Skeletal Tumourous conditions	Syndactyly (18%; see Fig. 38.23(a)), trigger thumb, Poland's syndrome (2%), camptodactyly** (7%; see Fig. 38.23(b)) Radioulnar synostosis (1%), carpal coalitions Include all vascular and neurological malformations
Type III: Duplication	Applies to whole limb, mirror hand, polydactyly (15%; see Fig. 38.23(c) and (d))
Type IV: Overgrowth	Hemihypertrophy and macrodactyly (1%)
Type V: Undergrowth	Brachydactyly (5%), radial hypoplasia (<1%), brachysyndactyly
Type VI: Constriction band syndromes	Involves amputation at any level (2%) with or without distal lymphoedema
Type VII: Generalised anomalies and syndromes	Clinodactyly*** (6%; see Fig. 38.23(e))

*This is abnormal development of the arms or legs but with hands and feet still present.
**Fixed flexion at one or both phalangeal joints.
***Abnormal bending of the fingers or toes.

(Canale ST, Beaty JH, Campbell WC. *Campbell's operative orthopaedics*, 12th edn. St Louis, MO: Elsevier/Mosby, 2013; and Flatt AE. *The care of congenital hand anomalies*, 2nd edn. St Louis, MO: Quality Medical, 1994.)

TABLE 38.11

Clinical photograph of complex syndactyly. Note both the flexion posture of the ring finger and the synonychia between the ring and little fingers

(From Charles A, Goldfarb MD, Jennifer A, Steffen BS, Christopher M, Stutz MD. Complex syndactyly: aesthetic and objective outcomes. *J Hand Surg* 2012; 37(10) 2068–2073, Copyright ©2012 American Society for Surgery of the Hand.)

FIGURE 38.23

of the hip or acetabular dysplasia is commonly seen in these patients.

Metatarsus adductus (MTA) is a transverse plane deformity in the tarsometatarsal joints, in which the metatarsals are deviated medially (see Fig. 38.24(a) and (b)). It is particularly seen in breech presentations and in oligohydramnios babies. In the mild form, the forefoot can be passively abducted to the midline and the condition resolves without treatment. A quick test for MTA is to place the heel of the neonate's foot between your index and middle fingers and to observe the lateral aspect of the foot from the plantar side for medial or lateral deviation from your middle finger. Medial deviation indicates MTA.[69]

Clubfoot (talipes equinovarus) (see Fig. 38.24(c)) is another relatively common condition. The four basic components can be remembered by the mnemonic CAVE:

Cavus
Adduction
Varus[y]
Equinus.[z]

---

[y] Varus is displacement or angulation towards the midline of the body; valgus is the opposite.
[z] In severe cases the foot looks like that of a horse.

(a) and (b) Metatarsus adductus (severe); (c) talipes equinovarus; and (d) congenital vertical talus

((a), (b) and (d) from Canale ST, Beaty J. *Campbell's operative orthopaedics*, 12th edn. St Louis, MO: Mosby, 2012; (c) from Kliegman RM, Stanton BMD. *Nelson textbook of pediatrics*, 19th edn. Philadelphia: Saunders, 2011.)

FIGURE 38.24

This varies in severity from mild positional clubfoot (passively correctable) to severe clubfoot with extreme, rigid hindfoot equinus. On examination, the foot appears small, with a flexible, soft heel that is internally rotated so as to make the soles of the feet face each other. All patients exhibit calf atrophy, and internal tibial torsion and shortening of the ipsilateral extremity may be seen.

Calcaneovalgus foot is seen in up to 30%–50% of newborns secondary to in utero positioning. The newborn typically presents with a dorsiflexed and everted foot; the dorsum may occasionally be in contact with the anterolateral surface of the lower leg. If there is a full passive range of motion present at birth, then no active treatment is required, but gentle stretching may be required if there is restriction of movement. In severe cases, casting may be considered.

Rocker-bottom foot (congenital vertical talus) is a rare foot deformity where the midfoot is dorsally dislocated on the hindfoot (see Fig. 38.24(d)). Although approximately 60% of cases are idiopathic, up to 40% are associated with an underlying neuromuscular condition or syndrome.[69] On examination, it is noted that the plantar surface of the foot is convex, with a prominent talar head along the medial border of the midfoot. The fore part of the foot is dorsiflexed and abducted relative to the hindfoot, and the hindfoot is in equinus and valgus. Examine closely for any coexisting neurological or musculoskeletal abnormalities (e.g. arthrogryposis and meningomyelocele). This does not respond to stretching, and usually requires surgery.

Hips

The hip examination is of critical importance to check for **developmental dysplasia of the hip (DDH)**. It has been estimated that approximately 15% of DDH is not detectable at birth, even by experienced examiners or ultrasonographers.[70] Careful repeated examination of the infant in the first year of life by a skilled practitioner is crucial. Be aware of the increased risk of DDH seen in breech deliveries, girls and babies who have a positive family history of this condition. The rationale and importance of repeated examination needs to be explained to parents prior to the examination. Examination of the hips is often best left until the end of the neonatal examination, as it can be distressing to the child (and parents!).[aa]

After inspecting the lower limbs, perform the Ortolani and Barlow tests (see below). Ensure that the baby is relaxed and undressed and lying supine. Examine each hip individually, with your free hand stabilising the contralateral side of the pelvis. Very little force is required for each of these manoeuvres. Forceful and repeated examinations can damage the femoral head. A high-pitched 'click' may be heard during these manoeuvres. This is often musculoskeletal or ligamentous in origin and is usually of no clinical significance. If the examination is equivocal, or the baby is at increased risk of DDH, then sonography at 6 weeks is recommended.

Ortolani test: this is performed to elicit the sensation of the dislocated hip being reduced. The hip is flexed to 90° with the knee resting in the palm of your hand. Place your index and middle fingers along the greater trochanter and your thumb on the inner thigh. Hold the leg in a neutral position. Gently abduct the hip while lifting the leg anteriorly. A positive Ortolani sign is when a 'clunk' is felt as the dislocated femoral head reduces into the acetabulum.

Barlow provocation test: this is performed to detect the unstable hip dislocating from the acetabulum. It is performed with your hands in the same positions as for the Ortolani test, with the hips flexed to 90°. The leg is adducted while posteriorly directed pressure is placed on the knee. A positive Barlow's sign occurs when a palpable 'clunk' or sensation of movement is felt as the femoral head exits the acetabulum posteriorly.

Central and peripheral nervous systems

Examine for tone and positioning taking into account the gestational age of the neonate. The normal term infant will usually position him- or herself with the hips abducted and slightly flexed, knees flexed, upper limbs adducted with flexion at the elbows and hands softly clenched (the well-known 'fetal position'). The hypotonic infant (and the preterm infant) often adopts a 'frog-like' position with abducted hips and extended elbows (see Fig. 38.25). Very premature infants (less than 30 weeks) will have very minimal flexor tone, and this will develop first in the lower limbs and then in the upper limbs (between 34 and 36 weeks' corrected age).[bb]

Another quick check for tone is to suspend the baby in a ventral position, lying supported over your hand and forearm (see Fig. 38.26). There should be some resistance to gravity in the normal baby, whereas the hypotonic baby will flop like a rag-doll. Bear in mind that following a feed even a normal term infant may appear slightly hypotonic, and repeat examination is suggested.

[aa] In fact, most parts of the neonatal examination seem best left to the end.

[bb] For babies up to at least 2 years of age, subtract the number of weeks the baby was premature from its age (and for longer in the extremely premature infant).

The 'frog-like' position in the extreme premature infant

FIGURE 38.25

Type 1 spinal muscular atrophy (Werdnig–Hoffmann disease). Clinical manifestations of weakness of limb and axial musculature in a 6-week-old infant with severe weakness and hypotonia from birth. Note the marked weakness of (a) the limbs and trunk on ventral suspension and (b) of neck on pull to sit

(From Volpe J. *Neurology of the newborn*, 5th edn. Philadelphia: Saunders, 2008, Figure 18.2, p 771.)

FIGURE 38.26

Developmental reflexes

Examination of the developmental (or primitive) reflexes can be disturbing for the baby and should join the queue at the end of the neonatal examination. The most commonly elicited reflex in newborns is the Moro reflex, but it is useful to check others including grasp, tonic neck and the Galant reflex. Again, explain the examination in detail to the parents and perform the various manoeuvres while they are present if possible. It is a great opportunity for parents to experience their baby's developmental maturity and responsiveness even if these reflexes are mediated at the brainstem or spinal cord level.

The following reflexes are usually all present in the normal term infant.[71]

- *The Moro reflex:* this can be elicited by suddenly allowing the infant to fall back from a semierect position to supine with the head supported in your hand (carefully, and preferably over a soft surface, just in case). The infant will abduct and extend the arms and open the hands, and then flex them. This is seen in newborns from about 32 weeks' gestation and usually disappears between 3 and 6 months of age. Warn the parents that this manoeuvre may be accompanied by an audible cry. Absence of this reflex usually signifies dysfunction of the central nervous system and is an ominous sign that mandates investigation. Unilateral absence may indicate brachial plexus palsy or fractures.
- *The stepping reflex:* this can be elicited by holding the infant vertically with the feet on a flat surface. The infant will then alternatively flex and extend the legs initiating a slow stepping

action. This is seen from about 32 weeks' gestation and disappears by around 1–2 months of age. The significance of this reflex is not entirely clear.[72]

- *The Galant reflex:* this is elicited by stroking gently down either side of the spine from the thorax to the sacrum while the baby is held in ventral suspension. The infant's trunk and hips will move towards the side of the stimulus. This gives some indication of segmental integrity from T2 to S1.[73] This reflex is usually present by 32 weeks' gestation and disappears by around 2–4 months of age.
- *The sucking reflex:* this is elicited by placing a gloved finger in the infant's mouth to evaluate the coordination and strength of the suck. A firm grip should be felt on the finger and a strong seal formed by the newborn's lips. This usually appears by 28 weeks' gestation and disappears by around 3–4 months of age.
- *The rooting reflex:* this is elicited by stroking along the infant's cheek towards the corner of the mouth. The head will turn towards the stimulus and the mouth will open. This is usually present by 34 weeks' gestation and disappears by around 3–4 months of age.
- *The grasp reflex/palmar grasp:* this is elicited by placing your index finger into the infant's palm. When you attempt to withdraw your finger, the infant should tighten his or her grasp—so much so that the term infant can be lifted off the bed for a few seconds. This reflex is usually present by 26 weeks' gestation, although fetal palmar reflex grasping of the umbilical cord is often seen on routine ultrasound examination from around 16 weeks' gestation.[74] The reflex usually disappears by around 3 months of age. The absence of this reflex usually reflects peripheral or spinal cord involvement, particularly if it is asymmetrical.[74]
- *The plantar grasp:* this is elicited by pressing your thumb against the sole of the infant's foot, just behind the toes. The infant should flex and adduct the toes. Alternatively, the infant can be held vertically and the feet stimulated by floor contact. Again, the toes should flex and adduct. This reflex is usually present by 30 weeks' gestation and disappears between 10 and 15 months of age. A reduced or negative plantar grasp reflex during early infancy can be a sensitive indicator of later development of spasticity.[74]
- *The asymmetric tonic neck reflex (ATNR):* this is elicited by turning the infant's head to the side. There should be extension of the upper extremity on the side to which the head and neck are turned and flexion of the contralateral upper extremity (the fencing posture). The lower extremity responds similarly, but is much less striking. This reflex is usually present by 35 weeks' gestation and disappears by around 6 months of age.[72] When this is seen as a resting posture, it is never normal.

Gestational age

The gestational age can be determined by fetal ultrasound, maternal menstrual cycle and postnatal neuromuscular and physical maturation. Although not performed routinely,[75] if there are doubts about the exact gestational age (e.g. late recognition of pregnancy), use the New Ballard Score (NBS)[75] for postnatal estimation of gestational age in neonates up to 1 week old.[76]

> **T&O'C ESSENTIALS**
>
> 1. Babies cannot cooperate with the examiner and their examination must be performed as the opportunity occurs.
> 2. The parents must be involved at all stages and nothing should be done without their being informed.
> 3. Parts of the examination may be performed while the mother nurses the baby.
> 4. Do not let the baby get cold or fall off the examination table.
> 5. Taking serial measurements and charting these results are essential for monitoring a baby's progress.

Continued

T&O'C ESSENTIALS continued

6. Always remember to look for asymmetry—a vital guide to abnormality.
7. Certain congenital abnormalities must always be looked for (e.g. hip dysplasia, spina bifida).
8. A below-normal temperature is a significant sign of acute illness.
9. If the baby's parent says that the baby is sick, take this very seriously.

OSCE REVISION TOPICS – THE NEONATAL HISTORY AND EXAMINATION

Use these topics, which commonly occur in the OSCE, to help with revision.

1. Take a history of the pregnancy from these new parents and any risk factors for their baby in their own history. (p 684)
2. Talk to this mother about the delivery of her baby. (p 685)
3. Chart this baby's size and weight and discuss the results. (p 689)
4. This neonate has some dysmorphic features. Please examine him. (pp 688, 706, 709, 718)
5. Examine this baby's primitive reflexes. (p 722)
6. Examine this baby's chest. She has had some problems with her breathing. (p 711)
7. This baby has a murmur. Please examine her. (p 712)
8. This baby's family think his feet look abnormal. Please examine him. (p 718)

References

1. Morris T. *Cultural aspects of birthing*, 2011. Sydney: NSW Government.
2. Weintrob N, Karp M, Hod M. Short- and long-range complications in offspring of diabetic mothers. *J Diabetes Complications* 1996; 10(5):294–301.
3. Fitzpatrick DL, Russell MA. Diagnosis and management of thyroid disease in pregnancy. *Obstet Gynecol Clin North Am* 2010; 37(2):173–193.
4. Smyth A, Oliveira GHM, Lahr BD et al. A systematic review and meta-analysis of pregnancy outcomes in patients with systemic lupus erythematosus and lupus nephritis. *Clin J Am Soc Nephrol* 2010; 5(11):2060–2068.
5. Namazy JA, Murphy VE, Powell H et al. Effects of asthma severity, exacerbations and oral corticosteroids on perinatal outcomes. *Eur Respir J* 2013; 41(5):1082–1090.
6. Lenke RR, Levy HL. Maternal phenylketonuria and hyperphenylalaninemia. An international survey of the outcome of untreated and treated pregnancies. *N Engl J Med* 1980; 303(21):1202–1208.
7. Hernandez-Diaz S, Smith CR, Shen A et al. Comparative safety of antiepileptic drugs during pregnancy. *Neurology* 2012; 78(21):1692–1699.
8. Jefferies AL. Selective serotonin reuptake inhibitors in pregnancy and infant outcomes. *Paediatr Child Health* 2011; 16(9):562–563.
9. Gilbert GL. 1: Infections in pregnant women. *Med J Aust* 2002; 176(5):229–236.
10. Cutland CL, Schrag SJ, Zell ER et al. Maternal HIV infection and vertical transmission of pathogenic bacteria. *Pediatrics* 2012; 130(3):e581–e590.
11. Montoya JG, Rosso F. Diagnosis and management of toxoplasmosis. *Clin Perinatol* 2005; 32(3):705–726.
12. Janakiraman V. Listeriosis in pregnancy: diagnosis, treatment, and prevention. *Rev Obstet Gynecol* 2008; 1(4):179–185.
13. Cherpes TL, Matthews DB, Maryak SA. Neonatal herpes simplex virus infection. *Clin Obstet Gynecol* 2012; 55(4):938–944.
14. Wong S, Ordean A, Kahan M. Substance use in pregnancy. *J Obstet Gynaecol Can* 2011; 33(4):367–384.
15. Apgar V. A proposal for a new method of evaluation of the newborn infant. *Curr Res Anesth Analg* 1953; 32(4):260–267.
16. Opiyo N, English M. What clinical signs best identify severe illness in young infants aged 0–59 days in developing countries? A systematic review. *Arch Dis Child* 2011; 96(11):1052–1059.
17. Bang AT, Bang RA, Reddy MH et al. Simple clinical criteria to identify sepsis or pneumonia in neonates in the community needing treatment or referral. *Pediatr Infect Dis J* 2005; 24(4):335–341.
18. Young Infants Clinical Signs Study Group. Clinical signs that predict severe illness in children under age 2 months: a multicentre study. *Lancet* 2008; 371(9607):135–142.
19. Robinson JN, Abuhamad AN. Abdominal wall and umbilical cord anomalies. *Clin Perinatol* 2000; 27(4):947–978, ix.
20. National Health Service. Newborn and infant physical examination screening: standards. 2008, updated April 2016. www.gov.uk/government/publications/newborn-and-infant-physical-examination-screening-standards.
21. Polin RA, Denson S, Brady MT. Strategies for prevention of health care-associated infections in the NICU. *Pediatrics* 2012; 129(4):e1085–e1093.
22. Babson SG, Benda GI. Growth graphs for the clinical assessment of infants of varying gestational age. *J Pediatr* 1976; 89(5):814–820.
23. Lubchenco LO, Hansman C, Boyd E. Intrauterine growth in length and head circumference as estimated from live births at gestational ages from 26 to 42 weeks. *Pediatrics* 1966; 37(3):403–408.
24. Dancis J, O'Connell JR, Holt LE. A grid for recording the weight of premature infants. *J Pediatr* 1948; 33(11):570–572.
25. Myrelid A, Gustafsson J, Ollars B, Annerén G. Growth charts for Down's syndrome from birth to 18 years of age. *Arch Dis Child* 2002; 87(2):97–103.
26. American Institute of Ultrasound in Medicine; American College of Radiology; Society for Pediatric Radiology; Society of Radiologists in Ultrasound. AIUM practice guideline for the performance of an ultrasound examination of the neonatal spine. *J Ultrasound Med* 2012; 31(1):155–164.
27. Kriss VM, Desai NS. Occult spinal dysraphism in neonates: assessment of high-risk cutaneous stigmata on sonography. *Am J Roentgenol* 1998; 171(6):1687–1692.
28. Moss C. Genetic skin disorders. *Semin Neonatol* 2000; 5(4):311–320.
29. Bruckner AL, Frieden IJ. Hemangiomas of infancy. *J Am Acad Dermatol* 2003; 48(4):477–493; quiz 494–496.
30. Kaplan M, Hammarman C. Neonatal hyperbilirubinaemia. In Polin RA, Yoder MC (eds) *Workbook in Practical Neonatology*, 4th edn, Ch 5. Philadelphia: Saunders, 2007.

31. Furdon SA, Clark DA. Scalp hair characteristics in the newborn infant. *Adv Neonatal Care* 2003; 3(6):286–296.
32. Davies DP, Ansari BM, Cooke TJ. Anterior fontanelle size in the neonate. *Arch Dis Child* 1975; 50(1):81–83.
33. Popich GA, Smith DW. Fontanels: range of normal size. *J Pediatr* 1972; 80(5):749–752.
34. Chen MY, Liu HM, Weng WC et al. Neonate with severe heart failure related to vein of Galen malformation. *Pediatr Neonatol* 2010; 51(4):245–248.
35. Brown RL. Samba San: the Japanese midwife. *Midwives Chron* 1970; 83(993):344–345.
36. Roth DA, Hildesheimer M, Bardenstein S et al. Preauricular skin tags and ear pits are associated with permanent hearing impairment in newborns. *Pediatrics* 2008; 122(4):e884–e890.
37. Fletcher MA. *Physical diagnosis in neonatology*. Philadelphia: Lippincott-Raven, 1998.
38. Roberts DG, Johnson CE, Carlin SA et al. Resolution of middle ear effusion in newborns. *Arch Pediatr Adolesc Med* 1995; 149(8):873–877.
39. Capasso A, Capasso L, Raimondi F et al. A nontraumatic and inexpensive clinical maneuver to check nasal patency at birth. *Pediatrics* 2001; 107(1):214.
40. Singh DJ, Bartlett SP. Congenital mandibular hypoplasia: analysis and classification. *J Craniofac Surg* 2005; 16(2):291–300.
41. Nwoku AL, Kekere-Ekun TA. Congenital ankylosis of the mandible. Report of a case noted at birth. *J Maxillofac Surg* 1986; 14(3):150–152.
42. Baumgart M, Lussi A. Natal and neonatal teeth. *Schweiz Monatsschr Zahnmed* 2006; 116(9):894–909.
43. Ballard JL, Auer CE, Khoury JC. Ankyloglossia: assessment, incidence, and effect of frenuloplasty on the breastfeeding dyad. *Pediatrics* 2002; 110(5):e63.
44. Koeller KK, Alamo L, Adair CF, Smirniotopoulos JG. Congenital cystic masses of the neck: radiologic–pathologic correlation. *Radiographics* 1999; 19(1):121–146; quiz 152–153.
45. Park YW. Evaluation of neck masses in children. *Am Fam Physician* 1995; 51(8):1904–1912.
46. Bamji M, Stone RK, Kaul A et al. Palpable lymph nodes in healthy newborns and infants. *Pediatrics* 1986; 78(4):573–575.
47. Haller JA, Kramer SS, Lietman SA. Use of CT scans in selection of patients for pectus excavatum surgery: a preliminary report. *J Pediatr Surg* 1987; 22(10):904–906.
48. Kelly DH, Shannon DC. Periodic breathing in infants with near-miss sudden infant death syndrome. *Pediatrics* 1979; 63(3):355–360.
49. Committee on Fetus and Newborn. American Academy of Pediatrics. Apnea, sudden infant death syndrome, and home monitoring. *Pediatrics* 2003; 111(4 Pt 1):914–917.
50. Duke T, Oa O, Mokela D et al. The management of sick young infants at primary health centres in a rural developing country. *Arch Dis Child* 2005; 90(2):200–205.
51. Sasidharan P. An approach to diagnosis and management of cyanosis and tachypnea in term infants. *Pediatr Clin North Am* 2004; 51(4):999–1021, ix.
52. Antia AU, Maxwell SR, Gough A, Ayeni O. Position of the apex beat in childhood. *Arch Dis Child* 1978; 53(7):585–589.
53. Perloff JK. *The clinical recognition of congenital heart disease*. Philadelphia: Saunders, 2003.
54. Gindes L, Hegesh J, Barkai G et al. Isolated levocardia: prenatal diagnosis, clinical importance, and literature review. *J Ultrasound Med* 2007; 26(3):361–365.
55. Le Mauviel L. Primary ciliary dyskinesia. *West J Med* 1991; 155(3):280–283.
56. Ainsworth S, Wyllie JP, Wren C. Prevalence and clinical significance of cardiac murmurs in neonates. *Arch Dis Child Fetal Neonatal Ed* 1999; 80(1):F43–F45.
57. Keane JF, Lock JE, Fyler DC, Nadas AS. *Nadas' pediatric cardiology*. Philadelphia: Saunders, 2006.
58. Bakr AF, Habib HS. Combining pulse oximetry and clinical examination in screening for congenital heart disease. *Pediatr Cardiol* 2005; 26(6):832–835.
59. de-Wahl Granelli A, Wennergren M, Sandberg K et al. Impact of pulse oximetry screening on the detection of duct dependent congenital heart disease: a Swedish prospective screening study in 39,821 newborns. *BMJ* 2009; 338:a3037.
60. Ravert P, Detwiler TL, Dickinson JK. Mean oxygen saturation in well neonates at altitudes between 4498 and 8150 feet. *Adv Neonatal Care* 2011; 11(6):412–417.
61. Takci S, Yigit S, Korkmaz A, Yurdakök M. Comparison between oscillometric and invasive blood pressure measurements in critically ill premature infants. *Acta Paediatr* 2012; 101(2):132–135.
62. Forgacs P. Crackles and wheezes. *Lancet* 1967; 2(7508):203–205.
63. Nath AR, Capel LH. Inspiratory crackles and mechanical events of breathing. *Thorax* 1974; 29(6):695–698.
64. Clark DA. Times of first void and first stool in 500 newborns. *Pediatrics* 1977; 60(4):457–459.
65. Loening-Baucke V, Kimura K. Failure to pass meconium: diagnosing neonatal intestinal obstruction. *Am Fam Physician* 1999; 60(7):2043–2050.
66. Wei C, Stevens J, Harrison S et al. Fractures in a tertiary neonatal intensive care unit in Wales. *Acta Paediatr* 2012; 101(6):587–590.
67. Canale ST, Beaty JH. *Campbell's operative orthopaedics: hand surgery*. St Louis, MO: Mosby, 2012.
68. Flatt AE. *The care of congenital hand anomalies*, 2nd edn. St Louis, MO: Quality Medical Pub, 1994.
69. Gore AI, Spencer JP. The newborn foot. *Am Fam Physician* 2004; 69(4):865–872.
70. Cady RB. Developmental dysplasia of the hip: definition, recognition, and prevention of late sequelae. *Pediatr Ann* 2006; 35(2):92–101.
71. Zafeiriou DI. Primitive reflexes and postural reactions in the neurodevelopmental examination. *Pediatric Neurology* 2004; 31(1):1–8.
72. Volpe JJ, Inder T, Darras B et al. *Neurology of the newborn*, 6th edn. Philadelphia, Elsevier, 2017.
73. Harris W. *Examination paediatrics*, 5th edn. Sydney: Elsevier Australia, 2017.
74. Futagi Y, Toribe Y, Suzuki Y. The grasp reflex and moro reflex in infants: hierarchy of primitive reflex responses. *Int J Pediatr* 2012; 2012:191562.
75. Ballard JL, Khoury JC, Wedig K et al. New Ballard Score, expanded to include extremely premature infants. *J Pediatr* 1991; 119(3):417–423.
76. Sasidharan K, Dutta S, Narang A. Validity of New Ballard Score until 7th day of postnatal life in moderately preterm neonates. *Arch Dis Child Fetal Neonatal Ed* 2009; 94(1):F39–F44.

SECTION 11
Women's health history and examination

CHAPTER 39
The obstetric history and examination

CHAPTER 40
The gynaecological history and examination

CHAPTER 41
The breasts history and examination

CHAPTER 39
The obstetric history and examination
Wendy Carseldine and Ian Symonds

Life is always a rich and steady time when you are waiting for something to happen or to hatch.
E B WHITE, Charlotte's Web

THE OBSTETRIC HISTORY

Obstetrics is the branch of medicine concerned with pregnancy and childbirth. It is derived from the Latin *obstetrix*, which literally means midwife: 'mid' meaning 'with' (Old English, still seen in 'mit' in German) and 'wife' meaning 'the woman'. The obstetric system is mostly concerned with normal processes, rather than a disease state. There are also two patients, and not one. Both of these factors differentiate it from other branches of medicine. It is important to understand the symptoms and signs of a normal pregnancy so as to understand what is pathological.[1-5]

EARLY PREGNANCY SYMPTOMS

(See Questions box 39.1.)

Amenorrhoea

Amenorrhoea is the absence of a menstrual period in a woman of reproductive age. In a woman presenting with amenorrhoea, pregnancy must be assumed until proven otherwise. A urinary or serum hCG level will confirm the presence of a pregnancy. The dating of pregnancy is done using the last external physical sign prior to pregnancy, which is the first day of the **last menstrual period** (LMP). This assumes that the patient's cycle length is 28 days and that ovulation thus occurs on day 14 (as ovulation occurs 14 days prior to the onset of menses). The estimated date of confinement (EDC), or due date, is calculated at 280 days, or 40 weeks from the LMP. When the cycle length varies

QUESTIONS TO ASK A WOMAN WHO MAY BE PREGNANT

1. When was the first day of your last menstrual period?
2. Was it normal in volume and length? (A light bleed may occur at the time of implantation and be confused with a period.)
3. Are your periods usually regular? What is the usual number of days from the first day of one period to the first day of the next period?
4. Are you currently sexually active?
5. Have you had previous pregnancies?
6. Have you had difficulty becoming pregnant or have you been using fertility treatment?
7. Have you been using any form of contraception? What have you used?
8. Have you performed a urine pregnancy test or had a blood test to confirm the pregnancy?
9. Have you had breast tenderness?
10. Have you been troubled by nausea?
11. How do you feel about the possibility of pregnancy?

QUESTIONS BOX 39.1

from 28 days, but remains regular, the EDC can be calculated accordingly. When the cycle length is irregular, the woman does not remember her LMP, she is breastfeeding or has ceased hormonal contraception immediately prior to the pregnancy, the date of the pregnancy should be confirmed with a pelvic ultrasound examination.

Another method of calculation of EDC is Naegele's rule. This is done by counting back 3 calendar months from the LMP and adding 7 days. For example, if the LMP is 15 May then the EDC will be 22 February. This rule also assumes a 28-day cycle.

> **MINOR SYMPTOMS IN PREGNANCY**
> - Hyperemesis gravidarum
> - Heartburn and acid regurgitation
> - Constipation
> - Back pain
> - Pubic symphysis pain
> - Vaginal discharge
> - Pruritus
> - Neuropathies
> - Tiredness
> - Breathlessness
> - Palpitations
> - Ankle oedema
>
> LIST 39.1

Breast changes

Although not diagnostic of pregnancy, breast tenderness and paraesthesia are common symptoms in the first weeks of pregnancy. As the pregnancy progresses the breasts enlarge and the subcutaneous veins become more prominent. The nipple area enlarges and the pigment darkens. Later in the pregnancy the nipple may produce colostrum, a thick yellow fluid.

Nausea and vomiting

The majority of women experience nausea in pregnancy and approximately half will experience vomiting. It is correlated with the rise of hCG levels and is usually present from 6–16 weeks' gestation. When a woman presents with very early or intractable vomiting, it is important to investigate with an ultrasound to rule out multiple pregnancy or gestational trophoblastic disease. In some cases it can lead to hyperemesis gravidarum[a] (see below).

MINOR SYMPTOMS IN PREGNANCY

Pregnancy is traditionally divided into three trimesters. The first trimester and its complications are considered 'gynaecological' by convention and are covered in Chapter 40, 'The gynaecological history and examination and basic investigations'. The following symptoms may occur at any stage of the pregnancy, but are more common in the second and third trimesters. (See List 39.1.)

Hyperemesis gravidarum

Hyperemesis gravidarum is intractable vomiting occurring in pregnancy, associated with increased hCG levels such as in multiple gestation and molar pregnancy. It is transient and usually resolves by 16 weeks' gestation. Hyperthyroidism should be excluded on initial investigations and treatment is guided by symptoms. Hyperemesis gravidarum can occur as early as 5 weeks' gestation.

Heartburn and acid regurgitation

Increased progesterone levels in pregnancy cause decreased gastrointestinal motility and slower gastric emptying. Levels of gastric acid secretion reduce; however, the oesophageal pressure is also reduced, leading to acid regurgitation.

Constipation

Constipation is a very common symptom in pregnancy, which is likely also to be associated with the effect of the progesterone. This is often worsened by iron supplementation. Haemorrhoids are a common side effect of the constipation, which usually resolve postnatally.

---

[a] 'Gravidus' means 'burdened' in Latin.

Back pain
As the uterine size increases, there is increasing lordosis in the lumbar spine and a relaxation of the musculature, contributing to back pain. As the fetal head descends into the pelvis, the pain may also occur in the vagina and buttocks and radiate into the upper legs.

Pubic symphysis pain
This is point tenderness over the pubic symphysis, which is usually exacerbated with movement. This is a result of ligament laxity as well as increasing uterine pressure. The pain can be relieved by rest, and simple analgesia may be useful.

Vaginal discharge
In the early stages of pregnancy the cervical mucus is thick, obstructs the cervical canal and creates a barrier to protect the uterine contents. During the early stages of labour, this mucous plug is expelled and is colloquially called 'the show'. There is an increase in vaginal discharge throughout pregnancy. It is usually thick and white, resulting from the increased lactic acid production from the glycogen in the epithelium of the vagina. Candidal vaginal infection is also common and if the discharge has more of a 'cottage cheese' appearance associated with itch then a culture should be performed and the infection treated with topical anti-yeast cream.

Pruritus
Itch is a common complaint in pregnancy. There are a number of pregnancy-related conditions that manifest with pruritus, including *intrahepatic cholestasis of pregnancy* with the itch often worse in the palms of the hands and soles of the feet. This is associated with abnormal liver function tests and an increased risk of fetal death in utero. Evaluation and treatment should be prompt and delivery should be considered from 37 weeks' gestation. *Pruritic urticarial papules and plaques of pregnancy (PUPPS)* is the most common dermatosis of pregnancy, which usually resolves soon after delivery and has no significant increase in fetal morbidity. The itch is likely to be on the abdomen, thighs, arms and buttocks.

Neuropathies
The most common neuropathy in pregnancy is carpal tunnel syndrome. This is often present in the third trimester, associated with increasing oedema and subsequent compression of the median nerve. Bell's palsy (unilateral lower motor neurone lesion of the facial nerve) has an increased incidence during pregnancy and the puerperium.[b] Compression and damage of the lumbar and sacral nerves are also associated with pregnancy and delivery.

Tiredness
This is most common in the first and third trimesters, affecting almost all pregnant women at some stage during their pregnancy. As the uterus enlarges, women feel uncomfortable and have increasing urinary frequency, causing sleep to become difficult.

Breathlessness
Dyspnoea is reported in up to 70% of pregnant patients. Most of this is physiological. Asthma exacerbations must be excluded in women in whom it is pre-existing.

Palpitations
Heart rate increases in pregnancy in response to the increasing blood volume and cardiac output requirements. There is poor correlation between symptoms and pathological arrhythmias; however, if the palpitations are persistent, they should be investigated with an ECG, Holter monitor and evaluation of electrolytes and thyroid function.

MAJOR SYMPTOMS IN PREGNANCY
The major symptoms in pregnancy are summarised in List 39.2.

Change in fetal movements
Fetal movements are a good indication of fetal wellbeing. They are usually first appreciated at 17–22 weeks' gestation (the 'quickening') and continue until delivery. Towards the end of the third trimester the movements are often not as vigorous, but should be as frequent.

---
[b] The Latin word for 'childbirth'.

> **MAJOR SYMPTOMS IN PREGNANCY**
> - Change in fetal movements
> - Vaginal bleeding
> - Rupture of membranes
> - Abdominal pain
> - Headache
> - Non-dependent oedema
>
> LIST 39.2

If the fetal movements are decreased, fetal evaluation with electronic heart rate monitoring and ultrasound should be undertaken and, once full term is reached, delivery should be considered.

Vaginal bleeding

Vaginal bleeding in pregnancy is never normal, but it is relatively common. In early pregnancy it may be associated with miscarriage or ectopic pregnancy or occur as a result of a subchorionic haematoma. In the second and third trimesters, vaginal bleeding may herald more sinister pathology. The three diagnoses that should be excluded include **placental abruption** (separation of the placenta from the uterine wall), **placenta praevia** (when the placenta is near or covering the cervical os) and **vasa praevia** (vessels containing fetal blood cross the cervical os). Non-pregnancy-related causes are also possible including trauma, malignancy and cervical polyp.

Investigation should include a full history, abdominal and vaginal examinations and bloods, including full blood count and Kleihauer (a test to assess the amount of fetal haemoglobin). Prompt resuscitation of the mother is required if there is significant haemorrhage.

Rupture of membranes

When the 'waters break', or rupture of the membranes (amnion and chorion) occurs, the colour of the liquor should be assessed. The liquor should be clear (not cloudy) and pale yellow in colour. Light bloodstaining may cause the fluid to become pink and is also acceptable. Cloudy, offensive, brown or green liquor should be addressed quickly. In the setting of ruptured membranes prior to 37 weeks' gestation, infection is often the cause and should be treated. At term, if the woman is group B *Streptococcus* (GBS) negative and otherwise uncomplicated, then a period of expectant management is usually allowed. If GBS is present, then antibiotic cover and consideration for induction of labour is recommended.

Abdominal pain

Throughout pregnancy, the uterine muscle contracts and relaxes. When this is a painless process, it is termed a Braxton–Hicks contraction. Once these become painful and regular, they are termed contractions. The nature of contractions is that they are intermittent and associated with uterine firmness, with the pain being in the abdomen and mid–lower back.

Constant or instantly severe abdominal pain in pregnancy should receive prompt assessment. Placental abruption, which may be concealed or associated with vaginal bleeding, can cause constant, severe pain. There is usually also frequent uterine activity with no period of relaxation. The other, potentially catastrophic causes of abdominal pain include uterine rupture, which is usually associated with previous uterine surgery or prolonged, obstructed labour. In all cases the mother and the fetus should be examined. Non-obstetric causes of abdominal pain include ruptured viscera and hepatic capsule oedema as well as causes seen outside of pregnancy.

Headache

Headache in pregnancy deserves special consideration as it may be the symptom of more ominous pathology such as cerebral irritation or haemorrhagic stroke associated with hypertensive disorders of pregnancy such as pre-eclampsia. Migraine can also manifest in pregnancy and should be treated initially with simple analgesia and hydration.

Oedema

Pedal and hand oedema in the third trimester is almost universal and transient in nature. More significant oedema that occurs over the course of a few days or affects the face should trigger evaluation of the blood pressure and urinalysis to exclude pre-eclampsia.

HISTORY

(See Questions box 39.2.)

QUESTIONS TO ASK WHEN PREGNANCY HAS BEEN CONFIRMED

Obstetric history
1. Have you been pregnant before? If so, how many times?
2. Have you had any miscarriages, ectopic pregnancies or terminations of pregnancy?
3. Did you go into labour prematurely? Did you have any problems with the delivery?
4. Were the babies delivered vaginally or by caesarean section?
5. Did you have any problem with high blood pressure or diabetes during your previous pregnancies?
6. Did you have problems with depression after the delivery?

Medical history
7. Do you currently have or have a history of any of the following?
    - Diabetes
    - Heart disease (especially congenital or valvular) or high blood pressure
    - Epilepsy
    - Kidney, thyroid, liver disease
    - Connective tissue disorders
    - Clotting or bleeding disorders
    - Chronic viral infection (hepatitis B or C, HIV)
    - Sexually transmitted diseases
8. Have you had any operations before? If so, were there any complications?
9. Do you suffer from anxiety, depression or other psychiatric illnesses?

Medications
10. Have you been taking any of the following?
    - Anticonvulsants
    - ACE inhibitors
    - Cytotoxic drugs
    - Statins
    - Anticoagulants
11. Have you been taking folic acid or a pregnancy multivitamin?
12. Do you have any allergies?

Family history
13. Do you have a family history of any genetic disorders?
14. Does anyone in your family suffer from blood clots?
15. Are there any other medical disorders that run in the family?

Social questions
16. Are you a smoker?
17. Do you drink alcohol? How many days a week do you drink and how much each day?
18. Do you take any recreational drugs? Which ones?
19. Are you working or studying? What type of work do you do?
20. How do you feel you will manage during the pregnancy and once the baby is born?
21. Do you have a partner? Are they supportive? Do you feel safe at home?
22. What supports do you have at home?

QUESTIONS BOX 39.2

Current pregnancy history

Firstly, the EDC should be confirmed and agreed upon with the woman. The antenatal screening tests should be checked: blood group and antibodies, rubella, syphilis, hepatitis B, hepatitis C, HIV serology, midstream urine culture and full blood count. If anaemia is present, serum ferritin and thalassaemia screening should also be performed. Glucose tolerance testing should be undertaken at around 28 weeks and group B streptococcus (GBS) should be screened for after 36 weeks.

First-trimester screening for aneuploidy and second-trimester morphological ultrasound examination results should be reviewed. The morphology, or fetal anomaly ultrasound, includes placental location and cervical length assessment to screen for placenta praevia and cervical shortening respectively. Cervical length is most accurately measured by transvaginal ultrasound. A shortened cervix is a risk factor for preterm delivery and treatment should be considered.

Reviewing the antenatal record also gives an overview of the examination findings over previous visits. Trends in blood pressure and fundal height over time give an indication of whether the pregnancy is progressing normally.

Past obstetric history

A detailed history of each prior pregnancy, regardless of outcome, should be obtained. Recurrent miscarriage (three or more first-trimester miscarriages or any second-trimester miscarriage) warrants investigation for underlying cause.

Past intrapartum and postnatal events such as preterm delivery, caesarean section, postpartum haemorrhage, shoulder dystocia and third/fourth-degree perineal tears should be noted and an appropriate screening, prevention and/or management plan formulated.

Past gynaecological history

Find out whether the patient has received human papillomavirus (HPV) vaccination. The antenatal period is an appropriate opportunity for a full maternal health check. This includes cervical screening history; whether it is up to date and normal. If there have been previous abnormal results, were they treated and how many times? If there has been more than one treatment for cervical abnormalities, or a cone biopsy, the woman should be considered for transvaginal ultrasound cervical length screening from 14 weeks' gestation.

It is important to ask about a history of sexually transmitted infections, especially *Chlamydia trachomatis*, *Neisseria gonorrhoeae* and herpes simplex virus (HSV), syphilis (*Treponema pallidum*) and human immunodeficiency virus (HIV) as these can be screened for and treated as they can potentially affect the fetus and newborn.

Past medical history

This should include all pre-existing medical conditions. Importantly, women should be questioned regarding a history of cardiac, respiratory, renal, endocrine and neurological disease. Commonly overlooked chronic conditions such as rheumatic fever and cardiac valve replacement, epilepsy, asthma, hypertension, diabetes, thromboembolic events or depression should be specifically asked about. Previous surgeries, particularly abdominal or pelvic procedures, should be noted and operative notes obtained in the event that a caesarean section is required so that intraoperative complications can be predicted.

It is routine for a screening tool for depression, for example the Edinburgh Depression Scale, to be administered at least once during the antenatal period. This is usually performed at the booking visit by the midwife. Antenatal depression is one of the strongest predictors of postnatal depression.

Treatment history

The treatment history is very important, especially in regard to the fetus. All medications have a pregnancy category rating (List 39.3).[6] All medications rated other than category A should be risk-assessed against the benefits and, if appropriate, changed after consultation with the patient. All women should be advised to take 0.5 mg of folic acid per day for 3 months prior to pregnancy and through the first trimester to reduce the risk of fetal neural tube defects. High-dose folic acid (5 mg/day) is recommended for high-risk groups of women—for example, type 1 diabetes, women on antiepileptic medication, those with a body mass index (BMI) >35 and those with a previous history of a fetus with a neural tube defect. Vitamin A supplements and

> ### PREGNANCY DRUG CATEGORY RATINGS
>
> **Category A**
> Drugs that have been taken by a large number of pregnant women and women of childbearing age without any proven increase in the frequency of malformations or other direct or indirect harmful effects on the fetus having been observed.
>
> **Category B1**
> Drugs that have been taken by only a limited number of pregnant women and women of childbearing age, without an increase in the frequency of malformation or other direct or indirect harmful effects on the human fetus having been observed. Studies in animals have not shown evidence of an increased occurrence of fetal damage.
>
> **Category B2**
> Drugs that have been taken by only a limited number of pregnant women and women of childbearing age, without an increase in the frequency of malformation or other direct or indirect harmful effects on the human fetus having been observed. Studies in animals are inadequate or may be lacking, but available data show no evidence of an increased occurrence of fetal damage.
>
> **Category B3**
> Drugs that have been taken by only a limited number of pregnant women and women of childbearing age, without an increase in the frequency of malformation or other direct or indirect harmful effects on the human fetus having been observed. Studies in animals have shown evidence of an increased occurrence of fetal damage, the significance of which is considered uncertain in humans.
>
> **Category C**
> Drugs that, owing to their pharmacological effects, have caused or may be suspected of causing harmful effects on the human fetus or neonate without causing malformations. These effects may be reversible. Accompanying texts should be consulted for further details.
>
> **Category D**
> Drugs that have caused, are suspected to have caused or may be expected to cause an increased incidence of human fetal malformations or irreversible damage. These drugs may also have adverse pharmacological effects. Accompanying texts should be consulted for further details.
>
> **Category X**
> Drugs that have such a high risk of causing permanent damage to the fetus that they should not be used in pregnancy or when there is a possibility of pregnancy.
>
> From Australian categorisation system for prescribing medicines in pregnancy, 2011, Therapeutic Goods Administration, used by permission of the Australian Government https://www.tga.gov.au/australian-categorisation-system-prescribing-medicines-pregnancy
>
> LIST 39.3

liver products should be avoided in pregnancy. Vitamin D supplementation should be considered after screening for deficiency, especially in high-risk groups, such as those with limited sunlight exposure or dark skin or who are obese.

Social history

Due to the harmful effects of both cigarette smoking and alcohol on the health of the fetus, both should be explored. Quit-smoking advice and referral should be made during the initial consultation as well as at each subsequent interaction. Quitting smoking decreases the risks of placental abruption, preterm delivery and fetal abnormalities. Although fetal alcohol syndrome is rare, women should be advised that there is no safe level of alcohol consumption in pregnancy.

Some workplaces have inherent risks for pregnant women, and these should be discussed. Specifically, contact with infectious diseases, radiation and potential abdominal trauma should be avoided. Many workplaces will also require a medical certificate if the woman wishes to work after 34 weeks' gestation. With the increasing weight, tiredness and general discomfort of advanced pregnancy, some work and exercise may not be possible. Appropriate advice regarding exercise, weight gain and manual work can be given on an individualised basis. In general terms, women with a

> **FACTORS INDICATING A RISK OF INHERITED GENETIC DISEASE IN THE FETUS**
>
> - Previous child affected
> - Either parent with a known genetic defect
> - Affected relative
> - Family history of sex-linked disease (e.g. Duchenne's muscular dystrophy)
> - Ethnicity (e.g. beta-thalassaemia in families of Mediterranean or Middle Eastern origin)
> - Consanguinity
>
> LIST 39.4

normal prepregnancy BMI should gain 10–15 kg throughout the entire pregnancy. This should be more if the woman is underweight and less if overweight or obese.

Food hygiene should be discussed during pregnancy in order to avoid both food poisoning and food-associated infectious diseases such as *Toxoplasmosis* (unwashed salads and fruit), *Listeria* (soft cheeses, uncooked meat, unpasteurised milk, pâté) and *Salmonella* (raw eggs, uncooked meat).

Pregnancy is a time of increased risk of domestic violence for some women. An initial 'screening' question such as whether the patient feels supported or safe at home may need to be followed by additional discussion if domestic violence is disclosed or suspected from signs of trauma on physical examination.

Family history

A family history of inherited disorders is important, especially if screening or diagnostic tests may be used in decision making for the patient (see List 39.4).

EXAMINATION ANATOMY

The **uterus** is centrally located in the pelvis and throughout the pregnancy grows directly superiorly. The gravid uterus is usually palpable abdominally (above the pubic symphysis) by 12–14 weeks' gestation, depending on the adiposity of the patient.

EXAMINATION

A suggested method for the examination is given in Text box 39.1.

> **The antenatal obstetric examination: a suggested method**
>
> This examination is a targeted examination designed to screen for abnormalities in both the mother and the fetus in the progression of the pregnancy. As with all other systems, it starts with an examination of general appearance. Special interest is taken in respiratory distress, increased oedema and pallor.
>
> **Position** the patient initially in a sitting position with the feet supported on the floor. Measure the blood pressure in the right arm.
>
> **Reposition** the patient to a semirecumbent position. Measure the symphyseal–fundal height and perform Leopold manoeuvres. Auscultate the fetal heart rate for at least 15 seconds. If the history or examination is suggestive of hypertension or pre-eclampsia, then reflexes, clonus and lower limb oedema should be assessed in this position prior to assisting the woman to sit again.
>
> Genital examination should be performed with a chaperone, after informed consent, only when indicated. Perform a urinalysis.
>
> Further investigation by electronic fetal heart rate monitoring and ultrasound should be considered if there are any concerns for fetal wellbeing.
>
> TEXT BOX 39.1

Positioning the patient

The blood pressure should be taken with the woman sitting with her feet on the floor. It should initially be measured on both arms and if it is equal should be measured on the right arm at subsequent visits.

Supine hypotension can complicate the examination once the pregnancy reaches the third trimester. For abdominal palpation, the woman should not lie flat if uncomfortable, but be at approximately 30°, with a pillow or bed head tilt. If the patient must lie flat, she should be placed with a slight left lateral tilt, using a pillow under the right hip/flank, to avoid venocaval compression.

General appearance

The woman should have her height and weight measured at her booking visit, and BMI calculated. The weight should be measured at subsequent visits in underweight, overweight and obese patients to monitor weight changes in pregnancy and guide treatment. Referral to a dietitian early in the pregnancy may be beneficial for these women. Those women with increased BMI should also be referred to anaesthetic services antenatally for assessment should the need arise for regional analgesia in labour or caesarean section.

All women should be examined for pallor and jaundice. Anaemia due to iron deficiency is common in pregnancy. Anaemia due to vitamin B_{12} or folate deficiency or thalassaemia can occur, but is less common. Jaundice may result from viral hepatitis, gallstones, drug-induced or pregnancy-related causes such as AFLP (acute fatty liver of pregnancy), obstetric cholestasis, pre-eclampsia or HELLP (Haemolysis, Elevated Liver enzymes, Low Platelets) syndrome.

Observations

Blood pressure should be measured at each antenatal visit or presentation. Physiological changes in the cardiovascular system of peripheral vasodilation and increased cardiac output give rise to profound haemodynamic changes during pregnancy. During the first and second trimester, the blood pressure usually falls for both systole and diastole. Diastolic blood pressure may be unrecordable owing to the decreased peripheral resistance of the maternal circulation. The blood pressure then returns to prepregnancy values in the third trimester.

The heart rate usually increases 10–20 beats per minute above baseline rate, although a persisting heart rate of over 100 b.p.m. should always be investigated for a cause.

The hands

Carpal tunnel syndrome is common in pregnancy, as discussed above. The tingling, numbness and pain can be recreated by pressing on the anterior aspect of the wrist. Anaemia can cause palmar crease pallor.

The face

Periorbital and generalised facial oedema can be a sign of pre-eclampsia. This can be difficult to determine if you have not examined the patient previously. Often when questioned the patient or her partner will volunteer a recent history of facial swelling.

The neck and chest

The pregnant woman's neck is commonly oedematous, which can make anaesthetic intubation problematic. The normal breast hypertrophy also makes ventilation under anaesthetic difficult. These anatomical changes are just two of the reasons a regional anaesthetic is preferred in the pregnant woman.

Initial antenatal visit examination should include examination of the thyroid for goitre or nodules. A routine breast examination can be performed; as well as screening for breast masses, the breasts can be assessed for nipple inversion, asymmetry or previous surgery. All of these factors may influence breastfeeding and an antenatal lactation consultation may be of benefit. Women should be encouraged to perform their own breast checks routinely and can be educated on the procedure at this time.

The abdomen: mother and fetal findings

The symphyseal–fundal height (SFH) is measured from the fundus of the uterus in the midline, to the symphysis pubis with a non-elastic measuring tape (Fig. 39.1). By 20 weeks the fundus of the uterus should be at the level of the umbilicus. After this, the SFH in centimetres should equate to the number of weeks' gestation of the pregnancy, with an allowable margin of up to 3 cm. It should be recorded at each visit and the trend can be observed over time. There can be discrepancy in the measurements if: the EDC is incorrectly calculated, the woman is overweight/obese, uterine fibroids are present, there is a multiple pregnancy, and there are abnormalities in either fetal growth or liquor volume. If there is any clinical concern over the SFH measurement, the woman should be referred for an ultrasound assessment.

Leopold manoeuvres (Fig. 39.2) can be used to palpate the gravid uterus in the second and third trimester to assess fetal lie, presentation, position and engagement into the maternal pelvis. Fetal lie is the relation of the fetal long axis to the maternal long axis, and is described as longitudinal, transverse or oblique. Fetal presentation describes the fetal part that is foremost within the maternal pelvis, or closest to it. Presentations include cephalic (head presenting) and breech (sacrum, knees or feet presenting). Malpresentations such as shoulder, brow, face or umbilical cord are also possible

Measurement of SFH.

Changes in fundal height with pregnancy. Weeks 10 to 12: uterus within pelvis; fetal heartbeat can be detected with Doppler. Week 12: uterus palpable just above symphysis pubis. Week 16: uterus palpable halfway between symphysis and umbilicus; ballottement of fetus is possible by abdominal and vaginal examination. Week 20: uterine fundus at lower border of umbilicus; fetal heartbeat can be auscultated with a fetoscope. Weeks 24 to 26: uterus changes from globular to ovoid shape; fetus palpable. Week 28: uterus approximately halfway between umbilicus and xiphoid; fetus easily palpable. Week 34: uterine fundus just below xiphoid. Week 40: fundal height drops as fetus begins to engage in pelvis

(From Seidel HM, Ball JW, Dains JE et al. *Mosby's guide to physical examination*, 7th edn. St Louis, MO: Mosby, 2011, Ch 18, pp 535–599.)

FIGURE 39.1

(Fig. 39.3). If the presenting part is unable to be identified, an ultrasound should be performed to confirm the presentation, especially after 36 weeks' gestation. Fetal position refers to the relation of fetal part to the right or left side. Most commonly, if the fetus is in a cephalic presentation the fetal occiput is described as being anterior (OA), posterior (OP) or transverse (ROT or LOT) (Fig. 39.4). Engagement is measured abdominally as the proportion of the fetal head that has descended into the maternal pelvis. It is expressed in fifths, and can be described as fifths palpable abdominally or as fifths in the pelvis. The fetal head may engage prior to labour or after the start of labour, especially in multiparous women.

Once the uterus has been palpated and the fetal orientation identified, the fetal heart rate should be auscultated. This is usually done over the anterior-most shoulder with either a Pinard stethoscope or an electronic Doppler fetal heart rate monitor. The heart rate should be between 110 and 160 b.p.m. in the third trimester. A faster heart rate may be heard if the fetus is active and auscultation should continue until it returns below 160 b.p.m. If a slower heart rate is auscultated, comparison should be made with the maternal heart rate to ensure it is not the maternal rate being detected. If it is not, the woman should be positioned into a left lateral position. If there is no recovery of the fetal heart rate over the following 30 seconds, immediate assistance should be sought.

During labour the fetal heart rate can be assessed either by intermittent auscultation or by continuous electronic fetal heart rate monitoring. The method will be determined by the risk factors present in the patient. Local electronic fetal heart rate assessment tools should be consulted. An example of these can be found at www.ranzcog.edu.au or www.rcog.org.uk.

The genitals

Examination of the external genitalia may reveal vaginal discharge or vulval lesions such as HSV. If the symptoms suggest further examination is warranted, this usually begins with a speculum examination (see Ch 40). The labia majora and minora are carefully parted and the speculum (usually a Graves speculum) is passed with gentle downward pressure along the posterior vaginal wall. Once the speculum has been inserted as far as it will easily go, the speculum can be opened until the cervix can be directly visualised. The cervix is usually

Leopold manoeuvres.

(a) First manoeuvre: place hand(s) over fundus and identify the fetal part. (b) Second manoeuvre: use the palmar surface of one hand to locate the back of the fetus; use the other hand to feel the irregularities, such as hands and feet. (c) Third manoeuvre: use thumb and third finger to grasp presenting part over the symphysis pubis. (d) Fourth manoeuvre: use both hands to outline the fetal head; with a head presenting deep in the pelvis, only a small portion may be felt

(From Seidel HM, Ball JW, Dains JE et al. *Mosby's guide to physical examination*, 7th edn. St Louis, MO: Mosby, 2011, Ch 18, pp 535–599.)

FIGURE 39.2

in the posterior aspect of the upper vagina, but may be more anterior or deviated laterally. The vaginal walls should be inspected during insertion of the speculum for lesions, discharge or bleeding areas.

Once the cervix is in view, it should be inspected for lesions, ectropion appearance and for any fluid coming through the os. This may be blood, liquor, pus or normal cervical discharge. Asking the patient to perform the Valsalva manoeuvre may elicit pooling of the liquor if the diagnosis of ruptured membranes is uncertain.

Vaginal examination is usually performed with the index and middle finger of the dominant hand of the examiner inserted gently into the vagina to assess the cervix. Examination of the cervix in pregnancy has five main features, which should each be assessed. In the antenatal period, this examination has a scoring system called the Bishop score (Table 39.1), where the

740   SECTION 11 WOMEN'S HEALTH HISTORY AND EXAMINATION

Fetal presentations and positions in labour

(Modified from Norwitz ER, Robinson J, Repke JT. The initiation and management of labor. In Seifer DB, Samuels P, Kniss D, eds. *The physiologic basis of gynecology and obstetrics*. Philadelphia: Lippincott Williams & Wilkins, 2001; Gabbe SG, Niebyl JR, Simpson JL et al. *Obstetrics: normal and problem pregnancies*, 6th edn. Ch 13, pp 267–286. Philadelphia: Elsevier Saunders. ©Elsevier, 2012.)

FIGURE 39.3

Cervical feature	Bishop score			
	0	1	2	3
Dilation	<1 cm	1–2 cm	3–4 cm	>4 cm
Length	4 cm	2–4 cm	1–2 cm	<1 cm
Consistency	Firm	Medium	Soft	
Position	Posterior	Central	Anterior	
Station	3	2	1, 0	>+1

(Goh J, Flynn M. *Examination obstetrics and gynaecology*, 3rd edn. Sydney: Elsevier Australia, 2011, Table 42.1.)

TABLE 39.1

cervix can be objectively described, usually when making decisions for induction of labour. The first feature is **cervical dilation**, which is measured in centimetres. This is how open the cervix is at the level of the internal os when the examination starts, not after manipulation. During the first stage of labour the cervix dilates to 'full' dilation at 10 cm, when the start of the second stage of labour begins. The second feature is **cervical length (effacement)**, which starts at 3–4 cm and effaces to become 'paper' thin. The third feature is **consistency**, which is described as soft, medium or firm. The prelabour cervix is firm, similar in consistency to the tip of the nose, and gradually softens as labour progresses. The fourth feature is the **cervical position**, which describes whether the cervix has started to move from the initial 'posterior' position, through to 'mid' position or has progressed to an 'anterior' position. The final feature is **station** of the presenting part. This is measured in centimetres above or below the ischial spines, which are located at approximately 5 and 7 o'clock in the vagina. During labour the vaginal examination should also include assessment of fetal head position, application to the cervix, caput and moulding.

The lower limbs

The lower limbs should be examined with the patient lying. Initial inspection should assess for oedema; often the patient should be asked to clarify whether the level of oedema is usual or increased. If oedema is present, the level of pitting should be checked from the ankle upwards on both sides. The calves and ankles can be palpated for tenderness consistent with deep vein thrombosis.

If hypertension is present, neurological signs are easily elicited in the lower limbs. Patella reflexes in pregnancy are usually normal to brisk and a tendon hammer is rarely required. Clonus is best assessed in the ankle joint by moving the foot in a quick upward motion to flex the joint. One or two beats are acceptable in pregnancy. Increased reflexes and/or clonus may reflect neurological irritation in the setting of pre-eclampsia and should be addressed in a timely fashion.

Fetal head positions.

LOA=left occiput anterior; LOT=left occiput transverse; LOP=left occiput posterior; ROA=right occiput anterior; ROT=right occiput transverse; ROP=right occiput posterior

(From *Dorland's medical dictionary for health consumers*. Philadelphia: ©2007 Saunders.)

FIGURE 39.4

Urinalysis

A midstream urine specimen should be collected at the first antenatal visit to exclude infection. At subsequent visits dipstick urinalysis should be performed if infection is suspected or there are signs/symptoms of pre-eclampsia to check for the presence of proteinuria.

Obstetric ultrasound: a systematic approach

First-trimester obstetric ultrasound can be used for dating of the pregnancy as described above. At 11–13 weeks' gestation the first-trimester screening for aneuploidy should be performed. This incorporates ultrasound assessment of the fetal nuchal thickness, hCG and PAPP-A blood tests and maternal demographics to give a risk assessment for trisomy 21, 13 and 18. Once this risk assessment has been performed the patient has the option for invasive diagnostic testing (chorionic villus sampling or amniocentesis) or non-invasive testing, which measures fetal DNA from a maternal blood sample.

At 18–20 weeks' gestation a full morphological assessment of the fetus is performed, including head, face, chest, heart, abdomen, limbs and spine being visualised. The placental location is also observed at

> ### T&O'C ESSENTIALS
>
> 1. Vaginal bleeding in pregnancy is never normal. Both pregnancy- and non-pregnancy-related causes should be explored.
> 2. Medical disorders can both affect pregnancy and be affected by pregnancy.
> 3. If a medication is being used (or being considered for use) in pregnancy or breastfeeding, always check the pregnancy category rating.
> 4. Supine positioning in pregnancy causes vena caval compression; use the left lateral or semirecumbent position to avoid hypotension and hypoperfusion of the uterus.
> 5. Fetal lie, presentation, position and engagement can be obtained from abdominal palpation.
> 6. Assessment of cervical dilation, effacement, position, consistency and fetal station is acquired by vaginal examination.

> ### OSCE REVISION TOPICS – THE OBSTETRIC HISTORY AND EXAMINATION
>
> 1. A multiparous woman presents for her routine antenatal visit at 37 weeks' gestation. Please explain how you would perform a routine examination. (pp 736–41)
> 2. A woman presents with severe nausea and vomiting at 8 weeks' gestation. Please describe your investigations and initial management. (p 730)
> 3. A primiparous woman presents to the delivery suite at 36 weeks' gestation with a severe frontal headache and a blood pressure of 170/110. Please take a history of the presenting illness. (pp 732–6)
> 4. At 41 weeks' gestation, a multiparous woman presents for cervical assessment for induction of labour. What are the five features assessed for the Bishop score? (p 740)
> 5. This 34-year-old woman presents at 38 weeks with spontaneous rupture of membranes. Please take a history and explain how you would perform the appropriate examination. (pp 732, 738–40)

this examination, with a further ultrasound to be performed at about 34 weeks if it is low-lying. If any abnormality is seen, then tertiary referral is usually sought for advice and management.

Further ultrasound assessment may be required to estimate the growth velocity of the fetus. The measurements used include head circumference, biparietal diameter, abdominal circumference and femur length. These are used to calculate an estimation of the fetal weight. Liquor volume is assessed by single deepest pool or amniotic fluid index (the sum of the pools in the four quadrants of the uterus). The placental location is again observed. Assessment of fetal wellbeing can also be performed using blood flow Doppler in the umbilical cord and middle cerebral artery.

References

1. Cunningham FG, Leveno KJ, Bloom SL et al. *Williams obstetrics*, 23rd edn. Sydney: McGraw Hill Medical, 2010.
2. Goh J, Flynn M. *Examination obstetrics and gynaecology*, 3rd edn. Sydney: Elsevier Australia, 2011.
3. Luesley DM, Baker PN. *Obstetrics and gynaecology: an evidence-based text for MRCOG*, 2nd edn. London: Hodder Arnold, 2010.
4. Nelson-Piercy C. *Handbook of obstetric medicine*, 4th edn. London: Informa Healthcare, 2010.
5. Sarris I, Bewley S, Agnihotri S. *Training in obstetrics and gynaecology: the essential curriculum*. London: Oxford University Press, 2009.
6. Therapeutic Goods Administration. The Australian categorisation system for prescribing medicines in pregnancy. www.tga.gov.au/hp/medicines-pregnancy.htm.

CHAPTER 40

The gynaecological history and examination

Ian Symonds

The good physician treats the disease; the great physician treats the patient who has the disease.
SIR WILLIAM OSLER (1849–1919)

Gynaecology is the field of medicine that includes disorders of the female genital tract and reproductive system. It also includes complications of early pregnancy such as miscarriage and ectopic pregnancy.

HISTORY

As with all areas of medicine a precise and comprehensive history is the most important component in making an accurate gynaecological diagnosis. The basic structure of the gynaecological history is similar to that for other systems, but with more emphasis on the patient's menstrual, sexual and past reproductive history. It is important to note the patient's age as this will influence the likely diagnosis for a number of presenting problems. Occupation may be relevant both to the level of understanding that can be assumed and to the effect of different gynaecological problems on the patient's life.

A method for the gynaecological history and examination is given in Text box 40.1.

Presenting symptoms

Ask the patient to describe the nature of her problem. Where there are multiple symptoms these may not be related to the same pathology and it is useful to address each of these in turn with appropriate open and closed questioning. Ascertain the timescale of the problem and, where appropriate, the circumstances surrounding the onset of symptoms and their relationship to the menstrual cycle. It is also important to discover the degree of disability experienced for any given symptom. In many situations, reassurance that there is no serious underlying pathology will provide sufficient 'treatment', because the actual disability may be minimal.

More detailed questions will depend on the nature of the presenting complaint. List 40.1 outlines some of the more common presenting symptoms encountered in the outpatient clinic. Further details for some of these are discussed below.

COMMON PRESENTING SYMPTOMS IN GYNAECOLOGY

- Disorders of menstruation
- Heavy menstrual bleeding
- Intermenstrual bleeding
- Oligomenorrhoea/amenorrhoea
- Postmenopausal bleeding
- Premenstrual syndrome
- Disorders of sexual function
- Dyspareunia
- Loss of libido
- Vaginismus
- Infertility
- Pain and/or bleeding in early pregnancy
- Pelvic/lower abdominal pain: acute and chronic
- Perimenopausal symptoms
- Symptoms of uterovaginal prolapse
- Urinary disorders
- Urinary incontinence
- Urinary urgency/frequency
- Voiding difficulties
- Vaginal discharge and genital tract infection
- Vulval pain/pruritis

LIST 40.1

The gynaecological history and examination: a suggested method

1. **History**
   - Presenting symptoms
     - Onset and duration of main complaint
     - Associated symptoms, relationship to menstrual cycle
     - Previous treatment and response
     - Specific closed questions
   - Previous gynaecological history
     - Previous investigations or treatment
     - Contraceptive history
     - Sexual history
     - Pap smear
     - Menstrual history
   - Previous pregnancies
     - How many (gravidity)
     - Outcome (parity)
     - Surgical deliveries (birth weight)
   - Past surgical and medical history
     - Previous abdominal surgery
     - Major cardiovascular/respiratory disease
     - Endocrine disease
     - Thromboembolic disease
     - Breast disease
   - Drug history and allergies
   - Social and family history
     - Home circumstances
     - Support
     - Smoking
     - Family history
2. **Examination**
   - General examination
     - General condition, weight, height
     - Pulse, blood pressure
     - Anaemia
     - Goitre
     - Breast examination (if indicated)
     - Secondary sex characteristics, body hair
   - Abdominal examination
     - Inspection: distension, scars
     - Palpation: masses, organomegaly, tenderness, peritonism, nodes, hernial orifices
     - Percussion: ascites
   - Pelvic examination
     - Explanation, comfort, privacy, chaperone
     - Inspection of external genitalia
     - Speculum examination, Pap smear, swabs
     - Bimanual examination
   - Rectal examination, if indicated

TEXT BOX 40.1

Menstrual history

A full menstrual history should be taken from all women of reproductive age, starting with the first day of the last menstrual period.

The length of the menstrual cycle is the time between the first day of one period and the first day of the following period. While there is usually an interval of between 26 and 32 days, occasionally the duration of the cycle may be as short as 21 days or as long as 42 days without necessarily indicating any underlying abnormality.

Normal menstruation lasts from 4 to 7 days, and normal blood loss varies between 30 and 80 mL. A change in pattern is often more noticeable and significant than the actual duration and volume of loss. Self-reported assessment of the amount of bleeding is subjective, with up to 50% of women who report excessive bleeding actually having a measured blood loss of less than 80 mL. Excessively prolonged or heavy regular periods are sometimes referred to as **menorrhagia**, but the term **heavy menstrual bleeding (HMB)** is now generally used to describe all excessive menstrual blood loss regardless of the regularity of the cycle (see below).

The cessation of periods for at least 12 months at the end of menstrual life is known as the **menopause**. Bleeding that occurs after this is described as **postmenopausal bleeding**. A history of irregular vaginal bleeding or blood loss that occurs after coitus or between periods should be noted.

Heavy menstrual bleeding

HMB is defined as menstrual loss of more than 80 mL per month or 'excessive menstrual loss leading to

> **CAUSES OF HEAVY MENSTRUAL BLEEDING**
>
> **Structural**
> - Uterine leiomyomata (fibroids)
> - Adenomyosis
> - Endometrial polyps
> - Endometrial hyperplasia
> - Endometrial cancer
>
> **Non-structural**
> - Disorders of ovulation (polycystic ovary syndrome, perimenopause, puberty)
> - Clotting disorders
> - Iatrogenic (intrauterine contraceptive device)
> - Dysfunctional bleeding (see above)
> - Hypothyroidism
>
> LIST 40.2

interference with the physical, emotional, social and material quality of life in a woman and which occurs alone or in combination with other symptoms.'[1] It affects about 10% of women. In most cases the cause is an imbalance in the mechanisms that regulate clotting at the endometrial level without any obvious structural pathology. However, it may be associated with a number of benign pathologies and, occasionally, with malignancy (see List 40.2).

Diagnosis

In practice, the diagnosis of HMB is made on the basis of symptoms, not measured blood loss. Symptoms of clotting, flooding (soiling of clothing), the use of a large amount of sanitary protection, bleeding lasting more than 7 days and treatment for anaemia are likely to indicate HMB. A change in the pattern of bleeding is more likely to be associated with a structural lesion. Malignancy is rare in women under the age of 40. A history of polycystic ovary syndrome (PCOS), diabetes, hypertension and/or obesity is associated with an increased risk of endometrial hyperplasia and malignancy.

All women with HMB should have a general examination for signs of anaemia and thyroid disease and a pelvic examination including a Pap smear (P). The finding of a pelvic mass is most likely to be associated with a diagnosis of fibroids (see Fig. 40.1) but can indicate malignancy.

A full blood count (FBC) should be requested for all patients with HMB. Additional investigation is mainly directed at excluding malignancy and usually includes a pelvic ultrasound scan. Endoscopic examination of the endometrial cavity (hysteroscopy) with endometrial biopsy is indicated when:

- there is a history of irregular or intermenstrual bleeding
- risk factors for endometrial cancer are present
- pelvic examination is abnormal
- there is no response to first-line treatment.

Young women under the age of 25 should have a partial coagulation screen to exclude Von Willebrand's disease.

Bleeding in early pregnancy

Any women of reproductive age presenting with abnormal vaginal bleeding should have the possibility of pregnancy considered. If a pregnancy test is positive, the cause of the bleeding can usually be determined by a combination of vaginal examination and ultrasound (see Table 40.1). The most common cause of bleeding in early pregnancy (before 20 weeks) is miscarriage, although hydatidiform and ectopic pregnancy may also present with bleeding. Miscarriage is the spontaneous termination of pregnancy prior to 20 weeks' gestation; it affects about 15–20% of pregnancies. It is important to remember that bleeding in pregnancy can result from the same lower genital tract lesions as in non-pregnant women.

Amenorrhoea and oligomenorrhoea

The onset of the first period, the **menarche**, commonly occurs at 12 years of age and can be considered to be abnormally early at 7 years. **Primary amenorrhoea** is the absence of menarche. The age at which the diagnosis is made depends on the presence or absence of other features of puberty. In the absence of other signs of puberty this is 14 years, but where there are other pubertal changes it is 16.

Secondary amenorrhoea is defined as the cessation of menses for 6 months or more in a woman who has previously menstruated. **Oligomenorrhoea** is the occurrence of five or fewer periods over 12 months. In practice, the distinction between the two can be somewhat arbitrary as they share many of the same causes.

Uterine fibroids.

(a) MRI image of uterine fibroids; (b) angiography of fibroid before embolisation and (c) after embolisation; (d) pedunculated subserous fibroid; (e) intramural fibroid; (f) angiography of fibroid before embolisation

(From Butori N. SSFSE sequence functional MRI of the human cervical spinal cord with complex finger tapping. *Eur J Radiol* 2009; 79(1):1–6.)

FIGURE 40.1

Diagnosis of bleeding in early pregnancy		
Symptoms and examination	**Ultrasound**	**Diagnosis**
Light vaginal bleeding with minimal pain; closed cervix	Viable intrauterine pregnancy	Threatened miscarriage
Heavy vaginal bleeding with cramping lower abdominal pain; open cervix	Products of conception in uterus with or without fetal heartbeat	Inevitable miscarriage
Heavy vaginal bleeding with cramping; open cervix, possibly with tissue	Products of conception in uterus, usually without fetal heartbeat	Incomplete miscarriage
Painless light bleeding or no symptoms; closed cervix	No fetal pole or fetal heartbeat in gestation sac >25 mm diameter	Missed miscarriage
Minimal bleeding after history of heavier bleeding and cramps; closed cervix	Empty uterus	Complete miscarriage (also consider ectopic pregnancy and very early viable pregnancy)
Mild-to-moderate bleeding; uterus large for dates, exaggerated pregnancy symptoms (e.g. hyperemesis)	Snowstorm appearance with or without gestation sac	Molar pregnancy
Light vaginal bleeding with unilateral abdominal pain; closed cervix; cervical excitation	No intrauterine pregnancy when hCG >1500; free fluid outside the uterus and/or an adnexal mass	Ectopic pregnancy

hCG=human chorionic gonadotrophin.

TABLE 40.1

Diagnosis

Amenorrhoea can be physiological or pathological (see List 40.3), with the most common causes being pregnancy, menopause and lactation. The possibility of pregnancy should be excluded in any woman of reproductive age by undertaking a urinary pregnancy test. Ask about recent emotional stress, changes in weight, menopausal symptoms and current medication. Relevant findings on examination are a low or high body mass index, hirsutism (PCOS), galactorrhoea and bitemporal hemianopia (pituitary tumours).

In cases of primary amenorrhoea look for features of secondary sex characteristics development, signs of imperforate hymen (P) and features of Turner's syndrome (short stature, wide carrying angle and widely spaced nipples).

The differential diagnosis is established by measurement of follicle-stimulating hormone (FSH), luteinising hormone (LH) and prolactin, and thyroid function tests. A pelvic ultrasound can provide additional evidence of polycystic ovary syndrome (POCS), ovarian tumours and abnormalities of the lower genital tract. In women with primary amenorrhoea, a karyotype should also be obtained.

Dysmenorrhoea

Dysmenorrhoea, or painful menstruation, is the most common of all gynaecological symptoms.

Primary dysmenorrhoea occurs in the absence of any significant pelvic pathology. It usually develops within the first 2 years of the menarche. The pain is typically described as central and cramping. Symptoms can be severely incapacitating, causing major disruption of social activities. The onset of symptoms is usually associated with the onset of menstrual blood loss but may begin on the day preceding menstruation. The pain occurs only in ovulatory cycles and often disappears or improves after the birth of the first child. Dysmenorrhoea may be associated with vomiting and diarrhoea. Pelvic examination reveals no abnormality of the pelvic organs.

Secondary or **acquired dysmenorrhoea** is more likely to be caused by organic pelvic pathology and usually has its onset many years after the menarche. Commonly associated pathologies include endometriosis (see Fig. 40.2), adenomyosis, pelvic infections and intrauterine lesions such as submucous fibroid polyps.

> ### CAUSES OF AMENORRHOEA
>
> **Primary**
> - Constitutional
> - Anatomical
>   - Imperforate hymen
>   - Transverse vaginal septum
>   - Müllerian agenesis: Mayer–Rokitansky–Küster–Hauser syndrome
> - Hypergonadotrophic hypergonadic
>   - Androgen insensitivity (XY)
>   - Turner's syndrome
>   - Gonadal dysgenesis
> - Hypogonadotrophic hypogonadic
>   - CNS lesions (tumours, infection, trauma)
>   - Kallmann's syndrome
>
> **Secondary**
> - Physiological causes
>   - Pregnancy
>   - Lactation
>   - Menopause
> - Pathological causes
>
> - Hypothalamic disorders
>   - Excessive weight loss or exercise
>   - Stress
>   - Chronic kidney disease
> - Pituitary disorders
>   - Prolactin-secreting tumours of the anterior pituitary (micro- or macroadenoma)
>   - Postpartum necrosis (Sheehan's syndrome)
>   - Antidopaminergic drugs
> - Ovarian disorders
>   - Premature ovarian failure
>   - Autoimmune disease
>   - Surgical removal of the ovaries
>   - Oestrogen- or testosterone-secreting ovarian neoplasms
> - Polycystic ovary syndrome
> - Failure of uterine response
>   - Surgical removal of the uterus
>   - Asherman syndrome
>   - Cryptomenorrhoea
>   - Cervical stenosis, as a result of surgical trauma or infection
>
> LIST 40.3

Investigations

A careful history is of great importance in this condition. Pelvic examination should be performed and, if this is abnormal, a pelvic ultrasound scan arranged. Laparoscopy is the gold standard investigation for the diagnosis of conditions such as endometriosis. It is performed in cases with primary dysmenorrhoea only if the condition is particularly resistant to therapy.

Acute abdominal pain

In women with a negative pregnancy test and acute pelvic pain, gynaecological disorders include pelvic inflammatory disease (PID), functional ovarian cysts, ovarian or peritoneal endometriosis and ovarian torsion. The most common gastrointestinal causes that can present with acute pelvic pain include appendicitis, acute sigmoid diverticulitis and Crohn's disease. In your assessment it is important to exclude those diagnoses that require urgent intervention: PID, ovarian torsion, ectopic pregnancy and appendicitis.

The history should include the onset site and the nature of the pain, the date of the last menstrual period and the presence of associated symptoms. On examination, identify the site of maximal tenderness and the presence of rebound tenderness and guarding. It is vital to always exclude pregnancy, particularly ectopic pregnancy.

Ovarian torsion usually occurs in the presence of an enlarged ovary. Women with torsion present with sudden onset of sharp, unilateral pelvic pain that is often accompanied by nausea and vomiting. The sonographic findings are variable. The ovary is enlarged and can be seen in an abnormal location above or behind the uterus. The absence of blood flow is an important sign, and a lack of venous wave form on Doppler ultrasound has a high positive predictive value.

Endometriotic patches on the surface of the ovary.

(From Symonds EM, Symonds IM. *Essential obstetrics and gynaecology*, 4th edn. Edinburgh: Churchill Livingstone, 2004.)

FIGURE 40.2

Risk factors for ectopic pregnancy

	Relative risk
Previous history of PID	4
Previous tubal surgery	4.5
Failed sterilisation	9
Intrauterine contraceptive device in situ	10
Previous ectopic pregnancy	10–15

PID = pelvic inflammatory disease.

TABLE 40.2

Causes of infertility

Cause	Primary infertility (%)	Secondary infertility (%)
Anovulation	32	23
Tubal disease	12	14
Endometriosis	11	10
Sperm quality problems	29	24
Other	14	21
Unknown	29	30

(Adapted from Bhattacharya S, Porter M, Amalraj E et al. The epidemiology of infertility in the North East of Scotland. *Hum Reprod* 2009; 24(12): 3096–3107.)

TABLE 40.3

However, the presence of arterial and venous flow does not exclude torsion and any cases where it is suspected clinically require laparoscopy to visualise the adnexa (ovaries and fallopian tubes). If the torsion is reversed early in the process, the ovary may be saved.

Approximately 1% of pregnancies are ectopic (occur outside the uterus) but the individual risk depends on the past history (see Table 40.2). Ectopic pregnancy presents classically with sudden onset of unilateral pain and irregular vaginal bleeding after a period of amenorrhoea. The presence of shoulder tip pain (due to diaphragmatic irritation) and peritonism are suggestive of rupture with intraperitoneal bleeding. In practice, it is rare for all three symptoms to be present and chronic presentation with atypical pain and bleeding are more common. Clinical examination findings include cervical excitation (increased pain on movement of the cervix during pelvic examination), adnexal pain and swelling with or without signs of hypovolaemic shock. The diagnosis is usually made by measurement of human chorionic gonadotrophin (hCG) levels and pelvic ultrasound and confirmed at laparoscopy (see Table 40.1).

Infertility

Approximately 80% of normally fertile couples will conceive within a year of unprotected intercourse; when conception does not occur within 12 months the couple can be considered at risk of infertility. The median prevalence of infertility in the developed world at 12 months of unprotected intercourse is 9%, although this varies significantly in relation to age in women. Infertility is called *primary* if the woman has not previously been pregnant and *secondary* if she has had one or more previous pregnancies. Table 40.3 summarises the common causes of infertility (note that it is not uncommon for more than one factor to affect fertility in a given couple). The initial consultation should include both partners. Key questions to ask are given in Questions box 40.1.

> **INITIAL ASSESSMENT OF THE INFERTILE COUPLE**
>
> 1. How long have you been trying to fall pregnant?
> 2. What methods of contraception did you use previously?
> 3. Have either you or your partner had a previous pregnancy together or with other partners?
> 4. If so, did you have any complications associated with the pregnancy?
> 5. Can you tell me about your periods and whether you have had any bleeding between your periods?
> 6. How often do you and your partner have sex? Are there any problems with pain during sex or ejaculatory/erection problems for your partner?
> 7. Have you ever had any sexually transmitted infections or has your partner ever had mumps orchitis (inflammation of the testes)?
> 8. Do you have any serious chronic illness or have you ever had surgery such as an appendectomy? Has your partner been treated for varicocele or undescended testes?
>
> QUESTIONS BOX 40.1

Diagnosis
Clinical examination findings of significance for women include those features potentially associated with causes of amenorrhoea (see above) and endometriosis. Male examination findings include testicular size, the presence of varicocele and thickening of the epididymis (see Ch 18). Initial investigations are determined by the history; for example, if this is suggestive of previous pelvic infection, an assessment of tubal patency would be a priority. Typically, initial baseline tests include semen fluid analysis, assessment of ovulation (such as a day 21 serum progesterone level) and assessment of tubal patency (such as hysterosalpingogram or laparoscopy).

Sexual history

The amount of detail required will depend on the presenting symptom. In women complaining of disorders of sexual function and suspected sexually transmitted infection (such as vaginal discharge, PID), a full sexual history should be obtained, as described in Questions box 40.2.

Always explain the reason you need to ask questions of such a personal nature. For example, 'From what you have told me I think some of these problems may have a sexual cause. Will it be all right if I ask you some personal questions?'

Previous gynaecological history

A detailed history of any previous gynaecological problems and treatments must be recorded. The amount of detail needed about previous pregnancies will depend on the presenting symptom. In most cases the number of previous pregnancies and their outcome (miscarriage, ectopic or delivery after 20 weeks) is all that is required.

For all women of reproductive age who are sexually active it is essential to ask about contraception. This is important not only to determine the possibility of pregnancy but also because the method of contraception used may itself be relevant to the presenting symptom. For women over the age of 25, ask about the date and result of the last cervical Pap smear.

Previous medical history

Take particular account of any history of medical disorders of the endocrine, urinary or cardiovascular systems. Make a record of all current medications and any known drug allergies.

Family and social history

A social history is important for all problems but is particularly relevant where the presenting difficulties relate to abortion or sterilisation. Ask about smoking, alcohol and other recreational drug use. A family history of breast or ovarian cancer or both, delayed puberty or premature menopause may be relevant where the patient has the same condition.

QUESTIONS TO ASK A PATIENT COMPLAINING OF SEXUAL DYSFUNCTION OR SUSPECTED SEXUALLY TRANSMITTED INFECTION[2]

1. What is the reason for your attendance today?
2. How long have you had these symptoms?
3. Do you suffer from any of the following?
   - Urethral and vaginal discharge
   - Abnormal vaginal or rectal bleeding
   - Genital and extragenital rashes, lumps or sores
   - Itching and/or discomfort in the perineum, perianal and pubic regions
   - Lower abdominal pain or dyspareunia
   - Difficulties/pain with micturition or defecation or during intercourse
4. When was the last time you had sexual intercourse?
5. Have you had unprotected intercourse?
6. How many sexual contacts have you had in the last 3–5 months? (All men should be asked whether they have ever had sex with another man in the past.)
7. What type of sexual activity did you practise? (Oral, anal, vaginal, use of toys)
8. Did you take any steps to prevent sexually transmitted infections, such as using condoms? If so, do you use this method consistently?
9. What is your relationship with your sexual contacts (regular, casual, known, unknown)?
10. Have any of your recent sexual contacts had any symptoms of sexually transmitted infection or infections?
11. Have you previously been tested for any sexually transmitted infections? If so, what was the date of the test, and the result?
12. Do you have a current or past history of injecting drug use? Sharing of needles or syringes? Body piercing and/or tattoos? If the last-named, where and when were these done and was sterile equipment used?
13. Have you had sex overseas with anyone other than with the person you were travelling with?
14. Have you ever worked in the sex industry or had sexual contact with a sex worker?
15. Have you been vaccinated for hepatitis A and B and HPV?
16. Are you taking any current medications?
17. Do you have a history of allergies, especially adverse reaction to penicillin?
18. What contraceptives do you use?
19. When was your last menstrual period?
20. When was your last cervical Pap smear? What was the result? Have you ever had an abnormal result?
21. Do you have any past medical and surgical history (including any overseas medical treatment and transfusions)?
22. What is your current alcohol, tobacco and other drug use?

(Adapted from NSW Sexually Transmissible Infections Programs Unit 2011. www.stipu.nsw.gov.au.)

QUESTIONS BOX 40.2

EXAMINATION

A general examination should always be performed at the first consultation, including assessment of pulse, blood pressure and temperature. Take careful note of any signs of anaemia. The distribution of facial and body hair is often important, as hirsutism may be a presenting symptom of androgen-producing tumours or PCOS. Also record the patient's body weight and height.

The intimate nature of the gynaecological examination makes it especially important to ensure that every effort is made to consider privacy and that the examination is not interrupted (see Text box 40.2). The examination should ideally take place in a separate area to the consultation. Allow the patient to undress in privacy and, if necessary, empty her bladder first. After she has undressed there should be no undue delay to the examination.

Examination of the breasts

Breast examination should be performed if there are symptoms or if the patient is over the age of 45. The presence of the secretion of milk at times not associated with pregnancy, known as galactorrhoea, may indicate the presence of pituitary disease. Palpation with the flat of the hand should be undertaken in each of the four quadrants of each breast to exclude the presence of any nodules. See Chapter 41 for further details on breast examination.

Examination of the abdomen

Inspection of the abdomen is undertaken as previously described in Chapters 14 and 18. In a patient presenting with gynaecological symptoms look for the presence of a mass as well as scars, striae and hernias. If there is a mass, try to determine whether it is fixed or mobile, smooth or regular, and whether it arises from the pelvis (you should not be able to palpate the lower edge above the pubic bone). Look for scars in the umbilicus from previous laparoscopies and in the suprapubic region where transverse incisions from caesarean sections and most gynaecological operations are found. Palpate the abdomen to assess for any guarding or rebound tenderness. Check the hernial orifices and feel for any enlarged lymph nodes in the groin. Percuss the abdomen to outline the limits of a tumour, detect the presence of a full bladder or recognise the presence of tympanic loops of bowel.

Pelvic examination

The pelvic examination should be performed *when indicated* as the final part of any complete physical examination.[4] It should not be considered an automatic and inevitable part of every gynaecological consultation.

Guidelines for intimate examination[3]

When conducting intimate examinations you should:

- Explain to the patient why an intimate examination is necessary and give the patient an opportunity to ask questions.
- Explain what the examination will involve, in a way the patient can understand, so that the patient has a clear idea of what to expect, including any potential pain or discomfort.
- Obtain the patient's permission before the examination and be prepared to discontinue the examination if the patient asks you to.
- Record that permission has been obtained.
- Keep discussion relevant and avoid unnecessary personal comments.
- Offer a chaperone. If the patient does not want a chaperone, you should record that the offer was made and declined. If a chaperone is present, you should record that fact and make a note of the chaperone's identity. If for justifiable practical reasons you cannot offer a chaperone, you should explain to the patient and, if possible, offer to delay the examination to a later date.
- Give the patient privacy to undress and dress and use drapes to maintain the patient's dignity. Do not assist the patient in removing clothing unless you have clarified with them that your assistance is required.
- Obtain consent prior to anaesthetisation, usually in writing, for the intimate examination of anaesthetised patients. If you are supervising students you should ensure that valid consent has been obtained before they carry out any intimate examination.

(Adapted from General Medical Council (2013). Intimate examinations and chaperones. Available at www.gmc-uk.org/guidance.htm.)

TEXT BOX 40.2

> **RULES FOR CONDUCTING A PELVIC EXAMINATION**
>
> When conducting a vaginal examination you should:
> - Explain that an intimate examination is needed and why.
> - Explain what the examination will involve.
> - Obtain the patient's permission.
> - Offer a chaperone or invite the patient to bring a relative or friend.
> - Allow the patient to undress in privacy.
> - Keep discussion relevant and avoid unnecessary personal comments.
> - Explain findings and encourage questions and discussion.
>
> LIST 40.4

You should consider what information will be gained by the examination, whether this is a screening or diagnostic procedure and whether it is necessary at this time. In a child or in a woman with an intact hymen, speculum and pelvic examinations are not usually performed unless as part of an examination under anaesthesia. Remember that a rough or painful examination rarely produces any useful information and, in certain situations such as tubal ectopic pregnancy, may be dangerous. Throughout the examination remain alert to verbal and non-verbal indications of distress from the patient.

It is essential to obtain informed consent and for male students and doctors to have a female chaperone (see List 40.4). The patient's privacy must be promised and ensured.

Wear gloves on both hands during vaginal and speculum examinations. Examine the patient either in the supine position or in the left lateral position with the knees drawn up and separated (see Fig. 40.3). The left lateral position is used when the woman cannot assume the lithotomy position or when a view of the anterior vaginal wall is required—for example, when a urinary fistula is suspected (see below). The perineum should be brightly illuminated by a lamp.

Examination of the external genitalia

Parting the lips of the labia minora with the left hand, look at the external urethral meatus and inspect the vulva for any discharge, redness, ulceration or old scars (see Table 40.4).

Bartholin's glands[a]

The Bartholin's glands lie in the posterior vaginal wall at the introitus (entrance) and secrete mucus-like fluid via a short duct into the vagina. They are normally the size of a pea but when the duct becomes blocked a cyst can form. These cysts may present acutely as an oval-shaped lump—in the posterior labia they may sometimes grow to the size of a golf ball or larger. They are usually unilateral and cause discomfort with walking, sitting and sexual intercourse. When the gland is infected, most commonly with skin or genitourinary bacteria (*Staphylococcus*, *Escherichia coli*), an abscess can develop. These abscesses arise more acutely than Bartholin's cysts and are particularly painful.

Speculum examination

Speculum examination should be performed before digital examination to avoid any contamination with lubricant. A bivalve speculum is most commonly used with the patient in the supine position as this enables a clear view of the cervix to be obtained. Where vaginal wall prolapse is suspected, a Sims' speculum should be used as an alternative with the patient in the left lateral position as this affords a better view of the anterior vaginal wall (see Fig. 40.6).

Part the labia minora with the left hand and insert the speculum into the introitus, initially with the widest dimension of the instrument in the anteroposterior orientation and turning gently to the transverse position as the tip passes the introitus, as the vagina is widest in this direction. When the speculum reaches the top of the vagina, gently open the blades to enable the cervix to be visualised. Note the presence of any discharge or bleeding from the cervix and any polyps or areas of ulceration. If the clinical history suggests possible infection (see Table 40.5), take swabs from the vaginal fornices and cervical os and place in a transport medium to look for *Candida*, *Trichomonas* and *Neisseria*; take a separate swab from the endocervix to look for *Chlamydia*.

---

[a] Caspar Bartholin Secundus (1655–1738), a professor of philosophy at Copenhagen at the age of 19, then professor of medicine, anatomy and physics. He described the glands in 1677.

Female reproductive anatomy.

(a) Lateral view, showing the relationship of the genitals to the rectum and bladder.
(b) Position for examination
(From Douglas G, Nicol F, Robertson C. *Macleod's clinical examination*, 12th edn. Edinburgh: Churchill Livingstone, 2009.)

FIGURE 40.3

Appearance of the vaginal wall
Ask the patient to bear down; a cystocele (descent of the bladder through the anterior vaginal wall) or rectocele (descent of the rectum through the posterior vaginal wall) or uterine prolapse may become apparent. Then ask the patient to cough; this may demonstrate stress incontinence. Note the presence of vaginal atrophy in older women.

Prolapse
Uterovaginal prolapse is the protrusion of the uterus and/or the vaginal walls beyond their normal anatomical confines. Prolapse commonly occurs in

Vulval skin conditions

Presentation	Condition
Itchy, erythematous rash (endogenous) Atopic/seborrhoeic Allergic or irritant induced (exogenous)	Dermatitis
Chronic irritation, results in thickening and hypertrophy of skin, erythema, excoriations Mucosa not involved	Lichen simplex chronicus
Itch, discomfort, white discharge, dyspareunia, dysuria Hypersensitivity reaction on vulva Requires positive culture to confirm diagnosis	Candidiasis
Whitened parchment-like plaques Classic hourglass appearance involving perianal skin Loss of labial/clitoral architecture, introital narrowing May have tearing or subepithelial haemorrhage/petechiae Mucosa not involved	Lichen sclerosus (see Fig. 40.4)
Lichen simplex chronicus difficult to differentiate from lichen planus Introitus of vagina involved Adhesions and erosions may occur; not responsive to surgical division Oral/gingival involvement possible	Lichen planus
Itchy, scaly red plaques not as well demarcated as elsewhere on the skin; examine hair/scalp and nails also	Psoriasis
Itching Different patterns may be associated with red velvety area or area of lichenification	Vulvar intraepithelial neoplasia
Itch, discharge, bleeding may be painful Associated lymphadenopathy Raised ulcerated lesion	Vulvar cancer (see Fig. 40.5)

TABLE 40.4

Common organisms causing lower genital tract infections

Condition	Causative organism	Symptoms	Signs
Bacterial vaginosis	Anaerobic organisms including *Gardnerella* spp	Smelly vaginal discharge Vulval irritation	A typical thin homogeneous vaginal discharge
Chlamydial vulvovaginitis	*Chlamydia trachomatis*	Asymptomatic or vaginal discharge Intermenstrual bleeding	Inflamed cervix Contact bleeding Tenderness on cervical movement
Genital herpes	Herpes simplex virus (HSV) type 2	Vaginal discharge Vulval pain Dysuria Urinary retention	Skin vesicles and multiple shallow skin ulcers Inguinal lymphadenopathy
Genital warts (condyloma acuminata)	Human papillomavirus	Pruritus Vaginal discharge	Papillomatous lesions over vulva, perineum and into vagina
Gonococcal vulvovaginitis	*Neisseria gonorrhoeae*	Vaginal discharge	Mucopurulent vaginal discharge
Trichomoniasis	*Trichomonas vaginalis*	Vaginal bleeding Vaginal soreness Pruritus	Green frothy, watery discharge
Vaginal candidiasis	*Candida albicans*	Increased or changed vaginal discharge associated with soreness and itching in the vulva area	White, curd-like collections attached to the vaginal epithelium

TABLE 40.5

Lichen sclerosus.

(Courtesy of Ruth Murphy, PhD, MBChB, FRCP, Nottingham, UK. In Murphy R. Lichen sclerosus. *Dermatol Clin* 2010; 28(4):707–715.)

FIGURE 40.4

Carcinoma of the vulva.

(From Arjona JE. Pregnancy following radical vulvectomy for carcinoma of the vulva: a case report and literature review. *Eur J Obstet Gynecol Reprod Biol* 2011; 158(1):113–114.)

FIGURE 40.5

women as a result of damage to the supporting structures of the vagina and uterus following childbirth, although it may occur in women even after delivery by caesarean section. It is not unusual for minor degrees of prolapse to be asymptomatic and detected only as an incidental finding on vaginal examination. Where symptoms do occur these are commonly a feeling of fullness in the vagina or being able to feel a swelling protruding beyond the vaginal introitus.

The diagnosis of prolapse is a clinical one based on the appearances at the time of examination (see Fig. 40.7). Swelling of the anterior vaginal wall is described as a **cystocele**. Where swelling of the lower posterior wall is present this is described as a **rectocele**, and swelling of the upper posterior vaginal wall or posterior fornix is an **enterocele**. Uterine prolapse is described in terms of movement of the cervix in relation to the level of the vaginal introitus. Complete prolapse of the uterus beyond the introitus is described as **procidentia** (see Fig. 40.8).

Cystic swellings in the vagina and vulva

Congenital cysts arise in the vagina from embryological remnants. The most common varieties are those arising from Gartner's duct (Wolffian duct remnants). They occur in the anterolateral wall of the vagina. They are usually asymptomatic and are found on routine examination.

Vaginal inclusion cysts arise from the inclusion of small particles or islands of vaginal epithelium under the surface. The cysts commonly arise in episiotomy scars and contain thick yellowish fluid.

Solid benign tumours of the vagina are rare but may represent any of the tissues found in the vagina. Thus, polypoid tumours may include fibromyomas, myomas, fibromas, papillomas and adenomyomas.

Appearance of the cervix

'Normal' cervical squamous epithelium has a smooth pink appearance with a circular external os placed centrally. In practice, in women of reproductive age the external os is more irregular and slit-like and there

Examination in the lateral semiprone positions with a Sims' speculum.

(From Symonds EM, Symonds IM. *Essential obstetrics and gynaecology*, 4th edn. Churchill Livingstone, 2004.)

FIGURE 40.6

is often a central area extending beyond the edge of the os that is a darker red and more velvety in appearance (see Fig. 40.9). This is sometimes called a cervical ectropion and represents an outgrowth of healthy columnar epithelium beyond the cervical canal. This is a normal variant, although it may be associated with an increase in clear vaginal discharge and, on occasion, contact bleeding. The columnar epithelium appears reddened because, unlike the stratified squamous epithelium of the ectocervix, there is only a single layer of columnar cells between the underlying capillaries and the surface. As the columnar epithelium is exposed to the acid pH of the vagina it tends to revert back to squamous epithelium in a process called squamous metaplasia. This sometimes traps islands of the mucus-secreting columnar epithelium below the surface of the new epithelium, leading to an accumulation of mucus in small retention cysts or Nabothian follicles.

In women with **cervicitis**, the cervix appears reddened and may be ulcerated, and there is a mucopurulent discharge as the endocervix is invariably involved. The diagnosis is established by examination and taking cervical swabs for culture.

Cervical intraepithelial neoplasia is not normally visible without the application of acetic acid or Lugol's iodine. The appearance of a raised or ulcerated lesion with irregular vessels on the surface is suggestive of cervical malignancy. Cervical polyps are common and may arise from the cervical canal or the external surface. Occasionally, an endometrial polyp may prolapse through the cervical canal and appear at the cervical os.

Pap smear

A Pap smear should be taken at least 6 weeks after pregnancy and not during menstruation. The age at which routine screening starts and the frequency of testing vary from country to country. In Australia from Dec 2017 initial testing of samples will be for the detection of HPV and cervical cytology will be performed only on HPV-positive specimens. The technique for collecting the sample will remain as below.

The procedure is as follows. After inserting the speculum as above, wipe away any discharge from the surface of the cervix and take a 360° sweep with a suitable spatula or brush pressed firmly against the cervix at the junction of the columnar epithelium of the endocervical canal and the squamous epithelium of the ectocervix. There are two methods by which cells are transferred onto a slide for staining and inspection by a cytologist:

1. In a conventional Pap smear, the specimen is spread immediately onto a clear glass slide in a thin, even layer. The slide is fixed with 95% alcohol alone or in combination with 3% glacial acetic acid.
2. In liquid-based cytology (LBC), the sampling device is transferred into the preservative solution vial by pushing the broom into the bottom of the vial 10 times, forcing the bristles apart. The solution is then passed through a filter, which traps the large squamous cells but allows smaller red cells, debris and bacteria to pass through. The squamous cells are then transferred to a slide.

The sensitivity of both methods for the detection of abnormal cells is similar, although the rate of unsatisfactory smears is lower in LBC. LBC also allows for testing for human papillomavirus and *Chlamydia* infection.

Clinical appearance of vaginal prolapse.

Cystocele   Urethrocele   Enterocele

(From Symonds EM, Symonds IM. *Essential obstetrics and gynaecology*, 4th edn. Edinburgh: Churchill Livingstone, 2004.)

FIGURE 40.7

Procidentia (third-degree uterine prolapse).

(From Lentz GM, Lobo RA, Gershenson DM. *Comprehensive gynecology*, 6th edn. Philadelphia: Elsevier Mosby, 2012, pp 453–474.)

FIGURE 40.8

Normal multiparous cervix.

NULLIPAROUS   MULTIPAROUS

(From Hacker NF, Gambone JC, Hobel CJ. *Hacker and Moore's essentials of obstetrics and gynecology*, 5th edn. Philadelphia: Saunders, 2010.)

FIGURE 40.9

Vaginal swabs

The indications for taking vaginal swabs are symptoms of vaginal discharge (see Table 40.6), irregular bleeding and PID. Swabs may also be taken to screen for sexually transmitted infection in asymptomatic women. Cervicitis is associated with purulent vaginal discharge, sacral backache, lower abdominal pain, dyspareunia and dysuria, although in many cases the symptoms are minimal. The proximity of the cervix to the bladder often results in coexistent trigonitis and urethritis, particularly in the case of gonococcal infections.

A high vaginal swab is taken as part of the speculum examination by dipping the tip of a culture swab moistened in culture medium in the posterior vaginal fornix and then placing the swab immediately back into a suitable culture medium. This procedure is used mainly to identify organisms such as *Candida* or *Trichomonas* and in the assessment of bacterial vaginosis.

Diagnosis of vaginal discharge

Features of discharge and associated symptoms	Possible causes
Thick, white, non-itchy	Physiological
Bloody	Menstruation, a miscarriage, cancer or a cervical polyp or erosion
Thick, white, cottage cheese discharge, vulval itching, vulval soreness and irritation, pain or discomfort	*Candida albicans*
Yellow-green, itchy, frothy, foul-smelling ('fishy' smell) discharge	*Trichomonas*
Thin, grey or green, discharge with a fishy odour	Bacterial vaginosis
Thick white discharge, dysuria and pelvic pain, friable cervix	Gonorrhoea

TABLE 40.6

Endocervical swabs are taken by inserting the tip of the swab into the external cervical os and rotating two or three times. Using standard culture medium as for the high vaginal swab, the swab can be tested for *Neisseria gonorrhoeae*. Testing for *Chlamydia* infection can also be done by swabbing the endocervix. However, instead of culturing the organism, the presence of *Chlamydia* DNA is tested for using polymerase chain reaction by placing the swab in a specialised collection fluid in a plastic vial. The same principle can be used to test a first-pass urine sample to diagnose *Chlamydia*, so an endocervical swab is no longer necessary to test for this infection.

Bimanual examination

This is performed by introducing the middle and index fingers of your examining hand into the vaginal introitus and applying pressure towards the rectum. At the same time, place your other hand on the patient's abdomen above the symphysis pubis (see Fig. 40.10). The intravaginal portion of the cervix is tipped by your examining fingers (it can be identified by its consistency, which has a similar texture to the cartilage of the tip of the nose). Note the size, shape, consistency and position of the uterus. The uterus is commonly preaxial or anteverted, but will be postaxial or retroverted in some

Bimanual examination.

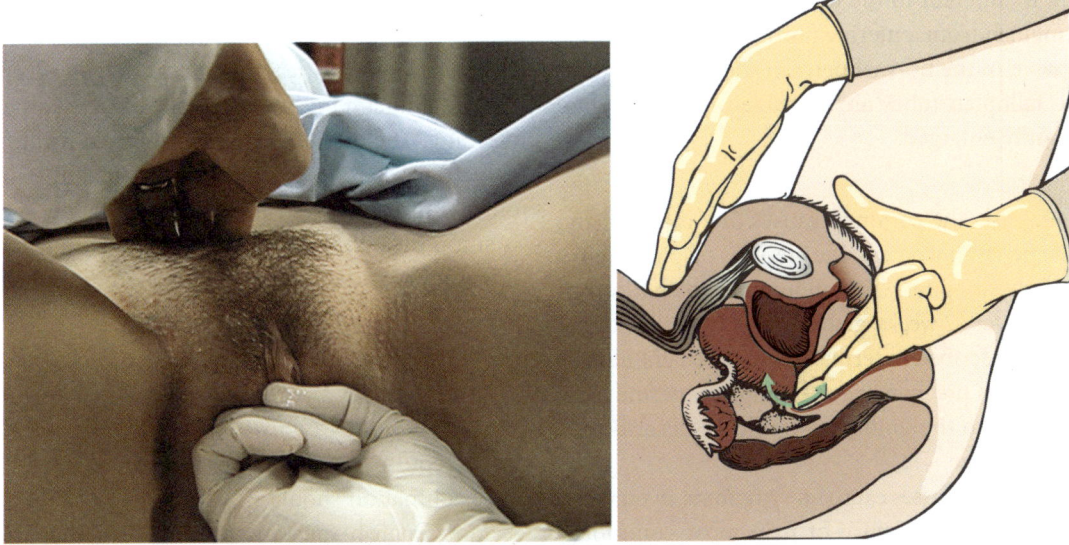

(From Seidel HM, Ball JW, Dains JE et al. *Mosby's guide to physical examination*, 7th edn. St Louis, MO: Mosby, 2011.)

FIGURE 40.10

Bimanual examination of (a) the pelvis and (b) the lateral fornix.

(From Symonds EM, Symonds IM. *Essential obstetrics and gynaecology*, 4th edn. Edinburgh: Churchill Livingstone, 2004.)

FIGURE 40.11

10% of women. Provided that the retroverted uterus is mobile, the position is rarely significant. It is important to feel in the pouch of Douglas for the presence of thickening or nodules (a feature of endometriosis), and then to palpate laterally in both fornices for the presence of any ovarian or tubal masses (see Fig. 40.11). An attempt should be made to differentiate between adnexal and uterine masses, although often this is not possible. For example, a pedunculated fibroid may mimic an ovarian tumour, whereas a solid ovarian tumour, if adherent to the uterus, may be impossible to distinguish from a uterine fibroid. The ovaries may be palpable in the normal pelvis if the patient is thin, but the fallopian tubes are palpable only if they are significantly enlarged.

Pelvic mass

Table 40.7 lists the common causes of a mass arising from the pelvis in women. The uterus is palpable above the symphysis pubis on abdominal palpation in pregnancy after 12 weeks' gestation and typically uterine masses are described in terms of the equivalent uterine enlargement in pregnancy. For example, a uterine mass extending up to the umbilicus would be described as '20 weeks' in size.

Many pelvic masses cause no symptoms, even when large in size. The presence of pain most commonly occurs only when there is bleeding within or from the lesion (for example, in the case of ovarian cysts) or when the lesion becomes infarcted (for example, as a result of torsion; see Fig. 40.12). If large enough, a mass may be associated with pressure symptoms on the adjacent organs, such as urinary frequency or changes in bowel habits.

The first step in evaluating a pelvic mass is an abdominal examination. Masses arising from the pelvis can be distinguished by failure to identify a gap between the mass and the symphysis pubis. The presence of scars from previous surgery or ascites should be noted.

On pelvic examination a pelvic space-occupying lesion may cause downward pressure leading to vaginal prolapse. A speculum examination is essential to exclude a primary cervical lesion such as advanced cervical cancer, although this will normally present earlier with bleeding. The mass can then be assessed by bimanual palpation. This allows a better estimate of the size and other clinical features—in particular, whether the mass is smooth or irregular, fixed or mobile, and whether it feels cystic or solid. Further assessment is normally undertaken using pelvic ultrasound.

Special circumstances

Keep in mind the following:

- Except in an emergency situation, a pelvic examination should not be carried out on a non-English-speaking patient without an interpreter. Be aware that examination may be more difficult for women with particular cultural or religious expectations.

Differential diagnosis of pelvic mass	
Origin of mass	**Clinical features**
Uterine	Central Uterus cannot be felt separately If uterus mobile, moves with uterus
Leiomyomata	Smooth, solid, may be single or multiple giving an irregular outline to the uterus Normally non-tender
Pregnancy	Uniform enlargement, soft and fluid-filled (the presence of fetal heart sounds is pathognomonic!)
Adenomyosis	Smoothly enlarged (rarely more than 12 weeks' size), globular shape and tender to palpation
Cancer of the corpus	Uniform enlargement, usually solid If tender, sarcoma more likely
Cervical cancer	Associated with an irregular mass arising from the cervix and extending into the vagina Often necrotic, with contact bleeding
Ovary/fallopian tubes	More likely to be adnexal than central
Inflammatory (tubo-ovarian abscess)	Tender, cervical excitation, ill-defined Solid or cystic, associated with systemic illness/fever
Ovarian cysts	May be solid (dermoid or fibroma) or cystic (epithelial tumours) Normally unilateral, smooth regular outline, mobile Tenderness suggests bleeding or torsion
Ovarian malignancy	More likely to be cystic fixed and associated with ascites
Endometriosis	May be associated with adnexal mass (usually ovarian endometrioma) More often diffuse change in the pelvis with fixed non-mobile uterus, nodules and thickening in the posterior fornix and tenderness

TABLE 40.7

Common complications of ovarian tumours causing symptoms.

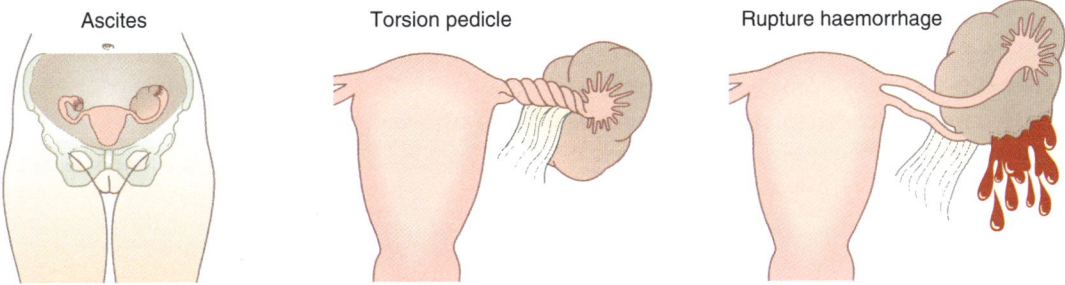

(From Symonds EM, Symonds IM. *Essential obstetrics and gynaecology*, 4th edn. Edinburgh: Churchill Livingstone, 2004.)

FIGURE 40.12

- Women who experience difficulty with vaginal examination should be allowed to disclose any underlying sexual difficulties or traumas. However, do not assume that all women who experience difficulty with pelvic examinations have a history of sexual abuse.

- Exceptional gentleness should be displayed in the examination of victims of alleged sexual assault. The woman should be given a choice about the gender of the doctor and be allowed to control the pace of, and her position for, the examination.

- The basic principles of respect, privacy, explanation and consent that apply to the conduct of gynaecological examinations in general apply equally to the conduct of such examinations in women who have temporary or permanent learning disabilities or mental illness.
- When examining an anaesthetised patient, treat the woman with the same degree of sensitivity and respect as if she were awake.

Rectal examination

Rectal examination may be indicated if there are symptoms such as a change in bowel habits or rectal bleeding, which may suggest bowel disease. It is occasionally used as a means of assessing a pelvic mass and in conjunction with a vaginal examination can provide additional information about disease in the rectovaginal septum.

OSCE REVISION TOPICS – THE GYNAECOLOGICAL HISTORY AND EXAMINATION

Use these topics, which commonly occur in the OSCE, to help with revision.

1. This woman has a history of heavy periods. Please take a full history from her and explain what further investigations you would like to perform. (pp 744–5)
2. This couple have been unable to conceive for 2 years. Please take a history and describe what features you would look for on examination that would be relevant to establishing a diagnosis. (pp 749–50, 752, 759–60)
3. This young woman presents with vaginal discharge 3 weeks after having unprotected intercourse with a new partner. Please take a full sexual history from her. (p 751)
4. Demonstrate how you would perform a pelvic examination and take a Pap smear using this manikin. (pp 753, 757, 759)
5. Explain how you would perform a pelvic examination for a woman with vaginal discharge. (pp 758–9)
6. This woman has a pelvic mass. Please examine her. (pp 760–1)

T&O'C ESSENTIALS

1. All women complaining of heavy periods should have a pelvic examination, full blood count and Pap smear.
2. Worrying features of uterine bleeding requiring further investigation include bleeding after the menopause, bleeding between periods and any abnormality of pelvic examination.
3. Pregnancy should be excluded in any women of reproductive age presenting with acute abdominal pain, abnormal bleeding or secondary amenorrhoea.
4. Atypical presentations are common in ectopic pregnancy.
5. The presence of a darker red area around the external cervical os on speculum examination is usually associated with an extension of the columnar epithelium onto the ectocervix and is a normal finding (ectropion).
6. Asymptomatic vaginal prolapse is common in multiparous women and does not require treatment.
7. Ovarian tumours can remain asymptomatic unless complicated by torsion, haemorrhage or rupture.

References

1. Critchley HOD, Munro MG, Broder M, Fraser IS. A five-year international review process concerning terminologies, definitions and related issues around abnormal uterine bleeding. *Semin Reprod Med* 2011; 29:377–382.
2. NSW Sexually Transmissible Infections Programs Unit. *NSW Health Sexual Health Services standard operating procedures manual.* Sydney: NSW STI Programs Unit, 2011.
3. General Medical Council Standards Committee. Maintaining boundaries: intimate examinations and chaperones, *GMC guidelines for intimate examination ethical practice.* London: GMC, 2013. www.gmc-uk.org/Maintaining_boundaries_Intimate_examinations_and_chaperones.pdf_58835231.pdf.
4. Deneke M, Wheeler L, Wagner G et al. An approach to relearning the pelvic examination. *J Fam Pract* 1982; 14:782–783. This study provides useful hints.

CHAPTER 41
The breasts: history and examination

Blessed is the physician who takes a good history, looks keenly at his patient and thinks a bit.

WALTER C ALVAREZ (1976)

Breast examination is a vitally important part of the general physical examination. In women aged 40 and older, a screening physical examination for breast cancer may be advised (e.g. monthly self-examination by the patient and yearly examination by the doctor), but there is no convincing evidence of the value of breast self-examination.[1]

EXAMINATION ANATOMY

The attachment of the female breast extends from the clavicle superiorly to the inframammary crease (sixth rib) inferiorly and from the sternum to the midaxillary line (see Fig. 41.1). The area covered is more rectangular than circular. The axillary tail is an extension of the superolateral part of the breast up towards the axilla. This tail extends along the lower border of the pectoralis major muscle and may abut the clavipectoral fascia, which separates this from the axillary lymph nodes.

Breast tissue has fatty, glandular and fibrous components, and the distribution is variable and depends on age and weight. Women in their twenties who are thin have very little fat. Most 80 year olds have very little fibroglandular tissue.

There is a surrounding superficial fascia attached to the skin and pectoral fascia by ligaments. The normal breast does not have a homogeneous feel but is somewhat lumpy.

There are a number of benign abnormalities of the breast that change the texture or appearance of the breast, including:
- fibroadenomas with overgrowth of connective tissue surrounding the ducts
- cysts with obstruction of collecting ducts (however, it is not simply due to obstruction; it is hormonally mediated as they are much less common in postmenopausal women not on hormone replacement therapy [HRT])
- intraductal papilloma, causing a nipple discharge on the affected side (clear or bloodstained)
- mammary duct ectasia, which causes nipple discharge.

HISTORY

The history is imperative. Essential questions to ask include the length of time any mass has been noticed, the presence of pain, any change in size or texture over time, relationship to the menstrual cycle, and any nipple discharge. Ask whether the patient has conducted regular self-examinations and has discovered a change in her breast. Ask about previous breast surgery, biopsies or cyst aspirations, or recurrent abscesses (e.g. granulomatous mastitis). Has the woman breastfed her babies and for how long? Was breastfeeding difficult or associated with breast infection (mastitis)? Has she had breast implants and have these caused any problems?

HINT BOX

Remember, pathological discharge is generally clear or bloodstained; spontaneous (i.e. not expressed), and uniduct. All other discharge—yellow/green/white, multiduct, bilateral or not spontaneous—is physiological.

Find out about risk factors for breast cancer, including any family history of breast or ovarian cancer (and age when affected), previous personal history of breast cancer, obesity, early menarche and late menopause, late first pregnancy, mantle radiation, heavy

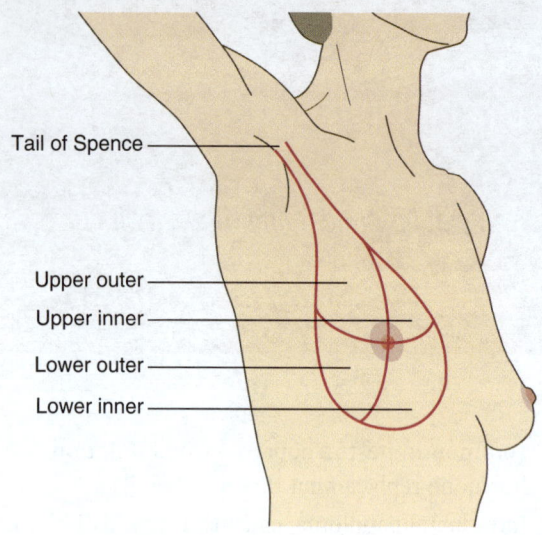

Breast anatomy

(From Douglas G, Nicol F, Robertson C. *Macleod's clinical examination*, 12th edn. Edinburgh: Churchill Livingstone, 2009.)

FIGURE 41.1

EXAMINATION

When it is done properly, the examination takes some time to perform (about 3 minutes per breast).[3] The need for examination must obviously be explained to the patient at the start. The patient should be offered a chaperone.

The examination is only just over 50% sensitive for carcinoma, but specificity is as high as 90%. The likelihood ratio (LR) of a positive examination is 14.1 and the LR of a negative examination is 0.47.[4]

Inspection

Ask the patient to sit up with the chest fully exposed. There is controversy about the value of inspection of the breasts as part of the examination, but advanced cancers may be obvious at this stage. Look at the *nipples* for retraction (due to cancer or fibrosis; in some patients retraction may be normal, so it is important to ask whether it is long-standing) and Paget's disease of the breast (where underlying breast cancer causes a unilateral rash or ulceration of the nipple). Asymmetry of breast size is common, and it is important to ask whether any asymmetry is new.

Next inspect the rest of the *skin*. Look for visible veins (which, if unilateral, suggest a cancer), skin dimpling and *peau d'orange* skin (where advanced, breast cancer causes oedematous skin pitted by the sweat glands). Look for erythema from mastitis (the area will be hot and tender).

A persistent erythematous plaque in the nipple area may be contact dermatitis or skin irritation, but if asymmetrical or it has not responded to treatment this may be malignant *Paget's disease of the breast*.

Ask the patient to *raise the arms above the head* and then lower them slowly. Look for tethering of the nipples or skin, a shift in the relative position of the nipples or a fixed mass distorting the breast (see Fig. 41.2).

Note whether there are any obvious visible masses in the axillae.

Next ask the patient to rest the hands on the hips and then press the hands against the hips (the pectoral contraction manoeuvre). This accentuates areas of dimpling or fixation.

Conditions unrelated to the breast may be found incidentally, such as pectus excavatum or carinatum, distended veins related to inferior vena caval (IVC)

alcohol use and use of oestrogens postmenopausally. A personal history of atypical hyperplasia (ductal or lobular) increases the risk of breast cancer. However, three-quarters of patients presenting with a breast cancer have *no* known risk factors.

Ask about genetic testing and mammography if relevant. The breast cancer genes *BRCA1* and *BRCA2* are associated with a strong risk of breast (and ovarian) cancer, as well as breast cancer in men. Patients with a strong family history of breast or ovarian cancer should be asked whether genetic testing has been carried out. Screening mammography is generally recommended for all women from the age of 50 years.[2]

Enlargement of the male breasts (gynaecomastia; p 476) is often a result of hormone or drug treatment (e.g. for carcinoma of the prostate or with aldactone). It is often tender. Bilateral enlargement is usually benign, but unilateral enlargement may be due to malignancy. As malignancy is more common in men with gynaecomastia, asymmetrical enlargement should arouse concern. Carcinoma of the male breast is over 100 times less frequent than female breast carcinoma. As there is less breast tissue present in men and the condition is often not thought of, disease tends to be locally advanced at the time of diagnosis.

Carcinoma of the right breast, showing elevation of the breast, dimpling of the skin and retraction of the nipple

FIGURE 41.2

Examination of the breast.

(a) Quadrants; (b) systematic examination

FIGURE 41.3

obstruction and signs of virilisation such as acne and hirsutism.

Palpation

Examine both the supraclavicular and the axillary regions for lymphadenopathy. It may be difficult, however, to distinguish an axillary fat pad from an enlarged lymph node.

Then ask the patient to lie down. The examination can be performed only if the breast tissue is flattened against the chest wall. It is helpful to have the patient place the hand behind the head for palpation of the lateral aspect of the breast and bring the elbow up level with the shoulder for palpation of the medial side of the breast.

There is no single correct way to palpate the breast, as long as all sections are palpated. We recommend palpation is performed gently with the pulps of the middle three fingers parallel to the contour of the breast supporting the breast with the other hand. The total examination should involve a rectangular area bordered by the clavicle, the sternum, the midaxillary line and the 'bra line'. Start in the axilla and palpate in a line down to the bra line inferiorly. Do not pinch the breast as you may mistakenly think you feel a mass. The pattern of palpation is like that of mowing a lawn, a series of vertical strips that cover the whole of the rectangle (see Fig. 41.3). Palpation may also be performed by quadrant, in a spiral fashion from the nipple outwards or in a 'flower petal' pattern radiating around the breast from the nipple outwards.

Palpation is more difficult when a breast implant is present. It is probably best to examine such a patient in a supine position and to keep the patient's ipsilateral arm down at the side.

Next feel behind the nipple for lumps.

Finish the examination of the breast with the patient sitting up as some lumps are easier to feel in this position. It is important to do this with two hands—that is, one (the left if right-handed) underneath and the right on top so that there is some flattening of the breast tissue.

Do not mistake normal breast structures for a mass.[5] You may feel a rib or costochondral junction normally on deep palpation. The inferior ridge of breast tissue (inframammary fold) may be felt and is symmetrical. You may feel normal rubbery-type plaques (fibroglandular tissue), especially in the upper outer quadrant. It is normal to feel firm breast tissue at the areola border, and the upper outer quadrant of the breast is often dense.

EVALUATION OF A BREAST LUMP

The following five points need to be carefully elucidated if a lump is detected.

1. *Position:* (see below).
2. *Size, shape and consistency:* a hard, irregular nodule is characteristic of carcinoma; a firm, smooth, very mobile, regular nodule is more likely to be a fibroadenoma, especially in a young woman.
3. *Tenderness:* suggests an inflammatory or a cystic lesion; breast cancer is usually not tender, although inflammatory breast cancer can be associated with tenderness.
4. *Fixation:* mobility is determined by taking the breast between the hands and moving it over the chest wall; in advanced carcinoma the lump may be fixed to the chest wall.
5. *Single or multiple lesions present:* multiple nodules suggest benign cystic disease or fibroadenosis.

Remember that lumps found on breast examination may not involve breast tissue; these include lipomas and sebaceous cysts.

Remember also that many normal breasts have palpable lumps and that, although benign lumps tend to be soft, moveable and regular, they can also have the characteristics of malignant lumps.[5] Causes of a lump in the breast are listed in Table 41.1.

In men with true gynaecomastia, a disc of breast tissue can be palpated under the areola. This is not present in men who are merely obese.

Document your findings using the 'clock system': envisage the breast like a clock with respect to the location of any lump or lesion indicated on the breast (e.g. 9 o'clock position) and the distance from the radial edge of the areola noted. The size of the mass and its other features must also be recorded (see above).

Causes of a breast lump

Non-tender	Tender
Cyst	Cyst
Carcinoma	Breast abscess
Fibrocystic disease*	Fibroadenosis
Fibroadenoma (benign highly mobile 'breast mouse')	Costal cartilage chondritis
	Inflammatory breast cancer

Uncommon causes:

Trauma, fat necrosis
Other cysts (e.g. galactocele)
Other neoplasms (e.g. duct papilloma)
Granulomatous mastitis (an inflammatory condition mimicking breast cancer)
Chest wall (e.g. lipoma, costal cartilage chondritis [causes tenderness but not a lump])

*Clinically lumps in the breast are often ridges of fibroglandular tissue that may become more prominent owing to changes in weight or hormonal influence. On imaging, the term 'fibrocystic change' is more commonly used to describe sonographic changes that are likely benign.

TABLE 41.1

T&O'C ESSENTIALS

1. A palpable breast mass is likely to be significant (called a dominant mass) if it is:
   - clearly three-dimensional
   - distinct from the surrounding tissue
   - asymmetrical compared with the other breast
   - persistent throughout a menstrual cycle
   - not smooth, well-demarcated or mobile.
2. A palpable breast mass is more likely to be malignant if it has the following characteristics:
   - Very firm.
   - Margins seem poorly defined or have an irregular edge.
   - Immobile or fixed.
   - Associated skin dimpling.
   - Associated retraction of the nipple, or nipple scaling.
   - Bloody nipple discharge history.
   - Draining lymph nodes are palpable.

OSCE REVISION TOPICS – THE BREASTS

Take a history from this woman who has found a lump in her breast. Explain what features you would look for on examination that would suggest malignancy. (p 766)

References

1. Riley M, Dobson M, Jones E, Kirst N. Health maintenance in women. *Am Fam Physician* 2013; 87(1):30–37. Describes current guidelines for screening for breast cancer and other cancers in women.
2. Kerlikowske K, Smith-Bindman R, Ljung BM et al. Evaluation of abnormal mammography results and palpable breast abnormalities. *Ann Intern Med* 2003; 139:274–284. Discusses how to approach interpreting mammogram reports and the next steps.
3. Fenton JJ, Rolnick SJ, Harris EL et al. Specificity of clinical breast examination in community practice. *J Gen Intern Med* 2007; 22(3):332–357. Screening breast examinations in clinical practice are highly specific but insensitive. A normal exam is reassuring.
4. Barton MB, Harris R, Fletcher SW. Does this patient have breast cancer? *JAMA* 1999; 282:1270–1280. The clinical breast examination has an overall specificity that is high (94%) but the sensitivity is poor (54%). Unfortunately, inter-observer variation seems to be high.
5. Pruthi S. Detection and evaluation of a palpable breast mass. *Mayo Clin Proc* 2001; 76:641–647. Most breast masses are benign but malignancy must be excluded. If cancer is suspected but mammography is negative, further testing is indicated.

SECTION 12
Specialty system history and examination

CHAPTER 42

The eyes, ears, nose and throat

CHAPTER 43

The skin and lumps

CHAPTER 44

The older person assessment

CHAPTER 45

Approaching infectious diseases

CHAPTER 42

The eyes, ears, nose and throat

Diagnosis is not the end, but the beginning of practice. MARTIN H FISCHER (1879–1962)

The examination of the eyes and ears, nose and throat is important for any medical patient because these small parts of the body may be involved in local or systemic disease.

EYES

Examination anatomy

The structure of the eye is shown in Fig. 42.1.[1] There are three layers that make up the eye ball:

- The **inner or neural layer** forms the retina itself and has inner and outer layers. The *outer layer* contains pigmented cells and the *inner layer*, which is continuous with the optic nerve, contains the photoreceptor *rod* (night and peripheral vision) and *cone* (central and colour vision) cells.

- The **central layer** is called the *uveal* tract. It forms the *iris* and *ciliary body* anteriorly and the *choroid* posteriorly. The choroid is a vascular structure. It supplies the optic nerve, the *fovea* (area of most acute vision) and the posterior two-thirds of the retina. The ciliary body produces the *aqueous humour*. This transparent fluid lies behind the cornea and fills the *anterior chamber* of the eye. The aqueous humour moves through the pupil and drains through a trabecular meshwork at the acute angle of the anterior chamber. The *lens* sits behind the cornea and is suspended from ligaments of the ciliary body.

- The **outer layer** is fibrous. The anterior part, the *cornea*, is transparent and the rest makes up the *sclera*. The main volume of the eyeball is filled with *vitreous humour*, which is a transparent gel.

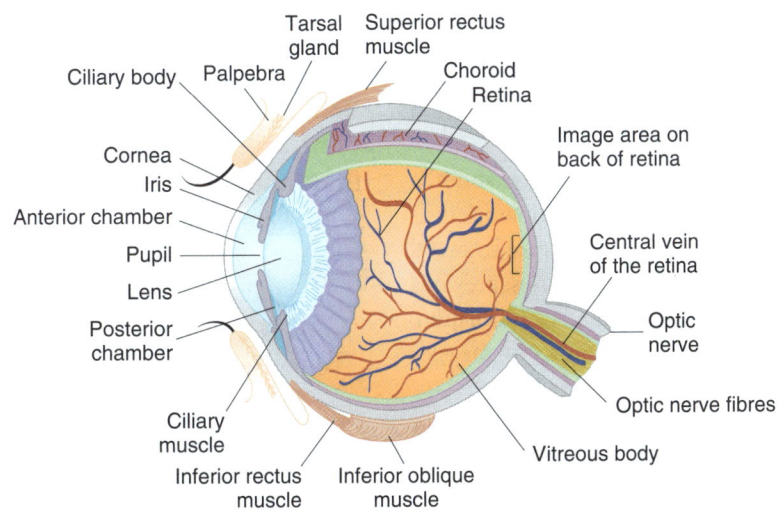

The structure of the eye

FIGURE 42.1

The anatomy of the optic nerve is described in Chapter 32.

The eyelids provide and distribute moisture to the corneas from three types of glands (two small and one large). The two types of small *lacrimal*[a] glands within the eyelids secrete tears and produce mucin and oil. These are sufficient to lubricate the eyelids and the cornea in normal circumstances. Emotion or a foreign body, however, will stimulate the large lacrimal glands that lie between the bony orbital wall laterally and the eyeball and the lateral rectus muscle medially. From each gland duct, big volumes of tears drain into the upper part of the lid. Tears either evaporate or are drained via the medial edge of the eye into the lacrimal canaliculi and on into the lacrimal sac, the lacrimal duct, the inferior nasal meatus and thence to the nose—and, if necessary, into a handkerchief. The conjunctiva is a mucous membrane that lines the eyelids and keeps them slippery on the inside.

History

Presenting symptoms include pain or discomfort and redness (see Table 42.2 and Questions box 42.1), loss or distortion of vision and watery eyes, and infection of the eyelids and associated structures. Loss of vision and other visual symptoms (see Table 42.1 and Questions box 42.2) are also discussed in Chapter 32.

Ask about symptoms of keratoconjunctivitis sicca (dry eyes). These include dryness, burning and irritation and usually become worse as the day goes on. They are made worse by smoke, allergens and low humidity (e.g. from air conditioning). The cause may be reduced tear production or increased tear evaporation (List 42.1).

More general questions include asking about a history of arthritis or known vasculitis, multiple sclerosis or thyroid disease; occupation and exposure to metal fragments or arc welding; use of contact lenses; previous history of vascular disease; diabetes or atrial fibrillation; and smoking. Conjunctivitis is a feature of measles (see Fig. 42.2).

Ask about previous eye problems or surgery including laser correction surgery. Have the intraocular pressures been measured recently?

---

[a] From the Latin word for tear, *lacrima*. Hence the famous phrase in *The aeneid* when Aeneas sees the depictions of the fall of Troy on the new walls of Carthage and becomes very emotional, saying '*Refum lacrimae sunt*'—there *are* tears for things.

QUESTIONS TO ASK THE PATIENT WITH A PAINFUL RED EYE

! denotes symptoms for the possible diagnosis of an urgent or dangerous problem.

1. Do you wear contact lenses? (Corneal ulceration)
2. Is it painful when you move your eyes? (Iritis or scleritis)
3. Are the lids stuck together in the morning? (Conjunctivitis)
! 4. Have you had an injury or worked with dust, metal grinders or welding equipment? (Injury, foreign body or flash burn)
5. Have you had arthritis or rashes? (Vasculitis)

QUESTIONS BOX 42.1

Take a drug history. Ask about eye drops and drugs such as corticosteroids (cataracts), anticholinergics (glaucoma from acute angle closure), amiodarone (corneal deposits), chloroquine and chlorpromazine (retinal toxicity) and ethambutol and isoniazid (optic neuropathy).

Examination method

Sit the patient at the edge of the bed. Stand well back at first, and note the following:

1. **Ptosis** (drooping of one or both upper eyelids).
2. The **colour of the sclerae**:
   - **yellow**, caused by deposits of bilirubin in jaundice
   - **blue**, which may be due to osteogenesis imperfecta, because the thin sclerae allow the choroidal pigment to show through; blue sclerae can also occur in families without osteogenesis imperfecta; blue-grey scleral discoloration occurs in patients with ochronosis (see Fig. 42.3(a)), resulting from the accumulation of homogentisic acid in connective tissue in this inherited condition;

Common causes of visual disturbance	
Symptom	**Common causes when answer is 'yes'**
Sudden partial or complete loss in one eye (important to distinguish from hemianopia)	**Transient:** retinal ischaemia (amaurosis fugax), retinal migraine, optic neuritis (may occur after exercise or a hot bath) **Prolonged:** retinal detachment, retinal embolus, diabetic retinopathy (sudden or gradual), temporal arteritis, trauma
Hemianopia	Visual cortical infarct, parieto-occipital infarct
Gradual loss of vision unilateral or bilateral	Cataract, macular degeneration, glaucoma (painless if chronic), tumour of base of skull (e.g. meningioma, pituitary adenoma)
Blurred vision	Refractive error, cataract, macular degeneration (usually a central scotoma)
Diplopia	**Monocular:** lens dislocation, cataract, astigmatism, hysteria **Binocular:** abnormal eye movements (e.g. ocular motor palsy)
Halos (distortion around the edges of bright lights)	Corneal oedema, acute glaucoma
Dry eyes (patient may feel something is in the eye)	Sjögren's syndrome, blepharitis (inflammation of eyelids [e.g. from eczema]), infection of eyelids
Eye pain and headache	Cluster headache or migraine
Pain on eye movement	Optic neuritis
Eye painful and red	**Diffuse with central sparing:** conjunctivitis (lids stuck together) **No central sparing:** iritis, acute glaucoma (cornea cloudy) **Pain on moving eye:** scleritis (e.g. systemic vasculitis) Foreign body, entropion (lower lid inverted) Corneal ulceration (herpes simplex, contact lens)
Floaters in visual fields	Vitreous degeneration (associated with age and myopia)

TABLE 42.1

> **CAUSES OF DRY EYES**
>
> 1. Reduced production: inflammation of the lachrymal glands from systemic illnesses such as rheumatoid arthritis and Sjögren's syndrome
> 2. Increased evaporation: enlarged palpebral fissure (Grave's disease), Bell's palsy
>
> LIST 42.1

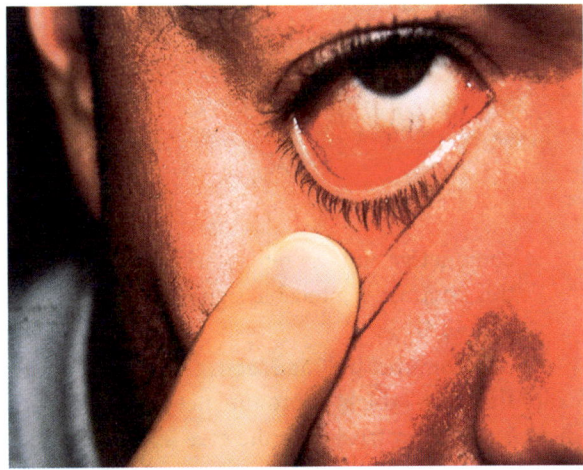

Conjunctivitis in a patient with measles

FIGURE 42.2

the concha of the ear is often affected (see Fig. 42.3(b)), as are the joints and heart valves

- **red**, from *iritis* or *scleritis*, which causes central inflammation; or *conjunctivitis*, which causes more peripheral inflammation often with pus; or *subconjunctival haemorrhage*, which causes influent blood as a result of trauma (see Table 42.2 and List 42.2)
- **scleral pallor**, which occurs in anaemia—pull down the lower lid and look for the normal contrast between the pearly white posterior

> **QUESTIONS TO ASK THE PATIENT WITH SUDDEN VISUAL LOSS**
>
> ❗ denotes symptoms for the possible diagnosis of an urgent or dangerous problem.
>
> 1. Does the abnormality persist when you close each eye in turn? (Visual field loss)
> 2. Was the sensation as if a curtain was drawn across your vision? Has your vision come back? (Amaurosis fugax)
> 3. Have you had previous strokes or fibrillation of your heart? (Retinal embolus, cortical infarct)
> ❗ 4. Has your eye been painful? (Acute glaucoma, iritis)
> 5. Have you injured your eye or head? (Trauma to eye or optic nerve)
> 6. Have you had preceding visual disturbance, e.g. flashing lights? (Migraine)
> 7. Have you had severe headache on the same side? (Temporal arteritis)
> 8. Have you had weakness or tingling in your arms or legs, or bowel or bladder disturbance? (Multiple sclerosis and optic neuritis)
> 9. Are you a diabetic? (Diabetic retinopathy with haemorrhage)
>
> **QUESTIONS BOX 42.2**

Ochronosis.

(a) Sclerae; (b) ears

FIGURE 42.3

conjunctiva and the red anterior part; loss of this contrast is a reliable sign of anaemia (see Fig. 42.4(b)).

Look from behind and above the patient for **exophthalmos**, which is prominence of the eyes. If there is actual protrusion of the eyes from the orbits, this is called **proptosis**. It is best detected by looking at the eyes from above the forehead; protrusion beyond the supraorbital ridge is abnormal. If exophthalmos is present, examine specifically for thyroid eye disease: lid lag (the patient follows your finger as it descends—the upper lid lags behind the pupil), chemosis (oedema of the bulbar conjunctiva), corneal ulceration and ophthalmoplegia (weakness of upward gaze). Look then for any corneal abnormalities, such as band keratopathy or arcus senilis.

Look for **corneal ulceration**, which may be obvious if severe. A strip coated with sterile fluorescein will stain corneal ulcers and make them easily visible. A branching (dendritic) ulcer is seen in herpes complex keratitis.

Proceed as for the **cranial nerve examination**—that is, testing *visual acuity*, *visual fields* and *pupillary responses* to light and accommodation. Interruption of the sympathetic innervation of the eye at any point results in *Horner's syndrome (partial ptosis and a*

Distinguishing among common causes of a red and painful eye			
Disease	**Distribution of redness**	**Corneal surface**	**Pupil**
Bacterial conjunctivitis	Peripheral conjunctiva Bilateral (central sparing)	Normal	Normal
Episcleritis	Segmental, often around cornea Unilateral	Normal	Normal
Acute iritis	Ciliary flush Unilateral	Dull (vision blurred)	Small, irregular shape, may be no light response
Glaucoma	Around cornea Unilateral	Dull	Mid-oval shape, no light response
Corneal ulcer	Around cornea Unilateral	Dull Fluorescein dye stains ulcer	Normal
Subconjunctival haemorrhage	Localised haemorrhage No posterior limit	Normal	Normal
Conjunctival haemorrhage	Localised haemorrhage Posterior limit present	Normal	Normal

TABLE 42.2

CAUSES OF UVEITIS

Iritis (anterior uveitis)

Viral

Idiopathic

Generalised disease
- Seronegative spondyloarthropathies
- Inflammatory bowel disease
- Diabetes mellitus
- Granulomatous disease (e.g. sarcoidosis)
- Infections (e.g. gonococcal, syphilis, toxoplasmosis, brucellosis, tuberculosis)

Choroiditis (posterior uveitis)

Idiopathic

Generalised disease
- Diabetes mellitus
- Granulomatous disease (e.g. sarcoidosis)
- Infections (e.g. toxoplasmosis, syphilis, tuberculosis, toxocaral infection)

The uveal tract consists of the anterior uvea (iris) and the posterior uvea (ciliary body and choroid).

LIST 42.2

T&O'C ESSENTIALS

Conjunctivitis

1. Viral conjunctivitis (adenovirus) often begins after an upper respiratory infection. It can be unilateral and is of sudden onset. There has often been contact with other infected people.
2. Bacterial conjunctivitis (e.g. Staph. aureus in adults) usually causes thick, discoloured (green or yellow) discharge. The eyelids may be stuck together.
3. Allergic conjunctivitis occurs in association with sneezing, itching and excessive tear production. Bilateral redness and chemosis (conjunctival oedema) are common.

constricted but reactive pupil). Perceptible *anisocoria* (inequality of the diameters of the pupils) has been found in 20% of healthy people. Remember also that elderly people quite often have imperceptible pupillary light reactions.

Test the **eye movements** (see Fig. 32.14, p 513). Look also for fatigability of eye muscles by asking the patient to look up at a hat-pin or finger for about half a minute. In myasthenia gravis the muscles tire and the eyelids begin to droop.

776 SECTION 12 SPECIALTY SYSTEM HISTORY AND EXAMINATION

(a) Normal sclera; (b) conjunctival pallor in an anaemic patient.

Note the contrast between the anterior and posterior parts in the normal eye

FIGURE 42.4

> **T&O'C ESSENTIALS**
>
> **Cataracts**
> 1. are very common in old age
> 2. have many causes and associations (List 42.3)
> 3. cause reduced visual acuity, poor night vision, diplopia and glare
> 4. surgery is indicated when loss of vision interferes with life, e.g. driving, reading.

Test **colour vision** if acuity is not poor. Ishihara test plates (where coloured spots form numbers) can be used. Red desaturation (impaired ability to see red objects) can occur with optic nerve disease. Red–green colour blindness affects 7% of males (X-linked recessive).

Test the **corneal reflex** (see also p 523).

Perform **fundoscopy**. Successful ophthalmoscopy requires considerable practice. It is important that it be performed in reduced ambient lighting so that the patient's pupils are at least partly dilated and you are not distracted. It can be easier to perform the examination, especially of the fundi, through the patient's spectacles. Otherwise, the patient's refractive error should be corrected by use of the appropriate ophthalmoscope lens. The patient should be asked to stare at a point on the opposite wall or on the ceiling and to ignore the light of the ophthalmoscope. Patients will often attempt to focus on the ophthalmoscope light and should be asked not to do this. Cataracts cause opacification of the lens and may make fundoscopy impossible. They are also associated with a reduced or absent light reflex.

Begin by examining the **cornea**. Use your right eye to examine the patient's right eye, and vice versa. Turn the ophthalmoscope lens to +20 and examine the cornea from about 20 centimetres away from the patient. Look particularly for corneal ulceration. Turn the lens gradually down to 0 while moving closer to the patient. Structures, including the *lens*, the *humour* and the *retina*, at increasing distance into the eye will swim into focus.

Examine the **retina** (see Fig. 42.5, also Fig. 32.10 on p 510 and pp 124–5). Focus on one of the retinal arteries and follow it into the optic disc. The normal disc is round and paler than the surrounding retina. The margin of the disc is usually sharply outlined but will appear blurred if there is papilloedema or papillitis, or pale if there is optic atrophy. Look at the rest of the retina, especially for haemorrhages and the retinal changes of diabetes mellitus or hypertension.

There are four types of **haemorrhages**: *streaky haemorrhages* near the vessels (linear or flame-shaped), large *ecchymoses* that obliterate the vessels, *petechiae*, which may be confused with microaneurysms, and *subhyaloid haemorrhages* (large effusions of blood that have a crescentic shape and well-marked borders; a fluid level may be seen). The first two types of haemorrhage occur in hypertensive and diabetic retinopathy. They may also result from any cause of raised intracranial pressure or venous engorgement,

Retinal photographs.

(a) Retinitis pigmentosa; (b) central retinal artery occlusion

(Courtesy of Lions Eye Institute.)

FIGURE 42.5

or from a bleeding disorder. The third type occurs in diabetes mellitus, and the fourth is characteristic of subarachnoid haemorrhage.

There are two main types of retinal change in diabetes mellitus: non-proliferative and proliferative. Non-proliferative changes include: (1) two types of haemorrhages occur specifically in diabetics—*dot haemorrhages*, which occur in the inner retinal layers, and *blot haemorrhages*, which are larger and occur more superficially in the nerve fibre layer; (2) *microaneurysms* (tiny bulges in the vessel wall), which are due to vessel wall damage; and (3) two types of exudates—*hard exudates*, which have straight edges and are due to leakage of protein from damaged arteriolar walls, and *soft exudates* (cottonwool spots), which have a fluffy appearance and are due to microinfarcts. Proliferative changes include *new vessel formation*, which can lead to retinal detachment or vitreous haemorrhage.

Hypertensive changes can be classified from grades 1 to 4:

Grade 1   'Silver wiring' of the arteries only (sclerosis of the vessel wall reduces its transparency so that the central light streak becomes broader and shinier)
Grade 2   Silver wiring of arteries plus arteriovenous nipping or nicking (indentation or deflection of the veins where they are crossed by the arteries)
Grade 3   Grade 2 plus haemorrhages (flame-shaped) and exudates (soft—cottonwool spots due to ischaemia, or hard—lipid residues from leaking vessels)
Grade 4   Grade 3 changes plus papilloedema.

It is important to describe the changes present rather than just give a grade.

Retinitis pigmentosa causes a scattering of black pigment in a criss-cross pattern (Fig. 42.5a). This will be missed if the periphery of the retina is not examined.

Inspect carefully for **central retinal artery occlusion** (Fig. 42.5b), where the whole fundus appears milky-white because of retinal oedema and the arteries become greatly reduced in diameter. This presents with sudden, painless unilateral blindness and is a medical emergency.

Central retinal vein thrombosis causes tortuous retinal veins and haemorrhages scattered over the whole retina, particularly occurring alongside the veins ('blood and thunder retina'). This presents with sudden painless loss of vision, which is not total.

In **retinal detachment**, the retina may appear elevated or folded. The patient describes a 'shade coming down', flashes of light or showers of black dots. A diagnosis requires immediate referral to try to prevent total detachment and irrevocable blindness.

White spots occur in **choroiditis** and when active have a fluffy edge (e.g. in toxoplasmosis, sarcoidosis).

Finally, ask the patient to look directly at the light. This allows you to locate and inspect the **macula**. Macular degeneration is the leading cause of blindness; central vision is lost. Drusen formation occurs in macular degeneration—small deposits are seen under the epithelium in the central retina. Macular degeneration may occur secondary to an atrophic or a neovascularisation process.

Palpate the orbits for tenderness. Auscultate the eyes with the bell of the stethoscope—the eye being tested is shut while the other is open and the patient is asked to stop breathing. Listen for a bruit that may be a sign of an arteriovenous malformation or a vascular tumour.

Feel for the preauricular node (adenoviral conjunctivitis).

Consider the possibility that the patient may have a glass eye. This should be suspected if visual acuity is zero in one eye and no pupillary reaction is apparent. Attempts to examine and interpret the fundus of a glass eye will amuse the patient but are always unsuccessful.

The causes of common eye abnormalities are summarised in List 42.3.

Diplopia

Most cases of diplopia (about 60%) are not due to a cranial nerve abnormality. It is important to have an approach to the problem that will help work out the cause.

First find out whether the diplopia is monocular (25%) or binocular. Monocular diplopia persists when one eye is covered. It is usually due to an eye problem such as astigmatism, dislocated lens, uneven contact lens surface or thick spectacles and some types of cataract. It disappears if the patient looks through a pin-hole. Although it is said to be due to hysteria, this is a very rare cause.

If the diplopia is binocular, consider the common causes:

1. Cranial nerve palsy (III, IV or VI)—look for ptosis, pupil changes (III), abnormal eye movements.
2. Eye muscle disease (myasthenia gravis)—worse later in the day, worse after prolonged upward gaze and associated with bilateral ptosis.
3. Thyroid ophthalmopathy—proptosis, lid lag, chemosis.
4. Trauma to the orbit—history or signs of trauma.
5. Internuclear ophthalmoplegia—associated neurological signs.

Left Horner's syndrome, with partial ptosis and miosis

FIGURE 42.6

Horner's syndrome

Examination anatomy

Interruption of the sympathetic innervation of the eye at any point (see Fig. 42.6) results in Horner's[b] syndrome (see List 42.4).

Clinical approach

The syndrome includes partial *ptosis* (as sympathetic fibres supply the smooth muscle of both eyelids) and a *constricted* pupil (unbalanced parasympathetic action) that reacts normally to light (see Fig. 42.6). Remember the other causes of ptosis (see Table 42.3).

Test for a difference (decrease) in the *sweating* over each eyebrow with the back of the finger (absence of this sign does not exclude the diagnosis).[c]

Horner's syndrome may be part of the *lateral medullary syndrome*.[d]

Next ask the patient to speak and note any hoarseness of the voice, which may be due to recurrent laryngeal nerve palsy from lung carcinoma or from a lower cranial nerve lesion.

---

[b] Johann Friedrich Horner (1831–86), a professor of ophthalmology at Zürich, described this in 1869.
[c] Enophthalmos, or retraction of the eye, which is often mentioned as a feature of Horner's syndrome, probably does not occur in humans. It may occur in cats. Horner's original paper was very specific about miosis and ptosis, but only casually mentioned that 'the position of the eye seemed very slightly inward'. Apparent enophthalmos results from a combination of ptosis and an elevated lower lid (upside-down ptosis).
[d] Occlusion of any of the following vessels may result in this syndrome: vertebral; posterior inferior cerebellar; superior, middle or inferior lateral medullary arteries.

CAUSES OF EYE ABNORMALITIES

Cataracts
1. Old age (senile cataract)
2. Endocrine (e.g. diabetes mellitus, steroids)
3. Hereditary or congenital (e.g. dystrophia myotonica)
4. Ocular disease (e.g. glaucoma)
5. Radiation
6. Trauma
7. Smoking

Papilloedema vs papillitis

PAPILLOEDEMA	PAPILLITIS
Optic disc swollen without venous pulsation	Optic disc swollen
	Acuity poor
Acuity normal (early)	Large central scotoma
Large blind spot	Pain on eye movement
Peripheral constriction of visual field	Onset usually sudden and unilateral
Colour vision normal	Colour vision affected (particularly red desaturation)
Usually bilateral	

Causes of papilloedema
1. Space-occupying lesion (causing raised intracranial pressure) or a retro-orbital mass
2. Hydrocephalus (large cerebral ventricles)
   - Obstructive (a block in the ventricle, aqueduct or outlet to the fourth ventricle—e.g. tumour)
   - Communicating
   - Increased formation of CSF (e.g. choroid plexus papilloma—rare)
   - Decreased absorption of CSF (e.g. tumour causing venous compression, subarachnoid space obstruction from meningitis)
3. Benign intracranial hypertension (pseudotumour cerebri) (small or normal-sized ventricles)
   - Idiopathic
   - The contraceptive pill
   - Addison's disease
   - Drugs (e.g. nitrofurantoin, tetracycline, vitamin A, steroids)
   - Head trauma
4. Hypertension
5. Central retinal vein thrombosis

Causes of optic atrophy
1. Chronic papilloedema or optic neuritis
2. Optic nerve pressure or division
3. Glaucoma
4. Ischaemia
5. Familial (e.g. retinitis pigmentosa, Leber's* disease, Friedreich's ataxia)

Causes of optic neuritis
1. Multiple sclerosis
2. Toxic (e.g. ethambutol, chloroquine, nicotine, alcohol)
3. Metabolic (e.g. vitamin B_{12} deficiency)
4. Ischaemia (e.g. diabetes mellitus, temporal arteritis, atheroma)
5. Familial (e.g. Leber's disease)
6. Infective (e.g. infectious mononucleosis)

Causes of retinitis pigmentosa
1. Congenital (associated with cataract and deaf-mutism)
2. Laurence–Moon–Biedl syndrome[†]
3. Hereditary trauma
4. Familial neuropathy (i.e. Refsum's disease[‡])

CSF = cerebrospinal fluid.
[*]Theodor von Leber (1840–1917), a Göttingen and Heidelberg ophthalmologist.
[†]John Laurence (1830–74), a London ophthalmologist; Robert Charles Moon (1844–1914), an American ophthalmologist; Arthur Biedl (1869–1933), a professor of physiology, Prague.
[‡]Sigvald Refsum (1907–91), a Norwegian physician.

LIST 42.3

> **CAUSES OF HORNER'S SYNDROME**
>
> 1. Carcinoma of the apex of the lung (usually squamous cell carcinoma)
> 2. Neck
>   - Malignancy (e.g. thyroid)
>   - Trauma or surgery
> 3. Lower trunk brachial plexus lesions
>   - Trauma
>   - Tumour
> 4. Carotid arterial lesion
>   - Carotid aneurysm or dissection
>   - Pericarotid tumours*
>   - Cluster headache
> 5. Brainstem lesions
>   - Vascular disease (especially the lateral medullary syndrome)
>   - Tumour
>   - Syringobulbia
> 6. Syringomyelia (rare)
>
> *Sweating unaffected, as tumour is localised to internal carotid artery.
>
> LIST 42.4

Important causes of ptosis

Cause	Associated features
Age-related stretching of the levator muscle or aponeurosis	Common, often asymmetrical
Orbital tumour or inflammation	Orbital abnormality
Constricted pupil, reduced sweating	Horner's syndrome
Eye 'down and out', dilated pupil	Third nerve palsy
Myasthenia gravis or dystrophia myotonica	Extraocular muscle palsies, muscle weakness
Congenital or idiopathic	

TABLE 42.3

Now look at the hands for clubbing and test for weakness of finger abduction. If any of these signs is present, perform a respiratory examination, concentrating on the apices of the lungs for signs of lung carcinoma.

Examine the neck for lymphadenopathy, thyroid carcinoma and a carotid aneurysm or bruit. Syringomyelia may rarely be a cause of this syndrome, so the examination should be completed by testing for dissociated sensory loss. Remember, syringomyelia may cause a bilateral Horner's syndrome.

Iritis

Iritis (anterior uveitis) presents with pain, photophobia and unilateral eye redness (see Table 42.2 and List 42.2). On examination of the eye, there is classically a ciliary flush with dilated vessels around the iris. *Hypopyon* refers to pus in the anterior chamber; a fluid level may be seen. The pupil is usually irregular. There may also be new vessel formation over the iris.

Iritis is associated with inflammatory arthropathies that are linked to HLA-B27 positivity, including ankylosing spondylitis, inflammatory bowel disease, reactive arthritis and Behçet's disease with an acute presentation. Chronic iritis can be linked to juvenile rheumatoid arthritis, as well as sarcoidosis and syphilis.

Keratitis is inflammation of the cornea and may be due to ulceration (often a result of herpes simplex infection) or injury (e.g. from metal fragments in grinders or flash burns in arc welders). Contact lens wearers who do not clean their lenses properly are also at risk. Severe proptosis or a facial nerve palsy that prevents lid closure can be a mechanical cause.

Scleritis presents similarly but with bilateral painful red eyes; it is also associated with the same HLA-B27 arthropathies. Eye movements are painful in scleritis.

Glaucoma

Primary open-angle glaucoma causes prolonged elevation of intraocular pressure and induces progressive visual loss. This begins in the peripheral visual fields and is painless.

Closed-angle (narrow-angle) glaucoma is due to a rapid pressure increase. Symptoms include severe eye pain, halos around lights and nausea; it is an ocular emergency. You may see a fixed mid-dilated pupil, conjunctival hyperaemia and corneal redness; intraocular pressure on measurement is increased. The condition occurs secondary to iris neovascularisation (e.g. new vessel formation in diabetes mellitus) or primarily from an anomalous iris (e.g. genetic). Acute

Nasociliary herpes zoster showing the distribution of the nerve

FIGURE 42.7

Herpes zoster, involving the eye, along the distribution of the ophthalmic branch of the fifth cranial nerve

(From Mir MA. *Atlas of clinical diagnosis*, 2nd edn. Edinburgh: Saunders, 2003.)

FIGURE 42.8

glaucoma can be precipitated by anticholinergic drugs (e.g. amitriptyline).

Shingles

Herpes zoster involving the first (ophthalmic) division of the trigeminal nerve may result in uveitis and keratitis and threaten vision. The tip of the nose, cornea and iris are all innervated by the nasociliary nerve (a branch of the trigeminal nerve; see Figs 42.7 and 42.8). The appearance of vesicles on the tip of the nose (Hutchinson's[e] vesicles) in a patient with herpes zoster indicates an increased risk of ophthalmic complication (LR+ 3.5).[2]

---

[e] Sir Jonathon Hutchinson (1828–1913). Among other appointments he was surgeon to Moorfields Eye Hospital. He was president of the Royal College of Surgeons in 1889, elected to the Royal Society in 1882 and knighted in 1908.

Eyelid

A number of conditions of the eyelid are worth remembering:

1. Stye of the eyelid (*hordeolum*) is an infection typically caused by *Staphylococcus aureus*; it is tender.
2. *Chalazion* is a slowly enlarging non-tender nodule of the eyelid (see Fig. 42.9), resulting from sterile inflammation of the meibomian glands if deep, or of the sebaceous glands if superficial.
3. *Dacrocystitis* is infection of a lacrimal gland or of the lacrimal duct (see Fig. 42.10).
4. *Orbital cellulitis* may spread to involve the eyelid (see Fig. 42.11).
5. *Ectropion* is a drooping of the lower lid when it loses its elasticity in old age and falls away from the sclera. This interrupts tear drainage, the eye

A chalazion; unlike styes, chalazions are not usually tender or painful

FIGURE 42.9

Orbital cellulitis

(Courtesy of Dr A Watson, Infectious Diseases Department, The Canberra Hospital.)

FIGURE 42.11

Dacrocystitis

(Courtesy of Dr A Watson, Infectious Diseases Department, The Canberra Hospital.)

FIGURE 42.10

becomes dry and tears spill over the patient's cheek.
6. *Entropium* is the opposite. Scarring or thickening of the lower lid leads to corneal abrasion from inverted lashes.

EARS

Examination anatomy

The ear is divided into three parts: the outer, middle and inner ear:

- The **outer ear** comprises the pinna, the external auditory canal and the eardrum (tympanic membrane), which are easily assessed with simple equipment (see Fig. 42.12). Glands in the skin of the auditory canal secrete cerumen.[f] As cells desquamate from the outer surface of the eardrum they combine with cerumen and migrate outwards to produce normal ear wax.
- The **middle ear** includes the inner layer of the tympanic membrane, the tympanic cavity (epimesohypotympanum), the ossicles (*malleus, incus* and *stapes*[g]), the *Eustachian* tube and the mastoid air cells. The Eustachian tube connects the middle ear with the nasopharynx. A branch of the facial nerve, the *chorda tympani*,[h] enters the tympanic cavity through its posterior wall and traverses the pars flaccida of the tympanic membrane, over the neck of the malleus adjacent to the mucosa, on its way back from receiving taste sensation from the front of the tongue.
- The **inner ear** (labyrinth) has vestibular (concerned with balance) and cochlear (concerned with hearing) parts. The vestibular part includes the semicircular canals that lie at right angles to each other. Movements of the head disturb the *endolymph*, a fluid that fills the canals. This stimulates hairs, which cause nerve

---

[f] From the Latin word for wax. *Cerula*, the diminutive, means a little piece of wax.
[g] From the Latin for hammer, anvil and stirrup.
[h] From the Latin for the string of a musical instrument and a drum.

CHAPTER 42 THE EYES, EARS, NOSE AND THROAT

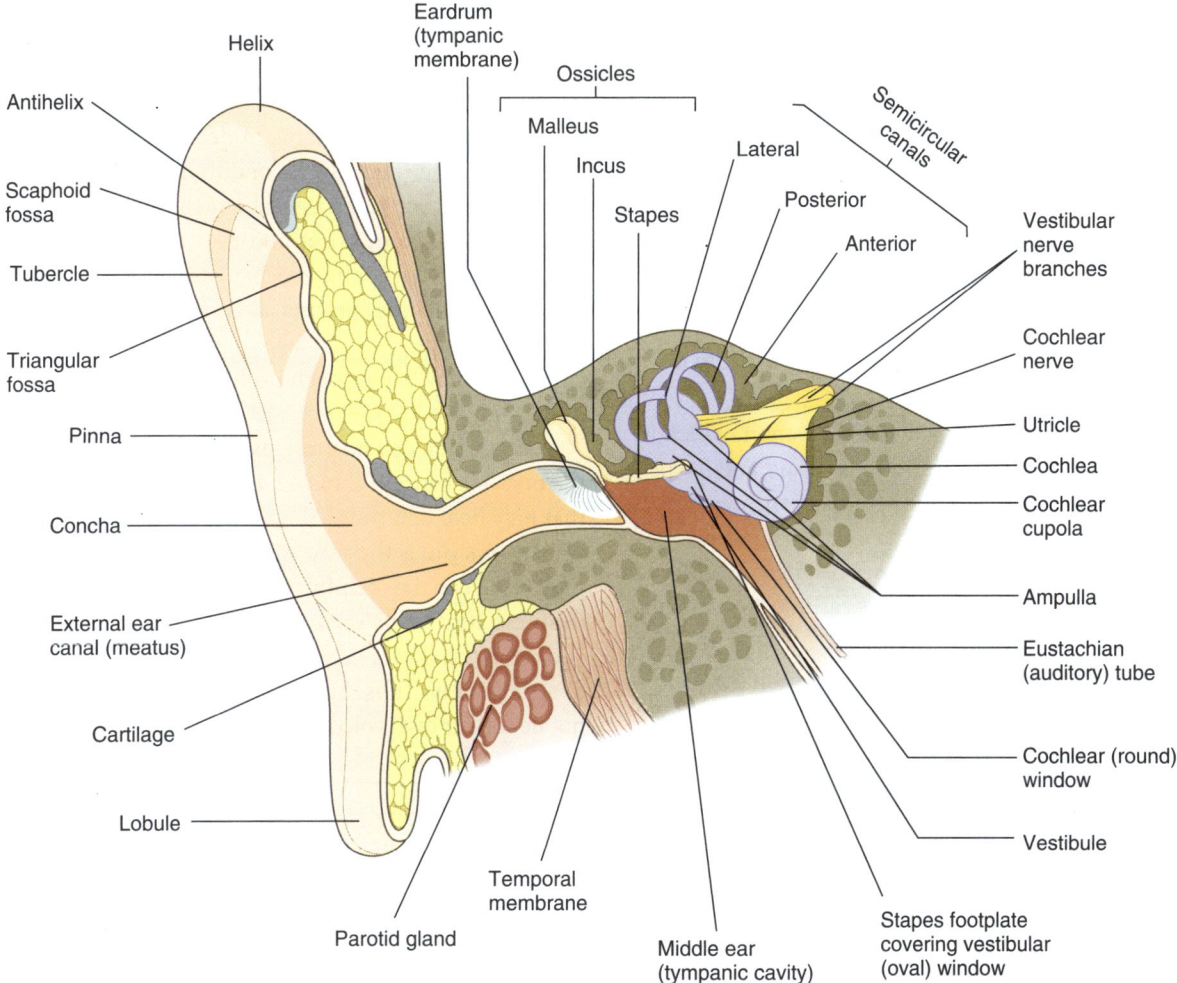

Cross-sectional anatomy of the ear showing the pinna, external auditory canal, middle and inner ear

FIGURE 42.12

impulses to travel in the vestibular part of the eighth nerve. Movement of the stapes on the *oval window* of the cochlear stimulates hair cells in the cochlear, which convert this movement into nerve impulses that travel in the cochlear part of the eighth nerve.

History

Patients may have symptoms from any of the three parts of the ear:

1. *Outer ear:* symptoms include itch, erythema and discharge (perforated drum and infection or otitis externa; see List 42.5). The pinna can be

> **COMMON SYMPTOMS OF EAR DISEASE**
> Deafness
> Vertigo
> Tinnitus
> Pain (otalgia)
> Discharge (otorrhoea)
> Itch
>
> LIST 42.5

damaged by trauma or affected by acquired or inherited diseases of cartilage. Otorrhoea is a more chronic scanty but offensive discharge. It may be due to a cholesteatoma. This is a growth of stratified squamous epithelium that begins in the middle ear or mastoid. It is a benign, slowly growing lesion that destroys bone and ear tissue as it grows. When perforation of the tympanic membrane occurs, cheesy white discharge can occur. It results in loss of hearing if the ossicles are involved. Accumulations of ear wax are a cause of deafness.

2. *Middle ear:* symptoms include infection, which is common in children, and causes pain and, if the eardrum ruptures, a purulent discharge. Otosclerosis is an inherited abnormality that affects the ossicles and causes deafness. Middle ear tumours and chronic middle ear infection are a cause of deafness.

3. *Inner ear:* deafness and balance problems including vertigo are the usual symptoms of inner ear disease. Tinnitus, which is usually described as a 'ringing in the ears', occurs with most types of inner ear disease. Drugs are a common cause (List 42.6).

Deafness may be due to a **conductive** problem because of abnormalities of the:

- outer ear
- eardrum
- ossicles, or

sensorineural, a result of abnormalities affecting the:

- inner ear
- acoustic nerve.

A patient who complains of deafness needs to be asked about the effect of the condition on work, family life and social activities. Ask about the severity of the deafness, the age of onset and the rapidity of onset. Also enquire what coping mechanisms have been tried. These may include hearing aids, sign language and support groups. People who have been deaf from childhood may have speech problems and educational difficulties.

For any patient who presents with deafness, consider the possible causes (Table 42.4) and ask the questions that may help determine the cause (see Questions box 42.3). Sometimes the way a patient speaks during the interview can be helpful. Patients with conductive deafness hear their own voices by bone conduction and often think they are speaking loudly but they tend to speak softly. Those with sensorineural deafness do not hear their own voices well and tend to speak loudly.

DRUG CAUSES OF TINNITUS

1. Antibiotics, especially aminoglycosides but also vancomycin, erythromycin and neomycin
2. Antimalarials: quinine, chloroquine
3. Benzodiazapines
4. Carbamazepine
5. Chemotherapeutic drugs: vincristine, carboplatin, cisplatin
6. Loop diuretics
7. Aspirin and non-steroidal anti-inflammatory drugs
8. Tricyclic antidepressants

LIST 42.6

QUESTIONS TO ASK THE PATIENT WITH DEAFNESS

1. How long has your hearing been a problem? (e.g. congenital)
2. Does your job or any of your hobbies expose you to noise?
3. Have you been treated with drugs that could damage your hearing? (Ask about salicylates, cisplatin and gentamicin)
4. Is there a history of deafness in your family? (e.g. otosclerosis)
5. Have you had recurrent ear infections? (Especially common in Aboriginal children)
6. Have you had problems with wax in your ears in the past?
7. Have you had any injury to your ears or head or a serious infection such as meningitis?
8. Have you also got ringing in your ears? (e.g. Ménière's disease)

QUESTIONS BOX 42.3

Causes of deafness

Conductive	Notes
Ear wax (cerumen)	Cerumen may completely block the external ear canal and reduce sound conduction
Perforation of eardrum (tympanic membrane)	A result of infection or trauma, reduces sound conduction to the ossicles
Otosclerosis	Bony overgrowth of the footplate of the stapes and reduces movement. There is often a family history of the condition
Colesteatoma	This is a mass of keratinising epithelial cells which expands and invades locally and can affect the cochlear, ossicles and tympanic membrane
Sensorineural	
Meniere's disease	Patient may have tinnitus, sensorineural hearing loss and vertigo
Presbycusis	Loss especially of high-frequency hearing in old age very common
Sudden sensorineural hearing loss	The cause is not known but it may respond to treatment with corticosteroids
Industrial (boilermaker's) deafness*	Chronic noise exposure or exposure to sudden extreme noise
Drug-induced	Ototoxic drugs include aminoglycoside antibiotics and some chemotherapeutic agents, aspirin and loop diuretics
Acoustic neuroma	Can also cause tinnitus and vertigo
Both	
Infection	Middle ear infection can interfere with tympanic membrane or ossicle function; viral cochleitis can cause sensorineural deafness
Head injury	Can damage the eardrum ossicles, cochlear or acoustic nerve

*Perhaps more common now in ageing popular musicians

TABLE 42.4

Tests of hearing can also provide information about the severity and anatomical site of hearing loss.

Sudden hearing loss (30 dB over 3 days) is an emergency. Causes include:
- viral infection
- bacterial meningitis
- migraine
- acoustic neuroma
- head injury
- drug reactions
- sarcoidosis, but
- 90% are idiopathic.

Examination method

Ear examination consists of inspection and palpation, otoscopy, tuning fork assessment, testing hearing and peripheral vestibular examination. In some cases lower cranial nerve assessment is indicated.

Inspect the position of the **pinna** and note its size and shape. Note any scars or swelling around the ears. Look for an obvious accessory auricle (separate piece of cartilage away from the pinna), cauliflower ears (haematomas from recurrent trauma, which obscure the normal anatomical features of the pinna) and bat ears (protrusion of the ears from the side of the head).

Look for **inflammation externally** and any obvious ear *discharge*. Inspect the auditory meatus and outer ear. There are four types of *otitis externa*, a condition associated with inflammation of the skin of the external canal:

1. *Acute localised otitis externa* involves the outer third of the auditory canal where the skin overlies cartilage and hair follicles are present. It is a form of furunculosis and is usually a result of *S. aureus* infection.

2. *Acute diffuse otitis externa* is often called swimmer's ear although it occurs in people who have not been swimming. Excessive moisture, heat and humidity, loss of protective cerumen and an increase in pH are responsible for skin

maceration and irritation. Infection may occur with *Pseudomonas aeruginosa*. The initial symptom is itching, which can progress to pain and is made worse by movement of the pinna. The appearance on examination ranges from mild erythema to severe erythema and swelling. There may be a small amount of white, clumpy discharge.

3. *Chronic otitis externa* is usually the result of repeated local irritation. This may be due to persistent drainage of a chronic middle ear infection but can also be caused by the insertion of foreign bodies into the ear (e.g. cotton swabs, ear picks). Itch is a more prominent symptom than pain. The appearance is of scaly erythematous dermatitis. It must be distinguished from other forms of dermatitis such as psoriasis, atopic dermatitis and seborrhoeic dermatitis.

4. *Malignant (invasive) otitis externa* is an aggressive and sometimes life-threatening condition. It affects elderly diabetics and immunocompromised patients. It begins in the external auditory canal and spreads slowly inwards. Untreated it can cause osteomyelitis of the base of the skull and reach the meninges and the brain. *Pseudomonas* infection is the most common cause but other organisms can be responsible. Deep otalgia is the most predominant symptom. The appearance at first is like that of severe chronic otitis externa. On examination there is discharge and the canal appears swollen and erythematous.

Then look for signs of **gouty tophi** (nodular, firm, pale and non-tender chalky depositions of urate in the cartilage of the ear, specific but not sensitive for gout).

Palpate the pinna for swelling or nodules. Pull it down gently; the manoeuvre is often painful when there is infection of the external canal.

Otoscope examination of the ears requires use of an earpiece that fits comfortably in the ear canal to allow inspection of the ear canal and tympanic membrane (see Fig. 42.13). This examination is essential for any patient presenting with an upper respiratory tract infection, any symptom related to the ears, dizziness, facial weakness or head injury. Always examine both ears!

Use of the otoscope

FIGURE 42.13

The correct technique is as follows. Ask the patient to turn his or her head slightly to the side, then pull the pinna up, out and back to straighten the ear canal and provide optimal vision. Stretch out the fingers of your hand holding the otoscope to touch the patient's cheek, to steady the instrument and to prevent sudden movements of the patient's head. When examining the patient's right ear, the otoscope is preferably held in a *downward position* with the right hand, while using the left hand to pull the pinna. An alternative position involves holding the otoscope upwards, but there is a risk that if the patient moves suddenly injury is more likely to occur.

Look at the **external canal** for any evidence of inflammation (e.g. redness or swelling) or discharge. There should be no tenderness unless there is inflammation. *Ear wax* is usually white or yellowish, and translucent and shiny; it can be moist or hard and impacted. It may obscure the view of the tympanic membrane. *Blood* or *cerebrospinal fluid* (watery, clear fluid) may be seen in the canal if there is a fracture at the base of the skull. In patients with herpes zoster, there may be *vesicles* (fluid-filled blisters) on the posterior wall around the external auditory meatus.

Inspect the **tympanic membrane** (eardrum) by introducing the speculum further into the canal in a forward but downward direction. The normal tympanic

CHAPTER 42 THE EYES, EARS, NOSE AND THROAT   787

The tympanic membrane as viewed through an otoscope

(From Mir MA. *Atlas of clinical diagnosis*, 2nd edn. Edinburgh: Saunders, 2003.)

FIGURE 42.14

Otitis media with hyperaemia of the tympanic membrane

(From Mir MA. *Atlas of clinical diagnosis*, 2nd edn. Edinburgh: Saunders, 2003.)

FIGURE 42.16

The detail of the tympanic membrane

(From Mir MA. *Atlas of clinical diagnosis*, 2nd edn. Edinburgh: Saunders, 2003.)

FIGURE 42.15

From the lower end of the handle a bright cone of light should be visible: the light reflex. The presence or absence of the light reflex is not a sensitive or a specific sign of disease. Note the colour, transparency and any evidence of *dilated blood vessels* (hyperaemia—a sign of otitis media; see Fig. 42.16). Look for *bulging* or *retraction* of the tympanic membrane. Bulging can suggest underlying fluid or pus in the middle ear. Retraction means a reduction in pressure in the middle ear and is a sign of a blocked Eustachian tube. Perforation of the tympanic membrane should be noted (see Fig. 42.17).

If a middle ear infection is suspected, **pneumatic auriscopy** can be useful. Use a speculum large enough to occlude the external canal snugly. Attach a rubber squeeze bulb to the otoscope. When the bulb is squeezed gently, air pressure in the canal is increased and the tympanic membrane should move promptly inwards. Absence of, or a decrease in, movement is a sign of fluid in the middle ear.

To test hearing, whisper numbers or words such as 'mark' or 'park' into one of the patient's ears while the other ear is distracted by movement of your finger in the auditory canal or the canal is occluded by pressure on the tragus. It is important to stand behind the patient to prevent lip reading. Then repeat the process with the other ear. With practice, the normal range of hearing is appreciated. If a patient says he or she is deaf, or the

membrane is a pearly grey colour. It is ovoid in shape and semitransparent (see Fig. 42.14). The upper fifth is called the *pars flaccida* and the lower four-fifths are called the *pars tensa* (see Fig. 42.15). The handle of the malleus is often visible near the centre of the latter.

Perforated tympanic membrane

(From Mir MA. *Atlas of clinical diagnosis*, 2nd edn. Edinburgh: Saunders, 2003.)

FIGURE 42.17

whisper test is positive, formal hearing testing (audiometry) is indicated.[3]

Traditionally, Rinne's and Weber's tests are performed if deafness is suspected, but these are not very useful screening tests:[3]

1. *Rinne's test:* place a vibrating 512 Hz tuning fork on the mastoid process. When the sound is no longer heard, move the fork close to the auditory meatus where, if air conduction is (as is normal) better than bone conduction, it will again be audible.
2. *Weber's test:* place a vibrating 512 Hz fork at the centre of the patient's forehead. Nerve deafness causes the sound to be heard better in the normal ear, but with conduction deafness the sound is heard better in the abnormal ear.

> **T&O'C ESSENTIALS**
>
> *If the patient or a relative says he or she is deaf then he or she is deaf. This can be confirmed by testing in 90% of cases.*

Sudden hearing loss requires urgent assessment and investigation.

Anatomy of the nose.

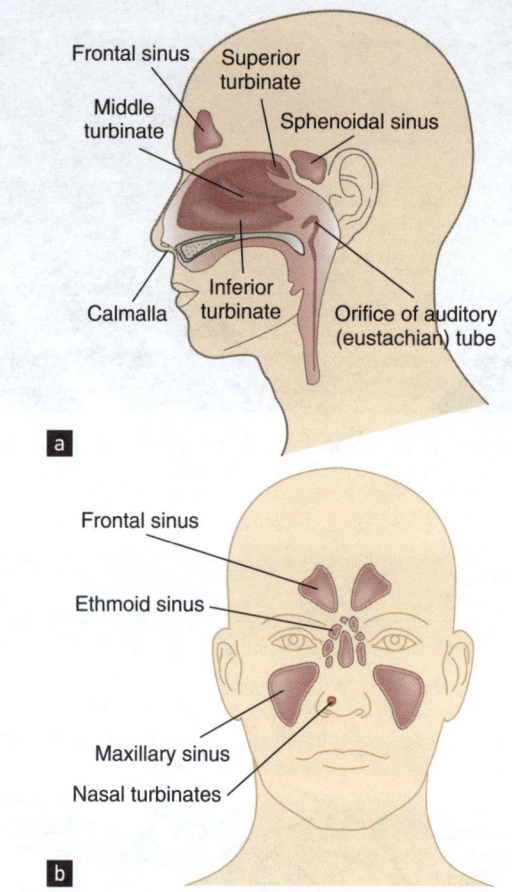

(a) Coronal view of paranasal sinuses; and (b) sagittal view of paranasal sinuses

FIGURE 42.18

NOSE AND SINUSES
Examination anatomy

The upper one-third of the nose is formed by the two nasal bones and the lower two-thirds are formed from cartilage (see Fig. 42.18). Cartilage divides the nose into its two cavities. The nasal bones articulate with the frontal bones and the maxilla. On the lateral walls of the nose the three pairs of nasal turbinates (superior, middle and inferior) cause turbulence as air enters the nose. This makes small particles drop onto the nasal mucosa, where cilia sweep them into the nasopharynx. The air is also warmed and humidified in the nose. Below each turbinate is a meatus named for the turbinate above it.

The frontal, maxillary and anterior ethmoid sinuses drain via the middle meatus. The posterior ethmoid sinus drains via the superior meatus. Drainage is assisted as a result of action of the ciliated epithelium. The maxillary sinus drains upwards against gravity through its ostium into the nasal cavity. This explains the importance of postural drainage for the treatment of bacterial sinusitis and why water drips from swimmers' noses when they bend over to dry their hair. The nasolacrimal duct drains into the inferior meatus. Drainage can be interrupted as a result of oedema (e.g. allergic rhinitis), mechanical obstruction (e.g. nasal polyps) or impaired ciliary function (Kartagener's syndrome).

The turbinates are vascular structures and their blood supply is under autonomic control. Sympathetic stimulation causes vasoconstriction and shrinkage of the turbinates. Parasympathetic stimulation causes vasodilation, swelling and sometimes obstruction of airflow and a watery discharge. The blood supply to the nose is from the internal and external carotid arteries. The blood vessels of the anterior nasal septum meet at *Little's*[i] *area*. This is about 2 centimetres from the nares (nostrils). Nose bleeds often come from this vascular area.

The nerve supply of the nose includes the olfactory nerve, which supplies the olfactory epithelium in the upper part of the nose. Fibres of the olfactory nerve pass through the cribriform plate of the ethmoid bone to reach the olfactory bulb in the brain. The rest of the inside of the nose is supplied by branches of the trigeminal nerve.

The vascular nasal mucosa produces mucus, which contains immunoglobulins. Mucus and the nasal hairs (*vibrissae*) trap particles and prevent them entering the lungs. The mucus is swept backwards by cilia and swallowed.

History

Common presenting problems include the following:

- *Nasal discharge (a runny nose):* consider allergy (watery discharge), a cold (coryza: more viscous discharge with or without fever and systemic symptoms) or sinusitis or a foreign body (purulent discharge)—see Questions box 42.4.
- *Blocked nose:* cold, foreign body, deviated nasal septum.
- *Epistaxis:* trauma (or nose picking), allergy, neoplasm or a cold. Ask about anticoagulation and use of antiplatelet drugs. Haematological malignancies and haemophilia are sometimes causes. Ask about the amount of blood loss, which can occasionally be severe. Have blood transfusions been required?
- *Anosmia or reduced sense of smell (often with apparent loss of taste):* consider mechanical obstruction due to polyps, infection or trauma if there is complete anosmia.
- *Symptoms of sinusitis:* 'sinus trouble again', cough, nasal congestion, sneezing, facial pain or headache worse with bending forwards, purulent discharge—see Table 42.5.
- *Big nose:* rhinophyma.

QUESTIONS TO ASK THE PATIENT WITH A BLOCKED NOSE

1. How long has your nose been blocked? (Acute problem suggests infection)
2. Are both sides of your nose affected or only one? (Deviation of nasal septum)
3. Have you had a problem with allergies?
4. Have you had polyps in your nose in the past?
5. Is the problem worse at different times of the year? (Allergic rhinitis)
6. Is it associated with sneezing? (Allergic rhinitis)
7. Have you had any injuries to your nose? Could there be anything in there? (Foreign body)
8. Are there any other symptoms? (Loss of sense of smell—polyps; headache and fullness in the head—sinusitis; fever)

QUESTIONS BOX 42.4

---

[i] William Little (1810–94), a surgeon at St Luke's hospital in New York, described this area in 1843.

Assessment for sinusitis

Sinusitis more likely	Sinusitis less likely
Maxillary toothache	Sore throat
Blocked nose	Itchy eyes
Purulent discharge	
Cough and sneezing	**Not helpful either way**
Headache	Malaise
Pain worse with bending	
Pain above the eye (frontal sinusitis)	
Periorbital pain (ethmoid sinusitis)	

TABLE 42.5

Examination method

Nose and sinus examination consists of inspection, palpation and testing the sense of smell. Inspect the **skin**. The patient concerned about a big nose may have a rhinophyma.[j] This enlargement and distortion of the skin of the nose is due to sebaceous gland enlargement. It is often associated with rosacea. Note any nasal deviation (best seen from behind the patient and looking down). Note any periorbital swelling (e.g. from sinusitis). Inspect the nares by pressing the tip of the nose upwards with the thumb.

Palpate the **nasal bones**. Then feel for facial swelling or signs of inflammation. Block each nostril to assess any obstruction by asking the patient to inhale. If there is a history of anosmia (loss of smell), test smell as described in Chapter 32 (cranial nerve I).

A saddle-nose deformity (collapse of the nasal septum) can occur in granulomatosis with polyangiitis (GPA) and relapsing polychondritis.

Examine **inside the nose** using a nasal speculum. This simple device with two blades can be used to open the nares. Hold the device in your left hand and introduce it into the patient's nose with the blades facing up and down. The blades should not rest or be pushed against the nasal septum. Use your other hand to steady and move the patient's head so that the inside of the nose can be seen. Your left index finger should rest against the patient's nose to steady the upper blade. Note:

1. deviation or perforation of the anterior septum

Bacterial ethmoidal sinusitis

(Courtesy of Dr A Watson, Infectious Diseases Department, The Canberra Hospital.)

FIGURE 42.19

2. the colour of the mucosa—usually a rich dark-red colour (darker than the oral mucosa) and smooth, moist and clean
3. the presence of bleeding, swelling or exudate
4. the presence of polyps—most often seen near the middle meatus
5. a foreign body
6. signs of bleeding at Little's area if epistaxis has occurred
7. the presence and nature of discharge (e.g. watery, purulent, bloody)
8. the size and colour of the turbinates.

Sinusitis

Sinusitis is inflammation of the paranasal sinuses. Pain and tenderness over the sinuses occurs, which in adults is classified as acute if less than 4 weeks in duration, subacute if 4–12 weeks in duration and chronic if greater than 12 weeks in duration. Most acute sinusitis is secondary to viral infection.[4]

Acute bacterial sinusitis (see Fig. 42.19) can occur after viral infection or in the setting of allergic rhinitis, in patients with anatomical abnormalities such as nasal septal deformity or polyps in the nose, or in immunocompromised patients. The most common

---

[j] From the Greek words meaning nose and an inflamed swelling.

bacterial causes of sinusitis are *Streptococcus pneumoniae* and *Haemophilus influenzae*. The four key clinical features suggesting that sinusitis may be bacterial are: (1) worsening symptoms after early improvement (a biphasic illness pattern), (2) purulent discharge from the nose, (3) tooth or facial pain over the maxillary sinus (especially if unilateral), and (4) tenderness over the maxillary sinus (unilaterally). Fever may occur.

Complications of acute bacterial sinusitis can include orbital cellulitis, meningitis, cavernous sinus thrombosis, brain abscess and osteolitis of the sinus bones. Therefore, if patients present with any of the following warning signs—periorbital oedema, visual changes or changes in mental status—you should be concerned about complicated bacterial sinusitis. Orbital cellulitis typically presents with erythema of the eyelid, oedema of the eyelid and proptosis. Periorbital cellulitis is a more benign condition caused by primary infection of the skin around the orbit.

Potential mimickers of acute bacterial sinusitis include GPA, carcinoma or lymphoma, sarcoidosis and, in immunocompromised or diabetic patients, fungal sinusitis. Chronic sinusitis presents with chronic sinus congestion, postnasal drip, cough, headache and bad breath.

Rhinocerebral mucormycosis is a fungal infection that destroys the sinuses. A black eschar may be seen on the nasal mucosa or palate.

Examination

There are two commonly used ways of illuminating the sinuses. The simpler method is to place a bright torch or proprietary transilluminoscope in the patient's mouth. The room must be completely dark and the patient must seal the lips around the device. Normal sinuses are visible through the skin of the face and appear as a warm glow. This method has the advantage that the two sides can be compared. The second method avoids the need to clean the torch between examinations. Place the torch over the infraorbital rim and shield your eyes from the light while peering into the patient's mouth to look for illumination of the hard palate.

MOUTH AND THROAT
Examination anatomy

The main structures of the oral cavity (see Fig. 42.20) are as follows:

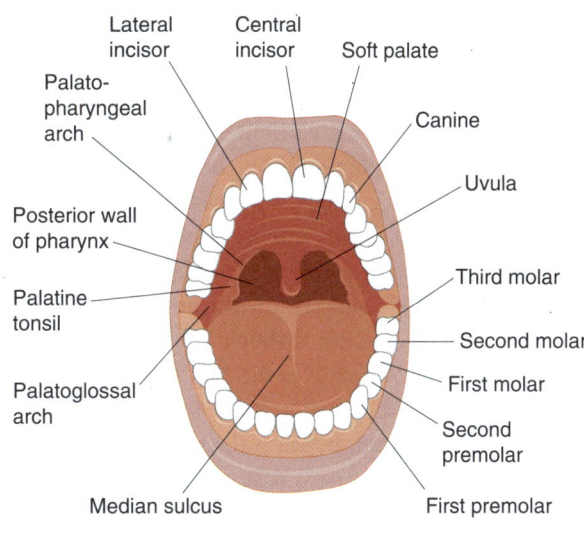

The mouth and throat

FIGURE 42.20

- The *lips* are covered in a thin epidermis and have numerous vascular papillae (the cause of their red colour).
- The *tongue* is attached to the hyoid bone. Its functions include eating and speech and it is the main area where taste is detected. It has a central sagittal median sulcus that ends posteriorly at the foramen caecum. The surface is rough because of its covering of papillae. The fungiform papillae are found on the tip and sides of the tongue. The largest papillae lie in front of the caecum and are called the circumvallate papillae. They divide the tongue into the posterior one-third and the anterior two-thirds.
- The *teeth*.
- The *hard palate* is a concave bony structure. Anteriorly its mucosa has raised folds called *rugae*. The *soft palate* is muscular and flexible. It ends at the uvula, which helps close off the nasopharynx during swallowing.
- The *taste buds* are found on the sides of the papillae. The chorda tympani, which is a division of the facial nerve, receives taste input from the anterior two-thirds of the tongue and the glossopharyngeal nerve from the posterior one-third. Salty taste is detected at the sides of the tongue, sweet taste at the tip of the tongue

and sourness and bitterness from the posterior third (glossopharyngeal nerve).
- The *salivary glands* lubricate the mouth and contain digestive enzymes including amylase. The largest are the parotid glands, which lie in front of the ears. They drain via Stensen's duct and through a papilla opposite the upper first molars. The submandibular glands are next in size. They are located below the angle of the mandible. They drain through Wharton's duct to papillae on either side of the frenulum below the tongue. The sublingual gland is found on the floor of the mouth beneath the tongue and drains through numerous small ducts.

History

The important symptoms of mouth and throat disease include the following:
- Pain in the mouth or throat (see Questions box 42.5).
- Ulceration (see Questions box 42.6).
- Bleeding: ask where the blood seems to be coming from (e.g. gums, throat or coughed up). Find out whether the patient is aware of a mass in the mouth or throat, whether there is bleeding anywhere else and whether he or she is taking antiplatelet or anticoagulant drugs.
- A mass or lump in the mouth: ask whether this is painful (infection) or not, how long it has been present and whether it has been bleeding (neoplasm).
- Dry mouth: ask about medications (e.g. antidepressants, antihistamines), previous radiotherapy (damage to salivary glands), dry eyes (sicca syndrome) and thrush (*Candida* infection is an association).
- Dysphagia: ask whether the patient has difficulty in swallowing only solids (oesophageal stricture or tumour) or liquids and solids (oesophageal motility problems). Is the problem associated with a sore throat (tonsillitis)?
- Dysphonia (difficulty with speech; see Questions box 42.7).

Examination method

Throat examination consists of inspection and palpation.

Inspect the **lips** for herpetic ulcers, Peutz–Jeghers syndrome, cyanosis and masses. The most common cause is a mucocele. These cystic painless lesions can be as large as a few centimetres in diameter. They are

QUESTIONS TO ASK THE PATIENT WITH PAIN IN THE MOUTH OR THROAT

1. Is the pain in your mouth? (Dental disease, ulcers)
2. What is the pain like? (Constant: toothache; only during exercise: angina; when eating: temporomandibular joint disease)
3. Is it painful when you swallow? (Tonsillitis, pharyngeal ulcers)
4. How long has it been there? (Acute problem suggests infection)
5. Have you had problems with your teeth?

QUESTIONS BOX 42.5

QUESTIONS TO ASK THE PATIENT WITH MOUTH ULCERS

1. Do you have more than one ulcer? (Multiple suggests systemic disease is possible, e.g. Crohn's disease)
2. Are they painful? (Painless suggests malignancy)
3. Have you had ulcers or lesions anywhere else: penis, vagina, anus? (Sexually transmitted infection, Crohn's disease)
4. Have you been unwell and are your lips involved? (Herpes simplex primary infection)
5. Have you had these many times before? (Aphthous ulcers)
6. Do you smoke or drink alcohol? (Malignant ulcers)

QUESTIONS BOX 42.6

> **QUESTIONS TO ASK THE PATIENT WITH HOARSENESS CAUSING DIFFICULTY WITH SPEECH (DYSPHONIA)**
>
> 1. How long have you been hoarse? (Short history suggests laryngitis)
> 2. Is it getting worse?
> 3. Have you had an injury to your neck?
> 4. Are you a smoker? (Laryngeal carcinoma, carcinoma of the lung and recurrent laryngeal nerve palsy)
> 5. Do you have to use your voice extensively? (Overuse, vocal cord papilloma)
> 6. Have you had a recent anaesthetic? (Intubation injury)
> 7. Have you had thyroid disease? (Hypothyroidism)
>
> QUESTIONS BOX 42.7

caused by traumatic damage or obstruction of a small salivary gland.

Look at the **buccal mucosa, palate and teeth**. Using a light, push the buccal mucosa out of the way with a tongue depressor. Note any signs of inflammation (e.g. redness, swelling). Look at the parotid duct opening (for inflammation). White painless plaques (leucoplakia) may be present on the gingivae, tongue or buccal mucosa. This is a precancerous condition. Lichen planus also causes a white painless lesion in the mouth. It has a reticulated pattern. Look for masses and ulcerated lesions. Inspect the teeth for obvious decay and infection.

Look at the **gingivae** for hypertrophy (associated with phenytoin use, leukaemia and pregnancy), bleeding and inflammation. Erythroplakia is a mucosal abnormality characterised by red granular papules that bleed easily. It has more malignant potential than leucoplakia.

Inspect the **tongue** first in the mouth, then ask the patient to poke it out to one side and then the other. Weakness of the tongue due to neurological or muscular disease may be seen. Look for masses and mucosal changes as with the rest of the mouth. The surface of the tongue may show localised red areas denuded of papillae surrounded by white or yellow margins and looking rather like a map. This is called *geographical tongue* and is quite benign. Elongation and pigmentation (from food or tobacco staining or certain microorganisms) of the papillae makes the tongue look black and hairy. This is also benign. A tongue with exaggerated fissures is called a *scrotal tongue*; it is also benign. Look for evidence of *Candida* infection (see Fig. 42.22). These white lesions cover an inflamed mucosa and may be the result of immunodeficiency or recent antibiotic use.

Inspect the **floor of the mouth** and under the tongue. Ask the patient to lift the tongue up onto the hard palate to give you a good view. Large veins may be visible under the tongue in elderly people. These are benign and are not a cause of bleeding. Inspect the mucosal surfaces for the abnormalities described above. There may also be a *ranula*.[k] This is a large mucus retention cyst. These can be quite large and although painless eventually interfere with eating and speech.

Inspect the hard and soft **palates** for similar mucosal lesions and the hard palate for petechiae. A common benign finding is a bony swelling of the posterior part of the hard palate. This occurs in the midline and is often lobulated. It is called a *torus palatinus*.[l]

Palpate the tongue with your gloved hand. Hold it with some gauze with one hand and feel with the other. The anterior two-thirds can usually be palpated without provoking the gag reflex. Feel for induration (hardening) of any lesion (a sign of malignancy).

Now palpate the floor of the mouth. Using both gloved hands, feel with your right index finger pointing downwards under the tongue and your left index finger under the chin and pushing upwards. Use the thumb and third finger of your left hand to push the patient's cheeks in between the teeth; this is a precaution that prevents your finger being bitten. Feel between your fingers for masses and tenderness. Feel the submandibular salivary glands.

Ask the patient to say 'Ah', then inspect the **oropharynx and uvula** (there is often a need to press a tongue depressor on the tongue to see properly—and using two tongue depressors can help even further). The tongue should be pushed forwards behind the front teeth. Applying the depressor too far back will cause

---

[k] From the Latin word for tadpole or little frog.
[l] From the Latin for a swelling or protuberance.

Buccal ulcer
(Courtesy of Dr A Watson, Infectious Diseases Department, The Canberra Hospital.)

FIGURE 42.21

Candidiasis
(Courtesy of Dr A Watson, Infectious Diseases Department, The Canberra Hospital.)

FIGURE 42.22

Koplik's spot (measles)
(Courtesy of Dr A Watson, Infectious Diseases Department, The Canberra Hospital.)

FIGURE 42.23

gagging; too far forward and the tongue will roll up and obscure the pharynx. Inspect the tonsils (note the size, shape and colour, and any discharge or membrane—they involute in adults and may not be seen). Enlarged tonsils with a covering of membrane or pus are typical of viral or bacterial tonsillitis. Enlargement may occur in patients with leukaemia and lymphoma.

Examine the **cervical lymph nodes**.

Abnormalities to look and feel for in the mouth and throat examination include:

1. angular stomatitis
2. the state of the teeth and gums
3. gum and tongue ulcers (herpes simplex, aphthous ulcers [see Fig. 42.21], candidiasis [see Fig. 42.22])
4. mucosal mass (consider malignancy)
5. parotid duct pus
6. Koplik's spot (measles; see Fig. 42.32)
7. tongue: smooth (iron, B_{12} deficiency), big (acromegaly, tumour), wasted and fasciculating (motor neurone disease), ulcers and white patches
8. tonsils: present or absent, inflamed or covered in pus; enlarged (lymphoma)
9. salivary glands: size and tenderness; squeeze to express pus through the salivary duct
10. the draining lymph nodes: tenderness and enlargement (see Fig. 42.24)
11. stridor and cough
12. the appropriate cranial nerves, if indicated.

Pharyngitis

A sore throat due to an exudative pharyngitis in adults is usually secondary to infection. The specific causes of pharyngitis include viruses in about 50% of cases (especially Epstein–Barr virus [EBV] in adolescents—1 in 13 cases) (see Good signs guide 42.1). About 10% of cases are due to the group A beta-haemolytic streptococci (see Fig. 42.25). *Neisseria gonorrhoea* is an

Submandibular abscess

(Courtesy of Dr A Watson, Infectious Diseases Department, The Canberra Hospital.)

FIGURE 42.24

Streptococcal throat

(Courtesy of Dr A Watson, Infectious Diseases Department, The Canberra Hospital.)

FIGURE 42.25

GOOD SIGNS GUIDE 42.1
Infectious mononucleosis (glandular fever)

Symptom or sign	Sensitivity or positive likelihood range (LR)
Sore throat and tiredness	Sensitivity range 0.81–83 (not specific)
Absence of any lymphadenopathy	LR +ve range 0.23–0.44
Posterior cervical lymphadenopathy	LR +ve 3.1
Inguinal or axillary lymphadenopathy	LR +ve 3
Petechiae on the palate	LR +ve 5.3
Splenomegaly	LR +ve range 1.9–6.6

uncommon cause of pharyngitis in adults, and primary human immunodeficiency virus (HIV) infection is an occasional cause; typically, there are sexual risk factors present in the history. The other two most important viruses are herpes simplex and adenovirus. Many cases of pharyngitis are of unknown cause. Clinically, there is redness of the pharynx with or without ulceration.

Clinical criteria help to determine whether or not pharyngitis may be due to beta-haemolytic streptococcus (the four-item Centor score):[6]

- absence of cough
- fever
- pharyngeal exudate
- anterior cervical adenopathy.

If all four criteria are present, this helps predict the presence of this infection, while the absence of the last three strongly suggests that the infection is *not* due to beta-haemolytic streptococcus.

Despite these criteria it is difficult to distinguish viral from bacterial pharyngitis in many cases. Antibiotic therapy should be reserved for patients who are at high risk of rheumatic fever and those who are very unwell.

Supraglottitis (epiglottitis)

Supraglottitis is a rare but important cause of sore throat.[7] This disease classically presents with a triad of sore throat, painful swallowing (odynophagia) and fever. The patient may uncommonly have stridor, which may be misdiagnosed as asthma; here there is inspiratory wheeze due to the inflammation above the epiglottis. Pooling of secretions is another clue to the diagnosis. Urgent medical attention is indicated to prevent airway obstruction.

COMMON INVESTIGATIONS

CT scans can be commonly used in the diagnosis of nasopharyngeal tumours and sinusitis (see Figs 42.26 and 42.27). They can help identify the spread of infection into the brain and orbits.

The visual fields can be mapped accurately with a visual field chart. Retinal photographs are often used for the screening of diabetic patients.

Nasopharyngeal carcinoma.

This CT scan shows a soft-tissue mass obstructing the right nasopharynx and right Eustachian tube

(From Haaga JR, Boll D, Dogra VS et al. *CCT and MRI of the whole body*, 5th edn. Maryland Heights MO: Mosby, 2008.)

FIGURE 42.26

Acute sinusitis.

This CT scan coronal view shows opacification of the right maxillary sinus; the left is almost completely opacified, with only a small air pocket visible

(From Zitelli BJ, Davis HW. *Atlas of pediatric physical diagnosis*, 5th edn. Philadelphia: Saunders, 2007.)

FIGURE 42.27

T&O'C ESSENTIALS

1. Important local and systemic disease will be missed unless the eyes and ears are examined as part of a general medical examination.
2. Accurate fundoscopy with the ophthalmoscope requires practice. Dilating the patient's pupils may be necessary to obtain an adequate view.
3. Subtle eye signs, such as Horner's syndrome, will be missed unless time is taken to stand back and compare the two sides.

OSCE EXAMPLES

A. EYE EXAMINATION

Mrs Baker has had painful eyes. Please examine her sclerae and conjunctivae.

1. Stand back to look. This is probably a spot diagnosis.
2. Look for scleral icterus. Proceed accordingly if present.
3. Look for conjunctival pallor or injection, or chemosis or subconjunctival haemorrhage.
4. Note the distribution of any redness (e.g. single red eye in iritis). Decide whether conjunctival injection is central (iritis) or spares the central region (conjunctivitis).
5. If there is conjunctival injection, ask for gloves before pulling down the lower lid. Note any ocular discharge (conjunctivitis).
6. If there is pallor, pull down the lower lid and compare the pearly white posterior part of the conjunctiva with the red anterior part.
7. If there is chemosis, look for proptosis and other signs of thyrotoxicosis.
8. Look at the iris (haziness indicates oedema or inflammation).
9. Look and test the pupils (e.g. small irregular pupil in iritis, dilated oval poorly reactive pupil in acute glaucoma).
10. Assess eye movements (painful in scleritis).
11. Fundoscopy (e.g. corneal ulceration looks black examining the red reflex).
12. Look for systemic evidence of vasculitis (e.g. urinalysis).

B. FUNDOSCOPY

Mr Abbott has diabetes. Please look in his fundi.

1. The pupils will probably have been dilated.
2. Use the ophthalmoscope in the approved manner.
3. Look for changes of hypertension or diabetes.

C. VISUAL LOSS

Ms Jenny Elder has experienced sudden loss of vision in one eye. Please examine her.

1. Test *each* eye for visual acuity, and fully assess the visual fields.
2. Assess each pupil's reaction to light and accommodation, and for an afferent pupillary defect (optic nerve damage).
3. Test eye movements and ask about any pain on movement (optic neuritis).
4. Examine the fundi. Note whether the disc is swollen and is abnormally pink or white (ischaemic optic neuropathy). Note any retinal fundal pallor (arterial occlusion), haemorrhages (venous occlusion) or an obvious embolus (at an arterial bifurcation).
5. Test colour vision (for optic nerve damage) if red–green test plates are available.
6. Auscultate for a carotid bruit (stenosis).
7. Take the pulse (atrial fibrillation) and blood pressure (hypertension).
8. Test the urine for blood or protein (vasculitis).

D. EAR EXAMINATION

Mr Li complains of a sore ear. Please examine his auditory canal and eardrum.

1. Note whether the patient looks unwell or feverish.
2. Look at the pinna and external auditory meatus for gouty tophi, dermatitis, cellulitis, signs of trauma (e.g. haematoma), scars (e.g. surgery) and discharge.
3. Look at both ears.
4. Ask the patient whether the ear is painful before using the otoscope to examine the canal and drum.
5. Look for erythema or blisters in the canal and for wax, pus or discharge from the drum.
6. Inspect the tympanic membrane (eardrum) for perforation, grommets or loss of the normal shiny appearance.

Continued

OSCE EXAMPLES continued

7. Test hearing, and perform Weber's and Rinné's tests.
8. Palpate the temporomandibular joint for tenderness and crepitus (referred pain).
9. Examine the throat for inflammation (referred pain).

E. THROAT EXAMINATION

Ms Peta Smith complains of recurrent sore throat. Please examine her.

1. Put on gloves and remove any dentures. Note any drooling or flushing or whether the patient appears ill.
2. Take a torch and ask the patient to open wide.
3. Inspect the mouth and pharynx using a tongue depressor. Note tonsillar enlargement and any erythema or other signs of inflammation.
4. Note whether the patient cannot open the mouth fully (trismus).
5. Feel the oral cavity and tongue gently with a gloved finger.

OSCE REVISION TOPICS – EYES, EARS, NOSE AND THROAT

Use these topics, which commonly occur in the OSCE, to help with revision.

1. This woman has experienced some loss of vision. Please take a history and then examine her. (pp 772, 797)
2. This woman complains of painful red eyes. Please examine her. (pp 772, 797)
3. This man has double vision. Please examine him. (p 506)
4. This man with diabetes mellitus has problems with his vision. Please examine his fundi. His pupils have been dilated. (pp 776, 797)
5. This woman has a sore throat. Please examine her. (pp 792, 798)
6. This woman reports that she has sinusitis again. Please examine her. (p 790)
7. This man has mouth ulcers. Please take a history and then examine him. (p 792)
8. This man has noticed a problem with deafness. Please take a history and then examine him (speak loudly). (p 783)

References

1. Robinett DA, Kahn DH. The physical examination of the eye. *Emerg Med Clin North Am* 2008; 26:1–16. An excellent summary of eye anatomy and examination.
2. McGee S. *Evidence-based clinical diagnosis*, 3rd edn. St Louis: Saunders, 2012.
3. Bagai A, Thavendiranathan P, Detsky AS. Does this patient have hearing impairment? *JAMA* 2006; 295(4):416–428.
4. Gwaltney JM, Sydnor A, Sande MA. Etiology and antimicrobial treatment of acute sinusitis. *Ann Otol Rhinol Larygol Suppl* 1981; 90(3 pt 3):68–71.
5. Ebell MH, Call M, Shinholser J, Gardner J. The Rational Clinical Examination Systematic Review. Does this patient have infectious mononucleosis? *JAMA* 2016; 315(14):1502–1509.
6. McIsaac WJ, Kellner JD, Aufricht P et al. Empirical validation of guidelines for the management of pharyngitis in children and adults. *JAMA* 2004; 291(13):1587–1595.
7. Cirilli AR. Emergency evaluation and management of the sore throat. *Emerg Med Clin North Am* 2013; 31(2):501–515.

CHAPTER 43
The skin and lumps

For one mistake made for not knowing, ten mistakes are made for not looking. J A LINDSAY

EXAMINATION ANATOMY

Fig. 43.1 shows the three main layers of the skin: the epidermis, dermis and subcutaneous fat. These layers can all be involved in skin diseases in varying combinations. For example, most skin tumours arise in the epidermis (see Fig. 43.2), some bullous eruptions occur at the dermoepidermal junction (DEJ), and lipomas are tumours of subcutaneous fat. The skin appendages, which include the sweat (eccrine and apocrine) glands, hair follicles (see Fig. 43.3) and the nails, are common sites of infection.

The eccrine glands are present everywhere except in the nail beds and on some mucosal surfaces. They are able to secrete over 5 litres of sweat per day. The apocrine glands are found in association with hair follicles but are confined to certain areas of the body, including the axillae, the pubis, the perineum and the nipples. They secrete a viscous fluid whose function is unclear in humans.

The nails are formed from heavily keratinised cells that grow from the nail matrix. The matrix grows in a semilunar shape and appears as the lunules in normal finger- and toenails. Hair is also the product of

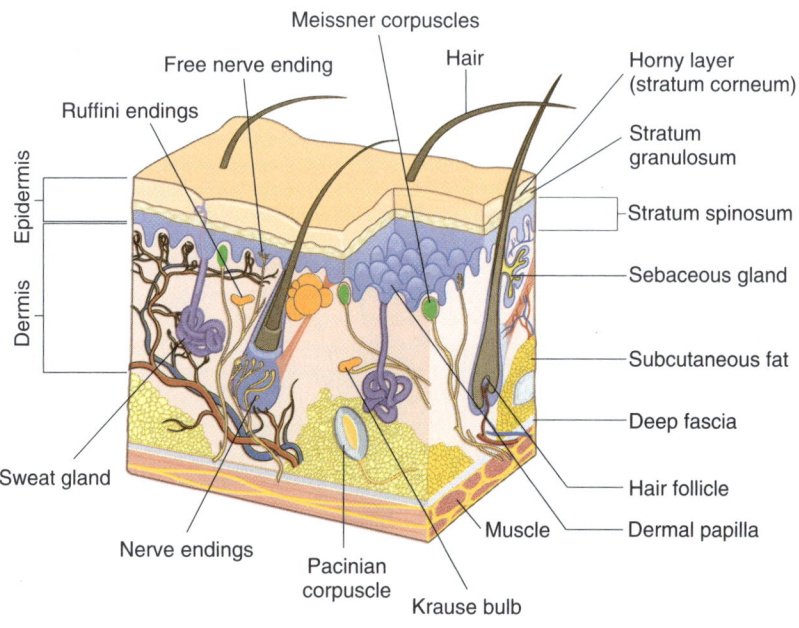

The layers of the skin

FIGURE 43.1

specialised epithelial cells and grows from the hair matrix within the hair follicle.

DERMATOLOGICAL HISTORY

For any patient with a rash or skin condition, it is important to determine when and where it began, its distribution, whether it has changed over time, its relationship to sun exposure or other environmental conditions and any treatments tried[1] (see Questions box 43.1). Ask whether pruritus is associated; localised pruritus is usually due to dermatological disease, but generalised pruritus can be present without a primary rash—such as in liver or renal disease and haematological malignancies. If an infestation is the suspected cause of pruritus it is useful to ascertain whether other household members are affected. Determine also whether pain or disturbed sensation has occurred; for example, inflammation and oedema can produce pain in the skin, whereas disease involving neurovascular bundles or nerves can produce burning or anaesthesia (e.g. leprosy, syphilis, cutaneous neural tumours). Constitutional symptoms such as fever, headache, fatigue, anorexia, weight loss and depression also need to be documented.

Ask about a past personal or family history of rashes, allergic reactions or medical conditions. Asthma, eczema or hay fever suggests atopy. Similarly, evidence of systemic disease in the past may be important in a patient with a rash (e.g. diabetes mellitus, connective tissue disease, inflammatory bowel disease).

A detailed social history needs to be obtained regarding occupation and hobbies, as chemical exposure and contact with animals or plants can all induce dermatitis. All medications that have been taken must be documented. Orally ingested or parenteral

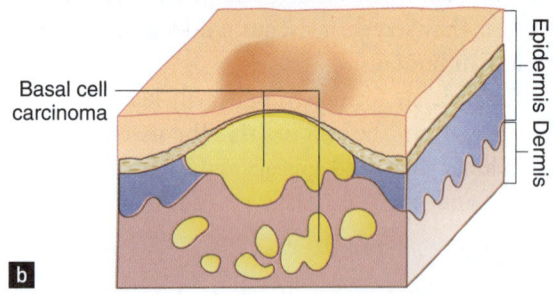

(a) Melanoma; (b) basal cell carcinoma

FIGURE 43.2

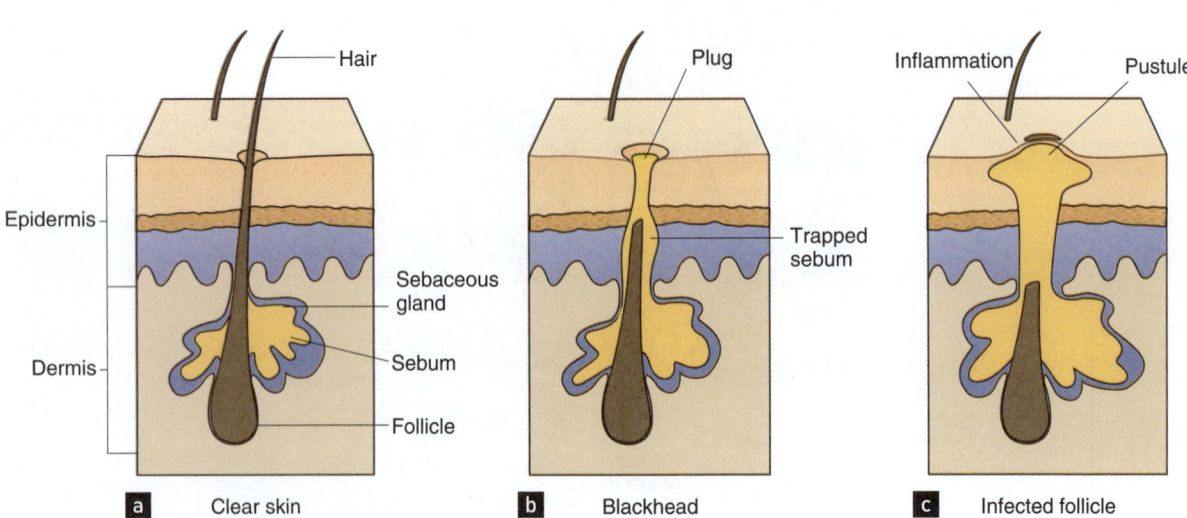

Common sites of infection in the skin

FIGURE 43.3

QUESTIONS TO ASK THE PATIENT WITH A RASH

1. How long have you had the rash?
2. Have you ever had it before?*
3. Is it getting worse?
4. What parts of your skin are affected (e.g. sun-exposed areas, areas in contact with clothing or chemicals)?
5. Was the rash flat or raised to begin with, or was it blistered?
6. Is the area itchy?
7. Does anything seem to make it better?
8. Has your diet changed recently?
9. What treatment have you tried for it?
10. Have you had a fever or any joint pains?
11. Have you had problems with allergies?
12. Are you taking any tablets or medicines? Are any of these new (in the last 6 weeks)?
13. Have you changed your soap, shampoo, deodorant or washing powder recently?
14. What sort of work do you do? Do you come into contact with chemicals at work or with your hobbies?
15. Have you travelled recently? Where to?
16. Has anyone you know got a similar rash?
17. Have you any other problems with your health?

*When a dermatologist cannot decide the cause of a rash this question can help. If the patient says that he or she has had the rash before, the clinician can then say with confidence 'Well, you've got it again'.

QUESTIONS BOX 43.1

Types of cutaneous drug reactions

1. Acne (e.g. steroids)
2. Hair loss (alopecia; e.g. cancer chemotherapy)
3. Pigment alterations: hypomelanosis (e.g. hydroxyquinone, chloroquine, topical steroids), hypermelanosis
4. Exfoliative dermatitis or erythroderma (p 814)
5. Urticaria (hives; e.g. non-steroidal anti-inflammatory drugs, radiographic dyes, penicillin)
6. Maculopapular (morbilliform) eruptions (see Fig. 43.4; e.g. ampicillin, allopurinol)
7. Photosensitive eruptions (e.g. sulfonamides, sulfonylureas, chlorothiazides, phenothiazines, tetracycline, nalidixic acid, anticonvulsants)
8. Drug-induced lupus erythematosus (e.g. procainamide, hydralazine, minocycline)
9. Vasculitis (e.g. propylthiouracil, allopurinol, thiazides, penicillin, phenytoin)
10. Skin necrosis (e.g. warfarin)
11. Drug-precipitated porphyria (e.g. alcohol, barbiturates, sulfonamides, contraceptive pill)
12. Lichenoid eruptions (e.g. antimalarials, beta-blockers)
13. Fixed drug eruption (e.g. sulfonamides, tetracycline, phenylbutazone)
14. Bullous eruptions (e.g. frusemide, nalidixic acid, penicillamine, clonidine)
15. Erythema nodosum or erythema multiforme (p 816)
16. Toxic epidermal necrolysis (e.g. allopurinol, phenytoin, sulfonamides, non-steroidal anti-inflammatory drugs)
17. Pruritus (e.g. opiates, antibiotics, ACE inhibitors, monoclonal antibodies)
18. Psoriasiform (e.g. lithium, beta-blockers)

TABLE 43.1

Maculopapular eruption

FIGURE 43.4

medications can cause a host of cutaneous lesions and can mimic many skin diseases (see Table 43.1).

GENERAL PRINCIPLES OF PHYSICAL EXAMINATION OF THE SKIN

The aim of this chapter is to provide an approach to the diagnosis of skin diseases.[2,3] Particular emphasis will be placed on cutaneous signs as indications of systemic disease. Other chapters have included the usual clues that can be used to arrive at a particular diagnosis. This chapter tries to unify the concept of 'inspection' as a valuable starting point in the examination of the patient. Text box 43.1 gives a suggested method for the dermatological examination.

Ask the patient to undress down to their undergarments and provide a gown for modesty. The whole surface of the skin and its appendages should

The dermatological examination: a suggested method

Even if the patient shows the examiner only a small single area of abnormality, proceed to examine all the skin, mucous membranes and nails (Fig. 43.5).

After obtaining good lighting conditions and asking the patient to disrobe, begin by looking at the **nails and hands**. Paronychia is an infection of the skin surrounding the nails. Other changes to note include pitting (psoriasis, fungal infections) and onycholysis (e.g. thyrotoxicosis, psoriasis). Dark staining under the nail may indicate a subungual melanoma. Linear splinter haemorrhages (e.g. vasculitis) or telangiectasias (e.g. systemic lupus erythematosus) may be seen in the nail bed.

A purplish discoloration in streaks over the knuckles may indicate dermatomyositis (Gottron's papules). Also look at the backs of the hands and forearms for the characteristic blisters of porphyria, which occur on the exposed skin. Papules and scratch marks on the backs of the hands, between the fingers and around the wrists may indicate scabies. Viral warts are common on the hands.

Look at the palms for Dupuytren's contracture, pigmented flat junctional moles (which have a high risk of becoming malignant) and xanthomata in the palmar creases.

Next look at the **forearms**, where lichen planus may occur on the flexor surfaces (characterised by small shiny, violaceous flat-topped polygonal papules) and psoriasis may be present on the extensor surfaces. Palpable purpura—raised bruising that indicates bleeding into the skin—may be seen on the arms and indicates vasculitis. Acanthosis nigricans can occur in the axillae.

Inspect the patient's **hair and scalp**. Decide whether or not the hair is dry and whether the distribution is normal. Alopecia may indicate male pattern baldness, recent severe illness, hypothyroidism or thyrotoxicosis. Patches of alopecia occur in the disease alopecia areata. Short broken-off hairs occur typically in systemic lupus erythematosus. In psoriasis there are silvery scales, which may be seen on the skin of the scalp. Metastatic deposits may rarely be felt as firm nodules within the skin of the scalp. Sebaceous cysts are common. The unfortunate examiner may find nits sticking to the head hairs.

Move down now to the **eyebrows** and look for scaling and greasiness, which are found in seborrhoeic dermatitis. A purplish erythema occurs around the eyelids in dermatomyositis (heliotrope rash). Xanthelasmata are seen near the eyelid.

Look at the **face** for rosacea, which causes bright erythema of the nose, cheeks, forehead and chin, and occasionally pustules and rhinophyma (disfiguring swelling of the nose). Acne causes papules, pustules and comedones involving the face, neck and upper trunk. The butterfly rash of systemic lupus erythematosus occurs across the cheeks but is rare. Spider naevi may be present. Ulcerating lesions on the face may include basal cell carcinoma, squamous cell carcinoma or, rarely, tuberculosis (lupus vulgaris).

Other tumours of the face include keratoacanthoma (a volcano-like lesion from a sebaceous gland) and congenital haemangiomas.

Look for the blisters of herpes zoster, which may occur strictly in the distribution of one of the divisions of the trigeminal nerve.

Inspect the **neck**, which is prone to many of the lesions that occur on the face. Rarely, the redundant loose skin of pseudoxanthoma elasticum will be seen around the neck.

Go on to inspect the **trunk**, where any of the childhood exanthema produce their characteristic rashes. Look for spider naevi. Campbell de Morgan spots are commonly found on the abdomen (and chest), as are flat, greasy, yellow-coloured seborrhoeic keratosis. They may also be pigmented (brown or black) or skin-coloured. Erythema marginatum (rheumatic fever) occurs on the chest and abdomen. Herpes zoster may be seen overlying any of the dermatome distributions.

TEXT BOX 43.1

CHAPTER 43 **THE SKIN AND LUMPS** 803

The dermatological examination: a suggested method *continued*

Sites of some important skin lesions of the limbs, face and trunk.

SLE = systemic lupus erythematosus

FIGURE 43.5

TEXT BOX 43.1

Continued

The dermatological examination: a suggested method *continued*

Metastases from internal malignancies may rarely occur anywhere on the skin. Neurofibromas are soft flesh-coloured tumours; when associated with more than five 'café-au-lait' spots (brownish, irregular lesions) they suggest neurofibromatosis. Pigmented moles are seen on the trunk and these should be assessed for signs of melanoma. The patient's buttocks and sacrum must be examined for bedsores, and the abdomen and thighs may have areas of fat atrophy or hypertrophy from insulin injections.

Go to the **legs**, where erythema nodosum or erythema multiforme may be seen on the shins. Necrobiosis lipoidica diabeticorum affects the skin over the tibia in diabetics. Pretibial myxoedema also occurs over the shins. Look for ulcers on either side of the lower part of the leg. Livedo reticularis is a net-like, red reticular rash that occurs in vasculitis, the antiphospholipid syndrome and with atheroembolism.

Inspect the **feet** for the characteristic lesion of reactive arthritis called keratoderma blennorrhagicum, where crusted lesions spread across the sole because of the fusion of vesicles and pustules. Look at the foot for signs of ischaemia, associated with wasting of the skin and skin appendages. Trophic ulcers may be seen in patients with peripheral neuropathy (e.g. diabetes mellitus). Always separate the toes to look for melanomas.

TEXT BOX 43.1

CONSIDERATIONS WHEN EXAMINING THE SKIN

1. Hair
2. Nails
3. Sebaceous glands—oil-producing and present on the head, neck and back
4. Eccrine glands—sweat-producing and present all over the body
5. Apocrine glands—sweat-producing and present in the axillae and groin
6. Mucosa

LIST 43.1

---

be carefully inspected (see List 43.1). The genitals are not routinely inspected unless directed by the patient or a specific pathology is being investigated.

When examining actual skin lesions, a number of features should be documented. First, the morphology of each lesion should be *described* precisely. Use the appropriate dermatological terminology (see Table 43.2), even though this may seem to make dermatological diseases more, rather than less, mysterious. As many dermatological diagnoses are purely descriptive, a good description will often be of considerable help in making the diagnosis. Second, the *distribution* of the lesions should be noted, as certain distributions suggest specific diagnoses. Third, the *pattern* of the lesions—such as linear, annular (ring-shaped), reticulated (net-like), serpiginous (snake-like) or grouped—also helps establish the diagnosis. Then *palpate* the lesions, noting texture, consistency, tenderness, temperature, depth and mobility.

Types of skin lesions are shown in Fig. 43.8 and a clinical algorithm for diagnosis is presented in Fig. 43.9. It is always important to keep in mind whether the skin changes are primary (i.e. caused by the disease itself) or secondary (i.e. caused by the patient—like excoriations [scratch marks]—or by the lesion's evolution—e.g. erosion or ulceration, crusting, eschar, fissuring or lichenification). Remember that if the history and clinical examination do not lead to a satisfactory explanation for a rash or lesion then a skin biopsy is a simple procedure of immense diagnostic utility.

HOW TO APPROACH THE CLINICAL DIAGNOSIS OF A LUMP

First, determine the lump's site, size, shape, consistency, mobility and tenderness. Next, evaluate in what tissue layer the lump is situated. If it is in the *epidermis or dermis* (e.g. epidermoid cyst, verruca), it should move when the skin is moved, but if it is in the *subcutaneous tissue* (e.g. neurofibroma, lipoma, lymph node), the skin can be moved over the lump. If it is in the *muscle or tendon* (e.g. tumour), then contraction of the muscle

Dermatological terms

Term	Definition	Descriptive terms	
Atrophy	Thinning of the skin with loss of normal markings	Annular	Ring-shaped (clear centre; e.g. tinea infection)
Bulla	A large collection of fluid below the epidermis (>1 cm)	Arcuate	Curved (e.g. secondary syphilis)
Crust	Dried serum, exudate, blood or pus	Circinate	Circular
Ecchymoses	Bruises	Confluent	Lesions that have coalesced (e.g. measles)
Excoriations	Lesions caused by scratching that results in loss of the epidermis	Discoid	Circular without a clear centre (e.g. lupus)
Keloid (see Fig. 43.6)	Persistent thickened scar that extends beyond the original wound margins	Eczematous	Inflamed scaly poorly defined plaques (e.g. atopic dermatitis)
Macule	A flat, non-palpable circumscribed alteration of skin colour (<1 cm)	Keratotic	Thickened from increased keratin (e.g. psoriasis, keratoacanthoma)
Nodule	A circumscribed palpable mass (>1 cm)	Lichenified	Thickening and roughening of the epidermis associated with accentuated skin markings
Papule	A circumscribed palpable elevation (<1 cm)	Linear	In lines (e.g. contact dermatitis)
Petechiae	Purpuric, non-blanching spots (<5 mm)	Papulosquamous	Plaques associated with scaling
Pigment alterations	Increased (hyperpigmentation) or decreased (hypopigmentation)	Reticulated	In a network pattern (e.g. cutaneous parasite)
Plaque	An elevated circumscribed thickened epidermis (>1 cm)	Serpiginous	Sinuous
Purpura	Purple, non-blanching spots (>5 mm)	Zosteriform (see Fig. 43.7)	Following a dermatomal distribution
Pustule	A visible collection of pus		
Scale	An accumulation of excess keratin (hyperkeratosis)		
Sclerosis	Fibrosis of subcutaneous tissues, which may involve the dermis		
Ulcer	Full thickness loss of epidermis, which may also include the dermis and subcutis		
Vesicle	A small collection of fluid below the epidermis (<1 cm)		
Wheal	An area of dermal oedema		

TABLE 43.2

or tendon will limit the lump's mobility. If it is in a *nerve*, pressing on the lump may result in pins and needles being felt in the distribution of the nerve, and the lump cannot be moved in the longitudinal axis but can be moved in the transverse axis. If it is in *bone*, the lump will be immobile.

Determine whether the lump is *fluctuant* (i.e. contains fluid). Place one forefinger (the 'watching' finger) halfway between the centre and the periphery of the lump. Place the forefinger from your other hand (the 'displacing' finger) diagonally opposite the watching finger at an equal distance from the centre of the lump. Press with the displacing finger and keep the watching finger still. If the lump contains fluid, the watching finger will be displaced in *both* axes of the lump (i.e. fluctuation is present).

Place a small torch behind the lump to determine whether it can be *transilluminated*. Light will be

Keloid

FIGURE 43.6

Zosteriform rash of the left buttock

(Courtesy of Dr A Watson, Infectious Diseases Department, The Canberra Hospital.)

FIGURE 43.7

transmitted through a cystic lump, which will appear to glow when transilluminated.

Note any associated signs of *inflammation* (i.e. heat, redness, tenderness and swelling[a]).

Look for similar lumps elsewhere, such as multiple subcutaneous swellings from neurofibromas or lipomas. Neurofibromas are smaller than lipomas. They look hard but are remarkably soft; they occur in neurofibromatosis type 1 (von Recklinghausen's[b] disease). They continue to increase in number throughout life and are associated with café-au-lait spots and occasionally spinal neurofibromas.

If an inflammatory or a neoplastic lump is suspected, remember always to examine the regional lymphatic field and the other lymph node groups.

CORRELATION OF PHYSICAL SIGNS AND SKIN DISEASE

There are many different skin diseases with varied physical signs (see Fig. 43.9). With each major sign the groups of common important diseases that should be considered will be listed.

Pruritus

Pruritus simply means itching, and is the most commonly reported skin symptom. It may be either generalised or localised. Scratch marks are generally present. Localised pruritus is usually caused by a dermatological condition such as dermatitis or eczema. Generalised pruritus may be caused by primary skin disease, systemic disease or psychogenic factors.

To determine the cause of the pruritus it is essential to examine the skin in detail (see List 43.2). Excoriations are caused by scratching, regardless of the underlying cause. Specific features of cutaneous diseases such as dermatitis, urticaria, scabies (see Fig. 43.10) or the blisters of dermatitis herpetiformis and bullous pemphigoid should be looked for.

When primary skin diseases have been excluded, a detailed history and examination should be undertaken

---

[a] These four cardinal signs were described by Celsus in the 8th volume of his medical book, which taught those who were interested surgical techniques. After performing surgery, readers were warned to look out for the four cardinal signs of postsurgical inflammation—'calor, rubor, dolor and tumor'. Modern surgeons have added loss of function to these signs.

[b] Frederich von Recklinghausen (1833–1910) was Virchow's assistant in Berlin and then a professor of pathology in Strasbourg from 1872. He described this disease in 1882 and haemochromatosis in 1889.

Types of skin lesion.

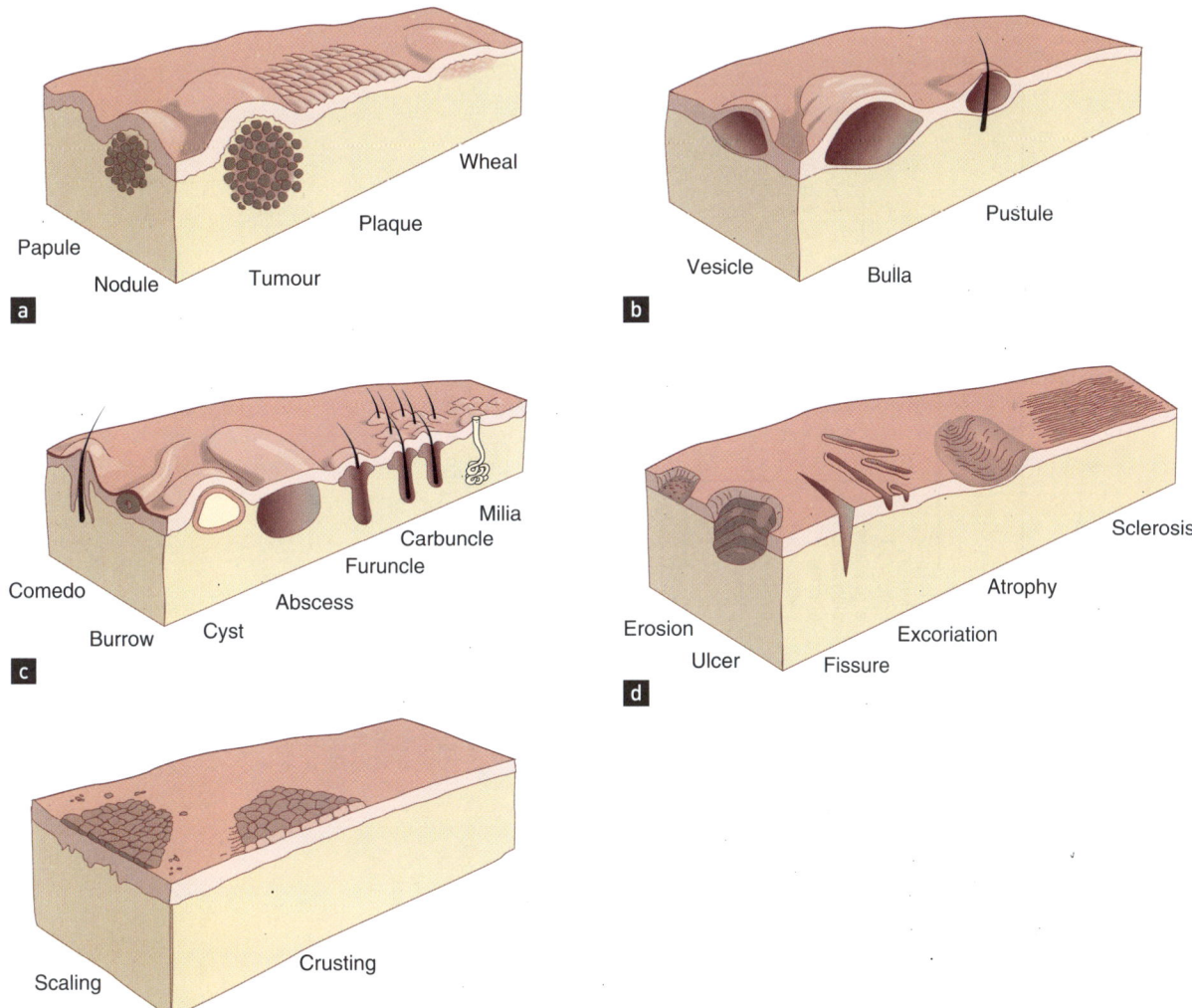

(a) Primary skin lesions, palpable with solid mass; (b) primary skin lesions, palpable and fluid-filled; (c) special primary skin lesions (milia are white papules due to keratin retention); (d) secondary skin lesions, below the skin plane; (e) secondary skin lesions, above the skin plane

(Adapted from Schwartz M. *Textbook of physical diagnosis*, 4th edn. Philadelphia: Saunders, 2002.)

FIGURE 43.8

to consider the various systemic diseases outlined in List 43.3.

Erythrosquamous eruptions

Erythrosquamous eruptions are made up of lesions that are red and scaly. They may be well demarcated or have ill-defined borders. They may be pruritic or asymptomatic.

When attempting to establish a diagnosis of an erythrosquamous eruption, the history is very important. Ask about the time course of the eruption, about a family history of similar skin diseases and whether or not there is a family history of atopy. The presence or absence of itching and the distribution of the lesions (often on the extensor surfaces of the limbs) also give clues about the diagnosis (List 43.4).

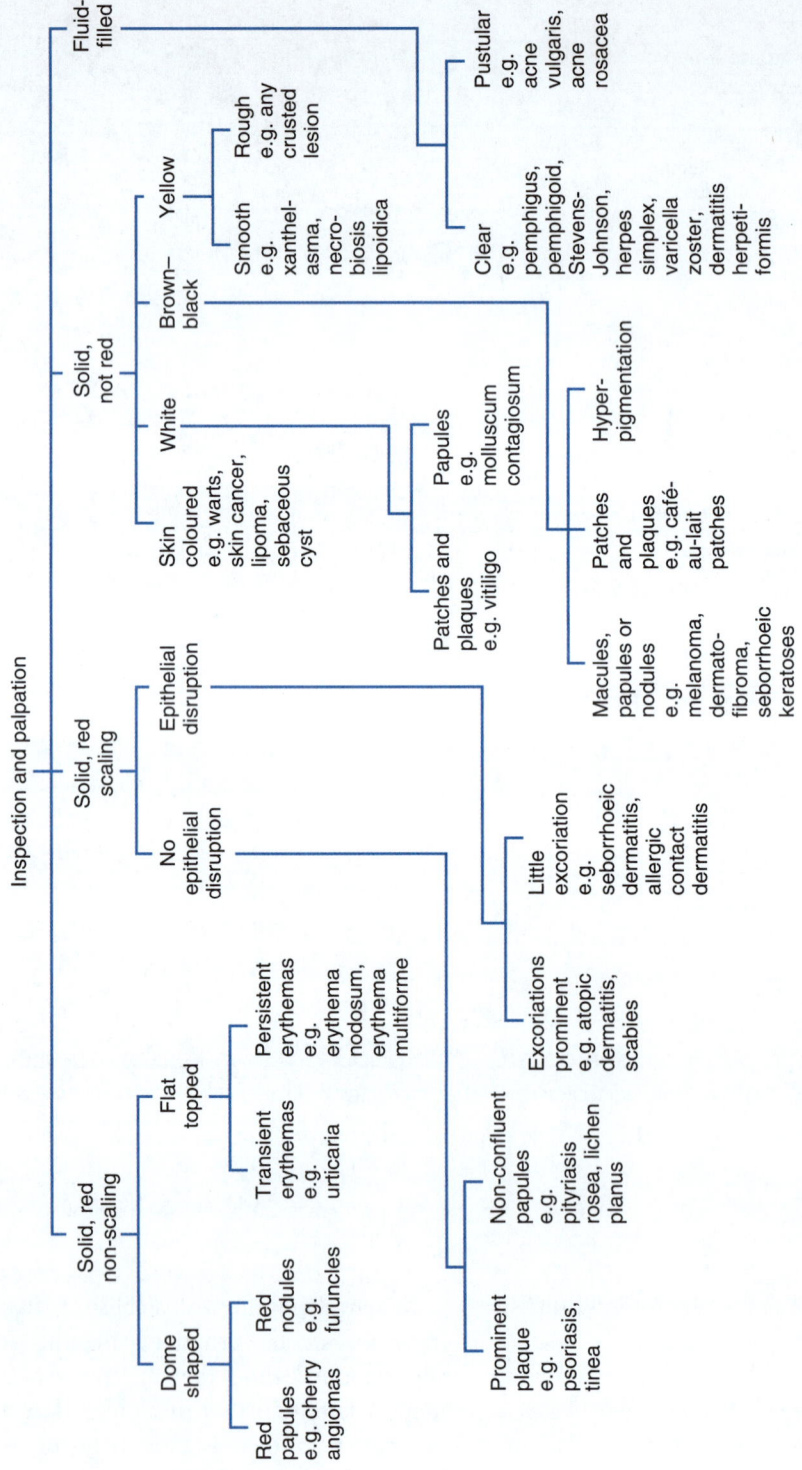

Diagnosis of skin disease: an algorithm

(Adapted from Lynch PJ. *Dermatology for the house officer*, 2nd edn. Baltimore: Williams & Wilkins, 1987.)

FIGURE 43.9

> **PRIMARY SKIN DISORDERS CAUSING PRURITUS**
>
> 1. Asteatosis (dry skin)
> 2. Atopic dermatitis (erythematous, oedematous papular patches on head, neck, flexural surfaces)
> 3. Psoriasis
> 4. Lichen planus
> 5. Urticaria
> 6. Scabies
> 7. Dermatitis herpetiformis
> 8. Bullous pemphigoid
>
> LIST 43.2

> **SYSTEMIC CONDITIONS CAUSING PRURITUS**
>
> 1. Cholestasis (e.g. primary biliary cirrhosis)
> 2. Chronic kidney disease
> 3. Pregnancy
> 4. Lymphoma and other internal malignancies
> 5. Iron deficiency, polycythaemia rubra vera
> 6. Endocrine diseases (e.g. diabetes mellitus, hypothyroidism, hyperthyroidism, carcinoid syndrome)
>
> LIST 43.3

Scabies.

Scattered fine papules with severe itching. Finger web involvement is common

(From Reeves JT, Maibach H. *Clinical dermatology illustrated: a regional approach*, 3rd edn. Sydney: McLennan & Petty, ©2000.)

FIGURE 43.10

> **CAUSES OF ERYTHROSQUAMOUS ERUPTIONS**
>
> 1. Psoriasis (salmon-pink plaques with silvery scale)
> 2. Atopic eczema (diffuse erythema with fine scaling)
> 3. Pityriasis rosea (pink, scaly, itchy macular lesions in a Christmas tree pattern; herald patch;* self-limited; young adults)
> 4. Nummular eczema (round patches of subacute dermatitis)
> 5. Contact dermatitis (irritant or allergic)
> 6. Dermatophyte infections (ringworm)
> 7. Lichen planus (violet-coloured, small, polygonal papules)
> 8. Secondary syphilis (flat, red, hyperkeratotic lesions)
>
> *The herald patch is a single lesion that looks like tinea corporis. It appears several days before the generalised eruption of pityriasis occurs.
>
> LIST 43.4

Asymptomatic lesions on the palms and soles are suggestive of secondary syphilis, whereas pruritic lesions on the anterior wrist would be more suggestive of lichen planus (see Figs 43.11 and 43.12) or scabies infestation. Lichen planus is occasionally associated with primary biliary cirrhosis and other liver diseases, chronic graft-versus-host disease and drugs (e.g. penicillamine, angiotensin-converting enzyme [ACE] inhibitors). Scattered lesions of recent origin on the trunk would be more suggestive of pityriasis rosea (see Fig. 43.13), whereas more widespread, diffuse and intensely pruritic lesions would be more suggestive of nummular eczema (see Fig. 43.14).

Erythematous lesions with a well-demarcated border and overlying silvery scale over the extensor surfaces are usually due to psoriasis (see Figs 43.15 and 43.16).

Blistering eruptions

There are a number of different diseases that will present with either vesicles or bullae (see List 43.5). Dermatitis can present as a blistering eruption, particularly allergic

Lichen planus, with polygonal flat-topped violaceous lesions

(From Reeves JT, Maibach H. *Clinical dermatology illustrated: a regional approach*, 2nd edn. Sydney: MacLennan & Petty Pty Ltd, ©1991.)

FIGURE 43.11

Pityriasis rosea, with scattered scaly oval lesions on the trunk and a larger 'herald' patch

(From Reeves JT, Maibach H. *Clinical dermatology illustrated: a regional approach*, 2nd edn. Sydney: MacLennan & Petty Pty Ltd, ©1991.)

FIGURE 43.13

Lichen planus, with development of lesions in an area of trauma—the 'Koebner' phenomenon

(From Reeves JT, Maibach H. *Clinical dermatology illustrated: a regional approach*, 2nd edn. Sydney: MacLennan & Petty Pty Ltd, ©1991.)

Figure 43.12

CAUSES OF BLISTERING ERUPTIONS

1. Traumatic blisters and burns
2. Bullous impetigo (due to a particular strain of *Staphylococcus aureus*)
3. Viral blisters (e.g. herpes simplex, varicella)
4. Bullous erythema multiforme
5. Bullous pemphigoid
6. Dermatitis herpetiformis
7. Pemphigus
8. Porphyria
9. Epidermolysis bullosa
10. Dermatophyte infections
11. Acute contact dermatitis
12. Necrotising fasciitis
13. Insect bites

LIST 43.5

contact dermatitis (see Fig. 43.17 and also Questions box 43.2).

Clinical features of bullous eruptions

Viral blisters such as those of herpes simplex virus infection (see Fig. 43.19) have a distinctive morphology (small grouped vesicles on an erythematous background, described as 'herpetiform').

Bullous pemphigoid is a rare autoimmune blistering disease usually affecting older patients. Blisters are widespread and tense, have a thick roof and tend not to rupture easily (see Fig. 43.20).

Pemphigus vulgaris is another autoimmune blistering disease (see Fig. 43.21). Patients are often younger than those affected by bullous pemphigoid, and the disease can be more severe. It has thin-roofed

(a) Nummular eczema—typical scattered coin-like lesions of indolent dermatitis; (b) nummular eczema, close-up view of typical lesions; (c) nummular eczema

((a) From Reeves JT, Maibach H. *Clinical dermatology illustrated: a regional approach*, 2nd edn. Sydney: MacLennan & Petty Pty Ltd, ©1991, with permission; (b) from Halberg M. Nummular eczema. *J Emerg Med* 2011; 43(5):e327–e328; (c) courtesy of Dr A Watson, Infectious Diseases Department, The Canberra Hospital.)

FIGURE 43.14

(a) Psoriasis—typical bright-red, scaly plaque with silvery scale over a joint; (b) psoriasis of the scalp in the hair line

((a) From Reeves JT, Maibach H. *Clinical dermatology illustrated: a regional approach*, 2nd edn. Sydney: MacLennan & Petty Pty Ltd, ©1991, with permission; (b) courtesy of Dr A Watson, Infectious Diseases Department, The Canberra Hospital.)

FIGURE 43.15

(a) Acute widespread pustular psoriasis. Often the eruption is bright red with bizarre patterns and pustules predominantly at the margins. (b) Pustular psoriasis of the hands

((a) From Reeves JT, Maibach H. *Clinical dermatology illustrated: a regional approach*, 2nd edn. Sydney: MacLennan & Petty Pty Ltd, ©1991; (b) from Hochberg M, Silman AJ, Smolen J et al. *Rheumatology*, 5th edn. Maryland Heights: Mosby, 2010.)

FIGURE 43.16

Allergic contact dermatitis from over-the-counter topical medication rubbed over congested sinuses

(Courtesy of Dr A Watson, Infectious Diseases Department, The Canberra Hospital.)

FIGURE 43.17

QUESTIONS TO ASK THE PATIENT WITH A BLISTERING ERUPTION

! denotes symptoms for the possible diagnosis of an urgent or dangerous problem.

1. Have you had blisters on the backs of your hands that break easily and are worse if you have been in the sun? (Porphyria cutanea tarda)
2. Have you had sores or blisters in your mouth that came on before the skin blisters? (Pemphigus vulgaris)
! 3. Did the inside of your mouth become ulcerated and painful suddenly? Have your eyes become painful? (Stevens–Johnson syndrome; see Fig. 43.18)
4. Was the blister on your lip or genitals, and was it preceded by itching or burning? (Herpes simplex)
! 5. Were the blisters preceded by some days of severe pain and burning in the areas where the blisters have broken out? (Herpes zoster)
6. Did you notice pink spots on the skin that were itchy before the blisters appeared? (Bullous pemphigoid)

QUESTIONS BOX 43.2

---

blisters that readily rupture and form erosions and crusts. The epidermis is fragile and can sometimes shear with lateral pressure (Nikolsky's[c] sign). Almost all patients will have oral mucosal involvement, and many will have other mucosal sites such as eyes and genitals affected.

Dermatitis herpetiformis is a cutaneous manifestation of gluten sensitivity characterised by a pruritic papules or vesicles favouring the extensor surfaces, back and buttocks.

---

[c] Pyotr Vasilyevich Nikolsky (1855–1940), a Kiev and Warsaw dermatologist. Nikolsky's sign also occurs in staphylococcal scalded-skin syndrome and toxic epidermal necrolysis.

Stevens–Johnson syndrome

(Courtesy of Dr A Watson, Infectious Diseases Department, The Canberra Hospital.)

FIGURE 43.18

Bullous pemphigoid

(From Schwarzenberger K. *General dermatology*. Philadelphia: Saunders, 2008.)

FIGURE 43.20

Primary herpes simplex virus infection in an adult; shows typical widespread distribution around the mouth

(From Reeves JT, Maibach H. *Clinical dermatology illustrated: a regional approach*, 2nd edn. Sydney: MacLennan & Petty Pty Ltd, ©1991.)

FIGURE 43.19

Porphyria cutanea tarda is a metabolic disorder characterised by clear or haemorrhagic tense blisters on the dorsal hands and other sun-exposed areas, hyperpigmentation and increased facial hair; hepatic insult from hepatitis C, alcohol, haemochromatosis and the oral contraceptive pill can induce symptoms (due to decreased uroporphyrinogen decarboxylase).

Erythroderma

Erythroderma is best thought of as the end stage of numerous skin conditions (see List 43.6). The erythrodermic patient has involvement of >90% of the skin with an erythematous inflammatory process, often with exfoliation. This represents that most unusual occurrence: a dermatological emergency.

An attempt should be made to determine the underlying cause of the erythroderma, and this is best done based on the history and examination. Specific treatment can then be directed at the underlying cause. Patients with erythroderma may develop systemic manifestations such as peripheral oedema, tachycardia, metabolic changes (including hypoalbuminaemia and extrarenal fluid loss) and disturbances in

Pemphigus vulgaris

(From Reeves JT, Maibach H. *Clinical dermatology illustrated: a regional approach*, 2nd edn. Sydney: MacLennan & Petty Pty Ltd, ©1991.)

FIGURE 43.21

Livedo reticularis and medical conditions	
Condition	Example
Haematological	Polycythaemia rubra vera, leukaemia, thrombocytosis
Hypercoagulable states	Antiphospholipid syndrome, factor V Leiden mutation, protein S or C deficiencies
Paraprotein	Multiple myeloma
Autoimmune diseases	Systemic lupus erythematosus, dermatomyositis, scleroderma, rheumatoid arthritis
Infections	Hepatitis C, syphilis, meningococcal disease, tuberculosis
Vasculitides	Polyarteritis nodosa, granulomatosis with polyangiitis
Endocarditis	
Cryoglobulinaemia, cryofibrinogenaemia	
Neurohumoral diseases	Carcinoid, phaeochromocytoma

TABLE 43.3

> **CAUSES OF ERYTHRODERMA**
> 1. Eczema
> 2. Psoriasis
> 3. Drugs (e.g. phenytoin, allopurinol)
> 4. Pityriasis rubra pilaris
> 5. Mycosis fungoides, leukaemia, lymphoma
> 6. Lichen planus
> 7. Pemphigus foliaceus
> 8. Hereditary disorders
> 9. Dermatophytosis
> 10. Toxic shock syndrome—generalised erythroderma
>
> LIST 43.6

thermoregulation. Therefore these patients require close medical supervision and monitoring until they have recovered from the acute phase of their illness.

The most common cause is eczema, which is usually of the atopic variety. These patients often have an intense pruritus. Some of them will develop a chronic unremitting erythroderma.

Livedo reticularis

This is a net-like pattern of blue or reddish blood vessels visible through the skin and is common particularly on the lower extremities (see Fig. 25.10 on p 416). It is usually the result of slow flow through subcutaneous vessels due to cold temperatures (physiological). Physiological livedo can be elicited by cooling the leg and will disappear on warming. Less commonly it can be secondary to an underlying disease (Table 43.3). There is no extravasation of blood, which distinguishes it from ecchymoses or purpura. Therefore it blanches upon pressure, unless vessel occlusion (e.g. thrombosis) with ischaemia has occurred.

Pustular and crusted lesions

The clinical appearance of a *pustular* lesion results from accumulation of neutrophils. Such collections usually indicate an infective process; however, sterile pustules may form as part of a number of skin diseases owing to the release of chemotactic factors following an immunological reaction.

A *crust* is dried serum, blood or pus that is found on the skin's surface. It may include bacteria (usually *Staphylococcus*); an example of where this occurs is a honey-yellow crust in impetigo.

It is essential to determine whether or not a pustular lesion (or a group of pustular lesions) represents a primarily infectious process or an inflammatory dermatological condition. For example, pustular lesions on the hands and feet may be due to tinea infection, a sterile primary pustular psoriasis or palmoplantar pustulosis (see List 43.7 and Questions box 43.3). Skin scrapings of desquamating skin flakes or a swab of pustule contents sent for microscopy and culture will help to differentiate infectious from inflammatory causes of pustules. If pustules, vesicles or crusts are herpetiform or haemorrhagic in morphology, swabs for herpes simplex and herpes zoster should be taken.

CAUSES OF PUSTULAR AND CRUSTED LESIONS

1. Acne vulgaris (comedones, papules, pustules, cystic lesions, ice-pick scars—no telangiectasias)
2. Acne rosacea (acne-like lesions, erythema and telangiectasias on central face—no comedones)
3. Impetigo
4. Folliculitis
5. Viral lesions
6. Pustular psoriasis
7. Drug eruptions
8. Dermatophyte infections
9. Sweet's syndrome (pustular dermatosis)

LIST 43.7

QUESTIONS TO ASK THE PATIENT WITH PUSTULAR LESIONS

1. Are you taking cortisone tablets? (Steroid acne)
2. Has your skin been painful or have you had a fever? (Pustular psoriasis)
3. Have you had psoriasis in the past?
4. Do you find your face becomes flushed easily, for example if you drink hot drinks? (Acne rosacea)
5. Are you a diabetic? (Cutaneous candidiasis)
6. Do you sweat excessively? (Folliculitis)

QUESTIONS BOX 43.3

Dermal plaques

Dermal plaques are localised thickenings of the skin that are caused by changes in the dermis or subcutaneous fat. These may be due to chronic inflammatory processes or scarring sclerotic processes (see List 43.8).

The pattern of involvement of the plaques, the age of the patient and other clinical features should enable a diagnosis to be established.

CAUSES OF DERMAL PLAQUES

1. Granuloma annulare (see Fig. 43.22)
2. Necrobiosis lipoidica
3. Sarcoidosis
4. Erythema nodosum
5. Lupus erythematosus
6. Morphoea and scleroderma
7. Tuberculosis
8. Leprosy

LIST 43.8

Granuloma annulare

(From James W. *Andrews' diseases of the skin: clinical dermatology*, 11th edn. Philadelphia: Saunders, 2011.)

FIGURE 43.22

Lupus pernio

(From Holmes J, Lazarus A. Sarcoidosis: extrathoracic manifestations. *Disease-a-month* 2009; 55(11):675–692.)

FIGURE 43.23

> ### CAUSES OF ERYTHEMA NODOSUM
> 1. Sarcoidosis
> 2. Streptococcal infections
> 3. Inflammatory bowel disease
> 4. Drugs (e.g. sulfonamides, penicillin, sulfonylurea, oestrogen, iodides, bromides)
> 5. Tuberculosis
> 6. Other infections (e.g. lepromatous leprosy, toxoplasmosis, histoplasmosis, *Yersinia*, *Chlamydia*)
> 7. Systemic lupus erythematosus
> 8. Behçet's syndrome
>
> LIST 43.9

Neutrophilic dermatoses are a group of conditions characterised by neutrophilic infiltrates without any identifiable infectious cause. Sweet's syndrome[d] (acute febrile neutrophilic dermatosis) is a condition involving painful red plaques and nodules that are well demarcated from surrounding skin. There is often an associated fever. Sweet's syndrome may be idiopathic or occur in association with haematological disease (myelodysplastic disorders and acute myeloid leukaemia), solid organ tumours, infections, inflammatory bowel disease, autoimmune disease, pregnancy and some drugs (e.g. granulocyte-stimulating factor).

There are a number of other neutrophilic dermatoses including pyoderma gangrenosum and Behçet's disease.

Lupus pernio (see Fig. 43.23) appears as violaceous papules and plaques on the nose, cheeks and ears. Despite its name this condition is not associated with systemic lupus erythematosus: it is a manifestation of cutaneous sarcoidosis. Lupus pernio on the nose is more commonly associated with pulmonary and upper respiratory tract sarcoidosis than with other forms of cutaneous sarcoidosis.

Erythema nodosum

This is the best known of the group of diseases classified as panniculitis (inflammation of the subcutaneous fat). Nodular vasculitis is another type of panniculitis causing painful nodules on the lower legs, usually on the calves. In contrast the lesions of erythema nodosum are usually found in the pretibial area and are erythematous, palpable and tender (p 278). Systemic symptoms may include fever, arthralgia, arthritis and malaise. A significant percentage of cases—more than one-third—are idiopathic; other common causes include upper respiratory tract infections (both streptococcal and viral), drugs such as the oral contraceptive and sulfonamides, inflammatory bowel disease, tuberculosis and sarcoidosis (see List 43.9).

Erythema multiforme (EM)

This is a distinctive inflammatory reaction of skin and mucosa. The characteristic skin lesion is a *target lesion* that has a well-defined border and consists of three distinct zones of colour change (see Fig. 43.24). The centre develops a dusky appearance over time and has been likened to a 'bulls eye'. The central zone can form a bulla or crust. When the mucosal membranes are significantly involved the condition is referred to as EM major; in the purely cutaneous form it is called EM minor. In most cases the condition is precipitated by viral infections, especially clinical or subclinical herpes simplex virus. Other causes include *Mycoplasma*

---

[d] Dr Robert Sweet from Plymouth, England, first described this in 1964.

Erythema multiforme; shows classic iris or target lesions, secondary to herpes simplex virus infection of the lips

(From Reeves JT, Maibach H. *Clinical dermatology illustrated: a regional approach*, 2nd edn. Sydney: MacLennan & Petty Pty Ltd, ©1991.)

FIGURE 43.24

Cellulitis

(Courtesy of Dr A Watson, Infectious Diseases Department, The Canberra Hospital.)

FIGURE 43.25

Erysipelas

(Courtesy of Dr A Watson, Infectious Diseases Department, The Canberra Hospital.)

FIGURE 43.26

pneumoniae, histoplasmosis and drugs. Sometimes no underlying cause will be established.

It is now known that this condition is a distinct disorder from *Stevens–Johnson*[e] *syndrome* (SJS) (see Fig. 43.18) and *toxic epidermal necrolysis* (TEN). These are two rare, potentially fatal variants within a continuous spectrum of adverse drug reactions. They are characterised by differing severity of mucocutaneous involvement, erythema and exfoliation. The medications most frequently implicated are antibiotics, anticonvulsants, allopurinol and non-steroidal anti-inflammatory drugs (NSAIDs). It is rare for SJS or TEN to be triggered by an infectious agent.

Cellulitis and erysipelas

Cellulitis (see Fig. 43.25) is inflammation of the deep dermis and subcutaneous tissue causing a unilateral erythematous lower limb. There may be associated lymphangitis and tender inguinal lymphadenopathy. In severe cases purple patches develop and may blister. It is usually due to beta-haemolytic *Streptococcus* or *Staphylococcus aureus* infection. In intravenous drug users it affects the upper limb (the usual sites of drug injection).

Erysipelas is a superficial variant of cellulitis caused primarily by beta-haemolytic *Streptococcus* that affects the dermis (see Fig. 43.26). It can occur on the face or the legs and consists of sharply demarcated erythema and a characteristic raised edge as a result of dermal involvement. There may be an obvious entry point for the organism, such as soft-tissue injury, tinea pedis, a varicose ulcer or a predisposing condition such as diabetes mellitus.

---

[e] Albert Mason Stevens (1884–1945), a New York paediatrician, and Frank C Johnson (1894–1934), an American physician.

Necrotising fasciitis is important to consider in the differential diagnosis. If there is severe pain, the skin is pale pink rather than floridly erythematous and the patient has signs of sepsis, consider necrotising fasciitis.

Folliculitis, furuncles and carbuncles

These conditions are all infections of hair follicles of varying severity.

Folliculitis is a very common disorder characterised by superficial inflammation of a hair follicle. Most cases are due to staphylococcal infection but they can be caused by other microorganisms (such as *Candida*, *Malassezia* or *Pseudomonas*) or topical medications, or be drug induced. If the infection becomes deeper, it becomes a *furuncle* (or boil) and if it spreads to involve a number of adjacent hair follicles it becomes a *carbuncle*. Lesions can occur anywhere on the skin but are commoner on the buttocks, neck and anogenital area. They are very painful and often associated with systemic symptoms. Staphylococcal organisms are usually responsible. The deep lesions heal by rupturing and exuding pus. They often leave a scar. Draining lymph nodes may be enlarged and tender.

The condition *hidradenitis suppurativa*, which especially affects obese young women, is associated with lesions similar to furuncles. The condition involves the apocrine glands in the axillae, the groin and the submammary areas and exhibits the pathognomonic double-ended comedone.

Other infections

Viral infections can lead to skin reactions. Measles is an example of an infection causing a *viral exanthem* (see Fig. 43.27). Many viruses including cytomegalovirus (CMV), Epstein–Barr virus (EBV), Coxsackie virus and the seroconversion illness after human immunodeficiency virus (HIV) infection can cause a similar rash. Patients with EBV infection treated with amoxicillin develop a characteristic rash (see Fig. 43.28). Meningococcal septicaemia causes a petechial rash, which can progress to purpura fulminans (see Fig. 43.29).

Impetigo is the most common cutaneous bacterial infection, characterised by honey-coloured golden crusting, vesicles and pustules on an erythematous base. *S. aureus* and *Streptococcus pyogenes* are the most frequent agents. Reactive arthritis caused by

Viral exanthema
(Courtesy of Dr A Watson, Infectious Diseases Department, The Canberra Hospital.)

FIGURE 43.27

Epstein–Barr virus infection after amoxicillin
(Courtesy of Dr A Watson, Infectious Diseases Department, The Canberra Hospital.)

FIGURE 43.28

genitourinary or gastrointestinal bacterial infection may be associated with *keratoderma blennorrhagicum*, in which tender hyperkeratotic nodules and plaques, sometimes with blisters or pustules, arise on the soles of the feet (see Fig. 43.30). Molluscum contagiosum is a common infectious viral disease of the skin characterised by discrete waxy dome-shaped papules, often with central umbilication (see Fig. 43.31).

Fungal skin infections include tinea, which often involves the foot (*tinea pedis*; see Fig. 43.32). It is caused by any of a number of dermatophyte species. Deep cutaneous infections caused by organisms such as

Petechial rash

(From Marks J, Miller J. *Lookingbill & Marks' principles of dermatology*, 4th edn. Philadelphia: Saunders, 2006.)

FIGURE 43.29

histoplasmosis, coccidioidomycosis and atypical mycobacterial species can present with ulceration, and are more common in immunosuppressed patients. Intertrigo is moist inflammation between skinfolds where skin rubs together; *Candida albicans* is often present (see Fig. 43.33).

Hyperpigmentation, hypopigmentation and depigmentation

The presence of hyperpigmentation can be a clue to underlying systemic disease (see List 43.10) but commonly develops after inflammation in skin. This pattern is called postinflammatory hyperpigmentation. Hypopigmentation (decreased pigment) may also occur after inflammation, or with pityriasis versicolor where *Malassezia* yeast creates azaleic acid, which destroys melanin. Depigmentation (complete loss of pigment) may be caused by vitiligo, which is associated with other autoimmune diseases such as type I diabetes mellitus, Hashimoto's thyroiditis and Addison's disease.

Flushing and sweating

Flushing of the skin may sometimes be observed, especially on the face, by the examiner. Some of the causes of this phenomenon are presented in List 43.11.

Keratoderma blennorrhagicum.

(a) Sole of foot; (b) toenails

(From Habif T. *Clinical dermatology*, 5th edn. St Louis MO: Mosby, 2009.)

FIGURE 43.30

Excessive sweating (hyperhidrosis) can be classified as primary or secondary. Primary hyperhidrosis is not associated with any systemic disorder and is the most common type. Secondary hyperhidrosis is associated with infection, tumours (e.g. phaeochromocytoma), hyperthyroidism, acromegaly, hypoglycaemia, menopause, autonomic dysfunction and drugs.

Molluscum contagiosum

(Black M. *Obstetric and gynecologic dermatology*, 3rd edn. St Louis MO: Mosby, 2008.)

FIGURE 43.31

Candida albicans

(From Male D, Brostoff J, Roth D, Roitt I. *Immunology*, 8th edn. Philadelphia: Saunders, 2012.)

FIGURE 43.33

Tinea pedis

(From Busam Klaus J, ed. *Dermatopathology—a volume in the series foundations in diagnostic pathology*. Philadelphia: Saunders, 2010.)

FIGURE 43.32

CAUSES OF DIFFUSE HYPERPIGMENTATION

Endocrine disease

Addison's disease (excess ACTH)
Ectopic ACTH secretion (e.g. carcinoma)
The contraceptive pill or pregnancy
Thyrotoxicosis, acromegaly, phaeochromocytoma

Metabolic

Malabsorption or malnutrition
Liver diseases (e.g. haemochromatosis, primary biliary cirrhosis, Wilson's disease)
Chronic kidney disease
Porphyria
Chronic infection (e.g. bacterial endocarditis)
Connective tissue disease (e.g. systemic lupus, scleroderma, dermatomyositis)

Racial or genetic

Other

Drugs (e.g. chlorpromazine, busulfan, arsenicals)
Radiation

ACTH = adrenocorticotrophic hormone.

LIST 43.10

CAUSES OF FACIAL FLUSHING

1. Menopause
2. Drugs and foods (e.g. nifedipine, sildenafil, monosodium glutamate [MSG])
3. Alcohol after taking the drug disulfiram (or alcohol alone in some people)
4. Systemic mastocytosis
5. Rosacea
6. Carcinoid syndrome (secretion of serotonin and other mediators by a tumour may produce flushing, diarrhoea and valvular heart disease)
7. Autonomic dysfunction
8. Medullary carcinoma of the thyroid

LIST 43.11

BENIGN SKIN TUMOURS

1. Warts
2. Molluscum contagiosum
3. Seborrhoeic keratoses
4. Dermatofibroma
5. Neurofibroma
6. Angioma
7. Xanthoma

LIST 43.12

Skin tumours

Skin tumours are very common and are usually benign (see List 43.12).[4] Most malignant skin tumours can be cured if they are detected early and treated appropriately (see List 43.13).

Skin cancer often occurs in those predisposed individuals (with the fair skin of Celtic or Northern European origin) who undergo chronic exposure to ultraviolet light. Skin cancers may present as flat scaly lesions or as raised scaly or smooth lesions. They may be large or small and they may eventually ulcerate. All non-healing ulcers should be considered to be skin cancer, until proven otherwise.

The earliest lesions are actinic (solar) keratoses, which are erythematous macules or papules surmounted by adherent scale (see Fig. 43.35). A small number of these may develop into Bowen's disease (*squamous cell*

MALIGNANT SKIN TUMOURS

1. Basal cell carcinoma
2. Squamous cell carcinoma
3. Bowen's* disease (squamous cell carcinoma confined to the epithelial layer of the skin—carcinoma in situ)
4. Malignant melanoma (which can be metastatic—see Fig. 43.34)
5. Metastatic deposits

*John Templeton Bowen (1857–1941), a Boston dermatologist.

LIST 43.13

Metastatic melanoma

(From O'Neill JK, Khundar R, Knowles L et al. Melanoma with an unknown primary: a case series. *J Plast Reconstr Aesthet Surg* 2010; 63(12):2071–2080.)

FIGURE 43.34

carcinoma [SSC] in situ). This is typically an opaque papule or plaque that is often eroded or scaly (see Fig. 43.36). Metastasis can occur.

Basal cell carcinoma (BCC) is characteristically a translucent papule with a depressed centre and a rolled border with ectatic capillaries (see Fig. 43.37). Different

Actinic keratosis, slightly eroded and scaly.

Higher on the forehead, additional granular keratosis could be easily palpated

(From Reeves JT, Maibach H. *Clinical dermatology illustrated: a regional approach*, 2nd edn. Sydney: MacLennan & Petty Pty Ltd, ©1991.)

FIGURE 43.35

Squamous cell carcinoma

(From Reeves JT, Maibach H. *Clinical dermatology illustrated: a regional approach*, 2nd edn. Sydney: MacLennan & Petty Pty Ltd, ©1991.)

FIGURE 43.36

(a) Basal cell carcinoma: noted the rolled edges; (b) pigmented basal cell carcinoma, with pearly quality and depressed centre, in a patient with sun-damaged skin

(From Pfenninger J. *Pfenninger and Fowler's procedures for primary care*, 3rd edn. Maryland Heights, MO: Mosby, 2010.)

FIGURE 43.37

Superficial spreading melanoma, still confined to the upper dermis

(© Dr Loren Golitz.)

FIGURE 43.38

Onychomycosis: fungal infection of the nails

(From Reeves JT, Maibach H. *Clinical dermatology illustrated: a regional approach*, 2nd edn. Sydney: MacLennan & Petty Pty Ltd, ©1991.)

FIGURE 43.39

subtypes include superficial, nodular, pigmented and sclerosing (morphoeic). These very rarely metastasise. Multiple BCCs may be associated with basal cell nevus syndrome (Gorlin's syndrome) with other cardinal signs including jaw cysts, palmar pits and bony abnormalities.

Malignant melanomas are usually deeply pigmented lesions that are enlarging and have an irregular notched border (see Fig. 43.38). There is often variation of pigment within the lesion. Sometimes melanomas lack pigment altogether and are referred to as amelanotic melanomas. Consider malignant melanoma if the lesion follows the **ABCDE** checklist:[5,6]

A symmetrical
B order irregularity
C olour variation
D iameter >6 millimetres
E volving (enlarging or changing) or **E** levated.

Patients with numerous large and unusual pigmented naevi (dysplastic naevus syndrome) are at an increased risk of developing malignant melanoma.[7]

THE NAILS

Systemic disease is commonly associated with changes in the patient's finger- and toenails and in the nail beds. The slow growth of the nails means that the temporal course of an illness may be seen in nail changes. Many of these findings have been described in other chapters, but important features of nail changes are dealt with here.

Fungal infection of the nails (**onychomycosis;** see Fig. 43.39) is the most common nail abnormality: it makes up 40% of all nail disorders and 30% of all cutaneous fungal infections. This infection is more common in people with diabetes, peripheral vascular disease and immunosuppression. The characteristic findings are thickened yellow nails, ridging, crumbling and deformity. The changes can be difficult to distinguish from psoriasis. A nail clipping should be taken to help confirm the diagnosis.

Acute paronychia is inflammation of the skin surrounding the nail; it can be acute or chronic. Acute paronychia is usually caused by *S. aureus* infection; other causes include ingrown nails, irritants, trauma (for example, from biting nails or sucking the thumb) or manicures. Chronic paronychia affects a number of fingers and causes red, swollen nail folds that have no cuticles. It leads to chronic ridging and dystrophy of the nail plate. The usual cause is chronic irritation from water or chemicals. Dermatophyes account for approximately 90% of fungal nail infections and *Candida* spp. make up the majority of the remainder. Candidal nail infection (diagnosed by microscopy and culture) suggests the possibility of chronic mucocutaneous

Nail involvement occurs in about 25% of patients with psoriasis

(From Reeves JT, Maibach H. *Clinical dermatology illustrated: a regional approach*, 2nd edn. Sydney: MacLennan & Petty Pty Ltd, ©1991.)

FIGURE 43.40

candidiasis, which is a rare condition associated with polyendocrinopathies.

Nail involvement occurs in about 25% of patients with psoriasis (see Fig. 43.40). The characteristic abnormality is pitting. This can also occur in fungal infections, chronic paronychia, lichen planus, alopecia areata and atopic dermatitis. Psoriasis is also the most common cause of onycholysis. Rarer changes in psoriatic nails include longitudinal ridging (onychorrhexis), proximal transverse ridging, subungual hyperkeratosis and yellow-brown discoloration (the 'oil drop' sign).

The presence of nailfold telangiectasias is an important sign in a number of systemic disorders, including systemic lupus erythematosus, scleroderma and Raynaud's phenomenon. These changes are not very specific and considerable variation in nailfold capillary shape is present in healthy people. In patients with dermatomyositis, nailfold telangiectasiae are associated with hypertrophy of the cuticle and small haemorrhagic infarcts. Raynaud's phenomenon is also associated with nail changes caused by the inadequate blood supply. These include brittleness, longitudinal ridging, splitting, flattening, onycholysis, koilonychia and a nail bed that is more erythematous than normal.

Clubbing is an important nail abnormality. It has been described in patients with HIV infection, and its severity seems proportional to the degree of immunosuppression. HIV infection is also associated with onychomycosis and longitudinal melonychia (dark line in the nail), secondary to treatment with zidovudine.

T&O'C ESSENTIALS

1. The time course of a skin condition may be a clue to the diagnosis.
2. A careful medical history may reveal a systemic illness that underlies the skin problem.
3. Questioning about contact with new soaps or deodorants may help explain a new rash.
4. Many rashes may be assumed to be the result of a new medication unless proven otherwise.
5. A thorough dermatological examination must include the whole surface of the skin, nails, hair and accessible mucosal surfaces.
6. Many common dermatological abnormalities can be diagnosed on inspection (as long as the student has enough experience to recognise them).
7. For any pigmented lesion consider the melanoma **ABCDE** checklist:
   A symmetrical (typically)
   B order irregular
   C olour irregular
   D iameter large
   E levated above the skin or Evolving

OSCE EXAMPLE – SKIN

Mr Talbot has a pigmented lesion on his chest. Please assess him.

1. Ask about sun exposure in childhood and as an adult.
2. Ask about any family history of melanoma (10% of melanomas have such a history).
3. Ask 'When was the lesion first noticed? Is it new?'
4. Ask 'Has the lesion changed in appearance?'
5. Ask 'Any itching or bleeding?'
6. Ask 'Has this lesion or any other pigmented lesion been biopsied or excised?'
7. Inspect the lesion: note whether symmetrical or not, regular or irregular border, raised or not, pigmentation uniform or variable and any ulceration or inflammation. Measure its size.
8. Inspect the skin all over the body including in the hair for other pigmented lesions. Inspect the draining lymph nodes if melanoma is suspected.
9. Present the ABCDE checklist.

References

1. Marks R. Diagnosis in dermatology. Tricks of the trade. *Aus Fam Physician* 2001; 30(11):1028–1032. A useful guide on clinical clues.
2. Ashton RE. Teaching non-dermatologists to examine the skin: a review of the literature and some recommendations. *Brit J Derm* 1995; 132:221–225. Presents a good scheme that can be used to describe any skin lesion.
3. Schwarzenberger K. The essentials of the complete skin examination. *Med Clin Nth Am* 1998; 82:981–999. Guidance on a thorough examination approach.
4. Preston DS, Stern RS. Nonmelanoma cancers of the skin. *N Engl J Med* 1992; 327:649–662. Provides useful information on discriminating between worrying and non-worrying lesions, and includes colour photographs.
5. Whitehead JD, Gichnik JM. Does this patient have a mole or a melanoma? *JAMA* 1998; 279:696–701. The ABCD checklist (asymmetry, border irregularity, irregular colour, diameter >6 millimetres) has a sensitivity over 90% and a specificity over 95% for identifying malignant melanoma.
6. Abbasi NR, Shaw HM, Rigel DS et al. Early diagnosis of cutaneous melanoma: rewriting the ABC criteria. *JAMA* 2004; 292:2771–2776. Changes (evolving) of symptoms or signs (size, shape, pruritus, tenderness, bleeding or colour) are additional evidence for the presence of melanoma.
7. Shenenberger DW. Cutaneous malignant melanoma: a primary care perspective. *Am Fam Physician* 2012; 85(2):161–168. An update on the clinical approach and management.
8. Bologna JL, Jorizzo JL, Schaffer JV. *Dermatology*, 3rd edn. Philadelphia: Saunders, 2012.

CHAPTER 44
The older person assessment

Old men forget. SHAKESPEARE, Henry V

Older patients make up an increasing proportion of people admitted to hospital, their length of stay is often long and they need special consideration because of their often varied and complicated multiple medical problems.[1]

There is lack of universal agreement on what constitutes the age cut-off that defines a geriatric patient. Only 140 years ago, old age was set above 50. Today in the Western world as people (and their doctors) age, the cut-off may be extended above 65[a] (what highly competent older doctor in practice would want to be classified as geriatric?). Arbitrary distinctions currently drawn between the young old (65–74), the middle old (75–84) and the oldest old (85+) do not necessarily reflect biological age. The number of oldest old is growing steadily; this change will increasingly challenge health systems and has major resource implications for the future.

Geriatric patients tend to report fewer symptoms but have more chronic diseases. Hence, disease presentation is more likely to be atypical, so spending time taking the history is critical. Emphasis must be placed on the big four matters of concern for older people:

- immobility
- instability
- impaired intellect or memory
- incontinence.

These can be assessed as part of an activities of daily living (ADL) index (see Lists 44.4 and 44.5).[2,3]

Any of these may be caused or worsened by polypharmacy, which is a very common problem in elderly patients.

> **THE COMPREHENSIVE GERIATRIC ASSESSMENT:**[1] **ASSESSMENT COMPONENTS (THE ABCs)**
>
> 1. Activities of daily living
> 2. Balance, frailty testing
> 3. Cognition
> 4. Depression, drugs (polypharmacy), dentition (including nutrition and weight change)
> 5. Environment: home situation, social support, financial issues, living will (advance care planning)
> 6. Falls risk (history of falls, 'get up and go' test, functional reach test)
> 7. Gait speed (faster walkers have better survival)
> 8. Hearing, vision
> 9. Incontinence (urine, stool), sexual function
>
> LIST 44.1

You need to find out about the risk of falls, mobility problems, ability to cope and risks to safety among other problems (see List 44.1 and Questions box 44.1). Functional and cognitive impairment are very important health problems to identify in older patients. Hearing and visual impairment, as well as cognitive decline, can impair history taking (see List 44.2).

HISTORY TAKING IN OLDER PERSONS: SPECIAL CONSIDERATIONS

1. *Presenting complaint:* a single complaint is unusual.
2. *Past history:* record the patient's immunisation status, especially for *Pneumococcus*, influenza and tetanus.

---

[a] Ask any relatives who are over 65 whether they think that they are old: 70 is the new 50!

SPECIFIC QUESTIONS TO ASK THE ELDERLY PATIENT

1. What do you think your main problems are at the moment?
2. What tablets are you taking? Do you have trouble remembering to take them? Have any of your medications changed recently? Do you think they have caused you any problems?
3. Are you able to walk without difficulty: (a) in the house; and (b) to the shops?
4. Do you exercise regularly?
5. Have you fallen over in the past year? What happened? Were you hurt? How many times have you fallen? Do you have arthritis or Parkinson's disease? (See List 44.3)
6. Have you had any fractures of your spine? Wrists? Hips?
7. Do you drive?
8. With whom do you live?
9. Do you have any trouble managing cooking, washing or banking?
10. Do you feel that you eat well? Do your teeth give you trouble? Do you take them out to eat? What sort of meals do you have at night? Who cooks them?
11. How is your vision? Have you had cataracts? Do you wear glasses?
12. How is your hearing? Have you got hearing aids? Do they work?
13. Do you worry that you will not be able to cope in the future? Have you thought how you will manage if your health gets worse?
14. During the past month have you been feeling down, depressed or hopeless? During the past month, have you been bothered by little interest or pleasure in doing things?[6]
15. Would you allow me to talk to any of your relatives or friends about your health issues?

QUESTIONS BOX 44.1

CHANGES TO STANDARD HISTORY-TAKING TECHNIQUE FOR OLDER PATIENTS

- Slow down the speed of the interview.
- Adjust your interview approach if the patient has hearing or visual impairment issues, or dementia.
- To maximise the interaction, when you talk to the patient make sure that he or she can see your face.
- Do not patronise the patient.
- With the patient's permission, involve a relative or friend (but not too many) to help with the interview.

LIST 44.2

3. *Medications:* many patients will be taking multiple medications for several diseases, not all of which they may really need (polypharmacy). A comprehensive list including reason for use is important in terms of planning management. Always ask about over-the-counter medications, laxatives and sleeping medications.

   Any new symptoms may be from polypharmacy.

4. *Social history:*
   - *Accommodation:* find out whether the patient lives in a house or flat or in some form of assisted or serviced accommodation and who else lives there. Ask about the health and mobility of other people in the house and the proximity of younger relatives and friends.
   - *Exercise:* exercise is safe in the elderly, in general, and improves flexibility, balance, endurance and strength, which can assist with

> ### RISK FACTORS FOR FALLS
>
> 1. A history of multiple previous falls (number, injuries)
> 2. Age over 80 years
> 3. Difficulty in getting up from a chair
> 4. Use of a walking stick or frame
> 5. Arthritis
> 6. Poor vision
> 7. Cognitive decline or depression
> 8. Muscle weakness
> 9. Parkinson's disease
> 10. Gait or balance problems (e.g. stroke)
> 11. Mechanical problems in the house (e.g. loose rugs, steep stairs)
> 12. Drug treatment (polypharmacy; particularly note sedatives, antidepressants, antihypertensives, anticholinergics)
>
> LIST 44.3

> ### LAWTON AND BRODY INSTRUMENTAL ACTIVITIES OF DAILY LIVING (IADL) SCALE[3]
>
> 1. Ability to use the telephone
> 2. Shopping
> 3. Food preparation
> 4. Housekeeping
> 5. Laundry
> 6. Transport
> 7. Medication management
> 8. Ability to handle finances
>
> Score 1 for each.
>
> 0 = total dependence, 8 = total independence for IADLs.
>
> (Lawton MP, Brody EM. Assessment of older people; self maintaining and instrumental activities of daily living. *Gerontologist* 1969; 9:179 © Oxford University Press.)
>
> LIST 44.4

maintenance of independent function as well as improving quality of life. It also reduces the risk of falls.
- *Smoking:* the details should be acquired as usual. Stopping smoking improves lung function even in people over the age of 60. Furthermore, advice to stop smoking is as successful in older patients as in younger ones.
- *Alcohol use:* alcohol intake is common and the details should always be recorded in the notes.
- *Abuse and neglect:* these can be problems in this age group. Careful questioning, often over a number of interviews, may help uncover such problems.[4]

5. *Review of systems:* concentrate especially on vision, hearing, chewing and dentition, weight changes, faecal and urinary incontinence, recurrent falls (see List 44.3), a history of fractures and foot disease, and chronic pain.
- Falls are an important cause of mortality in the elderly and are usually multifactorial: postural dizziness, poor vision, cognitive impairment, foot problems, impaired bone mineral density and gait problems can all contribute to or exacerbate the problem. A patient is more likely to have further falls if he or she has a history of three or more falls, or if during the past year a fall resulted in injury or if he or she currently has arthritis or Parkinson's disease.[5]
- Ask about the layout of the patient's house, including the number of steps and the presence of railings, for example, in the bathroom.
- Ask about depression, because this is a common problem in the elderly and needs to be recognised and treated.[6]

6. *Specific areas of enquiry:*
- *Instrumental activities of daily living (IADLs):* ask about using the telephone, shopping, preparing food, housekeeping, doing the laundry, driving, taking medicine and ability to handle finances (see List 44.4).
- *Physical activities of daily living (ADLs):* ask about bathing, dressing, toileting, transfer (i.e. getting in/out of bed or chair), continence and feeding (see List 44.5); these can be affected by many different chronic illnesses.
- *Driving:* older drivers share an increased risk of accidents with those under 25. Ask whether the patient still drives or has 'retired from driving'—a tactful way of approaching the loss of mobility and standing that comes with giving up a driver's licence. If the patient is

> **KATZ INDEX OF ACTIVITIES OF DAILY LIVING (ADLs)[2]**
>
> **Activity**
> 1. Bathing
> 2. Dressing
> 3. Toileting
> 4. Transferring
> 5. Continence
> 6. Feeding
>
> 1 point for each that can be done without help or supervision.
>
> Score:
> 6 = fully functional
> 4 = moderately impaired
> 2 = severely impaired
>
> Katz S, Down TD, Cash HR, Grotz RC. Program in the development of the index of ADL. *Gerontologist* 1970; 10:20, by permission of Oxford University Press.
>
> LIST 44.5

> **RISK FACTORS FOR URINARY INCONTINENCE IN THE ELDERLY**
>
> 1. Obesity
> 2. Parity
> 3. Gynaecological surgery
> 4. Diabetes mellitus
> 5. Smoking
> 6. Diuretic drugs, calcium channel blockers
> 7. Immobility
> 8. Recurrent urinary tract infections
> 9. Previous radical prostatectomy
> 10. Cognitive impairment
> 11. Immobility
>
> LIST 44.7

> **FACTORS SUGGESTING DRIVING ABILITY MAY BE IMPAIRED**
>
> 1. Passenger reports concern
> 2. Cognitive decline
> 3. Recent accidents or traffic offences
> 4. Driving of short distances (<100 km/week) and self-limited driving, e.g. not at night
> 5. Impaired mobility
> 6. Poor vision
> 7. Impulsive or aggressive behaviour
> 8. Use of alcohol or sedative drugs
> 9. History of syncope
>
> LIST 44.6

still driving ask about his or her confidence when driving and whether certain situations are now avoided, e.g. driving at peak hour or at night. The assessment of relatives who may have been terrified passengers is more accurate than self-assessment. Certain risk factors have been identified for impaired driving (see List 44.6).

- *Urinary incontinence:* up to 30% of older women and men are affected by urinary incontinence—risk factors are listed in List 44.7. Ask if it has been a problem and how it affects daily life. Consider the types:
  ○ urge incontinence—the feeling of an urgent need to urinate followed by incontinence
  ○ stress incontinence—loss of urine when straining, coughing or exercising
  ○ mixed urge and stress incontinence
  ○ overflow incontinence—constant dribbling of urine, which affects men with prostatic obstruction
  ○ functional incontinence, which occurs in people too immobile to reach a bathroom or who have cognitive problems.

  Ask about drugs that may exacerbate the problem (e.g. diuretics, alpha-blockers) and about previous surgery (e.g. radical prostatectomy), radiation treatment, prostate symptoms and urinary tract infections.

  Find out tactfully how the patient and those around them cope and what has been done to help the problem.

- *End-of-life and treatment decisions:* patients generally prefer this topic to be brought up actively by their doctor. It is worth encouraging the patient to place his or her preferences in writing about decisions such as 'do not resuscitate' orders and advance care planning.

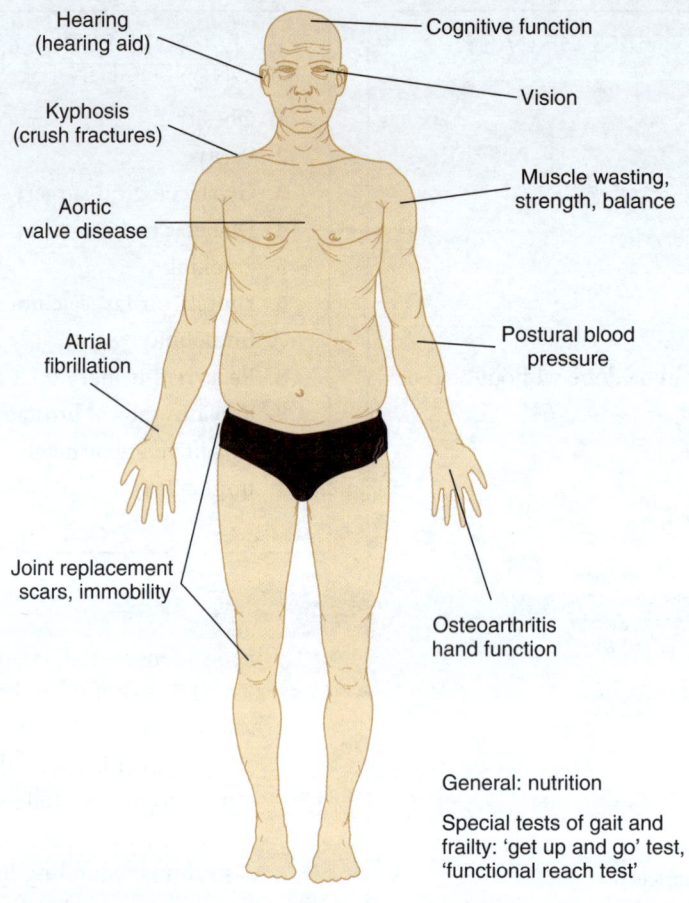

Examination of the geriatric patient: summary

FIGURE 44.1

PHYSICAL EXAMINATION IN OLDER PERSONS: SPECIAL CONSIDERATIONS

A complete examination is required as usual, but think about the following areas as you go about obtaining the data (see Fig. 44.1).

1. *General assessment:* check for postural blood pressure changes.

   Assess hydration, which may be impaired in older patients with cognitive dysfunction.

   Look at the patient's skin carefully for pressure sores. These are areas of injury to the skin or soft tissue and subcutaneous tissue as a result of localised pressure or shear injury and occur in immobile patients. Certain risk factors have been identified that increase the risk of a patient's developing pressure sores (List 44.8). Classify the severity and extent of the sores (Table 44.1).

   Look for evidence of bruises from falls or elder abuse. Look at the skin for any evidence of skin cancer.

   Measure the patient's weight and height to calculate the body mass index, as weight loss is common in the elderly.

2. *Heart:* if a systolic murmur is heard, consider whether this may be aortic stenosis, which, if severe, is likely to require evaluation.

   Ankle swelling may indicate venous insufficiency or antihypertensive drug use (e.g. calcium antagonists) rather than

> **RISK FACTORS FOR PRESSURE SORES**
>
> 1. Cognitive impairment
> 2. Immobility
> 3. Advanced age
> 4. Sensory impairment
> 5. Low body weight
> 6. Oedema
> 7. Incontinence
> 8. Hypoalbuminaemia
>
> LIST 44.8

Classification of bed sores

Stage	Description
I	Skin intact but non-blanching erythema
II	Partial thickness loss of skin. Shallow open ulcer, no slough or intact or burst blister
III	Full-thickness loss of tissue. Subcutaneous fat visible but not bone or muscle
IV	Full-thickness tissue loss and muscle or bone visible
Unstageable	Full-thickness but base covered in slough
Suspected deep tissue injury	Purple- or maroon-coloured area of intact skin or a blood-filled blister

TABLE 44.1

congestive cardiac failure. Ischaemic heart disease is common but often 'silent' in the elderly.

3. *Chest*: shortness of breath may be due to lung or cardiac disease, and these often coexist in the elderly.
4. *Gastrointestinal system*: look at the dentition and look for dry mouth, which may impair eating. Note signs of recent weight loss.

   A mass may be felt in the left lower quadrant in patients with constipation from hard stool; this will clear with treatment of the constipation.

   The aorta may be palpable in the thin elderly patient. This may be falsely interpreted as an aneurysm, but if the aorta seems significantly enlarged then an aortic aneurysm needs to be excluded. If the aneurysm is leaking, the classical presentation includes back pain, abdominal distension, shock and poor asymmetrical peripheral pulses in the legs.

   Perform a rectal examination and rule out faecal impaction, particularly if there is a history of faecal or urinary incontinence.

   An enlarged bladder may be felt in patients with acute urinary retention; this problem can present with delirium.

5. *Nervous system*: evaluation of mental status and cognitive function should be routine in older patients. If a patient is confused it is important to distinguish cognitive decline (dementia) from an acute confusional state (delirium; see Tables 46.5 and 46.6 on p 858).

   Primitive reflexes such as the glabellar tap (see Fig. 35.17 on p 599), palmomental reflex and grasp reflex are found in those of increasing age and may be evidence of dementia.

   Carefully assess gait (which may include gait speed over 8 metres with a stopwatch; normal gait speed in healthy elderly people ranges from 1.1 to 1.5 metres/second) and balance.[5]

   Further test gait with the 'get up and go' test (see Fig. 44.2): ask the patient to stand up out of a chair, walk 3 metres, turn around 180°, return to the chair and sit down. Assess the following:
   - Patient in the chair: does the patient have trouble getting out of a chair with or without arms?
   - Patient standing near the chair: is the patient unsteady?
   - Patient walking: is the gait abnormal— unsteady, Parkinsonian, hemiplegic, needs stick, frame, etc.?
   - Patient turning: is the patient slow or hesitant?
   - Patient sitting down: is the patient nervous or hesitant?

   Look for abnormalities in gait, balance and power. The test can be graded from 1 (normal) to 5 (severely impaired) but is usually timed (fixing the walking distance),

'Get up and go' test:
1. 'Stand up now for me and walk over to here.' 2. 'Now turn around and walk back.'
3. 'Now come and sit down again.' Difficulty in standing up from a chair indicates an increased falls risk

(From Douglas G, Nicol F, Robertson C. *Macleod's clinical examination*, 13th edn. Edinburgh: Churchill Livingstone, ©2013.)

FIGURE 44.2

comparing the time taken to age-adjusted normal values (however, these times appear to have limited diagnostic value).[7] Look carefully for lower leg weakness and test power if needed.[8,9]

Test for falls risk using the 'functional reach' test. Ask the patient to stand with his or her fist extended alongside a wall, then lean forwards as far as possible. The patient should be able to move the fist along the wall without taking a step or losing stability. Measure the length of movement. A distance of less than 15 centimetres suggests an increased falls risk.[10]

6. *Eyes and ears:* check the patient's vision and hearing as these may impair independent living. Does the patient have a hearing aid in place? (80% of 80 year olds have impaired hearing.) Hearing aids can be difficult to manage and patients need some enthusiasm to make them work, but there is some evidence that use of hearing aids reduces patients' sense of isolation. Hearing loss must not be confused with cognitive dysfunction. A whispered voice test may be useful for screening for hearing loss. Has the patient got cataracts interfering with vision?

7. *Rheumatological system:* examine for deformities and functional disabilities, including the feet.

8. *Breasts:* perform a breast examination in women, as the incidence of breast cancer greatly increases with age.

9. *Depression:* 5% of men and 7% of women over 60 have problems with depression. This can lead to lack of enthusiasm and engagement and must also not be confused with cognitive impairment.
   Ask: 'In the last month, have you been troubled by feeling little interest in doing things? Have you felt "low", "down" or depressed?' This simple questioning is very sensitive

(97%) but less specific (67%) for the diagnosis of depression.

10. *Cognitive function:* dementia affects 35% of people in their 90s. It can be defined as a decline in at least two cognitive areas:
    - memory
    - attention
    - language
    - visuospatial ability
    - decision making (executive function).

    Screening for dementia is not recommended as a routine but if there is any suspicion (e.g. concern by relatives, medical non-adherence, accidents or behavioural changes) then screening should be performed.[11]

Dementia screening

The mini-mental state examination (MMSE)[12] has a good evidence base but is protected by copyright; the Mini-Cog screening tool[13] is more readily available and is easy to use (see Ch 46, p 854).

OSCE REVISION TOPICS – ASSESSMENT OF THE GERIATRIC PATIENT

Use these topics, which commonly occur in the OSCE, to help with revision.

1. This 89-year-old man takes 11 regular medications. Take a drug history from him. (p 827)

2. This 77-year-old woman has some problems with her memory. Please take a history from her. (pp 546, 833, 854)

3. This 79-year-old man is having difficulty managing at home by himself. Please take a history from him. (p 828)

4. This elderly woman has had a number of falls recently and has fractured her wrist. Please take a history from her and perform an examination. (p 828)

References

1. Ellis G, Whitehead MA, O'Neill D et al. Comprehensive geriatric assessment for older patients admitted to hospital. *Cochrane Database Sys Rev* 2011; (7):CD006211.
2. Katz S, Down TD, Cash HR, Grotz RC. Progress in the development of the index of ADL. *Gerontologist* 1970; 10:20–30.
3. Lawton MP, Brody EM. Assessment of older people; self maintaining and instrumental activities of daily living. *Gerontologist* 1969; 9:179.
4. Lachs MS, Pillemer KA. Elder abuse. *N Engl J Med* 2015; 373(20):1947–1956. Like child abuse, clinicians should be alert to the possibility of elder abuse in patients who present with unexplained injuries.
5. Studenski S, Perera S, Patel K et al. Gait speed and survival in older adults. *JAMA* 2011; 305:50–58. Gait speed is a measure of frailty. Faster walkers have better survival.
6. Whooley MA, Avins AL, Miranda J, Browner WS. Case-finding instruments for depression: two questions are as good as many. *J Gen Intern Med* 1997; 12:439–445.
7. Schoene D, Wu SM, Mikolaizak AS et al. Discriminative ability and predictive validity of the timed up and go test in identifying older people who fall: systematic review and meta-analysis. *J Am Geriatr Soc* 2013; 61:202–208. 'Get up and go' test times have only poor-to-moderate diagnostic accuracy.
8. Nevitt MC, Cummings SR, Kidd S, Black D. Risk factors for recurrent nonsyncopal falls: a prospective study. *JAMA* 1989; 261:2663–2668. The history identifies those at higher risk of falls. Risk factors include three or more falls or a fall with injury in the previous year, arthritis, Parkinson's disease, difficulty in standing up from a chair or in performing a tandem walk.
9. Tinetti ME. Clinical practice. Preventing falls in elderly persons. *N Engl J Med* 2003; 348:42–49. Practical management advice.
10. Fleming KC, Evans JM, Weber DC, Chutka DS. Practical functional assessment of elderly persons: a primary-care approach. *Mayo Clin Proc* 1995; 70:890–910. Useful screening test advice is given. The 'functional reach' test is useful for predicting increased falls risk.
11. Lin JS, O'Connor E, Rossom RC et al. Screening for cognitive impairment in older adults: a systematic review for the U.S. Preventive Services Task Force. *Ann Intern Med* 2013; 159(9):601–612. Screening tests available for dementia include the Mini-Cog and the Clock Drawing Test.
12. Tangalos EG, Smith GE, Ivnik RJ et al. The mini-mental state examination in general medical practice: clinical utility and acceptance. *Mayo Clin Proc* 1996; 71:829.
13. Borson S, Scanlan JM, Chen P, Ganguli M. The Mini-Cog as a screen for dementia: validation in a population-based sample. *J Am Geriatr Soc* 2003; 51:1451.

CHAPTER 45
Approaching infectious diseases

As it takes two to make a quarrel, so it takes two to make a disease, the microbe and its host. CHARLES CHAPLIN (1856–1941)

We have selected two important presentations to be covered in this chapter to show how infectious diseases can be approached in a systematic manner.

PYREXIA OF UNKNOWN ORIGIN

Pyrexia of unknown origin (PUO) is defined as documented fever (>38°C) of more than 3 weeks' duration, where no cause is found despite basic investigations.[1] The most frequent causes to consider are tuberculosis, occult abscess (usually intra-abdominal), osteomyelitis, infective endocarditis, lymphoma or leukaemia, systemic-onset juvenile rheumatoid arthritis, giant cell arteritis and drug fever (drug fever is responsible for 10% of fevers leading to hospital admission[2]). In studies of fever of unknown origin,[3] infection is found to be the cause in 30%, neoplasia in 30%, connective tissue disease in 15% and miscellaneous causes in 15%; in 10% the aetiology remains unknown (see List 45.1). Remember: the longer the duration of the fever, the less likely there is to be

---

COMMON CAUSES OF PYREXIA OF UNKNOWN ORIGIN

Neoplasms
- Hodgkin's and non-Hodgkin's lymphoma, leukaemia, malignant histiocytosis
- Other tumours: hepatic, renal, lung, disseminated carcinoma, atrial myxoma

Infections
- *Bacterial*: e.g. tuberculosis, brucellosis and other bacteraemias, abscess formation (especially pelvic or abdominal), endocarditis, pericarditis, osteomyelitis, cholangitis, pyelonephritis, pelvic inflammatory disease, prostatitis, syphilis, Lyme disease, borreliosis, cat scratch disease, dental abscess
- *Viral*: e.g. infectious mononucleosis,* cytomegalovirus infection, hepatitis B or C, human immunodeficiency virus (HIV) infection, Ross River virus
- *Parasitic*: e.g. strongyloidiasis, schistosomiasis, malaria, Q fever, toxoplasmosis
- *Fungal*: e.g. histoplasmosis, cryptococcosis, blastomycosis

Connective tissue diseases
- Juvenile rheumatoid arthritis, adult Still's disease, systemic lupus erythematosus
- Vasculitis (e.g. giant cell arteritis, polyarteritis nodosa)
- Immunosuppressive drugs (occult infection)

Drug fever: e.g. anticonvulsants, antibiotics (e.g. minocycline), allopurinol, heparin

Miscellaneous
- Inflammatory bowel disease, acute alcoholic hepatitis, granulomatous disease (e.g. sarcoid), multiple pulmonary emboli, thyroiditis, adrenal insufficiency, phaeochromocytoma, familial Mediterranean fever and other hereditary periodic fever syndromes, haematoma, factitious fever

Uncertain

*Epstein–Barr virus is the cause of infectious mononucleosis.

LIST 45.1

an infectious aetiology. The majority of patients do not have a rare disease but rather a relatively common disease presenting in an unusual way.[4]

History

The history may give a number of clues in these puzzling cases. In some patients a careful history may give the diagnosis where expensive tests have failed. (See Questions box 45.1.)

The time course of the fever and any associated symptoms must be uncovered. Symptoms from the various body systems should be sought methodically. Examples include:

1. *gastrointestinal system*—diarrhoea, abdominal pain, recent abdominal surgery (inflammatory bowel disease, diverticular disease, cholangitis)
2. *cardiovascular system*—heart murmurs, dental procedures (infective endocarditis), chest pain (pericarditis)
3. *rheumatology*—joint symptoms, rashes, persistent back pain (spondylodiscitis may cause PUO and progress to quadriplegia)
4. *neurology*—headache (meningitis, cerebral abscess)
5. *genitourinary system*—history of renal disease or infection, dysuria
6. *respiratory system*—old tuberculosis (TB) or recent TB contact, chest symptoms.

Details of any recent overseas travel are important. Find out also about hobbies and exposure to pets. Occupational exposure may be important. Take a drug history. Find out whether the patient is involved in behaviour posing a risk of HIV infection. Patients who are already in hospital may have infected cannulas or old cannula sites. The new onset of fever in a hospitalised patient is an indication to remove a peripheral cannula (send the tip for culture).

Fever due to bacteraemia (the presence of viable bacteria in the bloodstream) is associated with a higher risk of mortality. Bacteraemia is present in up to 20% of hospital patients with acute fever.[5,6]

Examination

General

Look at the temperature chart to see whether there is a pattern of fever that is identifiable. Inspect the patient and decide how seriously ill he or she appears. Look for evidence of weight loss (indicating a chronic illness). Note any skin rash (see List 45.2). The details of the examination required will depend on the patient's history.[7]

GENERAL QUESTIONS TO ASK THE PATIENT WITH A FEVER

! denotes symptoms for the possible diagnosis of an urgent or dangerous problem.

1. How long have you had high temperatures?
2. Have you taken your own temperature? How high has it been?
! 3. Have you had shivers and shakes (rigors)? (Shaking chills suggest bacteraemia[4])
4. Has anyone you know had a similar illness?
5. What medications are you taking?
6. Have you had any recent illnesses?
7. Have you had any recent operations or medical procedures?
8. Have you travelled recently? Where to?
9. Did you take antimalarial prophylaxis and have the recommended vaccinations for your trip?
10. Have you any pets? Have they been sick lately?

QUESTIONS BOX 45.1

DIFFERENTIAL DIAGNOSIS OF PROLONGED FEVER AND RASH

1. *Viral*: e.g. infectious mononucleosis, rubella, dengue fever
2. *Bacterial*: e.g. syphilis, Lyme disease
3. *Non-infective*: e.g. drugs, systemic lupus erythematosus, erythema multiforme (which may also be related to an underlying infection)

LIST 45.2

Hands

Look for the stigmata of infective endocarditis or vasculitic changes. Note whether there is clubbing. The presence of arthropathy or Raynaud's phenomenon may point to a connective tissue disease.

Arms

Inspect for drug injection sites suggesting intravenous drug abuse (see Fig. 7.2 on p 123) as well as recent cannula sites. Peripheral cannulae are responsible for sepsis and death in hospitalised patients. The new onset of fever in a hospitalised patient is an indication to remove the peripheral cannula (send the tip for culture). Feel for the epitrochlear and axillary nodes (e.g. lymphoma, other malignancy, sarcoidosis, focal infections).

Head and neck

Feel the *temporal arteries* (over the temples for giant cell arteritis). In temporal arteritis these may be tender and thickened.

Examine the *eyes* for iritis or conjunctivitis (e.g. leptospirosis, measles, connective tissue disease e.g. reactive arthritis) or jaundice (e.g. ascending cholangitis, blackwater fever in malaria). Look in the fundi for choroidal tubercles in miliary tuberculosis, Roth's spots in infective endocarditis and retinal haemorrhages or the infiltrates of leukaemia or lymphoma.

Inspect the *face* for a butterfly rash (systemic lupus erythematosus, see Fig. 25.11 on p 416) or seborrhoeic dermatitis, which is common in patients with HIV infection.

Examine the *mouth* for ulcers, gum disease or candidiasis, and the teeth and tonsils for infection (e.g. abscess). Look in the *ears* for otitis media. Feel the *parotid glands* for evidence of infection.

Palpate the cervical lymph nodes. Examine for thyroid enlargement and tenderness (subacute thyroiditis).

Chest

Examine the chest. Palpate for bony tenderness. Carefully examine the respiratory system (e.g. for signs of pneumonia, tuberculosis, empyema, carcinoma) and the heart for murmurs (e.g. infective endocarditis, atrial myxoma) or rubs (e.g. pericarditis).

Abdomen

Examine the abdomen. Inspect for rashes, including rose-coloured spots (in typhoid fever—2- to 4-millimetre flat red spots, which blanch on pressure and occur on the upper abdomen and lower chest). Examine for evidence of hepatomegaly and ascites (e.g. spontaneous bacterial peritonitis, hepatic carcinoma, metastatic deposits), splenomegaly (e.g. haemopoietic malignancy, infective endocarditis, malaria), renal enlargement (e.g. renal cell carcinoma) or localised tenderness (e.g. collection of pus). Palpate for testicular enlargement (e.g. seminoma, tuberculosis). Feel for inguinal lymphadenopathy.

Perform a rectal examination, feeling for a mass or tenderness in the rectum or pelvis (e.g. abscess, carcinoma, prostatitis). Perform a vaginal examination to detect collections of pelvic pus or evidence of pelvic inflammatory disease. Look at the penis and scrotum for a discharge or rash.

Central nervous system

Examine the central nervous system for signs of meningism (e.g. chronic tuberculous meningitis, cryptococcal meningitis) or focal neurological signs (e.g. brain abscess, mononeuritis multiplex in polyarteritis nodosa).

Clinical scenarios for unexplained fever

Consider age, co-morbidities and the epidemiology, e.g. adult with a prosthetic heart valve (endocarditis), young female with a rash (systemic lupus), post neurosurgery on phenytoin (drug), middle-aged with easy bruising and fatigue (haematological malignancy), young migrant from Nepal (TB).

HIV INFECTION AND AIDS

The acquired immunodeficiency syndrome (AIDS), first described in 1981, is caused by the human immunodeficiency virus (HIV).[7–9] This is a T-cell lymphotrophic virus, which results in T4-cell destruction and therefore susceptibility to opportunistic infections and the development of tumours, notably Kaposi's[a] sarcoma and non-Hodgkin's lymphoma.

---

[a] Moritz Kohn Kaposi (1837–1902), a professor of dermatology in Vienna, described the sarcoma in 1892.

Table 45.1 Features of the HIV seroconversion illness (acute retroviral illness) and their frequency

Feature	%
Fever	95
Lymphadenopathy	75
Pharyngitis	70
Rash	70
Arthralgia/myalgia	55
Diarrhoea	32
Headache	30
Nausea and vomiting	25
Hepatosplenomegaly	15
Loss of weight	13
Thrush	10
Neurological symptoms	10

Questions Box 45.2 Questions to ask the patient with a recent diagnosis of HIV infection

1. Can you remember symptoms of a seroconversion illness?
2. Why was the diagnosis suspected?
3. How do you think you may have become infected?
4. Is your sexual partner(s) aware of your illness?
5. Are they taking precautions against infection?
6. Have you been tested for hepatitis?
7. Have you had a problem with chest or other infections?
8. Have you begun treatment?
9. What have you been told about your prognosis?

History

HIV infection should be suspected particularly if the patient falls into a high-risk group (e.g. men who have sex with men, intravenous drug user, sexual tourist, sexual partner of HIV-infected person, haemophiliac, blood transfusion or blood product recipient, prostitute or someone having sexual contact with one of these).

The patient may have had a seroconversion illness (50% of cases) (Table 45.1). Ask about: fever, lymphadenopathy, maculopapular rash, arthralgia, pharyngitis, nausea and vomiting, headache, weight loss and oral candidiasis.

Careful questioning (see Questions box 45.2) about the mode of infection is important but should be left to a subsequent consultation if the patient seems reluctant to discuss this. Patients may be unwilling to inform their sexual partners that they are infected. This puts the latter at risk of infection and there is a duty on the treating clinician's part to ensure that these people are informed, tested and protected (e.g. by condom use).

HIV infection is often present in combination with other sexually transmitted infections, such as syphilis and gonorrhoea, and with the hepatic viruses B and C. The incidence varies in different countries, but hepatitis C is uncommon in Australian HIV patients.

HIV should be strongly suspected in patients who present with TB, and TB should be suspected in HIV patients with a chronic respiratory illness. HIV infection has replaced TB as the great imitator of other illnesses. HIV testing should be routine in any unexplained infectious illness.

Ask about features of chronic HIV infection including:
- fever, night sweats
- enlarged lymph nodes
- fatigue
- weight loss
- chronic diarrhoea
- seborrhoeic dermatitis
- psoriasis
- fungal infections, e.g. tinea, onychomycosis
- apthous ulcers, gingivitis
- peripheral neuropathy
- anaemia, leucopenia, thrombocytopenia ('Have you got reduced red or white cells or platelets in your blood?')
- nephropathy ('Have you had kidney problems?').

Patients treated for HIV infection have an increased risk of cardiovascular disease. This is partly because of their chronic inflammatory condition and partly because of the development of metabolic risk factors as a side effect of their antiviral treatment. Cardiovascular disease has become the most common cause of death for treated HIV patients. Ask about cardiovascular risk factors: smoking, diabetes, hypertension etc. Has the patient had any diagnosis of heart disease?

Examination

Examine the patient as follows.

General inspection

Take the patient's temperature. The patient may appear ill and wasted owing to chronic ill-health or chronic opportunistic infection. *Mycobacterium avium* complex (MAC) presents with fever and weight loss.

Look at the skin for rashes:

- The maculopapular rash of acute HIV infection (5- to 10-millimetre maculopapular lesions on the face and trunk and rarely on the palms and soles).
- Herpes zoster (shingles, which may involve more than one dermatome in this disease and is more commonly seen in early rather than advanced HIV infection).
- Oral herpes simplex (cold sores) or genital herpes.
- Oral and flexural candidiasis (once the CD4 level is below $200/mm^3$).
- Molluscum contagiosum, impetigo, seborrhoea or other non-specific exanthems.
- Kaposi's sarcoma: red-purple vascular non-tender tumours. These present typically on the skin but can occur anywhere.
- Skin lesions resembling Kaposi's sarcoma may also be seen. These are called bacillary angiomatosis and are caused by *Bartonella henselae* and *Bartonella quintana* (see Figs 45.1 and 45.2).
- Severe psoriasis is common in HIV patients.

Adverse drug reactions are more common in patients with HIV infection and may be the cause of a rash. Look for hyperpigmentation. Patients taking the drug clofazimine for MAC infection usually become

Angry red nodule of bacillary angiomatosis

(Reeves JT, Maibach H. *Clinical dermatology illustrated: a regional approach*, 2nd edn. Sydney: MacLennan & Petty Pty Ltd, ©1991.)

FIGURE 45.1

Late nodules of Kaposi's sarcoma

(Reeves JT, Maibach H. *Clinical dermatology illustrated: a regional approach*, 2nd edn. Sydney: MacLennan & Petty Pty Ltd, ©1991.)

FIGURE 45.2

deeply pigmented. Areas of peripheral fat atrophy—lipodystrophy—on limbs, cheeks and buttocks may be seen in patients treated with protease inhibitor drugs. Some of these patients have fat redistribution with central obesity.

Oral candidiasis

((From McDonald FS, ed. *Mayo Clinic images in internal medicine*, with permission. © Mayo Clinic Scientific Press and CRC Press. Reproduced by permission of Taylor and Francis Group, LLC, a division of Informa plc.))

FIGURE 45.3

Hands and arms

Look for nail changes including onycholysis. Feel for the epitrochlear nodes; a node 0.5 centimetres or larger may be characteristic.[10] Note any injection marks.

Face

Inspect the mouth for:
- candidal plaques (see Fig. 45.3)
- angular stomatitis
- aphthous ulcers
- tongue ulceration (e.g. herpes simplex, cytomegalovirus or candidal infections) or gingivitis[11]
- periodontal disease.

Kaposi's sarcoma (see Fig. 45.4) may also occur on the hard or soft palate (in which case associated lesions are almost always present elsewhere in the gastrointestinal tract). Oral squamous cell carcinoma and non-Hodgkin's lymphoma are more common in AIDS.

Parotidomegaly is sometimes seen as a result of HIV-associated Sjögren's syndrome. These patients may have dry eyes and mouth for this reason.

Hairy leucoplakia is a unique raised or flat white, painless and often hairy-looking lesion typically present on the lateral surface of the tongue; it is caused by Epstein–Barr virus (EBV) infection in HIV-infected people and is almost diagnostic of HIV infection.

(a) Kaposi's sarcoma in the mouth.
(b) Kaposi's sarcoma on the foot

((a) From McDonald FS, ed. *Mayo Clinic images in internal medicine*, with permission. © Mayo Clinic Scientific Press and CRC Press. Reproduced by permission of Taylor and Francis Group, LLC, a division of Informa plc (b) Courtesy of Dr A Watson, Infectious Diseases Department, The Canberra Hospital.))

FIGURE 45.4

Palpate over the sinuses for tenderness (sinusitis). Examine the cervical and axillary nodes. There may be generalised lymphadenopathy, and all lymph node groups should be examined.

Chest

Note any tachypnoea or dry cough. Note chronic cough, either dry or productive of purulent sputum. On auscultation, crackles may be present at the bases owing to bronchiolitis obliterans. There are often, however, no chest signs despite the presence of pulmonary infiltrates on chest X-ray, due to *Pneumocystis jiroveci* (formerly *carinii*) or other opportunistic infections.

Retinal toxoplasmosis—old chorioretinal scar

(Courtesy of Dr Chris Kennedy & Professor Ian Constable, Lions Eye Institute.)

FIGURE 45.5

Cytomegalovirus retinitis

(Courtesy of Dr Chris Kennedy & Professor Ian Constable, Lions Eye Institute.)

FIGURE 45.6

Abdomen

Examine for hepatosplenomegaly (e.g. infection, lymphoma). Perform a rectal examination (e.g. perianal ulceration from herpes simplex) and a sigmoidoscopy looking for Kaposi's sarcoma or proctitis (e.g. cytomegalovirus, herpes simplex, amoebic dysentery or pseudomembranous colitis from antibiotic use). Examine the genitals for herpes simplex, warts, discharge or chancre.

Nervous system

Look for signs of meningism (e.g. cryptococcal meningitis). There may be focal signs due to a space-occupying intracranial lesion (e.g. toxoplasmosis, non-Hodgkin's lymphoma).

A syndrome similar to Guillain–Barré and a pure sensory neuropathy can occur. HIV infection itself, opportunistic infection or the drugs used in treatment can be responsible for peripheral sensorimotor neuropathy, polymyositis, radiculopathy, mononeuritis multiplex or a myelopathy.

Look in the fundi for soft exudates (common in AIDS patients), scars (e.g. toxoplasmosis—see Fig. 45.5) or retinitis (e.g. cytomegalovirus-induced retinitis with perivascular haemorrhages and fluffy exudates, which can cause blindness of rapid onset—see Fig. 45.6).[12] There may be signs of dementia (AIDS encephalopathy).

T&O'C ESSENTIALS

1. Persisting fever may be due to a common illness that has presented in an unusual way.
2. Careful history taking and examination will help direct the investigations in a febrile or possibly septic patient.
3. Recent travel or contact with other sick people or animals may suggest a specific line of investigation.
4. Systemic inflammatory response syndrome (SIRS) refers to two or more of the following four features: fever >38.3°C (or temperature <36°C), tachycardia (>90 beats/minute), tachypnoea (>20 breaths/minute) and an elevated white cell count. This may be due to acute infection (you must rule out sepsis), but can occur after burns or surgery or with other inflammatory diseases (e.g. thromboembolism, pancreatitis).
5. HIV infection should be suspected in a patient with tuberculosis or any unexplained infectious illness.
6. Questioning a patient with newly diagnosed HIV about the possible mode of infection and contacts is important from a public health point of view.

OSCE REVISION TOPICS – INFECTIOUS DISEASES

1. This woman has a prosthetic heart valve and has been unwell for 2 months. Please take a history from her and explain what examination you would perform. (p 835)

2. This man has recently been diagnosed with HIV infection. Please take a history from him. (p 837)

References

1. Hayakawa K, Ramasamy B, Chandrasekar PH. Fever of unknown origin: an evidence-based review. *Am J Med Sci* 2012; 344(4):307–316. The modern approach to diagnosis still relies on the history and physical examination initially.
2. Arbo M, Fine MJ, Hanusa BH et al. Fever of nosocomial origin: etiology, risk factors and outcomes. *Am J Med* 1993; 95:505–515.
3. Cunha BA, Lortholary O, Cunha CB. Fever of unknown origin: a clinical approach. *Am J Med* 2015; 128(10):1138.
4. Mourad O, Palda V, Detsky AS. A comprehensive evidence-based approach to fever of unknown origin. *Arch Intern Med* 2003; 163:545.
5. Coburn B, Morris AM, Tomlinson G, Detsky AS. Does this adult patient with suspected bacteremia require blood cultures? *JAMA* 2012; 308(5):502–511. Shaking chills but not fever alone suggests bacteraemia.
6. Bates DW, Cook EF, Goldman L et al. Predicting bacteremia in hospitalized patients: a prospectively validated model. *Ann Intern Med* 1990; 113:495–500.
7. Wood E, Kerr T, Rowell G et al. The rational clinical examination systematic review. Does this adult patient have early HIV infection? *JAMA* 2014; 312(3):278–285.
8. American College of Physicians and Infectious Diseases Society of America. Human immunodeficiency virus (HIV) infection. *Ann Intern Med* 1994; 120:310–319.
9. Nandwani R. Human immunodeficiency virus medicine for the MRCP short cases. *Br J Hosp Med* 1994; 51:353–356.
10. Malin A, Ternouth I, Sarbah S. Epitrochlear nodes as marker of HIV disease in sub-Saharan Africa. *BMJ* 1994; 309:1550–1551.
11. Weinert ML, Grimes RM, Lynch DP. Oral manifestations of HIV infection. *Ann Intern Med* 1996; 125:485–496. Details the 16 leading oral complications, based on an extensive literature review.
12. De Smet MD, Nessenbatt RB. Ocular manifestations of AIDS. *JAMA* 1991; 266:3019–3022. Provides a very good review of eye changes.

SECTION 13
Mental health history and examination

CHAPTER 46
The psychiatric history and mental state examination

CHAPTER 46
The psychiatric history and mental state examination

Law number four: the patient is the one with the disease. SAMUEL SHEM, The House of God

This chapter deals with the psychiatric history and the mental state examination. The practising clinician must have an understanding of psychiatric illness and know how to perform a psychiatric interview and a mental state examination. This is because there is considerable overlap between psychiatric and physical illness.

Psychiatric disorders (especially anxiety and depression) are common (one person in four will experience a mental illness in his or her lifetime) but most will fully recover. People suffering from these conditions often have medical problems or problems with drugs and alcohol. Appropriate management of these patients requires an understanding of the intercurrent psychiatric disorder and the effect of that disorder on the primary medical problem. A medical illness may, in some instances, present as a psychiatric illness. For example, some endocrine disorders, such as hypothroidism, may present with depression. On the other hand, some psychiatric disorders may present medically. Panic disorder (or acute anxiety) may be mistaken for an acute myocardial infarction. Furthermore, a patient's psychological state may interfere with the course of a medical illness; it may lead in some cases to exaggeration of the symptoms and in others to denial of the severity of physical symptoms. Medical illnesses, particularly chronic and/or life-threatening illnesses, have major psychological impacts and can be complicated by psychiatric symptoms (such as anxiety or depression) that can induce disability and affect recovery from illness.

THE HISTORY

The psychiatric history generally follows the same format as the standard medical history, and the principles described apply just as much here as in any history taking.[1] One should enquire about the history of the present illness, the past psychiatric and medical history, and the family and social history. However, the psychiatric history aims to elicit more detail about the patient's illness from a broad perspective, focusing not only on symptoms but also on the patient's social background, psychological functioning and life circumstances (a biopsychosocial approach). Within the psychiatric history, particular attention is paid to the developmental, personal and social history, although these factors are usually also relevant in the general medical history.

Every medical interview should aim to be therapeutic as well as diagnostic. The method of psychiatric history taking is somewhat different from the standard medical interview. In the course of the interview it is hoped that the patient will be able to talk about his or her concerns in detail, and their context. In doing so, patients should gain some relief from their distress by airing their problems. For this to take place, the clinician's attitude needs to be unhurried, patient and understanding. The psychiatric history also aims to gain an understanding of how the patient's problem arose from a biological, interpersonal, social and psychological perspective, so that the best management plan can be worked out. In this way, the psychiatric interview is similar to the general medical interview. These factors are also important in relation to any illness, especially if it is a chronic or life-threatening problem. Psychiatric and physical problems often coexist and each affects the other. A comprehensive medical interview should therefore encompass both physical and psychological concerns.

OBTAINING THE HISTORY

The clinician taking a psychiatric history wants the patient to tell his or her story in his or her own words. In this way the patient will be more likely to report the most important aspects of the illness. Of course, this technique also applies to the general medical interview. It is best achieved using a non-directive approach with open-ended questions. **Open-ended questions** are those to which the patient responds with a narrative (or a description about what has been happening) rather than a simple factual response. They give patients an opportunity to talk about their problems in their own words. **Closed questions**, on the other hand, are more likely to elicit 'yes' or 'no' responses. For example, in the assessment of a patient with depression, a closed question would be: 'Have you been depressed?' An open-ended question would be: 'Tell me about how you have been feeling.' At first glance it might appear that the open-ended question is less efficient, as it could take longer to find out about a range of symptoms. However, with a careful and judicious approach, open-ended questioning—by permitting the patient to tell the story—will enable the clinician to get a comprehensive history efficiently. This is not to say that targeted, more-closed questions must not be used—they are necessary to elicit information on certain symptoms.

It takes experience and practice to feel confident and unembarrassed when interviewing patients who have difficult psychiatric problems that may be associated with a certain stigma or where the questioning is about sexual or intimate problems. This is certainly not the place to make judgements about or appear shocked by what a patient is saying. Of course, appearing to be sympathetic about the patient's difficulties is necessary here, as it is with any medical interview.

While the patient is telling his or her story, you should begin to formulate hypotheses about the problem or diagnosis. These hypotheses are tested by asking more-focused questions later in the interview, at which point a diagnostic hypothesis can be rejected or pursued further. For example, a patient may describe tiredness and lethargy, an inability to concentrate and loss of appetite. These symptoms will suggest a diagnosis of depression. Follow-up questions should focus on this possibility. You should ask questions about other symptoms of depression such as: 'How have you been feeling in yourself?', 'What has your mood been like?' and 'How have you been sleeping?'

Introductory questions

The assessment of psychiatric symptoms should start with non-threatening questions. After introducing yourself, it can be useful to begin by asking about basic demographic information (age, marital status, occupation, whom the patient lives with) and then make the patient feel at ease by discussing some neutral topic. In some cases the presenting problem will be an obvious psychiatric or psychological one. For example, a patient may say, 'I've come to see you because I've been feeling very depressed'. However, even such an apparently definite psychiatric problem may have a medical cause, such as hypothyroidism or a recent serious medical illness. More often, the presenting problem will be a more general one, such as 'I have no energy and feel tired all the time'. This may be due to a depressive illness or it could have a medical cause such as anaemia. Remember that psychiatric and medical problems are intimately entwined. It is rare for an interview to focus purely on psychiatric problems.

History of the presenting illness

In assessing the history of the presenting illness, you need to cover a number of areas.

The problem

Find out the nature of the patient's problem, and the patient's perception of his or her difficulties. This can, of course, be difficult if the patient is psychotic and does not believe that a psychiatric problem exists at all. In these cases a corroborative history must be taken. For example, a manic patient may consider that there is nothing wrong and that his or her behaviour is reasonable, whereas the patient's partner is able to recognise that ordering an expensive new sports car when the family is impoverished is a problem.

A range of symptoms commonly found in psychiatric disorders needs to be reviewed in the course of assessing the history of the present illness. These include mood change, anxiety, worry, sleep patterns, appetite, hallucinations and delusions. A set of simple screening questions for each of the major diagnoses is listed within Table 46.1.

It is especially important to ask about symptoms of anxiety and depression (the most common psychiatric

Text continued on p 851

The common psychiatric disorders* and their screening questions

Mood (affective) disorders

Mood disorders have a pathological disturbance in mood (depression or mania) as the predominant feature. They are distinguished from 'normal' mood changes by their persistence, duration and severity, together with the presence of other symptoms and impairment of functioning.

Manic–depressive illness—bipolar disorder

Bipolar disorder is a broad term to describe a recurrent illness characterised by episodes of either mania or depression, with a return to normal functioning between episodes of illness.

(a) Mania A disorder demonstrated by change in mood (*elation*), thought form (*grandiosity*) and behaviour disturbance (*increased energy and disinhibition*). Frequently associated symptoms and signs: increased talkativeness, irritability, distractibility, decreased need for sleep, loss of inhibition (e.g. engaging in reckless behaviour such as spending sprees, sexual indiscretion or social overfamiliarity).	**Questions box 46.1** Questions to ask the patient with possible mania 1. Have you felt especially good about yourself? 2. Have you been needing less sleep than usual? 3. Do you feel that you are special or that you have special powers? 4. Have you been spending more than usual?
(b) Depression A disorder characterised by depressed mood (or loss of pleasure) and the presence of somatic (*sleep disturbance, change in appetite, fatigue and weight*), psychological (*low self-esteem, worry–anxiety, guilt, suicidal ideation*), affective (*sadness, irritability, loss of pleasure and interest in activities*) and psychomotor (*retardation or agitation*) symptoms.	**Questions box 46.2** Questions to ask the patient with possible depression 1. How have you been feeling in yourself? 2. What has your mood been like? 3. Have you been feeling sad, blue, down or depressed? 4. Have you lost interest in things you usually enjoy? 5. How have you been sleeping?

Anxiety disorders

Anxiety disorders are those in which the person experiences excessive levels of anxiety. Anxiety may be somatic (palpitations, difficulty breathing, dry mouth, nausea, frequency of micturition, dizziness, muscular tension, sweating, abdominal churning, tremor, cold skin) or psychological (feelings of dread and threat, irritability, panic, anxious anticipation, inner [psychic] tension, worrying over trivia, difficulty in concentrating, initial insomnia, inability to relax).

1. Generalised anxiety disorder (GAD) A chronic disorder characterised by a tendency to worry excessively about everyday things. It is accompanied by: symptoms of anxiety or tension; mental tension (*feeling tense or nervous, poor concentration, on edge*); physical tension.	**Questions box 46.3** Questions to ask the patient with possible anxiety 1. Have you been feeling nervy or tense? 2. Do you worry a lot about things? Find it hard to relax/switch off? 3. Do you worry about things most other people would not worry about?
2. Panic disorder A disorder characterised by episodes of panic occurring spontaneously in situations where most people would not be afraid. A panic attack is characterised by the presence of physical symptoms (*palpitations, chest pain, a choking feeling, a churning stomach, dizziness, feelings of unreality*) or fear of some disaster (*losing control or going mad, heart attack, sudden death*). They begin suddenly, build up rapidly and may last only a few minutes.	**Questions box 46.4** Questions to ask the patient with possible panic disorder 1. Have you ever had an attack of acute anxiety or panic (suddenly feeling very anxious and frightened, feeling something terrible could happen)? 2. Did this occur in a situation in which most people would not feel afraid? 3. Can these attacks happen at any time?
3. Agoraphobia (phobic anxiety) A disorder in which an individual avoids places (such as supermarkets or trains) in which they fear they may have a panic attack and cannot escape.	**Questions box 46.5** Questions to ask the patient with possible phobic anxiety 1. Do you avoid going out? 2. Do you avoid going to places or situations because you fear you may have an anxiety attack?

TABLE 46.1

Continued

The common psychiatric disorders* and their screening questions continued

4. Obsessive–compulsive disorder A disorder in which the person has either obsessions or compulsions that interfere with everyday life.	**Questions box 46.6** Questions to ask the patient with possible obsessive–compulsive disorder 1. Are there any rituals or habits that you have to carry out every day? 2. Do they cause you problems or make you anxious? 3. Do you find yourself having to do things even though they seem unnecessary, to stop yourself feeling anxious (compulsions)? 4. Do you ever have a thought going round in your head that you cannot get rid of?
Stress-related disorders	
1. Acute stress disorder Individuals may present shortly after a traumatic event with a range of symptoms, such as *anxiety, depression, disturbed sleep, problems with memory or concentration*. Images, dreams or flashbacks of the traumatic event may also occur.	**Questions box 46.7** Questions to ask the patient with possible acute stress disorder 1. Have you been having any problems following … ? 2. Have you been feeling especially anxious or worried? Or depressed? Finding you cannot get the events out of your mind? 3. Have you had trouble sleeping? 4. Do you have bad memories?
2. Post-traumatic stress disorder (PTSD) Onset of persistent problems within 6 months of a traumatic event of exceptional severity. The individual experiences *repetitive and intrusive re-enactments* of the trauma in images, dreams or flashbacks. *Sleep, concentration, memory, mood and attention may be disturbed*. Individuals may feel emotionally detached and avoid things that act as reminders of the traumatic event.	**Questions box 46.8** Questions to ask the patient with possible PTSD 1. Since … happened, have you been troubled by bad memories of it? 2. Have you been having nightmares? 3. Have you had trouble with sleep? 4. Have you had trouble with your memory? 5. Do you try to avoid any reminders of the event or situation? 6. Are you jumpy?
Schizophrenia and delusional disorders	
A condition characterised by disorders of content (presence of delusions), thought form (shown by difficulty in understanding the connections between the patient's thoughts), perception (hallucinations—predominantly auditory), behaviour (erratic or bizarre) and/or volition (apathy and withdrawal).	**Questions box 46.9** Questions to ask the patient with possible schizophrenia or delusions 1. Have you ever heard people speaking when there is no one around? 2. Do you ever hear voices speaking as if someone is there? 3. Have you heard your thoughts spoken out loud, as if by someone else? 4. Do you have any thoughts or beliefs that others might find unusual or strange? 5. Have you felt people may be against you? 6. Have you felt that the TV or radio sends you messages? 7. Do you ever feel as if someone is spying on you or plotting to hurt you? 8. Do you have any ideas that you don't like to talk about because you are afraid other people will not believe you or will think there is something wrong with you?
Organic brain disorders	
These are disorders in which there is brain dysfunction manifested by cognitive disturbances such as memory loss or disorientation; there may be behavioural disturbance as well.	

TABLE 46.1

The common psychiatric disorders* and their screening questions *continued*

1. Delirium (acute brain syndrome)
A disorder characterised by the acute onset of disturbed consciousness plus changes in cognition that are not due to a pre-existing dementia. It is a direct physiological consequence of a general medical condition (*substance intoxication or withdrawal, use of a medication, exposure to a toxin, or a combination of these factors*).
Delirium is characterised by fluctuating confusion and clouding of consciousness. This may be accompanied by *poor concentration, poor memory, disorientation, inattention, agitation, emotional upset, hallucinations, visions or illusions, suspiciousness and disturbed sleep* (*reversal of sleep pattern*).
Hypoactive delirium is characterised by withdrawal, slowing of thinking and behaviour, and a depression-like presentation.

Questions box 46.10
Questions to ask the patient with possible delirium
1. What day is it today?
2. How long have you been here?
3. What is the name of the place we are in?
4. Do you remember my name?
5. Are you having trouble staying awake?

Questions to ask the patient's attendant
6. Does …'s ability to concentrate vary from moment to moment?
7. Did these problems begin suddenly?

Mental state examination (see Table 46.4)

2. Dementia (chronic brain syndrome)
A generalised impairment of intellect, memory and personality with no impairment of consciousness.
Characterised by *loss of memory* (especially short-term memory), *loss of orientation and deterioration in social functioning and behaviour and emotional control* (may be easily upset—tearful or irritable).

Questions box 46.11
Questions to ask the patient with possible dementia
1. What day is it today?
2. How long have you been here?
3. What is the name of the place we are in?
4. Do you remember my name?

Mental state examination (see Table 46.4)

Other disorders
There are a number of other psychiatric disorders that may present with physical problems, or that may be seen in an emergency department with some complication (particularly after attempted suicide).

A. Eating disorders (anorexia nervosa and bulimia nervosa)

Here the sufferer (generally female) has a disturbed body image with an unreasonable fear of being fat, and makes extensive efforts to lose weight (strict dieting, vomiting, use of purgatives, excessive exercise). The patient may deny that weight or eating habits are a problem.
Bulimia nervosa is characterised by binge eating followed by vomiting or purging.
Anorexia nervosa is characterised by excessive dieting, but there may also be binges followed by vomiting or purging. Anorexic patients will be grossly underweight and may show signs of malnutrition. Amenorrhoea is generally present.
Binge-eating disorder (BED) is characterised by 3 months or more of eating more food, more rapidly than normally, often secretly. Patients feel lack of control of their eating, and guilt, self-disgust, and physical discomfort after overeating.

Questions box 46.12
Questions to ask the patient with a possible eating disorder
1. Do you worry about your weight?
2. Do you think that you are fat? *or* What are your feelings about your weight?
3. Do you diet? *or* What other things have you tried to control your weight?
4. Have you ever made yourself sick after a meal?

B. Somatoform disorders

1. Somatisation disorder
A disorder characterised by multiple physical complaints that cannot be satisfactorily explained by physical disease. An individual with this disorder will have unexplained complaints in several bodily systems (e.g. gastrointestinal, cardiac, respiratory, musculoskeletal, menstrual). Usually commences in teens or early adult life and there is a risk of iatrogenic complications.

Questions box 46.13
Questions to ask the patient with possible somatoform disorder
1. Do you have any other medical problems?
2. Have you had symptoms that your doctor has not been able to find a cause for?
3. Are you often sick?

TABLE 46.1

Continued

The common psychiatric disorders* and their screening questions *continued*

2. Somatic symptom disorder (hypochondriacal disorder) These patients fear they have a serious illness despite repeated medical reassurance and are preoccupied with physical symptoms. They often seek repeated medical opinions. In some cases the disorder becomes delusional (e.g. of parasitic skin infection).	**Questions box 46.14** Questions to ask the patient with possible somatic symptom disorder (hypochondriacal disorder[†]) 1. Have you been very worried about your health? 2. What do you think might be wrong? 3. What have your doctors told you?
3. Medically unexplained symptoms (MUS) (conversion disorder, hysteria) These patients usually present with a neurological abnormality that is not fully explained medically. Common symptoms include: blindness, gait disturbances, sensory loss, limb paralysis and loss of speech. There is usually a precipitating psychological stress event, and often a past history of similar episodes.	**Questions box 46.15** Questions to ask the patient with possible MUS disorder 1. What have you noticed has been wrong? 2. What tests have you had? 3. What have you been told about your illness?

Substance misuse

This category includes the misuse of alcohol, illegal drugs and prescription medications.

Personality disorders

In these disorders the individual, while not having specific symptoms, has behavioural disturbances and problems with impulse control, interpersonal relationships and mood. Typically there are problems involving many areas of personality. Individuals who have repeatedly and deliberately made self-harm attempts often have a personality disorder.[‡] They may also have unpredictable behaviour while in hospital, which may cause problems for staff.	**Questions box 46.16** Questions to ask the patient with a possible borderline personality disorder 1. Have you ever tried to harm yourself? 2. Have you ever had problems with relationships?

Neurasthenia (chronic fatigue syndrome)

This is a somewhat controversial inclusion in the current WHO classification of psychiatric disorders.

Puerperal mental disorders

This category includes peripartum depression and psychosis. Early recognition of this disorder is important for the mother and the baby. It needs to be distinguished from the more common 'postpartum blues'. Mothers may present with quite specific symptoms, such as excessive anxiety about the baby or feelings of failure as a mother and of inability to cope. There may be loss of ability to enjoy the baby and women often become isolated from others. In postpartum psychosis, the baby may be included in the mother's psychotic symptoms.	**Questions box 46.17** Questions to ask the patient with a possible puerperal mental disorder 1. Have you ever been worried that you might want to hurt your baby? 2. Have you ever thought of hurting yourself?

*Based on the WHO International Classification of Disease, 10th edn (ICD-10). ICD-11 will be published in 2018.
[†]Alfons Jakob (1884–1931), a professor of neurology in Hamburg from 1924, had more than 200 cases of neurosyphilis on his ward at a time; he died of osteomyelitis. Jakob described this cerebral atrophy in 1920 and before Hans Creutzeld (1885–1933).
[‡]Depression can be a cause of attempted self-harm but in this case it is not usually deliberate.

TABLE 46.1

disorders). A simple screening approach to determine whether the patient has depression is to ask him or her:[2]

- 'In the past month, have you felt down, depressed or hopeless?'
- 'Have you felt little interest or pleasure in doing things?'

If the patient answers 'yes' to either question, you need to explore the possibility of depression in detail (LR+, 2.9; LR–, 0.05).[2]

Screening is encouraged to reduce the high rate of undetected depression. Use of such screening questions in all patients (where there will be a low prevalence—i.e. a low pretest probability of depression) will lead to some false-positive responses so detailed follow-up questions are required to help confirm the results.[3]

The definitions of other symptoms are given in Table 46.2. It is important to ask about drug usage (legal and illegal) as well as alcohol and caffeine intake (which may be associated with anxiety disorders).

Precipitating events

Psychiatric illness can occur for no reason (e.g. bipolar disease episodes) but there is often an event that has precipitated the illness, even though this may not be obvious at the beginning. Such events include a range of experiences that may have affected the patient or a member of the patient's social network. Events such as physical illness, drug treatment or treatment non-adherence may be implicated as precipitants. Patients with psychiatric illnesses have a possibly undeserved reputation for non-adherence to treatment. It may be no more common than in non-psychiatric patients but when it occurs it can be a major contribution to relapse.

Risk

An assessment of the patient's risk of harm, either to others or to him- or herself, is essential: this will indicate any urgent steps that need to be taken to ensure safety and whether the patient needs to be treated involuntarily. Patients with psychotic illness may, in some circumstances, need to be treated involuntarily under the relevant legislation (e.g. *Mental Health Act*). Although the exact details for involuntary treatment are different under individual mental health laws, the essential features are generally that: (1) a person has

Assessment of suicide risk

Suicide may be the tragic outcome of psychiatric illness. Assessing the risk of suicide is an essential part of the psychiatric interview. Asking about this does *not* increase the risk or put the idea into the patient's head; it may reduce the risk, as the patient may feel relief in talking about his or her fears. The risk of suicide is assessed by asking directly whether the person has ever contemplated it.

1. Have you thought that life was not worth living?

   Or

2. Have you ever felt so bad that you have considered ending it all?

   If 'yes'

- Have you thought of killing yourself?
- Have you thought how you might do this?
- Have you made any plans for doing this?

TEXT BOX 46.1

a mental illness, and (2) the person is a danger to self or others. Assessment of danger to others is difficult, with the best predictor being a history of past threat or harm to others. It is best to err on the side of caution in such cases and seek advice from psychiatry colleagues and mental health services. Assessment of suicide risk needs to be made with sensitivity and using a direct approach, as shown in Text box 46.1.

Past history and treatment history

Both the past psychiatric history and the medical history should be assessed. The past medical history should be evaluated in the same way as the general medical history. An assessment should be made of stresses that may have contributed to past episodes of illness and that may have led to relapse. For the past psychiatric history, it is important to obtain not only the diagnosis but also the treatment the patient has had, and its outcome.

Ask about previous non-drug treatment including counselling, psychotherapy and electroconvulsive therapy (ECT), and whether the patient thought the treatment was effective. Was the patient ever admitted to a psychiatric unit, and for how long?

Symptoms of psychiatric illness

Affect	The observable behaviour by which a person's internal emotional state is judged.
Agitation (psychomotor agitation)	Excessive motor activity associated with a feeling of inner tension. The activity is usually non-productive and repetitious and consists of such behaviour as pacing, fidgeting, wringing the hands, pulling the clothes and inability to sit still.
Anxiety	The apprehensive anticipation of future danger or misfortune. It is associated with feelings of tension and symptoms of autonomic arousal.
Conversion symptom (hysteria)	A loss of, or alteration in, motor or sensory function. Psychological factors are judged to be associated with the development of the symptom, which is not fully explained by anatomical or pathological conditions. The symptom is the result of unconscious conflict and is not feigned.
Delusion	A false unshakable idea or belief that is out of keeping with the patient's educational, cultural and social background.
Depersonalisation	An alteration in the awareness of the self—the individual feels as if he or she is unreal.
Derealisation	An alteration in the perception or experience of the external world so that it seems unreal.
Disorientation	Confusion about the time of day, date or season (time), where one is (place) or who one is (person).
Flight of ideas	A nearly continuous flow of accelerated speech with abrupt changes from topic to topic that are usually based on understandable associations, distracting stimuli or plays on words. When severe, speech may be disorganised or incoherent.
Grandiosity	An inflated appraisal of one's worth, power, knowledge, importance or identity. When extreme, grandiosity may be of delusional proportions.
Hallucination	A sensory perception that seems real, but occurs without external stimulation of the relevant sensory organ. The term *hallucination* is not ordinarily applied to the false perceptions that occur during dreaming, while falling asleep (hypnagogic) or when awakening (hypnopompic).
Ideas of reference	The feeling that casual incidents and external events have a particular significance and unusual meaning that is specific to the person.
Illusion	A misperception or misinterpretation of a real external stimulus.
Mood	A pervasive and sustained emotion that colours the perception of the world.
Overvalued idea	An unreasonable belief that is held, but not as strongly as a delusion (i.e. the person is able to acknowledge the possibility that the belief may not be true). The belief is not one that is ordinarily accepted by other members of the person's culture or subculture.
Personality	Enduring patterns of perceiving, relating to and thinking about the environment and oneself.
Phobia	A persistent irrational fear of a specific object, activity or situation (the phobic stimulus) that results in a compelling desire to avoid it.
Pressured speech	Speech that is increased in amount, accelerated and difficult or impossible to interrupt. Usually it is also loud and emphatic. Frequently the person talks without any social stimulation and may continue to talk even though no one is listening.
Psychomotor retardation	Visible generalised slowing of movements and speech.
Psychotic	Psychotic can be used to mean a loss of contact with reality, but is generally used to imply the presence of delusions or hallucinations.

(Based on American Psychiatric Association. *Diagnostic and statistical manual of mental disorders*, 5th edn. Washington, DC: APA, 2013.)

TABLE 46.2

Classes of psychiatric drugs and their major indications	
Antianxiety (e.g. benzodiazepines, beta-blockers [control somatic symptoms])	For anxiety disorders, insomnia, alcohol withdrawal
Antipsychotic (e.g. atypical antipsychotics, phenothiazines, butyrophenones, major tranquillisers)	For schizophrenia, mania, delirium
Antidepressants (e.g. tricyclics, selective serotonin reuptake inhibitors [SSRIs] and serotonin–noradrenaline reuptake inhibitors [SNRIs])	For depression, anxiety disorders, obsessive–compulsive disorder
Mood-stabilising (e.g. lithium, anticonvulsants—carbamazepine, sodium valproate)	For prevention of manic depression or treatment of mania

TABLE 46.3

COMMON SIDE EFFECTS OF THE ANTIPSYCHOTIC DRUGS

1. *Anticholinergic*—dry mouth, blurred vision, urinary retention, erectile dysfunction, sedation, metabolic syndrome (weight gain, insulin resistance and hyperlipidaemia)
2. *Hypersensitivity reactions*—photosensitivity dermatitis, cholestatic jaundice, agranulocytosis (clozapine)
3. *Effects due to dopamine blockade*—Parkinsonianism, motor restlessness (akathisia), tardive dyskinesia, dystonia, gynaecomastia, malignant neuroleptic syndrome

LIST 46.1

Find out what drug treatment has been tried, the class (see Table 46.3) of psychiatric medication, its effectiveness and any side effects. The antipsychotic drugs in particular have common long-term side effects (see List 46.1).

Family history

Some mental illnesses have a genetic association and in other family situations behaviours are learned.

First, ask the patient tactfully whether anyone in the family has had any psychiatric or mental illness or has committed suicide. Also ask whether anyone in the family has had any treatment for psychological problems, such as anxiety, depression, agoraphobia,[a] eating disorders or drug and alcohol problems (these last few areas are often not considered by patients to be psychiatric or mental illnesses).

Second, try to gain an understanding of the patient's family origin. Drawing up a family tree is a useful way of finding this out. Factual details about each family member can be included in this family tree (age, mental state, health). In the psychiatric history one also needs to know what type of person each family member is, about any important family events (such as bereavements, separations) and how family members get on with each other. It is worth exploring the quality of care the patient received from each parent, and how controlling or protective each was. These two factors have been shown to be important in contributing to psychiatric illness. Ask about the quality of the parental relationship and the general family atmosphere.

Childhood abuse (emotional, physical or sexual)[4] may be an important predisposing event for many illnesses, and should be enquired about. This can be elicited by saying something like, 'Sometimes children can have had some unpleasant experiences—I wonder if you had any? Did anyone ever harm you? Or hit you? How about interfering with you sexually? Could you tell me more about that and what happened?'

Taking a detailed family history in this way sets the scene for the patient's developmental history, which should be taken next.

Social and personal history

Open-ended questions are again the best way to initiate discussion of personal and social history. Ask the patient something like, 'Could you tell me a bit about your background, your development, what sort of childhood you had, what are the important things you remember from your childhood?', and then allow the patient to tell his or her own story. During the course of this narrative, the patient may require some prompting to add information about important issues such as the birth history (schizophrenia is known to be associated with perinatal morbidity) and early development, and whether there were significant problems in early

---

[a] From the Greek, meaning 'fear of the market place'.

childhood, such as head injuries or serious infections. How did the patient cope with early separations, particularly when starting primary school and going on to secondary school (difficulty in separation may be a risk factor for panic disorder or abnormal illness behaviour)? The patient should be asked about peer relationships, friendships, school, academic ability, adolescence and teenage relationships. The adult history should focus predominantly on the quality of intimate relationships and the social support network, especially whether there are people in whom the patient can confide, and about significant events that may have occurred and about the patient's ability to cope with such events.

The patient's living circumstances should be asked about in the same way as for a medical history. There should also be a focus on the patient's occupation: not only on the type of job but also on how he or she copes with work or, if he or she does not work, how that is coped with.

Premorbid personality

An assessment should be made of the patient's premorbid personality. Ask the patient to describe him- or herself (e.g. 'How would your friends or family describe you?'). The personality can be described using the predominant trait, such as obsessional, nervy or highly strung; it is not necessary to use official systems to describe a patient's personality. In the assessment of premorbid personality it is important to evaluate both positive and negative aspects of the person, how he or she copes or responds to the strains of life, what type of interests he or she has, and what other strengths and weaknesses are present.

THE MENTAL STATE EXAMINATION

While assessing the patient, carefully make observations about appearance, behaviour, patterns of speech, predominant concerns, attitude to the examiner and ways of interacting. These observations are brought together in a systematic fashion in the mental state examination. This is not something that is 'done' at the conclusion of taking a history; it is an essential part of the total process of assessing the patient.[5]

However, there are a number of tests or specific tasks that need to be conducted in a formalised way as part of the mental state examination. These include assessing the patient's cognitive state (orientation, memory, attention, registration) and enquiring about perceptual disturbances and, in some cases, disorders of thought. The mental state examination provides valuable diagnostic information; with some disorders, it is this examination that gives most of the diagnostic clues.

The headings under which the mental state is recorded are shown in Table 46.4, together with some simple bedside tests for assessing cognitive function. Also shown in Table 46.4 are some abnormal features of the mental state examination that are commonly found in psychiatric disorders.

When cognitive dysfunction is suspected, as in patients with delirium or dementia,[6] a more detailed examination of cognitive function should be carried out. A widely used screening tool for doing this has been the mini-mental state examination (MMSE)™,[6] which assesses aspects of orientation, memory and concentration. The MMSE is copyright protected. Another useful screening tool is the simple three-step (3-minute) Mini-Cog™ test.[7] For this test, ask the patient to remember three words (repeat them up to three times to make sure that he or she has captured the words correctly). Next, ask the patient to draw a clock face with numbers and then draw the hands at a specified time (e.g. 11.10). Then ask the patient to repeat the original three words. Scoring is out of 5: 1 point for each word remembered and 2 for a correct clock face drawing (0 if not fully correct). A total score of 0–2 supports a diagnosis of dementia.

Some of the common causes of delirium and dementia are listed in Tables 46.5 and 46.6 respectively.

THE DIAGNOSIS

At the conclusion of the psychiatric history, which should include a general physical examination, a provisional diagnosis and formulation should be made. Essentially, the diagnostic formulation is a means of summarising, in a succinct yet comprehensive manner, your understanding of the patient's problem.

Psychiatric disorders generally arise through a combination of biological, psychological and psychosocial factors, and each of these needs to be considered when a patient's problem is being assessed (a biopsychosocial approach). The patient's problem

The mental state examination

	What is assessed, described or observed	Common findings indicating psychopathology	Types of illness
General description			
Appearance	A general description of the patient's appearance, including body build, posture, clothing (appropriateness), grooming (e.g. make-up) and hygiene. Note any physical stigmata (e.g. tattoos) and facial expression (depression, apprehension, worry, etc.).	Bizarre appearance	Psychotic disorders (schizophrenia, mania), personality disorder
		Unkempt, poorly groomed	Schizophrenia, depression, dementia or delirium
		Apprehensive, anxious	Anxiety disorders
		Over-bright clothing / disinhibited	Mania
		Scarred wrists, non-professional tattoos	Personality disorder
Behaviour	All aspects of the patient's behaviour. Note the appropriateness of the patient's behaviour within the interview context. Abnormal motor behaviour: mannerisms, stereotyped movements, tics. Variants of normal motor behaviour: restlessness, psychomotor change (agitation, retardation).	Uncooperative behaviour	Psychotic disorder, personality disorder, delirium, substance intoxication
		Manneristic behaviour	Psychotic disorder
		Stereotypical behaviour	Psychotic disorders, developmental disability, organic syndromes
		Bizarre behaviour	Psychotic disorders, substance intoxication, delirium
		Assaultive, threatening	Personality disorders, intoxication, neurological disorders, mania, delirium
		Restlessness	Akathisia from antipsychotic medication
		Psychomotor change (withdrawn)	Depression, delirium
Attitude towards examiner	The way the patient responds to the interviewer, the level of cooperation, willingness to disclose information. A range of attitudes and deviation from appropriateness may occur, ranging from hostility to seductiveness.	Uncooperative attitude, belligerence	Psychotic disorder, personality disorder, delirium, substance intoxication
		Seductiveness	Mania or hypomania, personality disorder
Mood and affect			
Mood	A relatively persistent emotional state: describe the depth, intensity, duration and fluctuations of mood. Mood may be neutral, euphoric, depressed, anxious or irritable.	Depressed	Depression
		Anxious / irritable	Depression / anxiety disorders
Affect	The way a patient conveys his or her emotional state. Affect may be full, blunted, restricted or inappropriate.	Depressed	Depression
		Blunted, restricted	Schizophrenia
Appropriateness	Are the patient's responses appropriate to the matter being discussed?	Inappropriate	Schizophrenia

TABLE 46.4

Continued

The mental state examination *continued*

	What is assessed, described or observed	Common findings indicating psychopathology	Types of illness
Speech	The tempo, modulation and quality of the patient's speech should be described here. Note should be made of dysphasia or dysarthria.	Increased tempo Slowed	Mania, acute schizophrenia Depression
Perceptual disturbances	The presence of hallucinations (auditory, visual, gustatory or tactile) should be noted. It is important to check whether they occurred with a clear sensorium. Hypnagogic or hypnopompic hallucinations are normal experiences. Other perceptual disturbances (e.g. illusions, depersonalisation or derealisation) should be noted.	Visual hallucinations Auditory Tactile/gustatory	Acute brain syndrome (delirium), epilepsy, alcohol withdrawal, drug intoxication Schizophrenia, delirium, organic states (hallucinosis) Epilepsy, schizophrenia
Thought			
Thought form	The process of the patient's thinking. This involves the quantity of ideas (pressured thought, poverty of ideas) and the way in which the ideas (thoughts) are produced. Are they logical and relevant, or are they fragmented and irrelevant? The link between ideas should be assessed—do they flow logically or are they disconnected and 'fragmented'? Are ideas connected by spurious concepts (rhyming, the way they sound—'clang' associations)?	Disorder of thought form Flight of ideas Poverty of ideas	Schizophrenia, mania, delirium Mania, schizophrenia Schizophrenia, depression, dementia
Thought content	The content of the patient's thoughts. Abnormalities range from preoccupation, obsessions and overvalued ideas to delusions. Themes should also be assessed: suicidal or homicidal thoughts or paranoid ideas. In the medical setting, preoccupation with illness (hypochondriacal thoughts) should be assessed, as well as thoughts of omnipotence—denying illness when it is present.	Delusions	Schizophrenia, mania, depression, delirium and other organic states
Sensorium and cognition			
Listed below are bedside tests for a basic assessment of cognitive function.			
Alertness and level of consciousness	The level of consciousness should be assessed. Clouding or fluctuating levels of consciousness should be noted.	Clouding	Delirium
Orientation	Orientation to time, place and person. Ask the day, date, month and year. Ask where he or she is. Ask for the names of his or her close family members.	Disorientation	Dementia, delirium

TABLE 46.4

The mental state examination *continued*

	What is assessed, described or observed	Common findings indicating psychopathology	Types of illness
Short-term memory	Short-term memory refers to the ability to retain information over a period of 3–5 minutes. Less than this refers to immediate recall. Ask the patient to recall a list of three objects after 3–5 minutes.	Loss of short-term memory Loss of immediate recall in delirium due to poor concentration	Dementia, delirium
Long-term memory	This refers to memory of remote events. Ask the patient to recall events of the previous few days, as well as events of a year ago.	Loss of long-term memory	Dementia
Concentration	Ask the patient to subtract 7 from 100 and keep subtracting 7, or spell 'world' backwards.	Poor concentration	Dementia, delirium
General knowledge and intelligence	Ask about some recent events. Intelligence can be gauged from the language used. Ask the patient to do some simple arithmetical tasks. Literacy should be assessed.	Poor general knowledge	Delirium, acute psychosis, dementia
Judgement and insight			
Judgement	The capacity to behave appropriately. Describe a hypothetical situation and ask how the patient would behave in it (e.g. 'What would you do if you smelt smoke while sitting in a cinema?').	Impaired judgement	Psychoses, dementia, personality disorders, delirium
Insight	Determine whether the patient is aware that he or she has a problem, and the level of understanding of this.	Lack of insight	Psychoses, dementia, delirium

TABLE 46.4

needs to be understood longitudinally, by defining biophysical factors that may have predisposed to the illness and, more immediately, may have precipitated the illness, and factors that may be contributing to the person remaining ill (perpetuating factors). A simple grid can be used for assessing the patient in this manner (see Table 46.7). Here biological, psychological or psychosocial factors that predispose to, precipitate or perpetuate the psychiatric illness are identified. Perpetuating factors are very important, particularly among medically ill patients, as it may be the medical or physical illness that maintains the patient's psychiatric problem. By the same token, psychological factors may perpetuate a patient's medical illness.

An example of such a formulation grid is shown in Table 46.8 for a 53-year-old man who becomes depressed after a myocardial infarction. He has a family history of depression (a genetic predisposing factor) and chronic low self-esteem (a psychological predisposing factor), which he coped with by succeeding in business. He has few friends and his marriage is unsatisfactory (a psychosocial factor). He had his infarct 1 week after he heard that he would not be promoted at work (a psychological factor) and his job was at risk (a psychosocial precipitant). His insecurity about work and his failing marriage, together with his low self-esteem, are maintaining his illness, as are the biological changes to the neurotransmitter system.

Common causes of delirium

Drug intoxication	Alcohol Anxiolytics Digoxin L-dopa 'Street drugs'
Withdrawal states	Alcohol (delirium tremens) Anxiolytic sedatives
Metabolic disturbance	Chronic kidney disease Liver failure Anoxia Cardiac failure Electrolyte imbalance Postoperative states
Endocrine disturbance	Diabetic ketosis Hypoglycaemia
Systemic infections	Pneumonia Urinary tract infection Septicaemia Viral infections
Intracranial infection	Encephalitis Meningitis
Other intracranial causes	Space-occupying lesions Raised intracranial pressure
Head injury	Subdural haemorrhage Cerebral contusion Concussion
Nutritional and vitamin deficiency	Thiamine (Wernicke's encephalopathy) Vitamin B_{12} Nicotinic acid
Epilepsy	Status epilepticus Postictal states

TABLE 46.5

Common causes of dementia

Hereditable Alzheimer's	Mutation of presenilin-1
Degenerative type	Senile dementia of Alzheimer's Dementia with Lewy bodies Parkinson's disease Frontotemporal dementia* Huntington's chorea
Vascular	Multi-infarct dementia Chronic kidney disease
Intracranial space-occupying lesions	Tumour Subdural haematomas
Traumatic	Head injuries Boxing encephalopathy
Infections and related conditions	Encephalitis Neurosyphilis HIV (AIDS dementia) Jacob–Creutzfeldt disease
Metabolic	Chronic kidney disease Hepatic failure
Toxic	Alcoholic dementia Heavy-metal poisoning
Anoxia	Carbon monoxide poisoning Cardiac arrest Chronic respiratory failure
Vitamin deficiency	Vitamin B_{12} Folic acid Thiamine (Wernicke–Korsakoff's syndrome)
Endocrine	Myxoedema, Addison's disease

AIDS = acquired immunodeficiency syndrome; HIV = human immunodeficiency virus.
*Motor neurone disease may precede or follow onset.

TABLE 46.6

A formulation grid

	Predisposing	Precipitating	Perpetuating
Biological			
Psychological			
Psychosocial			

TABLE 46.7

Understanding the patient in this manner helps you to plan an effective management approach that will focus on all the relevant factors, so that, for the patient in this example, a combination of antidepressants, marital counselling and assertiveness training (to build self-esteem) can be organised.

A good psychiatric history will provide a comprehensive understanding of the patient and will permit appropriate management to be planned. This is immensely rewarding for the clinician, and will also be of considerable benefit to the patient.

A completed formulation grid (see text)

	Predisposing	**Precipitating**	**Perpetuating**
Biological	Genetic predisposition	Acute myocardial infarct	Neurotransmitter changes
Psychological	Low self-esteem	Not promoted	Low self-esteem and insecurity
Psychosocial	Poor social support Dysfunctional marriage		Dysfunctional marriage

TABLE 46.8

PERSONALITY DISORDERS

A. **Eccentric thinking or behaviour**

1. **Paranoid**: pervasive and unjustified suspicion of others, hostile reactions to perceived insults
2. **Schizoid**: seemingly indifferent, cold in manner, not good at responding to social clues, prefer to be alone
3. **Schizotypal**: odd thinking, e.g. ability to influence others with powerful or magical thoughts, believe ordinary events have hidden meanings, may behave and dress eccentrically

B. **Unpredictable thinking and behaviours, emotional problems**

1. **Antisocial**: behaviour may include lying, stealing and aggression and violence. Little regard for the feelings or safety of others. Not remorseful. Often in legal difficulties.
2. **Borderline**: fragile self-image. Chaotic relationships with others, labile and intense emotions and mood, risky behaviour e.g. sexual activity and gambling. They may injure themselves and are at risk of suicide.
3. **Histrionic**: attention seeking and emotional behaviour, melodramatic. They can be sexually provocative.
4. **Narcissistic:*** inflated self-regard and need for attention.

C. **Anxious and fearful thinking and behaviours**

1. **Avoidant**: shy, sensitive to criticism, avoids encounters with others, particularly with strangers.
2. **Dependent**: fears being alone, excessively dependent on others, lacks self-confidence.
3. **Obsessive compulsive**: preoccupied with orderliness and rules. Controlling of self, situations and others; rigid values. This is a different condition from obsessive–compulsive disorder, which is an anxiety problem.

*Narkissos in Greek legend fell in love with his own reflection and pined away.

LIST 46.2

EXAMPLES OF IMPORTANT PSYCHIATRIC ILLNESSES

Some mental or possible mental disorders present as possible medical illnesses (see Table 46.1).

Patients with personality disorders have patterns of behaviour and thought that differ from that person's cultural norm. These characteristics are deeply entrenched and stable over long periods. They cause the patient considerable distress and usually begin in adolescence. The diagnosis requires evidence of problems across most areas of a person's life over many years. In some instances they may not be aware of the nature of their behaviour or interactions. List 46.2 sets out the current classification of these disorders.

Disorders that lead to physical illness

Eating disorders put patients at risk of physical illness and can be associated with a high mortality. There are three main types: binge eating and purging (bulimia nervosa), restricting without binge eating (anorexia nervosa), and binge-eating disorder (BED).

> **MEDICAL COMPLICATIONS OF BULIMIA NERVOSA**
>
> - Electrolyte changes and arrhythmias—a result of underweight and use of diuretics and purgatives
> - Oesophagitis
> - Mallory–Weiss oesophageal tears
> - Oesophageal rupture
> - Depression, anxiety, suicide risk
>
> LIST 46.3

> **MEDICAL COMPLICATIONS AND ASSOCIATIONS OF ANOREXIA NERVOSA**
>
> - Loss of bone density (more than 30% of patients)
> - Sinus bradycardia
> - Hypotension
> - Hypothermia
> - Electrolyte changes—hypokalaemia, hypomagnesaemia, hypophosphataemia
> - Cardiac arrhythmias including ventricular tachycardia associated with the long QT interval caused by electrolyte changes
> - Depression, anxiety, suicide risk
>
> LIST 46.4

1. **Bulimia nervosa** is a condition in which frequent (more than once a week) episodes of binge eating are followed by compensating behaviours that are promoted by fear of weight gain. These include induced vomiting, and use of laxatives, enemas or diuretics. Patients are at risk of the medical complications summarised in List 46.3.

    Examination findings include erosion of dental enamel from vomiting, parotid gland enlargement, xerosis (dryness of the mouth, eyes and skin) and scarring on the dorsum or knuckles of the hand used to induce vomiting (Russell's sign).[b,8] The sign is not present if an object such as a pencil or toothbrush is used to induce vomiting.

2. **Anorexia nervosa** is associated with a considerable mortality risk. It occurs predominantly in women. They aggressively restrict food intake because of a distorted body image and fear of gaining weight. Adolescent girls and young women are most commonly affected. The severe medical complications are slightly different from those of bulimia nervosa (List 46.4).

    Amenorrhoea is common but no longer required for the diagnosis. The examination findings include: emaciation, xerosis, brittle hair and nails, bradycardia, hypothermia, oedema and lanugo.[c]

3. **Binge-eating disorder** is defined as more-than-weekly episodes over 3 months or more of eating more food and eating more rapidly than normally. Patients feel lack of control of their eating. Unlike people who are merely greedy, these patients feel guilt and self-disgust after eating, often eat secretly to avoid embarrassment and feel physically uncomfortable after eating too much.

Schizophrenia

This psychotic illness is associated with an increased risk of death (2–3 times), of suicide (13 times) and of cardiovascular disease (twice). Patients have increased rates of cardiovascular risk factors including: hypertension, smoking, hyperlipidaemia, obesity and diabetes. They need medical assessment and help with these problems, some of which are exacerbated by their medication.

The condition begins usually in adolescence. At least two of the following symptoms are required for the diagnosis:
- hallucinations
- delusions
- disorganised or catatonic behaviour
- disorganised speech
- negative symptoms—a flattened affect, alogia, avolition.[d]

---

[b] Gerald Russell, b. 1928, a British psychiatrist who published the first description of bulimia nervosa in 1979.
[c] This is short, colourless, downy hair like that which covers unborn babies from the fourth month of gestation. It can also grow on people with malignancies. Lana means wool in Latin and lanugo means the downy hair that covers some plants and the cheeks of young people.
[d] Not talking, not doing anything spontaneously.

> **MEDICAL CONDITIONS THAT MAY RESEMBLE DEPRESSION**
>
> - Hypothyroidism
> - Androgen deficiency
> - Menopause
> - Parkinson's disease
> - Multiple sclerosis
> - Chronic illness—HIV infection, heart failure
> - Drug treatment—interferons, chemotherapeutic agents
>
> HIV=human immunodeficiency virus.
>
> LIST 46.5

The symptoms must interfere with work, study, relations with other people or self-care, and have been present for 6 months. (See Questions box 46.9.)

Depression

About a fifth of women and 10% of men experience depression during their lives. The peak age of onset is 40 for women and 55 for men. Depression is both more common in people with medical illnesses and adversely affects their recovery. Depression is a common reason for presentation to a doctor and a few simple questions can help the clinician decide whether depression is a major problem.

A number of medical conditions can resemble depression (see List 46.5).

Major depressive disorder

The current diagnosis of this requires that the patient has five of the following symptoms within a 2-week period including at least symptom 1 or 2:

1. Mood is depressed most of the time—reported either by the patient or by others—with feelings of hopelessness and sadness.
2. Greatly reduced interest in life, activities or pleasure most of the time.
3. Unintended loss or gain in weight or appetite.
4. Sleeping poorly or too much.
5. Agitation or psychomotor retardation every day.
6. Loss of energy and fatigue.
7. Inability to concentrate.
8. Feelings of worthlessness or guilt.
9. Recurrent thoughts of death and of suicide.

Persistent depressive disorder (dysthymia)

This is a less severe illness than major depressive illness. The criteria are similar but symptoms occur on most days rather than on nearly every day and over an extended period, often years. Thoughts of suicide are less prominent. Periods of more severe major depression are common.

Seasonal affective disorder

These patients have 3 successive years of major symptoms of depression beginning in the autumn or winter and resolving in spring. More women than men are affected.

Peripartum depression

This condition is no longer called postpartum depression as 50% of women develop their symptoms during pregnancy. Up to 15% of women are affected within 6 months of giving birth. It is considered a major depressive disorder.

Bipolar disorder

People affected by this relatively common mood disorder (1% of people) have periods of mania or hypomania (see Table 46.1), usually with a history of major depressive disorder. The onset is usually in early adult life. Most patients also have periods of depression. The features of an episode of mania include:
- abnormally euphoric or irritable mood
- pressured speech
- flight of ideas
- grandiosity (inflated self-importance)
- agitation
- disinhibited behaviour (spending sprees, sexual promiscuity)
- little need for sleep
- severe disruption of normal life.

Bipolar I disorder is diagnosed after one or more manic episodes lasting at least a week. Bipolar II disorder is diagnosed when patients have less severe symptoms of mania (hypomania) that last at least 4 days. These patients have episodes of major depression.

Anxiety disorders

Panic disorder

Up to 30% of people have a panic attack during their lives but panic disorder is much less common. Patients with panic disorder have recurrent and unexpected periods of extreme anxiety that builds up in minutes. The features include at least four of the following:

- sweating
- trembling
- a choking sensation
- breathlessness
- chest pain
- abdominal pain
- nausea
- dizziness
- feeling hot or cold
- paraesthesias
- a feeling of being separated from self
- fear of dying
- fear of losing control of oneself.

For the diagnosis to be made, attacks must be followed by a least a month of anxiety that another attack will occur. Because there are so many physical symptoms the condition may be diagnosed as a medical condition. Certain other medical conditions may need to be excluded including:

- hyperthyroidism
- phaeochromocytoma
- drug use
- myocardial infarction
- acute abdomen.

Generalised anxiety disorder (GAD)

Women are affected more than men. Some of the symptoms are like those of panic attacks but less dramatic in onset (see Table 46.1). They include:

- sweats
- abdominal pain
- palpitations and tachycardia
- chest pain
- breathlessness
- fatigue
- diarrhoea
- inability to sleep
- a feeling of muscle tension
- headache
- tremor.

Many patients have multiple unexplained physical symptoms.

A number of criteria are required for the diagnosis of GAD. These include:

- Anxiety that seems excessive about activities or events (e.g. work, school, social events) occurring on more days than not and for 6 months or more.
- Acknowledgment from the patient that the worry is difficult to control.
- The worry itself is associated with three or more of the following: restlessness, fatigue, irritability, insomnia, tiredness, difficulty in concentrating or muscle tension.
- The symptoms interfere with life—work or school.
- There is no other medical or drug cause for the symptoms.

Social anxiety disorder

This used to be called social phobia. The lifetime occurrence is about 2.5% of people. Patients with this condition have a persisting exaggerated fear of public performances (e.g. public speaking) or of unfamiliar social situations (e.g. meeting new people). The symptoms last for 6 months or longer. The anxiety is accompanied by physical symptoms such as breathlessness, flushing and palpitations. Patients realise their anxiety is excessive but may go to great lengths to avoid situations that bring them on. Their normal lives (work, etc.) are affected by their symptoms.

Post-traumatic stress disorder (PTSD)

PTSD occurs to people in response to seeing or directly experiencing traumatic events such as violence, threatened death, sexual assault or finding out about such an event happening to someone close. The diagnosis requires at least 1 month of symptoms that include upsetting memories of the events, nightmares or flashbacks. Patients avoid reminders and have a persisting change in mood and thoughts. There are changes in arousal: sleep disturbances, hypervigilance, startle reactions and sometimes risky behaviours.[9]

Risk factors for PTSD include: severe traumatic events, other stressors (loss of job, marriage failure), parental neglect, and history within the family or for the patient of another psychiatric illness. Many patients have other psychiatric problems including depression, anxiety and alcohol or drug problems. They are at increased risk of suicide, marriage failure and loss of employment.

Obsessive–compulsive disorder (OCD)

Obsession is defined as the occurrence of intrusive and persistent thoughts, impulses or images that cause distress (see Table 46.1). Compulsions are repetitive behaviours such as counting, inspecting, hand washing or saying ritualised phrases in order to offset the anxiety the obsession causes. These thoughts and actions cause difficulty with normal daily activities, waste time and cause distress. About 2% of women and men are affected.

OSCE REVISION TOPICS – THE PSYCHIATRIC HISTORY AND THE MENTAL STATE EXAMINATION

Use these topics, which commonly occur in the OSCE, to help with revision.

1. Please perform a mini-mental examination on this patient who has had recent memory problems. (p 855)
2. This woman has had recent problems with anxiety. Please take a history from her. (p 846)
3. This thin woman has been very concerned about being overweight. Please take a history from her. (p 849)
4. This man has been troubled by disturbing thoughts. Please take a history from him. (p 848)

T&O'C ESSENTIALS

1. The psychiatric interview can be therapeutic as well as diagnostic.
2. The mental state examination is a routine part of the assessment of a patient with suspected cognitive impairment.
3. It may take a number of interviews with a patient to gain his or her confidence.
4. Open-ended questions are more likely to produce accurate responses.
5. Depression is often overlooked. Ask the patient about current symptoms of depression in the setting of any chronic physical illness or alcohol abuse, or whether he or she has a past history of depression.
6. An acute decline in cognition suggests delirium, which usually has a medical cause.

References

1. Kopelman MD. Structured psychiatric interview: psychiatric history and assessment of the mental state. *Br J Hosp Med* 1994; 52:93–98. Know how to take a psychiatric history.
2. Arroll B, Khin N, Kerse N. Screening for depression in primary care with two verbally asked questions: cross sectional study. *BMJ* 2003; 327:1144–1146. Two questions help identify depression: one positive answer should be followed up.
3. Gilbody S, Sheldon T, Wessely S. Should we screen for depression? *BMJ* 2006; 332:1027–1030. Routinely screening for depression in practice is questioned because of the low pre-test probability.
4. Drossman DA, Talley NJ, Lesserman J et al. Sexual and physical abuse and gastrointestinal illness. *Ann Intern Med* 1995; 123:782–794. An excellent clinical summary of abuse in the genesis of illness and how to screen for abuse.
5. Johnson J, Sims R, Gottlieb G. Differential diagnosis of dementia, delirium and depression. Implications for drug therapy. *Drugs and Aging* 1994; 5:431–445. The differential diagnosis hinges on a careful clinical evaluation. Dementia is defined as a chronic loss of intellectual or cognitive function of sufficient severity to interfere with social or occupational function. Delirium is an acute disturbance of consciousness marked by an attention deficit and a change in cognitive ability.
6. Folstein MF, Folstein SE, McHugh PR. Mini Mental State. A practical method for grading the cognitive state of patients for the clinician. *J Psychiatr Res* 1975; 12:189–198. This is a useful instrument but is now copyright protected (see Wikipedia for details).
7. Borson S, Scanlan J, Brush M et al. The Mini-Cog: a cognitive 'vital signs' measure for dementia screening in multi-lingual elderly. *Int J Geriatr Psychiatry* 2000; 15(11):1021–1027. A useful and quick screening test for dementia.
8. Russell G. Bulimia nervosa: an ominous variant of anorexia nervosa. *Psychol Med* 1979; 9(3):429–448.
9. Spoont MR, Williams JW Jr, Kehle-Forbes S et al. Does this patient have posttraumatic stress disorder?: Rational clinical examination systematic review. *JAMA* 2015; 314(5):501–510.

SECTION 14
Acute care and end of life

CHAPTER 47
The acutely ill patient

CHAPTER 48
The pre-anaesthetic medical examination (PAME)

CHAPTER 49
Assessment of death

CHAPTER 47
The acutely ill patient

To be or not to be? That is the question. WILLIAM SHAKESPEARE, Hamlet

INITIAL ASSESSMENT

During your training, you will be expected to become expert in advanced life support and this training must be refreshed regularly. If you come across an obviously very ill patient, the first step is to ask, 'Are you okay?' If the patient is unresponsive on gentle shaking, quickly check whether the airway is patent and if he or she is breathing, then rapidly assess the circulation. This should all take no more than 10 seconds. Start cardiopulmonary resuscitation (CPR; see Fig. 47.1) if the patient is not breathing (or is just gasping) or has no pulse, and try to send someone else to call for help. Current guidelines emphasise the importance of adequate chest compressions during CPR (at least 100/minute, compressing the centre of the chest 5 centimetres with each downward compression, and no interruptions—remember to push hard and fast).[1]

If the patient is clearly responding appropriately to questions, and the skin is normal in colour as well as warm and dry, the patient is much less likely to need urgent intervention before appropriate history taking and a full examination are completed. If the patient's level of consciousness becomes impaired, recheck the **a**irway, **b**reathing and **c**irculation (**ABCs**), check the serum glucose (you must not miss hypoglycaemia) and obtain intravenous access immediately.

An acutely ill patient who presents to hospital may be able to give some history. Ask:
- What is wrong?
- What has happened?'
- Have you been injured? Are you in pain anywhere?

If possible, while beginning your physical assessment (see Fig. 47.2) ask about previous medical problems such as heart disease, diabetes, asthma or depression. If the patient is accompanied by others, ask these people if they have any more information. Look for an alert bracelet and for a list of medications in the patient's pockets.

LEVEL OF CONSCIOUSNESS

Assess the patient's **level of consciousness** using the AVPU system:

A lert (normal)
V erbal stimulus responsive
P ainful stimulus responsive
U nresponsive patient.

If the patient only responds to a painful stimulus or is unresponsive, assess him or her using the Glasgow Coma Scale (see Table 35.4, p 602).[2]

Gather key data, as summarised by the mnemonic **AMPLE**:

A llergies
M edication currently being taken and most recent medications taken
P ast medical history
L ast meal
E vents preceding the current incident.

If the patient is tachypnoeic, check pulse oximetry and start oxygen therapy unless there is a known contraindication.

If the patient is bradycardic or tachycardic, obtain an ECG.

DELIRIUM

Delirium is an acute change in cognitive function that occurs over hours or a few days. It is often associated with acute medical conditions and therefore is often seen in hospital patients. It is important that it be recognised and the cause removed or treated. Risk factors include:

Resuscitation.

(a) Head-tilt; (b) jaw-thrust and jaw-tilt manoeuvres to open the airway; (c) clearing the airway; (d) cardiopulmonary resuscitation

(Baker T, Nikolic G, O'Connor S. *Practical cardiology*, 2nd edn. Sydney: Elsevier, 2008.)

FIGURE 47.1

- pre-existing dementia or other neurological disease, e.g. Parkinson's disease
- severe illness, e.g. mechanical ventilation
- age over 65
- alcoholism.

The diagnosis should be considered in all patients with risk factors. Relatives or nursing staff may be concerned about the patient's being confused. Ask the staff or relatives about typical features (Questions box 47.1).

A diagnosis of delirium is confirmed if the answers to questions 1 and 2 are 'yes' and that to either or both 3 and 4 is also 'yes'.

If delirium seems confirmed, look into possible causes (List 47.1)

FURTHER EXAMINATION

(See List 47.2.)

Check the patient's blood pressure and other vital signs. Assess fluid status (see Ch 18). If the patient is hypotensive, consider an intravenous fluid challenge, and organise to regularly measure the heart rate, blood pressure, respiratory rate and hourly urinary output (if necessary by inserting a urinary catheter).

Assess the capillary refill time by depressing the finger- or toenail until it blanches and recording the

CHAPTER 47 THE ACUTELY ILL PATIENT

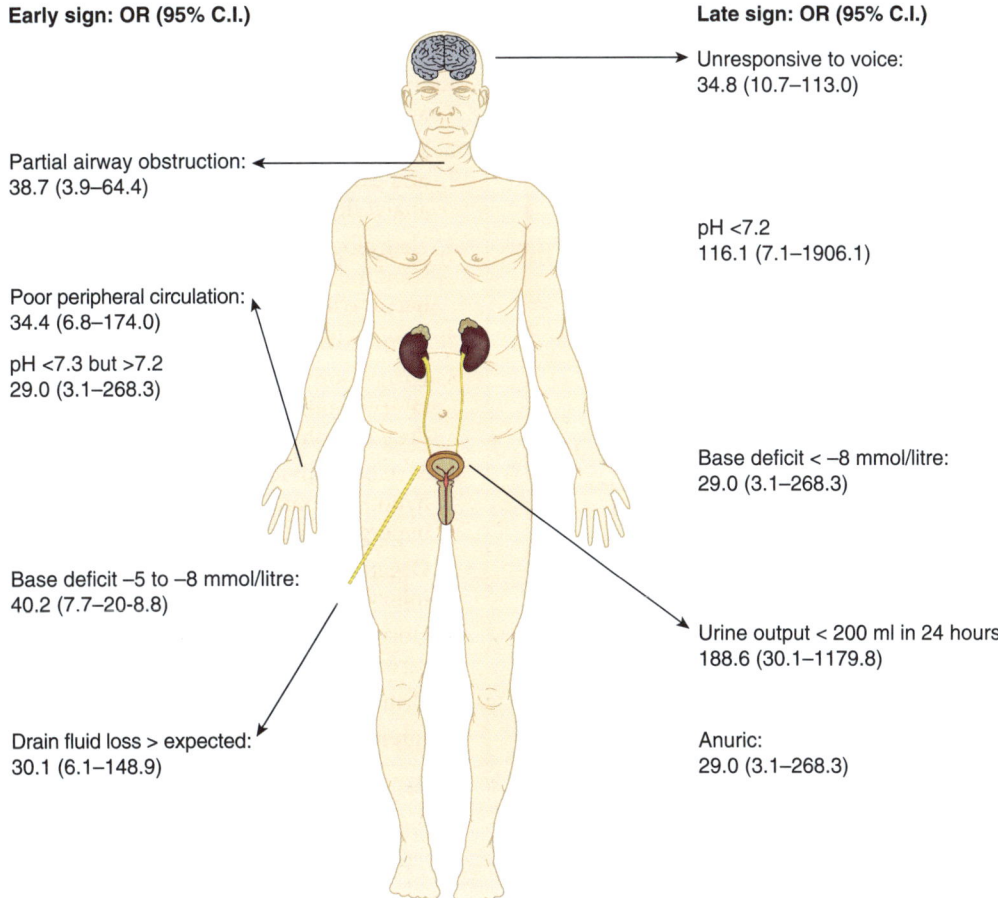

Assessment of the acutely ill patient: 'Top five' early and late signs of physiological deterioration with the odds ratio (OR) for death (95% confidence interval)

A = Airway
Obstructed? Look for injury

B = Breathing
1. Inspect chest for trauma
2. Look for chest wall movement
3. Is the patient using the accessory muscle of respiration?
4. Auscultate lungs for equal breath sounds

C = Circulation
1. Pulse: radial or femoral; rate and rhythm
2. Blood pressure
3. Perfusion: colour, temperature

D = Disability
1. Conscious state: Glasgow Coma Scale (see Table 35.4, p 602)
2. Pupillary responses
3. Abnormal movements: epileptiform
4. Localising signs (e.g. hyperreflexia)

Other
1. Signs of injury
2. Medical alert bracelet
3. Medication list in pocket

(Robertson LC. Recognizing the critically ill patient. *Anaesthesia and Intensive Care Medicine*, 2013; 14(1):11–14.)

FIGURE 47.2

QUESTIONS TO ASK RELATIVES OR STAFF ABOUT A PATIENT WHO MAY HAVE DELIRIUM

1. Has there been a recent change in the patient's mental state and has this been coming and going during the day or been worse at night?
2. Does the patient have difficulty in concentrating or following things said to him or her? Is he or she easily distracted?
3. Does he or she seem to have incoherent thinking with rambling conversation? Is there odd switching from one idea to another?
4. Does the patient seem alert, drowsy or comatose, or to have increased alertness (vigilance or agitation)?

QUESTIONS BOX 47.1

IMPORTANT CAUSES OF DELIRIUM

1. Infections—especially urinary tract infections and pneumonia
2. Surgery—postoperative delirium is common and exacerbated by anaesthetic drugs and analgesics
3. Neurological illnesses—stroke, seizures, subdural haematoma, intracranial haemorrhage
4. Myocardial infarction
5. Drugs—opioids, sedatives (including sleeping tablets), anticonvulsants, anti-Parkinsonian drugs, alcohol or drug withdrawal
6. Metabolic abnormalities—hypoxia, hyponatraemia, hypoglycaemia or hyperglycaemia, hypercarbia
7. Organ failure—heart failure, acute kidney injury
8. Hospital ward—sensory deprivation (intensive care ward), lack of sleep
9. Urinary retention

Combinations of these causes are common.

LIST 47.1

SIGNS OF A CRITICALLY ILL PATIENT

1. Respiratory signs
   - Stridor and intercostal recession
   - Threatened or obstructed airway (e.g. from injury or swelling; angio-oedema—see Fig. 47.4)
   - Abnormal respiratory rate >35 breaths/minute or <8 breaths/minute
   - No spontaneous respiratory effort
   - Respiratory distress: use of accessory muscles, unable to speak in sentences (e.g. severe asthma)
   - Abnormal oximetry: S_pO_2 <90% even with supplementary oxygen
   - Increasing P_aCO_2: blood gas measurements (indicates reduced respiratory effort)
2. Cardiovascular signs
   - Absent pulse
   - Heart rate <40 or >180 b.p.m.
   - Systolic blood pressure <100 mmHg (where blood pressure previously normal)
   - Poor peripheral perfusion (suggests tissue hypoxia)
   - Low urine output: <0.5 mL/kg/h (urinary catheter in situ)
   - ECG—asystole (no cardiac rhythm), ventricular fibrillation, fast ventricular tachycardia, complete heart block
3. Neurological signs
   - Airway threatened by absent gag reflex
   - Not obeying commands
   - Not responding to painful stimuli
   - Moving only one side in response to stimuli (stroke, cerebral haemorrhage)
   - Reduced respiratory rate
   - Sudden reduction in level of consciousness
   - Pupil size and reaction to light (pinpoint pupils suggest a pontine haemorrhage)
   - Recurrent seizures (tonic–clonic movements)
   - Glasgow Coma Scale score <10 (see Table 35.4, p 602)

LIST 47.2

Meningococcal rash

(Courtesy of Dr A Watson, Infectious Diseases Department, The Canberra Hospital.)

FIGURE 47.3

Angio-oedema

(Courtesy of Dr A Watson, Infectious Diseases Department, The Canberra Hospital.)

FIGURE 47.4

time it takes for the colour to become normal again, which is usually less than 2 seconds. A delayed capillary refill time occurs in hypovolaemic or cardiogenic shock.

Examine the patient's chest for any obvious evidence of tension pneumothorax—features include unilateral pleuritic chest pain, respiratory distress, decreased breath sounds and increased percussion over the affected side, tachycardia and hypotension, tracheal deviation (away from affected side), palpable subcutaneous emphysema and greatly distended neck veins.

Assess the patient for possible cardiac tamponade (features include dypspnoea, tachycardia, hypotension, distended neck veins, difficult-to-hear heart sounds, and pulsus paradoxus).

Examine the body for any evidence of obvious bleeding or other trauma.[3]

Look at the skin for a meningococcal rash (see Fig. 47.3). Angio-oedema (see Fig. 47.4) can occur in anaphylaxis.

Measure the patient's temperature. If it is elevated, consider taking blood and urine cultures.

The **systemic inflammatory response syndrome (SIRS)** refers to two or more of the following four features: fever >38.3°C (or temperature <36°C), tachycardia (>90 beats/min), tachypnoea (>20 breaths/min) and an elevated white cell count (although it may be suppressed).

SIRS may be due to acute infection but can also occur after burns or surgery or with other inflammatory diseases (e.g. thromboembolism, pancreatitis, vasculitis, autoimmune disease). Sepsis refers to the presence of infection in the setting of SIRS, so SIRS is sensitive but not specific for bacteraemia. Early identification of sepsis remains a clinical diagnosis, and immediate treatment with antibiotics saves lives.[4]

A useful prognostic score in sepsis is the quick sequential organ failure assessment (SOFA) score (1 point each for: a high respiratory rate—22 or higher per minute, low systolic blood pressure—100 mmHg or lower, and altered mentation; 2 or more indicates a poor outcome).[4]

OSCE EXAMPLE – EMERGENCY CARE

Mr Sherlock has had episodes of sudden loss of consciousness. Please examine him.

1. Assess the patient's level of consciousness, and test orientation in time, place and person.
2. Neurological examination: examine the patient's gait, then limbs and cranial nerves, looking for focal neurological signs (stroke, intracranial tumour).
3. Note whether there are tongue lacerations (seizures).
4. Auscultate for carotid bruits (carotid stenosis).
5. Take the patient's pulse (arrhythmias including atrial fibrillation or heart block) and blood pressure lying and sitting (postural hypotension).
6. Examine the praecordium (signs of new murmurs, tamponade).
7. Take the patient's temperature and assess for neck stiffness (sepsis, meningism).

References

1. Berg RA, Hemphill R, Abella BS et al. Part 5: adult basic life support: 2010 American Heart Association Guidelines for Cardiopulmonary Resuscitation and Emergency Cardiovascular Care. *Circulation* 2010; 122:S685–S705. Know how to do basic and advanced cardiac life support—and remain competent.
2. Easter JS, Haukoos JS, Meehan WP et al. Will neuroimaging reveal a severe intracranial injury in this adult with minor head trauma?: The Rational Clinical Examination Systematic Review. *JAMA* 2015; 314(24):2672–2681. Following head trauma, a patient may initially appear fine (Glasgow Coma Scale [GCS] scores ≥13) yet still have severe intracranial injury as documented by head CT scan. A history of being struck by a car (LR up to 4.3) or two or more vomiting episodes (LR 3.6) is worrying. Examine for physical signs of a skull fracture (LR 16). Watch for a decline of GCS score.
3. Joshi N, Lira A, Mehta N et al. Diagnostic accuracy of history, physical examination, and bedside ultrasound for diagnosis of extremity fractures in the emergency department: a systematic review. *Acad Emerg Med* 2013; 20(1):1–15. Physical examination is not sufficient to diagnose a limb fracture: an X-ray remains the gold standard.
4. Singer M, Deutschman CS, Seymour CW et al. The Third International Consensus Definitions for Sepsis and Septic Shock (Sepsis-3). *JAMA* 2016; 315(8):801–810.

CHAPTER 48
The pre-anaesthetic medical evaluation (PAME)

Whenever ideas fail, men invent words. MARTIN H FISHER (1879–1962)

An appropriate medical evaluation of the patient who has been admitted for elective surgery is always required. It includes a history and examination that is sufficient to uncover any likely major problems with anaesthesia or the procedure itself.

THE HISTORY

The first thing to find out, of course, is the presenting problem, what operation is intended and whether the surgery is expected to be performed under general or local anaesthesia. Clearly the assessment of a patient having a small lesion removed under local anaesthesia can be briefer than the assessment of a patient undergoing extensive bowel resection under general anaesthesia. As a rule, before any patient undergoes surgery under general anaesthesia or spinal anaesthesia, careful attention must be given to identifying whether he or she is at higher risk.

Cardiovascular history

The most important questions here relate to a history of ischaemic heart disease. Patients who have had a myocardial infarct in the preceding 3 months should not usually undergo elective surgery; the risks of further infarction or malignant arrhythmia and death are high during this period. A patient who has symptoms of angina that have recently become unstable is also at greater risk. A history of stable angina that has not changed for months or years is not a contraindication to most forms of surgery. The recent placement of a coronary stent may mean that cessation of antiplatelet drugs is not safe for 1 month after insertion of a bare metal stent and 6 months to 1 year after the insertion of a drug-eluting stent.

Symptoms of cardiac failure should be sought. Any patient with uncontrolled cardiac failure is at considerable risk of severe cardiac failure postoperatively. This is particularly true if large amounts of intravenous fluids are given during and after surgery while the patient's antifailure drugs (e.g. diuretics) are omitted.

Cardiac drugs should be asked about, particularly antianginal and antifailure drugs. It is important to attempt to ensure that the patient receives these drugs, particularly beta-blockers, on the day of the operation. The surgeon may require the patient to stop aspirin a week or more before surgery. This is usually a safe thing for the patient to do but may be a problem in the first month at least after a coronary angioplasty because of the risk of thrombosis of the stent in this early period. Previous coronary artery bypass grafting or angioplasty is not a contraindication to surgery.

A history of infective endocarditis or the presence of a prosthetic cardiac valve or complex congenital cardiac condition is an indication for antibiotic prophylaxis for any procedure that may result in bacteraemia—the circulation of bacteria in the bloodstream. These procedures include most types of dental work and surgery on the bowel or bladder and some gynaecological operations and vaginal delivery.

Patients who take oral anticoagulants such as warfarin or the new oral anticoagulants (dabigatran, apixaban or rivaroxaban) require special attention. When the drug is being used to protect the patient from embolic events associated with atrial fibrillation it may be reasonable, on the balance of risks, to have the drug stopped an appropriate period before surgery and resumed as soon as practical afterwards. If the patient takes the drug to protect a mechanical heart valve from clot, the drug should, in general, be replaced by intravenous unfractionated or subcutaneous fractionated heparin. The last dose of fractionated heparin can be given about 12 hours before surgery and the drug recommenced as soon as the surgeon feels it is safe. Many patients can administer the drug themselves at home. Patients with mechanical valves, especially in the mitral position, are at high risk of embolic events if their warfarin is stopped without replacement with some form of heparin.

The presence of a cardiac pacemaker or implanted defibrillator may be a problem if the surgeon intends to use a diathermy device.

The respiratory history

Enquire about a history of respiratory disease, particularly chronic obstructive pulmonary disease or severe asthma. Patients who have continued to smoke up to the time of their surgery have a much higher risk of postoperative chest infections than those who have not. Even stopping a few weeks before will reduce this risk. Severe respiratory disease is a relative contraindication to surgery. It may be difficult to reverse the anaesthetic and muscle relaxant drugs in such a patient, and he or she may require ventilation postoperatively. Doctors in charge of intensive care units are always happier to be warned that a patient may require ventilation postoperatively than to have it come as a surprise.

Drug therapy for respiratory disease must be asked about. Steroids may impair wound healing, and steroid doses may need to be increased during the operative period because of steroid-induced adrenal suppression.

Other

Enquire about any history of bleeding diathesis, diabetes mellitus, renal disease, hepatitis, jaundice or drug abuse. The control of blood sugar in diabetic patients can be difficult in the perioperative period, especially while normal diet is impossible. The fasting preoperative diabetic on insulin may need to be advised to have half the normal insulin dose on the morning of surgery. This may be important to avoid ketoacidosis.

Specific enquiries about *previous operations and anaesthetics*, particularly with reference to any complications, should be made. *Allergies* to anaesthetic agents or other drugs must be asked about. Attempt to distinguish a true allergy or anaphylaxis from an adverse effect such as vomiting after a morphine injection. Some operations involve the use of contrast media, and an allergy to iodine may be a contraindication to their use. This risk is now much less with the new non-ionic contrast media. There may occasionally be a *family history of anaesthetic complications* or deaths. This raises the possibility of malignant hyperthermia, which is an inherited disorder leading to fever and muscle destruction after administration of muscle relaxants.

Ask about exercise tolerance. How far can the patient walk? How many flights of stairs can the patient climb? Poor functional status is indicated by an inability to walk one or two blocks on the flat.

THE EXAMINATION

Examination according to the rapid screening method outlined in Chapter 51 represents the best approach. Record height, weight and vital signs (pulse rate, blood pressure, respiratory rate). The cardiovascular and respiratory systems must be fully examined. Patients with a short thick neck may be difficult to ventilate and intubate. It is better for the anaesthetist to be aware of this possible problem before the patient is given a muscle relaxant and is unable to breathe spontaneously. The presence of loose or fragile teeth must also be noted because of the risk of their dislodgement during attempted intubation.

If a previously undiagnosed symptom or sign of significance is uncovered, some further investigations may be required before surgery, and the operation may have to be deferred. For example, the discovery of a new and significant heart murmur, uncontrolled hypertension, respiratory failure, a bleeding diathesis, uncontrolled diabetes mellitus or renal failure should be brought to the attention of the surgeon and anaesthetist.

CHAPTER 49
Assessment of death

I'm not afraid of death; I just don't want to be there when it happens. WOODY ALLAN

We all die eventually, although most of us try not to ruminate on the subject. The certification of a patient's death is one of the legal responsibilities of a doctor. The experience can be distressing for the doctor as well as the patient's relatives. Students should be given the opportunity to observe senior colleagues performing these tasks and to learn what is required technically and emotionally. Clearly, the declaration that a patient has died must be correct, as well as sympathetically performed.

Death is not easy to define in absolute terms but generally means brain death—an irreversible loss of consciousness, usually but not always linked to an irreversible loss of spontaneous respiration.

ASSESSMENT

If you are called to assess an unresponsive patient, do *not* assume that the patient has died: start cardiopulmonary resuscitation (CPR) immediately (see p 868) and call for help, *unless* there is a confirmed and current advance care directive or resuscitation plan.

Do-not-resuscitate (DNR) orders

Most hospitals have specific policies in place about resuscitation. Patients have the right to make a *living will* or *advance directive* outlining their wishes concerning resuscitation; for example, a patient with a terminal condition can elect to refuse CPR or life support if cardiac arrest occurs. The directive, if known, should be honoured. Remember, however, that if the patient had changed his or her mind before collapsing and notified staff verbally, the current verbal decision rather than the written directive must be honoured (i.e. you should provide CPR or life support). Sometimes, directives may be more specific. For example, a directive may forbid intubation. It would be wrong in this case to deny the patient an attempt at cardioversion from ventricular fibrillation, but it may be reasonable not to proceed to more invasive resuscitation. If the patient is unknown to you, it is important to err on the side of caution and begin resuscitation.

Do not misdiagnose death

The dead patient is unresponsive, has no spontaneous respiratory movements, has no pulse or heart sounds, is very pale and usually the eyes are open and blankly staring. Red–purple discoloration in gravity-dependent areas occurs about half an hour after death, while rigor mortis (muscle stiffening) occurs hours later.

Note that death can be and has been diagnosed in error most often in patients on a ventilator. Important conditions to exclude before declaring a person is dead include:

- hypothermia
- near-drowning
- drug overdose (especially alcohol and tranquillisers)
- hypoglycaemia
- other causes of deep coma, or severe catatonia.

In these cases, some cardiac and respiratory activity will be present.

Examining a suspected death

List 49.1 summarises the physical examination to confirm death. After brain death there may still be spontaneous movements from the denervated spinal cord or peripheral nerves—examples include flexion of the neck, elbows and trunk (when dramatic, known as the 'Lazarus sign') or finger flexor movements.

Remember, certifying death has medicolegal consequences. As a doctor you will be required to examine the patient and record your findings in the medical record, including the date and time that life became extinct. Where possible, you should include the likely cause of death, and sign your name (legibly). You are required to notify the authorities of any unexpected or suspect death.

Brainstem death

Patients on a *mechanical ventilator* require additional testing to confirm that they are truly dead.

Potentially reversible causes must always be excluded (especially drugs; see above). There have been cases where brain death has been pronounced and the patient has later woken up.

Do not miss the rare **locked-in syndrome**. This can occur following an embolus blocking the basilar artery or some other local injury to the base of the pons. The unfortunate patient is not unconscious at all, but cannot move any face, limb or trunk muscles. You can identify the syndrome by asking the patient to blink once for 'yes' and twice for 'no'; voluntary blinking as well as vertical eye movements are not affected.

Testing protocols are based on the law, which vary by country and state (check the requirements in your state). Traditionally, testing is carried out by two different doctors on two separate occasions, typically 24 hours apart, to ensure that the state is irreversible (but the timing of repeat testing is dependent on the patient's age and likely cause of death). Testing typically includes a physical examination (as per List 49.1), an obvious lack of any response to suctioning the tracheal tube, plus an *ice-water (oculovestibular reflex) test*: no eye response to irrigation of ice-cold water into the ears. If the examination indicates brain death, a *medullary brainstem hypercapnia test* is performed, whereby the ventilator is ceased while giving 100% oxygen and the arterial CO_2 is permitted to rise above a preset threshold (>6.7 kPa). Seeing no respiratory effort after 8–10 minutes indicates that there is no medullary function.

INFORMING RELATIVES

Informing relatives is always difficult but is the responsibility of the certifying doctor. It is one of the hardest things doctors have to do. Give the news in person—this will usually be deeply appreciated. Break the bad news professionally and compassionately. Seek a private and quiet environment, speak clearly and concisely, be supportive, respect cultural and religious beliefs and engage the help of the team (e.g. nurse, social worker, and cleric). Relatives often want to know what happened, particularly if the death is unexpected. If the patient is well known to you, you may be able to provide that explanation; if not, you should suggest the relatives arrange to meet the consultant responsible for the patient to discuss the issues.

COMPLETING THE DEATH CERTIFICATE

The death certificate is a legal document. If the death was expected (and not suspect), you should complete the certificate as soon as possible. The World Health Organization (WHO) provides a certificate format that is applied internationally. Certify the disease that led directly to death (in part I of the form), as well as any other diseases that contributed (in part II of the form).

CONFIRMING DEATH: THE PHYSICAL EXAMINATION

Look
- Inspect the chest wall for any movement (nil).
- Look for any spontaneous movements (nil).
- Check the reflexes (eyes) for pupillary response to bright light (fixed, dilated, non-reactive).
- Assess the corneal reflexes (absent response to cottonwool).
- Assess the gag reflex (absent).

Feel
- Palpate the carotid or femoral artery (nil pulse over 1 minute).
- Check for a motor response to pain (nil after supraorbital pressure).

Listen
- Auscultate for heart sounds (nil over 1 minute).
- Auscultate for breath sounds (nil over 3 minutes).

LIST 49.1

POSTMORTEM

The relatives must agree to a postmortem (PM) before it can be undertaken unless mandated by law. There has been a major decline in the undertaking of postmortems in recent decades because of a reluctance to ask relatives and a community reluctance to agree. If the reasons for the request are communicated clearly and compassionately, many will sign the consent.

Remember, the information gleaned from a postmortem not uncommonly leads to significant surprises about the causes of death, and potentially can inform the profession, helping to prevent future diagnostic and treatment mistakes.

If the cause of death is uncertain, a postmortem becomes even more important, and certain events such as recent surgery or trauma mean the case should be referred to the coroner, who will usually insist on a postmortem examination.

ORGAN DONATION

In settings where there is brain death but mechanical ventilation can be continued, consent to organ donation should be explored and is ethical. The patient's wishes may be known (e.g. on the driver's licence or an organ donation register, or as a result of previous discussion between the patient and relatives). Organ donation may provide some comfort to grieving relatives.

SECTION 15
Adult history taking and examination in the wards and clinics

CHAPTER 50

Writing and presenting the adult history and physical examination

CHAPTER 51

A suggested method for a rapid screening adult physical examination

CHAPTER 50
Writing and presenting the adult history and physical examination

Medical education is not completed at the Medical School; it is only begun.
WILLIAM H WELCH (1850–1934)

Experience is never limited, and it is never complete. HENRY JAMES (1843–1916)

It is important that the medical record be kept succinct and relevant. The following approach is the one recommended by the authors. The detail of the history and examination and its record varies of course, depending on whether this is a first visit and on the complexity of the presenting problem. It is not necessary to ask every patient every question.

HISTORY

Personal information
Record the name, sex, date of birth and address. Write down the date and time of the examination.

Presenting (principal) symptoms (PS)
A short sentence identifies the major symptoms and their duration; it is often useful to quote the patient's own words.

History of present illness (HPI)
Don't record every detail; rather, prepare short prose paragraphs telling the story of the illness in chronological order. Describe the characteristics of each symptom. Note why the patient presents at this time. Also, describe any past medical problems that are related to the current symptoms. Include the relevant positive and negative findings on the system review here. Note how the diagnosis was reached, side effects and response to treatment. If there are many seemingly unrelated problems, summarise these in an introductory paragraph and present the history of each problem in separate paragraphs.

List current medications and doses and the indications for their use, if they are known, and any side effects, or known or measured therapeutic effects. For example, if the patient takes antihypertensive drugs ask whether blood pressure control has been satisfactory as far as the patient knows, or haemoglobin A_{1c} (HbA_{1C}) if the patient has diabetes mellitus. Finally, record your impression of the reliability of the history and, if the patient was unable to give the history, describe the source of this information.

Past history (PH)
List, in chronological order, past medical or surgical problems (sometimes called inactive problems), past medication use, if relevant, and any history of allergy (particularly drug allergy) or of drug intolerance. Find out what the problem with the drug was. The patient may know the results of certain previous important investigations (e.g. 'The scan showed I had clots in my lung'). A history of blood transfusions should be noted.

Social history (SH)
This may include recording the patient's occupation, schooling, hobbies, marital status, family structure, personal support system, living conditions and recent travel. The number and gender of sexual partners may be relevant. Smoking, alcohol and other recreational drug use should also be described. Ask about ability to perform the activities of daily living (ADL) if elderly. If a patient has a chronic illness, ask about the effect of this on his or life. If it is appropriate, ask about advance care planning.

Family history (FH)

Describe causes of mortality in the first-degree relatives and, if indicated, draw a family tree.

Systems review (SR)

All directly relevant information should be incorporated in the HPI or PH.

PHYSICAL EXAMINATION (PE)

Under each of the major systems, list the relevant positives and negatives using brief statements. (See Ch 51.)

PROVISIONAL DIAGNOSIS

Ask yourself the following questions when considering the differential diagnosis of a patient's major symptoms.

1. What is the likely diagnosis based on the patient's age, sex and background?
2. Are there other conditions that resemble the likely diagnosis but can present in the same way?
3. Is there a serious disorder, even if rare, that must not be missed?
4. Could the patient have a specific condition that often masquerades as (or mimics) other conditions (e.g. depression, drugs, diabetes mellitus, thyroid dysfunction, anaemia, malignancy, spinal cord disease, urinary infection, renal failure, alcoholism, syphilis, tuberculosis, HIV infection, infective endocarditis or connective tissue disease)?
5. Is the patient trying to really tell me that there is an emotional or psychological problem?

An example of a patient history is presented in Box 50.1.

PROBLEM LIST AND PLANS

Using a sentence or two, summarise the most important findings and then give a provisional diagnosis (PD) and differential diagnosis (DD).

Remember Occam's razor: choose the simplest hypothesis to explain any new observations. Also remember Sutton's law: the famous bank robber said he robbed banks because 'That's where the money is'—that is, consider a common diagnosis before resorting to a rare one to explain the symptoms and signs. Older patients are more likely to have multiple co-morbidities.

It is often useful to ask yourself whether the patient's problem is a diagnostic or management one (or both). For example, a patient with the new onset of dyspnoea presents both a diagnostic problem—'What is the cause of the breathlessness?' and a management problem—'How should the condition be treated?' The patient who presents with a worsening of previously diagnosed angina presents only a management problem—'How should the symptoms be treated?'

List all the active problems that require management. Outline the diagnostic tests and therapy planned for each problem.

Sign your name and then print your name and position underneath.

CONTINUATION NOTES

Date (and time) each progress note in the record. The SOAP (**S**ubjective, **O**bjective, **A**ssessment and **P**lans) format can be useful.

Subjective data refer to what the patient tells you; list relevant current problems and note any new problems. Have the patient's previous symptoms improved on the current treatment?

Objective data are physical or laboratory findings; relevant data for each active problem are summarised.

Assessment refers to the interpretation of any relevant findings for each problem.

Plans describe any interventions that will be started for each problem.

Many patient records are now kept in a computer file. Parts of this can be used to provide referral information for the patient to take to a specialist or if he or she is travelling. It is important that such files be kept up to date and especially that lists of medications that are no longer used are deleted from the current list before it is given to the patient.

PRESENTATION[1]

In their formal examinations and less formally on the wards, students and resident medical officers will often be expected to present the history and physical examination of a patient to an examiner or senior colleague. This is excellent training for clinical practice, as the need to discuss patients with colleagues or

An example of a medical history

Personal details
Mr W Witheridge, age 72, retired botanist.

Presenting symptoms
3 weeks of progressive exertional dyspnoea with 2 days of dyspnoea at rest.

History of present illness
Two nights of severe orthopnoea; unable to sleep except briefly while sitting in a chair.

Mild exertional shortness of breath for nearly 10 years.

Unable to walk 50 metres on the flat.

No associated chest tightness or pain.

No wheeze or cough.

No fever.

No recent change in medications.

No asthma or known lung disease. No other relevant positive symptoms on systems review.

Past cardiac history
Previous myocardial infarction 5 years ago, treated with thrombolytic drugs. No known valvular heart disease or history of rheumatic fever. Smoked 25 cigarettes a day until the time of his infarct—30 packet-years.

Risk factors for heart disease
Total cholesterol 6.7 mmol/L, a family history of ischaemic heart disease—his 55-year-old brother had hypertension for 30 years—inadequate control. Salt intake high, drinks 3-4 litres of fluid a day. Alcohol—25 g a week. There is no history of diabetes mellitus. Only occasional non-steroidal anti-inflammatory drugs.

Other symptoms
10 years of nocturia three times per night. He denies other urinary tract symptoms.

Current medications
Aspirin, 100 mg daily; metoprolol (a beta-blocker), 100 mg twice a day. No use of over-the-counter medications.

Past history
Gastric ulceration 3 years ago—successfully treated with a 14-day course of antibiotics and a proton pump inhibitor; no recurrence of symptoms. Appendectomy and tonsillectomy in his youth.

He has no drug allergies that he knows of and has never required a blood transfusion.

Social history
Lives in retirement with his wife, who is well.

Interests: gardening, history of medicinal plants. No other hobbies. No pets.

No recent overseas travel.

Family history
His father died of a myocardial infarct at age 64 years and his mother died of colon cancer at age 84 years. Both sons (42 and 39 years) are alive and well. No other relevant family history.

Physical examination
Breathless and uncomfortable at rest. Temperature 37°C. Respiratory rate—24 breaths per minute.

Cardiovascular
No cyanosis. No clubbing. No splinter haemorrhages.

Pulse rate 90 beats per minute and regular.

Blood pressure 180/110 mmHg, lying and standing.

Jugular venous pressure (JVP) not elevated.

Apex beat 2 cm displaced, dyskinetic.

Heart sounds (HS): S1 and S2 present and normal; S3 present.

Pansystolic murmur grade 3/6 maximum at the apex consistent with mitral regurgitation.

BOX 50.1

Continued

An example of a medical history *continued*

Chest
Trachea in the midline.
Expansion normal right and left.
Normal percussion note bilaterally.
Bilateral medium basal midinspiratory crackles and occasional expiratory wheeze over the right and left lung fields. No areas of bronchial breathing.

Abdomen
Well-healed appendix scar present.
Abdomen soft, no tenderness.
Liver not palpable, no other masses (spleen, kidneys).
No ascites.
Normal bowel sounds.
Rectal examination deferred (the patient was too unwell at the time of admission).

Legs
No calf tenderness.
No peripheral oedema.
Peripheral pulses present and equal.
No visible varicose veins.

Central nervous system (CNS)
Alert and orientated.
No neck stiffness.

Cranial nerves (assessed after initial treatment)
II—acuity and fields normal; fundi normal.
III, IV and VI—pupils equal, circular and concentric—react normally to light and accommodation; eye movements normal; no nystagmus.
V—sensation and motor function normal.
VII—muscles of facial expression normal.
VIII—hearing normal.
IX, X—no uvular displacement.
XI—normal power.
XII—no fasciculation or displacement of tongue.

Upper limbs
No wasting, fasciculations, tremor.
Tone normal.
Power normal (shoulders, elbows, wrists, fingers).
Reflexes normal and symmetrical.[1]

	Right	Left
Biceps	++	++
Triceps	++	++
Brachioradialis	++	++

Coordination normal.
Sensation—pain, proprioception normal.

Provisional diagnosis:
left ventricular failure secondary to ischaemic heart disease.

Differential diagnosis:
angina, pulmonary embolus, chronic obstructive pulmonary disease.

Investigations
Electrocardiogram
Chest X-ray
Full blood count
Electrolytes, creatinine, liver function tests
Echocardiogram

Comment
The aetiology of his cardiac failure is most likely to be ischaemic heart disease (previous infarct) or hypertension. He has signs of mitral regurgitation, which may be secondary to cardiac failure or, less likely, the cause. There is no known history of chronic lung disease, although he has been a chronic smoker. The history and examination are not very suggestive of pulmonary embolism.

---

1. The reflexes may be recorded as:
   O (absent)
   + (reduced)
   ++ (normal)
   +++ (increased)
   ++++ (exaggerated with clonus)

BOX 50.1

specialists arises frequently in both hospital and non-hospital practice.

A successful case presentation is both succinct and relevant. The examiner is most interested in what the patient's problems are now. One should aim to convey basic biographical information and an assessment of the patient's presenting problem in the first few sentences. It is often helpful to frame the presentation of the case as a diagnostic or management problem, or both.

The information will have been obtained from the patient by taking the history as set out above. The examination of the patient should be performed with particular attention to the areas most likely to be abnormal. This information must then be assembled into a form that can easily be conveyed to others. The following is a suggested method.

1. Begin with a sentence that tells your colleague about the essence of the patient and the clinical problem. For example, one might say 'Mr Jones is a 72-year-old retired cabinet minister who presents with 2 hours of chest pain which is not typically ischaemic'. This gives an idea about the patient himself and indicates that the problem is likely to be a diagnostic one.
2. One should then go on to explain in what way the pain is atypical of ischaemia and whether it has features suggestive of any other diagnosis.
3. Once the presenting symptom or problem has been described, relevant past history should be discussed. In a patient with chest pain this would include any previous cardiac history or investigations, and a summary of the patient's risk factors for ischaemic heart disease.
4. Present a list of the patient's current medications.
5. Important previous health problems should be outlined briefly. This retired cabinet minister might also have a history of intermittent claudication and of chronic obstructive pulmonary disease. These facts will affect possible treatment for ischaemic heart disease, e.g. the use of beta-blockers.
6. Present the physical examination in two parts.
   a. Abnormal and important normal examination findings in the presenting system—in this patient's case this would mean giving the pulse rate and blood pressure but not details of normal heart sounds. If there was a history of claudication, the examination of the peripheral pulses should be presented even if it is normal.
   b. Abnormal findings in the rest of the examination.
7. Offer the most likely diagnosis and the differential diagnosis.
8. Suggest a plan for investigation and treatment.
9. Much more detail will have been obtained in the assessment of the patient than should be presented routinely, but further details may be asked for by your colleague. These may include information about the patient's living conditions and the availability of support from the family. This may determine how soon the patient can be sent home from hospital after treatment.

By the end of your presentation your colleague should know what you think is wrong with the patient and what you intend to do about it.

Reference

1. Kroenke K. The case presentation: stumbling blocks and stepping stones. *Am J Med* 1985; 79:605–608.

CHAPTER 51

A suggested method for a rapid screening adult physical examination

A good teacher knows the rules; a good pupil, the exceptions. MARTIN H FISHER (1879–1962)

To all students of medicine who listen, look, touch and reflect: may they hear, see, feel and comprehend. JOHN B BARLOW (1986)

Begin by positioning the appropriately undressed patient in bed. Use this opportunity to make a spot diagnosis if this is possible. Look particularly for any of the diagnostic facies or body habits. Decide whether the patient looks ill or well. Note whether there is any dyspnoea or other distress. Take the blood pressure. Repeat the measurement a few minutes later if the first reading is abnormal.

KEY TO CHAPTER 51	
CNS	central (and peripheral) nervous system
CVS	cardiovascular system
ENDO	endocrine system
GIT	gastrointestinal system
HAEM	haematological system
INF	infectious diseases
RENAL	renal system
RESP	respiratory system
RHEUM	rheumatological system

HANDS AND ARMS

Begin by picking up the patient's right hand and examine the nails for clubbing (RESP, CVS, GIT) and for the stigmata of infective endocarditis (CVS) or chronic liver disease (GIT) (Fig. 51.1). The nail changes suggesting chronic renal disease or iron deficiency must also be spotted (RENAL, HAEM). Note any evidence of arthropathy (RHEUM). Examine the other hand.

Take the patient's pulse, and note the rate and regularity or irregularity (CVS). While this is being done the arms can be inspected for bruising or scratch marks (GIT, HAEM, RENAL). Determine the state of hydration (GIT, RENAL, CVS). Go on and examine for axillary lymphadenopathy (HAEM).

FACE

Look at the eyes for jaundice (GIT, HAEM) or exophthalmos (ENDO). Look at the face for evidence of a vasculitic rash (RHEUM). Inspect the mouth for mucosal ulcers (RHEUM, GIT, HAEM, INF) and the tongue for glossitis (nutritional deficiencies) or cyanosis (RESP, CVS) or macroglossia (ENDO).

FRONT OF THE NECK

Feel the carotid pulses and at 45° pay careful attention to the state of the jugular venous pressure (CVS). Feel gently for the position of the trachea (RESP). Then palpate the supraclavicular lymph nodes (HAEM, GIT).

CHEST

Examine the front of the chest for scars and deformity. Note any spider naevi (GIT) or hair loss (GIT, ENDO). Palpate the chest wall and auscultate the heart (CVS). Then percuss and auscultate the chest (RESP) and examine the breasts.

BACK OF THE CHEST AND NECK

Sit the patient up and lean him or her forwards. After inspection, test chest expansion of the upper and lower lobes of the lungs. Percuss and auscultate the back of

The detailed examination of most of the body systems begins with the hands of the patient

FIGURE 51.1

the chest (RESP). Feel for cervical lymphadenopathy (RESP, GIT, HAEM). Then examine formally for a goitre from behind (ENDO). Test for sacral oedema (CVS, RENAL).

ABDOMEN

Lay the patient flat on one pillow. Inspect the abdomen from the side and then palpate for organomegaly and other abdominal masses. Percuss for shifting dullness if this is appropriate and auscultate over the abdomen. Palpate for inguinal lymphadenopathy and hernias, and in men palpate the testes (GIT, RENAL).

LEGS

Look for peripheral oedema (CVS, RENAL) and leg ulcers (HAEM, RHEUM, CVS, CNS). Feel all the peripheral pulses (CVS).

NEUROLOGICAL EXAMINATION

Find out whether the patient is right- or left-handed. Begin with examination of the higher centres and cranial nerves. Test orientation and note any speech defect. Ask about any noticed problem with the sense of smell (I). Then examine the visual acuity, visual fields, the fundi (II), the pupils and eye movements (III, IV, VI). Screen for the other cranial nerves by testing pain sensation over the face (V), the strength of upper and lower facial muscles (VII), whispered voice hearing (VIII), the palatal movement ('Ah') (IX, X), poking out the tongue (XII) and rotation of the head (XI).

Next look for wasting and fasciculation in the upper limbs. Test tone, power (shoulders, elbows, wrists and fingers) and the biceps, triceps and brachioradialis reflexes. Assess finger–nose movements. Then test pinprick sensation on the tip of the shoulder, outer and inner forearms and on the median, ulnar and radial areas of the hands.

Go to the lower limbs. Test gait: ask the patient to walk several paces, turn around rapidly and walk back. Then test heel–toe walking (cerebellum), ability to stand on the toes (S1) and heels (L4, L5) and squatting (proximal muscles). Finally look for Romberg's sign (posterior columns). Next, test hip and knee flexion and extension, and dorsiflexion and plantar flexion of the feet in bed. Then do knee, ankle and plantar reflexes and heel–shin tests. Test pinprick sensation on the middle third of the thighs, both sides of the tibia, the dorsum of the feet, the little toes, on the buttocks and three levels on the trunk on both sides.

COMPLETING THE EXAMINATION

Thorough physical examination may include a rectal or pelvic examination, analysis of the patient's urine, a temperature reading and measurement of height and weight and calculation of the BMI.

Particular details of the examination will be altered depending on what is found. An important guide to the areas where examination should be particularly directed, apart from the history, is the general inspection. A minute spent standing back to inspect the patient before the detailed examination begins is never wasted.

Now this is not the end.
It is not even the beginning of the end.
But it is, perhaps, the end of the beginning.

WINSTON CHURCHILL
Speech at the Lord Mayor's Day Luncheon,
London, 10 November 1942

Index

Page numbers followed by "f" indicate figures, "t" indicate tables, and "b" indicate boxes.

A

a wave, 90–91
abdomen
    acute
        after blunt trauma, 274
        differential diagnosis of, 273f
        examination of, 272–274, 273b, 281b
    auscultation of, 260–261, 260f, 312
    bloating of, 225–226
    in cardiac examination, 106
    chronic constrictive pericarditis and, 123
    CT of, 289–290, 291f, 293t
    diabetes mellitus and, 469
    distension of, 245–246, 245f
    examination of, paediatric, 674t
    in gastrointestinal examination, 244–261
    in genitourinary examination, 310–312
    in gynaecological examination, 752
    in haematological examination, 343
    inspection of, 244–248
    intra-abdominal masses of, 249b
    masses in, 248f, 253–257, 255b
    pain in, 217–218
    palpation of, 248–257, 310, 311b
    percussion of, 257–258, 311–312
    in pregnancy, 737–738, 738f, 740f
    regions of, 249f
    in respiratory examination, 188
    RVF and, 120
    sample questions for, 621b
    scars of, 245, 245f
    short stature and, 474
    skin lesions on, 247
    striae of, 460f
    ultrasound of, 287–289
        densities in, 289t
        terminology for, 289t
    veins in, 246, 246f
    X-ray of, 285–287, 286t
abdominal reflex, 575f
abdominal wall, 256–257, 257b
abdominojugular reflux test, 91
abducens nerve, 503t, 510–521
    paediatric examination of, 653
    palsy, 518

ABI *see* ankle-brachial index
abnormal limb movements, in neonatal examination, 699–700
abscesses
    brain, 614f
    submandibular, 795f
abuse, elder, 33
acalculia, 543
acanthosis nigricans, 231–232, 232f
accessory nerve, 503t, 532f, 533–534, 534f
    palsy, 534
accommodation, 512
Achilles tendon, xanthomata in, 113
achondroplasia, 47f, 473–475
acid regurgitation, 219–220
    in pregnancy, 730
acquired immunodeficiency syndrome (AIDS), 836
acromegalic facies, 42f
acromegaly, 456–458, 456f–457f
ACTH *see* adrenocorticotrophic hormone
action plan, 14–15
active movement, 373–374
activities, in HEADSSS assessment, 620t
activities of daily living (ADL), 31–32, 826, 828, 829b
acute aortic dissection, 122
acute arterial occlusion, 114
acute cardiac tamponade, 123
acute coronary syndrome, 62, 63t, 121
acute inflammatory polyradiculoneuropathy, 583–584
acute otitis media (AOM), 647
acute pericarditis, 122
acute respiratory infection, 168
acute stress disorder, 847t–850t
acutely ill patient, assessment of, 867–872, 869f
Addison's disease, 461, 461f, 483
adduction, 386
adenomyosis, 761t
adenoviral conjunctivitis, 778
adherence, of elderly patients, 32
ADL *see* activities of daily living
adrenal insufficiency, causes of, 461b

adrenals, 458–461
    tumour, 484f
adrenocorticotrophic hormone (ACTH), 454
advance care planning, in history taking, 33
advance directive, 875
advance health directives, 33
adverse reactions, 13
affect, 852t
affective disorders, 847t–850t
age-appropriate visual acuity charts, 654f
agitation, 852t
agoraphobia, 847t–850t
agraphaesthesia, 544f, 545
agraphia, 543
AIDS *see* acquired immunodeficiency syndrome
airway, unconscious patients and, 601–602
airways disease, 166–168
alanine transaminase (ALT), 285
alcohol use, 17–18, 18b
    in HEADSSS assessment, 620t
allergy, to drugs, 13
alleviating factors, 8
alopecia, 414
amaurosis fugax, 505
ambiguous genitalia, in neonatal examination, 717
amblyopia, 507
amenorrhoea, 729–730, 745–747, 748b, 860
amiodarone facies, 42f
AMPLE mnemonic, 867
anaemia, 307, 350–354
    causes of, 353b
    iron-deficiency, 352f
    megaloblastic, 354f
    pallor and, 44–45
    palms and, 236
    pernicious, 340
    in physical examination, 44–45
    questions for patient with, 331b
    sickle cell, 351f
    spherocytic, 351f
anal examination, paediatric, 678
anal fissure, 265
analgesics, 18–19

INDEX

aneurysm
    cerebral, 614f
    dissecting, 63
    ventricular, 152f
angina, 60–61, 62b
    classification of, 62t
    locations of symptoms of, 62f
    typical, 62
angio-oedema, 871f
angular stomatitis, 243f
anisocoria, 511
ankle
    jerk, 456f, 570, 571f
    power testing for, 568, 568f–569f
    swelling of, 64
ankle oedema, 112b
ankle-brachial index (ABI), 113
ankyloglossia, 710f
ankylosing spondylitis, 411, 432, 432f
anorectum, 230
anorexia nervosa, 847t–850t, 860
    complications of, 860b
anoscopy, 266
anosmia, 504, 789
antenatal obstetric examination, 736b
anterior uveitis, 780
anthropometric measurements, in general physical examination, 624
antineutrophil cytoplasmic antibodies (ANCA), 429
antinuclear antibody (ANA), 429
antipsychotic drugs, side effects of, 853b
anus
    carcinoma of, 265
    pruritus of, 265
anxiety, 852t
    disorders, 847t–850t, 862
    dyspnoea and, 64, 168
    questions for patient with, 25b
aorta, 230
    coarctation of, 83, 141, 141f, 153f
    palpation of, 255–256
aortic regurgitation, 84, 128t, 131–135, 135f, 136t
    echocardiogram of, 157, 157f
    eponymous signs of, 134t
aortic stenosis (AS), 128t, 130–131, 132f–133f
    echocardiogram of, 157
    severe, 131t
    syncope and, 67
apex beat, 74, 93, 93f–94f
    chest palpation and, 182
    chronic constrictive pericarditis and, 123
    LVF and, 119
Apgar value, 687t
apical (Pancoast's) tumour, 198
apical thrills, 95
Apley scratch test, 386, 389f
Apley's grinding test, 402–403, 403f
apnoeas, 711

apocrine glands, 804b
apparent leg length, 639
appendicitis, 274, 274t
appetite, 218, 439
apprehension test, 386, 388f
apraxia, 545, 546f
aqueous humour, 771
arcus senilis, 89, 89f
Argyll Robertson pupils, 467
arms
    arteries in, 109
    drift, 550–551, 550f
    in gastrointestinal examination, 237–238
    in genitourinary examination, 307–309, 309f
    paediatric examination of, 635–639
arrhythmia, 67
arterial pulse, 81–84
    character of, 84, 90t
    LVF and, 119
    radial-radial delay in, 83
    radiofemoral delay in, 82–83, 84f
    rate of, 83
    rhythm of, 83, 84f
    RVF and, 120
    vessel wall in, 84
    volume of, 84
arterial ulcer, 115f
arteries
    in arms, 109
    carotid, 537f
        bruits, 537
    dorsalis pedis, 113, 114f
    femoral, 113
    in legs, 109
    popliteal, 113, 113f
    posterior tibial, 113, 114f
    temporal, 507f
    transposition of, 143
arteritis
    giant cell, 422f
    temporal, 491–492
arthritis, 335–337
    calcium hydroxyapatite, 413
    calcium pyrophosphate, 413
    enteropathic, 412
    functional assessment in, 369t
    gouty, 412–413, 412f–413f
    mutilans, 376
    psoriatic, 412, 432, 433f
    reactive, 411–412
    rheumatoid, 408–410
        ACR criteria for, 429t
        examining for, 409b, 409f
        X-ray of, 431f, 433f
    X-ray of, 430
    see also monoarthritis; osteoarthritis; polyarthritis
AS see aortic stenosis
asbestos exposure, 171b

ascites, 258–260, 258t, 260b, 287, 310
ASD see atrial septal defect
ashleaf macules, 644f
Ashrafian's sign, 134t
aspartate aminotransferase (AST), 285
assessment, of acutely ill patient, 867–872, 869f
assessment of function, 51
astereognosis, 545
asterixis, 178, 236–237, 237f, 307
asthma, 168
    bronchial, 194–195
    pulse rate and, 178
asymmetric tonic neck reflex (ATNR), 723
atelectasis, 192
atrial fibrillation, 65, 83
atrial septal defect (ASD), 139–140, 140f, 153f
    echocardiogram of, 158
atrophy, 372–373, 641t, 805t
AUDIT-C, 18
auditory dysphasia, 540
aura, 493, 494b
auscultation, 665–666
    of abdomen, 260–261, 260f, 312, 675–676
    chest, 184–188, 185f, 186b
    chronic constrictive pericarditis and, 123
    in common structural heart diseases, 671, 672t
    dynamic, 104t
    in lungs, 673–674
    LVF and, 120
    of neck, 105–106, 106f
    of praecordium, 95–97, 95f–96f
    RVF and, 120
    of thyroid, 447
Austin Flint murmur, 131–135, 134t
autoagglutination, 351f
autoimmune antibodies, 429–430
autoimmune polyglandular syndromes, 462t
AVPU mnemonic, 867
axillary freckling, 642–644, 645f

B

Babinski, Josef, 570–571
bacillary angiomatosis, 838, 838f
back
    in cardiac examination, 106
    in genitourinary examination, 312, 312f
    in paediatric examination, 639–640, 640f
    pain, 365–366
        in pregnancy, 731
bacterial vaginosis, 755t
'bad breath', 50
Baker's cyst, 402, 402f
ballotting, 253, 311, 311f
bamboo spine, 432
band keratopathy, 310
Barlow provocation test, 721

Bartholin's glands, 753
basal cell carcinoma, 821–823, 822f
Beau's lines, 48f
Becker's sign, 134t
bed sores, classification of, 831t
bedside manner, 3–5
Bell's palsy, 528, 528f
Bell's phenomenon, 527
benign joint hypermobility syndrome (BJHS), 636
benign paroxysmal positional (positioning) vertigo (BPPV), 529
BEST CARE, mnemonic, 620–622
biceps jerk, 554–555, 555f
bicipital tendinitis, 386
bigeminy, 83
bilateral hallux valgus, 405–406, 405f
biliary pain, 218
bilirubin
    pathway, 270f
    urinalysis and, 269
bimanual examination, 759–760, 759f–760f
binge-eating disorder (BED), 847t–850t, 860
biochemistry, of gastrointestinal system, 285
biphasic stridor, 664t
bipolar disorders, 847t–850t, 861
Bishop score, 739–740, 740t
Bitot spot, 239f
bladder, 256
bleeding, 330–332
    in early pregnancy, 745, 747t
    excess, test for, 350
    gastrointestinal, 224–225, 225t, 276–277
blood
    loss, in gastrointestinal bleeding, 276–277
    peripheral film, 350, 351f–352f, 354f
    in stools, 267–268
    tests
        for renal disease, 319
        for renal dysfunction, 319
    in urine, 321, 322b
blood glucose, 482–483
    of unconscious patients, 604
blood pressure (BP), 84–88
    acute coronary syndrome and, 121
    chronic constrictive pericarditis and, 123
    classification of, 86t
    in genitourinary examination, 313
    high, 88
    normal, 84–86
    in paediatric examination, 633–634, 634f, 634t
    postural, 88, 88f
    sphygmomanometer and, 86–88, 86f
    systolic, 84–86
    variations in, 88
blot haemorrhages, 468, 468f
Blumer's shelf, 266
blunt trauma, acute abdomen after, 274

BMI *see* body mass index
body habitus, 45–46, 46b
body habitus abnormalities, 666, 666b
body mass index (BMI), 624
body, of unconscious patients, 604
body system, 37
bodygram, 680, 681f
bones, 150
    disease, 483–484
    nasal, 788
    tenderness, 342–343
bony swelling, 373
borborygmi, 260
Bouchard's nodes, 376, 378f
boutonnière deformity, 375–376, 377f
bow legs, 637, 638f
bowel, 256
    changes in, 439
    dilation of, 286
    gas pattern in, 286
    inflammatory disease of, 277–279
    obstruction, 218, 273–274, 273t, 287f–288f
    sounds, 260, 675
BPPV *see* benign paroxysmal positional (positioning) vertigo
brachial plexus, 562–566, 563t, 564f
    lesion, 565b, 565t
brachioradialis (supinator) jerk, 555, 556f
brachycephaly, 704
bradycardia, 83, 85t
bradykinesia, 598, 598f
bradypnoea, 174–175
brain
    abscess, 614f
    functional areas of, 500f
brainstem death, 876
Braxton-Hicks contraction, 732
breast changes, in pregnancy, 730
breast examination, 752
    anatomy of, 763, 764f
    history of, 9b–12b
breasts, 763–767, 766b–767b
    cancer, 763–764
    carcinoma, 765f
    inspection of, 764–765
    lumps, 766–767, 766t
    palpation of, 763b, 765–766
    quadrants of, 765, 765f
breath, 240–241
breathing
    abnormal patterns of, 170t
    COPD and, 175–176
    sounds of, 184–187
        added, 186–187
        bronchial, 186, 186b
        intensity of, 186
        quality of, 186
    of unconscious patients, 601–602
breathlessness *see* dyspnoea

Broca's area, 540–541
bronchial asthma, 194–195
bronchiectasis, 194, 212f
bronchiolitis, 673
bronchitis, chronic, 196
bronchopneumonia, 191
Brown-Séquard syndrome, 588, 590f
Brudzinski's sign, 501
bruising, 308–309, 335
bruits, 105–106, 106f, 261
    carotid, 310, 537
    renal, 312
buccal ulcer, 794f
Buerger's test, 113
buffalo hump, 459, 460f
bulge sign, 400–401
bulimia nervosa, 847t–850t, 860
    complications of, 860b
bullae, 641t, 805t
bullous pemphigoid, 813f
burrows, 641t
bursitis, 424, 424f

C

cachexia, 45
café-au-lait spots, 642–644, 645f
CAGE questions, 17
calcaneovalgus foot, 720–721
calcification, 286–287
    pancreatic, 289f
calcinosis, 418
calcium hydroxyapatite arthritis, 413
calcium metabolism, 469–471
calcium pyrophosphate arthritis, 413
Campbell de Morgan spots, 238
camptodactyly, 719f
Campylobacter jejuni, 583–584
cancer, breast, 763–764
Candida albicans, 755t, 820f
candidiasis, 243, 755t, 794f, 838, 839f
cannon a waves, 91
capillary refill time, in neonatal examination, 711–712, 712b
Caplan's syndrome, 410
caput Medusae, 246–247, 247f
caput succedaneum, 704
carcinoma
    of anus, 265
    basal cell, 821–823, 822f
    breast, 765f
    of lungs, 198–199
    nasopharyngeal, 796f
    squamous cell, 822f
cardiac cachexia, 77
cardiac cycle, 98f
cardiac dullness, 184
cardiac dyspnoea, 63–64
cardiac failure, 119–121
cardiac valves, 74, 76f

INDEX

CARDIO mnemonic, 712–713
cardiomyopathy
    dilated, 139
    hypertrophic, 137–139
        echocardiogram of, 158
        syncope and, 67
    restrictive, 139
cardiopulmonary resuscitation (CPR), 867, 868f
cardiothoracic diameter, 149
cardiovascular disease, correlation of physical signs disease and, 119–144, 143b–144b
cardiovascular examination, 74–108, 107b–108b
    abdomen in, 106
    back in, 106
    extending of, 145–158, 159b
        chest X-ray, 147–151
        physical, 147–158
    face in, 89
    general appearance in, 76–79
    hands in, 79–81
    method of, 145b–147b
    neck in, 89–92
    positioning in, 75–76, 78f
cardiovascular history, 59–73, 71b–72b
    drug and treatment, 70
    family, 71
    past, 70–71
    presenting symptoms in, 59–68, 61b
    social, 71
cardiovascular system (CVS), 146f
    alcohol in, complications of, 18b
    examination anatomy of, 74–75, 74f–75f
    in neonatal examination, 711–715, 712t
    in paediatric examination, 663–674, 666b, 668t
    systemic hypertension and, 124–125
    systems review questions of, 9b–12b
cardioverter-defibrillator box, 93
CARE mnemonic, 684–685
carotid arteries, 89–90, 90f
    anatomy of, 537f
    bruits, 310, 537
carpal tunnel syndrome, 380, 380b, 425, 737
Castell method, 344–345, 345f
Castell spot, 344–345, 345f
casts, 323, 323f
cataracts, 776b
cavernous sinus, 454f
central cyanosis, 713, 714t
    causes of, 44b
    in physical examination, 41–44, 41f
central nervous system, 125
central scotoma, 509
central sleep apnoea, 169
cephalohaematoma, 698f, 704
cerebellar disease, 551, 596b

cerebellar examination, paediatric, 655–658, 656f
cerebellar tumour, 613f
cerebellopontine angle tumour, 525f
cerebellum, examination of, 595–597, 595f–596f, 596b–597b
cerebral aneurysm, 614f
cerebral atrophy, 614f
cerebral hemispheres, 543–547
cerebral palsy, 655–657
cervical cancer, 761t
cervical dilation, 739–740
cervical length (effacement), 739–740
cervical lymph nodes, examination of, 794
cervical rib syndrome, 563, 565b
cervicitis, 757
cervix, 266
    appearance of, 756–757
    multiparous, 758f
chalazion, 781, 782f
Charcot-Marie-Tooth disease, 592b
Charcot's joint, 463, 466f
chest
    auscultation of, 184–188, 185f, 186b
    barrel, 180f
    expansion, 182, 674
    funnel, 180, 181f
    in gastrointestinal examination, 243–244
    in genitourinary examination, 310
    inspection of, 180–182
    in neonatal examination, 711–715
    palpation of, 182–184
    percussion of, 184, 185f
    pigeon, 180, 181f
    in pregnancy observation, 737
    in respiratory examination, 180–188
    sample questions for, 621b
    short stature and, 474
    signs, in respiratory disorders, 191t
    wall
        lesions of, 180–181
        movement of, 181
        paediatric examination of, 673
        pain in, 63
chest pain, 59–63, 121–122, 665, 665b
    causes of, 59t–60t
    differential diagnosis of, 60t
    in respiratory history, 168
chest X-ray, 147–151, 148f, 159b
    checklist of, 206–210
    frontal film of, 148–150
    lateral film of, 150
    in respiratory examination, 206
child abuse
    physical examination for, 678–681, 679b–680b, 681f
    risk factors for, 680t
Chlamydia trachomatis, 755t
chlamydial vulvovaginitis, 755t
cholecystitis, 63

cholesterol measurements, 68–69
chorda tympani, 782
chorea, 70, 496–497, 600, 601b
choroid, 771
choroiditis, 777
chronic bronchitis, 196
chronic constrictive pericarditis, 123
chronic fatigue, 24–25
chronic fatigue syndrome, 847t–850t
chronic kidney disease (CKD), 300–303, 302t
    cause of, 309b
    classification of, 302t
    coronary artery disease and, 69
    examination of, 317–326, 317b–318b, 317f, 326b
chronic obstructive pulmonary disease (COPD), 166–168, 195–196, 195t
    in wheeze, 168
chronic subjective dizziness (CSD), features of, 27b
chronic venous disease, 116, 116f
Chvostek's sign, 471
circinate balanitis, 411f
circulation
    paediatric examination of, 668–671, 668t
    unconscious patients and, 602
circumflex artery, 74, 76f
cirrhosis, 275t
CKD *see* chronic kidney disease
claudication
    distance, 67–68
    intermittent, 67–68
clicking, 395–396
clinical assessment, 34
clinical examinations, 38
    evidence-based, 51–54
    see also objective structured clinical examination
clinodactyly, 719f
closed questions, 846
clotting, 330–332
clubbing, 79, 235, 668
    causes of, 79, 80b
    finger, 81f
    proper examination for, 79–80
    in respiratory examination, 178, 178f
clubfoot, 719–720, 720f
clunk test, 386
CMV *see* cytomegalovirus
coagulation abnormalities, 331
cochlear nerve, in paediatric examination, 654–655
colic, renal, 218
colitis, ulcerative, 277–279
collateral ligaments, 401–402, 401f
colon, 230
colonoscopy, 284
colour, of urine, 319, 319t
colour vision, 776
coma, 601–602

comedones, 641t
community-acquired pneumonia (CAP), causes of, 192
complete blood count (CBC), 350
compliance, 32
comprehensive geriatric assessment, 826b
computed tomography (CT) scan
    of abdomen, 289–290, 291f, 293t
    of adrenal tumour, 484f
    in haematological imaging, 358, 358f–359f
    of interstitial lung disease, 213f
    of osteoporosis, 485f
    in respiratory examination, 206
    in rheumatological examination, 430
conductive dysphasia, 541
condylomata acuminata, 265, 266f, 755t
confetti hypopigmentation, 644f
confidentiality, 33
congenital cysts, 756
congenital heart disease, 713t
    acyanotic, 139–141
    classification of, 142b
    cyanotic, 142
    'grown-up', 143
congenital vertical talus, 720f, 721
congestive cardiac failure, 310
conjugate gaze, 518–521
conjunctivitis, 773, 775b
    with measles, 773f
consciousness, 501
    level of, 602, 867
consolidation, 190–192, 208f
constipation, 223–224
    in pregnancy, 730
    questions for patient with, 223b
consultation
    initial, 5
    sequence, 3b
continuous murmurs, 102–103, 102t
conversion symptom, 852t
coordination test, 556–557, 571
COPD *see* chronic obstructive pulmonary disease
cornea, 771
    examination of, 776
    reflex, 523, 776
    ulceration of, 774
coronary arteries, 74, 76f
coronary artery disease
    drug and treatment history of, 70
    risk factors for, 68–70, 69b
Corrigan's sign, 134t
cough, 163–165, 163b, 663, 663b
    character of, 177
    differential diagnosis of, 163, 164b, 164t
    impulse test, 116
Courvoisier's law, 253–254, 254t
CPR *see* cardiopulmonary resuscitation
crackles, 187, 674, 715

cranial nerve examination, 774–775
cranial nerves (CN), in paediatric examination, 653–655
craniosynostosis, 645–647, 704
crescent sign, 402
CREST syndrome, 416, 418f
critically ill patient, signs of, 870b
Crohn's disease, 279
cross-arm test, 386
cross-cover test, 515–517, 516f
cross-cultural history taking, 28
cruciate ligaments, 401–402, 401f
crusts, 641t, 805t
CT scan *see* computed tomography (CT) scan
cubital fossa, lesion in, 559–561
Cullen's sign, 247, 248f
cultural awareness, 28
cultural safety, 28
cultural sensitivity, 28
current treatment, in respiratory history, 169–171
Cushing's syndrome, 458–461, 460f, 483
    causes of, 458b
    questions for patient with, 459b
    signs guide for, 459t
CVS *see* cardiovascular system
cyanosis, 41–44, 41f, 177, 355
    causes of, 44b
cystocele, 756, 758f
cytomegalovirus (CMV), retinitis, 840, 840f

D

dacryocystitis, 708f, 781, 782f
dactylitis, 376
Dalrymple's sign, 450
de la Tourette's syndrome, 601
De Musset's sign, 134t
deafness, 496, 784, 788b
    causes of, 531, 785t
    questions for, 784b
death
    assessment of, 875–877
    brainstem, 876
    certificate, 876
    confirming, 876b
    diagnosing, 875
    examining, 875–876
deep expiration, in dynamic manoeuvres, 104–105, 105f
deep venous thrombosis (DVT), 115, 331–332
defibrillators, 154f
deforming polyarthropathy, 375b
deformity, 373, 375
dehydration, 47, 47b, 47f
delirium, 32–33, 847t–850t, 867–868
    causes of, 858t, 870b
    hypoactive, 847t–850t
    questions for patient with, 870b

delivery, 685–687
    questions for patient regarding, 685b, 687b
deltoid wasting, 385–386
delusion, 852t
delusional disorders, 847t–850t
dementia, 32–33, 847t–850t
    causes of, 858t
demyelinating disease, 582
dental decay, as coronary artery disease risk factor, 70
depersonalisation, 852t
depression, 19, 847t–850t, 861, 861b
    in HEADSSS assessment, 620t
    questions for patient with, 25b
derealisation, 852t
dermatitis, as vulval skin condition, 755t
dermatitis herpetiformis, 231f, 281f
dermatomes
    of head and neck, 523f
    of lower limbs, 572, 575f
    of upper limb and trunk, 559, 560f
dermopathy, late diabetic, 463
detrusor underactivity, 300
developmental assessment, 658–660, 661t
developmental reflexes, in neonatal examination, 722–723
DEXA *see* dual-energy X-ray absorptiometry
dextrocardia, 712
diabetes mellitus, 463–469
    abdomen and, 469
    causes of, 464b
    coronary artery disease and, 69
    examination of, 465b, 465f
    face and, 467–469
    general inspection of, 463
    lower limbs and, 463–467
        inspection of, 463–466
        neurological examination for, 466–467
        palpation of, 466
    neck and shoulders and, 469
    questions for, 464b
    retinopathy in, 468f
    ulcers in, 463, 466f
    upper limbs and, 467
    urinalysis for, 469
diabetic (neuropathic) ulcer, 115f, 117b
diagnosis
    death, 875
    definition of, 38
    of lump, 804–806
    of psychiatric disorders, 854–858
    see also differential diagnosis
diagnostic facies, 40
diagnostic hypotheses, 6
diagnostic testing
    in endocrine examination, 480–484
    in nervous system examination, 611
dialysis, 302

diaphragm, 149, 174
diarrhoea, 222–223
    questions for patient with, 222b
diastolic murmurs, 102
diastolic obstructive murmurs, 670
diastolic pericardial knock, 100
diastolic regurgitant murmurs, 670
diastolic thrill, 95
diet, 16
differential diagnosis, 22
    of acute abdomen, 273f
    of chest pain, 60t
    of cough, 163, 164b, 164t
    of deforming polyarthropathy, 375b
    of dyspnoea, 167b–168b
    evidence-based history taking and, 33–34
    of foot drop, 577b
    of groin lump, 262b
    in liver palpation, 252b
    of lymphadenopathy, 333b
    of prolonged fever, 835b
    of rash, 835b
    of scrotal mass, 314, 315f
    of syncope, 66b
    of thickened tethered skin, 418b
difficult breathing (dyspnoea), 665
digital infarcts, 418f
diplopia, 512–514, 778
dipping, 259–260
discoid lupus rash, 414–415
discomfort, radiation of, 8
disease
    airways, 166–168
    bones, 483–484
    cardiac, chest X-rays in, 150–151
    liver, 274–275
    mitral valve, 152f
    motor neurone, 562f, 583
    myeloproliferative, 355–357, 356b
    pericardial, 122–123
    skin, 806–823, 808f
    vascular, 580–582, 581f, 582t
    see also specific disease types
dislocation, 373
disorientation, 852t
dissecting aneurysm, 63
distal interphalangeal joints, 375–376, 377f
distal myopathy, 591
distension, abdominal, 245–246, 245f
distraction test, 402–403
Dix-Hallpike manoeuvre, 529–530, 529f
dizziness, 66–67, 66b, 495, 665, 666b
    non-specific, in history taking, 26–27
    questions for patient with, 493b
DNR orders see do-not-resuscitate (DNR) orders
doctor-patient relationship, 3–4
doll's eye phenomenon, 603
dominant lobe signs, 543–544

donation, organ, 877
do-not-resuscitate (DNR) orders, 875
Doppler echocardiography, 137
dorsalis pedis artery, 113, 114f
dorsiflexion, 406
dot haemorrhages, 468, 468f
double-impulse apex beat, 94
Down's syndrome, 473–475
driving, 828–829, 829b
drop-arm test, 386
drugs
    adverse reactions to, 13
    allergy to, 13
    in HEADSSS assessment, 620t
    history, 12–14, 13f
    psychiatric, 853t
    side effects, in elderly people, 32, 32t
    street, 14
    see also medication
dry eyes, 772
    causes of, 773b
dry mouth, 792
dual-energy X-ray absorptiometry (DEXA), 484
Duchenne-Erb palsy, 697f, 697t
duodenum, 255
Dupuytren's contracture, 236, 236f, 383
Duroziez's sign, 134t
DVT see deep venous thrombosis
dwarfism, 475
dynamic auscultation, systolic murmurs and, 104t
dynamic left ventricular outflow tract obstruction, 131
dynamic manoeuvres, 104–105, 104t
dysarthria, 540
dysdiadochokinesis, 556–557, 557f, 595–596
dyskinesia, 600–601
dyskinetic apex beat, 94
dysmenorrhoea, 747–748
dysphagia, 220–222, 221b, 276, 792
dysphasia, 540–542, 540b
dysphonia, 169, 177, 540, 543, 792, 793b
dysplasia, developmental, of hip, 718f, 721
dyspnoea, 63–64, 165–168
    cardiac failure and, 119
    causes of, 119b, 166b
    differential diagnosis of, 167b–168b
    left ventricular failure in a patient with, 120t
    questions in, 167b
    signs of, 174–175
dysprosody, 542
dysraphism, 698
dystonia, 600–601
dystrophia myotonica, 591–593, 594f

E

ear, nose, and throat (ENT) examination, paediatric, 647–650, 648f–650f

ear wax, 786
eardrum, paediatric examination of, 648, 649f
early diastolic murmurs, 102t
ears, 771–799, 796b–798b
    anatomy of, 783f
    discharge from, 785–786
    disease of, symptoms of, 783b
    examination anatomy of, 782–783
    examination method for, 785–788
    external canal of, 786
    history of, 783–785
    inner, 782–783
    middle, 782
    in neonatal examination, 707–708, 708f
    outer, 782
    sample questions for, 621b
    of unconscious patients, 603
eating disorders, 847t–850t, 859–860
eating, in HEADSSS assessment, 620t
Ebstein's anomaly, 141
EBV see Epstein-Barr virus (EBV) infection
ecchymoses, 337, 337f, 805t
eccrine glands, 804b
ECG see electrocardiogram
echocardiography, 151–158
    colour flow mapping of, 153–156
    continuous wave Doppler, 153
    Doppler, 137
    of hypertrophic cardiomyopathy, 158, 158f
    important indications for, 154b
    information available from, 156–158
    M mode, 151–153, 155f
    pulsed wave Doppler, 153
    sector scanning, 153
    two-dimensional, 153
ectopic pregnancy, 749, 749t
ectropion, cervical, 756–757
eczema, nummular, 811f
education, in HEADSSS assessment, 620t
education level, 15
effusion, 373
Ehlers-Danlos syndrome, 277, 278f
Eisenmenger's syndrome, 142
ejection murmur, 670
elbow
    epicondylitis, 423, 423f
    power testing of, 552, 553f
elder abuse, 33
elderly patient, 31–33
    activities of daily living in, 31–32
    adherence of, 32
    drug side effects in, 32t
    mental state of, 32–33
    polypharmacy, 32
    specific problems in, 33
    systems review questions in, 9b–12b
electrocardiogram (ECG), 92f
electrolyte abnormalities, 323–324

elephantiasis, 112f
elevation, 386
embolic stroke, 611f
embolism
    arterial, 332
    venous, 331–332
emergency care, 872b
emotion-handling skills (NURS), 23, 24b
emphysema, 211f
    generalised, cause of, 196
employment, in HEADSSS assessment, 620t
encephalopathy, hepatic, 275–276
endocarditis, infective, 123
endocrine disease, correlation of physical signs and, 463–479, 478b–479b
endocrine examination, 444–462, 462b, 480–484, 481b–482b, 481f, 486b
    diagnostic testing in, 480–484
    extending of, 480–484
    method for, 480, 480b
endocrine history, 439–443, 443b
    family history, 443
    presenting symptoms in, 439–441, 440b
    social history, 443
endocrine system
    glands of, 445f
    sample questions for, 621b
    systems review of, 9b–12b
end-of-life and treatment decisions, 829
endolymph, 782–783
endometriosis, 761t
endoscopy, of gastrointestinal system, 284–285
enterocele, 756, 758f
enzymes, of liver, 285
epicardial coronary arteries, 74
epicondylitis, elbow, 423, 423f
epidermoid cysts, 647
epiglottitis, 795
epilepsy, 492–494, 494b
    questions for patient with, 493b
    temporal lobe, 494
episcleritis, 278–279, 279f
epistaxis, 789
Epstein-Barr virus (EBV) infection, 818f
Epstein's pearls, 709, 710f
Epworth sleepiness scale, 169, 169b
erectile dysfunction, 441
    as coronary artery disease risk factor, 69
erosions, 641t
erythema, 372–373
erythema nodosum, 278f
erythema toxicum, 701f
estimated date of confinement (EDC), 729–730
Eustachian tube, 782
euvolaemia, 324
evidence-based clinical examination, 51–54
evidence-based history taking and differential diagnosis, 33–34

exacerbating factors, 8
examination anatomy
    of breast, 763, 764f
    of CVS, 74–75, 74f–75f
    of ears, 782–783
    of eyes, 771–772, 782–783
    of gastrointestinal tract, 229–230, 229f
    of genitourinary system, 306, 307f–308f
    of haematological system, 335, 336f
    of hernias, 261–262
    of lower limbs, 109–113
    of mouth, 791–792
    of nervous system, 500, 500f
    of nose, 788–789
    of peripheral nervous system, 549–550
    of respiratory system, 174, 175f–176f
    rheumatological, 370–372, 370b, 371f–372f, 372b, 380b
    of throat, 791–792
excoriations, 308–309, 641t, 805t
exercise, 16
    isometric, 105
    respiratory rate on, 188
exophthalmos, 449–450, 450b, 774
expansile impulse, 256f
expiratory stridor, 664t
expiratory wheeze, 664t
expressive (anterior) dysphasia, 540–541
extension, 386, 388f
external canal, 786
external rotation, 386
eyelids, 772
    conditions of, 781–782
eyes, 771–798, 796b–798b
    abnormalities, 778
        causes of, 779b
    dry, 367–368, 368b
    examination anatomy of, 771–772
    examination method for, 772–778
    examination of, 505b
    history of, 772
    movements of, 512–515, 513f, 520f, 775
    muscles, 512f
    in neonatal examination, 704–707, 706b, 708f
    painful, 775t
    red, 368, 773
        causes of, 775t
        questions for, 772b
    sample questions for, 621b
    structure of, 771, 771f
    of unconscious patients, 603, 603f

F

FABER test, 397
face
    in cardiac examination, 89
    in gastrointestinal examination, 238–243
    in genitourinary examination, 309–310

    in haematological examination, 340–341, 342f
    hyperparathyroidism and, 470
    in neonatal examination, 704–709
    in paediatric examination, 650–652, 651t
    in Paget's disease, 477–478
    pain, 490–492
    in Parkinson's disease examination, 598–599, 599f
    in pregnancy observation, 737
    in respiratory examination, 178–179
    of unconscious patients, 603–604
facial angiofibromas, 641–642, 643f
facial nerve, 503t, 525–528, 526f–527f
    in paediatric examination, 654
facial nerve palsy, 528, 698f
facial sensation, 523
facies, 40, 40b, 41f–44f
    amiodarone, 42f
    lipodystrophic, 42f
    mitral, 89
    moon-like, 459, 460f
    myopathic, 43f
    myotonic, 43f
faeces, 268–269
    changes of, with jaundice, 270t
    see also stool
Fagan's nomogram, 53, 53f
faints, 492–494, 665, 666b
Fallot's syndrome, 142
falls, risk factors for, 826, 828b
false negative, 52
false positive, 52
family history, 19, 19b, 20f
    in endocrine examination, 443
    in gastrointestinal examination, 227
    in genitourinary examination, 304
    in gynaecological examination, 750
    in haematological examination, 334
    in mental health examination, 853
    in neurological examination, 498, 498t
    in pregnancy, 736
    in rheumatological history, 369
family tree, preparing, 20f
fasciculations, 551
    differential diagnosis of, 551b
fat atrophy, diabetes mellitus and, 466
fat deposition, 476
fat hypertrophy, diabetes mellitus and, 466
fatigue, 67, 368
    causes of, 26b
    in history taking, 24
fatty casts, 323
FBC see full blood count
feet, peripheral neuropathy in, monofilament testing for, 466–467, 467f
Felty's syndrome, 335–337, 410
female genitalia, in neonatal examination, 717
female reproductive anatomy, 754f

femoral arteries, 113
FET *see* forced expiratory time
fetor, 241, 241*b*
fetor hepaticus, 241
fetus
    factors indicating risk of inherited genetic disease in, 736*b*
    head positions of, 741*f*
    movements, change in, 731–732
FEV *see* forced expiratory volume
fever
    prolonged, 835*b*
    questions for, 835*b*
    rheumatic, 420
    types of, 50*t*
fibromyalgia syndrome, 426, 426*f*
fine-motor skill, developmental examination in, 659
finger
    jerks, 556, 556*f*
    power testing of, 553, 554*f*
finger agnosia, 543
finger-nose test, 556, 556*f*
Finkelstein's test, 424, 424*f*
first impressions, 39–45, 39*f*
fissures, 641*t*
fistula-in-ano, 265
fits, 492–494
fixed extension deformity, 373–374
fixed flexion deformity, 373–374
fixed splitting, 97
flapping tremor, 178
flexion, 386
flight of ideas, 852*t*
flow volume curve, 204–205, 205*f*
fluent aphasia, 540–541
fluid status, acutely ill patient and, 868
fluid thrill, 259
folliculitis, 818
fontanels, in neonatal examination, 704, 706*b*, 706*f*
foot
    calcaneovalgus, 720–721
    clubfoot, 719–720, 720*f*
    rocker-bottom, 720*f*, 721
foot drop, 577*b*, 578*f*
foot-tapping test, 571
forced expiratory time (FET), 203
forced expiratory volume (FEV), 204
forced vital capacity (FVC), 204
formulation grid, 858*t*–859*t*
fovea, 771
free peritoneal gas, 286*f*
friction rub
    abdominal, 260–261
    pericardial, 103
    pleural, 187
Friedreich's ataxia, 596–597, 597*b*
'frog-like' position, in premature infant, 721, 722*f*

Froment's sign, 562
frontal lobe function, 546–547
full blood count (FBC), 350
functional activity, 31–32
functional impairment, 395–396
fundi, 124
    in genitourinary examination, 313
    in haematological examination, 346
fundoscopy, 509, 510*f*, 776
funnel chest, 711
FVC *see* forced vital capacity

G

gag reflex, 533
gait
    disorders, 577, 579*b*
    disturbances of, 496
    in Parkinson's disease examination, 597–598
    testing of, 566
galactorrhoea, 441
Galant reflex, 723
gallbladder, 230
    CT of, 293*f*
    enlargement of, 256*b*
    palpation of, 253–254
gallop rhythm, 98–99
gallstones, 293*f*
GALS screening test, 428*b*–429*b*
gamma glutamyl transpeptidase (GGT), 285
gastric dilation, 288*f*
gastrointestinal bleeding, 224–225, 225*t*, 276–277
gastrointestinal contents, 268–269
gastrointestinal disease, correlation of physical signs and, 272–281
gastrointestinal examination, 229–271, 271*b*, 282–290, 282*b*–284*b*, 282*f*, 294*b*
    abdomen in, 244–261, 245*f*
    arms in, 237–238
    chest in, 243–244
    extending of, 284–285
    face in, 238–243
    general appearance in, 230–235
    hands in, 235–237
    mouth in, 240–243
    nails in, 235
    neck in, 243–244
    positioning in, 230, 230*f*
gastrointestinal history, 217–228, 227*b*–228*b*
    family history, 227
    past history, 227
    presenting symptoms in, 217–226, 217*b*
    social history, 227
    treatment history, 226–227
gastrointestinal system
    abdomen, paediatric examination of, 674–676, 674*t*
    auscultation of, 675–676
    inspection in, 675

    palpation in, 676
    percussion in, 676
    positioning the patient in, 674–675
    alcohol in, complications of, 18*b*
    biochemistry of, 285
    examination anatomy of, 229–230, 229*f*
    imaging of, 285–290
    mental state and, 234–235
    in neonatal examination, 715–717, 716*f*
    skin and, 231–234, 231*f*–233*f*, 233*t*–234*t*
    systems review of, 9*b*–12*b*
gastro-oesophageal reflux disease (GORD), 63, 219–220
    questions for patient with, 220*b*
gegenhalte, 551
general appearance
    in cardiovascular examination, 76–79
    in gastrointestinal examination, 230–235
    in genitourinary examination, 306
    in haematological examination, 335
    in physical examination, 37–38
    in respiratory examination, 174–177
general physical examination, 622–681, 623*b*
generalised anxiety disorder (GAD), 847*t*–850*t*, 862
genes, breast cancer, 764
genetic factors, increased risk to patient from, 19*b*
genital herpes, 755*t*
genital tract infections, lower, 755*t*
genital warts (condyloma acuminata), 755*t*
genitalia
    female, examination of, 753, 755*t*
    male, 313–314, 313*f*, 314*b*
    in neonatal examination, 717
    of pregnancy, 738–740
genitourinary examination, 306–316, 315*b*–316*b*
    abdomen in, 310–312
    arms in, 307–309, 309*f*
    back in, 312, 312*f*
    blood pressure in, 313
    chest in, 310
    extending of, 317–326, 326*b*
    face in, 309–310
    family history in, 304
    fundi in, 313
    general appearance in, 306
    hands in, 306–307, 309*f*
    legs in, 312
    neck in, 310
    past history in, 304
    social history in, 304
genitourinary system
    alcohol in, complications of, 18*b*
    examination of, 306, 309*b*
    anatomy of, 306, 307*f*–308*f*
    history of, 297–305, 304*b*–305*b*
    in paediatric examination, 676–678, 677*f*
    presenting symptoms in, 297–303, 297*b*

sample questions for, 621b
systems review of, 9b–12b
treatment in, 304
genu valgum (knock-knees), 373, 637–639, 638f
genu varum (bow legs), 373, 637, 638f
geographical tongue, 793
Gerhard's sign, 134t
gestational age, 723
'get up and go' test, 831, 832f
GFR *see* glomerular filtration rate
giant a waves, 91
giant cell arteritis, 422f
Gilbert's disease, jaundice from, 41
gingival fibromas, 644f
gingival hyperplasia, 310
glands
    of endocrine system, 445f
    lacrimal, 772
    salivary, 239–240, 240b, 792
    submandibular, 240, 241f
Glasgow Coma Scale, 602, 602t
glaucoma, 780–781
glomerular filtration rate (GFR), 302, 302t
glossitis, 242, 242f
glossopharyngeal nerve, 503t, 531–533, 532f
    paediatric examination of, 655
    palsy, 533
glossopharyngeal neuralgia, 531–533
glucagonoma, 231f
glucose, blood, 482–483
glycosuria, 321b
goitre, 444, 446f–447f
    causes of, 448b
gonadotrophins, 454
gonococcal vulvovaginitis, 755t
GORD *see* gastro-oesophageal reflux disease
gout, 412, 413b, 434
    X-ray of, 434f
gouty tophus, 413f, 786
Gower's sign, 655, 656f
Gowers, William, 553–554
grandiosity, 852t
granular casts, 323
granular keratosis, 822f
granuloma annulare, 815f
grasp reflex, 546, 723
Graves' disease, 449
gravida, 15
grip strength, 381
groin
    hernias in, 262–264
    lump, 262b
gross-motor skills, developmental examination in, 659
growth charts
    from birth to 5 years, 624, 625f–632f
    for term infants, 690f–695f
growth hormone (GH), 454
grunt, 664t, 673

Guillain-Barré syndrome, 583–584
gum hypertrophy, 240–241, 241b
gynaecological history and examination, 743–762, 744b, 752b, 762b
    family and social history, 750
    in pregnancy, 734
    presenting symptoms in, 743, 743b
gynaecology, 743
gynaecomastia, 244, 244f, 476, 476f, 764
    causes of, 477b

H

haemangiomas
    of infancy, 700, 702f
    infantile, 641, 642f, 643t
haemarthrosis, 435f
haematemesis, 224
    questions for patient with, 226b
haematochezia, 224, 268
haematological disorders, 329
haematological examination, 335–358, 347b, 348f, 360b
    abdominal, 343–345, 345t
    axillary nodes in, 339–340, 340f–341f
    bone tenderness in, 342–343
    cervical and supraclavicular nodes in, 341–342, 342f
    epitrochlear nodes in, 339, 339f
    extending of, 350–358
        acute leukaemia in, 354–355
        anaemia in, 350–354, 353b
        chronic leukaemia in, 355
        haematology tests in, 350
        lymphoma in, 357–358, 357t, 358f
        multiple myeloma in, 358
        myeloproliferative disease in, 355–357, 356b
        pancytopenia in, 354
        peripheral blood film in, 350, 351f–352f, 354f
    face in, 340–341, 342f
    family history in, 334
    forearms in, 339
    fundi in, 346
    general appearance in, 335
    haematological imaging in, 358, 358f–359f
    hands in, 335–337, 337f
    inguinal nodes in, 345, 345f
    legs in, 345–346
    method of, 348b–349b
    past history in, 333–334
    presenting symptoms in, 329–333, 330b
    social history in, 334
    treatment history in, 333
haematological history, 329–334, 334b
haematological imaging, 358, 358f–359f
haematological system
    anatomy of, 335, 336f
    systems review of, 9b–12b

haematology tests, 350
haematopoietic system, alcohol in, complications of, 18b
haematuria, 298, 299b, 322b
haemochromatosis, 463
haemoglobinuria, 322b
haemolytic anaemia, 41
haemophilia, 331, 332b, 433f
Haemophilus influenzae type B, 611
haemoptysis, 165
    causes of, 165t
    haematemesis and nasopharyngeal bleeding from, 166t
haemorrhage
    pulmonary, 211f
    retinal, 776–777
    splinter, 80, 82f
    subarachnoid, 491–492
    subconjunctival, in neonatal examination, 707f
haemorrhagic stroke, 612f
haemorrhagic telangiectasia, 232, 233f, 340–341
haemorrhoids, 267
    in pregnancy, 730
    thrombosed external, 264
hair, 45
    distribution, changes in, 439–440
    paediatric examination of, 644
hallucination, 852t
Hamman's sign, 103
hand hygiene, 689f
handedness, 501, 608
hands
    in cardiac examination, 79–81
    claw, 562
        differential diagnosis of, 562b
    in gastrointestinal examination, 235–237
    in genitourinary examination, 306–307, 309f
    muscle wasting in, 566
        differential diagnosis of, 563b
    in physical examination, 48–49, 48f
    in pregnancy observation, 737
    in respiratory examination, 177–178
    systemic sclerosis in, 419f
    telangiectasia of, 418f
    washing, 38–39, 39f
hard exudates, 468, 468f
hard palate, 791
Harrison's sulcus, 180
HDL *see* high-density lipoprotein
head
    dermatomes of, 523f
    examination of, 644–647, 646f–647f
    large, 645
    lymph node groups of, 662f
    in neonatal examination, 703
    in neurological examination, 536–537
    sample questions for, 621b

head *continued*
  shape of, 645, 646f
  small, 644–645
  of unconscious patients, 603–604
head circumference
  for-age, growth charts in, 625f–632f
  measurement of, 644
    in neonatal examination, 689, 690f–695f
head impulse (thrust) test (HIT), 517, 518f
headache, 490–492
  cluster, 490–491
  coital, 490–491
  migraine, 490–491
  of pregnancy, 732
  questions for patient with, 491b
  signs guide for, 492t
  tension-type, 492
HEADSSS assessment, 620t
head-tilt manoeuvre, 868f
hearing
  developmental examination in, 659
  loss of, 785
heart, 149–150, 151f
  normal four-chamber view of, 156f
  normal long-axis view of, 155f
  paediatric examination of, 668–671, 668t, 671t–672t
  in respiratory examination, 188
heart murmurs, 100–105, 100t, 127b
  in area of greatest intensity, 101f, 103
  Austin Flint, 131–135
  character of, 669–670
  continuous, 102–103, 102t
  diastolic, 102
  diastolic obstructive, 670
  diastolic regurgitant, 670
  ejection, 670
  innocent, 126, 670, 671t
  intensity of the loudness of, 670
  loudness of, 103–104, 670
  in neonatal examination, 712
  pathological, 670–671
  pitch of, 103–104
  systolic, 100, 156f
  systolic regurgitant, 670
  timing of, 100–103, 102t, 670–671
heart sounds
  abnormalities of, 97–100
  alterations in intensity of, 97
  extra, 98–99
  first, 96
  fourth, 99
  second, 96–97
  splitting of, 97–98
  third, 98–99
heart valves, prosthetic, 100, 137
  physical signs of, 138t
heartburn, 219–220
  of pregnancy, 730

heavy menstrual bleeding, 744–745, 745b
Heberden's nodes, 376, 378f
heel-shin test, 571, 571f
heel-toe walking, 578f
HeLP mnemonic, 684–685, 686t
hemianopia, 509
hemiballismus, 600
hemiplegia, 580–582
Henoch-Schönlein purpura, 345–346, 346f
hepatic encephalopathy, 275–276
hepatic flap, 236–237
hepatojugular reflux, 91
hepatomegaly, 250
hepatosplenomegaly, 252b
hernias, 261–264, 273
  epigastric, 264
  examination anatomy of, 261–262
  femoral, 262
  in groin, 262–264, 262b
  incisional, 264
  inguinal, 262, 263f–264f
  umbilical, 716f
herpes simplex virus infection, 813f
herpes simplex virus, type 2, 755t
herpes zoster, 63, 503, 504f, 523f
  nasociliary, 781f
  shingles and, 781
hiccupping, 306
hidradenitis suppurativa, 818
high-density lipoprotein (HDL), 68–69
higher centre dysfunction, 540, 544b
hila, 149
Hill's sign, 134t
hips
  developmental dysplasia of, 718f, 721
  in neonatal examination, 721
  power testing for, 566–567, 566f–567f
hirsutism, 475, 476f
  causes of, 475b
history taking, 23b
  advance care planning in, 33
  advanced, 22–36
  clinical assessment in, 34
  common general symptoms in, 24–27
  concluding the consultation in, 34–35
  cross-cultural, 28
  in elderly patient, 31–33
  essentials, 35b
  evidence-based, 33–34
  general principles of, 3–21, 3b
    doctor-patient relationship, 3–4
    past history, 14–15
    sequence, 5b
    skills in, 20–21, 20b
  for geriatric patients, 827b, 828
  for maintenance of good health, 29–30, 30b
  medically unexplained symptoms in, 26
  patient confidentiality in, 33

  personal, 23–27
  reproductive history, 27
  self-harming in, 29
  sexual history, 27
HIV *see* human immunodeficiency virus
hoarseness, 169, 177, 793b
hobbies, 16, 16b
Hodgkin's disease, 340–341, 357–358, 358f
Homans' sign, 115
home, in HEADSSS assessment, 620t
Hoover's sign, 182, 183f
hormone production, 454
Horner's syndrome, 179, 778–780, 778f
  causes of, 780b
HPO *see* hypertrophic pulmonary osteoarthropathy
human immunodeficiency virus (HIV), 836–840
  examination of, 838–840, 838f–840f
  history of, 837–838, 837t
  questions for, 837b
  UMN lesions and, 582
hyaline casts, 323
hydration, 46–48
hydrocephalus, 645, 698, 699b
hydropneumothorax, 209f
hyperbilirubinaemia, 703b
hypercalcaemia, causes of, 470b
hypercholesterolaemia, 68–69
hyperemesis gravidarum, 730
hyperkalaemia, 323
hyperkeratosis, 376–377
hyperlipidaemia, 68–69
hypernatraemia, 324
hyperoxygenation test, 714
hyperparathyroidism, 469b
  body and lower limbs and, 470
  face and, 470
  general inspection of, 469
  primary, 469–470, 484
  questions for, 470b
hyperpigmentation, 701f
hyperpyrexia, 50
hypertension, 633–634
  CKD and, 310
  complications of, 125
  as coronary artery disease risk factor, 69, 70b
  idiopathic intracranial, 491–492
  malignant, 125
  M-mode measurements in patient with, 155f
  portal, 275
  pulmonary, 125–126, 188
  systemic, 125
hypertensive retinopathy, 125f
hyperthyroidism, 448–451, 449f, 482, 730
  causes of, 451b
  questions for patient with, 448b

INDEX   I-11

hypertrophic cardiomyopathy, 128t, 139f
    syncope and, 67
hypertrophic pulmonary osteoarthropathy (HPO), 178
hyperventilation, 169, 306
hypoactive delirium, 847t–850t
hypocalcaemia, 470
    causes of, 471b
    questions for, 470b
hypoglossal nerve, 503t, 534–536, 535f
    paediatric examination of, 655
    palsy, 536
hypoglycaemia, 494
hypoglycaemia stimulation test, 482
hypokalaemia, 324
hyponatraemia, 324
hyponychial angle, 79–80
hypoparathyroidism, 470–471
hypopituitarism, causes of, 455b
hypopyon, 780
hypotension, 634
    acute abdomen and, 274
hypothermia, 50
hypothetico-deductive approach, 22
hypothyroidism, 451–453, 452f, 482
    causes of, 451b
    neurological associations of, 453b
    questions for patient with, 452b
    signs guide for, 452t
hypotonia, 595
hypovolaemia, 47–48
hysteria, 852t

I

IADL see instrumental activities of daily living
ice-water test, 876
ideas of reference, 852t
ILD see interstitial lung disease
ileus, generalised, 287f
illness
    effect of, 12
    presenting, 7–12
    viral, 352f
illness anxiety disorder, 26, 26b
illusion, 852t
imaging
    of gastrointestinal system, 285–290
    haematological, 358, 358f–359f
    of kidneys and scrotum, 325, 325f–326f
    neurological, 611, 611f–615f
    in rheumatological examination, 430–434
immune system, paediatric examination of, 660–663, 660b, 662f–663f
immunisations, 15
incontinence, urinary, 300
incus, 782

individual joints, rheumatological examination of, 374–406
    ankles, 403–406, 404f, 405b, 407b
    elbows, 383–384, 383f
    feet, 403–406, 404f, 405b, 407b
    hands, and wrists, 374–383, 374f, 375b–377b, 378f, 383b
    hips, 395–399, 396f, 397b, 398f
    knees, 399–403, 399f, 399t
    neck, 388–392, 390f–392f
    sacroiliac joints, 392–395, 393b, 394f
    shoulders, 384–388, 385f, 387f
    temporomandibular joints, 388, 389f
    thoracolumbar spine, 392–395, 393b, 394f
infants
    term, growth charts for, 690f–695f
    upper motor neurone weakness in, 696b
infection
    acute respiratory, 168
    bacterial, 352f
    HIV, 836–840
    lower genital tract, 755t
    recurrent, 333, 333b
    sinusitis and, 790–791
    of skin, 463
    urinary tract, 298–300, 300t
        risk factors for, 299b
infectious diseases examination, 834–841, 840b–841b
    HIV infection and AIDS, 836–840
        examination of, 838–840, 838f–840f
        history of, 837–838, 837b, 837t
    pyrexia of unknown origin (PUO), 834–836
        clinical scenarios for unexplained fever, 836
        common causes of, 834b
        examination of, 835–836, 835b
        history of, 835, 835b
infectious mononucleosis, 795t
infective endocarditis, 123
infertility, 749–750, 749t, 750b
inflammatory bowel disease, 277–279
inguinal canal, 230, 264f
inguinal hernias, 262, 263f
    in neonatal examination, 717
inguinal ligament, 262f
injury, acute, to kidneys, 300
    causes of, 301b
innocent murmurs, 670, 671t
insomnia, 25
inspiratory stridor, 664t
instrumental activities of daily living (IADL), 828b
insulin tolerance test (ITT), 482
intercostal muscles, 174
intermittent claudication, 67–68
internal carotid artery, 580–581

internal rotation, 386, 388f
internuclear ophthalmoplegia, 515f, 584
inter-observer agreement, 53–54, 54b
interphalangeal depth ratio, 79–80
interphalangeal joint, 406
interphalangeal movements, 380, 382f
interpreter, 28
interstitial lung disease (ILD), 168, 196–197, 196b
    computed tomography of, 213f
intra-abdominal masses, 249b
intracranial pressure, raised, headache and, 491–492
intravenous drug addict's forearm, 123f
introductory questions, 846
involuntary movements, 496–497
    of unconscious patients, 602
ion channelopathies, 67
iritis, 278–279, 279f, 411, 411f, 780
irritable bowel syndrome, 224, 224b
ischaemic heart disease, 68
ischaemic ulcer, 115f, 117b
isometric exercise, 105

J

Jacksonian epilepsy, 494
Janeway lesions, 80–81, 82f
jaundice, 89, 225, 310, 335, 700
    changes in urine and faeces with, 270t
    gallbladder enlargement with, 256b
    in physical examination, 40–41
    questions for patient with, 226b
jaw jerk, 524, 524f
jaw-thrust manoeuvre, 868f
jaw-tilt manoeuvre, 868f
jerky limb movements, in neonatal examination, 699–700
jittery limb movements, in neonatal examination, 700
joint crepitus, 374
joint position sense pathways, 558f
joints
    Charcot's, 463, 466f
    deformity, 365
    instability of, 365
    morning stiffness in, 365
    pain in, 363
    peripheral, 363–365, 363b, 364f, 365b–366b
    referral patterns of, 364f
jugular chain, 341–342, 343f
jugular vein, 74
jugular venous pressure (JVP), 77f–78f, 90–92, 91f–92f, 92b, 188, 310
    acute coronary syndrome and, 121
    chronic constrictive pericarditis and, 123
    pulsation, 90
    RVF and, 120

K

Kaposi's sarcoma, 838, 839f
Kartagener's syndrome, 712
Kayser-Fleischer rings, 238–239, 239f
keloid, 805t, 806f
keratoconjunctivitis sicca, 772
    causes of, 773b
keratoderma blennorrhagicum, 818, 819f
Kernig's sign, 501, 608
ketoacidosis, diabetic, 463
ketonuria, 320–321, 321b
key grip, 381, 382f
kidneys, 230
    imaging of, 325, 325f–326f
    palpation of, 252–253, 255f
    percussion of, 258
    polycystic, 310
        adult, 311b
    transplanted, 310
    see also chronic kidney disease
Killip class, 121
kinesia paradoxica, 598
Klinefelter's syndrome, 476, 477f
Klumpke palsy, 697f, 697t
knee
    absent, ankle jerks and, extensor plantar response plus, 590, 590t
    jerk, 570, 570f
    power testing for, 567–568, 567f–568f
knock-knees, 637–639, 638f
koilonychia, 335
Koplik's spot, 794f
Korotkoff sounds, 87, 87f
Korsakoff's psychosis, 545
Kussmaul's breathing, 463
Kussmaul's sign, 91
kyphoscoliosis, 93, 180
kyphosis, thoracic, 473

L

laboratory testing, 429–430
labour, 685–687
    questions regarding, 685–687
Lachman test, 401–402, 401f
lacrimal gland, 772
LAD see left anterior descending (LAD) artery
Landolfi's sign, 134t
language, 28
large for gestational age (LGA), 696
large v waves, 91–92
Lasègue's test, 393
laser scars, 468
late diabetic dermopathy, 463
late systolic murmur, 100–102, 102t
lateral bending, 392
lateral medullary syndrome, 581–582, 582b, 778
Lazarus sign, 875
left anterior descending (LAD) artery, 74

left lateral position, in dynamic manoeuvres, 104, 104f
left ventricular failure (LVF), 119–120
left-right disorientation, 543
legs
    arteries in, 109
    in genitourinary examination, 312
    in haematological examination, 345–346
    length, 397
    paediatric examination of, 635–639
    Paget's disease and, 478
    in respiratory examination, 188
    ulcers, 117b
leiomyomata, 761t
length, in neonatal examination, 689, 690f–695f
length/height-for-age, growth charts in, 625f–632f
lens, 771
Leopold manoeuvres, 737–738, 739f
lethargy, 226, 440
leucoerythroblastic film, 351f
leuconychia, 235, 235f
leucoplakia, 242, 242f
    hairy, 839
leukaemia
    acute, 352f, 354–355
    chronic, 355
    chronic myeloid, 355
Levine's grading system, 103
lichen planus, 755t
    with 'Koebner' phenomenon, 810f
    with polygonal flat-topped violaceous lesions, 810f
lichen sclerosus, 755t, 756f
lichen simplex chronicus, 755t
ligaments, 401–402, 401f, 402t
    inguinal, 262f
light reflex, 511
light-touch testing, 559, 574f
likelihood ratio (LR), 52–53
limb examination, 109–118, 117b–118b
limb length discrepancies, measurement for, 639, 639f
limbs
    in neonatal examination, 718–721, 719t
        abnormal movements in, 699–700
    weakness in, 496
limp, 395–396
Lincoln's sign, 134t, 135f
lipodystrophic facies, 42f
lipoedema, 109
lips, 791
    inspection of, 792–793
Listeria monocytogenes, 611
Little's area, 789
livedo reticularis, 416f
liver, 229–230
    CT of, 293f
    cysts in, 291f

    disease, 274–275
    dullness, 184
    enzymes of, 285
    metastasis to, 292f
    palpation of, 250–251, 250f
    percussion of, 250, 251f, 257–258
living conditions, 15
living will, 875
LMN see lower motor neurone
locked-in syndrome, 876
locking, 375
loose nuchal skin, in neonatal examination, 709, 710f
loss of function, 375
lower limbs
    dermatomes of, 572, 575f
    diabetes mellitus and, 463–467
        inspection of, 463–466
        neurological examination for, 466–467
        palpation of, 466
    examination anatomy of, 109–113
    examination of, 111b, 610
    hyperparathyroidism and, 470
    motor system of, 566–571
    paediatric examination of, 635–639
    peripheral nerves of, 575–577
    peripheral nervous system examination of, 566–577
    position sense of, 574f
    power, 569, 569f
    of pregnancy, 740
    reflexes of, 570–571
    sensory system testing of, 572–574
    of unconscious patients, 604
    vibration sense in, 573f
lower motor neurone (LMN)
    lesions, 535f, 582, 583b
    weakness, 496
lower segment lengths, measurement of, 633
LP see lumbar puncture
LR see likelihood ratio
lumbar hyperlordosis, 639–640
lumbar puncture (LP), 611
lumbar spinal stenosis, 67–68
lump, 799–825
    diagnosis of, 804–806
lungs, 174
    anatomy of, 175f
    carcinoma of, 198–199
    collapse of, 192
    disease, interstitial, computed tomography of, 213f
    fields, 149–150
    function assessment of, 203–206
    lobes of, 176f
    lower lobe expansion of, 183f
    in neonatal examination, 714–715
    paediatric examination of, 671–674

segments of, 207f
upper lobe expansion of, 182f
lupus pernio, 816, 816f
LVF *see* left ventricular failure
lymph nodes
axillary, 339–340, 340f–341f
cervical, 243–244, 244f, 341–342, 342f
characteristics of, 339b
epitrochlear, 339, 339f
inguinal, 256, 345, 345f
malignant, 345b
supraclavicular, 341–342, 342f
lymphadenopathy, 660, 660b
causes of, 340b, 344b
differential diagnosis of, 333b
with significant disease, 340t
lymphangitis, 342, 344f
lymphatic system, paediatric examination of, 660–663, 660b, 662f–663f
lymphoedema, 112f
lymphoma, 357–358, 357t, 358f

M

MAC *see* Mycobacterium avium complex
macrocephaly, 645
macroglossia, 242, 457f
macula, examination of, 777–778
macules, 641t, 805t
maculopapular eruptions, 801f
magnetic resonance imaging (MRI), 14
of brain pituitary, 484f
of multiple sclerosis (MS), 612f
in rheumatological examination, 430
main d'accoucheur, 471
major depressive disorder, 861
malabsorption, 279–281
malaria, 352f
malignant melanoma, 823, 823f
malignant skin lesions, 641–642
malleus, 782
malnutrition, 238b
mania, 847t–850t
manic-depressive illness-bipolar disorder, 847t–850t
Marfan's syndrome, 79f, 89, 154f
high-arched palate and, 89
marital status, 15
massive pulmonary embolism, 63
maternal health, 684–685, 685t
Mayne's sign, 134t
McMurray's test, 403, 403f
MCV *see* mean cell volume
mean cell volume (MCV), 350–354
measles, 794f
with conjunctivitis, 773f
mechanical ventilator, death and, 876
meconium, in neonatal examination, 686
mediastinal compression, 197–198
mediastinal crunch, 103

mediastinum, 149, 174
medical history, in pregnancy, 734
medically unexplained symptoms (MUS), 26, 27b, 847t–850t
medication, in neurological history, 497–498, 498b
medulla, anatomy of, 532f
medullary brainstem hypercapnia test, 876
melaena, 224–225, 268
melanoma, metastatic, 821f
membranes, rupture of, 732
Ménière's disease, 495
meningocele, 699f
meningococcal rash, 871f
meningomyelocele, 698t
meniscal tear, 434f
meniscus sign, 208f
menorrhagia, 744
MENs syndromes *see* multiple endocrine neoplasias (MENs) syndromes
menstrual history, 15, 303, 744–750
menstruation, 441
mental health
of elderly patients, 32–33
gastrointestinal system and, 234–235
neurological history and, 497
risk, 851
systems review of, 9b–12b
mental health examination, 845–863, 855t–857t, 863b
family history in, 853
social history in, 853–854
meralgia paraesthetica, 425, 575
metabolic syndrome, 442, 442t
metacarpophalangeal (MCP) joints, 375–379, 379f
metacarpophalangeal movements, 380, 382f
metastases
liver, 292f
pulmonary, 210f
metastatic melanoma, 821f
metatarsalgia, 425, 426b
metatarsus adductus (MTA), 719, 720f
metopic synostosis, 704
microaneurysms, 468, 468f
microangiopathic haemolysis, 351f
microcephaly, 644–645
micrographia, 599
micturition syncope, 66
midbrain, anatomy of, 511f
mid-diastolic murmurs, 102, 102t
midsystolic ejection murmur, 100, 102t
mid-upper arm circumference, in general physical examination, 624
migraine, 490–491
miliae, 700, 701f
mini-mental state examination (MMSE), 854
miosis, 510–511
mitral facies, 43f

mitral regurgitation (MR), 103t, 128t, 129f, 157f
acute, 129–130
chronic, 128–129
loudness of, 103t
mitral stenosis, 126–128, 127f, 128t
mitral valve
disease, 152f
leaflets, 155f
prolapse, 130, 130f
echocardiography of, 156f
mixed connective tissue disease, 420
M-mode measurements
normal long-axis, 155f
in patient with hypertension, 155f
MMSE *see* mini-mental state examination
molluscum contagiosum, 820f
monoarthritis, causes of, 364b
monofilament testing, for peripheral neuropathy, 466–467, 467f
mononeuritis multiplex, 585b
monoplegia, 580
mood, 19, 852t
disorders, 847t–850t
Moro reflex, 722
Morton's 'neuroma', 425–426
motion, 373–374
motor examination, 655–658, 656f
motor neurone
disease, 562f, 583
lesion of, 549f
see also lower motor neurone; upper motor neurone
motor system
of lower limb, 566–571
spinal cord compression and, 586b
of upper limbs, 550–557
mottling, 703, 703f
mouth, 791–795, 791f
dry, 367–368, 368b
examination anatomy of, 791–792
examination method for, 792–794
in gastrointestinal examination, 240–243
history of, 792
lesions, 241b
in neonatal examination, 709, 710f
paediatric examination of, 648–649
pain in, 792b
sample questions for, 621b
ulcers of, 242–243, 243b, 243f, 792b
of unconscious patients, 603–604
movement disorders, 497t
MR *see* mitral regurgitation
MRI *see* magnetic resonance imaging
MS *see* multiple sclerosis
mucormycosis, rhinocerebral, 469
mucosal neuromas, of tongue, 470, 471f
mucosal ulcers, 310
mucus, 224
Muehrcke's nails, 306

Mueller's sign, 134t
multiple endocrine neoplasias (MENs) syndromes, 470
multiple myeloma, 342–343, 358
multiple sclerosis (MS), 582, 584–585, 585b
    MRI of, 612f
Münchhausen's syndrome, 29
murmurs *see* heart murmurs
Murphy's sign, 253
muscle
    of eyes, 512f
    intercostal, 174
    strength, 552
    stretch reflex, 553, 554t
    wasting, 373
        in hands, 566
    weakness, 549–550
muscle disease, 496
muscular dystrophy, 591
    fascioscapular, 592f
musculoskeletal disease, 408–427
musculoskeletal system
    in neonatal examination, 718–721
    systems review of, 9b–12b
Mustard procedure, 143
myasthenia gravis, 593–594, 594f
Mycobacterium avium complex (MAC), 838
Mycobacterium tuberculosis, 611
mydriasis, 510–511
myelocele, 699f
myelocystocele, 699f
myelofibrosis, 352f
myelomeningocele, 699f
myocardial infarction, 121
    chest pain and, 60
myocardial ischaemia, 168
myocardium, 74
myoglobinuria, 322b
myopathic facies, 43f
myopathy, 590–591, 591b–592b, 592f–593f
myotonic facies, 43f
myxoedema, 109, 451–453, 452f
    causes of, 451b
    neurological associations of, 453b
    questions for patient with, 452b
    signs guide for, 452t

N

Nabothian follicles, 756–757, 758f
Naegele's rule, 730
naevus flammeus, 700
naevus simplex, 701f
nails, 823–824, 824b–825b
    changes in, 440–441
    in gastrointestinal examination, 235
    Muehrcke's, 306
    in physical examination, 48–49, 48f, 49t
    Plummer's, 449, 449f
    with psoriasis, 824f
    yellow nail syndrome and, 193, 193f
narrow pulse pressure, 634–635
nasal speculum, 790
nasopharyngeal bleeding, 166t
nasopharyngeal carcinoma, 796f
National Health and Medical Research Council (NHMRC), 17
National Institute on Alcohol Abuse and Alcoholism (NIAAA), 17
nausea, 218–219
    in pregnancy, 730
neck
    in cardiac examination, 89–92
    dermatomes of, 523f
    diabetes mellitus and, 469
    examination of, 647
    in gastrointestinal examination, 243–244
    in genitourinary examination, 310
    lymph node groups of, 662f
    in neonatal examination, 709, 710f
    in neurological examination, 536–537
    Paget's disease and, 478
    in pregnancy observation, 737
    sample questions for, 621b
    stiffness, 501, 608
    swellings in, 445b
    of unconscious patients, 603
necrobiosis lipoidica diabeticorum, 463–466, 466f
necrotising fasciitis, 818
Neisseria gonorrhoeae, 755t
Neisseria meningitidis, 611
Nelson's syndrome, 461
neonatal history and examination, 684–725, 723b–724b
    gestational age and, 723
    head-to-toe assessment in, 696–723
        abnormal limb movements, 699–700
        ambiguous genitalia, 717
        cardiovascular system, 711–715
        chest, 711–715
        developmental reflexes, 722–723
        eyes, 704–707, 706b, 708f
        face, 704–709
        female genitalia, 717
        gastrointestinal system, 715–717, 716f
        head, 703
        hips, 721
        inguinal region, 717
        limbs, 718–721, 719t
        lungs, 714–715
        mouth, 709, 710f
        musculoskeletal system, 718–721
        neck, 709, 710f
        nervous system, 721–723
        penis, 717
        posture, 696–697
        scrotum, 717
        skin, 700–703
        skull, 698–699
        spine, 698–699
        spontaneous movements, 696–697
        temperature, 703
        urogenital system, 715–717
    measurements in, 689–696
    method for, 688b
    physical examination in, 687–723
    preparation for, 688–689, 689f
nephropathy, diabetic, 469
nephrotic syndrome, 321b
nerves
    cranial, 501–537, 502f, 503t, 608–609
        examination of, 774–775
        fifth, 781f
    eighth (vestibulocochlear), 529–531, 609
    eleventh (accessory), 532f, 533–534, 534f, 609
    entrapment, 367
    entrapment syndromes, 424–426
    femoral, 575, 576f
    fifth (trigeminal), 521–525, 522f, 524f, 609
    first (olfactory), 504
    fourth (trochlear), 510–521, 609
    lateral cutaneous, 575, 576f
    lesions, multiple cranial, 536–537, 537b
    median, 559–561
    ninth (glossopharyngeal), 531–533, 532f, 609
    peripheral
        of lower limb, 575–577
        thickened, 585, 585b, 592b
        of upper limb, 559–566
    peroneal, 576–577, 577f
    radial, 559, 561f
    root, 563t
        compression, 565t
    sciatic, 575–576, 576f
    second (optic), 505–510, 506f, 608, 608f
    seventh (facial), 525–528, 526f–527f, 609
    sixth (abducens), 510–521, 609
    tenth (vagus), 531–533, 532f–533f, 609
    third (oculomotor), 510–521, 609
        lesion, 517
    twelfth (hypoglossal), 534–536, 535f, 609
    ulnar, 561–562
nervous system
    alcohol in, complications of, 18b
    examination anatomy of, 500, 500f
    in neonatal examination, 721–723
nervous system examination, 606b–608b, 606f
    diagnostic testing in, 611
    HIV infection and, 840
neurasthenia, 847t–850t
neurofibroma, subcutaneous, 502f
neurofibromatosis type 1 (NF1), 642–644, 645f
neurological conditions, inherited, 498t

neurological examination, 500–539, 538b–539b, 652–655
    extending of, 608–610
    family history in, 498, 498t
    general signs in, 501
    head in, 536–537
    medication history in, 497–498, 498b
    neck in, 536–537
    past history in, 497
    presenting symptoms in, 489–497
    social history in, 498
    summary of, 606–611, 615b
neurological history, 489–499, 489b, 498b–499b
neurological imaging, 611, 611f–615f
neurological symptoms, 375
neurological syndromes and disease, physical signs and, correlation of, 580–605, 604b
neurological system
    sample questions for, 621b
    systems review of, 9b–12b
neuropathic ulcer, 115f, 117b
neuropathy, 367
    peripheral, 583, 583f, 584b
    in pregnancy, 731
neutrophilic dermatoses, 816
NHMRC *see* National Health and Medical Research Council
NIAAA *see* National Institute on Alcohol Abuse and Alcoholism
Nikolsky's sign, 700
nitrite, 321
nodular scleritis, 410f
nodules, 641t, 805t
nominal dysphasia, 541
non-ejection systolic click, 99
non-fluent aphasia, 540–541
non-pitting oedema, 109
non-steroidal anti-inflammatory drugs (NSAIDs), 12–13
non-verbal clues, 6
nose, 771–798, 796b–798b
    anatomy of, 788f
    blocked, 789
    examination anatomy of, 788–789
    examination method for, 790
    examination of, 504, 648, 791
    history of, 789
    in neonatal examination, 708–709
    sample questions for, 621b
nostrils, of unconscious patients, 603
NSAIDs *see* non-steroidal anti-inflammatory drugs
nuclear scans
    in rheumatological examination, 431
    of thyroid nodules, 482f
nummular eczema, 811f
NURS *see* emotion-handling skills

nutritional status, 279–281
nystagmus, 514–515, 514b

O

OA *see* osteoarthritis
obesity, 45, 46b
    central, 459, 460f
    dyspnoea and, 168
objective scepticism, 14
objective structured clinical examination (OSCE), 38
    introduction to, 55–56, 55f
observation
    in developmental assessment, 659
    in general physical examination, 622–624
obsessive-compulsive disorder (OCD), 847t–850t, 863
obstetric examination, 729–742, 742b
    anatomy in, 736
    general appearance of, 736–737
    observations of, 737
    patient position of, 736
obstetric history, in pregnancy, 734
obstetric ultrasound, for pregnancy, 741–742
obstructive sleep apnoea (OSA), 169
obstructive ventilatory defect, 204
occipital nodes, 341–342
occipital plagiocephaly, 645
occiput-to-wall distance, 473, 473f
occupation, 16, 16b
ochronosis, 774f
Ochsner's clasping test, 559–561, 562f
oculomotor nerve, 503t, 510–521
    lesion, 517
    paediatric examination of, 653
    palsy, 517, 519f
oculovestibular reflex test, 876
odynophagia, 276
oedema, 109
    alveolar pulmonary, 152f
    ankle, 64, 112b
    causes of, 112b
    interstitial pulmonary, 151f
    non-pitting, 109
    pitting, 109, 111f
    in pregnancy, 732
    RVF and, 120
oesophageal spasm, 63
older person
    assessment of, 826–833, 833b
    comprehensive geriatric assessment, 826b
    history taking in, 826–829, 827b–829b
    physical examination in, 830–833, 830f, 831b, 831t, 832f
    questions for, 827b
olfactory nerve, 503t, 504, 789
    paediatric examination of, 653
oligomenorrhoea, 745–747

omphalitis, 716f
180° examination, 657–658, 657f
one-and-a-half syndrome, 520–521
onychogryphosis, 48f
onycholysis, 376–377, 449, 449f
onychomycosis, 823f
open-ended questions, 846
opening snap, 99
ophthalmoscope, 509
opposition strength, 381, 382f
optic nerve, 503t, 505–510, 506f
optic nerve, examination of, paediatric, 653
oral candidiasis, 839f
orbital cellulitis, 781, 782f
orbits, palpation of, 778
organ donation, 877
organic brain disorders, 847t–850t
orientation, 501, 608
oropharynx, 649–650
    inspection of, 793–794
orthopnoea, 64, 64b
Ortolani test, 721
OSA *see* obstructive sleep apnoea
OSCE *see* objective structured clinical examination
Osler's nodes, 80–81
osteoarthritis (OA), 376, 378f
    X-ray of, 430f
osteomalacia, 471–473
    causes and risk factors for, 472b
    examination for, 473
    questions for, 473b
osteoporosis, 471–473, 485f
    causes and risk factors for, 472b
    examination for, 473
    questions for, 473b
    screening of, in elderly patients, 33
otitis externa, 785–786
    acute diffuse, 785–786
    acute localised, 785
    chronic, 786
    malignant, 469, 786
otorrhoea, 783–784
otoscope examination, 786, 786f
otoscopy, 647–648, 648f
ovarian cysts, 761t
ovarian torsion, 748–749
ovarian tumours, complications of, 761f
ovary, endometriotic patches on, 749f
overflow incontinence, 300
overseas travel, 16
overvalued idea, 852t
oximetry, pulse, 205–206, 206f
oxycephaly, 704
oxygen saturation (SpO_2), 205–206

P

pacemaker, 93, 154f
    sound, 100

I-16 INDEX

paediatric history and examination, 619–683, 682b
  general physical examination, 622–681, 623b
    blood pressure, 633–634, 634f, 634t
    cranial nerves, 653–655, 654f
    developmental assessment, 658–660, 661t
    ear, nose and throat, 647–650, 648f–650f
    face and dysmorphology, 650–652, 651t–652t
    gastrointestinal system, 674–676, 674t
    genitourinary system and Tanner staging, 676–678, 677f
    head, 644–647, 646f–647f
    heart and circulation, 668–671, 668t, 671t–672t, 672b
    lungs, 671–674, 672b, 673t
    lymphatic and immune system, 660–663, 660b, 662f–663f
    measurements for, 624–633, 625f–632f
    motor and cerebellar examination, 655–658, 656f–657f
    neurological, 652–655
    observation for, 622–624
    preparing for, 622
    pulse and respiratory rates, 634–635, 635f–636f
    respiratory and cardiovascular system, 663–674, 663b, 664t, 665b–666b, 667t
    specific, 635–652
    suspected child abuse, 678–681, 678t, 679b–680b, 679f, 681f
    tall and short stature, 633
    temperature, 635, 636t
    upper and lower limbs (legs and arms), 635–639, 637f–640f, 641t, 642f–645f
    vital signs, 633–635
  principles of, 619
  taking of, 619–622, 620t
    history-taking sequence, 620–622, 621b
Paget's disease, 476–478, 478f, 764
  back and, 478
  general inspection for, 477
  head and face in, 477–478
  legs and, 478
  neck in, 478
pain, 373–375
  abdominal, 217–218, 748–749
    in pregnancy, 732
  in abdominal wall, 257
  back, 365–366
    in pregnancy, 731
  biliary, 218
  chest wall, 63
  in eyes, 775t
  facial, 490–492

  in joint, 363
  limb, 366–367
  loss of sensation of, 561f, 572f
  in mouth, 792b
  pancreatic, 218
  pathways of, 557f
  pleural, 62–63, 168
  pubic symphysis, in pregnancy, 731
  radiation of, 8
  in rheumatological history, 363–365
  testing, 557–558, 558f
  in throat, 792b
  see also chest pain
palate
  hard, 791
  high-arched, 89
  soft, 791
palatine tonsils, 650
pallor, 44–45, 335
palmar crease pigmentation, 461f
palmar creases, 335
palmar erythema, 235–236, 235f
palmar grasp, 723
palmar surfaces, 377
palmar xanthomata, 81
palmomental reflex, 546
palms, 235–236
palpable arteries, 74, 75f
palpation, 665–666
  of abdomen, 248–257, 249f, 310, 311b, 676
  of aorta, 255–256
  of breast, 765–766
  of chest, 182–184
  of gallbladder, 253–254
  of kidneys, 252–253, 255f
  of liver, 250–251, 250f
  of nasal bones, 790
  of pancreas, 255
  of pinna, 786
  of praecordium, 93–95, 95f
  of ribs, 184
  of spleen, 251–252, 254f
  of testis, 314
  of thyroid, 446–447, 446f
  of tongue, 793
  of trachea, 179f
palpitations, 64–65, 65b, 65t, 665, 666b
  in pregnancy, 731
palsy
  Bell's, 528, 528f
  bulbar, 536t
  eleventh nerve, 534
  fifth nerve, 524–525
  ninth nerve, 533
  pseudobulbar, 536t, 543
  seventh nerve, 528
  sixth nerve, 518
  supranuclear, 520, 521f

  tenth nerve, 533
  third nerve, 517, 519f
  twelfth nerve, 536
pancreas, 230
  calcification in, 289f
  pain, 218
  palpation of, 255
pancytopenia, 354
panhypopituitarism, 454–456
  questions for patient with, 454b
panic disorder, 847t–850t, 862
pannus, 370
pansystolic murmurs, 100, 102t
Pap smear, 757
papillomavirus, human, 755t
papules, 641t, 805t
para, 15
paraesthesias, 404
paraparesis, 597b
paraplegia, 478, 580
parasternal impulse, 94–95, 94f
parathyroid hormone, bone diseases and, 484
parathyroidectomy, 310
paratonia, 551
paravalvular leak, 137
parietal lobe function, 543–545
Parinaud's syndrome, 520
Parkinson's disease, 496–497, 551
  causes of, 599, 600b
  examination of, 597–599
parotid enlargement, 239–240, 240f
paroxysmal nocturnal dyspnoea (PND), 64
pars flaccida, 786–787
pars tensa, 786–787
passive movement, 373–374
past history
  gastrointestinal history, 227
  haematological history, 333–334
  mental health examination, 851–853
  in neurological history, 497
patches, 641t
patellar apprehension test, 402
patellar tap, 400–401, 401f
patent ductus arteriosus, 141, 141f, 158
pathological murmurs, 670–671
patient
  acutely ill, 867–872, 869f
  cachectic, 77
  with chronic illness, 29
  confidentiality, 33
  critically ill, 870b
  elderly, 31–33
  geriatric
    examination of, 830f
    special considerations for, 826–829
  personal questions to consider asking, 24b
  with rare disease, 29
  relatives of, 876

INDEX I-17

'uncooperative or difficult', 28–29
  see also elderly patient
patterns of irregularity, 83, 84f
PE see pulmonary embolism
peak flow meter, 203, 204f
pectus carinatum, 180, 181f, 711
pectus excavatum, 93, 180, 181f, 711, 711f, 764–765
pelvic examination, 312, 752–762, 753b
pelvic floor, 267
pelvic mass, 760, 761t
Pemberton's sign, 188, 447–448
pemphigus vulgaris, 810–812, 814f
penile length, 677
penis, in neonatal examination, 717
pen-touching test, 561f
peptic ulcer disease, 218
percussion, 665–666, 674
  of abdomen, 257–258, 311–312, 676
  auscultatory, 311–312
  of chest, 184, 185f
  of kidneys, 258
  of liver, 251f, 257–258
  of praecordium, 95
  of spleen, 258, 258f
  of thyroid, 447
pericardial disease, 122–123
pericarditis, 310
  acute, 122
perifollicular haemorrhages, scurvy with, 46f
periorbital purpura, 239, 240f
peripartum depression, 861
peripheral arterial embolism, 114
peripheral blood film, 350, 351f–352f, 354f
peripheral blood smear, 350
peripheral cyanosis
  causes of, 44b
  in physical examination, 41–44, 41f
peripheral joints, 363–365, 363b, 364f, 365b–366b
peripheral nerves
  of lower limb, 575–577
  of upper limb, 559–566
peripheral nervous system examination, 548–579, 579b
  anatomy of, 549–550
  approach to, 550
  inspection of, 550
  of lower limbs, 566–577
  of upper limbs, 550–566
peripheral neuropathy, 309, 583, 583f, 584b
peripheral vascular disease, 68b, 113, 114f, 117b
  intermittent claudication and, 67–68
peristalsis, 247
peritonitis, 272t
persistent depressive disorder, 861
personal history, 853–854
personal history taking, 23–27
personality, 852t

personality disorders, 847t–850t, 859b
Perthes' test, 116
petechiae, 237, 237f, 805t
  causes of, 338b
  in neonatal examination, 700–703, 703f, 707f
petechial rash, 819f
Peutz-Jeghers syndrome, 231, 232f, 792–793
pH, of urine, 320
Phalen's wrist flexion test, 380
pharyngitis, 794–795
phobia, 852t
phobic anxiety, 847t–850t
physical examination, general principles of, 37–56, 54b–55b
  evidence-based clinical examination, 51–54
  first impressions in, 39–45
  objective structured clinical examination (OSCE), 38, 55–56, 55f
  preparing the patient for, 51
  start of, 38–39, 38b
physical fitness, lack of, dyspnoea and, 168
physical signs, respiratory disease and, correlation of, 190–200, 200b
physiotherapy, 14
pigeon chest, 711
pigment alterations, 805t
pigmentation, 231
  changes in, 441
pigmented scars, diabetes mellitus and, 463
pinna, palpation of, 786
pitting, 376–377
pitting oedema, 109, 111f
pituitary, 453–458, 484f
pituitary testing, 480–482
pityriasis rosea, 810f
placenta praevia, 732
placental abruption, 732
plagiocephaly, 704
plantar flexion, 406
plantar grasp, 723
plaques, 641t, 805t
platelets, 330, 331t
pleura, 174
pleural effusion, 192–193, 208f
pleural pain, 168
pleurisy, 62–63
Plummer's nails, 449, 449f
PM see postmortem
PND see paroxysmal nocturnal dyspnoea
pneumatic auriscopy, 787
pneumonia, 191t
  bacterial, 168
  classification of, 190–191
  community acquired, causes of, 192
  lobar, 190–192
  viral, 168

pneumonitis, 168
pneumothorax, 168, 193–194, 209f
  tension, 194
polyarthritis
  causes of, 365b
  patterns of, 366b
polycystic kidney disease, 298b, 311b
polycythaemia, 340, 342f, 355–356, 356b
polydactyly, 719f
polymyalgia rheumatica, 366–367
polymyositis, 366–367
polypharmacy, 32, 32t
polyuria, 441
pons, anatomy of, 522f
popliteal artery, 113, 113f
popliteal artery, entrapment, 67–68
porphyria cutanea tarda, 233f, 234
portal hypertension, 275
port-wine stains, 700
positional plagiocephaly, 645
positioning, in gastrointestinal examination, 230, 230f
postauricular node, 341–342, 343f
posterior tibial artery, 113, 114f
posterior triangle nodes, 341–342, 343f
postmortem (PM), 877
postprandial fullness, 218
postprimary tuberculosis, 197
postsplenectomy, 351f
post-traumatic stress disorder (PTSD), 847t–850t, 862–863
postural blood pressure, 88, 88f
postural hypotension, 47–48, 88, 88b
postural syncope, 66
posture
  in neonatal examination, 696–697
  in physical examination, 45–46
  of unconscious patients, 602
power testing, 552–553, 566–569
practical test, 381
praecordium, 74, 92–106
  auscultation of, 95–97, 95f–96f
  inspection of, 92–93
  palpation of, 93–95, 95f
  percussion of, 95
preauricular node, 341–342, 778
precipitating events, 851
pregnancy, 685–687
  breathlessness in, 731
  current history, 734
  drug category ratings, 735b
  early, bleeding in, 745, 747t
  intrahepatic cholestasis of, 731
  major symptoms in, 731–732, 732b
  minor symptoms in, 730–731, 730b
  questions for patient regarding, 685b, 729b
premorbid personality, 854

presenting symptoms, 7
    in cardiovascular examination, 59–68
    in endocrine history, 439–441
    in gastrointestinal history, 217–226, 217b
    in haematological history, 329–333, 330b
    in neurological history, 489–497
    in respiratory history, 163–168, 163b
    in rheumatological history, 363–368
pressure loaded apex beat, 94
pressure sores, risk factors for, 831b
pressured speech, 852t
presyncope, 66–67
presystolic murmur, 102, 102t
primary hyperparathyroidism, 484
primary skin lesions, 641t
primary tuberculosis, 197, 210f
procidentia, 758f
prognathism, 457f
prolactin, 454
prolonged expiration, 673
prolonged inspiration, 673
proprioception, 558–559
    loss of, 551
    testing, 558–559
proptosis, 774
prostate, 266
protein, in urine, 320
proteinuria, 320b
Proteus mirabilis, 320
proximal interphalangeal (PIP), 375–376, 377f
proximal myopathy, 591
proximal weakness, 591b
pruritic urticarial papules and plaques of pregnancy (PUPPS), 731
pruritus, 225
    ani, 265
    in pregnancy, 731
pseudoathetosis, 600
pseudobulbar palsy, 543
pseudo-cyst, pancreatic, 290f
pseudogout, 434
pseudohypoparathyroidism, 471, 472f
pseudopseudohypoparathyroidism, 471
pseudoxanthoma elasticum, 277, 277f
psoas sign, 274
psoriasis, 811f
    as vulval skin condition, 755t
psoriatic arthritis, 404–405, 405f
psoriatic nail, 376–377, 378f
psychiatric disorders, 847t–850t
    diagnosis of, 854–858
    examples of, 859–863
    symptoms of, 852t
psychiatric history, 845–863, 863b
psychiatric interview, history taking and, 24
psychomotor agitation, 852t
psychomotor retardation, 852t
psychotic, 852t

ptosis, 511, 772
    causes of, 780t
pubic symphysis pain, in pregnancy, 731
pubic tubercle, 262f
puerperal mental disorders, 847t–850t
pull to sit, in 180° examination, 657f, 658
pulmonary embolism (PE), 122, 199–200
    risk factors for, 199b
pulmonary haemorrhage, 211f
pulmonary hypertension, 188
    causes of, 126
pulmonary mass, 209f
pulmonary metastases, 210f
pulmonary oedema, 310
pulmonary regurgitation, 137
pulmonary stenosis, 137
    valvar, 137f
pulmonary venous congestion, 151f
pulsation, 90
pulse
    acute coronary syndrome and, 121
    asthma and, 178
    bisferiens, 131–135
    chronic constrictive pericarditis and, 123
    deficit, 83
    paediatric examination of, 634–635, 635f
    peripheral vascular disease and, 113
    regularly irregular, 83
    see also arterial pulse
pulse oximetry, 205–206, 206f, 635
pulsus alternans, 84, 119f
pulsus paradoxus, 87–88
PUO *see* pyrexia of unknown origin
pupillary reflex, 511f
pupils
    Argyll Robertson, 467
    examination of, 511–512
    in neonatal examination, 704–706, 707f
purpura, 337, 337f, 805t
    causes of, 338b
    drug, 346f
    Henoch-Schönlein, 345–346, 346f
    periorbital, 239, 240f
    thrombocytopenic, 337f
pustules, 641t, 805t
pyoderma gangrenosum, 279f
pyrexia of unknown origin (PUO), 834–836

Q

quadrantanopia, 509
quadrants, of breast, 765, 765f
quadriceps muscle wasting, 466
quadriplegia, 580
Queen Square hammer, 553–554, 554f
questions
    for anaemia, 331b
    for blocked nose, 789b
    CAGE, 17
    closed, 846

    for constipation, 223b
    for cough, 163, 163b
    Cushing's syndrome, 459b
    for deafness, 784b
    for delirium, 870b
    for delivery, 685b, 687b
    for diabetic patient, 464b
    for dialysis, 303b
    for diarrhoea, 222b
    for difficulty swallowing, 221b
    for dizziness, 493b
    for dysphonia, 793b
    for dyspnoea, 167b
    for epilepsy, 493b
    for fever, 835b
    for gastro-oesophageal reflux disease, 220b
    for haematemesis, 226b
    for haemophilia, 332b
    for headache, 491b
    for HIV infection and AIDS, 837b
    for hyperparathyroidism, 470b
    for hyperthyroidism, 448b
    for hypocalcaemia, 470b
    for hypothyroidism, 452b
    introductory, 6, 6b, 846
    for jaundice, 226b
    for joint pain, 363b
    for labour, 685–687
    for mouth ulcers, 792b
    for muscle weakness, 548b
    for neurological problem, 491b
    for older person, 827b
    open-ended, 5, 846
    for osteomalacia, 473b
    for osteoporosis, 473b
    for pain in mouth or throat, 792b
    for panhypopituitarism, 454b
    for pregnancy, 685b, 729b, 733b
    for rash, 801b
    for red eye, 772b
    for renal failure, 298b
    for stroke, 490b
    for sudden visual loss, 774b
    systems review, 9b–12b, 19–20
    for transient ischaemic attack, 490b
    for vomiting, 219b
Quincke's sign, 134t

R

radial deviation, 379f
radial pulse, 81–82, 82f
radial-radial delay, 83
radicular symptoms, 390
radiofemoral delay, 82–83, 84f
rapid breathing (tachypnoea), 665
rapidly alternating movements, 556–557
rapport, establishing, 3–5, 4f

rash, 372–373
    differential diagnosis of, 835b
    of discoid lupus, 414–415
    meningococcal, 871f
    questions for, 801b
    SLE, 416f
rattle, 664t
Raynaud's phenomenon, 367, 367b, 414
RBCs *see* red blood cells
RCA *see* right coronary artery
receptive (posterior) dysphasia, 540
rectal examination, 264–268, 265f, 274, 312, 762
    paediatric, 678
rectocele, 756
rectum
    mass in, 267b
    prolapse, 264–265
rectus sheath divarication, 257f
red blood cells (RBCs), 321–323
    abnormalities of, 329–330, 331b
red cell casts, 323
reflexes
    abdominal, 572–574, 575f
    anal, 574
    corneal, 523, 776
    cremasteric, 574
    gag, 533
    grasp, 546
    light, 511
    of lower limbs, 570–571
    palmomental, 546
    plantar, 570–571, 571f
    primitive, 546
    spinal cord compression and, 586b
    spine, 574
    superficial, 572
    of upper limb, 553–556
    vestibulo-ocular, 517
rehabilitation, 14
Reiter's disease, 410–411
Reiter's syndrome, 434f
relative afferent pupillary defect (RAPD), 511–512
relatives, informing of, 876
renal biopsy, 319
renal bruits, 312
renal calculus, 300, 322f
renal colic, 218
renal failure, 297, 302–303
renal function, test of, 319
renal masses, 310, 311b
renal syndromes, 299t
reproductive history, 27
reproductive system, systems review of, 9b–12b
respiration, in dynamic manoeuvres, 104
respiratory disease, physical signs and, correlation of, 190–200, 200b

respiratory disorders, 191t
respiratory distress, 190, 190b, 665, 667t
    in neonates, 715t
respiratory examination, 174–189, 188b–189b, 201–213, 213b
    abdomen in, 188
    chest in, 180–188
        auscultation, 184–188, 185f, 186b
        inspection of, 180–182, 180f–182f
        palpation, 182–184, 183f
        percussion, 184, 185f
    chest X-ray in, 206
    computed tomography scan in, 206
    examination anatomy in, 174, 175f–176f
    extending of, 203–210
    face in, 178–179
    general appearance in, 174–177
        chronic obstructive pulmonary disease (COPD), characteristic signs of, 175–177
        cough, character of, 177
        cyanosis, 177
        dyspnoea, 174–175
        hoarseness, 177
        sputum, 177
        stridor, 177, 177b
    hands in, 177–178
        clubbing, 178, 178f
        flapping tremor (asterixis), 178
        pulse rate, 178
        staining, 178
        wasting and weakness, 178
    heart in, 188
    legs in, 188
    method for, 201b–203b
    Pemberton's sign in, 188
    positioning in, 174
    respiratory rate, on exercise, 188
    temperature in, 188
    trachea in, 179–180, 179b, 179f
respiratory failure, 190, 190b
respiratory history, 163–173, 173b
    current treatment in, 169–171, 170b
    family history, 173
    occupational history, 171–172, 171b, 171t–172t
    past history, 171
    presenting symptoms in, 163–168, 163b
        breathlessness (dyspnoea), 165–168, 166b–168b
        chest pain, 168
        cough, 163–165, 163b, 164t
        haemoptysis, 165, 165t–166t
        sputum, 163–165
        wheeze, 168
    social history, 172
respiratory infection, acute, 168
respiratory noises, 663, 664t

respiratory rate
    on exercise, 188
    paediatric examination of, 634–635, 636f, 671, 672b, 673t
respiratory system, 201f
    examination anatomy of, 174, 175f–176f
    paediatric examination of, 663–674, 663b, 664t, 666b
    systems review of, 9b–12b
resting tremor, 598
restrictive ventilatory defect, 204
resuscitation, 868f
reticulocyte count, 350
retina, 771
    detached, 468
    diabetes mellitus and, 468
        non-proliferative changes in, 468
        proliferative changes in, 468, 469f
    examination of, 776
    haemorrhages, 776–777
    photographs of, 777f
retinal artery occlusion, central, 777
retinal toxoplasmosis, 840f
retinal vein thrombosis, central, 777
retinitis
    cytomegalovirus-induced, 840
    pigmentosa, 777
retinopathy, hypertensive, 124f
reversed splitting, 97–98
rheumatic fever, 70, 420
rheumatism, soft-tissue, 421–424
rheumatoid factor, 429
rheumatoid nodules, 381–383, 406f
rheumatoid vasculitis, 376–377, 378f
rheumatological disease, 408–427, 427b
rheumatological examination, 370–407, 407b
    anatomy in, 370–372, 370b, 371f–372f, 372b, 380b
    extending, 428–435, 435b
    general inspection for, 370–372
    imaging in, 430–434
    individual joints, assessment of, 374–406
        ankles, 403–406, 404f, 405b, 407b
        elbows, 383–384, 383f
        feet and, 403–406, 404f, 405b, 407b
        hands, and wrists, 374–383, 374f, 375b–377b, 378f, 383b
        hips, 395–399, 396f, 397b, 398f
        knees, 399–403, 399f, 399t
        neck, 388–392, 390f–392f
        sacroiliac joints, 392–395, 393b, 394f
        shoulders, 384–388, 385f, 387f
        temporomandibular joints, 388, 389f
        thoracolumbar spine, 392–395, 393b, 394f
    joint examination and, 372–374
        feel, 373
        look, 372–373
        measure, 374
        move, 373–374, 374b

rheumatological history, 363–369, 363b, 369b
    family history, 369
    past history, 368–369
    presenting symptoms in, 363–368
        back pain, 365–366
        dry eyes and mouth, 367–368, 368b
        limb pain, 366–367
        peripheral joints, 363–365, 363b, 364f, 365b–366b
        Raynaud's phenomenon, 367, 367b
        red eyes, 368
        systemic symptoms, 368
    social history, 369, 369t
    treatment history, 368
rhinocerebral mucormycosis, 791
    diabetes mellitus and, 469
ribs, palpation of, 184
rib-to-pelvis distance, 473
rickets, 474f, 475
right coronary artery (RCA), 74
right ventricular failure (RVF), 120–121
Rinné's test, 530, 531f, 788
risk factors
    for falls, 826, 828b
    for mental health, 851
    for osteoporosis and osteomalacia, 472b
    for pressure sores, 831b
    for pulmonary embolism (PE), 199b
    for urinary tract infection, 299b
risus sardonicus (tetanus), 43f
Ritter's disease of newborn, 700
rocker-bottom foot, 720f, 721
Romberg test, 577, 578f
rooting reflex, 723
Rosenbach's liver pulsation sign, 134t
rotation, 392
rotator cuff syndrome, 421–422, 422f
Roth's spot, 124f
Rovsing's sign, 274
rubeosis, diabetes mellitus and, 467–468, 468f
rugae, 791
RVF *see* right ventricular failure

S

sacral dimple, 699f
saddle sensation, 574
safety, from injury and violence, in HEADSSS assessment, 620t
salivary gland, 792
sarcoidosis, 199, 199b
satiation, early, 218
saturation, oxygen, 205–206
scale, 805t
scaling, 641t
scalp hair, in neonates, 705t
scaphocephaly, 704
scapulae, winging of, 565f

scarf sign, in 180° examination, 657f, 658
scars, 372–373, 641t
    abdominal, 245, 245f
    pigmented, diabetes mellitus and, 463
Schamroth's sign, 79–80, 81f
Scheuermann's disease, 639–640
schizophrenia, 847t–850t, 860–861
Schober's test, 392, 395f
sciatica, 392
sclerae, 774f
    colour of, 772–774
    normal, 776f
scleral icterus, 40, 239f
scleral pallor, 773–774
scleroderma *see* systemic sclerosis
scleroedema diabeticorum, 469
scleromalacia, 409
sclerosis, 805t
scoliosis, 640, 640f
scratch marks, 237, 308–309, 335
scratch test, 261
scrotum
    examination of, 313f
    imaging of, 325, 326f
    inspection of, 313–314
    mass, differential diagnosis of, 314, 315f
    in neonatal examination, 717
    transillumination of, 315f
scurvy, with perifollicular haemorrhages, 46f
seasonal affective disorder, 861
sebaceous glands, 804b
sebaceous hyperplasia, 701f
secondary sexual development, 455t
secondary skin lesions, 641t
seizures, 493–494
    abnormal movements suggesting, 492t
    absence, 494
    focal, 493–494
    generalised tonic-clonic, 494
    psychogenic non-epileptic, 495b
self-harm, 29, 620t
sensation, disturbed, 496
sensitivity, of sign, 52, 52t
sensory abnormalities, interpretation of, 559
sensory loss, dissociated, 589, 591f
sensory system testing
    of lower limbs, 572–574
    of upper limb, 557–559
sepsis, 50
sequential organ failure assessment (SOFA) score, 871
seronegative spondyloarthritides, 410–412
serum alkaline phosphatase (SAP), 285
sexual development, secondary, 455t
sexual history, 19, 27, 303, 750, 751b
sexual infantilism, 474
sexual maturity, classification of, 678t
sexuality, in HEADSSS assessment, 620t
shagreen patch, 644f

Sherman's sign, 134t
shifting dullness, 258, 259f
shingles, 781
shock, causes of, 45b
short neck, 647
short stature, 633
    syndromes associated with, 473–475
        abdomen and, 474
        chest and, 474
        general inspection for, 473–474
shoulder abduction relief test, 392
shoulder suspension, in 180° examination, 657f, 658
shoulders
    diabetes mellitus and, 469
    frozen, 422
    girdle examination, 564b
    power testing of, 552, 552f
    syndromes, 421–422
SIC mnemonic, 684
sick sinus syndrome, 67
Simmonds' test, 406
sinus tachycardia, 65
sinuses, 788–791
sinusitis, 179, 790–791
    acute, 796f
    assessment of, 790t
    bacterial ethmoidal, 790f
SIRS *see* systemic inflammatory response syndrome
6-minute walking test (6MWT), 206
Sjögren's syndrome, 368b
skin, 799–825
    blistering eruptions on, 809–813, 810b, 812b, 812f
    changes in, 440–441
    common sites of infection in, 800f
    depigmentation, 819, 820b
    dermatological history of, 800–801, 801b, 801f, 801t
    dermatological terms, 805t
    disease, 806–823, 808f
        algorithm, 808f
        blistering eruptions, 809–813, 810b, 812b, 812f
        carbuncles and, 818
        cellulitis and, 817–818, 817f
        crusted lesions and, 814–815, 815b
        dermal plaques, 815–816, 815b
        erysipelas and, 817–818, 817f
        erythema multiforme, 816–817, 817f
        erythema nodosum, 816, 816b
        erythroderma, 813–814, 814b
        erythrosquamous eruptions, 807–809, 809b, 810f–812f
        flushing and, 819, 821b
        folliculitis and, 818
        furuncles and, 818
        livedo reticularis, 814, 814t
        other infections and, 818–819

pruritus, 806–807, 809b, 809f
pustular and, 814–815, 815b
sweating and, 819, 821b
Ehlers-Danlos syndrome and, 278f
erythrosquamous eruptions on, 807–809, 809b, 810f–812f
examination anatomy of, 799–800, 799f–800f
gastrointestinal tract and, 231–234, 231f–233f, 233t–234t
hyperpigmentation, 819, 820b
hypopigmentation, 819, 820b
infection of, diabetes mellitus and, 463
inspection of, in diabetes mellitus, 463
layers of, 799f
lesions of, 247, 641, 641t, 803f
lump, 804–806
in neonatal examination, 700–703
paediatric examination of, 640–644, 641t, 642f–645f
physical examination of, 801–804, 802b–804b, 803f, 805t, 807f–808f
pigmentation of, 231, 308–309
reactions, cutaneous drug, 801t
sample questions for, 621b
tags, 264, 457f
thickened tethered, 418b
tumours, 821–823, 821b
skinfold measurements, in general physical examination, 624, 624f
skull, in neonatal examination, 698–699
SLE see systemic lupus erythematosus
sleep apnoea, 169
small for gestational age (SGA), 696
small intestine, 230
smell, 50–51
first nerve and, 504
of urine, 319
smoking, 16, 17b
as coronary artery disease risk factor, 69
staining from, 178
snapping, 375, 395–396
snore, 664t
snort, 664t
SnOut, 52
snuffle, 664t
social anxiety disorder, 862
social history, 15–19, 15b
endocrine history, 443
gastrointestinal history, 227
in genitourinary examination, 304
in gynaecological examination, 750
haematological history, 334
mental health examination, 853–854
in neurological history, 498
in pregnancy, 735–736
in rheumatological history, 369, 369t
social support, 15
soft exudates, 468, 468f
soft palate, 791

soft tissue, 150
soft-tissue rheumatism, 421–424
somatic symptom disorder, 26, 26b, 847t–850t
somatisation disorder, 847t–850t
somatoform disorder, 847t–850t
sores, bed, 831t
spatial neglect, 545, 546f
specificity, of sign, 51–52, 52t
speculum examination, 753–757, 757f
speech, 540–547, 547b, 608
examination of, 541–542, 541b, 542f
neurological history and, 497
sphygmomanometer, 86–88, 86f
spider naevi, 237–238, 238f
SpIn, 52
spina bifida cystica, 698, 699f
spina bifida occulta, 639
spinal accessory nerve, paediatric examination of, 655
spinal column, 388–389
spinal cord
central cavity in, 589
compression, 585, 586b, 587f, 587t
subacute combined degeneration of, 588–589
syndromes, 588–590, 588f–590f
tumour, 615f
spinal muscular atrophy, type 1, 722f
spinal stenosis, 367
spine
bamboo, 432
in neonatal examination, 698–699
spinothalamic pathway testing, 557–558
spirometry, 204, 204f
spleen, 230
palpation of, 251–252, 254f
percussion of, 258, 258f
splenomegaly, 253f
cause of, 344b
portal hypertension and, 275
splinter haemorrhage, 80, 82f
SpO$_2$ see oxygen saturation
spontaneous movements, in neonatal examination, 696–697
spontaneous pneumothorax, 63
Spurling test, 391
sputum, 163–165, 177
squamous cell carcinoma, 822f
squamous metaplasia, 756–757
squatting, 665
squatting to standing, 105
stability, 374
stadiometer, 473
standing to squatting, 105
stapes, 782
Staphylococcus, 373
Staphylococcus aureus, 810b
Staphylococcus scalded skin syndrome, 700
κ–statistic, 53–54

stature, changes in, 441
steatorrhoea, 268
stepping reflex, 722–723
stertor, 664t
stethoscope bell, in physical examination, 38, 39f
Stevens-Johnson syndrome, 813f, 817
stiffness, 375
Still's murmur, 669
Stokes-Adams attacks, 67
stomach, 255
stomach contents, of unconscious patients, 604
stool
blood in, 267–268
see also faeces
strabismus, 515
straight leg raising, 393
street drugs, 18–19
streptococcal throat, 795f
Streptococcus pnueumoniae, 611
Streptococcus pyogenes, 818
stress incontinence, 300
stress-related disorders, 847t–850t
stridor, 168, 177, 177b, 673, 714
wheezes and, 187
stroke, 489–490
embolic, 611f
haemorrhagic, 612f
hemiplegia and, 580–582
questions for patient with, 490b
structural hyperkyphosis, 639–640, 640f
stupor, 602
Sturge-Weber syndrome, 502
subcutaneous emphysema, 181
subcutaneous nodules, 381–383, 383f
subluxation, 373
submandibular abscess, 795f
submandibular gland, 240, 241f
submandibular nodes, 341–342
submental node, 341–342, 343f
substance misuse, 847t–850t
subvalvular obstruction, 131
sucking reflex, 723
suicide, in HEADSSS assessment, 620t
suicide risk, 851b
summation gallop, 99
superficial and profundus flexor tendons, 380, 382f
superior vena cava obstruction, 198, 198f
supraclavicular nodes, 341–342, 343f
supraglottitis, 795
supranuclear palsy, 520, 521f
supraspinatus tendinitis, 386
supravalvular obstruction, 131
supraventricular tachycardia (SVT), 65
sutures, head, in neonatal examination, 704
SVT see supraventricular tachycardia

I-22 INDEX

swallowing, 220
  difficulty, questions for patient with, 221b
swan neck, 375–376, 377f
sweating, changes in, 439
swelling, 373, 375
  neck, 445b
  in rheumatological history, 363–365
swimmer's ear, 785–786
sympathetic confrontation, 23
symphyseal-fundal height (SFH), 737
symptoms
  associated, 8
  character of, 8
  common general, history taking, 24–27
  current, 7–8
  onset of, 7–8
  presenting, 7
  of psychiatric disorders, 852t
  severity of, 8
  site of, 7
  timing of, 8
  see also presenting symptoms
synacthen test, 483
syncope, 66–67
  differential diagnosis of, 66b
  drugs and, 67b
syndactyly, 719f
syndrome of inappropriate antidiuretic hormone (SIADH), 324b
synovitis, 373
syringomyelia, 589, 780
systemic exertion intolerance disease (SEID), 24
systemic hypertension, causes of, 125
systemic inflammatory response syndrome (SIRS), 50, 840b, 871
systemic lupus erythematosus (SLE), 44f, 368, 414–416
  examining for, 415b, 415f
  rash, 416f
systemic sclerosis, 234, 416–419
  examining for, 417b, 417f
systems review, 9b–12b, 19–20
systolic blood pressure, 84–86
systolic bruits, 477
systolic ejection click, 99
systolic flow ejection murmurs, 669
systolic murmurs, 100
systolic regurgitant murmur, 670
systolic thrill, 95
systolic-click murmur syndrome, 130

T

tachycardia, 83, 85t
  sinus, 65
  ventricular, 65
tachypnoea, 174–175
talipes equinovarus, 719–720, 720f
tall stature, 633

Tanner staging, in puberty, 678, 678t, 679f
tape measure, 374
tapping apex beat, 94
tarsal joint, 568
tarsal tunnel syndrome, 425
taste buds, 791–792
teeth, 240–241
telangiectasia, 641t
  haemorrhagic, 232, 233f, 340–341
  of hands, 418f
temperature
  chest infection and, 188
  in neonatal examination, 703
  paediatric examination of, 635, 636t
  pathways, 557f
  in physical examination, 49–50, 49t
  testing, 557–558
  of unconscious patients, 604
temporal lobe function, 545
Tenckhoff catheter, 310
tenderness, 373
tendon xanthomata, 81
tenosynovitis
  de Quervain's, 424f
  of wrist, 423–424
tenovaginitis, 375
tension pneumothorax, 194
  acutely ill patient and, 871
testis, 256
  in neonatal examination, 717
  palpation of, 314
tests of function, 373–374
tetanus, 43f
tetralogy of Fallot, 142
Thomas's test, 396–397
thoracic kyphosis, 473
thoracoplasty, 180–181
thrills, 95
throat, 771–798, 791f, 796b–798b
  examination anatomy of, 791–792
  examination method for, 792–794
  history of, 792
  paediatric examination of, 648–649
  pain in, 792b
  sample questions for, 621b
  Streptococcal, 795f
thrombocytopenia, 335–338, 337f
thrombophilia, test for, 350
thrombosis
  arterial, 332
  venous, 331–332, 332b
thumb movements, 380, 381f
thyroglossal cysts, 647
thyroid, 444–453, 446f
  anatomy of, 444f
  auscultation of, 447
  function testing, 482
  nodules, 447b, 482f
  palpation of, 446–447, 446f

percussion of, 447
  signs guide for, 445t
thyroid-stimulating hormone (TSH), 454, 482
thyrotoxicosis, 448–451, 449f, 476
  causes of, 451b
  questions for patient with, 448b
TIA *see* transient ischaemic attack
tic douloureux, 522–523
tics, 601
tinea pedis, 820f
Tinel's sign, 380
tinnitus, drug causes of, 784b
tiredness, pregnancy and, 731
toe-finger test, 571
toeing in, 639, 639f
toeing out, 639
tone, in Parkinson's disease examination, 598
tone testing, 551–552, 566
tongue, 241–242, 791
  fasciculations of, 535f
  geographical, 793
  mucosal neuromas of, 470, 471f
  scrotal, 793
  of unconscious patients, 603–604
top-to-toe checklist, 621b
torticollis, 391, 534
torus palatinus, 793
toxic epidermal necrolysis (TEN), 817
toxoplasmosis, retinal, 840f
TR *see* tricuspid regurgitation
trachea
  paediatric examination of, 673
  palpation of, 179f
  in respiratory examination, 179–180, 179b, 179f
tracheal displacement, 179b
tracheal tug, 176–177, 179
traction apophysitis, 400
transient ischaemic attack (TIA), 489–490, 494
  hemiplegia and, 580–582
  questions for patient with, 490b
Traube space, 343–344
Traube's sign, 134t
trauma, blunt, acute abdomen after, 274
treatment history, 12–14, 13f
  gastrointestinal history, 226–227
  in genitourinary system, 304
  haematological history, 333
  in mental health examination, 851–853
  in rheumatological history, 368
tremor, 496–497, 496t, 598
  flapping, 178
  non-physiological, 599b
Trendelenburg test, 116
triceps jerk, 554f–555f, 555
Trichomonas vaginalis, 755t
trichomoniasis, 755t

tricuspid regurgitation (TR), 128t, 136, 136f
　　echocardiogram of, 157–158
tricuspid stenosis, 135–136
trigeminal nerve, 503t, 521–525, 522f, 524f
　　paediatric examination of, 653–654
　　palsy, 524–525
trigeminy, 83
trigger finger, 375
trigonocephaly, 704
trisomy 21, 475
trochlear nerve, 503t, 510–521
　　paediatric examination of, 653
Trousseau's sign, 471
true leg length, 639
TSH see thyroid-stimulating hormone
tuberculosis (TB), 197
　　miliary, 197
　　postprimary, 197
　　primary, 197, 210f
tuberous sclerosis (TS), 641–642, 643f
tuboeruptive xanthomata, 81, 82f
tumour plop, 99–100
tumours
　　adrenal, 484f
　　apical (Pancoast's), 198
　　cerebellar, 613f
　　cerebellopontine angle, 525f
　　spinal cord, 615f
turbinates, 789
Turner's syndrome, 473–474, 474f, 647, 647f, 710f
turricephaly, 704
tussive syncope, 66
two-point discrimination, 545, 545f
tympanic membrane, 787f
　　detail of, 787f
　　hyperaemia of, otitis media with, 787f
　　inspection of, 786–787
　　perforated, 788f
tympanic thermometry, 635
type 1 respiratory failure, 671, 672b
type 2 respiratory failure, 671, 672b

U

ulcerative colitis, 277–279
ulcers, 641t, 805t
　　aphthous, 243f
　　buccal, 794f
　　diabetes mellitus and, 463, 466f
　　mouth, 242–243, 243b, 792b
　　peptic, 218
ulnar deviation, 375, 375b, 377f, 379f
ultrasound
　　abdominal, 287–289
　　　densities in, 289t
　　　indications for, 287–288
　　　terminology for, 289t
　　in haematological imaging, 358
　　of kidneys and scrotum, 319, 325f–326f

　　in rheumatological examination, 431
　　of thyroid nodule, 483f
umbilical cord, 687, 687f
umbilical hernia, 716f
UMN see upper motor neurone
unconsciousness, 601
underweight, 45
upper limbs
　　dermatomes of, 559, 560f
　　diabetes mellitus and, 467–469
　　examination of, 609–610
　　motor system of, 550–557
　　paediatric examination of, 635–639
　　peripheral nerves of, 559–566
　　peripheral nervous system examination of, 550–566
　　reflexes of, 553–556
　　sensory system testing of, 557–559
　　of unconscious patients, 604
upper motor neurone (UMN)
　　facial weakness, 526f
　　lesions, 580–582, 580b, 583b
　　spasticity, 580
　　weakness, 496, 551, 696b
upper segment lengths, measurement of, 633
uraemia, 300
uraemic fetor, 306
uraemic frost, 308–309
uraemic tinge, 306
urethral meatus, in neonatal examination, 717
urethrocele, 758f
urge incontinence, 300
urinalysis, 269, 274
　　for diabetes mellitus, 469
　　for pregnancy, 741
urinary incontinence, 300, 829, 829b
urinary obstruction, 300
urinary tract infection (UTI), 298–300, 300t
　　risk factors for, 299b
urine, 319–323
　　appearance of, change in, 298
　　blood in, 321, 322b
　　changes of, with jaundice, 270t
　　chemical analysis of, 320–321
　　examination of, 319
　　glucose and ketones in, 320–321, 321b
　　gravity of, 319–320
　　pH of, 320
　　polyuria and, 441
　　protein in, 320
　　sediment, 321–323, 322t
　　smell of, 319
　　of unconscious patients, 604
urobilinogen, 269
urogenital system, in neonatal examination, 715–717
uterine fibroids, 746f
UTI see urinary tract infection

uveal tract, 771
uveitis, causes of, 775b
uvula, inspection of, 793–794

V

v wave, 90–91
vaccines
　　contraindications to, 30b
　　recommendations for, 31t
vagina
　　bleeding, in pregnancy, 732
　　cystic swellings in, 756
vaginal discharge, 759t
　　in pregnancy, 731
vaginal examination, 274
vaginal inclusion cysts, 756
vaginal prolapse, 754–756, 758f
vaginal swabs, 758–759
vagus nerve, 503t, 531–533, 532f–533f
　　paediatric examination of, 655
　　palsy, 533
valgus, 373
Valsalva manoeuvre, 91, 105
κ–value, 53–54, 54t
valve calcification, 149
valve cusps, 157f
valve disease
　　of left heart, 126–135
　　mitral, 152f
　　of right heart, 135–137
valve lesion, features of, 128t
varicocele, 314
varicose veins, 115–116
varus, 373
vascular disease, 580–582, 581f, 582t
vascular malformations, 641, 643t
vasculitides, 420–421, 421t
vasculitis, 308–309
vasovagal syncope, 66
veins
　　abdominal, 246, 246f
　　distended, 247f
　　prominent, 181
venous hums, 261
venous staining, 111f
venous system, 110f
venous ulcer, 114f, 117b
ventilatory defect
　　obstructive, 204
　　restrictive, 204
ventral suspension, in 180° examination, 657f, 658
ventricular ectopic beat, 64
ventricular septal defect (VSD), 128t, 135, 139, 140f
　　echocardiogram of, 158
ventricular tachycardia, 65
vertebrobasilar artery, 581–582
vertigo, 495, 495t

vesicles, 641t, 805t
vesico/urethral fistula, 300
vessel wall, 84
vestibular nerve, examination of, paediatric, 654–655
vestibulocochlear nerve, 503t, 529–531
vestibulo-ocular reflex (VOR), 517
vibration testing, 558, 558f
viral exanthema, 818, 818f
Virchow's triad, 115
virile facies, 44f
vision
    colour, 776
    developmental examination in, 659
    loss of, 774b
visual acuity, 506
visual disturbances, 496
    causes of, 773t
visual fields, 506–507
    charts, 608, 608f
    defects of, 508f
    testing, 507f
vital signs, in physical examination, 40
vital signs, paediatric examination of, 633–635
    blood pressure, 633–634, 634f, 634t
    pulse and respiratory rates, 634–635, 635f–636f
    temperature, 635, 636t
vitamin A deficiency, 280f
vitamin B_{12} deficiency, 340, 588–589
vitamin K deficiency, 45
vitiligo, 461, 461f
vitreous humour, 771
vocal fremitus, 674
vocal resonance, 187–188
vocal (tactile) fremitus, 182–184
volume-loaded apex beat, 94
vomiting, 218–219
    in pregnancy, 730
    questions for patient with, 219b
vomitus, 269
von Graefe's sign, 450

von Willebrand's disease, 331–332
VSD *see* ventricular septal defect
vulva
    cystic swellings in, 756
    skin conditions of, 755t
vulvar cancer, 755t, 756f
vulvar intraepithelial neoplasia, 755t

W

waist-hip ratio (WHR), 45
Waldeyer's ring, 340–341
walking frame, 31f
Wallenberg's syndrome, 581–582, 582b
warmth, 373
wasting, 178, 231
'water hammer', 133
waterbrash, 220
Watson's water hammer pulse, 134t
WBCs *see* white blood cells
weakness, 178
webbed neck, 647, 647f
Weber's test, 530, 531f, 788
weight, 231
    change, 218, 439
    in neonatal examination, 689, 690f–695f
    in physical examination, 45–46
weight-for-age, growth charts in, 625f–632f
Wenckebach phenomenon, 83
Werdnig-Hoffmann disease, 722f
Wernicke's area, 540–541
wheal, 641t, 805t
wheelie-walker, 31f
wheeze, 168, 673
    stridor and, 187
white blood cells (WBCs), 323
white cell casts, 323
WHR *see* waist-hip ratio
wide pulse pressure, 634–635
WIPER, 38b
World Health Organization (WHO), guidelines, in hand washing, 38–39

wrist
    extension, 380, 380f
    flexion, 380, 380f
    lesion at (carpal tunnel), 559
    power testing of, 552–553, 553f
    tenosynovitis of, 423–424
writing, 599, 600t

X

x descent, 90–91
xanthelasmata, 89, 89f, 239
xanthomata, in Achilles tendon, 113
X-ray
    abdominal, 285–287, 286t
    of alveolar pulmonary oedema, 152f
    of ankylosing spondylitis, 432f
    of aortic coarctation, 153f
    of arthritis, 430
    of ASD, 153f
    chest
        checklist of, 206–210
        in respiratory examination, 206
    of gout, 434f
    of interstitial pulmonary oedema, 151f
    of Marfan's syndrome, 154f
    of mitral valve disease, 152f
    of osteoarthritis, 430f
    of osteoporosis, 485f
    of psoriatic arthritis, 433f
    of pulmonary venous congestion, 151f
    of rheumatoid arthritis, 431f, 433f
    of ventricular aneurysm, 152f
    see also chest X-ray

Y

yellow nail syndrome, 193, 193f

Z

Z deformity, 375–376, 377f
zosteriform rash, 806f